D1271171

# The Cleveland Clinic Cardiology Board Review

# The Cleveland Clinic Cardiology Board Review


EDITORS

**BRIAN P. GRIFFIN, MD**
Department of Cardiovascular Medicine
The Cleveland Clinic Foundation
Cleveland, Ohio

**CURTIS M. RIMMERMAN, MD**
Department of Cardiovascular Medicine
The Cleveland Clinic Foundation
Cleveland, Ohio

**ERIC J. TOPOL, MD**
Department of Cardiovascular Medicine
The Cleveland Clinic Foundation
Cleveland, Ohio



Lippincott Williams & Wilkins
a Wolters Kluwer business
Philadelphia • Baltimore • New York • London
Buenos Aires • Hong Kong • Sydney • Tokyo

*Acquisitions Editor:* Fran Destefano
*Developmental Editor:* Annette Ferran
*Production Editor:* Dave Murphy
*Manufacturing Manager:* Benjamin Rivera
*Design Coordinator:* Terry Mallon
*Compositor:* TechBooks
*Printer:* Quebecor World Taunton


**530 Walnut Street**
**Philadelphia, PA 19106 USA**
**LWW.com**



Printed in the USA

---

**Library of Congress Cataloging-in-Publication Data**

The Cleveland Clinic cardiology board review / editors, Brian P. Griffin, Curtis M. Rimmerman, Eric J. Topol.
p. ; cm.
Includes bibliographical references and index.
ISBN 0-7817-5942-0 (alk. paper)
1. Cardiology–Examinations, questions, etc. 2. Cardiology–Outlines, syllabi, etc. I. Griffin, Brian P., 1956– . II. Rimmerman, Curtis M. III. Topol, Eric J., 1954– . IV. Title: Cardiology board review.
[DNLM: 1. Cardiovascular Diseases–Examination Questions. 2. Cardiovascular Diseases–Outlines. WG 18.2 C635 2007]
RC669.2.C5544 2007
616.1'20076–dc22

2006026932

---

Care has been taken to confirm the accuracy of the information presented and to describe generally accepted practices. However, the authors, editors, and publisher are not responsible for errors or omissions or for any consequences from application of the information in this book and make no warranty, expressed or implied, with respect to the currency, completeness, or accuracy of the contents of the publication. Application of this information in a particular situation remains the professional responsibility of the practitioner.

The authors, editors, and publisher have exerted every effort to ensure that drug selection and dosage set forth in this text are in accordance with current recommendations and practice at the time of publication. However, in view of ongoing research, changes in government regulations, and the constant flow of information relating to drug therapy and drug reactions, the reader is urged to check the package insert for each drug for any change in indications and dosage and for added warnings and precautions. This is particularly important when the recommended agent is a new or infrequently employed drug.

Some drugs and medical devices presented in this publication have Food and Drug Administration (FDA) clearance for limited use in restricted research settings. It is the responsibility of the health care provider to ascertain the FDA status of each drug or device planned for use in their clinical practice.

To purchase additional copies of this book, call our customer service department at (800) 638-3030 or fax orders to (301) 223-2320. International customers should call (301) 223-2300.

Visit Lippincott Williams & Wilkins on the Internet: at LWW.com. Lippincott Williams & Wilkins customer service representatives are available from 8:30 am to 6 pm, EST.

10 9 8 7 6 5 4 3 2 1

To our families
BG, CR, EJT

# Contents

# Contributors

**HANNA AHMED** Cleveland Clinic, Cleveland, Ohio

**CHRISTINE L. AHRENS, PHARM D** Cleveland Clinic, Cleveland, Ohio

**DREW S. ALLEN, DO** Resident, Internal Medicine, Cleveland Clinic, Cleveland, Ohio

**SOUFIAN ALMAHAMEED, MD** Cardiology Fellow, Cardiology, Cleveland Clinic Florida, Weston, FL

**CRAIG R. ASHER, MD, FACC** Director, Cardiology Fellowship Program, Cardiology Staff, Department of Cardiology, Cleveland Clinic Florida, Weston, Florida

**JOHN R. BARTHOLOMEW, MD** Section Head, Vascular Medicine, Department of Cardiovascular Medicine, Cleveland Clinic, Cleveland, Ohio

**GREGORY G. BASHIAN, MD** Fellow, Department of Cardiovascular Medicine, Cleveland Clinic, Cleveland, Ohio

**ANTHONY A. BAVRY, MD, MPH** Interventional Fellow, Department of Cardiovascular Medicine, Cleveland Clinic, Cleveland, Ohio

**DEEPAK L. BHATT, MD, FACC, FSCAI, FESC, FACP** Associate Director, Cleveland Clinic Cardiovascular Coordinating Center, Staff, Cardiac, Peripheral, and Carotid Intervention, Associate Professor, Department of Medicine, Cleveland Clinic, Cleveland, Ohio

**SORIN J. BRENER, MD** Associate Professor, Department of Medicine, Case Western Reserve University, Staff Cardiologist, Director, Angiography Core Laboratory, Department of Cardiovascular Medicine, Cleveland Clinic, Cleveland, Ohio

**RICHARD C. BRUNKEN, MD, FACC, FAHA** Director of Molecular Cardiac Imaging, Department of Molecular and Functional Imaging/Gb3, Cleveland Clinic, Cleveland, Ohio

**J. DAVID BURKHARDT, MD, FACC** Staff, Cardiovascular Medicine, Cardiac Electrophysiology and Pacing, Cleveland Clinic, Cleveland, Ohio

**MATTHEWS CHACKO, MD** Interventional Fellow, Department of Cardiovascular Medicine, Cleveland Clinic, Cleveland, Ohio

**MICHAEL S. CHEN, MD** Fellow, Interventional Cardiology, Department of Cardiovascular Medicine, Cleveland Clinic, Cleveland, Ohio

**APARNA CHERLA, MD** Cardiology Fellow, Department of Cardiology, Cleveland Clinic Florida, Weston, Florida

**RYAN D. CHRISTOFFERSON, MD** Fellow, Department of Cardiovascular Medicine, Cleveland Clinic, Cleveland, Ohio

**HSUAN-HUNG CHUANG, MBBS, M MED (INT MED), MRCP, TESTAMUR (NBE), FAMS** Associate Consultant, The National Heart Centre, Singapore

**MINA K. CHUNG, MD** Staff, Cardiovascular Medicine, Cardiac Electrophysiology and Pacing, Cleveland Clinic, Cleveland, Ohio

**JENNIFER E. CUMMINGS, MD** Staff, Cardiovascular Medicine, Cardiac Electrophysiology and Pacing, Cleveland Clinic, Cleveland, Ohio

**ROSS DOWNEY, MD, MS** Fellow, Department of Cardiovascular Medicine, Cleveland Clinic, Cleveland, Ohio

**BRENDAN DUFFY, MD** Interventional Fellow, Department of Cardiovascular Medicine, Cleveland Clinic, Cleveland, Ohio

**STEPHEN ELLIS, MD** Director, Sones Cardiac Laboratories, Cardiovascular Medicine, Cleveland Clinic, Cleveland, Ohio

**JODI M. FINK, PHARM D** Transplantation Clinical Specialist, Department of Pharmacy, Cleveland Clinic, Cleveland, Ohio

**GARY S. FRANCIS, MD** Professor of Medicine, Department of Cardiology, Cleveland Clinic Lerner College of Medicine of Case Western Reserve University, Head, Clinical Cardiology Section, Department of Cardiology, Cleveland Clinic, Cleveland, Ohio

**MARIO JORGE GARCIA, MD, FACC** Professor, Department of Medicine, Cleveland Clinic Lerner College of Medicine of Case Western Reserve University, Director of Cardiac Imaging, Department of Cardiology, Cleveland Clinic, Cleveland, Ohio

**STEVEN M. GORDON, MD** Associate Professor, Department of Medicine, Cleveland Clinic Lerner College of Medicine of Case Western Reserve University, Chairman, Department of Infectious Diseases, Cleveland Clinic, Cleveland, Ohio

**CELESTE GRANT, MD** Heart Failure Fellow, Department of Cardiovascular Medicine, Cleveland Clinic, Cleveland, Ohio

**ADAM W. GRASSO, MD, PHD** Cardiology Fellow, Department of Cardiovascular Medicine, Cleveland Clinic, Cleveland, Ohio

**BRIAN P. GRIFFIN MD, FACC** Director, Cardiovascular Training Program, Department of Cardiovascular Medicine, Cleveland Clinic, Cleveland, Ohio

**RICHARD A. GRIMM, DO, FACC** Director, Echocardiography Laboratory, Section of Cardiovascular Imaging, Department of Cardiovascular Medicine, Cleveland Clinic, Desk F-15, Cleveland Clinic, Cleveland, Ohio

**CHRISTIAN GRING, MD** Fellow, Department of Cardiovascular Medicine, Cleveland Clinic, Cleveland, Ohio

**ROBERT E. HOBBS, MD** Associate Professor, Department of Medicine, Cleveland Clinic Lerner College of Medicine of Case Western Reserve University, Staff Physician, Department of Cardiovascular Medicine, Cleveland Clinic, Cleveland, Ohio

**JULIE C. HUANG, MD** Associate Staff, Department of Cardiovascular Medicine, Cleveland Clinic, Cleveland, Ohio

**CARLOS A. HUBBARD, MD, PHD** Cardiovascular Fellow, Cardiovascular Medicine, Cleveland Clinic, Cleveland, Ohio

**FREDERICK A. HUEPLER, JR. MD** Director, Diagnostic Cath Lab, Department of Cardiovascular Medicine, Cleveland Clinic, Cleveland, Ohio

**FREDRICK J. JAEGER, DO** Cardiac Pacing and Electrophysiology, Department of Cardiovascular Medicine/Desk F15, Cleveland Clinic, Cleveland, Ohio

**BRIAN K. JEFFERSON, MD** Fellow, Department of Cardiovascular Medicine, Cleveland Clinic, Cleveland, Ohio

**SREENIVAS KAMATH, MD** Staff Physician, Department of Cardiology, Cleveland Clinic, Cleveland, Ohio

**ANNE KANDERIAN, MD** Cardiology Fellow, Department of Cardiology, Cleveland Clinic, Cleveland, Ohio

**SAMIR R. KAPADIA, MD** Associate Professor, Department of Medicine, Cleveland Clinic Lerner College of Medicine of Case Western Reserve University, Director, Interventional Cardiology Fellowship, Department of Cardiovascular Medicine, Cleveland Clinic, Cleveland, Ohio

**JUHANA KARHA, MD** Interventional Fellow, Department of Cardiovascular Medicine, Cleveland Clinic, Cleveland, Ohio

**ALLAN L. KLEIN, MD, FRCP(C), FACC, FAHA, FASE** Professor, Department of Medicine, Cleveland Clinic Lerner College of Medicine of Case Western Reserve University, Director, Cardiovascular Imaging Research, Department of Cardiovascular Medicine, Cleveland Clinic, Cleveland, Ohio

**RAGHU KOLLURI, MD, MS** Clinical Fellow, Department of Vascular Medicine, Cleveland Clinic, Cleveland, Ohio

**RICHARD A. KRASUSKI, MD** Director, Adult Congenital Heart Services, Department of Cardiology, Cleveland Clinic, Cleveland, Ohio

**OMOSALEWA O. LALUDE, MD** Assistant Professor, Division of Cardiology, Department of Internal Medicine, Texas Tech University Health Sciences Center, El Paso, Texas

**MICHAEL S. LAUER, MD** Professor, Departments of Medicine, Epidemiology, and Biostatistics, Cleveland Clinic Lerner College of Medicine of Case Western Reserve University, Cardiologist, Department of Cardiovascular Medicine, Cleveland Clinic, Cleveland, Ohio

**HARRY M. LEVER, MD** Staff Physician, Cardiovascular Medicine, Cleveland Clinic, Cleveland, Ohio

**A. MICHAEL LINCOFF, MD** Professor, Department of Medicine, Cleveland Clinic Lerner College of Medicine of Case Western Reserve University, Director, Cleveland Clinic Cardiovascular Coordinating Center, Department of Cardiovascular Medicine, Cleveland Clinic, Cleveland, Ohio

**ANJLI MAROO, MD** Senior Fellow, Department of Cardiology, Section of Interventional Cardiology, Cleveland Clinic, Cleveland, Ohio

**MICHAEL A. MILITELLO, PHARM D** Cardiology Clinical Specialist, Department of Pharmacy, Cleveland Clinic, Cleveland, Ohio

**SOUNDOS MOUALLA, MD** Fellow, Department of Cardiovascular Medicine, Cleveland Clinic, Cleveland, Ohio

**JOSEPH V. NALLY, JR., MD** Clinical Professor, Department of Medicine, Cleveland Clinic Lerner College of Medicine of Case Western Reserve University, Staff Nephrologist, Department of Nephrology and Hypertension, Cleveland Clinic, Cleveland, Ohio

**ANDREA NATALE, MD** Medical Director, Center for Atrial Fibrillation/EP Lab, Section Head, Pacing and Electrophysiology, Cardiovascular Medicine, Cleveland Clinic, Cleveland, Ohio

**GIAN M. NOVARO, MD, MS** Director, Echocardiography Laboratory, Staff Cardiologist, Department of Cardiology, Cleveland Clinic Florida, Weston, Florida

**RAVINDRAN A. PADMANABHAN, MD, MRCP** Fellow, Department of Infectious Diseases, Cleveland Clinic, Cleveland, Ohio

**DIMPI PATEL, DO** Electrophysiology Research Fellow, Section of Electrophysiology and Pacing, Cleveland Clinic, Cleveland, Ohio

**TARAL N. PATEL, MD** Fellow, Department of Cardiovascular Medicine, Cleveland Clinic, Cleveland, Ohio

**RUSSELL ERIC RAYMOND, DO** Interventional Cardiology, Department of Cardiology, Cleveland Clinic, Cleveland, Ohio

**CURTIS MARK RIMMERMAN, MD, MBA, FACC** Associate Professor, Department of Cardiovascular Medicine, Division of Medicine, Cleveland Clinic Lerner College of Medicine of Case Western Reserve University, Cleveland, Ohio, Gus P. Karos Chair of Clinical Cardiovascular Medicine, Medical Director, Westlake, Lakewood, and Avon, Cleveland Clinic, Westlake, Ohio

**MICHAEL B. ROCCO, MD** Assistant Professor, Department of Medicine, Cleveland Clinic Lerner College of Medicine of Case Western Reserve University, Staff Physician, Department of Cardiovascular Medicine, Cleveland Clinic, Cleveland, Ohio

**L. LEONARDO RODRIGUEZ, MD, FACC** Cardiovascular Imaging Center, Department of Cardiology, Cleveland Clinic, Cleveland, Ohio

**BRET A. ROGERS, MD** Clinical Fellow, Department of Cardiovascular Medicine, Cleveland Clinic, Cleveland, Ohio

**ELLEN MAYER SABIK, MD** Staff, Cardiovascular Medicine, Imaging Section, Cleveland Clinic, Cleveland, Ohio

**WALID SALIBA, MD** Staff, Director of EP LAB, Cardiovascular Medicine, Department of Pacing and Electrophysiology, Cleveland Clinic, Cleveland, Ohio

**DANIEL SAURI, MD** Imaging Fellow, Department of Cardiovascular Medicine, Cleveland Clinic, Cleveland, Ohio

**MARTIN J. SCHREIBER, JR., MD** Chairman, Department of Nephrology and Hypertension, Cleveland Clinic, Cleveland, Ohio

**ROBERT A. SCHWEIKERT, MD** Staff Physician, Department of Cardiovascular Medicine, Section of Electrophysiology and Pacing, Cleveland Clinic, Cleveland, Ohio

**CRISTIANA G. SCRIDON, MD** Cardiology Fellow, Department of Cardiology, Cleveland Clinic Florida, Weston, Florida

**AMY L. SEIDEL, MD** Fellow, Department of Interventional Cardiology, Emory University School of Medicine, Atlanta, Georgia

**MEHDI H. SHISHEHBOR, DO, MPH** Cardiology Fellow, Cardiovascular Medicine, Cleveland Clinic, Cleveland, Ohio

**CONRAD SIMPFENDORFER, MD, FACC** Staff, Department of Cardiovascular Medicine, Section of Interventional Cardiology, Cleveland Clinic, Cleveland, Ohio

**SRIKANTH SOLA, MD** Assistant Professor, Department of Medicine, Cleveland Clinic Lerner College of Medicine of Case Western Reserve University, Associate Staff Cardiologist, Department of Cardiology, Cleveland Clinic, Cleveland, Ohio

**RANDALL C. STARLING, MD, MPH** Vice-Chairman, Dept. of Cardiovascular Medicine, Head, Section of Heart Failure & Cardiac Transplant Medicine, Medical Director, Kaufman Center for Heart Failure, Cleveland Clinic, Cleveland, Ohio

**JAMES K. STOLLER, MD, MS** Professor, Department of Medicine, Cleveland Clinic Lerner College of Medicine of Case Western Reserve University, Vice Chair, Division of Medicine, Section Head, Respiratory Therapy, Staff, Pulmonary, Allergy, and Critical Care Medicine, Cleveland Clinic, Cleveland, Ohio

**WILLIAM J. STEWART, MD, FACC, FASE** Associate Professor of Medicine, Department of Cardiovascular Medicine/DeskF15, Cleveland Clinic, Cleveland, Ohio

**WAI HONG WILSON TANG, MD** Assistant Professor, Department of Medicine, Cleveland Clinic Lerner College of Medicine of Case Western Reserve University, Staff Cardiologist, Department of Cardiovascular Medicine, Cleveland Clinic, Cleveland, Ohio

**DAVID O. TAYLOR, MD** Professor of Medicine, Department of Cardiovascular Medicine, Cleveland Clinic, Cleveland, Ohio

**PATRICK J. TCHOU, MD** Co-Section Head, Cardiac Electrophysiology and Pacing, Department of Cardiovascular Medicine, Cleveland Clinic, Cleveland, Ohio

**SERGIO G. THAL, MD** Fellow, Cardiac Electrophysiology and Pacing, Department of Cardiovascular Medicine, Cleveland Clinic, Cleveland, Ohio

**ERIC J. TOPOL, MD** Professor, Department of Genetics and Medicine, Chairman, Department of Cardiovascular Medicine, Cleveland Clinic Lerner College of Medicine of Case Western Reserve University, Cleveland, Ohio

**E. MURAT TUZCU, MD** Professor, Department of Medicine, Division of Cardiology, Cleveland Clinic Lerner College of Medicine of Case Western Reserve Univerisity, Director, Structural Heart Disease Intervention, Department of Cardiovascular Medicine, Cleveland Clinic, Cleveland, Ohio

**DONALD A. UNDERWOOD, MD** Associate Professor, Department of Medicine, Cleveland Clinic Lerner College of Medicine of Case Western Reserve University, Staff Cardiologist, Director, Electrocardiography, Cleveland Clinic, Cleveland, Ohio

**OUSSAMMA WAZNI, MD** Staff, Cardiovascular Medicine, Cardiac Electrophysiology and Pacing, Cleveland Clinic, Cleveland, Ohio

**RICHARD D. WHITE, MD** Professor and Chair, UF Jacksonville Department of Radiology, Jacksonville, Florida

**BRUCE L. WILKOFF, MD** Professor, Department of Cardiovascular Medicine, Cleveland Clinic Lerner College of Medicine of Case Western Reserve University, Director, Cardiac Pacing and Tachyarrhythmia Devices, Department of Cardiovascular Medicine, Cleveland Clinic, Cleveland, Ohio

**JAMES B. YOUNG, MD** George and Linda Kaufman Chair, Chairman, Division of Medicine, Cleveland Clinic Lerner College of Medicine of Case Western Reserve University, Cleveland, Ohio

**JOHN S. ZAKAIB, MD** Chief Cardiovascular Medicine Fellow, Department of Cardiovascular Medicine, Cleveland Clinic, Cleveland, Ohio

# Preface

This book aims to provide a concise but comprehensive overview of Cardiovascular Medicine. As such, it was specifically written to meet the needs of those preparing for certification or recertification examinations in Cardiovascular Medicine. It is based on a review course that we have organized at Cleveland Clinic over the last 7 years. This course has proven popular not only with those preparing for examinations but also with clinical cardiologists, internists, and nurse practitioners. This book would not be possible without the input and support of many individuals specifically the faculty and fellows in Cardiovascular Medicine and related disciplines at Cleveland Clinic who wrote the individual chapters and questions. We also wish to thank the Cardiovascular Graphics group at Cleveland Clinic under the leadership of Robin Moss who provided inestimable assistance to this book and to the course over the years. As with all our endeavors, this book would also have been impossible without the support of our families to whom this book is dedicated. We hope that you enjoy the book and that you find it useful.

*Brian Griffin*
*Curtis Rimmerman*
*Eric Topol*

# Fundamentals

# Cardiovascular Physiology: Pressure–Volume Loops

# 1

***Aparna Cherla Craig R. Asher***

An understanding of the factors that influence cardiac performance in normal and pathologic states is essential for the Cardiology Boards. The determinants of cardiac function, including preload, afterload, and contractility, and the effect of various disease states and medications on these variables can be studied comprehensively with the use of Frank–Starling and force–tension curves and pressure–volume loops.

## DETERMINANTS OF MYOCARDIAL PERFORMANCE

Myocardial performance is determined by contractility, heart rate, preload, and afterload. Each of these parameters can be defined and measured clinically and is affected by many variables.

### Preload

Preload is the hemodynamic load or stretch on the myocardial wall or fiber at the end of diastole just before contraction begins. There are several experimental and clinical measures of left ventricular (LV) preload. These include (a) end diastolic pressure (EDP), (b) end diastolic volume (EDV), (c) wall stress or tension at end diastole, and (d) end diastolic muscle or sarcomere length. Clinically, EDV provides the most meaningful measure of ventricular preload.

Factors that affect preload include factors that determine the venous return to the heart. Preload is influenced by total blood volume, body position (↓ upright, ↑ supine), venous tone, atrial contraction (↑), skeletal muscle contraction (↑), intrapericardial pressure (tamponade impairs ventricular filling and ↓ preload), and intrathoracic pressure (↑ intrathoracic pressure ↓ venous return).

### Afterload

Afterload is the mechanical force on the ventricle during ejection, determined by the resistance against which the myocardium is contracting. It is also defined as the tension in the myocardium during active contraction. Although there are several measures of afterload, the most commonly used are (a) aortic pressure, (b) total or systemic peripheral vascular resistance, (c) arterial impedance, (4) myocardial peak wall stress (affected by LV geometry), and (e) LV pressure.

Myocardial peak wall stress is related to the amount of force and work the muscle does during contraction. During systole, the muscle contracts and generates force, which is transduced into intraventricular pressure. This depends on the amount of muscle and the geometry of the chamber.

Wall stress is the force per unit cross-sectional area of muscle and is related to intraventricular pressure according to Laplace's law:

$$\textit{Laplace's law:}\quad \text{wall stress} \sim \frac{\text{pressure} \times \text{radius}}{2 \times \text{wall thickness}}$$

Peak wall stress relates to the amount of force and work done by the muscle during contraction. Therefore, this is used as an index of afterload.

Effective arterial elastance (Ea) is also an index of afterload. This is closely related to total peripheral resistance (TPR) and will be defined later.

Under pathologic conditions, when either the mitral valve is incompetent or the aortic valve is stenotic, afterload is determined by additional factors besides the properties of the arterial system.

### Contractility

Contractility refers to the intrinsic "strength" of the cardiac muscle. When loading conditions (preload and afterload) remain constant, an increase in contractility augments cardiac performance, whereas a depression in contractility lowers cardiac performance. As will be described later, ejection fraction is the most commonly used surrogate for contractility. However, it is not always an equivalent measure of contractility.

### Pressure–Volume Loops

The mechanical events that occur during the cardiac cycle consist of changes in pressure in the ventricular chamber, which results in subsequent changes in ventricular volumes. If the ventricular volumes during one cardiac cycle are plotted against simultaneous pressures within the ventricle, a pressure–volume loop is constructed as shown in Figure 1–1. Generally pressure–volume loops are constructed in the cardiac catheterization laboratory with high-fidelity catheters (e.g., Millar catheters).

The end-diastolic pressure–volume relationship (EDPVR) describes the diastolic filling properties of the ventricle similar to the way the end-systolic pressure–volume relationship (ESPVR) describes the systolic filling changes in the ventricle. Together these two pressure–volume relationships are the primary components of the pressure–volume loop. ESPVR represents the properties of the cardiac muscle at the point of maximal activation (systole), unlike the EDPVR, which represents the properties at the end of maximal relaxation (diastole). ESPVR is determined by the mechanical and structural features of the cardiac muscle. ESPVR is linear, unlike EDPVR, which is nonlinear.

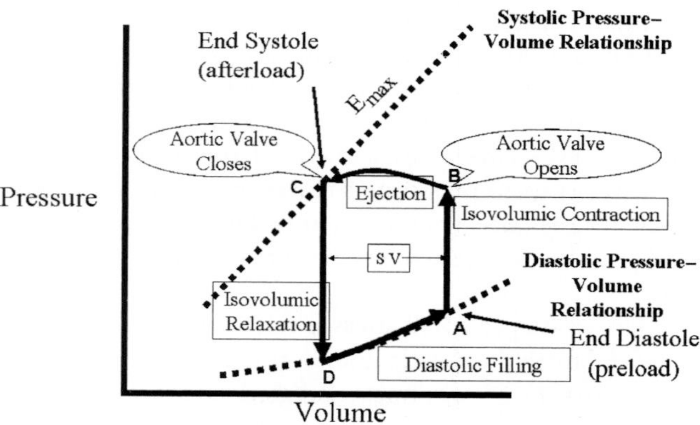


**Figure 1–1** Pressure–volume loops. Time A is the onset of systole. This is followed by the period of isovolumic contraction (change in pressure with no change in volume). The aortic valve opens at point B and the point of maximal ventricular activation is reached at point C. This is followed by a period of isovolumic relaxation (change in pressure with no change in volume). The mitral valve opens at point D, followed by the filling of the LV. Systole includes the time period of isovolumic contraction and ejection (point A to C). Diastole includes the period of isovolumic relaxation and filling (point C to A). The dotted lines represent the end-systolic and end-diastolic pressure-volume relationships, which represent the boundaries of the pressure–volume loops.

## PHYSIOLOGIC MEASUREMENTS RETRIEVABLE FROM THE PRESSURE–VOLUME LOOP

### Volumes

The maximum volume in the ventricle during the cardiac cycle is the end-diastolic volume (EDV). The minimum volume is the end-systolic volume and is the ventricular volume at the end of systolic ejection. Stroke volume (SV) is found from

$$(SV) = EDV - ESV$$

### Pressure Axis

As shown in Figure 1–1, point B represents the point at which the ventricle begins to eject blood into the vasculature (with an open aortic valve). At this time, the ventricular pressure just exceeds aortic pressure. During the ejection phase, aortic and ventricular pressures are nearly equal, so the point of greatest pressure on the loop represents the greatest pressure in the aorta and is equal to the systolic blood pressure (SBP). End-systolic pressure ($P_{es}$) is the pressure on the pressure–volume (*PV*) loop at the end of systole and is only slightly less than the maximal pressure (SBP). Point D, following isovolumic relaxation, represents the pressure in the left atrium (LAP) at the time the mitral valve opens. End-diastolic pressure is represented at the end of diastole (point A) and is influenced by the compliance of the chamber.

### Compliance

Compliance is the change in volume for a given change in pressure or, in mathematical terms, the reciprocal of the derivative of EDPVR. EDPVR is nonlinear and hence compliance varies with volume. Change in volume for a given change in pressure is greater at low volumes (greater compliance) than at higher volumes (lower compliance). Changes in compliance are related to structural and pressure changes of the heart, pericardium, and thorax.

### Elastance

Elastance is a measure of myocardial performance or intrinsic contractility. Defined as the linear relationship between the change in pressure for a given change in volume at end systole on the ESPVR, elastance can be described by the slope, $E_{max}$ or $E_{es}$.

### Stroke Work

Stroke work represents the work of the heart during each heart beat and is represented by the area of the pressure–volume loop.

### Contractility

Contractility refers to the "intrinsic strength" of the cardiac muscle, and is independent of external conditions imposed by either the preload or afterload (i.e., the venous, atrial, or arterial) systems. $E_{es}$ or $E_{max}$ of the ESPVR is considered an index of contractility.

## FACTORS THAT AFFECT VENTRICULAR CONTRACTILITY

Factors that affect ventricular contractility include:

1. Drugs that alter the calcium/actin–myosin coupling mechanism, which can alter the contractility (negative and positive inotropes, sympathetic stimulation, circulating catecholamines) (Table 1–1)
2. Changes in the number of myofilaments participating in the contraction process (ventricular hypertrophy, loss of myocytes after myocardial infarction)

Ejection fraction (EF) is a clinical index of contractility. The disadvantage of EF is that it is dependent on arterial properties or loading conditions. However, based on the ease of measurement and because it does vary with changes in contractility, EF remains the most widely used index of contractility.

## DIFFERENTIATING CARDIAC OUTPUT AND EJECTION FRACTION

Ejection fraction is calculated as the percentage of volume ejected *per beat* by the ventricle (SV/EDV), whereas cardiac output (CO) represents a measure of SV × HR ejected *per minute.*

## FRANK–STARLING LAW OF THE HEART AND FRANK–STARLING CURVES

Cardiac performance increases as preload is increased. However, there is a nonlinear relationship between end-diastolic pressure (EDP, a measure of preload) and CO, as shown in Figure 1–2.

**TABLE 1–1**
**SUMMARY OF MECHANISMS OF ACTION OF COMMONLY USED CARDIOVASCULAR DRUGS AND THEIR PHYSIOLOGIC EFFECTS**

| Drug | Receptors or Mechanisms of Action | Physiologic Effects |
|---|---|---|
| Phenylephrine | $\alpha$ | ↑ afterload, usually no change in HR |
| Isoproterenol | $\beta 1$ and $\beta 2$ | ↑ contractility, ↑ HR, ↓ afterload |
| Norepinephrine | $\alpha > \beta 1$<br>No $\beta 2$ | Marked ↑ afterload, modest ↑ CO |
| Epinephrine | $\beta 1$, $\beta 2$, and $\alpha$ ($\alpha > \beta 2$ at high dose) | Low doses ↑ CO, ↓ SVR, Variable effects on MAP; higher doses ↑ SVR, ↑ CO |
| Dobutamine | $\beta 1 > \beta 2, \alpha$ | ↑ CO, ↓ SVR, ↑ HR with or without a small reduction in BP |
| Dopamine | Dopa (low doses, <4)<br>$\beta 1$ (intermediate, 4–10)<br>$\alpha$ (high doses, >10) | At moderate doses, ↑ contractility, ↑ HR ↑ CO; high doses (>10 μg/kg) cause vasoconstriction and ↑ SVR |
| Nitroprusside | Arterial, venous dilator | ↓ preload, ↓ afterload |
| Nitroglycerin | Venous ≫ arterial dilator | ↓ preload ≫ ↓ afterload |
| Hydralazine | Direct arterial vasodilator | ↓ afterload, no effect on preload |
| Phentolamine | $\alpha$ antagonist | ↓ afterload, ↑ contractility, ↑ HR |
| Furosemide | Diuretic | ↓ preload |
| Milrinone | Phosphodiesterase inhibitor | Similar to dobutamine, no change in HR, ↓ pulmonary vascular resistance |

HR, heart rate; CO, cardiac output; SVR, systemic vascular resistance; MAP, mean arterial pressure.

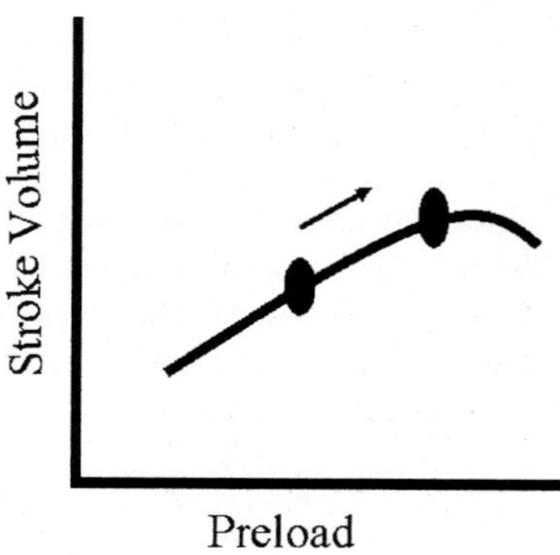


**Figure 1–2** Frank–Starling curves. As preload increases, stroke volume increases.

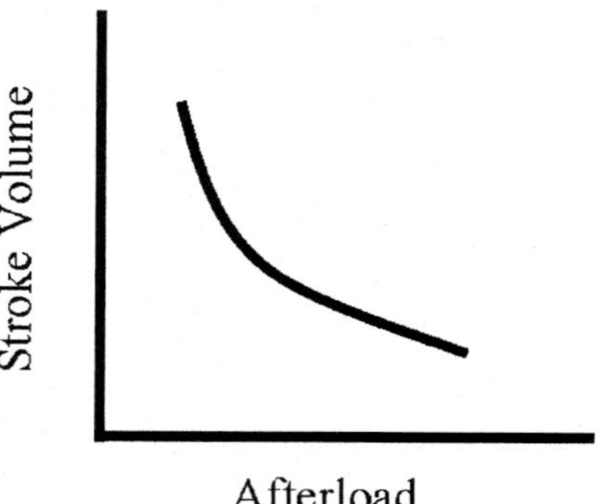


**Figure 1–3** Force–tension curves. As afterload is reduced, stroke volume increases.

In addition to preload, ventricular contractility and afterload can influence Frank–Starling curves. When the ventricular contractile state is increased, CO or SV for a given EDP increases (the curve shifts upward and to the left). When the contractile state is depressed, CO decreases (the curve shifts downward and to the right). When arterial resistance (afterload) increases, CO decreases for a given EDP (the curve shifts downward and to the right), whereas CO increases when arterial resistance decreases (the curve shifts upward and to the left).

## FORCE–VELOCITY RELATIONSHIP AND FORCE–TENSION CURVES

As afterload is reduced, the velocity of shortening increases (Fig. 1–3). When afterload is zero, the velocity of shortening is maximal ($V_{max}$). As with the Frank–Starling relationship, preload and contractility also influence the force–velocity relationship. As preload increases for a given afterload, CO or SV increases (the curve shifts upward and to the right), whereas CO decreases if preload is decreased (the curve shifts downward and to the left). When ventricular contractile state increases, then, for a given afterload, CO increases (the curve shifts upward and to the right). When contractile state is depressed, CO decreases (the curve shifts downward and to the left).

## METHODS OF MEASURING CARDIAC PERFORMANCE

Methods of measuring cardiac performance include the following:

- Chamber size (volume, area): LV angiography, echocardiography (two-dimensional or three-dimensional), gated nuclear, MRI, CT
- Chamber pressure (fluid-filled catheter): ($dP/dt$), LVEDP, LV systolic pressure
- Blood velocity: Doppler echocardiography ($V_{max}$, $dP/dt$)
- Myocardial velocity: Doppler tissue imaging, MRI

## SIMPLE SUMMARY OF THE ACTIONS OF THE AUTONOMIC NERVOUS SYSTEM

Following is a simple summary of the actions of the autonomic nervous system:

$\alpha 1$ stimulation: ↑ afterload, ↑ preload
$\beta 1$ stimulation: ↑ contractility, ↑ HR
$\beta 2$ stimulation: ↓ afterload

## VALVULAR HEART DISEASE AND PRESSURE–VOLUME LOOPS

The pressure–volume loops in various valvular diseases are depicted in Table 1–2 and Figure 1–4.

**TABLE 1–2**
**VALVULAR HEART DISEASE: PRESSURE–VOLUME LOOPS**

| Valve Condition | Afterload | Preload | Contractility (Early) | Contractility (Late) |
|---|---|---|---|---|
| Aortic stenosis | ↑ | ↔ | ↑ | ↓ |
| Aortic regurgitation | ↑ | ↑ | ↔ | ↓ |
| Mitral regurgitation | ↓ | ↑ | ↑ | ↓ |
| Mitral stenosis | ↔ | ↓ | ↔ | ↔ |

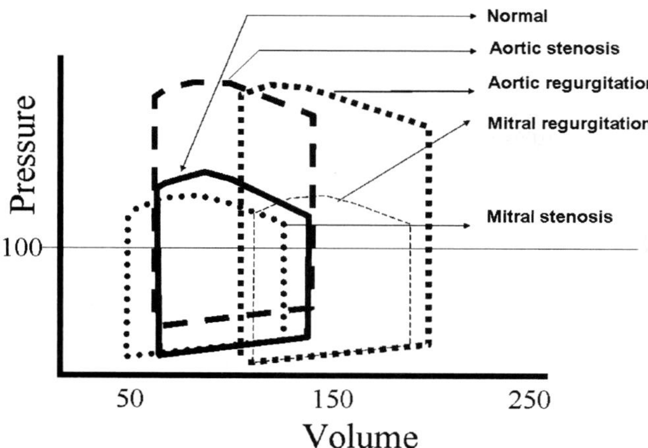


**Figure 1–4** PV loops in various valvular disease states, with curves as depicted here for aortic and mitral regurgitation representing decompensated states.

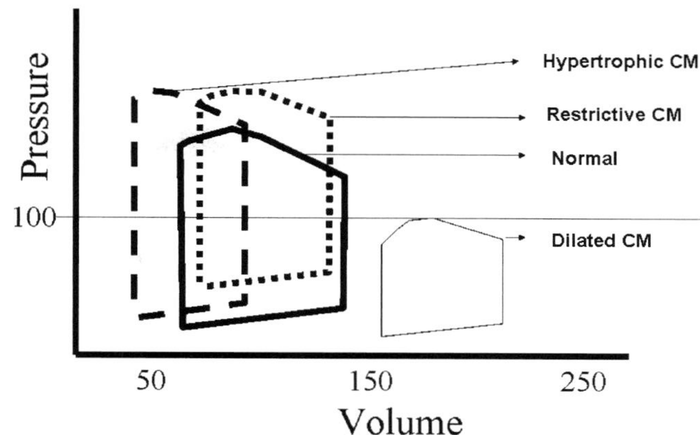


**Figure 1–5** PV loops in various cardiomyopathies (CM).

**TABLE 1–3**

**CARDIOMYOPATHY: PRESSURE–VOLUME LOOPS**

| Condition | ESV | EDV | Contractility |
|---|---|---|---|
| Dilated | ↑ | ↑ | ↓ |
| Hypertrophic | ↓ | ↓ | ↑ |
| Restrictive | ↓ or ↔ | ↓ or ↔ | ↓ or ↔ |

ESV, end-systolic volume; EDV, end-diastolic volume.

## CARDIOMYOPATHY AND PRESSURE–VOLUME LOOPS

The pressure–volume loops in various cardiomyopathies are depicted in Table 1–3 and Figure 1–5.

## QUESTIONS

1. What medication will cause the following changes? (The arrows indicate the direction of change in stroke volume.)

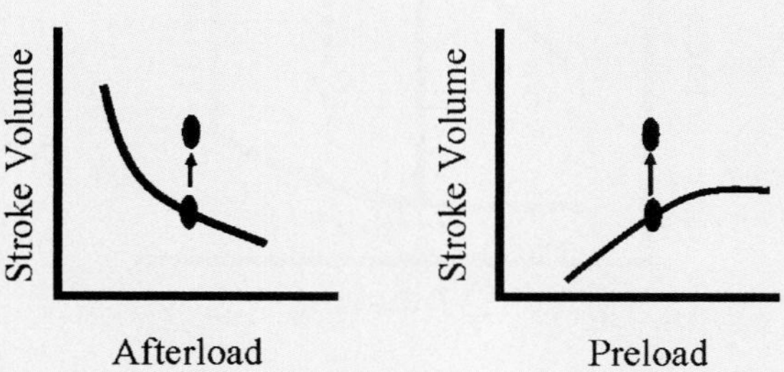


a. Isoproterenol
b. Digitalis
c. Phentolamine
d. Norepinephrine
e. Epinephrine (high dose)

Answer is b: Digitalis increases contractility without affecting preload or afterload.

2. What medication will take a patient from point A to point B on the following curves?

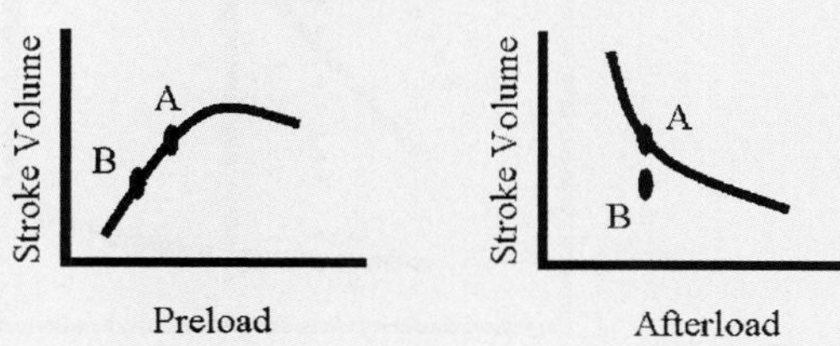


a. Propranolol
b. Isoproterenol
c. Norepinephrine
d. Furosemide
e. Hydralazine

Answer is d: Furosemide is a diuretic and hence decreases preload.

3. A patient with congestive heart failure is started on a new medication and the pressure–volume loop moves from I to II. What drug was started?

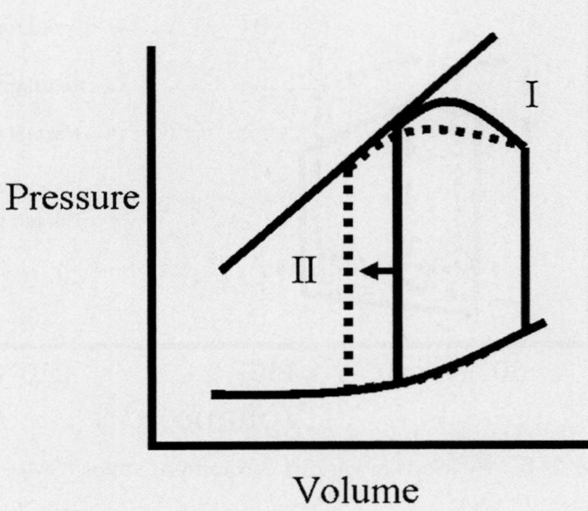


a. Digitalis
b. Hydralazine
c. Epinephrine
d. Norepinephrine
e. Isoproterenol

Answer is b: Hydralazine is a direct arteriolar vasodilator and decreases afterload. Preload and contractility remain unchanged.

**4.** What medication will cause the following change in the pressure–volume loops (from the solid loop to the dotted lines)?

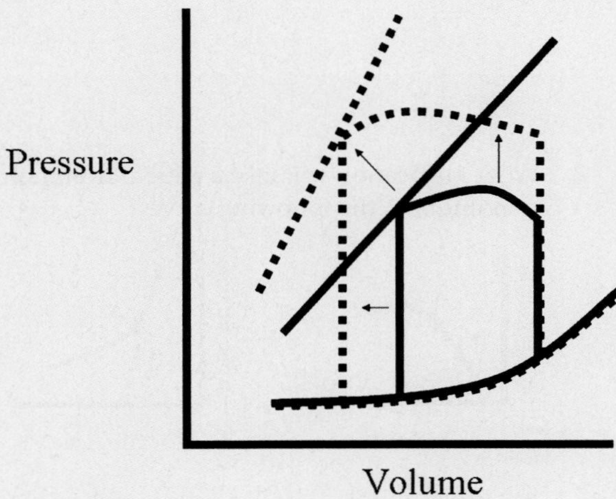


a. Norepinephrine
b. Digitalis
c. Isoproterenol
d. Hydralazine
e. Epinephrine (low dose)

Answer is a: Norepinephrine increases afterload by its effects on the $\alpha 1$ receptors. It also increases contractility by its action on the $\beta 1$ receptors.

**5.** What medication will cause the following change (solid loop to dotted line)?

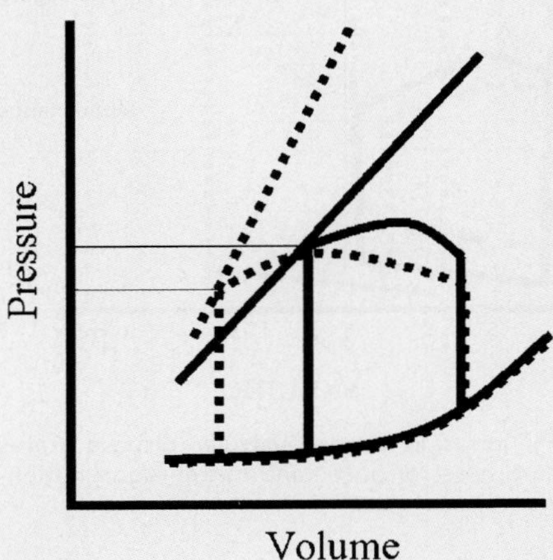


a. Norepinephrine
b. Digitalis
c. Isoproterenol
d. Hydralazine
e. Phenylephrine

Answer is c: Isoproterenol increases contractility. It also increases heart rate and decreases afterload by its action on $\beta 1$ and $\beta 2$ receptors.

**6.** What medication, administered acutely, will shift the pressure–volume loop as outlined below (from the solid line to the dotted line)?

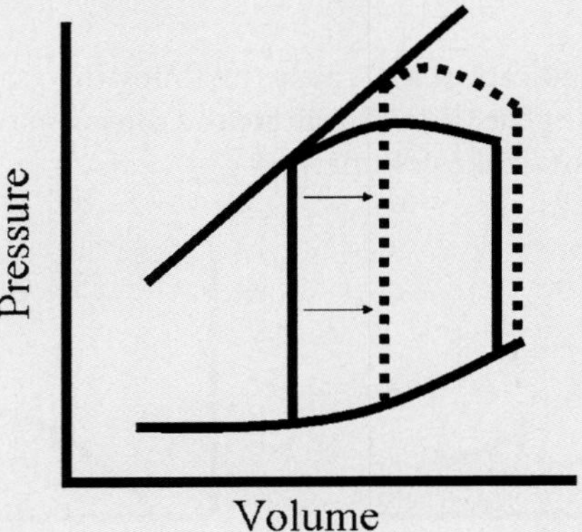


a. Phenylephrine
b. Captopril
c. Hydralazine + nitrates
d. Digitalis + Intravenous fluids (IVF)
e. Epinephrine

Answer is a: Phenylephrine ($\alpha$-agonist). It increases afterload more than it increases preload.

# Basic Cardiac Electrophysiology

2

*Sergio G. Thal*  *Patrick J. Tchou*

The aim of this chapter is to cover the main aspects of basic cardiac electrophysiology, developed in a review fashion for the Cardiovascular Medicine Board Examination. The information is organized as follows:

1. Basic action potential and ion channel implications
2. Electrical activity coupling mechanisms
3. Conduction system anatomy
4. Local electrophysiology characteristics of various conduction system components

## MEMBRANE ACTION POTENTIAL

The initiation of the cell membrane action potential (AP) is the first event in a process that ends with a cardiac contraction. Grossly, myocardial cells can be divided into those dependent on sodium ions ($Na^+$) or calcium ions ($Ca^{2+}$) to drive action potential depolarization.

### Sodium-Dependent Cells (Fig. 2–1)

Each AP starts with net movement of ions across the cell membrane. In a steady state, the membrane is polarized near −90 mV. The transmembrane ionic current is the result of the balance between many inward and outward ionic currents. The sodium channel is voltage sensitive. This means that the probability of the channel being open for transport of the sodium ion increases with increase of transmembrane voltage (toward zero). When a cell receives depolarizing current, sodium channels open and increase the inward current. When the inward current exceeds the total outward current, a rapid opening of sodium channels occurs that overwhelms any outward current, resulting in the rapid upstroke portion of the AP termed Phase 0 (Fig. 2–2).

Sodium channels are characterized by a protein that works as a voltage-gated system. The active portion of this channel is the $\alpha$ subunit, which consists of a 2,000–amino acid glycoprotein. Properties of these channels include the following:

- Selective permeation
- Gating (activation and inactivation)
- Drug binding (local anesthetics)
- Susceptibility to many different neurotoxins

### Levels of $Na^+$ Channel Activity Regulation

1. Transcriptional regulation of $Na^+$ channel proteins is a mechanism to control $Na^+$ channel expression at a genomic level. This pattern of regulation can be influenced by feedback originating in the tissue electrical activity. The exact mechanism of this gene regulation remains incompletely understood.
2. Phosphorylation/dephosphorylation of the $\alpha$ subunit
3. Glycosylation. The regulation mechanism affects all channel subunits.

Abnormalities of the sodium channel can result in both the long QT syndrome as well as the Brugada syndrome.

Phase 1 (see Fig. 2–2) starts with the opening of a rapid outward potassium ($K^+$) current called $I_{to}$. This determines a fast early repolarization with a prominent notch shape that approximates the membrane potential to 0 mV.

These channels are characterized by outward movement of $K^+$ ions, which constitutes the principal source of membrane repolarization early during the action potential. The channels inactivate soon after activation, although not as rapidly as the sodium current does. A dynamic interaction of four $\alpha$ subunits and an apparatus composed of a

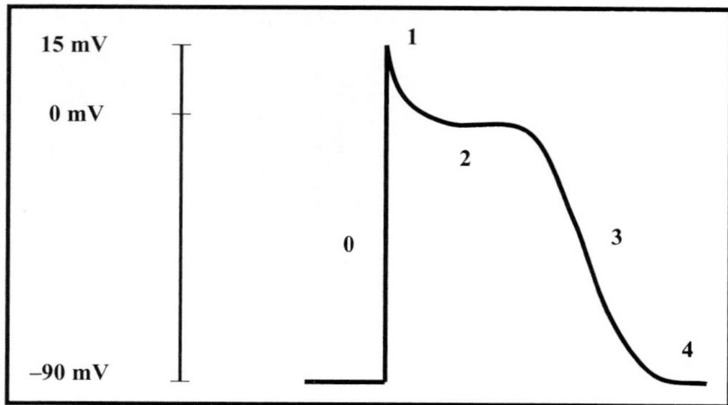


**Figure 2–1** Action potential (sodium channel tissue). Action potential model of a sodium tissue. Numbers 0, 1, 2, 3, 4 delineate the different phases of the action potential.

cytoskeleton and signaling complexes mainly form the $K^+$ pore. During the AP, these $K^+$ channels activate in response to membrane depolarization and inactivate in a timed manner. The channels are regulated by:

- Angiotensin II, which reduces $I_{to}$ fast velocity
- $\alpha$-Adrenergic stimulation, which reduces $I_{to}$ fast velocity
- Hyperthyroidism, which increases $I_{to}$ current density
- Aldosterone, which mediates a receptor-specific down-regulation of $I_{to}$

In human pathophysiology, these channels provide an early repolarization current that can drive the transmembrane voltage toward resting membrane potential when the sodium current is dysfunctional. Thus, in Brugada syndrome, in which there is an abnormality in the sodium current that results in depressed sodium conductance, the $I_{to}$ current may cause full repolarization in a portion of the myocardium early during the AP, resulting in a large voltage gradient between the repolarized part and parts that have more normal AP. Such gradients have been demonstrated in isolated tissue preparations to be capable of initiating re-entrant wavefronts. These re-entrant wavefronts can initiate polymorphic ventricular tachycardia or ventricular fibrillation.

The next portion of the AP, termed Phase 2 or the plateau phase (see Fig. 2–2), is the result of the balance of two different ion currents. During Phase 0, at the level of −40 mV, $Ca^{2+}$ channels open, creating an inward $Ca^{2+}$ current. This

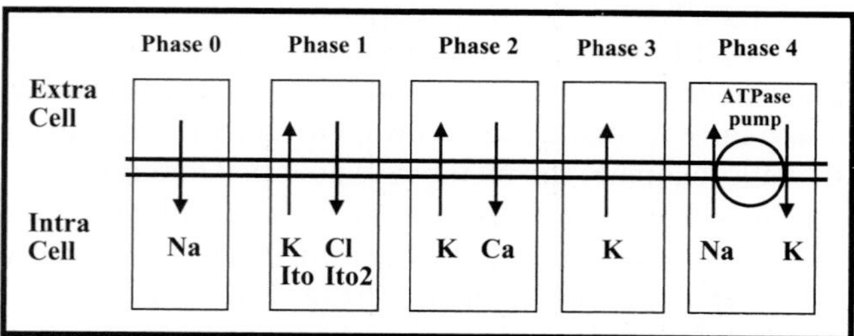


**Figure 2–2** Main ion channel activities in action potential phases. Na: sodium; K: potassium; Cl: chloride; Ca: calcium.

current, acting as an antagonist to the outward $K^+$ current, exerts its action by stabilizing transmembrane potential during the plateau phase. This phase concludes as the $Ca^{2+}$ current declines by inactivation of L-type $Ca^{2+}$ channels. These channels are also the critical initiators of cardiac excitation–contraction coupling through the initial increase in intracellular $Ca^{2+}$, which triggers the release of $Ca^{2+}$ from the sarcoplasmic reticulum, which in turn provides a contraction signal to the cellular contractile elements. At a level of −40 mV of membrane potential, these channels rapidly activate, reaching a peak in approximately 2 to 7 milliseconds. Inactivation of the channel depends on time, membrane potential, and $Ca^{2+}$ concentration.

Phase 3 (see Fig. 2–2), the repolarization phase, is dominated by the outward current of $K^+$ through the so-called "delayed rectifier" $K^+$ channels, which are responsible for the return of the cell membrane to its resting polarized state. Two types of delayed rectifiers are important in the repolarization of human ventricular myocardium, a rapidly activating $I_{Kr}$ and a more slowly activating $I_{Ks}$ that peaks late in the AP, during Phase 3. Abnormalities in either of these two types of delayed rectifier $K^+$ channels can cause the long-QT syndrome.

Phase 4 (see Fig. 2–2) constitutes a stable polarized membrane. This stabilization of membrane AP after the descending Phase 3 is achieved mainly by the action of the voltage-regulated inward rectifiers ($I_{K1}$). These channels behave differently than the delayed rectifiers, which open in response to depolarization. The inward rectifier $K^+$ channels are opened at near resting membrane potential, stabilizing the resting membrane potential near the $K^+$ equilibrium potential, but close in response to depolarization, facilitating the action potential, hence the description of "inward rectifying."

## Myocardial Tissues That Have Calcium-Dependent AP versus Tissues with Sodium Channels (Fig. 2–3)

The main differences between these two types of myocardial tissue can be found in Phases 4 and 0 of the action potential. Calcium-dependent tissues are the principal cellular component of the specialized conduction system and the sinus node. These cells have the ability to generate a spontaneous action potential based on the differential characteristic of Phase 4. This difference is produced by ion currents that affect $Na^+$ and $K^+$ concentrations, called $I_f$, which activate at membrane potentials below −40 mV, and the K rectifier currents. These currents confer an unstable electrical property, causing these cells to develop spontaneous diastolic depolarization and automatic onset of action potentials in a rhythmic fashion. Once spontaneous diastolic activity raises the membrane potential to a value of −40 mV, opening of the slow $Ca^{2+}$ channels results in an inward $Ca^{2+}$ current (L-type Ca) that generates the slow action potential upstroke (Phase 0). $Na^+$ channels possess

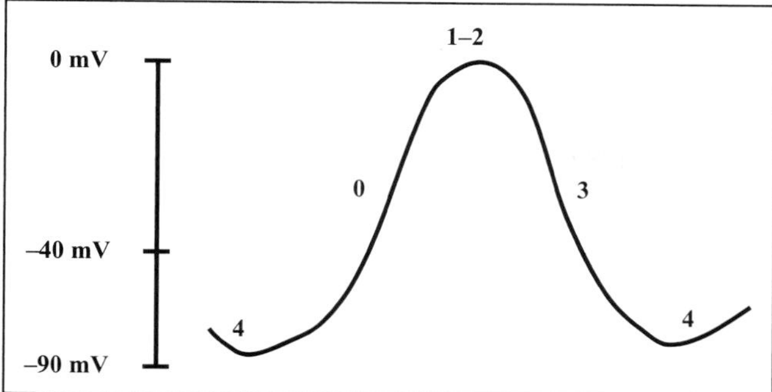


**Figure 2–3** Action potential (calcium channel tissue). Action potential model of a calcium tissue. Numbers 0, 1, 2, 3, 4 delineate the different phases of the action potential.

a small if any role in the action potential generation in these particular cells.

## ELECTRICAL COUPLING CELLS (GAP JUNCTION)

GAP junction channels are the functional units that produce direct ionic communication between cardiac cells and play a major role in the propagation of the action potential from one myocardial cell to the next. The molecular unit of the GAP junction is a protein called connexin. The oligomerization of six connexins forms a connexon, and two connexons form the final channel called the GAP junction. Among the 20 different subtypes of connexins identified in the human genome, connexin-43 is the most abundant in myocardial cells. Besides the genomic regulation of channel expression, they are also affected by the activity of protein kinase activity, low intracellular pH, and dephosphorylation.

GAP junction channels are not uniformly distributed within cardiac tissues. They are almost absent in the sinus node, are found in low concentration in various areas of the atrioventricular node, and demonstrate significant expression in the faster conducting atrial and ventricular muscle as well as His–Purkinje fibers. In these cells, the distribution of the conexons is not uniform. They are more concentrated along the ends of the myocytes than along the sides of the cell, thus giving a directional propensity for action potential propagation. This gives rise to anisotropic propagation of depolarization, with faster conduction velocities along the muscle fiber orientation compared to the slower transverse fiber–orientated velocities.

## CONDUCTION SYSTEM ANATOMY AND PHYSIOLOGY

The sinus node is located beneath the epicardial surface of the crista terminalis, at its junction with the high right atrium. It possesses a spindle-shaped structure and measures an average 10 to 20 mm in the long axis and 2 to 3 mm in the transverse axis. It is composed of a cumulus of small cells called P cells; the main component of the natural pacemaker. They are grouped in elongated clusters and are centrally located within the sinus node. Transitional cells called T cells surround the P cells and transmit the impulse generated by the P cells to the surrounding atrium. The final synchronized activity of the sinus node is achieved via the presence of GAP junctional channels that electrically couple the depolarization of P cells. At the periphery of the node, strands of nodal cells interdigitate with atrial cells, forming lateral connections and transferring the pacemaker impulse to the atrial cells. This organization is believed to be important to impulse propagation from a small source (the nodal cells) to a large reservoir (the atrial myocardium), preventing excessive dampening of the pacemaker current within the nodal cells by the large reservoir of atrial myocardium.

Cells within the sinus node demonstrate spontaneous diastolic depolarization, initiating action potentials in a repetitive fashion. These action potentials are calcium channel dependent and possess a similar morphology to those of the atrioventricular nodal cell, characterized by a slow Phase 0 upstroke velocity. Sinus node cells do not possess the gap junction protein connexin-43. Therefore, electrical coupling at the node center is poor, reflected as a low measured conduction velocity. The periphery is associated with an increase in conduction velocity. This characteristic is most likely important in isolating the sinus node from the potential suppressive hyperpolarizing influence of the atrial myocardium.

Normal sinus node function is affected by age. In the young, the intrinsic heart rate is faster, but vagal tone predominates at rest, causing slowing of the heart rate. In the elderly, resting autonomic tone tends to shift away from vagal predominance to sympathetic outflow. Thus, the extrinsic sinus rate at rest, the rate as modified by autonomic tone, tends to be similar within the ages of adulthood.

The impulse generated at the sinoatrial node is next transmitted to the atrioventricular node (AVN) through atrial myocytes. There is anatomic evidence for the presence of three atrionodal pathways traversing the right atrium. A fourth pathway, called Bachmann's bundle, derived from the anterior atrionodal pathway, directs impulse propagation to the left atrium via the interatrial septum. Anatomically, these so-called pathways do not demonstrate any specialized conduction tissue. Rapid conduction along these intra- and interarterial paths appears to be correlated with fiber size and orientation rather than the presence of specialized conduction tissue.

The AVN is a fusiform structure located subendocardially along the annular regions of the interatrial septum, with its distal end, the compact node, at the superior corner of the triangle of Koch. The triangle of Koch is defined by the insertion of the septal leaflet of the tricuspid valve, the tendon of Todaro, and the line that connect the os of the coronary sinus and the tricuspid annulus. The body and proximal end (the tail) of the atrioventricular (AV) node are directed posteriorly along the tricuspid annulus. A second tail extends from the body of the AV node along the mitral annulus. The so-called slow pathway of the AV node corresponds to the tail of the AV node, whereas the fast pathway involves atrial inputs into the distal compact node. Similar to the sinus node, transitional cells surround this structure. Circulation to the AV node is provided in nearly 90% of individuals by branches of the right coronary artery extending superiorly from the crux into the trigone area along the AV annulus.

The His bundle is the anatomic structure that connects the compact AV node to the bundle branches. At the junction between the distal AV node and the proximal His bundle, the cells undergo a gradual change from possessing nodelike action potentials to having His–Purkinje action potentials. That is the APs change from having slow upstrokes dependent on $Ca^{2+}$ current to fast upstrokes dependent on $Na^{+}$current. The branches from the anterior and posterior descending arteries provide circulation to this portion of the conduction system and confer a better security margin for ischemic damage. The His bundle penetrates the AV ring at the central fibrous body and then arches anteriorly and inferiorly along the crest of the septal myocardium that forms the lower edge of the membranous ventricular septum. As it courses along the crest, left-sided fibers in the His bundle drop over the crest into the left ventricle, forming the posterior, septal, and anterior fascicles of the left bundle branch. The His bundle then continues its course over the right ventricular septum as the right bundle branch. The right bundle brunch adopts a subendocardial trajectory over the right side of the interventricular septum and transmits the cardiac impulse to the Purkinje fibers located at the apical portions of the right ventricle. The bundle branches spread into a smaller Purkinje bundle and then into finer fibers that terminate at the myocardium. This branching structure of the His–Purkinje system failitates a near-synchronous arrival of the sinus impulse at the myocardial endocardial surface.

Electrophysiologically, the AVN can differentiated into three portions: atrionodal, compact node, and nodo-His. The compact node area presents a response characterized by an action potential with a slow rate of rise during its upstroke and a low amplitude. The other two zones have transitional characteristics between the compact node zone and the atrial and His bundle potentials, respectively.

Calcium-type APs characterize the main AVN cellular type. Differentiating the AVN from the sinus node, GAP junctions play an important role in AVN conduction. Connexin-45 is present in this portion of the conduction system, though at a low level. It has also been demonstrated that the expression of connexin-45 constitutes the molecular basis of AVN dual pathways.

## BIBLIOGRAPHY

**Beardslee MA, Tadros PN, Laing JG, et al.** Dephosphorylation and intracellular redistribution of ventricular connexin43 during electrical uncoupling induced by ischemia. *Circ Res.* 2000;87(8):656–662.

**Boyett MR, Kodama I.** The sinoatrial node, a heterogeneous pacemaker structure. *Cardiovasc Res.* 2000;47(4):658–687.

**Coppen SR.** Diversity of connexin expression patterns in the atrioventricular node: vestigial consequence or functional specialization? *J Cardiovasc Electrophysiol.* 2002;13(6):625–626.

**de Carvalho A, de Almeida D.** Spread of activity through the atrioventricular node. *Circ Res.* 1960;8:801–809.

**DiFrancesco D, Mazzanti M, Tromba C.** Properties of the hyperpolarizing-activated current (if) in cells isolated from the rabbit sino-atrial node. *J Physiol.* 1986;377:61–88.

**Douglas P, Zipes MJJ.** *Cardiac Electrophysiology. From Cell to Bedside.* 4th ed. Philadelphia: WB Saunders; 2004.

**Gourdie RG, Green CR, Rothery S, Germroth P, Thompson RP.** The spatial distribution and relative abundance of gap-junctional connexin40 and connexin43 correlate to functional properties of components of the cardiac atrioventricular conduction system. *J Cell Sci.* 1993;105(4):985–991.

**Irisawa H.** Cardiac electrophysiology: past, present and future. Part II. Membrane currents in cardiac pacemaker tissue. *Experientia.* 1987; 43:1131–1135.

**Kwak BR, De Jonge HR, Lohmann SM, et al.** Differential regulation of distinct types of gap junction channels by similar phosphorylating conditions. *Mol Biol Cell.* 1995;6(12):1707–1719.

**Makowski L, Phillips WC, Goodenough DA.** Gap junction structures. II. Analysis of the x-ray diffraction data. *J Cell Biol.* 1977;74(2):629–645.

**Morley GE, Delmar M.** Intramolecular interactions mediate pH regulation of connexin43 channels. *Biophys J.* 1996;70(3):1294–1302.

**Nikolski VP, Lancaster MK, Boyett MR, Efimov IR.** Cx43 and dual-pathway electrophysiology of the atrioventricular node and atrioventricular nodal reentry. *Circ Res.* 2003;92(4):469–475.

**Trabka-Janik E, Lemanski LF, Delmar M, Jalife J.** Immunohistochemical localization of gap junction protein channels in hamster sinoatrial node in correlation with electrophysiologic mapping of the pacemaker region. *J Cardiovasc Electrophysiol.* 1994;5(2):125–137.

## QUESTIONS

1. Which of the following is *not* a characteristic of sodium channels?
   a. Selective permeation
   b. Pump electrolytes exchange mechanism
   c. Gating
   d. Drug binding
   e. Susceptibility to many different neurotoxins

Answer is b: Sodium channels are characterized by a protein that works as a voltage-gated sodium channel. The active portion of this channel is the $\alpha$ subunit, which consists of a 2,000–amino acid glycoprotein. The other choices are all properties of these channels.

2. Which of the following is *not* a characteristic of Phase 1 of the action potential?

a. Phase 1 starts with the opening of a rapid outward $K^+$ ion current called $I_{to}$.
b. These $K^+$ channels activate in response to membrane depolarization.
c. These $K^+$ channels inactivate in a time-dependent manner.
d. $\alpha$-Adrenergic stimulation increases $I_{to}$ maximum current.
e. Aldosterone mediates a receptor-specific downregulation of $I_{to}$.

Answer is d: Phase 1 starts with the opening of a rapid outward $K^+$ ion current called $I_{to}$. This determines a fast early repolarization. These $K^+$ channels activate in response to membrane depolarization and inactivate in a time-dependent manner. These channels may be regulated by the following means:

- Angiotensine II reduces $I_{to}$ maximum velocity.
- $\alpha$-Adrenergic stimulation reduces $I_{to}$ fast velocity.
- Hyperthyroidism increase $I_{to}$ current density.
- Aldosterone mediates a receptor-specific downregulation of $I_{to}$.

**3.** Which of the following is *not* a characteristic of calcium channels?

a. During Phase 0, at the level of −40 mV, $Ca^{2+}$ channels open, creating an inward $Ca^{2+}$ current.
b. This current acts as an agonist to the outward $K^+$ current.
c. Phase II concludes as $Ca^{2+}$ current declines by inactivation of L-type $Ca^{2+}$ channels.
d. Inactivation of the channel depends on time, membrane potential, and Ca concentration.
e. Intracellular $Ca^{2+}$ concentration acts as a critical initiator of cardiac excitation–contraction coupling.

Answer is b: During Phase 0, at the level of −40 mV, $Ca^{2+}$ channels open, creating an inward $Ca^{2+}$ current. This current act as an antagonist to the outward $K^+$ current. Phase II concludes as $Ca^{2+}$ current declines by inactivation of L-type $Ca^{2+}$ channels, letting the plateau phase subside. These channels are also the critical initiators of cardiac excitation–contraction coupling through the initial increase in intracellular $Ca^{2+}$ concentration that triggers the release of $Ca^{2+}$ from the sarcoplasmic reticulum, which in turn provides a contraction signal to the contractile elements of the cell. Inactivation of the channel depends on time, membrane potential, and Ca concentration.

**4.** Which of the following is the main mechanism by which resting membrane potential (Phase 4 of the action potential) is maintained?

a. Delayed rectifier $K^+$ channels
b. Voltage-regulated inward rectifiers
c. These channels open in response to depolarization.
d. These channels open after reaching the resting membrane potential.
e. These potassium channels stabilize the resting membrane potential near the sodium equilibrium potential.

Answer is b: The stabilization of resting membrane potential after the descending Phase 3 of the action potential is achieved mainly by the action of the voltage-regulated inward rectifiers ($I_{K1}$). These channels behave differently than the delayed rectifiers, which open in response to depolarization. The inward rectifier $K^+$ channels are opened near resting membrane potential, stabilizing the resting membrane potential near the $K^+$ equilibrium potential, but close in response to depolarization, facilitating the action potential, hence the description as "inward rectifying."

**5.** Which of the following statements about GAP junctions is wrong?

a. GAP junction channels are the functional units that allow direct ionic communication between cardiac cells.
b. GAP junctions play a major role in the propagation of the action potential.
c. The molecular unit of the GAP junction is a protein called connexin.
d. Connexin-43 is the most abundant in cardiac conduction system cells.
e. Connexin-43 may be affected by the activity of protein kinase, low intracellular pH, and dephosphorylation.

Answer is d: GAP junction channels are the functional units that allow direct ionic communication between cardiac cells and play a major role in the propagation of the action potential from one cell to the next. The molecular unit of the GAP junction is a protein called Connexin. The oligomerization of six connexins form a connexon, and two connexons form the final channel called the GAP junction. Among the 20 different subtypes of connexins identified in the human genome, connexin-43 is the most abundant in myocardial cells. Besides the obvious genomic regulation of the expression of these channels, they may also be affected by the activity of protein kinase activity, low intracellular pH, and dephosphorylation.

# Cardiac Biochemistry

# 3

***Matthews Chacko*** ***Marc S. Penn***

The biochemistry of cardiac tissue involves tightly regulated interactions among ions, proteins, receptors, second messenger systems, and various cellular structures as well as extracardiac influences. Several abnormalities involving neurohormonal pathways as well as derangements of the contractile apparatus of the cardiac myocyte have been demonstrated in cells isolated from failing hearts. This chapter reviews some of the salient features of the biochemistry of the cardiac myocyte.

## CARDIAC CONTRACTILITY AND CALCIUM HOMEOSTASIS

The cardiac myocyte is an interconnected network of myofibrils surrounded by sarcoplasmic reticulum. Each myofibril is comprised of sarcomeres made up of thick myosin filaments and thin actin filaments that form the basic contractile unit of the cardiac myocyte (Fig. 3–1). The active sites of the actin filaments are covered in the resting state by two regulatory proteins, tropomyosin and troponin. Intracellular $Ca^{2+}$ is the most important determinant of myocardial contractility and relaxation (1). Once contraction ensues, calcium ($Ca^{2+}$) entry through L-type $Ca^{2+}$ channels triggers an exponential release of $Ca^{2+}$ from the sarcoplasmic reticulum (SR) through ryanodine receptors (2). Calcium then binds troponin, leading to a conformational alteration of tropomyosin, exposing the actin active site, facilitating a "sliding" interaction between the actin filaments and the myosin heads as well as the hydrolysis of ATP (adenosine triphosphate), thus providing energy for contraction (3). Following a cycle of excitation–contraction coupling, diastolic relaxation is initiated by cytosolic $Ca^{2+}$ sequestration in the sarcoplasmic reticulum (SR) by the SR-$Ca^{2+}$ ATPase (SERCA2a) pump (~75%) and exportation extracellularly by the $Na^+/Ca^{2+}$ exchanger (~25%) located on the sarcolemmal membrane (4,5). Abnormalities with this mechanism may be partly responsible for the diastolic dysfunction seen in congestive heart failure (CHF) (6). Phospholamban, a regulatory protein, exerts an inhibitory effect on SERCA2a, limiting its ability to remove cytosolic $Ca^{2+}$ following contraction (7). Calcium dysregulation including reduced SR $Ca^{2+}$ release, elevated diastolic $Ca^{2+}$ levels, and delayed $Ca^{2+}$ efflux parallel the systolic and diastolic dysfunction seen in the failing myocardium (8,9), with key derangements being with SERCA2a (5,6,10) and phospholamban (11–13) activity.

## β-ADRENERGIC SIGNALING

Three β-adrenergic receptor subtypes have been characterized, $\beta_1$, $\beta_2$, and $\beta_3$. Catecholamines act to increase myocardial contractility primarily through $\beta_1$-adrenergic receptor stimulation leading to G protein–mediated adenyl cyclase activation and cyclic adenosine 3′5′ monophosphate (cAMP) generation, which triggers protein kinase A (PKA)–dependent phosphorylation of voltage-gated L-type $Ca^+$ channels, ryanodine receptors, and phospholamban, which de-represses SERCA2a, leading to excitation–contraction coupling and positive inotropy (Fig. 3–2) (14–16). $\beta_2$-Adrenergic receptors as well as muscarinic cholinergic receptors, through an inhibitory G protein, provide negative control of adrenergic stimulation by inactivating adenyl cyclase, thereby limiting the generation of cAMP (17). The role of $\beta_3$-adrenergic receptors is poorly defined, but there is some evidence that $\beta_3$-adrenergic receptors maintain coronary vasomotor tone through the nitric oxide pathway (18). β-Arrestins also serve to restrict cAMP generation by increasing cAMP degradation and desensitizing the β-receptor (19). Derangements in chronic β-adrenergic signaling that have been implicated in the pathogenesis of CHF include β-adrenergic receptor (β-AR) downregulation, β-AR uncoupling from second messenger systems, upregulation of β-adrenoreceptor kinase (βARK1), and altered calcium trafficking (20–25). β-Receptor blockade can restore calcium homestasis and upregulate SERCA2a, ultimately improving cardiac performance with long-term treatment (26).

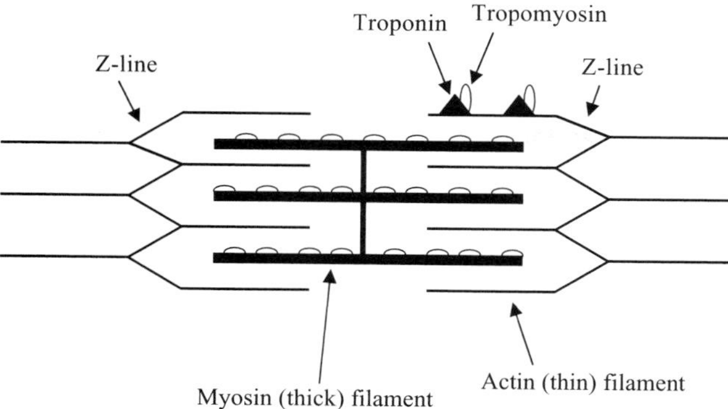


**Figure 3–1** Sarcomere anatomy.

## DIGITALIS AND THE $Na^+$-$K^+$ATPase

Digitalis, a cardiac glycoside derived from the foxglove plant, has been used for centuries to treat heart failure and atrial fibrillation. Digitalis functions by inhibiting the sodium pump ($Na^+/K^+$ATPase) found in the cardiac cell membrane (27,28). The $Na^+/K^+$ATPase works constitutively, using energy from the hydrolysis of ATP to maintain a high intracellular $K^+$ concentration and a high extracellular $Na^+$ concentration (29). $Ca^{2+}$ is removed from the cytosol into the extracellular fluid by a sodium–calcium exchange (NCX1) pump driven by the pre-existing $Na^+$ gradient (30). Inhibiting the $Na^+/K^+$ATPase promotes enhanced $Na^+/Ca^{2+}$ exchange, leading ultimately to increased intracellular $Ca^{2+}$ being available to the contractile apparatus, potentially leading to increased myocardial contractility.

## PHOSPHODIESTERASE INHIBITION

Phosphodiesterase inhibitors (PDIs) such as milrinone affect contractility by inhibiting phosphodiesterase 3 (PDE3), increasing intracellular cAMP and $Ca^{2+}$, which leads to increased inotropy (31). PDIs also have vasodilating properties that are important in unloading the failing ventricle (32). Unfortunately, the gain in cardiac performance is tempered by increased arrhythmogenesis, myocardial oxygen consumption, and cardiac death, mitigating its usefulness beyond being a bridge to cardiac transplantation in end-stage CHF (33,34).

## RENIN–ANGIOTENSIN SYSTEM

The renin–angiotensin system (RAS) has a detrimental role in the pathogenesis of heart failure. Beyond its influences on blood pressure and salt and water regulation, it has stimulatory effects on the sympathetic nervous system, direct effects on myocardial hypertrophy, and indirect effects on myocardial contractility. Numerous large randomized clinical trials have demonstrated the symptom relief and survival benefit in patients with CHF treated with

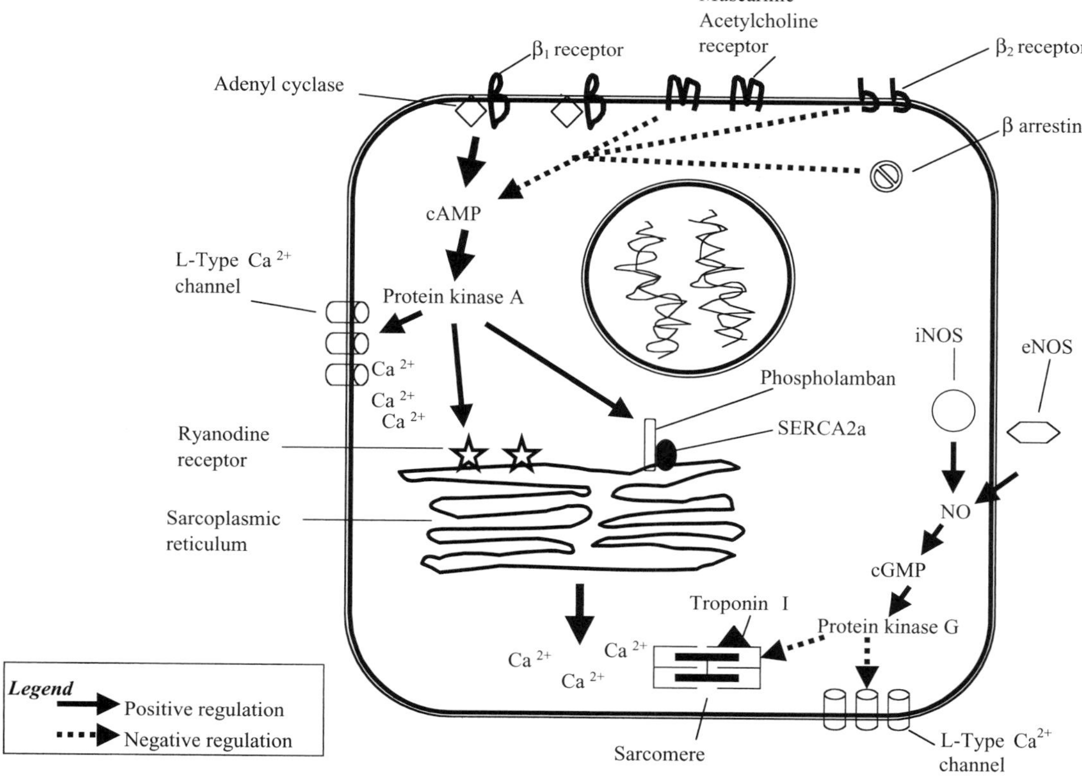


**Figure 3–2** $\beta$-Adrenergic and nitric oxide regulation of the cardiac myocyte.

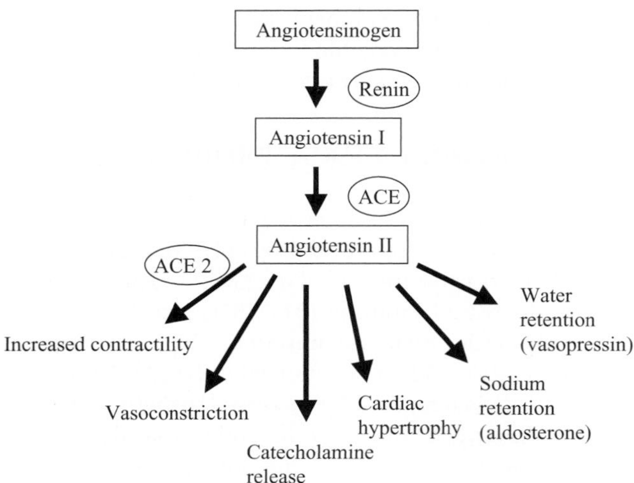


**Figure 3–3** Renin–angiotensin system.

angiotensin-converting enzyme (ACE) inhibitors (35–37). Angiotensinogen is cleaved to angiotensin I by the renally produced enzyme renin in response to renal hypoperfusion. Angiotensin I is then cleaved by ACE into the potent vasoconstrictor angiotensin II. Angiotensin II stimulates catecholamine release, increases cardiac hypertrophy, regulates blood pressure (angiotensin II receptors), and increases blood volume by stimulating aldosterone and vasopressin release, enhancing sodium and water retention (Fig. 3–3) (38). ACE inhibitors also increase the generation of bradykinin (thought to mediate the cough associated with ACE inhibitors), which is a nitric oxide synthase (NOS) agonist and may attenuate $\beta$-adrenergic contractility through nitric oxide (NO) signaling (39). Bradykinin degradation may also have untoward effects on myocardial contractility that are offset by ACE inhibition (40).

ACE-2 is an ACE isoform that is thought to be an important regulator of cardiac contractility. It catalyzes the cleavage of angiotensin I to angiotensin 1-9 and of Angiotensin II to Angiotensin 1-7. ACE-2 is not inhibited by ACE inhibitors, nor is bradykinin a by-product of its activity (41–43). ACE-2 is upregulated within the myocardium with angiotensin II receptor blockade (44). ACE-2 deficiency diminishes cardiac contractility and upregulates hypoxia-induced genes, suggesting its role in RAS modulation following ischemia-mediated cardiac injury (45).

## NITRIC OXIDE

Nitric oxide (NO) plays an important role in the endothelium-dependent functions of coronary vasomotor tone and thrombogenesis, but it also has direct effects on myocardial relaxation. NO is generated by the enzyme nitric oxide synthase (NOS), which has three isoforms: eNOS (endothelial), iNOS (inducible), and nNOS (neuronal). NO affects myocardial relaxation through effects on excitation–contraction coupling, regulation of adrenergic signaling, and mitochondrial metabolism (46). Attenuation of $\beta$-adrenergic stimulation by NO (Fig. 3–2) is mediated by cyclic guanosine 3′5′-monophosphate (cGMP)–dependent phosphodiesterase EII regulation of cAMP levels, protein kinase G-mediated downregulation of L-type $Ca^{+}$ channels (47,48), and the desensitization of troponin I to calcium (49). NO may also influence myocardial relaxation by enhancing the activity of the delayed rectifier $K^{+}$ current (50) as well as cGMP-mediated inhibition of phospholamban and its negative control over SERCA2a (51).

## REFERENCES


1. Morgan JP. Abnormal intracellular modulation of calcium as a major cause of cardiac contractile dysfunction. *N Engl J Med.* 1991; 325:625.
2. Lehnart SE, Wehrens XH, Kushnir A, et al. Cardiac ryanodine receptor function and regulation in heart disease. *Ann N Y Acad Sci.* 2004 (May);1015:144–159.
3. Guyton AC. Textbook of Medical Physiology.8th ed. Philadelphia: WB Saunders; 1991:68–72.
4. Schulze DH, Muqhal M, Lederer WJ, et al. Sodium/calcium exchanger (NCX1) macromolecular complex. *J Biol Chem.* 2003; 278(31):28849–28855.
5. Arai M, Matsui H, Periasamy M. Sarcoplasmic reticulum gene expression in cardiac hypertrophy and heart failure. *Circ Res.* 1994; 74:555–564.
6. Schmidt U, Hajjar RJ, Helm PA, et al. Contribution of abnormal sarcoplasmic reticulum ATPase activity to systolic and diastolic dysfunction in human heart failure. *J Mol Cell Cardiol.* 1998;30:1929–1937.
7. Schmidt AG, Zhai J, Carr AN, et al. Structural and functional implications of the phospholamban hinge domain: impaired SR $Ca^{2+}$ uptake as a primary cause of heart failure. *Cardiovasc Res.* 2002; 56(2):248–259.
8. Whitmer JT, Kumar P, Solaro RJ. Calcium transport properties of cardiac sarcoplasmic reticulum from cardiomyopathic Syrian hamsters (BIO 53.58 and 14.6): evidence for a quantitative defect in dilated myopathic hearts not evident in hypertrophic hearts. *Circ Res.* 1988;62:81–85.
9. Gwathmey JK, Slawsky MT, Hajjar RJ, et al. Role of intracellular calcium handling in force-interval relationships of human ventricular myocardium. *J Clin Invest.* 1990;85:1599–1613.
10. Mercadier JJ, Lompre AM, Duc P. et al. Altered sarcoplasmic reticulum Ca2(+)-ATPase gene expression in the human ventricle during end-stage heart failure. *J Clin Invest.* 1990;85:305–309.
11. Kadambi VJ, Ponniah S, Harrer JM, et al. Cardiac-specific overexpression of phospholamban alters calcium kinetics and resultant cardiomyocyte mechanics in transgenic mice. *J Clin Invest.* 1996;97:533–539.
12. Hajjar RJ, Schmidt U, Kang JX, et al. Adenoviral gene transfer of phospholamban in isolated rat cardiomyocytes. Rescue effects by concomitant gene transfer of sarcoplasmic reticulum Ca(2+)-ATPase. *Circ Res.* 1997;81:145–153.
13. Hajjar RJ, Schmidt U, Matsui T, et al. Modulation of ventricular function through gene transfer in vivo. *Proc Natl Acad Sci USA.* 1998;95:5251–5256.
14. van der Heyden MA, Wijnhoven TJ, Opthof T. Molecular aspects of adrenergic modulation of cardiac L-type $Ca^{2+}$ channels. *Cardiovasc Res.* 2005;65(1):28–39.
15. Gao MH, Ping P, Post S, et al. Increased expression of adenylyl cyclase type VI increases $\beta$-adrenergic receptor-stimulated production of cAMP in neonatal rat myocytes. *Proc Natl Acad Sci USA.* 1998;95:1038–1043.
16. Freeman K, Lerman I, Kranias EG, et al. Alterations in cardiac adrenergic signaling and calcium cycling differentially affect the progression of cardiomyopathy. *J Clin Invest.* 2001;107:967.

17. Dorn GW, Molkentin JD. Manipulating cardiac contractility in heart failure: data from mice and men. *Circulation.* 2004;109:150–158.
18. Dessy C, Moniotte S, Ghisdal P, et al. Endothelial beta3-adrenoceptors mediate vasorelaxation of human coronary microarteries through nitric oxide and endothelium-dependent hyperpolarization. *Circulation.* 2004;110(8):948–954.
19. Perry SJ, Baillie GS, Kohout TA, et al. Targeting of cyclic AMP degradation to beta 2-adrenergic receptors by beta-arrestins. *Science.* 2002;298(5594):834–836.
20. Bristow MR, Minobe W, Rasmussen R, et al. Beta-adrenergic neuroeffector abnormalities in the failing human heart are produced by local rather than systemic mechanisms. *J Clin Invest.* 1992;89:803–815.
21. Bristow MR, Ginsburg R, Minobe W, et al. Decreased catecholamine sensitivity and beta-adrenergic-receptor density in failing human hearts. *N Engl J Med.* 1982;307:205–211.
22. Akhter SA, Skaer CA, Kypson AP, et al. Restoration of beta-adrenergic signaling in failing cardiac ventricular myocytes via adenoviral-mediated gene transfer. *Proc Natl Acad Sci USA.* 1997; 94:12100–12105.
23. Rockman HA, Chien KR, Choi DJ, et al. Expression of a beta-adrenergic receptor kinase inhibitor prevents the development of myocardial failure in gene-targeted mice. *Proc Natl Acad Sci USA.* 1998;95:700–705.
24. Harding VB, Jones, LR, Lefkowitz RJ. Cardiac $\beta$ARK1 inhibition prolongs survival and augments $\beta$-blocker therapy in a mouse model of severe heart failure. *Proc Natl Acad Sci USA.* 2001;98: 5809.
25. Engelhardt S, Hein L, Dyachenkow V, et al. Altered calcium handling is critically involved in the cardiotoxic effects of chronic beta-adrenergic stimulation. *Circulation.* 2004: 109(9):1154–1160.
26. Plank DM, Yatani A, Ritsu H, et al. Calcium dynamics in the failing heart: restoration by beta-adrenergic-receptor blockade. *Am J Physiol Heart Circ Physiol.* 2003;285(1):H305–H315.
27. McDonough AA, Velotta JB, Schwinger RH, et al. The cardiac sodium pump: structure and function. *Basic Res Cardiol.* 2002; 97(suppl 1):I19–I24.
28. Gheorghiade M, Adams KF, Colucci WS. Digoxin in the management of cardiovascular disorders. *Circulation.* 2004;109:2959–2964.
29. Smith TW, Antman EM, Friedman PL, et al. Digitalis glycosides: mechanisms and manifestations of toxicity: part I. *Prog Cardiovasc Dis.* 1984;26:495–530.
30. Hilgemann DW. New insights into the molecular and cellular workings of the cardiac $Na^+/Ca^{2+}$ exchanger. *Am J Physiol Cell Physiol.* 2004;287(5):C1167–C1172.
31. Yano M, Kohno M, Ohkusa T, et al. Effect of milrinone on left ventricular relaxation and Ca(2+) uptake function of cardiac sarcoplasmic reticulum. *Am J Physiol Heart Circ Physiol.* 2000;279(4): H1898–H1905.
32. Sonnenblick EH, Grose R, Strain J, et al. Effects of milrinone on left ventricular performance and myocardial contractility in patients with severe heart failure. *Circulation.* 1986;73(3 pt 2):III162–III167.
33. Chatterjee K, De Marco T. Role of nonglycoside inotropic agents: indications, ethics, and limitations. *Med Clin North Am.* 2003;87(2):391–418.
34. Cuffe MS, Califf RM, Adams JF Jr, et al. Short-term intravenous milrinone for acute exacerbation of chronic heart failure: a randomized controlled trial. *JAMA.* 2002;287(12):1541–1547.
35. Pfeffer MA, Braunwald E, Moye LA, et al. Effect of captopril on mortality and morbidity in patients with left ventricular dysfunction after myocardial infarction. Results of the survival and ventricular enlargement trial. The SAVE Investigators. *N Engl J Med.* 1992;327(10):669–677.
36. The SOLVD Investigators. Effect of enalapril on survival in patients with reduced left ventricular ejection fractions and congestive heart failure. *N Engl J Med.* 1991;325(5):293–302.
37. The CONSENSUS Trial Study Group. Effects of enalapril on mortality in severe congestive heart failure. Results of the Cooperative North Scandinavian Enalapril Survival Study (CONSENSUS). *N Engl J Med.* 1987;316(23):1429–1435.
38. Paul M, Pinto YM, Schunkert H, et al. Activation of the renin-angiotensin system in heart failure and hypertrophy: studies in human hearts and transgenic rats. *Eur Heart J.* 1994;15:63–67.
39. Wittstein IS, Kass DA, Pak PH, et al. Cardiac nitric oxide production due to angiotensin-converting enzyme inhibition decreases beta-adrenergic myocardial contractility in patients with dilated cardiomyopathy. *J Am Coll Cardiol.* 2001;38(2):429–435.
40. Krombach RS, McElmuray JH 3rd, Gay DM, et al. Bradykinin degradation and relation to myocyte contractility. *J Cardiovasc Pharmacol Ther.* 2000;5(4):291–299.
41. Boehm M, Nabel EG. Angiotensin-converting enzyme 2—a new cardiac regulator. *N Engl J Med.* 2002;347(22):1795–1797.
42. Crackower MA, Sarao R, Oudit GY, et al. Angiotensin-converting enzyme-2 is an essential regulator of heart function. *Nature.* 2002;417(6891):822–828.
43. Donoghue M, Hsieh F, Baronas E, et al. A novel angiotensin-converting enzyme-related carboxypeptidase (ACE2) converts angiotensin I to angiotensin 1-9. *Circ Res.* 2000;87(5):E1–E9.
44. Ishiyama Y, Gallagher PE, Averill DB, et al. Upregulation of angiotensin-converting enzyme 2 after myocardial infarction by blockade of angiotensin II receptors. *Hypertension.* 2004;43(5): 970–976.
45. Burrell LM, Risvanis J, Kubota E, et al. Myocardial infarction increases ACE2 expression in rat and humans. *Eur Heart J.* 2005; 26(4):369–375.
46. Massion PB, Feron O, Dessy C, et al. Nitric oxide and cardiac function: ten years after, and continuing. *Circ Res.* 2003;93:388–398.
47. Han X, Kobzik I, Balligand JL, et al. Nitric oxide synthase (NOS3)-mediated cholinergic modulation of $Ca^{2+}$ current in adult rabbit atrioventricular nodal cells. *Circ Res.* 1996;78:998–1008.
48. Gallo MP, Ghigo D, Bosia A, et al. Modulation of guinea-pig cardiac L-type calcium current by nitric oxide synthase inhibitors. *J Physiol.* 1998;506(pt 3):639–651.
49. Layland J, Li JM, Shah AM. Role of cyclic GMP-dependent protein kinase in the contractile response to exogenous nitric oxide in rat cardia myocytes. *J Physiol.* 2002;540:457–467.
50. Bai CX, Namekata I, Kurokawa J, et al. Role of nitric oxide in $Ca^{2+}$ sensitivity of the slowly activating delayed rectifier $K^+$ current in cardiac myocytes. *Circ Res.* 2005;96(1):64–72.
51. Zhang Q, Scholz PM, He Y, et al. Cyclic GMP signaling and regulation of SERCA activity during cardiac myocyte contraction. *Cell Calcium.* 2005;37(3):259–266.


## QUESTIONS

1. Following a cycle of excitation-contraction coupling in cardiac muscle, cytosolic $Ca^{++}$ is sequestered in the sarcoplasmic reticulum *primarily* by what entity?

   a. $Na^+/Ca^{++}$ exchanger
   b. L-Type Ca++ channels
   c. Phospholamban
   d. SERCA2a
   e. Ryanodine receptors

Answer is d: The active sites of the actin filaments are covered in the resting state by two regulatory proteins, tropomyosin and troponin. Intracellular $Ca^{2+}$ is the most important determinant of myocardial contractility and relaxation. Once contraction ensues, calcium ($Ca^{2+}$) entry through L-type $Ca^{2+}$ channels triggers an exponential release of $Ca^{2+}$ from the sarcoplasmic reticulum (SR) through ryanodine receptors. Calcium then binds troponin leading to a conformational alteration of tropomyosin exposing the actin active site which facilitates a "sliding" interaction between the actin filaments and the myosin heads as well as the hydrolysis of ATP providing energy for contraction. Following a cycle of excitation-contraction coupling, diastolic relaxation is initiated by cytosolic $Ca^{2+}$ sequestration in the sarcoplasmic reticulum (SR) by the SR-$Ca^{2+}$ ATPase (SERCA2a) pump (~75%) and exportation extracellularly by the $Na^+/Ca^{2+}$ exchanger (~25%) located on the sarcolemmal membrane. Phospholamban, a regulatory protein, exerts an inhibitory effect on SERCA2a limiting its ability to remove cytosolic $Ca^{2+}$ following contraction.

2. Down-regulation of adrenergic signaling system in failure is due to all the following except:
   a. G-protein mediated adenyl cyclase activation and cAMP generation through $\beta$-1 over-stimulation
   b. Beta Adrenoreceptor Kinase ($\beta$-ARK) up-regulation
   c. Beta Adrenoreceptor ($\beta$-AR) uncoupling from second messenger systems
   d. Altered $Ca^{++}$ trafficking
   e. Beta blocker therapy

Answer is e: Catecholamines increase myocardial contractility primarily through $\beta_1$-adrenergic receptor stimulation leading to G-protein-mediated adenyl cyclase activation and cyclic adenosine 3′5′ monophosphate (cAMP) generation which triggers protein kinase A (PKA)-dependent phosphorylation of voltage-gated L-type $Ca^+$ channels, ryanodine receptors and phospholamban which derepresses SERCA2a leading to excitation-contraction coupling and positive inotropy. Derangements in chronic $\beta$-adrenergic signaling that have been implicated in the pathogenesis of CHF include $\beta$-adrenergic receptor ($\beta$-AR) down-regulation, $\beta$-AR uncoupling from second messenger systems, up-regulation of $\beta$-AR kinase ($\beta$ARK1) and altered calcium trafficking. $\beta$-blocker therapy can restore calcium homeostasis and up-regulate SERCA2a ultimately improving cardiac performance with long-term treatment.

3. Digitalis is a cardiac glycoside that does all of the following except:
   a. indirectly activates a $Na^+/Ca^{++}$ exchanger found in the cardiac cell membrane
   b. inhibits the $Na^+/K^+$ ATPase found in the cardiac cell membrane
   c. increases chronotropy by increasing intracellular $Ca^{++}$
   d. leads to a sodium gradient across the cardiac cell membrane that is favorable for $Ca^{++}$ influx
   e. increases parasympathetic tone

Answer is c: Digitalis inhibits the $Na^+/K^+$ ATPase found in the cardiac cell membrane which maintains a high intracellular $K^+$ concentration and high extracellular $Na^+$ concentration. $Ca^{2+}$ is removed from the cytosol into the extracellular fluid by a sodium-calcium exchange pump driven by the pre-existing $Na^+$ gradient. Inhibiting the $Na^+/K^+$ ATPase promotes enhanced $Na^+/Ca^{2+}$ exchange ultimately leading to increased intracellular $Ca^{2+}$ available to the contractile apparatus increasing myocardial contractility. Chronotropy would not be increased with digitalis and in fact it is often used for the opposite effect of heart rate control in patients with atrial fibrillation.

4. Regarding the role of nitric oxide (NO) and cardiac function, which of the following is false:
   a. Bradykinin is a nitric oxide synthase (NOS) antagonist and may increase myocardial contractility.
   b. NO mediates endothelium-dependent coronary vasodilation
   c. NO has three isoforms: iNOS (inducible), eNOS (endothelial) and nNOS (neuronal).
   d. NO leads to cGMP-mediated attenuation of $\beta$–adrenergic stimulation and myocardial relaxation

Answer is a: Nitric oxide (NO) plays an important role in the endothelium-dependent functions of coronary vasomotor tone but also has direct effects on myocardial relaxation. NO is generated by the enzyme nitric oxide synthase (NOS) which has three isoforms: eNOS (endothelial), iNOS (inducible) and nNOS (neuronal). NO impacts myocardial relaxation through effects on excitation-contraction coupling, regulation of adrenergic signaling and mitochondrial metabolism. Bradykinin is a Nitric Oxide Synthase (NOS) agonist, not antagonist, and may decrease myocardial contractility.

5. Regarding the Renin-Angiotensin system, which if the following is false:
   a. Chronic renal hypoperfusion leads to catecholamine release, hypertension, cardiac hypertrophy and salt and water retention
   b. Angiotensin Converting Enzyme (ACE) inhibitors work by inhibiting Angiotensinogen cleavage to Angiotensin I
   c. ACE-2 is not inhibited by Angiotensin Converting Enzyme (ACE) inhibitors
   d. Bradykinin is thought to mediate the cough associated with ACE inhibitors

Answers is b: Angiotensinogen is cleaved to angiotensin I by renin in response to renal hypoperfusion. Angiotensin I is then cleaved by Angiotensin Converting Enzyme (ACE) into the potent vasoconstrictor angiotensin II. Angiotensin II stimulates catecholamine release, cardiac hypertrophy, regulates blood pressure and increases blood volume by stimulating aldosterone and vasopressin release enhancing sodium and water retention. ACE inhibitors also increases bradykinin generation which is thought to mediate the cough associated with ACE inhibitors. ACE 2 is an ACE isoform thought to be an important regulator of cardiac contractility and is not inhibited by ACE inhibitors.

# Cardiac Anatomy

4

***Robert E. Hobbs***

The heart is a muscular organ, pyramidal in shape, consisting of two parallel-valved pumps, located within the middle mediastinum, two thirds to the left of the centerline. The base of the heart is oriented superiorly, whereas the apex points leftward, anteriorly, and slightly inferiorly. The cardiac apex is located at the fifth intercostal space near the mid-clavicular line. The heart is enclosed by the fibrous pericardium, which is bordered by the diaphragm inferiorly, the sternum and ribs anteriorly, the pleurae laterally, and the esophagus, descending aorta, and vertebrae posteriorly.

The average adult heart measures 12 cm from base to apex, 8 to 9 cm in width, and 6 cm deep, approximating the size of a clenched fist. The heart weighs approximately 325 ± 75 g in men, and 275 ± 75 g in women, accounting for 0.45% of body weight in males and 0.40% in females.

Viewed from the front, visible structures include the superior and inferior vena cavae draining into the right atrium, the right ventricle (the most anterior chamber of the heart), the main pulmonary artery that courses superiorly and posteriorly before bifurcating, the left atrial appendage, a small portion of the left ventricle visible to the left of the left anterior descending coronary artery, and the ascending aorta (Fig. 4–1). The right heart forms the largest part of the anterior surface, whereas the left heart is largely posterior. The epicardial surface of the heart usually is covered with fat, proportional to age and the amount of body fat. Beneath the epicardial fat, the interventricular grooves separate the right and left ventricles, and contain arteries, veins, nerves, and lymphatics. The atrioventricular grooves, which separate the atria from the ventricles, are located at the base of the heart. The interatrial grooves mark the borders between the atria. Posteriorly, the crux ("cross") is the intersection of the atrioventricular, interatrial, and interventricular grooves. The acute cardiac margin is the junction of the inferior and anterior walls of the right ventricle. The obtuse margin is the rounded lateral wall of the left ventricle.

The heart is composed of four chambers. The right and left atria are weakly contractile reservoirs that receive blood from the body and the lungs. They are positioned above the ventricles and are separated by the atrioventricular (tricuspid and mitral) valves. The right and left ventricles are muscular pumping chambers separated from each other by the interventricular septum. The ventricles eject blood through the semilunar (pulmonic and aortic) valves to the pulmonary artery and aorta, respectively.

The shape of the heart and position of the valves are maintained by an internal fibrous skeleton. The cardiac skeleton consists of four valve annuli (or rings), the membranous septum, and the right and left fibrous trigones. The right fibrous trigone, also known as the central fibrous body, is located between the aortic, mitral, and tricuspid valves. It houses the His bundle and is the strongest component of the cardiac skeleton.

## THE PERICARDIUM

The pericardium is a fibrous sac surrounding the heart and great vessels and containing 10 to 50 cc of pericardial fluid (Fig. 4–2). It maintains the position of the heart within the mediastinum, lubricates the cardiac surfaces, and provides a barrier against infection. Inferiorly, the pericardium is anchored to the central tendon of the diaphragm. Anteriorly, it is attached by ligamentous connections to the posterior sternum. Superiorly, the pericardium extends to the level of the second intercostal space, and laterally it is attached to the pleurae. The pericardium encloses the heart, portions of the vena cavae, most of the ascending aorta, the main pulmonary artery, and the four pulmonary veins. The pericardium consists of two layers. The inelastic fibrous pericardium is the outermost layer. The serous pericardium forms a thin mesothelial layer on the cardiac surface (the visceral pericardium or the epicardium) and lines the inferior surface of the fibrous pericardium (the parietal layer).

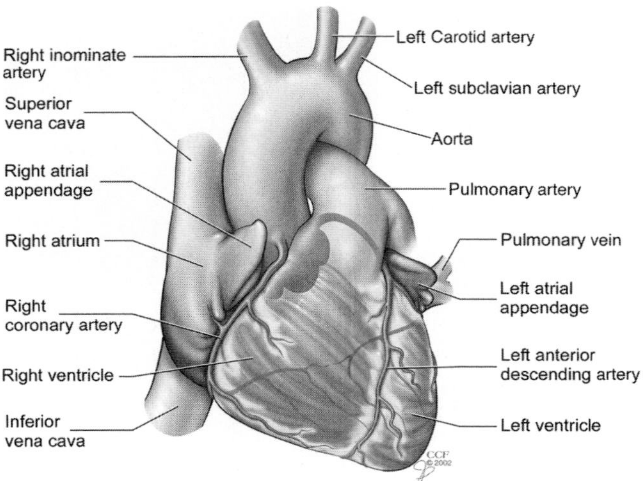


**Figure 4–1** Frontal view of the heart and great vessels.

The visceral pericardium covers the heart and contains the coronary arteries and veins, autonomic nerves, lymphatics, and fat. Posteriorly, the pericardium folds upon itself to create several distinct sinuses. The oblique sinus is a pericardial reflection along the vena cavae and the pulmonary veins. The transverse sinus is a pericardial reflection located between the aorta, pulmonary artery, and atria. The ligament of Marshall is a pericardial fold containing the remnant of the embryonic left superior vena cava.

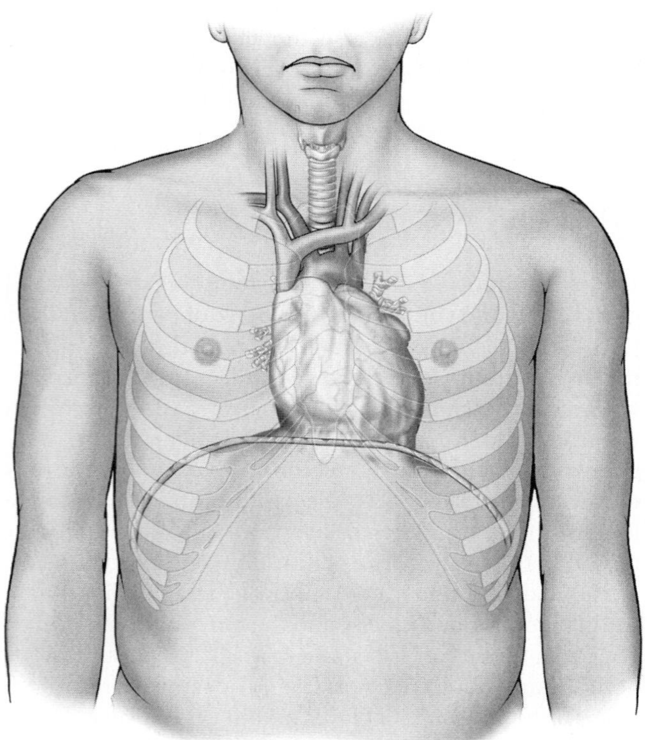

**Figure 4–2** Frontal view of the pericardium.

## CARDIAC CHAMBERS

### Right Atrium

The right atrium is a low-pressure capacitance chamber that receives blood from the superior vena cava, inferior vena cava, and coronary sinus (Fig. 4–3). The right atrial volume is approximately 75 to 80 mL, and its free-wall thickness is 1 to 3 mm. The superior vena cava enters the superior aspect of the right atrium and directs its blood flow toward the tricuspid valve. The inferior vena cava returns blood from the lower body, and its eustachian valve directs blood flow toward the foramen ovale or fossa ovalis. The coronary sinus returns most of the blood from the heart itself through an orifice partially guarded by the thebesian valve (valve of the coronary sinus). When the eustachian or thebesian valves are large and fenestrated, it is described as a Chiari net. Thebesian veins drain cardiac blood into the right atrium via multiple small orifices. The fossa ovalis, representing a closed foramen ovale, forms a 1.5- to 2.0-cm depression on the interatrial septum. A patent foramen ovale is found in up to one third of adults. The crista terminalis is a C-shaped muscular ridge on the right atrial free wall that separates the smooth posterior portion of the right atrium from the muscular anterior portion. The pectinate ("comb") muscles arise from the crista terminalis and course as bands anteriorly on the right atrial free wall. The right atrial appendage is a large triangular structure that overlies the right coronary artery and contains pectinate muscles. In the lower medial portion of the right atrium, Koch's triangle overlies the atrioventricular node and the proximal His bundle.

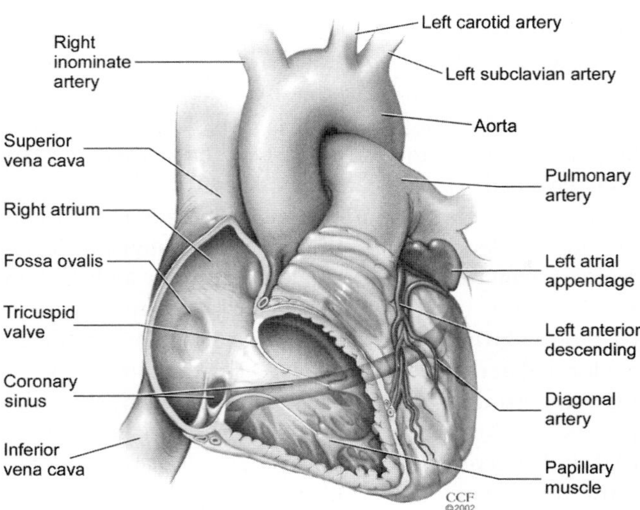


**Figure 4–3** Frontal cutaway view of the right atrium and right ventricle.

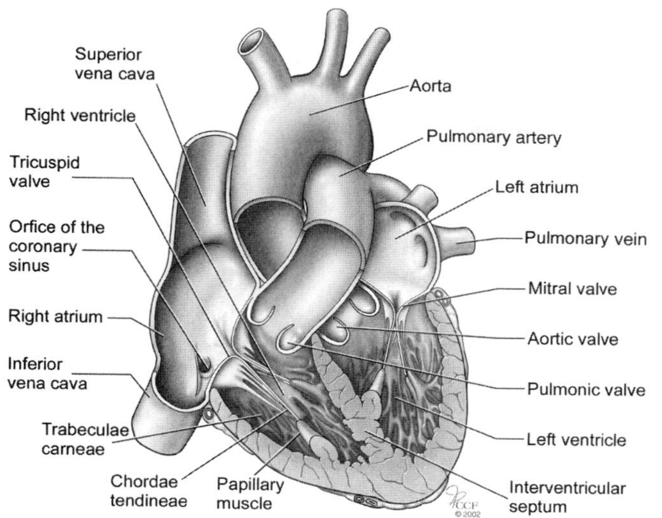


**Figure 4–4** Coronal section of the heart and great vessels.

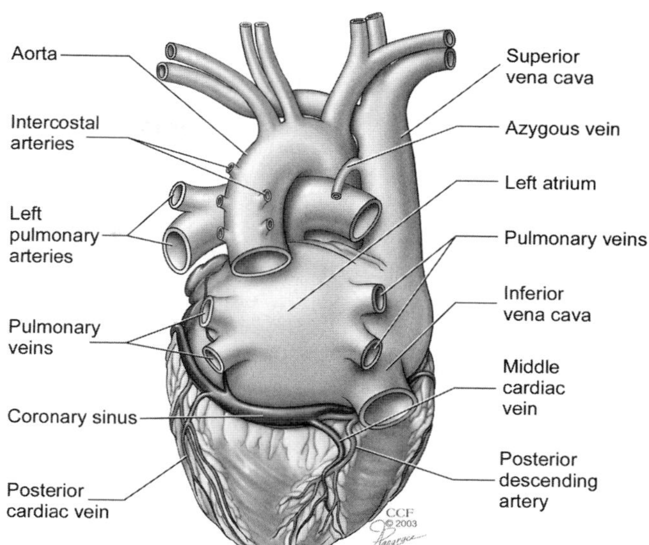


**Figure 4–5** Posterior view of the heart and great vessels.

The tendon of Todaro is a fibrous band located between the valves of the inferior vena cava and the coronary sinus.

## Right Ventricle

The right ventricle is the most anterior chamber of the heart (Fig 4–4). It is the smaller of the two ventricular chambers, separated from the left ventricle by the interventricular septum, which bulges into the right ventricle. It is triangular shaped when viewed from the right, and crescent shaped when viewed in cross section from the left. The right ventricular free wall is approximately 3 to 4 mm thick, or about one third the thickness of the left ventricle. The right ventricle consists of an inlet portion, a trabeculated apical portion, and a smooth right ventricular outflow tract (infundibulum or conus portion). The walls of the right ventricle contain a latticework of muscle fibers called trabeculae carneae. The right ventricular apex is heavily trabeculated, more so than the left ventricle. The infundibulum (outflow tract or conus) portion of the right ventricle is smooth walled to the pulmonic valve. The right ventricle contains three papillary muscles, although the septal papillary muscle occasionally may be absent. Chordae tendineae (fibrous cords) extend upward from the papillary muscles and attach to the leaflet edges and to the ventricular side of the tricuspid valve. Chordae from one papillary muscle often attach to more than one tricuspid leaflet, and some chordae arise from the septum. The crista supraventricularis (supraventricular crest) separates the inflow and outflow portions of the right ventricle. It consists of a septal band on the ventricular septum and a parietal band on the right ventricular free wall. The moderator band is an intracavity muscular bridge that connects the distal septum with the right ventricular free wall at the anterior papillary muscle. Blood enters the right ventricle via the tricuspid valve, turns upward at a 45- to 60-degree angle, and passes through the pulmonic valve into the main pulmonary artery.

## Left Atrium

The left atrium is the left upper posterior chamber of the heart (Fig. 4–5). It is cuboidal shaped, smaller than the right atrium (volume, 55 to 65 mL), but with thicker walls (3 mm) and higher pressure. It receives oxygenated blood from the lungs via four pulmonary veins (two from each lung). Unlike the right atrium, the left atrium has smooth interior walls and does not have bands of pectinate muscles except in the left atrial appendage. The left atrial muscle extends a variable distance within the pulmonary veins to prevent reflux during atrial contraction. The left atrial appendage, overlying the left circumflex coronary artery, is smaller, longer, more tortuous, and less triangular than the right atrial appendage, often containing two or more lobes. Left atrial contraction generates a stroke volume of 20 to 30 mL.

## Left Ventricle

The left ventricle is a high-pressure, muscular chamber, 2.5 to 3 times thicker than the right ventricle (see Fig. 4–4). It is ellipsoid, or cone shaped when viewed from the right, and ring or doughnut shaped when viewed in cross section from the left. It is longer and narrower than the right ventricle, measuring approximately 7.5 cm in length and 4.5 cm in width. Structurally, the left ventricle consists of the inflow tract, the apical zone, and the left ventricular outflow tract. The anterior mitral leaflet separates the left ventricle into the posterior inflow tract and the anterior outflow tract.

The septum consists of a large inferior muscular portion and a small superior membranous portion. The septum is thickest at the midportion and thinnest at the membranous portion near the aortic valve. The membranous septum has atrioventricular and intraventricular portions divided by the septal tricuspid leaflet. The His bundle is located within the interventricular portion of the membranous septum.

The left ventricular free wall measures approximately 8 to 12 mm, and is thicker at the base than at the apex. It is composed of three layers: the endocardium, the myocardium, and the epicardium (or visceral pericardium). The outer two thirds of the myocardium contains compact layers of muscle that twist and spiral inward from apex to base during contraction. The inner third of the myocardium consists of a latticework of trabeculae carneae that are more intricate than right ventricular trabeculations. The septal surface of the left ventricle is smooth.

Two papillary muscles, the larger anterolateral and the smaller posteromedial, arise from the free wall and have a variable number of heads. They anchor the chordae tendineae of the mitral valve, which are thicker than tricuspid valve chordae. Chordae tendineae restrict valve excursion during ventricular systole, thereby preventing the mitral valve leaflets from prolapsing into the left atrium. Most chordae arise from the heads of the papillary muscles, but some arise from the free wall. Chordae from one papillary muscle may diverge and attach to both mitral leaflets. False chordae occur in half of normal hearts, and may connect walls, papillary muscles, and the septum, but are not attached to the mitral leaflets. They often cross the left ventricular outflow tract, and can be identified by echocardiography. Many false chordae contain extensions of left ventricular conducting fibers.

Blood enters the left ventricle via the mitral valve and is ejected at a 90- to 120-degree angle through the aortic valve. The ejection phase is shorter in the left ventricle, but the pressure is greater compared with right ventricular contraction.

## CARDIAC VALVES

### Tricuspid Valve

The tricuspid valve is the largest of the heart valves, and maintains forward flow of blood through the right heart (Fig. 4–6). The functional components of the tricuspid valve include the three leaflets, commissures, annulus, chordae tendineae, papillary muscles, and the right ventricle. The leaflets are named for their anatomic position: anterior, posterior, and septal. The anterior leaflet, which is the largest and most mobile, partially separates the right ventricular inflow and outflow tracts. The posterior leaflet is the smallest, whereas the septal leaflet is the least mobile and is occasionally absent. The valve leaflets are attached

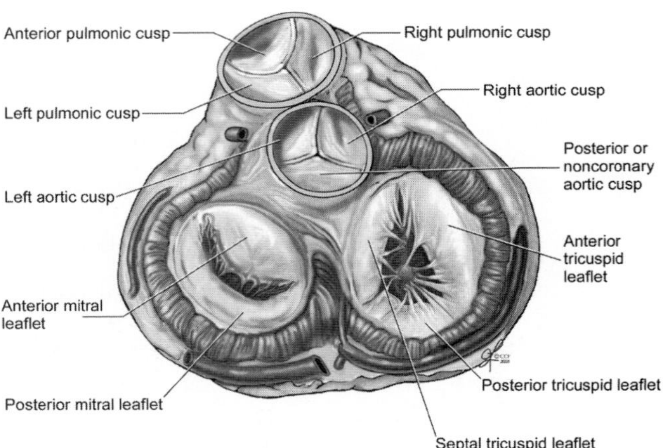


**Figure 4–6** Cross-sectional view of the cardiac valves.

to a discontinuous fibrous annulus that has a "D" shape. Chordae tendineae (tendinous cords) are attached to the edges and undersurface of each leaflet and are anchored by the papillary muscles and the interventricular septum.

### Pulmonic Valve

The pulmonic valve is the most anterior valve of the heart, located between the right ventricular outflow tract and the main pulmonary artery (see Fig. 4–6). It is the mirror image of the aortic valve, containing right, left, and anterior cusps (or leaflets) that are thinner than those of the aortic valve. The pulmonary sinuses are partially embedded within the right ventricular infundibulum. During systole the valve opens to form a rounded, triangular-shaped central orifice.

### Mitral Valve

The mitral valve is named after the miter, a tall ornamental hat worn by bishops and abbots (Figs. 4–6, 4–7). The valve,

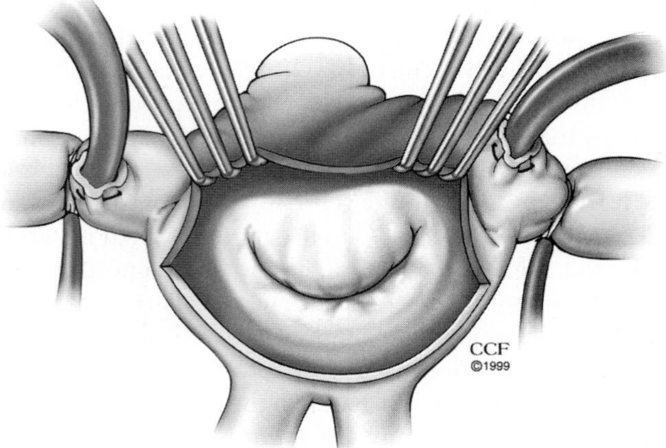


**Figure 4–7** Surgical view of the atrial surface of the mitral valve.

located between the left atrium and the left ventricle, maintains the forward flow of blood in the left heart. The mitral valve has six components: leaflets, commissures, annulus, chordae tendineae, papillary muscles, and left ventricle. When viewed from the side, the valve is funnel shaped, with the leaflets forming an apex protruding into the left ventricle. There are two mitral leaflets, the anterior and the posterior, which have similar surface areas but different shapes. The anterior leaflet is semicircular or oval shaped, broader but narrow transversely. It partially separates the left ventricular inflow tract from the left ventricular outflow tract. The posterior leaflet is crescent shaped, longer and narrower, half the height but twice the length of the anterior leaflet. It attaches over two thirds of the posterior valve circumference. The posterior leaflet has two or more indentations forming three scallops (the middle usually is the largest). During atrial contraction, the valve forms an ellipsoid orifice. During ventricular contraction, the atrial side of the leaflets coapt, preventing regurgitation of blood into the atrium. Two commissures, the anterolateral and the posteromedial, separate the two leaflets. The chordae tendineae prevent the mitral valve from prolapsing into the left atrium during ventricular systole. Approximately 100 primary, secondary, and tertiary chordae attach to the free edge and underside of the valve and are anchored by two papillary muscles in the left ventricle. Some of the posterior leaflet chordae arise from the left ventricular free wall. Unlike the tricuspid chordae, mitral chordae do not have insertions into the septum. The mitral valve is surrounded by a saddle-shaped fibrous ring, the mitral annulus, which anchors the valve. It is connected to the tricuspid annulus by the right fibrous trigone (central fibrous body), forming part of the fibrous skeleton of the heart.

### Aortic Valve

The aortic valve, located between the left ventricle and the aorta, is thicker and stronger than the pulmonic valve (Figs. 4–6, 4–8). It consists of three semilunar (half-moon) cusps located within the sinuses of Valsalva, three commissures, and an annulus. The three semilunar cusps, left, right, and noncoronary (or posterior), are pocketlike structures. The valve has a triangular-shaped central orifice when fully opened during systole. In diastole, blood fills the pocketlike cusps, causing the valve to close by coapting on the ventricular surfaces of the cusps. The nodules of Arantius are small fibrous mounds at the center of the free edge of each cusp. Three commissures radiate from the center of the valve, giving the appearance of a "peace sign." Approximately 1% to 2% of aortic valves are bicuspid.

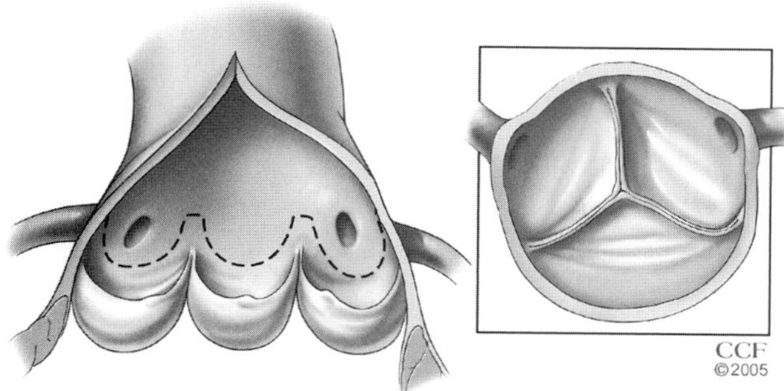


**Figure 4–8** Side and top views of the aortic valve.

## GREAT VESSELS

### Vena Cavae

These large veins return blood from the body to the right atrium (see Fig. 4–1). The superior vena cava is formed by the juncture of the left and right innominate veins. The azygos vein enters the superior vena cava in the mid-thorax. Half of the superior vena cava is contained within the pericardium. The superior vena cava enters the upper portion of the right atrium, where its blood flow is directed toward the tricuspid valve. The inferior vena cava is larger than the superior vena cava. It receives blood from the lower body, and from the abdominal viscera via the hepatic veins. Only 1 to 2 cm of the inferior vena cava is enclosed by the pericardium. The inferior vena cava enters the right atrium on the lower lateral free wall, where its blood flow is directed by the eustachian valve toward the fossa ovalis.

### Pulmonary Arteries

The main pulmonary artery is the most anterior cardiac vessel, located entirely within the pericardium (see Fig. 4–1). It arises from the base of the right ventricle, courses superiorly and posteriorly below the aortic arch, where is bifurcates into the left and right pulmonary arteries. The right pulmonary artery is slightly larger and longer than the left, dividing into a superior ascending branch and an inferior descending branch. The left pulmonary artery passes over the left mainstem bronchus and subdivides into a variable number of branches that parallel bronchial bifurcations. The left pulmonary artery is connected to the descending thoracic aorta by the ligamentum arteriosum (ductal artery ligament), a remnant of the ductus arteriosus.

### Pulmonary Veins

Four pulmonary veins, the right and left, superior and inferior, return oxygenated blood from the lungs to the left atrium (see Fig. 4–5). Occasionally, five or six pulmonary veins may be found. Atrial muscle extends for 1 to 3 cm within the pulmonary veins, and functions as a sphincter to prevent reflux of blood during atrial systole.

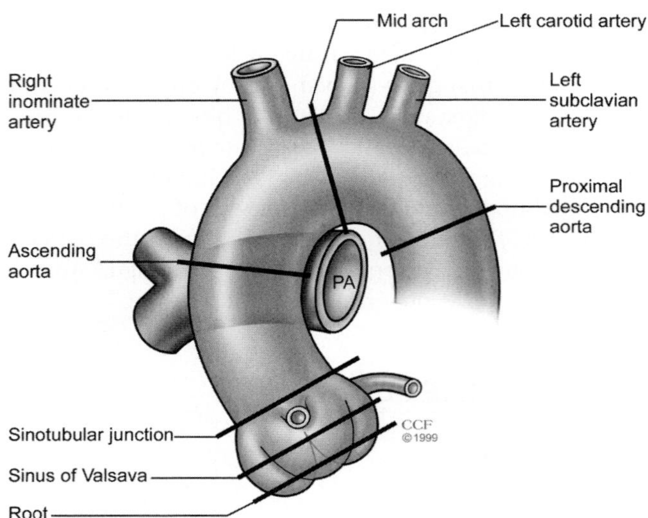


**Figure 4–9** Aortic valve, thoracic aorta, and arch vessels.

## The Aorta

The aorta arises from the aortic fibrous ring and passes superiorly and to the right as the ascending aorta (Fig. 4–9). The proximal aorta (aortic root) is dilated and contains the aortic valve and the sinuses of Valsalva. The coronary arteries, the first two branches of the aorta, arise from the left and the right sinus of Valsalva, respectively. The aortic root measures approximately 3 cm at the annulus. The sino-tubular junction, at the top of the sinuses of Valsalva, separates the aortic root (sinus portion) from the tubular ascending aorta. The proximal two thirds of the ascending aorta is located within the fibrous pericardium. In the upper thorax, the aorta courses to the left and posteriorly, forming the transverse aortic arch. Three large vessels arise from the transverse aortic arch: the right innominate (brachiocephalic) artery, the left carotid artery, and the left subclavian artery. The aorta passes over the left pulmonary artery and then descends through the posterior mediastinum to the left of the midline. The ligamentum arteriosum (ductal artery ligament) is the remnant of the ductus arteriosus that is connected to the left pulmonary artery. In the thorax, the aorta gives rise to 12 pairs of intercostal arteries, the anterior spinal artery, and several bronchial arteries. It passes through the diaphragm, where it narrows to approximately 1.75 cm, and bifurcates into the iliac arteries at the level of the fourth lumbar vertebra.

## Coronary Arteries

The coronary arteries are the first branches of the aorta, located on the surface of the heart in the atrioventricular and interventricular grooves between the cardiac chambers. They are often covered with fat, which is proportional to body fat and aging. The coronary arteries deliver oxygenated blood to the underlying heart muscle.

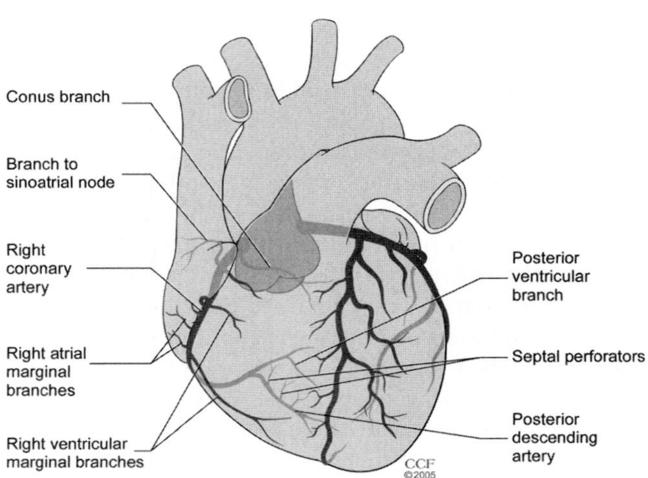


**Figure 4–10** Right coronary artery, left anterior oblique view.

The right coronary artery is located in the right atrioventricular groove. It forms a C-shaped structure when viewed from the left, and an L-shaped structure when viewed from the right (Figs. 4–10, 4–11). The right coronary artery bifurcates at the crux of the heart into a posterior descending branch and an atrioventricular branch. The posterior descending artery (PDA) follows the posterior interventricular groove and provides blood supply to the inferior (diaphragmatic) portion of interventricular septum. The atrioventricular branch passes beyond the crux of the heart, where it gives off branches that perfuse the posterolateral left ventricular myocardium. A dominant right coronary artery provides a posterior descending branch, an atrioventricular branch, and posterior ventricular or posterolateral branches. A codominant (balanced) right coronary artery provides a posterior descending branch but does not perfuse the posterior left ventricular myocardium. A nondominant right coronary artery is a small vessel that does not reach the crux of the heart and does not have posterior descending, atrioventricular, or posterior ventricular

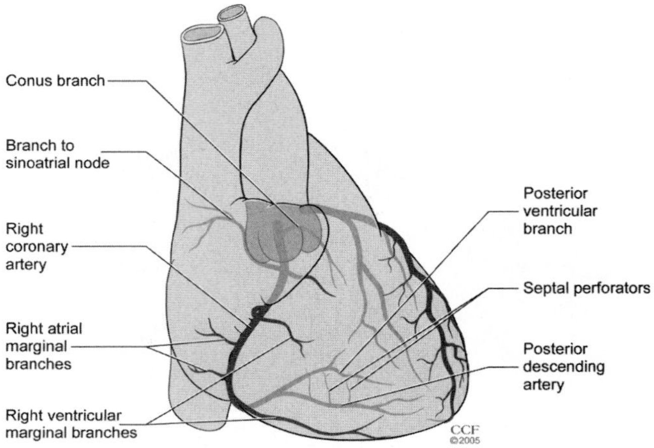


**Figure 4–11** Right coronary artery, right anterior oblique view.

branches. The size of the right coronary artery is inversely proportional to the size of the circumflex branch. The first branch of the right coronary artery is the conus branch, which perfuses the right ventricular outflow tract. It has a "hook" or "question mark" shape when viewed from the right. Fifty percent of hearts have a separate origin of the conus branch from within the right sinus of Valsalva. The second branch of the right coronary artery is the branch to the sinoatrial node. This thin vessel courses superiorly and posteriorly, supplying blood to the right atrium and the sinoatrial node. It has the appearance of a "tree branch" or an "antler" when viewed angiographically. The right coronary artery has a variable number of right atrial marginal branches and right ventricular marginal branches that arise perpendicularly from the main vessel. The atrioventricular nodal artery arises from the atrioventricular branch at the crux of the heart and courses superiorly.

The left main trunk varies from 3 to 10 mm in diameter and from 1 to 4 cm in length (Figs. 4–12, 4–13). Occasionally the left main trunk is absent, whereby the left anterior descending branch and the left circumflex branch arise from separate but adjacent orifices within the left sinus of Valsalva. The left main trunk trifurcates in 30% of hearts into the left anterior descending, a ramus branch, and the left circumflex branch.

The left anterior descending branch, located in the anterior interventricular groove, supplies blood to the anterolateral wall of the left ventricle and most of the interventricular septum. It reaches the cardiac apex in 80% of hearts. The left anterior descending provides four to seven septal perforators, which supply blood to the anterior interventricular septum, and two to three diagonal branches, which perfuse the anterolateral wall of the heart.

The left circumflex coronary artery arises from the left main trunk and supplies blood to the lateral wall of the heart and to the left atrium. The branches of the circumflex sometimes are referred to as obtuse marginal branches. A different classification system describes these branches in relation to their position on the left ventricle: high lateral, lateral, posterolateral, posterior ventricular, and posterior descending. The size of the left circumflex is inversely proportional to the size of the right coronary artery.

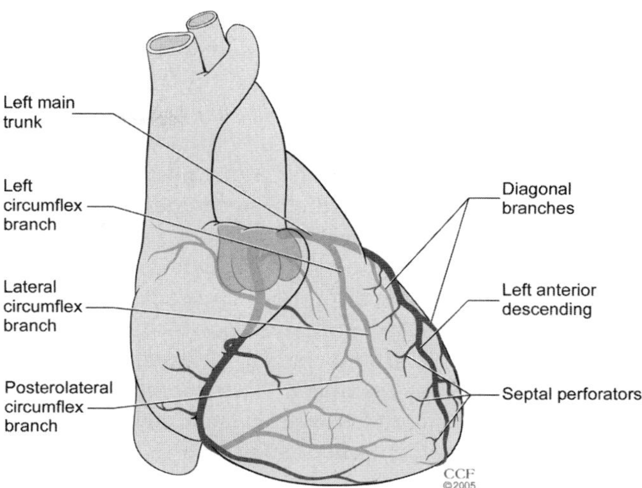


**Figure 4–13** Left coronary artery, right anterior oblique view.

## Cardiac Veins

The venous system of the heart consists of the coronary sinus, cardiac veins, and the thebesian venous system (Fig. 4–14). The cardiac veins generally follow the anatomic course of the coronary arteries, and return blood to the right atrium via the coronary sinus. The great cardiac vein parallels the left anterior descending coronary in the

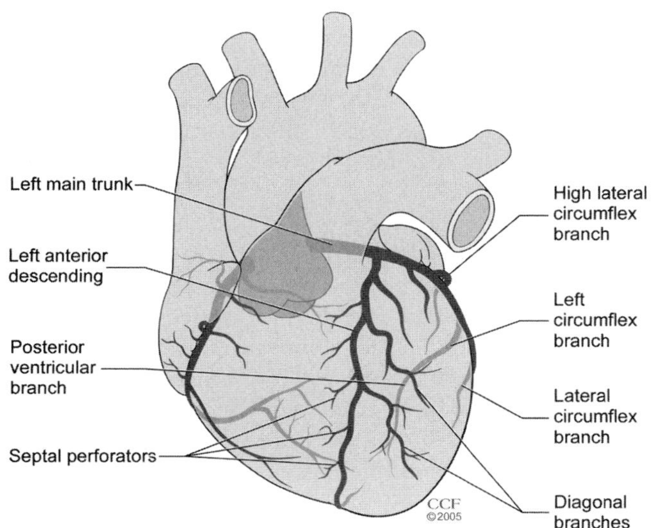


**Figure 4–12** Left coronary artery, left anterior oblique view.

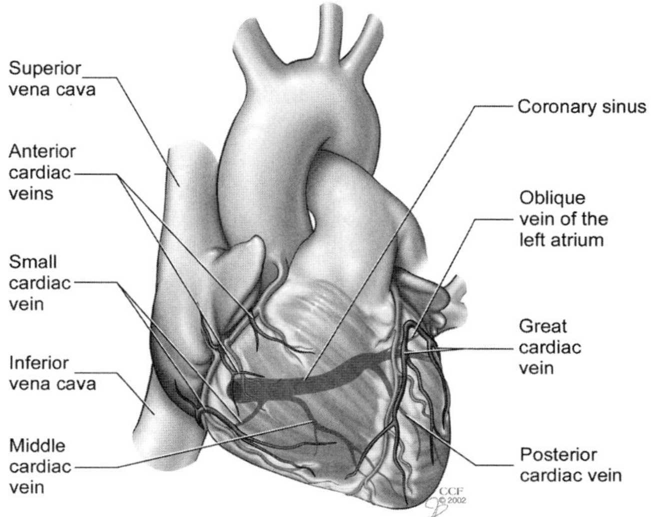


**Figure 4–14** Frontal view of the cardiac veins.

anterior interventricular groove. It drains upward from the apex toward the base and then passes leftward and posteriorly, paralleling the left circumflex artery, and entering the coronary sinus at its origin. The posterior vein of the left ventricle drains into the distal end of the coronary sinus. The middle cardiac vein, located in the posterior interventricular groove adjacent to the posterior descending coronary artery, drains into the distal coronary sinus. The small cardiac vein parallels the course of right coronary artery and drains into the distal coronary sinus. There are 3 to 12 smaller anterior cardiac veins, some of which drain directly into the right atrium. Many small thebesian veins drain directly into cardiac chambers, most commonly the right atrium and right ventricle. Venous anatomy is extremely variable, with multiple venous anastomoses. The coronary sinus is the largest cardiac vein, measuring approximately 2 to 5 cm in length and 3 to 5 mm in diameter. It is located in the posterior atrioventricular groove, and drains into the right atrium.

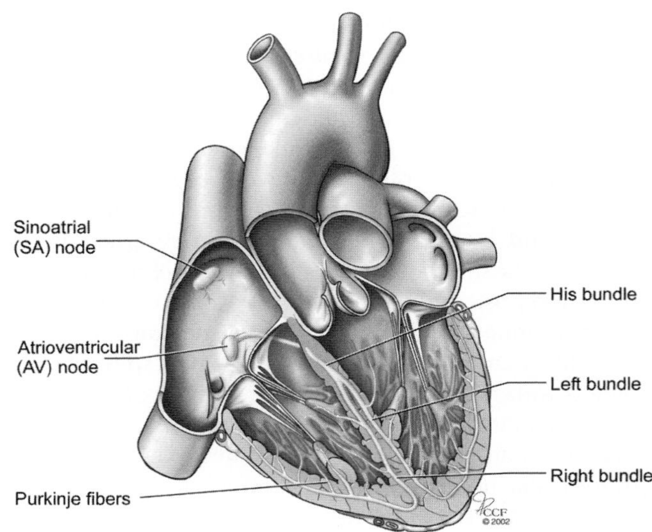


**Figure 4–15** Cardiac conducting system.

### Cardiac Lymphatic System

A plexus of lymphatic channels is located throughout the myocardium of all four cardiac chambers, draining outward from the endocardium toward the epicardium. Larger lymphatic channels follow the paths of the coronary arteries and veins and coalesce to forms a large lymphatic trunk that courses over the left main coronary artery and below the left pulmonary artery, where it drains into pretracheal lymph nodes and then into the thoracic duct.

## THE CONDUCTING SYSTEM

The conducting system consists of the sinoatrial node, the atrioventricular node, the His bundle, the right and left bundles, and the Purkinje fibers (Fig. 4–15). The components of the conducting system consist of modified myocardial cells that either have spontaneous automaticity or conduct electrical impulses throughout the myocardium to initiate contraction. The sinoatrial and the atrioventricular nodes have spontaneous automaticity, whereas the other components conduct electrical impulses rapidly.

The sinoatrial (SA, sinus) node is a histologically distinct structure located in the roof of the right atrium between the superior vena cava and the right atrial appendage. It spontaneously depolarizes 60 to 90 times a minute, functioning as the heart's intrinsic pacemaker. Sinus node depolarization is more rapid in children and during exercise. The blood supply to the sinoatrial node consists of a central artery arising from the right coronary artery in 60% of hearts and from the left circumflex branch in 40%. There are no histologically distinct pathways between the sinoatrial and atrioventricular nodes. Conduction spreads via ordinary atrial myocardium rather than specialized bundles of conducting fibers.

The atrioventricular (AV) node is located inferomedially within the right atrium, beneath Koch's triangle, above the septal leaflet of tricuspid valve, near the orifice of the coronary sinus. The atrioventricular node regulates the number of impulses that pass to the ventricles. It also has spontaneous depolarization, usually occurring at a rate of 40 to 60 per minute. Atrioventricular nodal function is modulated by the autonomic nervous system, parasympathetics via the vagus nerve and sympathetics via the sympathetic trunk. The atrioventricular node has a dual blood supply arising from the atrioventricular branch of the dominant coronary artery and the first septal perforator of the left anterior descending. Impulses from the atrioventricular node pass to the His bundle located in the upper portion of the interventricular septum. Abnormal bypass tracks are strands of muscular tissue connecting the atrium and ventricle, bypassing the atrioventricular node, originally described by Kent, Mahaim, and James.

The His bundle is a continuation of the AV node within the central fibrous body, which conducts electrical impulses rapidly. At the top of the muscular interventricular septum, the His bundle divides into the right and left bundles.

The right bundle courses down the septum, passes across the right ventricle within the moderator and septal bands towards the anterior papillary muscle, and extends upward to the right ventricular outflow tract. The left bundle courses down the septum and fans out into multiple conduction fibers to the papillary muscles and the rest of the left ventricle. False chordae may contain conduction fibers from the left bundle. The bundle branches have a dual blood supply arising from septal perforators of the left anterior descending and the posterior descending arteries.

Purkinje fibers are a terminal network of electrical conducting fibers, which initiate cardiac contraction in the myocytes. Muscular contraction starts in the papillary muscles, then spreads from the endocardial to epicardial segments of the apex upward to the outflow tract.

## INNERVATION OF THE HEART

The heart receives parasympathetic and sympathetic afferent and efferent nerves. Preganglionic sympathetic nerves are located in upper thoracic spinal cord. Second-order neurons are found in cervical sympathetic ganglia. Postganglionic fibers terminate in the heart and great vessels. Parasympathetic fibers are located within the vagus nerves. They synapse with second-order neurons in ganglia located on the wall of the heart and great vessels. Sympathetic and parasympathetic fibers are contained within two cardiac nerve bundles. These nerve fibers course down the atrioventricular groove as the right coronary plexus and down the interventricular groove as the left coronary plexus.

## BIBLIOGRAPHY

**Agur AM, Dalley AF.** *Grant's Atlas of Anatomy*. 11th ed. Philadelphia: Lippincott Williams & Wilkins; 2004.
*Atlas of Human Anatomy*. Springhouse, PA: Springhouse; 2001.
**Chung KW.** *Gross Anatomy*. 5th ed. Philadelphia: Lippincott Williams & Wilkins; 2004.
**Gosling JA, Harris PF, Whitmore I, Willan PLT.** *Human Anatomy Color Atlas and Text*. 4th ed. Edinborough: Mosby, 2002.
**Malouf J, Edwards WD, Tajik AJ.** Functional anatomy of the heart. In: Fuster V, Alexander RW, O'Rourke RA, Roberts R, King SB, Nash IS, Prystowsky EN, eds. *Hurst's The Heart*. 11th ed. New York: McGraw-Hill; 2004:45–86.
**Marieb EN, Mallatt J, Wilhelm PB.** *Human Anatomy*. 4th ed. San Francisco: Benjamin Cummings; 2005.
**Netter FH, Hansen JT.** *Atlas of Human Anatomy*. 3rd ed. Carlstadt, NJ: ICON Learning Systems; 1997.
**Rohen JW, Yokochi C, Lutjen-Drecoll E.** *Color Atlas of Anatomy: A Photographic Study of the Human Body*. 5th ed. Philadelphia: Lippincott Williams & Wilkins; 2002.
**Sauerland EK, Grant JCB.** *Grant's Dissector*. 12th ed. Philadelphia: Lippincott Williams & Wilkins; 1999.
**Stranding S.** *Gray's Anatomy*. 39th ed. Philadelphia: Elsevier; 2004.
**Zuidema GD.** *The Johns Hopkins Atlas of Human Functional Anatomy*. 4th ed. Baltimore: The Johns Hopkins University Press; 1997.

## QUESTIONS

1. Which of the following structures are not found in the right atrium?
   a. Tendon of Todaro
   b. Moderator band
   c. Koch's triangle
   d. Pectinate muscle

Answer is b: The moderator band, located in the right ventricle, is a muscular bridge that connects the distal septum and the right ventricular free wall at the anterior papillary muscle. The tendon of Todaro is a fibrous band located between the valves of the inferior vena cava and coronary sinus in the right atrium. Koch's triangle is located in the lower medial portion of the right atrium, overlying the AV node and the proximal His bundle. Pectinate muscles arise from the crista terminalis and course as bands on the right atrial free wall.

2. Which of the following statements about the pericardium is false?
   a. The pericardium contains 80 to 90 mL of pericardial fluid.
   b. It is connected to the diaphragm, sternum, and pleurae.
   c. It encloses the entire main pulmonary artery.
   d. The ligament of Marshall is a pericardial fold that contains the remnant of the embryonic left superior vena cava.

Answer is a: The pericardium contains 10 to 50 mL of pericardial fluid. It is attached to the central tendon of the diaphragm, posterior sternum, and laterally to the pleurae. It encloses the heart, portions of the vena cavae, most of the ascending aorta, the main pulmonary artery, and pulmonary veins. The ligament of Marshall is a pericardial fold containing the remnant of the embryonic left superior vena cava.

3. Which of the following statements about coronary arteries is true?
   a. The conus branch arises from a separate orifice in the aorta in 10% of patients.
   b. The left main trunk trifurcates into a left anterior descending, ramus branch, and left circumflex in 75% of patients.
   c. The sinoatrial nodal artery usually arises from an atrial branch of the left circumflex coronary artery.
   d. A dominant right coronary artery gives rise to a posterior descending artery, an AV branch, an artery supplying the AV node, and a posterior ventricular branch.

Answer is d: A dominant right coronary artery usually is a large vessel that crosses the crux of the heart to perfuse the posterolateral aspect of the left ventricle. The conus branch arises from a separate orifice in the aorta in 50% of patients. The sinoatrial nodal artery arises from the right coronary artery in 60% of patients and from the left circumflex in 40%. The left main trunk gives rise to a ramus branch in 30% of patients.

4. Which of the following statements about false chordae is true?
   a. False chordae are found in 1% of normal hearts.

b. False chordae connect the upper septum with the mitral valve leaflets.
c. False chordae often contain conducting fibers.
d. False chordae are identified only at autopsy.

Answer is c: Many false chordae contain extensions of left ventricular conducting fibers. They are found in 50% of normal hearts. False chordae may connect walls, papillary muscles, and the septum, but are not attached to mitral valve leaflets. They often cross the left ventricular outflow tract and can be identified by echocardiography.

5. Which of the following statements about the tricuspid valve is true?

a. It has three leaflets: anterior, lateral, and posterior.
b. It is the largest heart valve.
c. It is the most anterior heart valve.
d. The posterior leaflet is the largest and most mobile.

Answer is b: The tricuspid valve is the largest heart, whereas the pulmonic valve is the most anterior. The tricuspid valve consists of three leaflets, anterior, septal, and posterior. The anterior leaflet is the largest and most mobile. The posterior leaflet is the smallest, whereas the septal leaflet is the least mobile and occasionally absent.

# Cardiac Physical Examination

5

*Craig R. Asher* *Cristiana Scridon*

Over the years, the skill of the cardiologist examining a patient at the bedside has diminished, due in part to the availability, safety, and accuracy of echocardiography. However, the cardiology boards expect a high level of understanding of physical diagnosis. Most of the testing of physical diagnosis is indirect. Many of the questions are structured with a brief history and physical exam that provide clues about the diagnosis or answer. Often these are subtle clues that will not be appreciated by the unprepared. This chapter provides many of the pearls of physical diagnosis that are important for taking the boards.

## ESSENTIAL FACTS—TESTABLE INFORMATION

### Arterial Pulse (Fig. 5–1)

#### *Normal Pulse*

- Described by upstroke, magnitude, and contour.
- Composed of percussion (left ventricular) and tidal waves (reflected wave from periphery).
- Graded 0 to 4.
- Normal pulse pressure ~30 to 40 mm Hg (systolic minus diastolic blood pressure).
- Anacrotic notch is the systolic upstroke in the arterial pulse (ascending limb).
- Dicrotic notch is the diastolic downstroke of arterial pulse at aortic valve closure.

#### *Pulsus Alternans*

- Alternating strong and weak pulsations in sinus rhythm.
- Reflects myocardial dysfunction though not necessarily decompensation due to alterations in preload, afterload, and contractility with each beat.

#### *Pulsus Paradoxus*

- Exaggeration of normal inspiratory fall of systolic blood pressure (SBP) >10 mm Hg.
- Causes include cardiac tamponade, chronic lung disease/acute asthma, massive pulmonary embolism, right ventricular (RV) infarction, heart failure, tension pneumothorax, pregnancy, obesity, and *rarely* constrictive pericarditis.
- Mechanisms include: (a) increased venous return to the right heart during inspiration, with shift of the septum to the left resulting in decreased left ventricle (LV) stroke volume; and (b) increased pulmonary venous reservoir with decreased left-sided filling during inspiration.
- May have tamponade *without* pulsus paradoxus with high left ventricular end-diastolic pressure (AR, LV dysfunction), atrial septal defect (ASD, shunting to the left atrium during inspiration/expiration), or right ventricular hypertrophy (RVH) and pulmonary hypertension.

#### *Double-Peaked Pulse*

- Increased amplitude pulse with two *systolic* peaks.
- Results from accentuated percussion wave and tidal wave with aortic regurgitation.
- Most common cause is severe aortic regurgitation (AR, bisferiens) with or without aortic stenosis (AS), though may also occur with hypertrophic obstructive cardiomyopathy (HOCM, bifid, "spike and dome"), hyperdynamic states (i.e., patent ductus arteriosus, arteriovenous malformations).

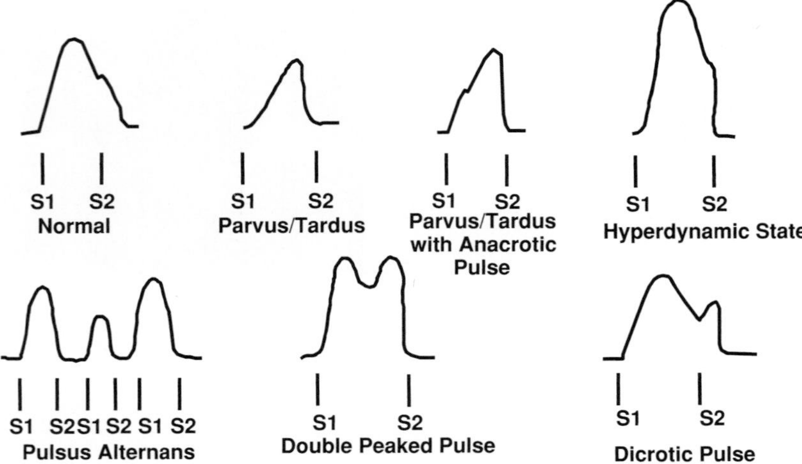


**Figure 5–1** Typical arterial pulse waveforms.

### *Pulsus Tardus and Parvus*

- Tardus (slow upstroke) and parvus (low amplitude).
- Caused most commonly by aortic stenosis, though may be absent even in the setting of severe AS in elderly with stiff carotid vessels.
- Associated with an anacrotic pulse.

### *Anacrotic Pulse*

- Notch on the upstroke of the carotid pulse (anacrotic notch). May not be palpable.
- Two distinct waves can be seen, *slow initial upstroke* and *delayed peak,* which is close to S2.
- Present in aortic stenosis.

### *Dicrotic Pulse*

- Accentuated upstroke with second peak after dicrotic notch in diastole.
- Second peak occurs in *diastole,* after S2, differentiating it from a bisferiens pulse.
- Occurs in patients with low cardiac output (CO) and high systemic vascular resistance (SVR) or high CO and low SVR (in both cases, the systolic pressure is low).

Other miscellaneous signs/findings related to arterial pulse include the following.

### *Osler Sign*

- Obliteration of brachial pulse by BP cuff with sustained palpable and rigid radial artery.
- Invasive BP measurements will not correlate with cuff pressures, and *pseudohypertension* may be diagnosed.

### *Pulse Deficit*

- Difference in the heart rate by direct cardiac auscultation and the distal arterial pulse rate when in atrial fibrillation.
- Due to short diastoles with short RR interval, the contraction may not be strong enough to generate enough stroke volume to periphery and thus the peripheral pulse may underestimate the heart rate.

### *Radial-to-Femoral Delay*

- Generally, radial and femoral pulse occur at nearly the same time (femoral slightly earlier).
- Because of obstruction of arterial flow due to *coarctation,* the femoral pulse may be delayed.
- Confirmed by decrease in lower-extremity pressure compared to upper-extremity pressure in the supine position.

### *Supravalvular AS*

- Results in blood directed toward the *right* side and greater right-sided compared to left-sided pulses and pressures (including inequality of carotid pulses).

### *Pressure/Pulse Difference in Two Arms (> 10 mm Hg systolic)*

- Due to obstruction involving aorta, innominate, and subclavian arteries by arteriosclerosis, embolism and arteritis; cervical rib or scalenus anticus syndrome, thoracic outlet syndrome, subclavian steal syndrome, supravalvular AS, or aortic dissection.
- Due to previous subclavian flap repair of a coarctation of the aorta or systemic-to-pulmonary artery shunts.

Signs of *severe aortic regurgitation* due to high stroke volume detected by pulse abnormalities include the following.

### *Hill Sign*

- Extreme augmentation of SBP in the femoral artery compared with the brachial artery (~40 mm Hg).
- Reliable sign for the detection of severe chronic AR.
- Results from a summation of waves traveling distally in the aorta.

### *Traube Sign*

- "Pistol shot."

### Corrigan Pulse

- "Water-hammer" pulse.
- Large-amplitude upstroke and downstroke due to high cardiac output and low resistance.

### Duroziez Sign

- Systolic/diastolic murmur in the femoral artery.

## Jugular Venous Pulse

### Basic Principles

- Pressure and waveforms should be evaluated.
- Adjust level of head/torso until pulsations optimally visualized, generally around 45 degrees.
- *Internal* jugular preferable to external jugular and *right* internal jugular preferable to left.
- Jugular venous pulse (JVP) decreases with inspiration in normal patients.

### Jugular Venous Pressure

- Measured as vertical height above the sternal angle (junction of manubrium and sternum)—considered to be 5 cm above the right atrium (RA) in all positions.
- $\geq$9 cm $H_2O$ is considered elevated.
- Conversion: 1.36 cm $H_2O$ = 1 mm Hg.
- Abdominal jugular reflux can be tested to confirm or determine elevated venous pressure. More than 10 to 30 seconds of right upper quadrant (RUQ) pressure results in elevation of pressure 4 cm or more and elevation is sustained for > 10 seconds following release of pressure. Must avoid straining, which will cause a false positive.

### Jugular Venous Waveforms (Fig. 5–2)

- "a" wave (positive wave)—atrial contraction (atrial systole).

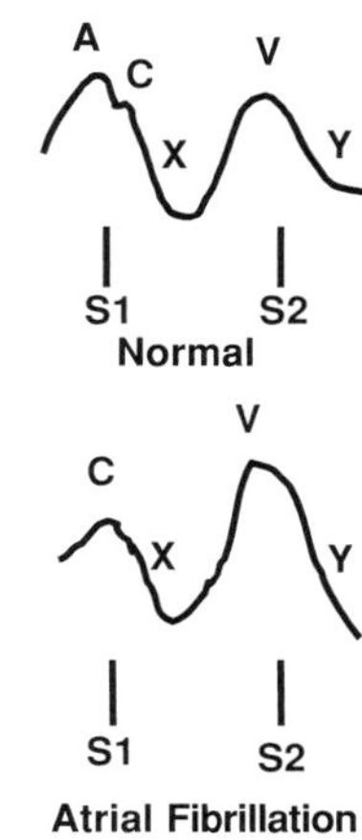


**Figure 5–2** Components of the normal jugular venous waveform.

- "x" descent (negative wave)—atrial relaxation during ventricular systole with descent of the RA.
- "v" wave (positive wave)—RA filling in systole.
- "y" descent (negative wave)—opening of the tricuspid valve and filling of the RV in diastole.

### Disease States (Fig. 5–3)

- Atrial fibrillation—loss of "a" wave, resulting in just one positive wave.
- Complete heart block or atrioventricular (AV) dissociation—cannon "a" wave due to contraction against a closed tricuspid valve.
- Tricuspid stenosis (RVH, pulmonary hypertension, sometimes severe LVH)—giant "a" waves and slow "y" descent for TS.
- Severe tricuspid regurgitation (TR) or ASD—prominent "v" wave and rapid "y" descent.

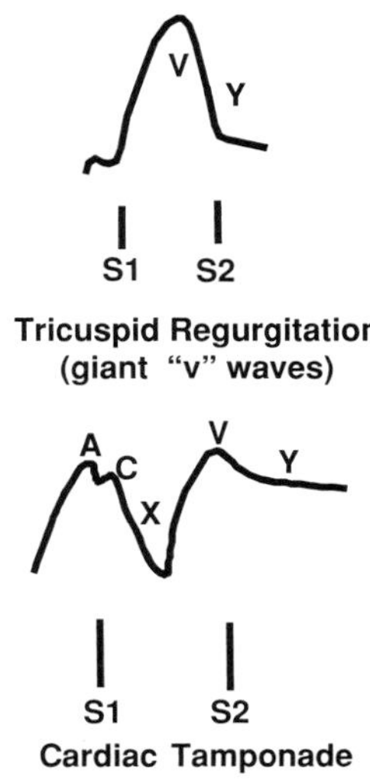


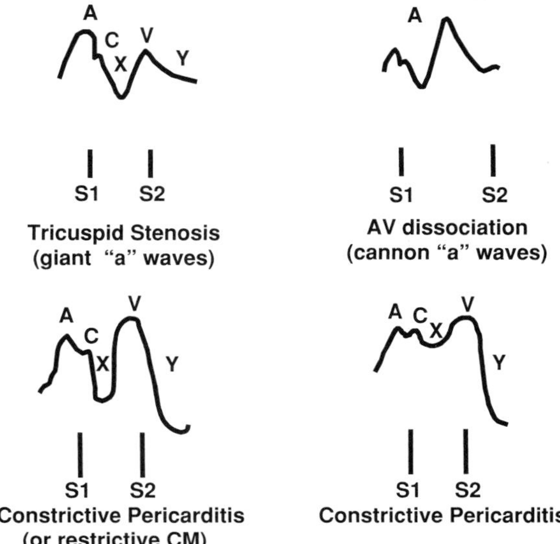


**Figure 5–3** Abnormal venous pulse wave patterns.

- Constrictive pericarditis—prominent "y" descent (predominant filling during early diastole) and sometimes prominent "x" descent giving W-shaped waveform along with elevated jugular venous pressure and Kussmaul sign.
- Restrictive cardiomyopathy—prominent "x" and "y" descent may also be present.
- Cardiac tamponade—prominent "x" wave and loss of the "y" descent representing loss of filling in diastole along with elevated jugular venous pressure.
- Superior vena cava (SVC) obstruction—elevated JVP but *not pulsatile*.

Other miscellaneous signs/findings include the following.

- Kussmaul sign—paradoxical rise in jugular venous pressure during inspiration, due to increased resistance of RA filling during inspiration. *Classical finding in constrictive pericarditis*. May also occur with RV infarct, severe TR, pulmonary embolism (PE), restrictive cardiomyopathy, and extremely rare and practically absent with tamponade.

## Precordial Motion

### *Principles*

- The apical pulsation is not always the point of maximal impulse (PMI) (i.e., in rheumatic mitral stenosis, the PMI may be produced by the right ventricle).
- The normal apex moves toward the chest wall in early systole and is best palpated in the fourth or fifth left intercostal space just medial to the midclavicular line.
- It is 1 to 2 cm in size and lasts less than half of systole.

### *Hypertrophy*

- LVH results in an apical impulse that is sustained and not diffuse.
- RVH or pulmonary hypertension results in a left parasternal heave or lift that is sustained and not diffuse.
- Hypertrophic cardiomyopathy causes a double or triple systolic outward motion.

### *Dilation*

- LV enlargement results in a diffuse, leftward apical impulse.
- RV enlargement results in a diffuse impulse occurring in the parasternal region.

### *Disease States*

- LV aneurysms may produce diffuse outward bulging and a rocking effect.
- Constrictive pericarditis may be characterized by systolic retraction of the chest (instead of outward motion)
- Hyperactive precordium in volume overload (severe aortic and mitral regurgitation, large left-to-right shunt).

## First Heart Sound

### *Examination*

- Ventricular systole begins with *closure* of the mitral (first) and tricuspid (second) valves.
- Best heard with the diaphragm of the stethoscope at the apex for the mitral and left sternal border for the tricuspid valve.
- Opening sounds of the mitral and tricuspid valves are pathologic sounds.

### *Intensity*

- Mitral closure is generally louder than tricuspid closure.
- S1 is generally louder than S2 at the apex and left sternal border and softer than S2 at the left and right second interspaces.
- S1 (particularly M1) is increased with:
  Short PR interval (due to wide separation of leaflets at onset of ventricular systole).
  MS with mobile leaflets.
  Hyperdynamic LV function or increased transvalvular flow due to shunts (increased force of leaflet closure).
  TS or ASD (T1 increased).
- S1 is decreased with:
  Long PR interval (leaflets close together at onset of ventricular systole).
  MS with immobile leaflets.
  Severe AR (due to mitral preclosure from jet hitting mitral valve and high LVEDP).
  Mitral regurgitation (MR) due to prolapse or flail (poor coaptation of leaflets).
  Severe LV dysfunction with poor cardiac output (decreased force of leaflet closure).
- S1 is variable with:
  Atrial fibrillation (AF).
  Complete heart block and AV dissociation.

### *Splitting*

- Occurs due to right bundle branch block (RBBB) (S2 also split), LV pacing, pre-excitation, or Ebstein anomaly.
- Reverse splitting of S1 is rare, can be caused by delayed M1 closure due to severe MS, LBBB, RV pacing.
- Split S1 must be differentiated from an S4 gallop heard best at the apex with the bell of the stethoscope and an ejection sound (pulmonic or aortic) heard at the base of the heart.

## Second Heart Sound

### *Examination*

- Ventricular systole ends with *closure* of the aortic (first) and pulmonic (second) valves.
- Heard best with the diaphragm of the stethoscope in the second left and right intercostal spaces near the sternum.

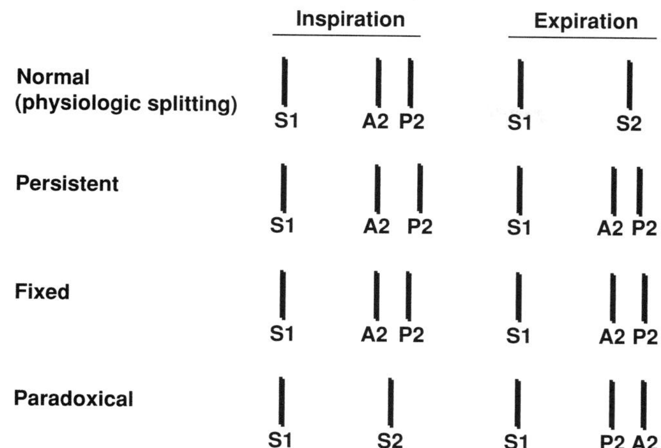


Figure 5–4 Types of S2 splitting, including physiologic and pathologic.

### Intensity

- Aortic closure, heard best at the second right intercostal space adjacent to the sternum, is generally louder than pulmonic closure, heard best at the left intercostal space adjacent to the sternum.
  S2 (A2) is increased with hypertension (HTN), dilated aorta.
  S2 (A2) is decreased with AS.
  S2 (P2) is increased with pulmonary HTN, dilated pulmonary artery (PA).
  S2 (P2) is decreased with pulmonary stenosis (PS).

### Splitting (Fig. 5–4)

- Normally, A2 and P2 separate during inspiration and come together during expiration (physiologic splitting). This occurs because the RV ejection period is longer than the LV ejection period and because of decreased impedance of the pulmonary vascular bed.
- Splitting of the S2 may also be referred to as physiologic or pathologic splitting.
- Pathologic splitting:
  *Fixed* splitting—wide splitting that does not vary with respiration due to minimal change in volume in right heart during inspiration and expiration.
  Conditions—ASD, PS, RV failure.
  *Persistent* splitting—widening in the usual splitting that occurs throughout the respiratory cycle. Splitting occurs with both inspiration and expiration but is not fixed. This is due to:
  1. P2 delayed—RBBB, pulmonary HTN, RV dysfunction, PS, dilated PA.
  2. A2 early—severe MR, ventricular septal defect (VSD), WPW (LV preexcitation).

  *Paradoxical* splitting—splitting that occurs with expiration (P2 followed by A2) and disappears on inspiration.
  1. A2 delayed—LBBB, AS, LV dysfunction, HOCM, dilated aorta, ischemia.
  2. P2 early—WPW (RV preexcitation).

## Third Heart Sound

### Examination and Intensity

- Mechanism related to the deceleration of flow during early filling.
- Physiologic in young adults, though may disappear with standing. Almost all adults lose S3 after age 40 years.
- Best heard with light pressure of the bell of the stethoscope (low frequency) in left lateral decubitus position at the apex.
- Right-sided S3 can be heard at left sternal border and may increase with inspiration.
- Most commonly heard in conditions of high flow across an AV valve.
- S3 follows an opening snap and pericardial knock in timing.
- S3 corresponds with the "y" descent of the atrial waveform or the Doppler E wave on an echocardiogram.
- An S3 is rare with significant MS.

## Fourth Heart Sound

### Examination and Intensity

- Caused by resistance and deceleration of ventricular filling during atrial contraction and movement of the valve and noncompliant ventricle.
- S4 is usually pathologic (atrial gallop), though it can be heard uncommonly in young people.
- S4 is heard best with the bell of the stethoscope and occurs just before S1, after the P wave on the EKG, and is equivalent to the A wave on the Doppler echocardiogram.
- A left-sided S4 is heard best in the left lateral decubitus position at the apex during expiration and a right-sided S4 is heard at the left sternal border to mid-sternum best with inspiration.
- Common pathologic states associated with a left-sided S4 include aortic stenosis, hypertension, HCM, and ischemic heart disease. Right-sided S4 is heard with pulmonary hypertension and pulmonic stenosis.
- S4 gallop not heard in atrial fibrillation.
- When S3 and S4 are heard simultaneously, such as may occur with tachycardia and prolonged PR intervals, a "summation gallop" is present.
- A quadruple rhythm with a distinct S3 and S4 may be heard with tachycardia.

## Extra Heart Sounds

### Diastole (Fig. 5–5)

#### Opening Snap (OS)

- Pathologic sound generated by abrupt movement in early diastole due to mitral or tricuspid stenosis.

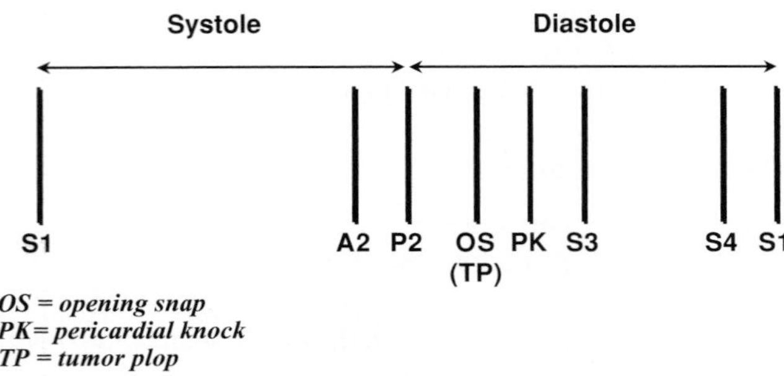


Figure 5–5 Diastolic heart sounds in sequence of occurrence during the cardiac cycle.

- OS is a high-pitched sound best heard medial to the apex with the diaphragm of the stethoscope.
- If the valve is not mobile or MR is present, an OS may not occur.
- An interval of less than 70 milliseconds is consistent with severe MS. However, this interval is affected by other factors such as left atrial and left ventricular pressure and compliance.
- S2–OS interval may not be useful with rapid heart rates or with AS, AR, or MR.
- A tumor plop has about the same timing as an OS.
- An OS precedes a pericardial knock or S3 in timing.
- A right-sided OS is best heard at the left sternal border and varies with respiration.

Diastole Others

- A tumor "plop" occurs at about the same time as an OS. It is due to the movement of a tumor such as a myxoma into the atrium during diastole.
- A pericardial knock occurs earlier than an S3 and later than an OS. It is best heard with the diaphragm at the apex and may vary with respiration. It is due to the rapid early filling that occurs with constrictive pericarditis.

### *Systole*

Ejection Sounds (ES)

- ES occur in early systole, following valve opening.
- ES occur before the upstroke of the carotid.
- ES are high pitched and heard best with the diaphragm.
- *Aortic* ES occur most often with opening of a bicuspid aortic valve and may be heard at the sternum, LSB, or apex. They are also heard with dilated aorta. They do not vary with respiration.
- *Pulmonic* ES may be heard with PS increasing during *expiration* and diminishing during inspiration (the only right-sided sound that decreases with inspiration). They are also heard with dilated PA.

Nonejection Clicks (Mid-Late Systolic) (Fig. 5–6)

- Predominantly due to mitral valve prolapse (MVP)with myxomatous mitral valve.

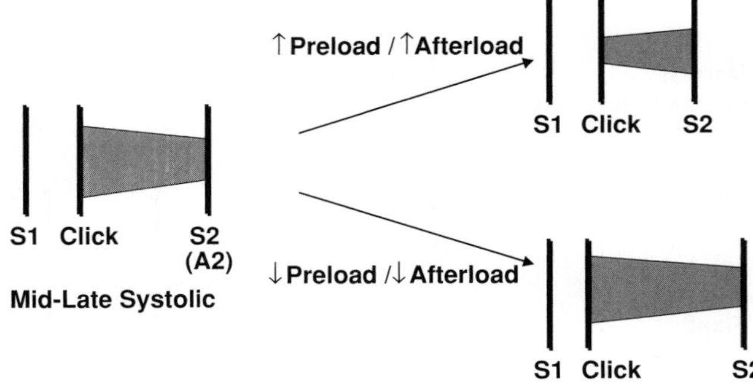


Figure 5–6 Mitral valve click-murmur response to different loading conditions, including preload and afterload.

- Clicks due to MVP are due to tensing of the chordae during systole.
- Clicks are best heard with the diaphragm at the apex.
- Other uncommon causes include atrial septal aneurysms, tumors, or nonmyxomatous mitral valve disease.
- Clicks may be single or multiple and may vary over time.
- Maneuvers that decrease LV volume of afterload move the click closer to S1 and maneuvers that increase LV volume or afterload move the click away from S1.

Pericardial Friction Rubs and Other Extra Sounds

- High-pitched and scratchy sounds.
- Best heard with the patient leaning forward following expiration.
- Three components may be heard, though often only one or two components are heard: (a) atrial systole; (b) ventricular systole; (c) rapid ventricular filling.

### *Pacemaker Sounds*

- *Pacemaker sounds* are extra high-frequency sounds heard during contraction of the chest wall muscles with pacing before the first heart sound.

### *Prosthetic Heart Sounds*

- Intensity of the opening and closing sounds vary according to the type and design of the prosthetic valve.
- With ball-cage valves, both the opening and closing clicks are loud.
- With bileaflet or tilting disc valves, the closing sound is louder than the opening sound.
- With aortic valve prosthesis, diastolic (AR) murmurs are abnormal.
- With mitral valve prosthesis, holosystolic (MR) murmurs are abnormal.

## Systolic Heart Murmurs

### *Ejection (Fig. 5–7)*

Aortic Valvular Stenosis

- *Location*—heard best with the diaphragm at the right second or left second interspace.

| Feature | Valvular | Subvalvular | Hypertrophic |
|---|---|---|---|
| Effect of Valsalva maneuver on systolic murmur | ↓↓ | ↓ | ↑ |
| Murmur of aortic regurgitation | Common | Common | Uncommon |
| Fourth heart sound | Common | Uncommon | Common |
| Paradoxical splitting | Common | Uncommon | Common |
| Carotid pulse | ↓ | Normal or ↓ | ↑ |

**Figure 5–7** Features that help to differentiate causes of left ventricular outflow tract obstruction.

- *Character*—mainly harsh, with a crescendo/decrescendo configuration. In elderly patients there is a high-pitched musical murmur that may be heard (Gallavardin) radiating to the apex.
- *Radiation*—into the neck and great vessels, though it may be toward the apex in elderly patients, but not beyond the apex.
- *Intensity*—related to the stroke volume and therefore may or may not reflect the severity of stenosis.
- *Severity*—severe AS is suggested with an increase in ejection time (longer duration and delayed peaking).
- *Maneuvers*—AS murmur may decrease following Valsalva and increases post–PVC.
- *Associated findings:*

  Prominent "a" waves (decreased RV compliance because of septal hypertrophy—Bernheim effect).

  "Parvus and tardus" carotid upstroke with anacrotic pulse, though not always true in elderly patients with stiff vessels.

  Thrill over the carotid pulse (shudder).

  Apical impulse is sustained, nondisplaced.

  Early ejection sound heard with congenital stenosis.

  Second heart sound is single (P2) or may be paradoxically split.

  A2 intensity decreased with severe AS.

  Palpable and audible S4.

  Reduced pulse pressure.
- *Variations*—Congenital supravalvular AS is heard best at the first or second right interspace and is associated with relatively decreased left-sided pulse.

#### Aortic Sclerosis

- *Location*—second right upper sternal border with the diaphragm.
- *Character*—soft.
- *Radiation*—does not radiate widely.
- *Intensity/severity*—related to flow, early peaking.
- *Associated findings*—no associated findings of AS—normal S2 and no radiation to the carotids.

#### Hypertrophic Cardiomyopathy

- *Location*—left ventricular outflow tract (LVOT) obstruction murmur is heard best along the left sternal edge.
- *Character*—harsh.
- *Radiation*—LVOT obstruction murmur may be widely transmitted though not to the base of the neck.
- *Intensity/severity*—related to the degree of obstruction.
- *Maneuvers*—hemodynamic changes that affect LV volume, contractility, and vascular resistance help differentiate HCM from AS:

  Standing decreases AS and increases HOCM.

  Valsalva (straining phase) increases the murmur of HOCM and decreases or does not change the murmur of AS.

  Amyl nitrite increases the murmur of HOCM and AS.

  Post–PVC the murmur of HOCM and AS is increased.
- *Associated findings:*

  Increased "a" wave (decreased RV compliance secondary to septal hypertrophy).

  Brisk carotid upstrokes, sometimes bifid, "spike and dome."

  Sustained LV apical impulse, double or triple (presystolic and double systolic outward thrust).

  S2 paradoxical split.

  S4 gallop.

#### Pulmonic Stenosis

- *Location*—heard best in the pulmonic area.
- *Character*—harsh crescendo/decrescendo and low or medium pitched
- *Radiation*—directed to the left shoulder and neck.
- *Intensity/severity*—depends on stroke volume and reflected by duration of murmur and time to peak and also the degree of splitting of S2.
- *Maneuvers*—increases with inspiration.
- *Associated findings:*

  "a" wave increased.

  Sustained sternal lift or heave.

  Absent or decreased P2.

  Widely split S2.

  Early pulmonic ejection sound that decreases with inspiration.

  Right-sided S4.

#### Innocent and Functional (in Children—Still's Murmur)

- *Location*—left or right sternal border.
- *Character*—soft, brief, midsystolic.
- *Radiation*—no radiation.
- *Intensity/severity*—related to stroke volume but usually soft.
- *Maneuvers*—may change in intensity or disappear with different positions, such as standing.
- *Associated findings:*

  Relatively smaller aortic size.

  Left ventricular false tendons.

### *Regurgitant*

#### Mitral Regurgitation

- *Location*—usually heard best with the diaphragm at the apex.
- *Character*—blowing, high-pitched.

- *Radiation*—typically into left axilla, unlike with AS.
- *Intensity/Severity*—variable related to BP, loading conditions, mechanism and acuity.
- *Maneuvers*—may increase with expiration and during isometric handgrip.
- *Variations*—MR due to posterior prolapse may be anteriorly directed toward the left sternal border and neck. MR may not be holosystolic; following a click it may be mid- or late systolic and it may be early systolic with acute MR (rapid equalization of pressures).
- *Associated findings*—displaced apical impulse, decreased S1, S3 present, S2 (P2) may be increased when pulmonary hypertension occurs.

#### Tricuspid Regurgitation (TR)

- *Location*—heard best along the lower sternal border but also along the right sternal border.
- *Character*—blowing, high-pitched.
- *Radiation*—to the right side, not beyond the axilla as in MR.
- *Intensity*—may increases with inspiration (Carvallo sign), though sometimes even severe TR is not loud and may not increase with inspiration (RV failure when RV volume does not change).
- *Severity*—may not be related to intensity. Always with elevated JVP.
- *Variations*—if RV is severely dilated, occupying the left precordium, then TR may be heard toward the apex.
- *Associated findings*—left parasternal lift (due to RV hypertrophy). Elevated JVP with large "v" wave and rapid "y" descent, pulsatile liver, right-sided S3, diastolic flow rumble, narrow split S2 and increased P2 if due to pulmonary hypertension.

#### Ventricular Septal Defect

- *Location*—around the lower sternum.
- *Character*—harsh, high-pitched.
- *Radiation*—toward sternum and not to axilla.
- *Intensity*—generally loud, but depends on the size of the shunt.
- *Severity*—usually accompanying thrill, though the intensity of murmur is not proportional to the degree of shunt (loud, restrictive murmur is generally small, and soft, nonrestrictive murmur is generally a large shunt).
- *Maneuvers*—does not increase with inspiration as TR does. Decreased intensity with amyl nitrite.
- *Variations*—depends on relative pressures of LV and RV, may be early systolic ejection. If heard best in first and second left intercostal spaces and radiating to the left clavicle, suspect supracristal defect.
- *Associated findings*—thrill, S2 is usually normal.

## Diastolic Heart Murmurs

### *Mitral Stenosis*

- *Location*—localized around apex, best in left lateral decubitus position.
- *Character*—low-pitched diastolic rumble heard best with the bell, crescendo in late diastole with presystolic accentuation (heard in normal sinus rhythm or atrial fibrillation).
- *Radiation*—no.
- *Severity*—related to duration of murmur. A2–OS interval may be related to severity.
- *Maneuvers*—increased with amyl nitrite, due to the tachycardia.
- *Variations*—early to mid-diastolic rumble may be heard without stenosis, due to increased flow (i.e., large VSD, PDA).
- *Associated findings*—S1 may be increased. OS present with decreased OS–A2 interval, increased P2 and left parasternal lift.

### *Aortic Regurgitation*

- *Location*—left or right sternal border.
- *Character*—blowing, high-pitched decrescendo, heard best with the diaphragm, begins with A2. Best heard sitting, leaning forward in expiration.
- *Radiation*—if heard best and with radiation to right sternal border, suspect *aortic root* disease. *Leaflet* abnormalities heard on left chest and radiation to apex.
- *Intensity*—related to the difference between the aortic diastolic pressure and the left ventricular end diastolic pressure. This intensity is affected by the acuity of the AR.
- *Severity*—severity cannot be determined by the duration of murmur, though a holodiastolic murmur is associated with severe AR. Acute severe AR may result in a brief and soft early diastolic murmur. Associated findings are important in determining severity.
- *Variations*—leaflet perforation may cause musical murmur. Acute AR with early diastolic murmur.
- *Associated findings*—aortic systolic ejection murmur, Austin–Flint murmur that is a low rumbling apical diastolic murmur with late presystolic accentuation resembling MS, soft S1 (premature closure), paradoxically split S2, S3 present, displaced hyperdynamic apical impulse, wide pulse pressure with decreased diastolic pressure and large volume pulses that may be bisferiens. Positive Hill sign. Diastolic MR may occur.

### *Pulmonic Regurgitation (PR)*

- *Location*—localized to second or third left intercostal space.
- *Character*—high-pitched and blowing, early diastolic decrescendo and generally brief beginning with P2 if due to pulmonary hypertension (Graham Steel's) and lower-pitched in the absence of pulmonary hypertension beginning after P2.
- *Radiation*—very localized.
- *Intensity*—increases with inspiration.
- *Severity*—"to-and-fro" murmur with severe PR.
- *Associated findings*—loud S2 and no peripheral signs of AR.

### *Tricuspid Stenosis*

- *Character*—very localized at the lower left sternal border or xiphoid area.
- *Quality/pitch*—higher in frequency and starts earlier than MS, crescendo in late diastole with presystolic accentuation though best heard with the bell.
- *Radiation*—localized.
- *Intensity*—increases with inspiration.
- *Severity*—related to the duration of the murmur.
- *Maneuvers*—OS also increases with inspiration.
- *Variation*—short, early to mid-diastolic rumble may be heard without stenosis, due to increased flow such as with ASD.
- *Associated findings*—large "a" wave and slow "y" descent; splitting of S1 and loud S1/T1 may occur. Hepatomegaly, ascites, edema.

## Continuous Heart Sounds

- Encompass part or all of systole and diastole but *must extend through S2* without discontinuation.
- A holosystolic and holodiastolic murmur together is not a continuous murmur because it does not go through the second heart sound.
- Continuous murmurs occur because of a continuous gradient between chambers or vascular structures (aorta–PA, artery–artery, artery–vein, vein–vein).
- Benign continuous sounds include a venous hum and mammary soufflé.
- Pathologic continuous murmurs include patent ductus arteriosus, coronary fistula, pulmonary arteriovenous fistulas, and coarctation of the aorta.

### *Patent Ductus Arteriosus*

- Heard in left second interspace near the sternum with radiation to the left clavicle.
- Harsh, loud, machinery-like quality, sometimes associated with a thrill.
- Increases with peak intensity around S2 and then gradually wanes and may not encompass all of diastole.
- When pulmonary hypertension develops, diastolic portion gets shorter. With severe pulmonary systolic hypertension, the diastolic component is absent.

### *Coronary Artery Fistulas*

- May empty into the right atrium, right ventricle, left ventricle, or pulmonary artery, so the location of the murmur will differ.

### *Venous Hum*

- A benign sound heard mostly in children.
- Heard in the supraclavicular fossa (best on the *right)* in the *sitting* position.
- Variable quality but may be humming or roaring.
- Loudest component in *diastole.*
- Can be brought out by movements of the head and abolished by compression and supine position.

### *Pericardial Friction Rub*

- Heard to the left of the sternum with a scratchy, high-pitched sound.
- Increases when the patient leans forward and exhales.
- Three components: atrial systole, ventricular systole (most prominent component), and ventricular diastole.

### *Mammary Souffle*

- Innocent murmur heard during late pregnancy or lactation.
- Loudest in *systole.*
- Firm pressure will obliterate the murmur.

## Dynamic Auscultation (Fig. 5–8)

### *Respiration*

- In general, right-sided murmurs and sounds increase with inspiration, and left-sided murmurs and sounds decrease.
- *Exceptions include:*
  TR may not increase with inspiration when there is RV failure.
  Click of mitral valve prolapse moves closer to S1, and the murmur may be longer and accentuated with inspiration.
- Inspiratory click of pulmonic stenosis decreases with inspiration.

### *Valsalva*

- Inspiration followed by forced exhalation.
- *Phase II during straining* is detected at the bedside—there is a *decrease* in venous return and BP and reflex tachycardia.
- During the strain phase *the only murmurs that increase* are that of *HOCM* and the *MR murmur associated with MVP,* which gets longer and may increase in intensity.
- Right-sided murmurs return to baseline levels within two to three beats after *Valsalva release.*

### *Hemodynamic Maneuvers*

- Raising legs while supine augments venous return and *augments most* left- and right-sided heart sounds. The murmur of *HOCM is diminished.*
- Squatting results in increased venous return and systemic resistance. Most right- and left-sided murmurs increase. The murmur of *HOCM is diminished.*
- Hand grips increase BP and HR. AS murmur is unchanged or may decrease, most other left-sided murmurs increase. *HOCM murmur decreases,* and click and murmur of *MVP are delayed and decreased in intensity.*

### *Pharmacologic Agents*

- Amyl nitrite results in marked transient preload and afterload (BP) reduction and subsequent increase in heart rate.
- Best for distinguishing:
  AS (augmented) vs. MR (diminished).
  MS (augmented) vs. Austin Flint (diminished).
  MVP click murmur gets longer.

| Murmur | Respiration | | | Standing | Squatting | Handgrip | Post–PVC | Amyl nitrite | Phenyl ephrine |
|---|---|---|---|---|---|---|---|---|---|
| | Insp | Exp | Valsalva | | | | | | |
| Aortic stenosis | ↓ | ↑/- | ↓ | ↓ | ↓/- | ↓/- | ↑ | ↑ | ↓ |
| Mitral regurgitation | ↓ | ↑/- | ↓ | ↓ | ↑ | ↑ | - | ↓ | ↑ |
| Mitral valve prolapse | ↑ | ↓ | ↑ | ↑ | ↓ | ↓ | - | ↑ | ↓ |
| Hyperthrophic obstructive cardiomyopathy | ↑ | ↓ | ↑ | ↑ | ↓ | ↓ | ↑ | ↑ | ↓ |
| Tricuspid regurgitation | ↑ | ↓ | ↓ | ↓ | ↑ | - | - | ↑ | - |
| Pulmonic stenosis | ↑ | ↓ | ↓ | ↓ | ↑ | ↑ | ↑ | ↑ | - |
| Mitral stenosis | ↓ | ↑/- | ↓ | ↓ | ↑ | ↑ | - | ↑ | ↓ |
| Tricuspid stenosis | ↑ | ↓ | ↓ | ↓ | ↑ | ↑ | - | ↑ | - |
| Aortic regurgitation | ↓ | ↑ | ↓ | ↓ | ↑ | ↑ | -/↑ | ↓ | ↑ |
| Pulmonic regurgitation | ↑ | ↓ | ↓ | ↓ | ↑ | ↓/- | - | ↑ | - |
| Ventricular septal defect | ↓/- | ↑/- | ↓ | ↓ | ↑ | ↑ | ↑ | ↓ | ↑ |

**Figure 5–8** Dynamic auscultatory changes in specific cardiac conditions.

*Post–PVC*

- The pulse pressure with *HCM decreases* (Brockenbrough phenomenon) and that of *AS increases.*

## SPECIFIC DISEASES

### Acute MI

- Tachycardia.
- S1 soft.
- S2 paradoxically split.
- S3 gallop.
- S4 (decreased LV compliance during ischemia)
- Systolic murmur of mitral regurgitation (papillary muscle dysfunction/LV dilatation).

### RV Infarction

- Increased "a" wave.
- Kussmaul sign (increased venous pressure in inspiration because of decreased RV compliance).
- Hypotension
- S3, S4.
- Systolic murmur of TR (papillary muscle dysfunction).
- Clear lungs.

### Dilated CM

- Increased JVP, "a," "v" waves.
- Low pulse amplitude, narrow pulse pressure, pulsus alternans.
- Apical impulse laterally displaced, often diffuse.
- S2 paradoxically split in presence of LBBB or due to prolonged LV ejection time, S2 (P2) increased in PHTN
- S4, S3 or summation gallop in tachycardia.
- Mitral/tricuspid regurgitation murmur.

### Restrictive CM

- Increased JVP, rapid "y" descent.
- Kussmaul sign.
- Narrow pulse pressure.
- S3 or S4.
- Atrioventricular valvular regurgitation murmur.
- Hepatomegaly, edema, ascites.

### Cardiac Tamponade

- Increased JVP.
- Hypotension (Beck's triad: increased JVP, quiet heart sounds, and hypotension).
- Tachycardia.
- Pulsus paradoxus.

- Prominent "x" descent, "y" descent diminished/absent.
- Pericardial rub may be present.

## Constrictive Pericarditis

- Increased JVP.
- Rapid "x" and "y" descent.
- Kussmaul sign.
- Systolic retraction of the apical impulse—Broadbent sign.
- Pericardial knock.
- Hepatomegaly, edema, ascites.

## Pulmonary Hypertension

- Prominent "a" waves.
- Left parasternal systolic lift.
- P2 loud, can be transmitted throughout the precordium.
- S2 persistently split.
- Right S4 or S3.
- Pulmonic ejection sound.
- Pulmonic regurgitation.
- Tricuspid regurgitation.

## Type A Aortic Dissection

- Unequal/absent pulses.
- New high-pitched diastolic murmur, best heard along the right sternal border (RSB).
- Pericardial rub (if rupture into pericardial sac).

## ASD

- Large "v" waves.
- Hyperdynamic RV systolic lift.
- P2 increased.
- S2 *fixed split*.
- Pulmonic vascular ejection sound.
- Mid-systolic ejection murmur.
- Early low-pitched diastolic rumble of tricuspid origin.
- Pulmonary regurgitation.
- Association with Holt–Oram syndrome (hand–heart).
- Lutembacher syndrome: ASD ostium secundum + mitral stenosis.

## VSD

- S2 normal.
- S2 widely split (larger defect).
- LV $S_3$ (larger defect).
- Systolic murmur of variable intensity and duration.
- Thrill.

## PDA

- Brisk and bounding pulses.
- Apical impulse displaced, diffuse.
- S2 difficult to hear because of the murmur, but usually normal.
- S3.
- Continuous murmur "machinery" heard below the left clavicle, peaking near S2.
- Diastolic component of the murmur disappears with shunt reversal.
- "Differential cyanosis" = cyanosis/clubbing of the toes with shunt reversal.

## BIBLIOGRAPHY

**Braunwald E.** *Heart Disease: A Textbook of Cardiovascular Medicine*. 5th ed. Philadelphia: WB Saunders; 1997.

**Hurst JW.** The examination of the heart: the importance of initial screening. Emory Univ J Med.1991;5:135165.

**Hurst JW.** *The Heart*. 8th ed. New York: McGraw-Hill; 1994.

**Topol E.** Physical examination. In: *Textbook of Cardiovascular Medicine*. Philadelphia: Lippincot–Raven Publishers; 1998: 293–332.

## QUESTIONS

1. Which of the following statements about the assessment of the severity of a valvular abnormality are *not* true?
   a. Severe acute aortic regurgitation results in a holodiastolic murmur.
   b. Severe aortic stenosis results in a long-duration and late-peaking systolic ejection murumur.
   c. An S2–OS interval of less than 70 milliseconds is consistent with severe mitral stenosis with normal heart rates and absence of other left-sided valve disease.
   d. Severe aortic stenosis may be present with a soft murmur.
   e. The duration of a tricuspid stenosis murmur correlates with the severity of stenosis.

The answer is a: The severity of AS is best determined by the duration and time to peak of the murmur. Long-duration and late peaking are consistent with severe AS. The intensity of an AS murmur is dependent on the stroke volume, so a soft murmur may occur with severe AS and LV dysfunction. Similarly, the duration of TS or MS murmurs are helpful in determining severity, as is the duration of the S2–OS interval. However, the S2–OS interval is also affected by heart rate and other valvular lesions that affect LA and LV pressure. Severe acute AR may be a short-duration murmur due to the rapid elevation in LVEDP.

2. Which of the following statements about distinguishing an Austin–Flint murmur from a mitral stenosis (MS) murmur is *not* true?
   a. S1 is usually diminished with an Austin–Flint murmur and not with an MS murmur.
   b. An opening snap is not present with an Austin–Flint murmur.
   c. An S3 may be present with an Austin–Flint murmur but not generally with an MS murmur.
   d. Amyl nitrite increases the intensity of an MS murmur and increases the intensity of an Austin–Flint murmur.

The answer is d: The Austin–Flint murmur that occurs with severe AR is thought to occur as a result of mitral valve preclosure and is a diastolic rumble similar to that of MS. When an Austin–Flint murmur is present, S1 will be diminished, S3 may be present, and an OS will be absent. With severe MS, S1 will be increased with mobile leaflets, an OS will be present, and S3 is usually absent. Amyl nitrite will result in a decrease in the intensity of the Austin–Flint murmur due to decreased afterload and preload and an increase in the MS murmur due to increase in heart rate.

3. Which of the following statements about systolic clicks is *not* true?
   a. With severe pulmonary valve stenosis, the pulmonary artery ejection sound decreases in intensity with inspiration.
   b. An aortic valve ejection click occurs with a bicuspid aortic valve.
   c. Systolic clicks due to atrial septal aneurysms and nonmyxomatous valve disease may occur.
   d. The systolic click of MVP moves closer to S1 with the Valsalva maneuver.
   e. The systolic click of MVP moves closer to S2 with standing.

The answer is e: Systolic ejection clicks may occur with pulmonary valve stenosis and aortic stenosis, particularly with a bicuspid valve. Other causes of systolic clicks include atrial septal aneurysms and nonmyxomatous mitral valve disease. The mid-systolic click of MVP is affected by maneuvers that alter volume. With a reduced LV volume such as with Valsalva and standing, the click moves closer to S1 and the murmur gets longer.

4. Which of the following will *not* cause a continuous murmur?
   a. An right coronary sinus to the right atrial fistula.
   b. A stenotic and regurgitant aortic valve.
   c. A venous hum.
   d. An aorta-to-pulmonary artery connection.
   e. A high-grade coarctation of the aorta.

The answer is b: A continuous murmur must extend uninterrupted through S2. An aorta–pulmonary connection such as a PDA, a coronary sinus-to-RA connection such as with a ruptured sinus of Valsalva, a severe coarctation, and a venous hum all result in continuous murmurs. The combination of a systolic and diastolic murmur of AS and AR is not considered a continuous murmur.

5. Which of the following about differentiating AS from HCM on examination is true?
   a. The murmur of AS decreases and the murmur of HCM increases with amyl nitrite.
   b. Post–PVC, the pulse pressure of HCM decreases and that of AS increases.
   c. The murmur of AS and HCM decrease with standing.
   d. With Valsalva, the murmur of AS and HCM decrease.

The answer is b: Amyl nitrite results in an increase in the murmur of AS and HOCM. Valsalva (straining phase) and standing result in an increase of the murmur of HOCM and decreases the murmur of AS. Post–PVC, the murmur of AS and HOCM increases but the pulse pressure of HOCM decreases (Brockenbrough phenomenon) while that of AS increases.

# 6 Clinical Epidemiology and Biostatistics for the Clinical Practitioner

***Michael S. Lauer***

An ability to read the medical literature intelligently is an essential skill for the competent clinical practitioner. Acquiring this skill is challenging because of the high volume of medical articles published and the increasing sophistication of modern epidemiologic and statistical methods.

Topics that will be covered in this chapter include:

1. Exposures and outcomes
2. Types of clinical studies
3. Types of statistical errors
4. Data presentation: reporting of outcomes
5. Confounding and interaction
6. Multivariable regression and pitfalls
7. Bias and its consequences
8. External validity: assessments of causation and validity
9. Issues related to:
   a. Randomized treatment/prevention trials
   b. Studies of diagnostic tests
   c. Prognostic (survival) studies
   d. Case-control studies
   e. Economics
   f. Clinical prediction guides
   g. Systematic review articles and meta-analyses

## CURRENT CONCEPTS AND ESSENTIAL FACTS

### Exposures and Outcomes

At the heart of virtually all clinical studies is an attempt to link an "exposure" with an "outcome." When reading an article, you should ask yourself what exactly the exposure and outcome variables are and whether their association is of interest to you.

For exposure, the "independent" variable, examples include:

1. A treatment strategy (or lack thereof)
2. A patient characteristic (such as age, gender, or cholesterol level)
3. A diagnostic test result (such as ejection fraction)

Outcome, the "dependent" variable, examples include:

1. A treatment outcome (such as death, myocardial infarction, need for revascularization)
2. A clinical event during follow-up (such as death or myocardial infarction)
3. A "gold standard" finding (such as evidence of coronary disease on an angiogram)

### Types of Clinical Studies

Various types of clinical studies are reported in the literature, including the following.

#### *Case Reports*

Case reports, although they may be fun to read, but rarely provide the kind of high-level evidence needed to influence clinical practice.

#### *Case Series*

Case series report on a group of patients who show a certain finding. Although there may be a clear-cut exposure and an

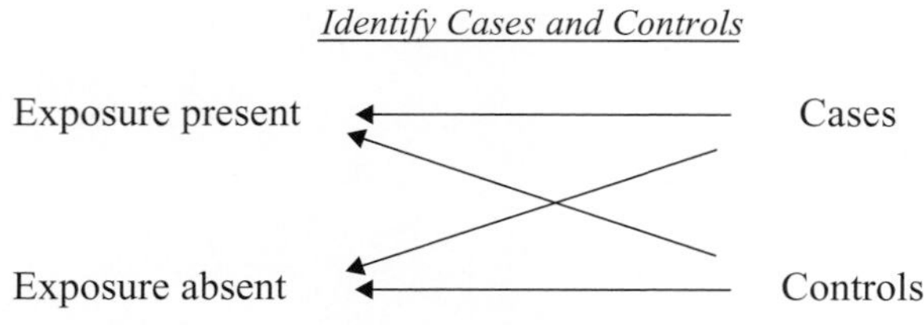


**Figure 6–1** Case-control study diagram.

outcome variable, the absence of a comparison group limits any conclusions that can be drawn. Case reports and case series are best thought of as hypothesis-generating studies.

### *Cohort Study*

The cohort study is a fundamentally strong study design in which:

1. An inception cohort is clearly defined.
2. An exposure variable is defined.
3. The cohort consists of individuals with and without the exposure variable present at the time of inception.
4. The cohort is followed over time for the occurrence of a clearly and objectively defined outcome.
5. The occurrence of the outcome is compared in individuals with and without the exposure variable.

### *Case-Control Study*

A case-control study (Fig. 6–1) is a somewhat weaker study design than a cohort study. In a case-control study,

1. A "case" group of subjects with a given outcome is identified.
2. A "control" group of subjects, without the outcome, is identified.
3. The occurrence of an exposure variable is compared between the case group and the control group.

### *Studies of Diagnostic Tests*

In studies designed to assess the value of a diagnostic test, a group of patients suspected of having a certain disease (outcome) undergo the diagnostic test, and then the results of the diagnostic test are compared against an accepted standard.

### *Cost-Effectiveness Studies*

Cost-effectiveness studies usually take the form of a cohort study in which (a) the cost of an intervention is measured, (b) the outcomes of performing or not performing an intervention are compared, or (c) the cost of preventing an outcome is measured; typically, this last is recorded as dollars per year of life saved or dollars per quality-adjusted year of life saved (QALY).

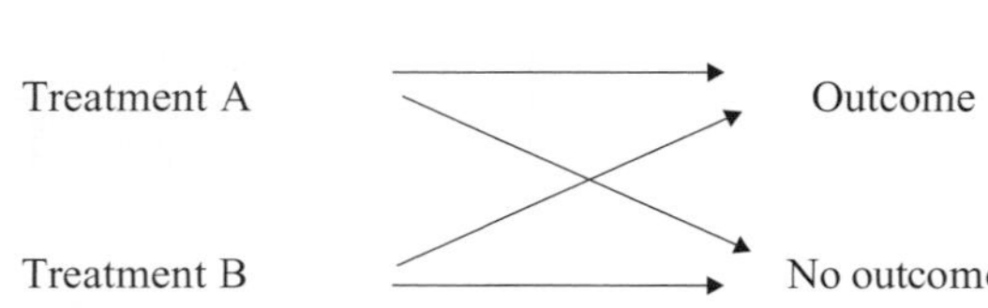


**Figure 6–2** Randomized trial diagram.

### *Randomized Controlled Trials*

Randomized controlled trials (Fig. 6–2) are the gold standard for assessing a treatment or prevention measure. In these studies,

1. A cohort of patients at risk for an outcome is defined.
2. Determination of which patients receive treatment or prevention is made entirely at random.
3. An outcome is measured after a predetermined follow-up period.

In effect, a randomized controlled trial is a kind of cohort study, except that the exposure variable is determined by the investigator, not by nature, using a randomization technique.

### *Prospective-versus-Retrospective Studies*

In prospective-versus-retrospective studies, prospective data are obtained and coded at the time they are first available and, in the case of cohort studies, prior to the outcome. Retrospective data are obtained at a later time, often after the outcome has occurred.

Prospective studies are much less likely to be subject to observation bias or problems with missing data.

## Statistical Tests

Statistics is the science by which observations made of a sample are assessed with respect to their likely validity in the entire universe.

### *Type I and Type II Errors*

Commonly reported statistics include two types of statistical error analysis. In *Type I errors,* an association between an exposure and an outcome is in fact a spurious one that has resulted from random chance. The "*p* value" refers to the likelihood that an observed association is due to chance alone. In *Type II errors,* on the other hand, the lack of an observed association between an exposure and an outcome is in fact due to chance because the sample size was not large enough to detect an association if one in fact exists. This is one of the most common errors reported in clinical literature.

### *Hypothesis Testing*

Statistical tests also aim to determine whether a "null hypothesis" should be rejected, where the null hypothesis is that no association exists between the exposure and the outcome. Today many clinical researchers are moving away from this sort of *hypothesis testing* and more toward estimation of effects along with confidence intervals, discussed below.

### *Comparisons of Continuous Variables*

*Continuous variables* are variables that can have an infinite number of values, such as age, height, blood pressure, or cholesterol level. They are described using means, standard deviations, ranges, quartiles, quintiles, deciles, and so on.

When continuous variables are normally distributed (i.e., described by a Gaussian or bell-shaped curve), *t* tests are generally used to compare the means of two groups and ANOVA is used to compare means of three or more groups.

When the continuous variables cannot be assumed to be normally distributed, then *nonparametric testing,* such as the Wilcoxon rank-sum, which compares median values and distributions of two groups, or the Kruskall-Wallis test, which compares medians and distributions of three or more groups, is often used.

To compare the strength of a presumed linear association between two continuous variables (e.g., left ventricle mass versus blood pressure), researchers often use *tests of correlation* (*r* value), such as Pearson or Spearman tests. In these tests, the square of the *r* value describes how much the variability of one variable can be attributed to the other.

### *Comparisons of Categorical Variables*

Variables that can only have a finite set of values (e.g., gender, presence or absence hypertension, use of a certain medication) are called *categorical variables*. For most samples, these kinds of variables are compared using the chi-square test. However, if the sample size is very small, researchers may instead use the Fischer exact test.

## Data Presentation and Reporting of Outcomes

The statistical tests discussed above tell only part of the story. The *strengths* of associations can be described in a number of ways.

### *Number of Outcomes*

Knowing the number of outcomes is essential to determining the strength of a study. In general, studies with <25 outcome occurrences are suspect. Studies with >100 outcomes may be compelling.

### *Absolute Event Rates*

Absolute event rates are generally considered the most honest way to present data. How many outcomes were associated with exposures? How many outcomes occurred among those not exposed? Be suspicious if raw data are not provided. A careful reading of the raw data will enables a reader to distinguish between "statistical significance" and "clinical significance." It is the latter that we really care about.

### *Relative Risk or Risk Ratio*

Relative risk or risk ratio (*RR*) is the proportion of event rates according to exposure, or

$$RR = \frac{O_E/N_E}{O_0/N_0}$$

where

$O_E$ = number of patients with exposure who had the outcome
$N_E$ = number of patients with exposure
$O_0$ = number of patients without exposure who had the outcome
$N_0$ = number of patients without exposure

A risk ratio of 1.0 implies no association; a value >1 implies an increased risk, and a value <1 implies a protective effect.

### *Relative Risk Reduction*

Relative risk reduction (*RRR*) is defined as the proportional reduction in rates, or

$$RRR = \frac{\left(\frac{O_0}{N_0} - \frac{O_E}{N_E}\right)}{\left(\frac{O_0}{N_0}\right)}$$

### *Absolute Risk Reduction*

Absolute risk reduction (*ARR*) is the difference between absolute event rates, a more honest way of presenting data, or

$$ARR = \frac{O_0}{N_0} - \frac{O_E}{N_E}$$

### *Number Needed to Treat*

Number needed to treat (*NNT*) is the number of patients who would need to be exposed in order to prevent one outcome, or

$$NNT = \frac{1}{ARR}$$

### *Confidence Interval*

The confidence interval (*CI*) is a measure of uncertainty; given a 95% confidence interval, we can be 95% sure that the true measure lies somewhere within the interval.

### *Odds Ratio*

Odds are another way of describing the frequency of an event. For any given population in which *O* outcomes occur among *N* subjects,

$$Odds = \frac{O/N}{1-(O/N)}$$

In effect, this is the probability of an event occurring divided by the probability that the event will not occur. The odds ratio compares odds between exposed and unexposed groups.

It is very important that you not confuse odds ratios with risk ratios (or relative risks). Generally, odds ratios and risk ratios are similar only if the outcome event rates are low (i.e. <10%).

### Hazard Ratio

The hazard ratio is used specifically in survival studies. The hazard is the instantaneous probability of an event occurring given that a subject has survived a for certain period of time without experiencing that event. The hazard ratio compares the hazards of exposed and unexposed groups.

### Attributable risk

Attributable risk measures the relative contribution of a given exposure to an outcome in a population. Thus, if we assume that the association is causal and we then remove the exposure, the attributable risk tells us by how much the outcome event rate should be reduced. Attributable risk (*AR*) is calculated as

$$AR = \frac{P(RR-1)}{P(RR-1)+1}$$

where $P$ is the prevalence of exposure (or $N_E/[N_E+N_O]$) and $RR$ is the relative risk as described above.

### Kaplan–Meier Event Rates

Kaplan–Meier event rates are a graphical way of showing time free of an event. This method takes into account variable follow-up times (or censoring), an issue that is common in studies of outcomes of chronic diseases.

An example showing how these terms are calculated is now shown. Imagine a clinical trial in which 10,000 patients are randomized in a 1:1 manner to either drug A or drug B (that is 5000 are assigned drug A and 5000 are assigned drug B). Suppose that 2500 of the drug A patients experience events, whereas 2000 of the drug B patients have events. Thus we have:

- Drug A: 5,000 patients
- Drug B: 5,000 patients
- Events with drug A: 2,500

  Absolute event rate: 2,500/5,000 = 0.50

- Events with drug B: 2,000

  Absolute event rate: 2,000/5,000 = 0.40

- Absolute rates, drug A and drug B: 0.50 and 0.40
- Risk ratio for drug B: 0.40/0.50 = 0.80
- Absolute risk reduction: 0.50 − 0.40 = 0.10
- Relative risk reduction: (0.50 − 0.40)/0.50 = 0.20
- Number needed to treat: 1/0.10 = 10
- Absolute rates, drug A and drug B: 0.50 and 0.40

| | Disease Present | Disease Absent | Totals |
|---|---|---|---|
| Test Positive | $A$ = true positives | $B$ = false positives | $T^+$ |
| Test Negative | $C$ = false negatives | $D$ = true negatives | $T^-$ |
| | $D^+$ = prevalence (N) | $D^-$ = (1 − prevalence)($N$) | $N$ = total |

**Figure 6–3** A 2 × 2 table.

- Odds for drug B: 0.40/(1 − 0.40) = 0.67
- Odds for drug A: 0.50/(1 − 0.50) = 1.00
- Odds ratio of drug B to drug A: 0.67/1.00 = 0.67

### Terms Related to Studies of Diagnostic Tests

Studies of diagnostic tests often rely on 2 × 2 tables that relate diagnostic test findings to the presence or absence of disease as assessed by a given standard. Figure 6–3 shows an example for which

$$\text{Sensitivity } (Sens) = A/D^+ = \text{positive for disease}$$
$$\text{Specificity } (Spec) = D/D^- = \text{negative for health}$$

Thus,

$$A = \text{true positive} = Sens(D^+) = Sens(\text{prevalence})(N)$$
$$B = \text{false positive} = (1 - Spec)(D^-)$$
$$= (1 - Spec)(1 - \text{prevalence})(N)$$

Here, positive predictive value = true positives/all positives = $A/(A+B)$, which is what we as clinicians really care about.

Substituting the above terms, we get the clinical version of *Bayes' theorem*, namely,

$$PPV = \frac{Sens(\text{prevalence})(N)}{Sens(\text{prevalence})(N) + (1 - Spec)(1 - \text{prevalence})(N)}$$
$$= \frac{Sens(\text{prevalence})}{Sens(\text{prevalence}) + (1 - Spec)(1 - \text{prevalence})}$$

where *PPV* is the positive predictive value.

Implications of Bayes' theorem include:

1. *PPV* depends on sensitivity, specificity, and prevalence; the last is sometimes referred to as the *pretest likelihood* of disease.
2. *PPV* is most different from prevalence when the latter has a value near 0.50; that is, a diagnostic test is most useful the more uncertain one is of the diagnosis.

If one varies the cutoff point for a positive test, the specificity and sensitivity will vary in an inverse way. In other words, the better the sensitivity, the worse is the specificity, and vice versa. A plot of sensitivity versus (1 − specificity) yields the receiver operating characteristic (*ROC*) curve, where the area under the curve (*AUC*) is a measure of the overall ability of the test to distinguish between patients with and without disease (Fig. 6–4).

The likelihood ratio (*LR*) enables us to relate pretest odds of disease to posttest odds:

$$LR+ = \frac{Sensitivity}{1 - Specificity}$$

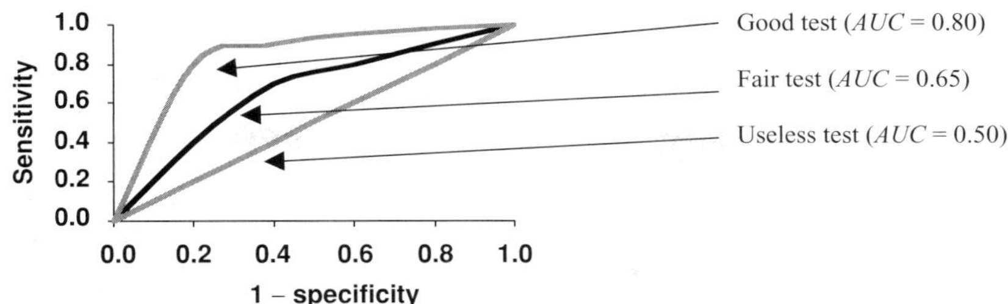


**Figure 6–4** ROC curve.

where $LR+$ is the positive likelihood ratio, and

$$Odds_{\text{post}} = LR(Odds_{\text{pre}})$$

where

$$Odds_{\text{pre}} = \frac{prevalence}{1 - prevalence} \quad \text{and} \quad Odds_{\text{post}} = \frac{PPV}{1 - PPV}$$

In general, for a test to be clinically useful, the positive likelihood ratio ($LR+$) should be at least 10, whereas the negative likelihood ratio ($LR-$) should be $<0.1$.

In a similar fashion, the negative predictive value ($NPV$) is the ratio of true negatives to all negatives:

$$NPV = \frac{D}{D+C}$$
$$= \frac{(specificity)(1 - prevalence)}{(specificity)(1 - prevalence) + (1 - sensitivity)(prevalence)}$$

Analogously, $LR-$ is

$$LR- = \frac{specificity}{1 - sensitivity}$$

The negative likelihood ratio relates the pretest odds of not having disease to the posttest odds of not having disease.

## Confounding and Interaction

Even if an association between an exposure and an outcome is not due to random chance, it may not be a clinically meaningful one if confounding is present. A *confounding factor* is said to exist if the factor has an association with both the exposure and the outcome but is not a causative link between them. As an example, consider alcohol intake as the exposure, lung cancer as the outcome, and smoking as the confounder. Smoking is a confounding factor with regard to the association between alcohol intake and lung cancer (Fig. 6–5).

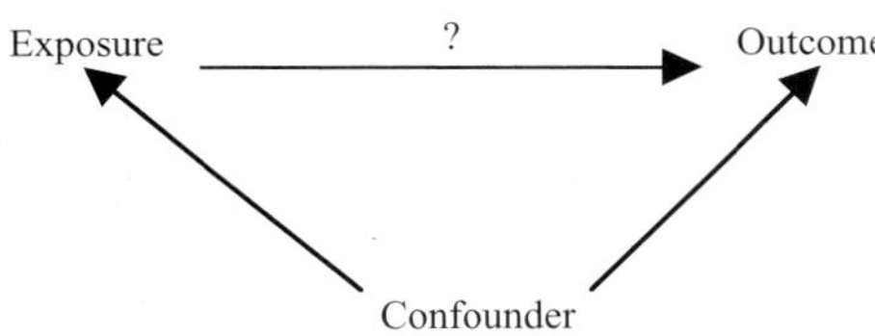


**Figure 6–5** Confounding-factor diagram.

Researchers have several ways to deal with confounding.

### *Dealing with Confounding by Altering Study Design*

The study design can be adjusted by:

- Restriction: Keep patients with confounders out of the study.
- Matching: Keep confounding factors balanced between those who are and those who are not exposed; this technique works better for cohort studies than for case-control studies.
- Randomization: If done properly and if sample size is large enough, randomization can assure balance of both observed and *unobserved* confounders.

### *Dealing with Confounding in the Analyses of the Study*

Confounding can be avoided by:

- Restriction: Keep patients with confounders out of the analyses.
- Stratification: Assess the association between exposure and outcome according to the presence or absence of possible confounders (discussed in more detail below).
- Multivariable methods: Discussed below.

#### Assessing Confounding by Stratified Analyses

Scenario a:

- Whole-population risk ratio ($RR$) = 3.0.
- Stratum with confounder C present, $RR = 3.0$.
- Stratum with confounder C absent, $RR = 3.0$.
- No confounding is present.

Scenario b:

- Whole-population $RR = 3.0$.
- Stratum with confounder C present, $RR = 1.0$.
- Stratum with confounder C absent, $RR = 1.0$.
- Complete confounding is present.

Scenario c:

- Whole-population $RR = 3.0$.
- Stratum with confounder C present, $RR = 1.5$.
- Stratum with confounder C absent, $RR = 1.5$.

- Partial confounding is present.
- This is the most common scenario.

### Interaction

Interaction (also known as "effect modification") is an interesting situation in which the strength of an association between an exposure and an outcome is related to another factor. Such a scenario might be

- Whole-population $RR = 3.0$
- Stratum with interaction factor I present, $RR = 5.0$
- Stratum with interaction factor I absent, $RR = 2.0$

Interaction can also be assessed using multivariable regression analysis by incorporating "interaction" terms into the analyses.

One of the most common errors in clinical research is failure to consider potential interactions.

## Uses and Pitfalls of Multivariable Regression

Multivariable regression is used (a) to assess multiple confounders simultaneously, and (b) to estimate the likelihood of an outcome given multiple possible predictors.

### Linear Regression

Linear regression is used when the outcome variable is continuous:

$$Y = \alpha + \beta_1 x_1 + \beta_2 x_2 + \beta_3 x_3 + \cdots + \beta_i x_i$$

where $x_1$ is the exposure of interest; $x_2, x_3, \ldots, x_i$ are potential confounders; and the $\beta$ coefficients are parameter estimates of the associations between each covariate $x$ and outcome $Y$.

### Logistic Regression

Logistic regression is used when the outcome variable is binary (yes/no):

$$\text{Log } Odds = \alpha + \beta_1 x_1 + \beta_2 x_2 + \beta_3 x_3 + \cdots + \beta_i x_i$$

### Cox Proportional Hazards Regression

Cox proportional hazards regression is used when the outcome is a hazard ratio, which is an assessment of time free of an outcome. Thus, the outcome includes not only whether an event occurs but also the length of observation before an event either does or does not occur. This is expressed as

$$\text{Log hazard ratio} = h_0(\beta_1 x_1 + \beta_2 x_2 + \beta_3 x_3 + \cdots + \beta_i x_i)$$

where $h_0$ is the theoretical hazard for subjects with all $x = 0$.

### Common Errors in Using Multivariable Regression

- Model overfitting: more than one covariate per 10 outcome events—a very common and serious mistake
- Inappropriate linear assumption: when a logarithmic, inverse, or quadratic model would yield a better fit
- Violation of the proportional hazards assumption, which maintains that the hazard ratio between exposed and unexposed groups remains constant over time
- Failure to account for interactions
- Inappropriate variable selection: here knowledge of the biology of the question is really essential.
- Collinearity: covariates associated with one another
- Failure to look for and account for outliers and/or excessively influential observations

## Bias and Its Consequences

Statistical bias is a systematic problem by which exposed and nonexposed subjects are either selected for study inclusion differently and/or have their outcomes assessed differently.

*Selection bias* occurs when the exposure of interest affects whether a subject is included in a study. A typical example is referral bias, under which patients with particularly severe illnesses are more likely to be studied at a tertiary care center. This can lead to an invalid comparison with an unexposed group (a problem of internal validity) or difficulty generalizing results to the population at large (a problem of external validity).

*Observation bias* occurs when the exposure of interest has an affect, conscious or not, on how the outcome is measured. A way of avoiding this is "blinding" patients and investigators as to the nature of the exposure variable. Observation bias can result in an invalid comparison between exposed and unexposed patients, which is a problem of internal validity.

*Recall bias* may be a problem in case-control studies, in which patients with an outcome are more likely to recall an exposure than those without the outcome. A typical example is recall of pregnancy exposures among women who give birth to children with congenital defects.

*Verification bias* may be a problem in studies of diagnostic tests, in which the result of the diagnostic test directly affects the clinician's decision to refer a patient for the "gold standard" test. A typical example: patients with an abnormal stress study are more likely to be referred for coronary angiography. Verification bias results in an overestimation of sensitivity and an underestimation of specificity.

A key question to ask is "Are there differences in the way exposed and unexposed subjects are selected or evaluated?" If the answer is yes, then bias is likely to be present.

## Causality and Validity

Randomized trials can establish *causality,* that is, that a particular treatment or prevention strategy specifically causes a certain outcome. Other types of clinical studies can only establish *association,* not cause.

Criteria have been established by which to judge whether an association is likely to be causal. These criteria include:

1. Strength of association
2. Dose–response relationship
3. Temporal relationship (exposure always precedes outcome)
4. Biologic plausibility
5. Consistency with other studies

Another important area to consider in evaluating research studies is *validity*. An observed association between an exposure and an outcome in a given population is likely to have *internal validity* if, after use of appropriate methods, it is not due to chance, confounding, or bias.

*External validity* refers to both the likelihood of a cause–effect association as noted above and the likelihood that the observed association is relevant to other populations not studied.

### Issues Related to Specific Types of Studies (Taken from ACP Journal Club Criteria)

#### *Randomized Trials*

- Adequate randomization must be achieved. Look for "Table 1" and the type of randomization method used.
- Follow-up should include at least 80% of the study population.
- Consider the outcome measures chosen. Are they objective and clinically relevant? Are they subject to bias? For cardiology studies, all-cause death is the best outcome.

#### *Studies of Diagnosis*

- There should be a reasonable spectrum of patients.
- The "gold standard" should be interpreted without knowledge of the results of the test of interest (source of observation bias).
- Each participant should get both the test being studied and the gold standard test, with performance on the gold standard being independent of the results of the diagnostic test (i.e., no verification bias).

#### *Studies of Prognosis*

- The inception cohort should consist entirely of people who are free from the outcome.
- Follow-up should include at least 80% of the study population.
- Consider the outcome measures chosen.

#### *Case-Control Studies*

- The key to validity is how controls were chosen.
- Controls should come from the same person–time pool as cases.
- If a control had had the outcome, would he or she have become a case for the study?

#### *Studies of Economics*

- Comparisons involving real patients are best.
- Costs should be measured in terms of resources used, not charges.
- Incremental costs of one intervention over another should be included.
- Sensitivity analyses should be performed.

#### *Clinical Prediction Rules*

- Should be validated either in a different data set or by using modern validation techniques, such as bootstrapping
- Should consider treatment, diagnosis, prognosis, causation

#### *Systematic Review Articles*

- The article should identify the search methods used.
- Only quality source materials should be chosen.
- If the review includes meta-analysis, appropriate techniques to consider variations in study quality, sample sizes, and publication bias should be used.

## CURRENT CONTROVERSIES IN RESEARCH

1. The peer review method: Issues include
   a. Assessment of reviewers
   b. Dealing with bias and conflicts of interest
   c. Creating uniform standards
2. Investigator concerns
   a. Conflicts of interest
   b. Drug and device company control over data and publication
   c. Ethical issues, particularly regarding safety of human subjects
   d. Informed consent and documentation
   e. Complex regulations regarding research practice
3. Statistical and analytical methods
   a. Getting away from $p$ values
   b. Equivalency trials
   c. New types of databases (object oriented, "metadata," XML)
   d. Controlling for bias and confounding with propensity analysis
   e. Nonproportional hazards
   f. Validation with bootstrapping and similar techniques
   g. Optimal model selection methods; information theory

4. Public policy concerns
   a. How to keep up
   b. Proliferation of journal summary publications
   c. Development of guidelines and their dissemination
   d. Timing of publication and meeting presentations
   e. The impact of the media
   f. Associations between medical societies and editors; maintenance of editorial independence
   g. Electronic versus paper information

## BIBLIOGRAPHY


American College of Physicians Journal Club Series.

**Elwood M.** *Critical Appraisal of Epidemiological Studies and Clinical Trials.* New York: Oxford University Press; 1998.

**Gordis L.** *Epidemiology.* 2nd ed. Philadelphia: WB Sauders;. 2000.

**Guyatt G, Rennie D, eds.** *Users' Guides to the Medical Literature: A Manual for Evidence-Based Clinical Practice.* Chicago: American Medical Association; 2002.

**Woodward M.** *Epidemiology: Study Design and Data Analysis.* New York: Chapman & Hall/CRC Press; 1999.


## QUESTIONS

**1.** A study finds that in the largely white community of Olmstead County, Minnesota, drug B is effective for controlling blood pressure compared to placebo. As a physician working in a practice caring mainly for African American patients, your concern is that this study may lack

a. Control for bias
b. Internal validity
c. Consideration of the effects of chance
d. External validity
e. Failure to consider interaction

Answer is d: external validity. Just because the finding is true among Caucasians, it may not be true among African Americans.

**2.** A new diagnostic test for coronary disease is compared against cardiac catheterization among 100 patients who had both studies performed. Coronary disease is present in 50 patients, among whom 45 had a positive test. Among the patients without coronary disease, 25 had a positive test. Which of the following is true?

a. The sensitivity is 90%.
b. The specificity is 50%.
c. The sensitivity is likely to be <90%.
d. The sensitivity is likely to be <50%.
e. The positive likelihood ratio is 2.

Answer is c: The sensitivity is likely to be <90%. This is an example of verification bias, in which sensitivity is overestimated and specificity is underestimated.

**3.** A study of 10,000 people without a history of myocardial infarction (MI) is done to see what effect a high uric acid level has on risk. An elevated level is present in 2,000, among whom 100 have an MI during 5 years of follow-up. Among the people without an elevated uric acid level, 200 have an MI during the same period. The odds ratio for an MI given an elevated uric level compared to those without an elevated level is

a. 0.50
b. 2.00
c. 0.25
d. 2.05
e. 5.25

Answer is d: 2.05. Remember, $Odds = P/(1 - P)$. Thus the odds for patients with an elevated uric acid level are $0.05/(1 - 0.05)$ and the odds for patients without an elevated uric acid level are $0.025/(1 - 0.025)$.

**4.** In the above study, if we assume that there is a causative link between uric acid and MI, the attributable risk is

a. 0.13
b. 0.17
c. 0.25
d. 2.00

Answer is b: 0.17. Attributable risk is $Prev(RR - 1)/[Prev(RR - 1) + 1]$. The prevalence is 0.2 and the relative risk is 2.0.

**5.** A study of a new electrocardiograph (ECG) technology looks at the ability of the ECG finding to predict sudden death. Among 300 patients studied, 25 had sudden death. The unadjusted relative risk for the ECG finding for prediction of sudden death is 3.0. After adjustment for age, gender, left ventricular ejection fraction, nuclear findings, diabetes, hypertension, and cholesterol level in a multivariable Cox regression analysis, the adjusted relative risk is 2.5. Which of the following is true?

a. The ECG finding is a valid, independent predictor of death.
b. Confounding is present.

c. Model overfitting occurred.
d. The finding is statistically significant but not clinically significant.
e. Bias was not adjusted for.

Answer is c: Model overfitting occurred. There were only 25 outcome events, meaning that at most two or three covariates can be considered in a regression model.

# Cardiac Neoplasms

7

***Sreenivas Kamath***

Primary cardiac tumors are rare and occur in 1 per 1,000 to 1 per 100,000 individuals in unselected autopsy series at tertiary care centers. Approximately 75% of cardiac tumors are histologically benign and the remainder are malignant, in almost all case sarcomas.

## CARDIAC MYXOMAS

Myxomas are the most common type of primary cardiac tumor in adults, accounting for approximately 25% of the cardiac neoplasms and 50% of the benign primary cardiac tumors. The cellularity of these lesions was controversial, and some thought they represented thrombus rather than neoplasia. However, extensive analysis has confirmed that these lesions represent a primary neoplastic process. They occur at all ages and do not show any sex preference.

Approximately 75% of cardiac myxomas are solitary and the most common location is the left atrium, attached to the atrial septum in the vicinity of the fossa ovalis. Cardiac myxomas may arise from any endocardial surface within the heart and, thus, may be located in other cardiac chambers or on the cardiac valves (Table 7–1).

Approximately 10% of cardiac myxomas are determined to be familial. Familial myxomas have autosomal dominant transmission or are part of a syndrome that involves multiple abnormalities including pigmented nevi, primary adrenal cortical disease with or without Cushing's syndrome, pituitary tumors, and testicular tumors. A set of findings has been referred to as the NAME syndrome (Nevi, Atrial myxoma, Myxoid neurofibroma, and Ephelides), or the LAMB syndrome (Lentigines, Atrial Myxoma, and Blue nevi), or the Carney syndrome, which includes myxomas arising in a noncardiac location (breast or skin), nonmyxomatous extracardiac tumors (e.g., pituitary adenoma), skin pigmentation, and hyperendocrine states. In contrast to sporadic myxomas, familial or syndrome myxomas tend to occur in younger individuals, are multicentric, demonstrate an apical location, and are more likely to have postoperative recurrences.

The classic triad of symptoms secondary to a myxoma include heart failure due to valvular obstruction, stroke due to embolism, and constitutional rheumatologic symptoms thought to be due to tumor secretion of cytokines such as interleukin-6. The most common clinical presentation resembles that of mitral valve disease, more commonly as stenosis as a result of tumor prolapse into the mitral orifice during diastole or regurgitation as a consequence of injury to the valve by tumor-induced trauma. The rare ventricular myxomas may cause outflow tract obstruction and thus mimic subaortic or subpulmonic stenosis. On auscultation, a characteristic low-pitched sound, termed a "tumor plop," may be audible during early or mid-diastole. Cardiac myxomas may produce syncope, transient ischemic attack (TIA), or stroke from embolism. They may also present with peripheral or pulmonary emboli or many noncardiac symptoms and signs including fever, weight loss, malaise, cachexia, arthralgias, rash, anemia, polycythemia, leucocytosis, elevated ESR, and low or high platelets. A myxoma does not undergo malignant transformation.

ECHO (both M-mode and two-dimensional Echocardiography (ECHO)) is very useful not only in the diagnosis of cardiac myxomas, but also in determining the site of tumor attachment and size, both of which provide important preoperative information. Myxoma may have clear spaces (cysts), and highly reflective patches (bone) (Fig. 7–1).

In summary:

- Cardiac myxomas are the most common primary cardiac tumor.
- Most are sporadic; 10% familial: these can be multicentric, can recur after surgery, and may be part of a syndrome.
- The most common site is the left atrium, attached to the atrial septum in the vicinity of the fossa ovalis.

**TABLE 7–1**
**LOCATION OF CARDIAC MYXOMAS**

| Location | % |
|---|---|
| Left atrium | 80 |
| Right atrium | 15 |
| Right ventricle | 5 |
| Left ventricle | 5 |

- The classic triad of symptoms includes heart failure due to obstruction, stroke due to embolism, and constitutional rheumatologic symptoms.

## OTHER BENIGN CARDIAC TUMORS

### Cardiac Papillary Fibroelastoma

Papillary fibroelastoma is the most common tumor involving the cardiac valves. The vast majority of (80%) of papillary fibroelastomas occur in the left heart. The aortic valve is the most commonly affected, but other valves or other noncardiac structures may also be involved (Fig. 7–2).

Papillary fibroelastomas are generally small, single nodular tumors that occur most often on the valvular surfaces and may be mobile, resulting in embolization. Unlike vegetations, fibroelastomas are more often found on the downstream side of the valve (left ventricular side of the mitral valve, aortic side of the aortic valve) as papillary fronds attached by a short stalk. Occasionally they are attached to the ventricular septum or near the left ventricular (LV) outflow tract. The most feared complication of a fibroelastoma is an embolic event, such as stroke or coronary embolization. The current clinical approach to cardiac papillary fibroelastomas larger than 1 cm, especially if mobile, is excision. Surgery is performed especially when the patient is young, has a low surgical risk, and has a high cumulative risk of embolization.

In summary:

- Papillary fibroelastomas are the most common tumor involving the cardiac valves.

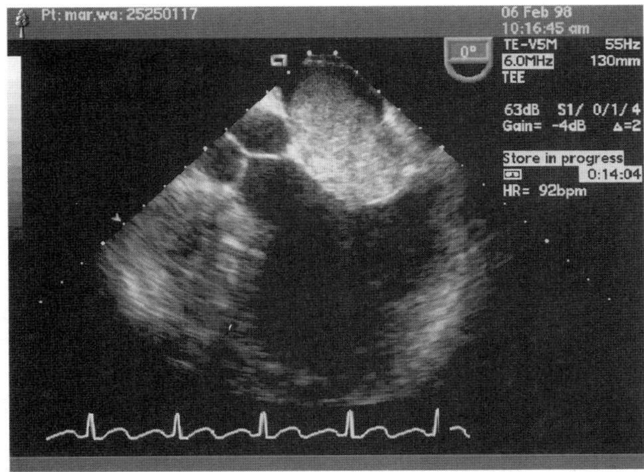


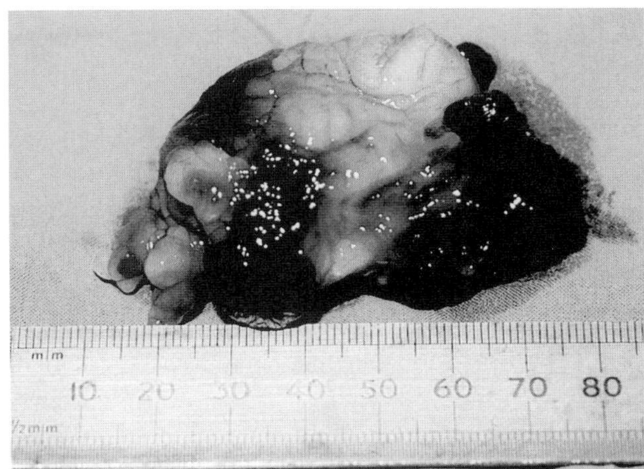


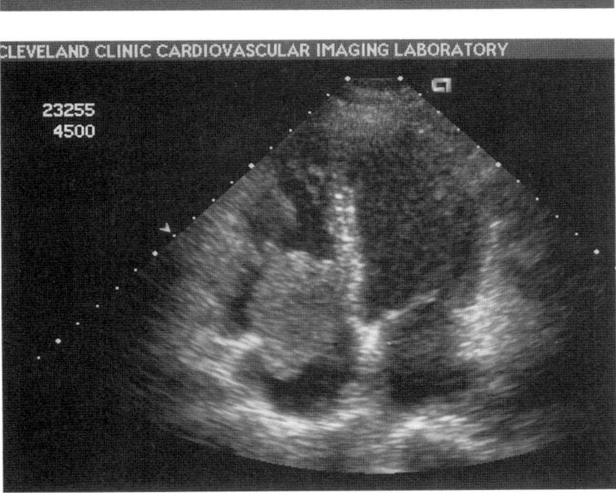


**Figure 7–1** **A:** Left atrial myxoma. **(B)** Surgical specimen, left atrial myxoma (same as part **A**). **(C)** Right atrial myxoma.

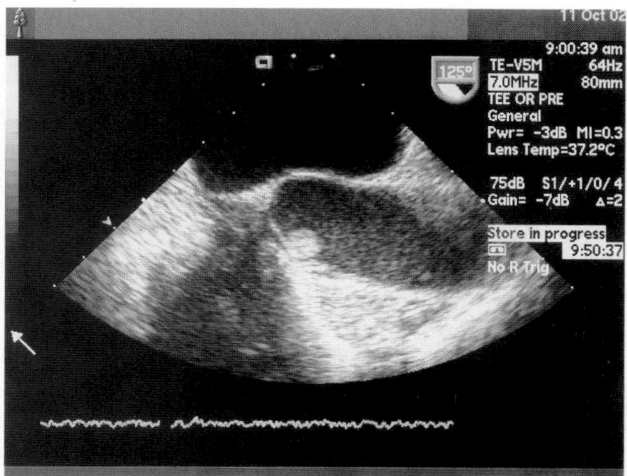


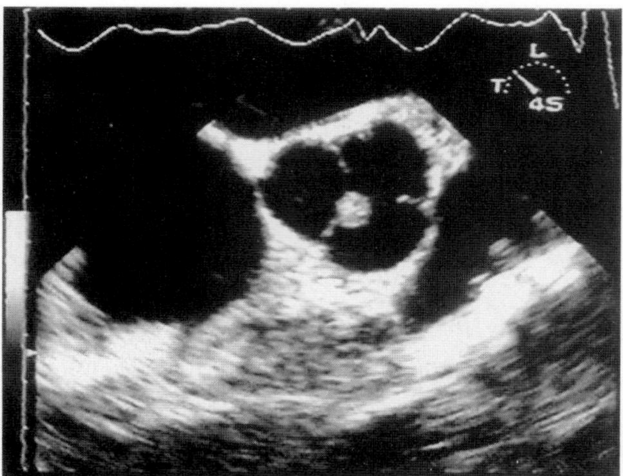


**Figure 7–2** **A,B.** Aortic valve papillary fibroelastoma.

- They are the second most common primary cardiac tumor.
- The large majority are found in the left heart, commonly involving the aortic valve.
- They have significant embolic potential, hence surgery is indicated if they are larger than 1 cm.

## Cardiac Fibroma

Cardiac fibroma is associated with sudden death, more commonly in children than in adults. Usually, there is only a single mass. Fibromas are benign tumors that are typically located in the LV free wall, in the ventricular septum, or at the apex. Therefore, they can lead to signs and symptoms of mechanical obstruction that may mimic valvular stenosis, congestive heart failure, restrictive or hypertrophic cardiomyopathy, or malignant arrhythmias. Calcification of a cardiac tumor strongly suggests that it is a fibroma, although myxomas and sarcomas may also be calcified (Fig. 7–3).

In summary:

- Fibromas are usually solitary, and they are more common in children.
- They are commonly located in the LV free wall, in the ventricular septum, or at the apex.
- Calcification is common.

## Cardiac Lipomas

Cardiac lipomas are relatively common and rarely cause symptoms. They may grow to large size and can present with symptoms due to mechanical interference with cardiac function, arrhythmias, conduction disturbances, or an abnormality of the cardiac silhouette, most commonly detected on chest x-ray.

*Lipomatous hypertrophy* of the interatrial septum presents as a cardiac mass that may be mistaken for a tumor. It typically involves the superior and inferior fatty portions of the atrial septum, sparing the fossa ovalis region.

## Cardiac Rhabdomyomas

Cardiac rhabdomyomas are probably hamartomatous growths, are multiple in about 90% of cases, and present in the right ventricle (RV) or RV outflow tract and even in the pulmonary artery. They may be associated with tuberous sclerosis, adenoma sebaceum, and benign kidney tumors. Cardiac rhabdomyomas are the most common primary cardiac tumor of infancy and childhood, but they may regress spontaneously after birth.

## Cardiac Hemangiomas

Cardiac hemangiomas are very rare benign tumors that typically arise from the endothelium and are usually intramural, often in the intraventricular septum or AV node. They may cause complete heart block or cardiac tamponade due to hemopericardium. More commonly found in the right heart chambers, they are red, hemorrhagic, generally sessile or polypoid, ranging in size from 2 to 4 cm in diameter.

## Mesotheliomas of the AV node

Mesotheliomas of the AV node are thought to originate from the remnants of mesothelium. They may occur in any age group, more commonly in females, almost always located near the AV node, and hence are frequently associated with partial or complete heart block.

# MALIGNANT CARDIAC TUMORS

Malignant cardiac tumors account for approximately 25% of primary cardiac tumors. The most frequent malignant

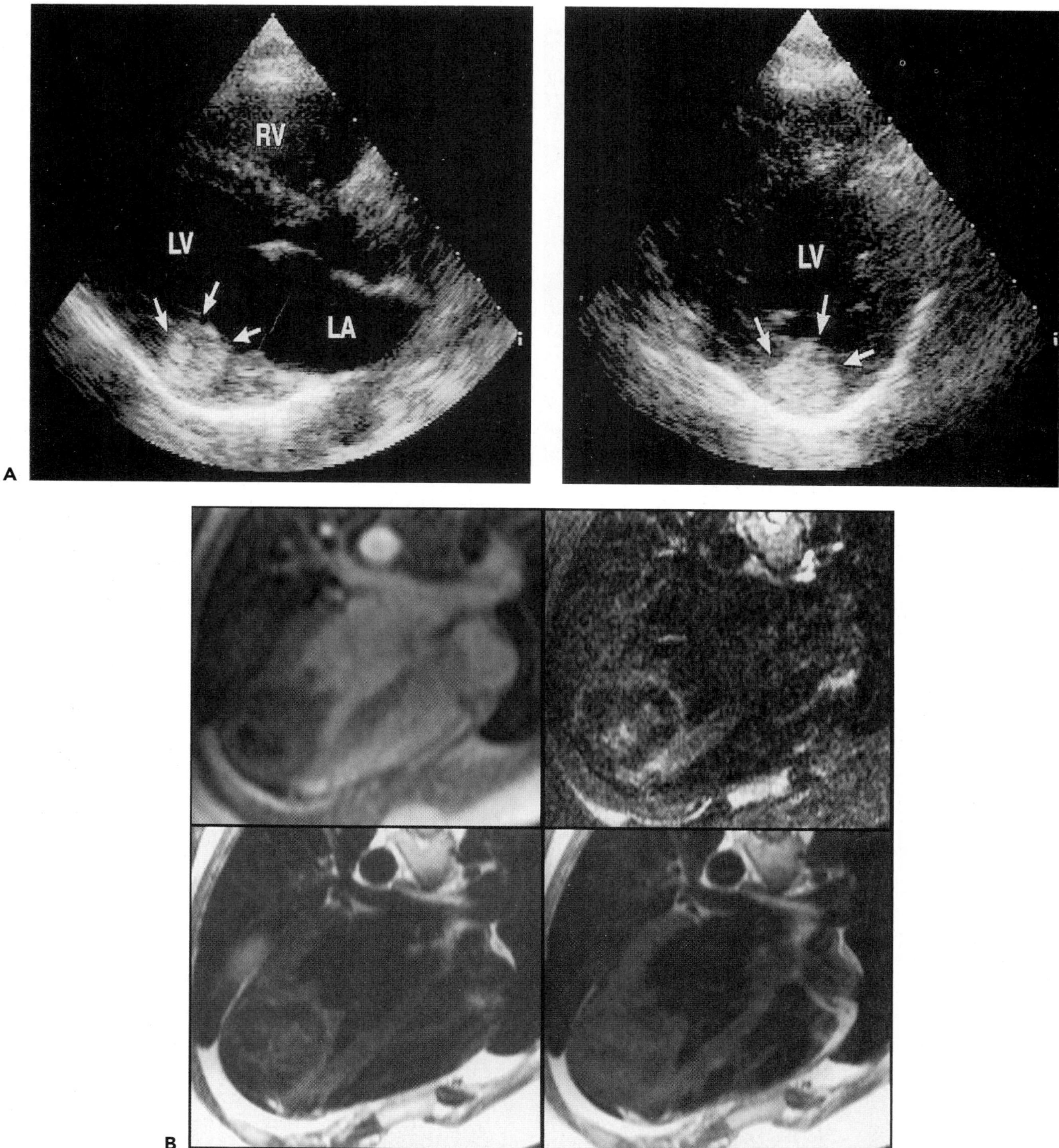


Figure 7–3 A: Left ventricular fibroma. (B) MRI, left ventricular fibroma.

primary cardiac tumor is angiosarcoma. Angiosarcoma is more common in adults than in children, with a greater male preponderance, with 80% right atrial location. Extensive involvement of the pericardium is common, hence the most common presentation is pericardial effusion ± tamponade. Because of their rapid growth, invasion of the pericardial space and obstruction of the cardiac chambers or venae cavae are common.

Other malignant tumors include rhabdomyosarcoma, mesothelioma, and fibrosarcoma, in order of frequency of

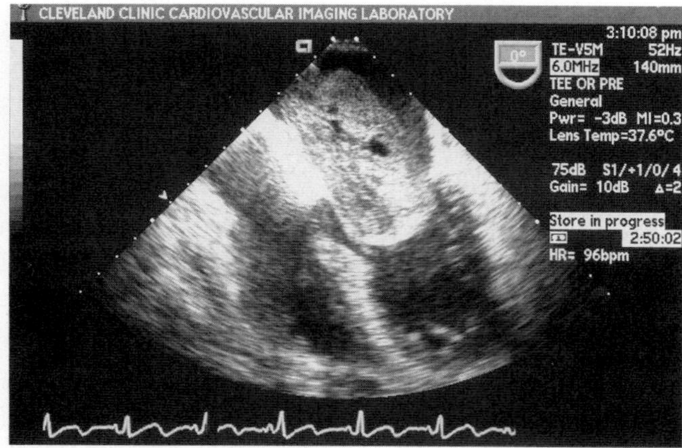


**Figure 7–4** Left atrial sarcoma.

occurrence. Generally, malignant cardiac tumors are associated with a poor prognosis, as these tumors have often spread too extensively for surgical excision (Fig. 7–4).

## METASTATIC TUMORS

Tumor metastases to the heart are several times more common than primary tumors. Most frequently, they are from the lung, lymphoma, breast, leukemia, stomach, melanoma, liver, and colon, in order of frequency. The malignancy with the greatest frequency of cardiac involvement is melanoma (60% to 70% cardiac involvement with metastatic diagnosis). However, in absolute numbers, cardiac metastases are most common in carcinoma of the breast and lung, reflecting the higher incidence of these cancers. Autopsy series suggest that 15% to 30% of lung cancer patients demonstrate some pericardial/cardiac involvement. Cardiac metastases almost always occur in the presence of a widespread primary tumor and with evidence of metastasis within the thoracic cavity. Rarely, cardiac metastases may be the initial presentation of an extracardiac tumor (Fig. 7–5).

Metastases reach the heart via the bloodstream or lymphatics (melanoma, lymphoma, and breast), or invasion of venous structures (renal, hepatocellular, adrenal, uterine), or direct invasion (lung, breast, esophageal). The pericardium is most often involved, followed by myocardial involvement of any chamber, and rarely endocardium and cardiac valves.

Tumors can also affect the cardiac structures, as is seen in *carcinoid heart disease.* Metastatic carcinoid tissue in the liver produces serotonin, which causes abnormalities. The tricuspid valve is involved in carcinoid heart disease in 90% of cases. The classic findings include thickening of the

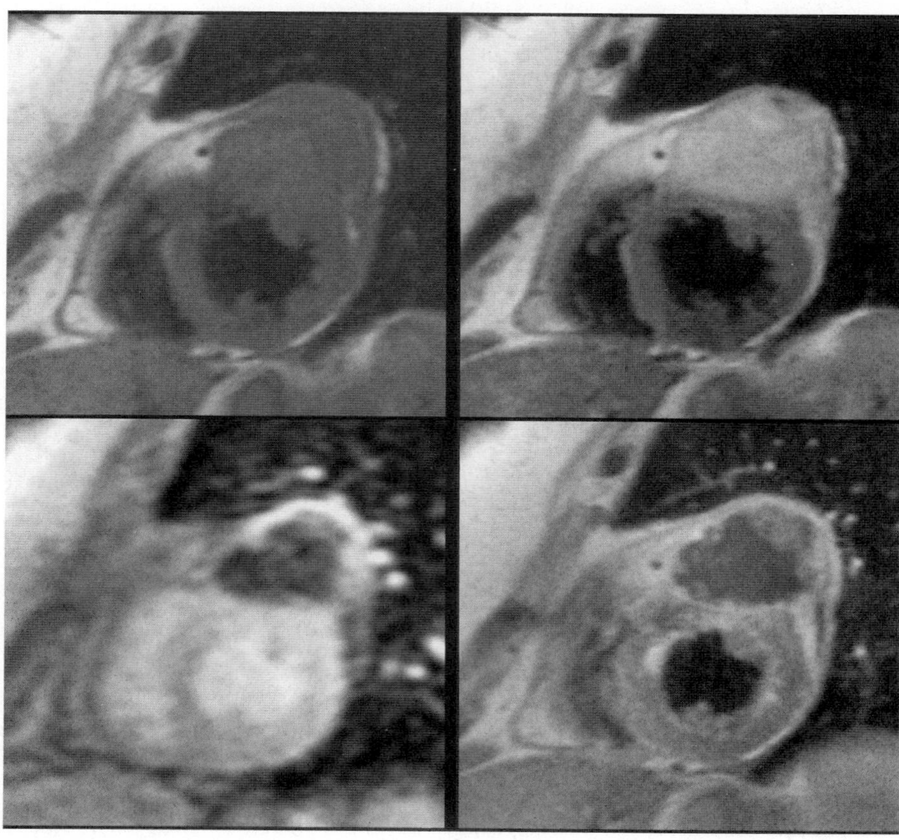

**Figure 7–5** MRI, pericardial metastasis.

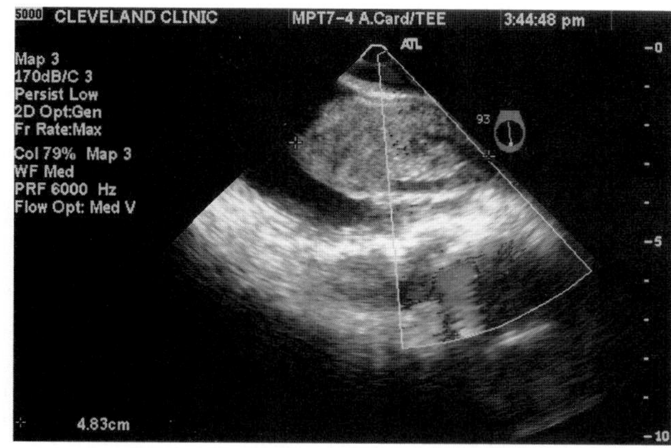


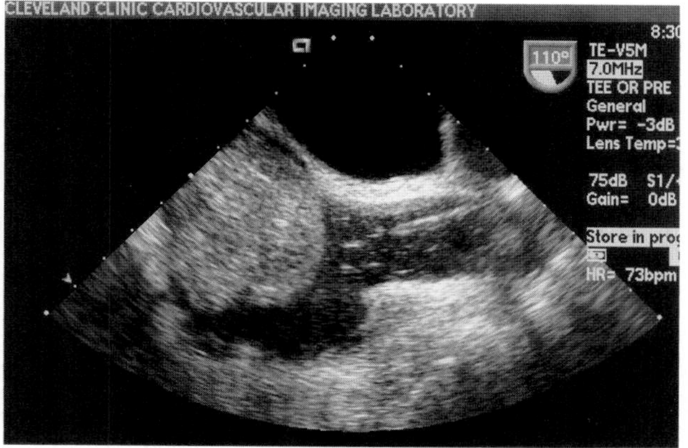


**Figure 7–6** **A: (B)** Inferior vena cava/right atrial tumor, renal cell carcinoma.

tricuspid leaflets, with an appearance of the valve frozen in both systole and diastole. Left-sided involvement is rare in carcinoid disease, possibly due to a lower concentration of the active molecules (serotonin, bradykinin, or other substances secreted by the tumor) after passage through the lungs.

A specific type of cardiac involvement by tumor that should be recognized is extension of *renal cell carcinoma* up the inferior vena cava with potential right atrial enlargement. Pulmonary embolization can occur, and in some cases the initial diagnosis of this tumor is made after detection of a right atrial mass on echocardiography (Fig. 7–6).

There may be multiple nonspecific presenting symptoms. The patient may present with dyspnea, signs of acute pericarditis, cardiac tamponade, rapid increase in the cardiac silhouette on chest x-ray (CXR), new-onset tachyarrhythmia, and congestive heart failure.

Echocardiography is useful for the diagnosis of pericardial effusion/tamponade and the visualization of larger masses. CT, MRI, and radionuclide imaging may provide important anatomic information.

Since most patients with cardiac metastases have widespread disease, therapy is generally directed at the primary tumor. However, removal of a malignant pericardial effusion by pericardiocentesis, a pericardial window, or sclerosing therapy may palliate symptoms and delay or prevent recurrence of the effusion.

In summary:

- Cardiac metastases are 20 to 40 times more common than primary tumors.
- Malignant melanoma has the highest propensity for metastases.
- Lung and breast cancer are more commonly encountered.

## BIBLIOGRAPHY

**Abraham KP, Reddy V, Gattuso P.** Neoplasms metastatic to the heart: review of 3314 consecutive autopsies. *Am J Cardiovasc Pathol.* 1990;3:195–198.

**Burke A, Virmani R.** Tumors of the heart and great vessels. In: *Atlas of Tumor Pathology.* Third Series. Fasicle 16. Washington, DC: Armed Forces Institute of Pathology; 1996.

**Carney JA, Gordon H, Carpenter PC, et al.** The complex of myxomas, spotty pigmentation and endocrine overactivity. *Medicine.* 1985;64:270–283.

**Lie JT.** The identity and histogenesis of cardiac myxomas: a controversy put to rest. *Arch Pathol Lab Med.* 1989;113:724–726.

**McAllister HA Jr, Fenoglio JJ Jr.** Tumors of the cardiovascular system. In: *Atlas of Tumor Pathology.* Second Series. Fasicle 15. Washington, DC: Armed Forces Institute of Pathology; 1978.

**Sun JP, Asher CR, Yang XS, et al.** Clinical and echocardiographic characteristics of papillary fibroelastoma: a retrospective and prospective study in 162 patients. *Circulation.* 2001;103(22):2687–2693.

**Vidaillet HJ, Seward JB, Fyke E, Tajik AJ.** NAME syndrome (nevi, atrial myxoma, myxoid neurofibroma, ephelides): a new and unrecognized subset of patients with cardiac myxoma. *Minn Med.* 1984;67:697–6.

## QUESTIONS

**1.** Regarding cardiac myxoma, all of the following statements are true except:

a. It can arise anywhere within the heart.
b. It is the most common primary cardiac tumor.
c. Approximately 75% occur in the left atrium.
d. Most are familial.
e. Myxomas may be associated with syncope, TIA, or stroke.

Answer is d: Cardiac myxoma is the most common primary cardiac tumor, accounting for 50% of primary cardiac tumors in adults. Though it can be found anywhere in the heart, the most common location is the left atrium attached to the atrial septum near the fossa ovalis. Myxomas can present with the classic triad of symptoms including heart failure, embolism, or rheumatologic symptoms. Most myxomas are nonfamilial (approximately 90%), with about 10% familial that may be part of a syndrome.

**2.** True statements about papillary fibroelastoma include all the following except:

a. They have a fronded appearance.
b. They have a benign histology.
c. The vast majority arise on the right side.
d. They can have significant embolic potential.
e. They are the most common tumor involving the cardiac valves.

Answer is c: Cardiac papillary fibroelastoma is the second most common primary cardiac tumor and is the most common tumor of the cardiac valves. The majority involve the left heart, commonly the aortic valve. They have embolic potential, hence surgery is recommended for fibroelastomas of large size.

**3.** Which of the following statements regarding myxoma is true?

a. Apical location of myxoma has high risk for recurrence.
b. Most myxomas are located in the right atrium.
c. Myxomas have a high tendency for malignant transformation.
d. Myxoma are rarely attached to the atrial septum.

Answer is a: Cardiac myxomas are commonly located in the left atrium, attached to the atrial septum. They do not have a malignant potential. Familial myxomas, accounting for about 10% of myxomas, tend to be located apically, with more chance for recurrence after resection.

**4.** What of the following malignancies has the highest likelihood of cardiac metastasis?

a. Lung cancer
b. Renal cell carcinoma
c. Melanoma
d. Breast cancer
e. Colon cancer

Answer is c: The malignancy with the highest likelihood of cardiac metastasis is melanoma, though in absolute numbers, cardiac metastases are more common, with lung and breast cancers reflecting the higher incidence of these cancers.

**5.** A 61-year-old man is admitted with fatigue, shortness of breath, diarrhea, and increasing abdominal girth. The following TTE findings are suggestive of which condition?

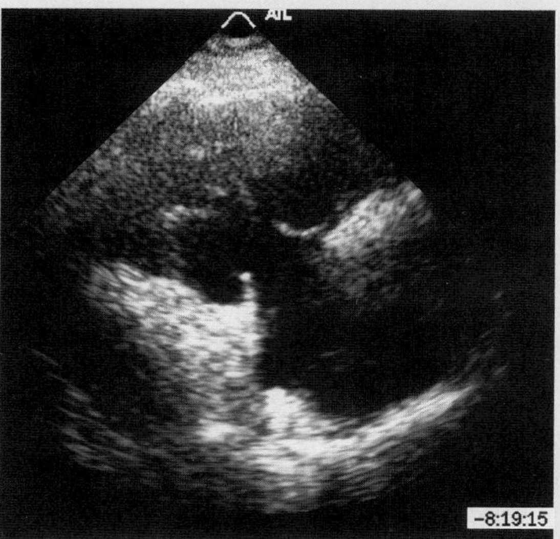


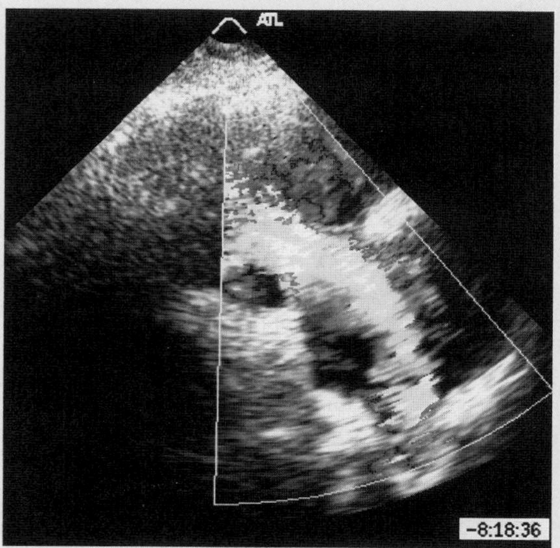


a. Rheumatic valvular disease
b. Carcinoid syndrome
c. Constrictive pericarditis
d. Restrictive cardiomyopathy

Answer is b: The tricuspid valve findings in this case are classic for carcinoid involvement of the tricuspid valve. The findings include thickening of the tricuspid leaflets, best seen on RV inflow view, with an appearance of the valve frozen open in both systole and diastole, without any doming of the leaflet. The color flow Doppler indicates that the Tricuspid Regurgitation (TR) is severe.

# Fundamentals of Doppler Echocardiography

# 8

***Anne Kanderian*** ***L. Leonardo Rodriguez***

## BASIC PRINCIPLES OF ULTRASOUND

Sound waves are mechanical vibrations produced by a source that are transmitted through a medium such as air. As sound waves travel through a medium, the particles of the medium are packed or compressed, alternating with being spaced apart (called *rarefaction*). Sound waves can be represented graphically as sine waves (Fig. 8–1). The wavelength ($\lambda$) is the distance between two similar areas along the wave path and is measured in millimeters. The frequency ($f$) is the number of wavelengths per unit time. Frequency is expressed in hertz (Hz), which is equivalent to cycles per second. The velocity of sound in a medium ($c$) is the wavelength multiplied by the frequency:

$$c = \lambda f$$

Therefore, wavelength and frequency are inversely related. The amplitude of the sound wave (loudness) is measured in decibels (dB). The decibel is a logarithmic unit used to describe a ratio. When the decibel is used to give the sound level for a single sound rather than a ratio, then a reference level must be chosen.

As the density of a medium increases, the velocity of sound through that medium also increases. In human tissue, the velocity of sound is 1,540 m/s (Table 8–1). Humans hear sound waves with frequencies between 20 Hz and 20 kHz. Ultrasound is defined as sound with frequencies higher than 20 kHz. Diagnostic medical ultrasound uses transducers with frequencies between 1 and 20 MHz.

## INTERACTION OF ULTRASOUND WITH TISSUE

The path of an ultrasound beam in a homogenous medium is a straight line; however, when the beam travels through a medium with two or more interfaces or in a medium that is not homogenous, the path is altered. The alteration can be in the form of reflection, scattering, refraction, or attenuation.

When the ultrasound beam encounters a boundary between two different media, part of the ultrasound is reflected back toward the transducer and part continues into the second medium. The amount of *reflection* of the ray depends on the difference in acoustic impedance between the two media. The amount of ultrasound reflected back is constant, but the amount received back at the transducer varies with the angle of the ultrasound beam to the tissue interface. Because the angles of incidence and reflection are equal, optimal return of the reflected ray occurs when the beam is perpendicular (90 degrees) to the tissue interface.

*Scattering* occurs when the ultrasound beam strikes smaller structures (less than one wavelength in the lateral dimension). This results in the ultrasound beam being radiated in all directions, with a minimal amount returning to the transducer. Scattering of ultrasound produced from

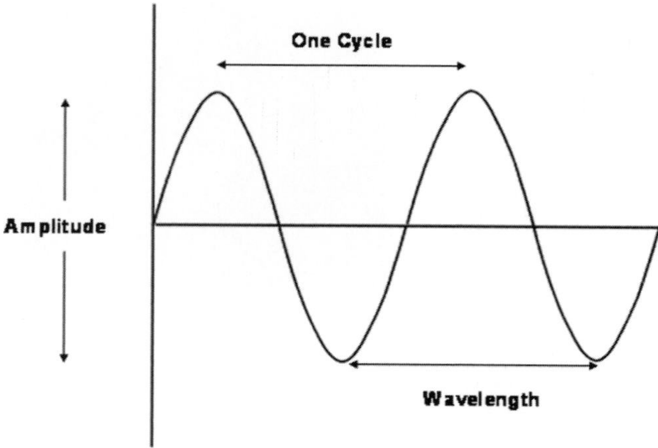


**Figure 8–1** Figure of sound wave.

moving red blood cells is the principle behind Doppler echocardiography.

When the speed of sound differs in the two media, the acoustic impedance is different, and the ultrasound waves in the second medium are deflected from their original orientation. This is known as *refraction*. Because blood and most tissues have similar sound velocities, this is not a prominent effect in echocardiography.

When ultrasound travels through a biologic medium, some of it is absorbed into heat. This process whereby the ultrasound signal strength is reduced is called *attenuation*. The degree of absorption of ultrasound depends on the frequency of the ultrasound and on the differences in acoustic impedances between the two media. Lower ultrasound frequencies penetrate deeper into the tissue. Air has a high acoustic impedance, which causes significant attenuation if there is any air between the transducer and the body tissue. Water-soluble gel is applied on the transducer to minimize contact with air and hence attenuation.

**TABLE 8–1**
**VELOCITY OF SOUND THROUGH DIFFERENT MEDIA**

| Material | Velocity of Sound (m/s) |
|---|---|
| Air | 330 |
| Fat | 1,450 |
| Water | 1,480 |
| Human soft tissue | 1,540 |
| Brain | 1,540 |
| Liver | 1,550 |
| Kidney | 1,560 |
| Blood | 1,570 |
| Muscle | 1,580 |
| Lens of eye | 1,620 |
| Bone | 4,080 |

## TRANSDUCERS

The ultrasound transducer is the small hand-held probe that transmits acoustic energy and receives the returning echoes. It converts one form of energy to another by means of a piezoelectric crystal, which converts electrical energy into sound energy. Piezoelectric elements lack a center of symmetry and are anisotropic. When an electric current is applied, the polarized particles within the crystal are aligned, causing the crystal to expand and produce a mechanical effect. This is known as the *direct piezoelectric effect*. An alternating current causes the crystal alternately to compress and expand, which produces an ultrasound wave by compressions and rarefactions.

Piezoelectric crystals are also able to generate an electric current when their shapes are altered while being struck by ultrasound waves. The transducer functions as a transmitter, transmitting a burst of ultrasound, and also as a receiver, receiving the ultrasound signals that are reflected by the internal tissue interfaces. The burst of pulse usually lasts for only 1 to 6 microseconds.

The frequency of a transducer is determined by the nature and thickness of the piezoelectric element.

Image formation is based on the interval of time between ultrasound transmission of a structure and the arrival of its reflected signal. Structures that are deeper inside tissues have longer flight times (Fig. 8–2). The depth ($d$) of a certain structure is determined by the speed of sound in blood and the time delay between transmission and reception:

$$d = ct/2$$

The factor 2 appears because $t$ includes the time to and from the object. Knowing that the speed of sound in blood is 1,540 m/s,

$$d = 77t \text{ cm} \quad (t \text{ in ms})$$

*Resolution* of the imaging system is defined as the smallest distance between two points at which they can be distinguished by the system as separate entities. *Axial resolution* refers to the ability to differentiate between points lying along the path or axis of the beam. *Lateral resolution* refers to the ability to differentiate between points that are side by side relative to the beam.

Axial resolution is related to the ultrasound's wavelength or frequency, and to the duration of the transmitted pulse.

Lateral resolution, which is the ability to differentiate between points that are lateral to the beam, is dependent on the distance of the specular reflector to the transducer. This is a function of the beam width, which is defined as the diameter of the beam at a particular point. In the *near field*, the beam is maintained as a cylinder with a diameter comparable to the transducer. However, at points farther away from the transducer, the beam diverges and widens into a cone. This area is called the *far field*. Beam width is a function of transducer size, shape, frequency, and focusing. When the transducer is bigger, the near field is longer.

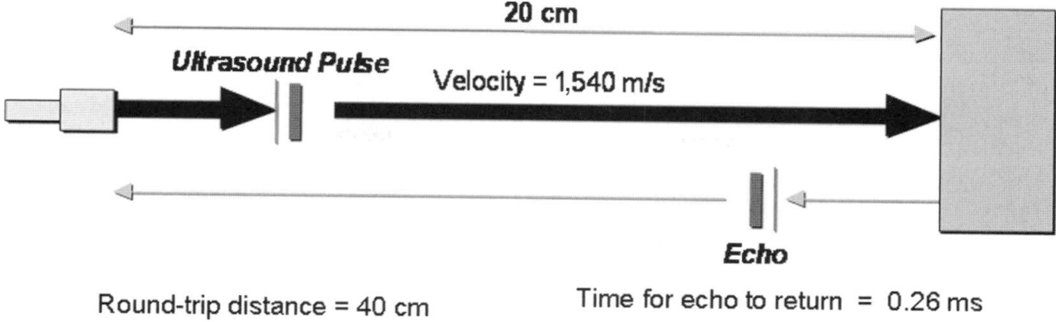


**Figure 8–2** The time for the ultrasound beam to return to the transducer from a particular structure is a measure of the structure's distance from the transducer.

The lateral resolution is also dependent on the gain of the system. Specular reflectors that are along the center of the beam produce stronger echoes than those that are at the beam margins. When the gain or sensitivity is set low, the echoes from the beam margins that are lower in amplitude may not be recorded, which makes the beam appear narrower. With higher gain, the echoes at the margins are recorded, and the beam width is greater.

## IMAGING MODALITIES

There are several imaging modalities in echocardiography. A mode and B mode have only historical importance.

M mode (motion) displays axial information along a single scan line, displaying depth on the vertical axis and time on the horizontal axis. This provides high temporal resolution, rapid sampling rates, and the ability to visualize wall or valve motion. M mode can also provide information on dimensional measurements such as chamber size or endocardial thickening (Fig. 8–3).

Two-dimensional echocardiographic imaging is generated by sweeping the ultrasound beam through an arc across a particular area of the heart.

Electronic sweeping is accomplished by the use of phased array transducers. Transducer arrays are groups of individual transducers or transducer elements. Linear arrays are composed of a group of transducers or transducer elements that are lined up next to each other in a straight row. The transducers are then pulsed individually or in groups. This requires a large window, which limits their use in cardiac imaging. The phased arrays contain multiple element transducers that sweep the ultrasound beam electronically through an arc. When the transducers are exited in sequence, the ultrasound wave generated propagates at an angle to the transducer, which sweeps the beam from side to side.

A focused transducer is used to decrease the amount of diversion in the far field of the ultrasound beam. By placing a concave acoustic lens on the surface of the transducer or by altering the curvature of the transducer, the ultrasound beam is narrowed at a point away from the transducer. The focal zone is the area where the beam is narrowest and the amount of divergence is decreased. The phased array transducer can also focus the beam electronically by altering the shape of the wavefront according to the timing of firing of the individual transducer elements.

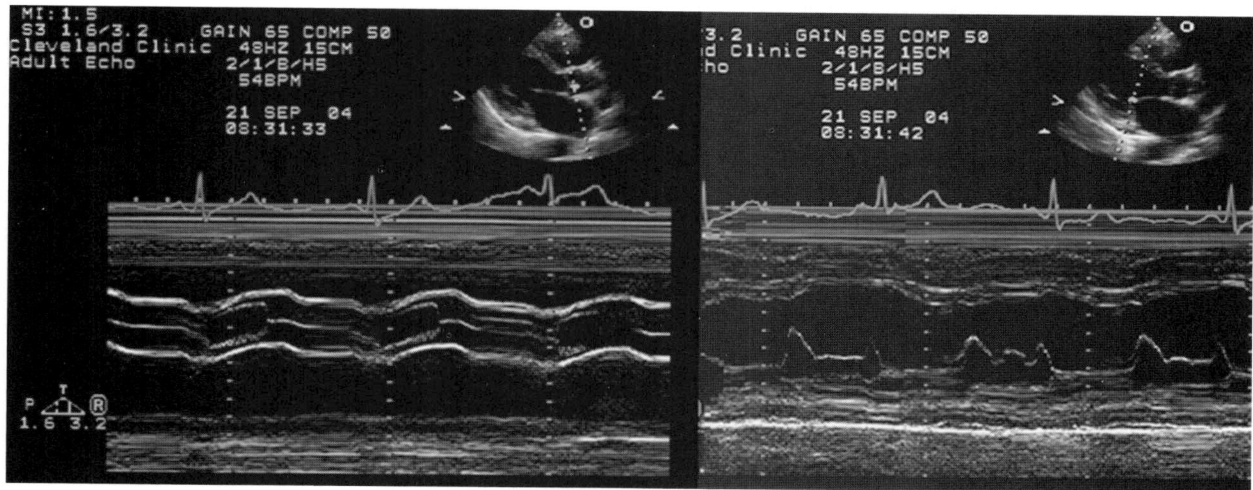


**Figure 8–3** M-mode display.

Two-dimensional echocardiography displays ultrasound data in a spatial orientation relative to time. This leads to a limitation in the amount of data that can be collected in a period of time. The pulse duration (*PD*) is the time needed for the pulse to travel from the transducer to the tissue and back. This is dependent on the depth of that tissue and the speed of sound in that tissue:

$$PD = 2d/c$$

The pulse repetition frequency (*PRF*) is the rate at which individual pulses are transmitted (per second) and is equal to $c/2d$. Knowing that the speed of sound in human tissue is 1,540 m/s, this translates to

$$PRF = 77/d \text{ pulses/ms}$$

The pulse repetition frequency in M mode is about 1,000 to 2000/s and 3,000 to 5,000/s in two-dimensional studies. The number of lines per sweep depends on the time taken to produce one scan line and the time set for each sweep. The frame rate is the number of images formed per second. In cardiac applications, the frame rate is typically >30 frames/s. A higher frame rate is needed to visualize valvular motion well. However, increasing the frame rate leads to fewer scan lines per frame, resulting in less data acquired per frame and therefore decreased image quality.

Serial processing occurs when one scan line is produced for each ultrasound pulse. This method limits the frame rate. With phased array transducers, it is possible to send out several scan lines simultaneously in different directions. Through parallel processing, the data from each scan line are analyzed separately, which increases the frame rate.

The echoes that are received by the tissues produce vibrations within the piezoelectric crystal that translate into a small voltage. To form a final image, the electrical signal goes through complex signal processing. The signals are initially amplified by a radiofrequency amplifier and are compressed logarithmically in order to be displayed in varying shades of gray.

The *dynamic range* (expressed in decibels) refers to the ratio of the amplitude of the largest signal displayed to the amplitude of the smallest signal detected above the noise of the system. Noise is a combination of all signals that reach the transducer from structures that do not lie on the ultrasound beam axis. These signal amplitudes are compressed into shades of gray. The gray scale can display both the strong and weak echoes in various shades of gray. The dynamic range consists of the number of levels of gray in an image and can be adjusted.

The echo images are obtained in a polar coordinate system and are converted into a video image by means of a digital scan converter.

Because structures that are deeper produce weaker echoes than structures that are closer to the transducer (because of attenuation), the electrical energy produced by these echoes are even less. In order to display those electrical signals, time gain compensation is employed. Greater amplification is applied for echoes returning at longer intervals from the initial pulse, which corresponds to the depth of the structure. Since attenuation can vary in people, the time gain compensation can be individually adjusted by the user for these variations. Near-field gain can be set lower while far-field gain can be gradually increased.

## HARMONIC IMAGING

When a sound pulse of frequency *fo* propagates through the tissues, nonlinear interactions occur, generating a pulse with frequencies at multiples of the fundamental frequency *fo*: 2*fo* (second harmonic), 3*fo*, (Figs. 8–4A and 8–4B). This is caused by minor changes in the density of tissue water that affects how sound travels, producing a very slight change in the shape of the wave as it propagates.

It is important to keep in mind that harmonic generation increases with the distance of propagation and that there is a nonlinear relation between fundamental frequency energy and harmonic frequency energy. These aspects of harmonic imaging help to understand why they are useful

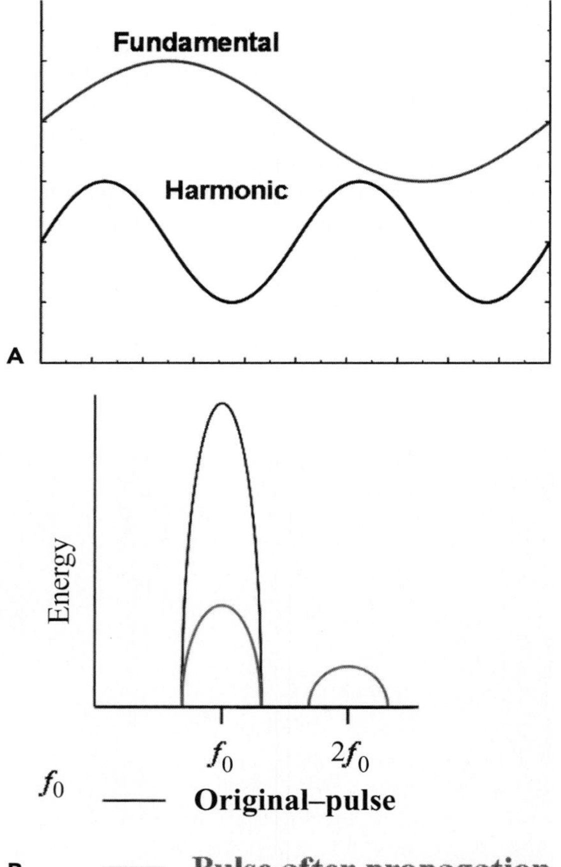


**Figure 8–4** **A:** Tissue harmonic imaging utilizes pulse frequencies at multiples of the fundamental frequency $f_0$. **B:** Harmonic frequencies are of lower energy than the fundamental frequency.

to reduce near-field artifacts (low harmonic energy close to the transducer) and also to reduce side-lobe artifacts.

The energy of these harmonic frequencies returning from the tissue is significantly less than the fundamental frequency. In order to benefit from harmonic imaging, the fundamental frequency needs to be filtered out, so that only the harmonic frequencies are passed to the demodulator.

Second harmonic tissue imaging is now used routinely in adult echocardiography. The benefits can be striking, particularly in patients with difficult images. In general, there is an improved signal-to-noise ratio with brighter tissue and superior endocardial definition.

Another use of harmonic imaging is contrast echocardiography. New contrast agents have been manufactured with very small (1- to 5-$\mu$m) bubbles capable of crossing the pulmonary capillary bed. The contrast effect is produced by microbubbles having different acoustic impedances than blood, causing the reflection and scattering of ultrasound. The ultrasound causes compressions and rarefactions of the microbubbles with a resonant frequency that is inversely related to the diameter of the microbubble. This interaction between ultrasound and microbubbles also generates harmonic frequencies. Compared to tissue, the microbubbles are strong reflectors, so tuning the ultrasound receiver to the second harmonic frequency will display the contrast agent preferentially within the image.

The approved indication for contrast imaging is for left ventricle opacification. In patients with very limited views, the use of contrast can significantly improve endocardial definition. Its main application is in patients with suspected wall motion abnormalities, stress test, or when left ventricular (LV) thrombus is suspected. The use of contrast agents for myocardial perfusion, although promising, is still investigational. Myocardial perfusion and viability are also potential uses of this technique, although they are not yet approved for clinical use.

## THREE-DIMENSIONAL ECHOCARDIOGRAPHY

While two-dimensional (2-D) echocardiography is now the standard ultrasound imaging modality, efforts are being made to enhance three-dimensional (3-D) ultrasound imaging. This may provide better detail of cardiac structures and functions. Different approaches are used for 3-D imaging. One approach is to construct a 3-D display by using conventional 2-D imaging with a multiplanar transducer. Tomographic slices of the heart are obtained and constructed into a 3-D image.

Another approach is to obtain real-time 3-D data. This requires the use of a matrix array transducer that is composed of a square array of thousands of elements. The sector can then be oriented in any direction and, by using parallel processing, a pyramidal scan can be produced. Three-dimensional echo is already commercially available. This technique appears to have an advantage for volumetric calculations and in complex congenital disease.

## DOPPLER ECHOCARDIOGRAPHY

Doppler echocardiography utilizes the Doppler principle to determine the presence, velocity, character, and timing of blood flow within the cardiovascular system. The Doppler principle states that the frequency reflected on a moving object is a higher observed frequency than when it moves away from the observer. The *Doppler shift* ($Fd$) is the difference in frequency between the received frequency ($Fr$) and the transmitted frequency ($Ft$):

$$Fd = Fr - Ft$$

In the same way, the backscatter of signal from small moving objects such as red blood cells produces a change in frequency of the signal, creating a Doppler effect. The Doppler shift is related to the velocity of the moving source ($V$):

$$Fd \alpha V => Fd = V/\lambda$$

Knowing that $\lambda = c/f$, and that the speed of sound tends to remain constant in tissue, change in the transmitted frequency will alter the wavelength. Therefore,

$$\lambda = c/Ft = V/Fd$$

Rearranging this expression produces

$$Fd = V \cdot Ft/c$$

In actuality, the ultrasound beam may be at an angle to the direction of blood flow. Using trigonometry, the true velocity is equal to the measured velocity divided by the cosine of the angle $\theta$. Therefore,

$$Fd = Ft \cdot V \cdot \cos\theta/c$$

where $V$ is the true velocity of blood flow. To adjust for the sound being reflected, the equation is multiplied by 2, which produces the final Doppler equation:

$$Fd = 2Ft \cdot V \cdot \cos\theta/c$$

Since it is the velocity of the moving object that is of interest, rearranging the equation produces

$$V = Fd \cdot c/(2Ft \cdot \cos\theta)$$

The angle that the ultrasound beam makes with the direction of blood flow is important. When the beam is parallel to the direction of flow, the angle is 0 degrees and $\cos 0 = 1$. When the beam is perpendicular to the direction of flow, the angle is 90 degrees and $\cos 90 = 0$, which means that there is no Doppler shift. Angles $<$20 degrees result in change of $<$6% in the recorded velocity. Thus, the effect of the beam angle on Doppler shift becomes more important when the angle is greater. For example, if the angle is 60 degrees, $\cos 60 = 0.5$, which leads to a 50% velocity error. This is important when calculating velocities in areas with abnormal blood flow, as in valvular stenosis.

**TABLE 8–2**
**COMPARISION OF CONTINUOUS-WAVE, PULSED-WAVE, AND COLOR DOPPLER**

| Continuous Wave | Pulsed Wave | Color Doppler |
|---|---|---|
| Ultrasound transmitted and received continuously | Ultrasound transmitted intermittently; two crystals; received after an interval (pulse velocities superimposed on a repetition frequency) | Doppler display color coded; one crystal; 2-D image |
| Records all blood velocities along beam | Records blood velocity at particular axis region of interest/sample volume | Useful for spatial mapping of Doppler signals (i.e., regurgitant jets or intracardiac shunt) |
| Records maximum velocity; useful for obtaining gradients | Useful for assessing low-velocity flow | Useful for quantification of regurgitant lesions |
| Smooth spectral signal defining onset and end of flow | Aliasing occurs when velocity of interest exceeds Nyquist limit | Aliasing appears as color reversal |

The difference between the transmitted and backscattered signals received by the transducer is determined by comparing the two waveforms. The frequency content is analyzed by fast Fourier transform. The display generated is known as a *spectral analysis*, with time displayed on the $x$ axis and frequency shift or blood velocity on the $y$ axis. Frequency shifts toward the transducer are displayed above the baseline, whereas frequency shifts away from the transducer are below the baseline. There are multiple frequencies for every given point in time, and each amplitude is displayed corresponding to its brightness (by gray or color scale). Therefore the spectral display produces information on the direction of blood flow, the velocity (or frequency shift), and the signal amplitude.

Three different modalities are used in Doppler echocardiography: continuous-wave Doppler, pulsed Doppler, and color Doppler flow mapping. Each modality is processed differently (Table 8–2).

Continuous-wave Doppler occurs when the sound beam is continuously transmitted and received. The transducer contains two crystals, one for continuous transmission and a second for continuous reception of the ultrasound signal. The spectral signal that is displayed is smooth in contour, displaying the maximum velocity and defining the onset and end of flow. The velocity curve is filled in because lower velocities are also recorded. This modality is useful for calculating high-frequency shifts or velocities encountered in stenotic or regurgitant lesions. The disadvantage is that because the wave is continuous, all signals along the ultrasound beam are recorded simultaneously. Thus the detected Doppler shift may have occurred at any point along the scan line (Fig. 8–5A).

In pulsed Doppler echocardiography, pulses of ultrasound are transmitted intermittently. This allows the pulse to traverse to a desired depth and, after a specific time delay, the backscattered signals are received by the transducer (Fig. 8–5B). As mentioned above,

$$d = ct/2 \qquad \text{and} \qquad PD = 2d/c$$

The Doppler shift or velocity at the depth of interest is based on the time delay that is required. This is useful in assessing low-velocity flows such as in transmitral flow. However, this may not be a reflection of the maximum velocity that is produced. The pulse repetition frequency is the interval that the transducer waits after a signal before it sends out the next signal. Because the time interval is dependent on the depth of interest, the pulse repetition frequency is also dependent on the depth. From earlier,

$$PRF = 77/d$$

In pulsed Doppler echo, the sample volume is the depth of interest. Pulsed Doppler echo samples the returning signal repeatedly, and there is a limit to the frequency shift (or velocity) that can be displayed unambiguously. The frequency of the ultrasound is determined by sampling the waveform for at least twice the wavelength. This requires sampling the pulse at twice the rate. The maximum detectable frequency shift is called the *Nyquist limit,* which is one half the pulse repetition frequency.

When the velocity of interest is higher than the Nyquist limit, the signal wraps around into the reverse channel and then back to the forward channel. This is known as *signal aliasing* (Fig. 8–5D). Various methods can be used to resolve aliasing, such as using continuous-wave Doppler ultrasound, shifting the baseline, increasing the pulse repetition frequency, or using a lower-frequency transducer.

Color Doppler flow mapping differs from pulsed Doppler echo in that multiple sample volumes (or *multigates*) are evaluated along each scan line. The 2-D image obtained from sweeping the scanning line across the echo sector is superimposed on color-coded velocity patterns. Flow toward the transducer is displayed in red, whereas flow away from the transducer is displayed in blue. The shade of color that is displayed indicates the velocity up to the Nyquist limit. As velocity increases, aliasing may occur. This is displayed by reversal of color.

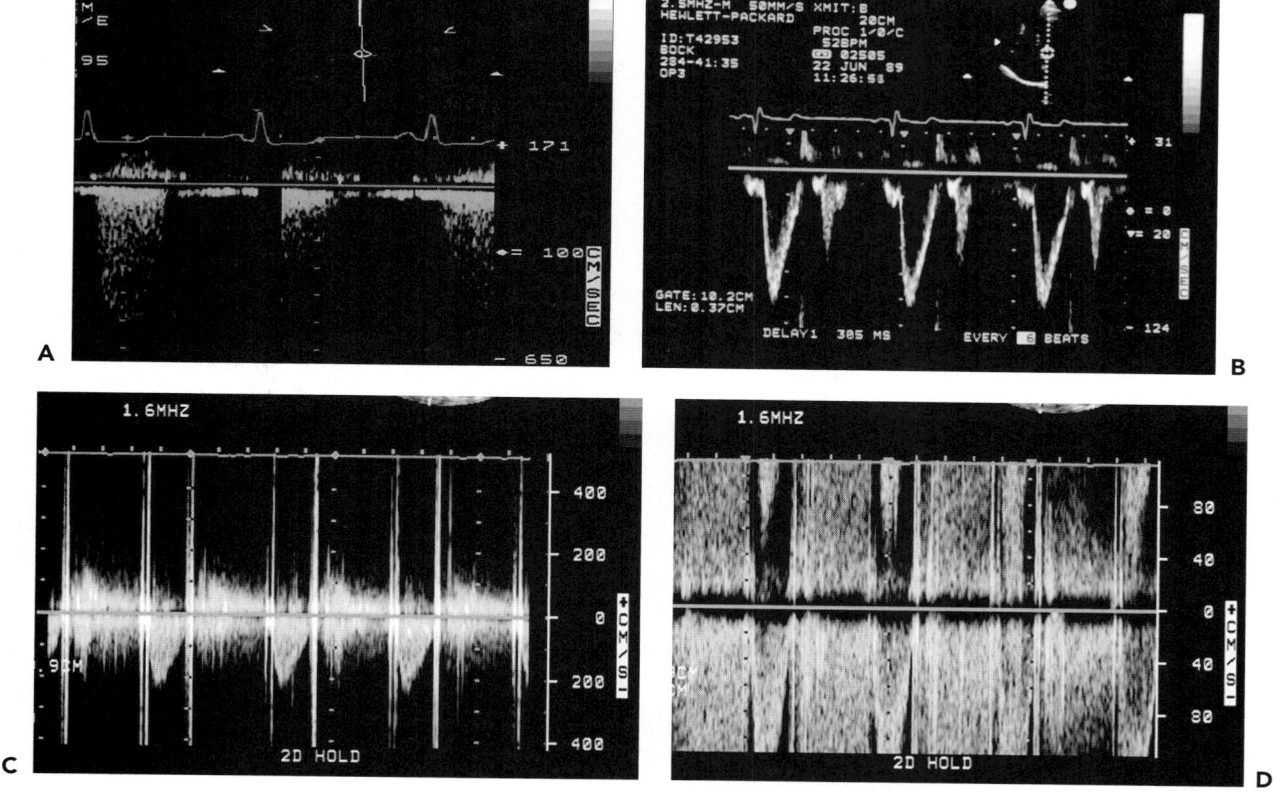


**Figure 8–5** **A:** Continuous-wave Doppler. **B:** Pulsed-wave Doppler. **C, D:** High velocities—continuous-wave **(C)** versus pulsed-wave **(D)** Doppler with aliasing.

## IMAGING ARTIFACTS

Imaging artifacts can be produced, which can either display structures that are not there, fail to display structures that are actually there, or form an image of a structure that is different in shape or size from what it actually is. Side lobes occur when the ultrasound energy disperses laterally from the main ultrasound beam and are produced from the edges of the transducer elements. The side lobes may reflect or backscatter signals and produce an artifactual image as though it were originating from the center of the ultrasound beam. The amplitude of these waves is generally much lower and as a result may not produce a strong image artifact. The extraneous beams produced from phased array transducers are termed *grating lobes* and the problem then is more serious. These affect the lateral resolution of the transducer.

Beam-width artifacts occur when structures that are in the far field of the ultrasound beam produce images that are superimposed on structures that are in the center of the ultrasound beam. This can produce artifactual images creating distorted images or the display of artifactual structures such as the appearance of vegetations on a valve leaflet, an intracardiac mass, or an aortic dissection. This also affects lateral resolution.

Reverberation artifacts are produce when ultrasound waves are being bounced back and forth between two or more highly reflective surfaces. This produces multiple linear echo signals that appear as parallel lines. This limits evaluation of structures within the far field and may also display abnormal structures.

Acoustic shadowing may occur when structures with high density block transmission of the ultrasound. This can be seen with calcified or prosthetic valves. This presents a problem when trying to image structures that are distal to these dense structures, because no reflected signals return to the transducer. In these cases, an alternate window is necessary to visualize structures of interest.

When an echo signal from a previous pulse reaches the transducer on the next pulse cycle, range ambiguity can occur. This causes deeper structures to appear as though they are closer to the transducer. By increasing the depth setting, the pulse repetition frequency decreases, which eliminates range ambiguity.

## PRINCIPLES OF FLOW

*Blood flow* is defined as the volume of blood moved per unit time. Flow is related to the pressure, the radius of the vessel, and the viscosity of blood. In steady flow, the fluid particles move along parallel lines to the vessel wall. This is described as laminar flow. Turbulent flow occurs when blood cells move in different directions at different velocities. This can occur in stenotic valves, regurgitant valves, or intracardiac shunts.

The velocity of blood flow changes when there is a change in size of the vessel diameter. This is expressed by the *Bernoulli principle,* which is based on the conservation of energy (kinetic and pressure energy). The kinetic energy from the blood flow is proportional to the density and the square of the blood flow velocity. When there is a change in the blood flow velocity, the kinetic energy (*KE*) also changes.

$$KE = {}^1\!/_2 \rho v^2$$

Because total energy is conserved, the total energy at point 1 ($P_1$) must equal the total energy at point 2 ($P_2$).

$$P_1 + KE_1 = P_2 + KE_2$$
$$=> P_1 + {}^1\!/_2 \rho (v_1)^2 = P_2 + {}^1\!/_2 \rho (v_2)^2$$
$$=> P_1 - P_2 = {}^1\!/_2 \rho [(v_2)^2 - (v_1)^2]$$

It is important to realize that some of the energy lost when going from point 1 to point 2 is due to energy required to overcome forces caused by changes in flow rate over time. This is caused by the vessel being pulsatile (flow acceleration), as well as energy lost because of viscous friction. Therefore, the complete Bernoulli equation is

$$\Delta P = {}^1\!/_2 \rho [(v_2)^2 - (v_1)^2] + \rho (dv/dt)dx + R(v)$$

The energy lost to viscous resistance ($R(v)$) and flow acceleration is negligible and can be eliminated from the Bernoulli equation. The velocity across stenotic lesions (such as valves) is much higher than the velocity proximal to the stenosis. The velocity proximal to the mitral valve is typically 0.2 m/s, and it is 0.8 m/s for the aortic valve. Because these numbers are small, $(v_1)^2$ can usually be dropped from the equation, except when $v_1 > 1$ m/s, such as in severe aortic regurgitation or subaortic obstruction. Using appropriate units of measurement, the value ${}^1\!/_2 \rho$ is approximately 4. Therefore, the simplified Bernoulli equation is often used to calculate the pressure gradient across the valve:

$$\Delta P = 4(v_2)^2$$

Blood flow also must obey the principle of conservation of mass. The average velocity of blood at a particular point ($v$) is defined as the flow rate ($Q$) divided by the cross-sectional area ($A$) across the vessel at that point:

$$v = Q/A$$

Knowing that the volume of blood entering the vessel is the same as the volume leaving (conservation of mass), the volume flow rate ($Q$) remains constant:

$$Q = v_1 \times A_1 = v_2 \times A_2$$

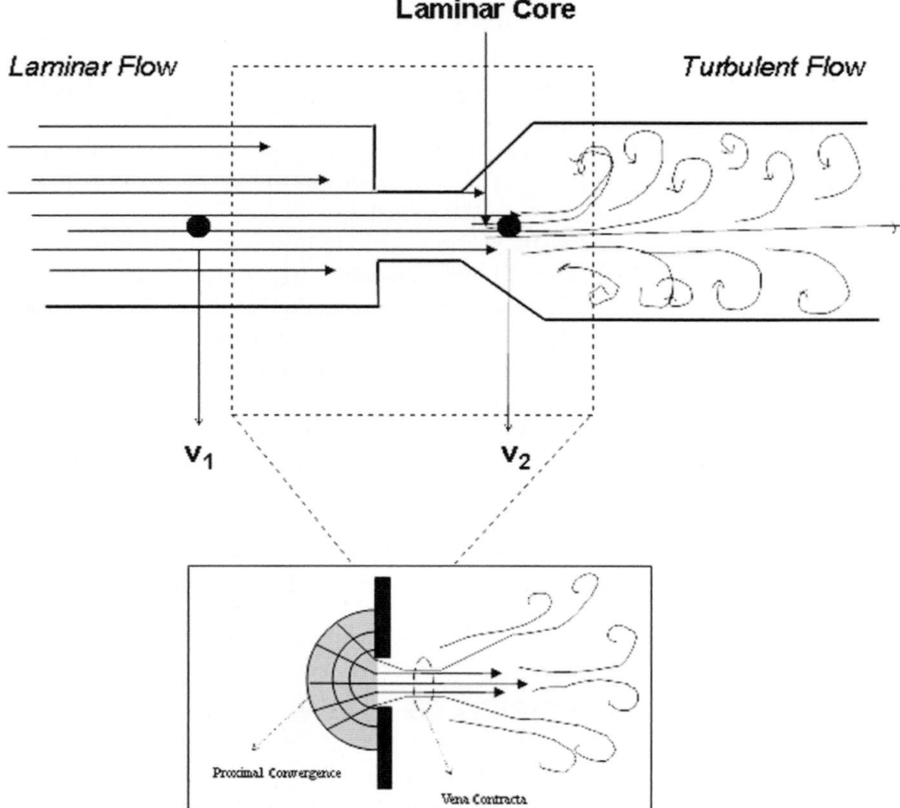


**Figure 8–6** Flow through a stenotic lesion (e.g., valve).

This equation is referred to as the *continuity equation*. Therefore, as the vessel size increases, the cross-sectional area increases, causing the velocity to decrease, resulting in a decrease in kinetic energy. In stenotic lesions, the cross-sectional area decreases, causing the velocity to increase. The increase in velocity causes the parallel streamlines to converge and is called *convective acceleration* (Fig. 8–6).

Applying the continuity equation, one can calculate the area across a stenotic lesion (such as the aortic valve). This requires knowing the velocities proximal to the valve and across the valve in addition to the area proximal to the valve ($r$ = radius, $d$ = diameter at point 1).

$$A_2 = A_1 \times (v_1/v_2)$$
$$=> A_2 = \pi r^2/2 \times (v_1/v_2)$$
$$=> A_2 = \pi d^2/4 \times (v_1/v_2)$$
$$=> A_2 = 0.785d^2 \times (v_1/v_2)$$

For example,

$$A_{\text{aortic valve}} = 0.785 d^2_{\text{LV outflow tract}} \times (V_{\text{LV outflow tract}}/V_{\text{aortic valve}})$$

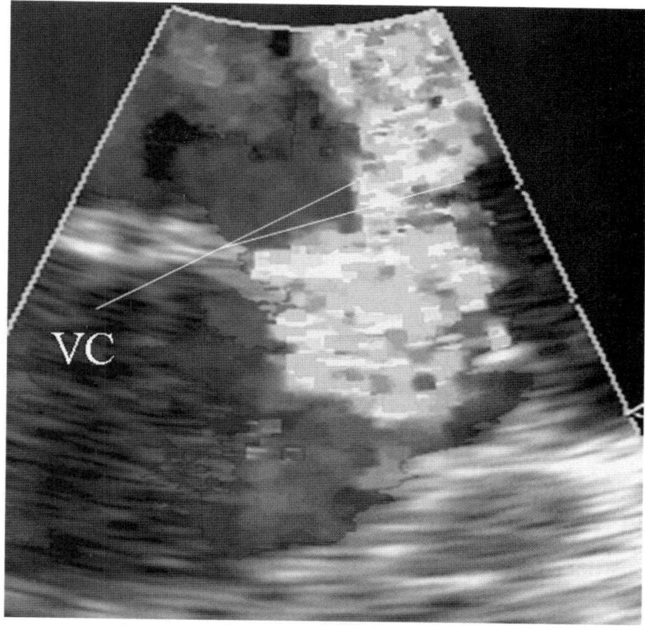


**Figure 8–7** Vena contracta (VC)—the point of maximal velocity and minimal cross-sectional area.

## BASIC PRINCIPLES OF JETS

As flow approaches a restricted orifice, flow accelerates, achieving maximal velocity at the orifice or slightly distal from the obstruction. The point of maximal velocity and minimal cross-sectional area is called the *vena contracta* (Fig. 8–7). The location of the vena contracta depends on the geometry of the orifice and can occur downstream from the orifice. After exiting the orifice, flow remains laminar for about five orifice diameters before becoming turbulent. Downstream the flow loses velocity and reattaches to the wall, recovering part of the pressure. This phenomenon of pressure recovery has implications in prosthetic valves and helps to explain some of the discrepancies between Doppler-derived gradients and those measured with catheters.

So far we have discussed conservation of mass and energy. A jet also follows the conservation of momentum. Momentum equals mass multiplied by velocity. Jet momentum ($M$) is

$$M = \rho \times Q \times v$$

where $\rho$ = density, $Q$ = flow rate, and $v$ = velocity. Knowing that $Q = A \times v$, where $A$ is the orifice area,

$$M = \rho \times A \times v^2$$

The momentum is the best predictor of jet appearance by color flow mapping. Jet flow can also be affected by the *Coanda effect*. This occurs when the jet attaches to and flows around nearby structures such as the atrial wall. These confined jets typically look smaller when imaged by color Doppler and may underestimate the severity of the regurgitation.

## BIBLIOGRAPHY


**Feigenbaum H.** *Echocardiography*. 5th ed. Philadelphia: Lea & Febiger; 1994.

**Otto C.** *The Practice of Clinical Echocardiography*. 2nd ed. Philadelphia: WB Saunders; 2002.

**Otto C.** *Textbook of Clinical Echocardiography*. 3rd ed. Philadelphia: Elsevier Saunders; 2004.

**Weyman A.** *Principles and Practice of Echocardiography*. 2nd ed. Philadelphia: Lea & Febiger; 1994.


## QUESTIONS

**1.** All of the following statements regarding the Doppler equation are true except:

a. In order to obtain the true velocity of blood flow at a certain point, the beam needs to be parallel to the direction of blood flow.

b. The measured velocity of blood is overestimated when the beam is at a greater angle to the direction of blood flow.

c. There is no Doppler shift when the beam is perpendicular to the direction of blood flow.

d. The true velocity of blood flow is equal to the measured velocity divided by the cosine of the angle the beam makes with the direction of blood flow.

Answer is b: The true velocity of blood flow is equal to the measured velocity divided by the cosine of the angle the beam makes with the direction of blood flow. The Doppler equation enables us to measure the velocity based on knowing the frequency shift, the transmitted frequency, and the speed of sound in blood. When the beam is parallel to the direction of blood flow, the angle is 0 degrees and $\cos 0 = 1$, therefore the true velocity is equal to the measured velocity. However, when the beam is perpendicular to the direction of blood flow, the angle is 90 degrees; $\cos 90 = 0$, so there is no Doppler shift. The greater the angle between the beam and the direction of blood flow, the greater is the error in measuring the velocity of blood flow. In actuality, the measured blood flow will be underestimated in this scenario, and the true velocity will actually be higher than what is reported. Therefore, it is essential to keep the beam parallel to the direction of blood flow in order to minimize velocity errors, because it is important to assess the velocity of blood flow in cases such as valvular stenosis. Angles that are <20 degrees may be acceptable, because there is less velocity error.

**2.** Continuous-wave Doppler echocardiography is useful for all of the following except:

a. Determining peak velocity across the aortic valve
b. Determining the pressure gradient across the aortic valve
c. Determining precise location of flow obstruction
d. Assessing the presence of dynamic left ventricular outflow tract obstruction

Answer is c: Continuous-wave Doppler is a useful modality for determining peak flow velocity and is used for high velocities such as in stenotic and regurgitant lesions. Therefore, it is used for determining peak velocity and pressure gradient across the aortic valve. It is also used in assessing whether there is dynamic left ventricular outflow tract (LVOT) obstruction, which is observed in hypertrophic cardiomyopathy. Provocative maneuvers such as Valsalva or use of inhaled amyl nitrate increases the obstruction across the LVOT, which is manifested by a higher peak velocity and is determined by continuous-wave Doppler. Continous-wave Doppler measures the highest velocity along the scan line but does not allow spatial location.

**3.** All of the following are used to resolve aliasing except:

a. Decreasing the pulse repetition frequency
b. Using continuous-wave Doppler ultrasound
c. Using a lower-frequency transducer
d. Shifting the baseline

Answer is a: Aliasing occurs when the signal wraps around into the reverse channel and then back to the forward channel. This occurs when the velocity of interest is higher than the Nyquist limit. The Nyquist limit is the maximum detectable frequency shift and is equal to one half the pulse repetition frequency. To resolve aliasing, the Nyquist limit needs to be raised, which means increasing the pulse repetition frequency.

**4.** Which of the following is true?

a. The modified Bernoulli equation is used to calculate the area of a stenotic valve.
b. The velocity of blood remains constant.
c. The continuity equation is used to calculate the area of a stenotic valve.
d. The continuity equation only requires knowing the velocities proximal to and across the valve.

Answer is c: The velocity of blood flow changes when there is a change in the size of the vessel diameter, as can occur across a stenotic valve. The Bernoulli principle is based on the conservation of energy, and the modified Bernoulli equation is used to calculate the pressure gradient across the valve. The continuity equation is based on the principle of conservation of mass, and that the volume of blood entering a vessel is equal to the volume leaving, implying a constant flow rate (area × velocity). As the vessel size increases, the cross-sectional area increases, causing the velocity to decrease. The continuity equation therefore allows us to measure the area across a stenotic valve and requires knowing the velocities proximal to and across the valve as well as the area of the vessel proximal to the valve (e.g., LVOT area [or diameter]) when calculating the area across the aortic valve).

**5.** Which of the following is true regarding contrast echocardiography?

a. Harmonic imaging is used in contrast echocardiography.
b. Contrast agents typically use microbubbles that are 50 mm in dimension.
c. Commercial microbubbles are used for determining the presence of an atrial septal defect or a patent foramen ovale.
d. Contrast echocardiography is a standard modality in determining myocardial perfusion.

Answer is a: Contrast echocardiography is dependent on contrast agents that use bubbles that are small (1 to 5 mm) and are able to cross the pulmonary capillary bed, in order to better visualize the left ventricle. The main indication for using contrast is to improve endocardial definition to assess for wall motion abnormalities or presence of a left ventricular thrombus. Its use in myocardial perfusion is still investigational. The interaction between ultrasound and the microbubbles generates harmonic frequencies, so tuning the ultrasound receiver to the second harmonic frequency will preferentially display the contrast agent, which is a stronger reflector than tissue.

# Nuclear Cardiac Imaging: A Primer

9

*Gregory G. Bashian* *Richard C. Brunken*

Nuclear cardiac imaging contributes significantly to the care of patients with known or suspected heart disease. More than 6 million nuclear cardiac imaging procedures are performed annually in the United States, and the number of studies will grow further as more hospitals and physicians' offices acquire this imaging technology. The information afforded by noninvasive nuclear imaging techniques is valuable, not only for the detection and localization of coronary artery disease, but also for risk stratification and the assessment of myocardial viability. In order to understand the clinical role and utility of nuclear imaging studies, one must first understand the physics and physiology of the various imaging techniques. The goal of this chapter is to review the fundamentals of nuclear imaging and relate them to their specific clinical role.

## PERFORMING NUCLEAR IMAGING

The goal of a nuclear imaging study is to visualize a physiologic process in vivo using instruments (e.g., gamma cameras) that are capable of recording the naturally occurring emissions of a radioactive tracer. Different radioactive agents trace different physiologic processes, and the specific tracer used for imaging is determined by the type of information the clinician desires. The ideal tracer should be nontoxic and emit radiation with energies appropriate for imaging without imparting an excessively high radiation dose to the patient. The ideal imaging agent should *depict* the physiologic process of interest *without disturbing* it. Finally, it should be readily available and relatively inexpensive in order to be feasible for routine clinical use. Most radioactive tracers used for cardiac nuclear imaging are administered intravenously, but some may be administered as inhaled gases.

As radioactive tracers spontaneously decay, they emit packets of high-frequency electromagnetic energy, or *photons*. Some of the emitted photons are *attenuated* (absorbed or deflected) before they leave the body, and cannot be used for imaging. The photons that exit the body are captured with gamma cameras and used to create an image. Image quality improves as the number of scintillation events, or counts, in the picture increases. Thus, it is important to use a high enough dose of the radioactive tracer and to image for a long enough period of time to achieve satisfactory image quality.

A gamma camera usually has a *lead collimator*, a piece of metal with a "honeycomb" of openings that serves to focus the incident photons (Fig. 9–1). Most collimators used for cardiac imaging have holes that are parallel to each other (*parallel-hole collimators*). Photons that travel perpendicular to the camera pass through the holes and are used to create the image. Photons that approach at an angle are stopped by the septa and are not incorporated into the image. Collimator performance depends on the length and diameter of the holes, as well as the thickness of the septa. In general, spatial resolution improves as the ratio of the hole diameter to length decreases. Thus, the resolution of the collimator is improved at the cost of a decrease in efficiency, and collimator selection reflects this trade-off between spatial resolution and count sensitivity. *High-resolution* collimators provide better spatial resolution but lower sensitivity (maximum number of counts entering the camera per unit time) than other collimators, because more counts are absorbed by the collimator and not the crystal. "General-purpose" or *high-sensitivity* collimators are

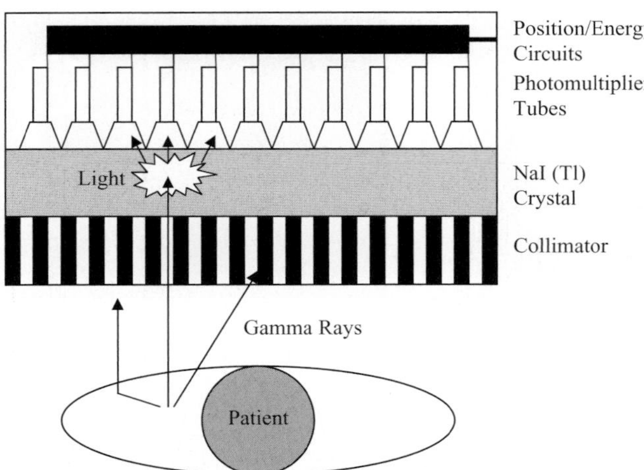


**Figure 9–1** Schematic representation of a gamma camera. Photons emitted by decay of the radiotracer of interest in the target organ can travel directly to the camera, or be scattered by interposed tissue. Photons that strike the lead collimator are absorbed and do not reach the crystal. The photons that pass through the collimator strike the crystal and interact with it, producing flashes of visible light. The photomultiplier tube closest to the gamma-ray interaction receives the greatest amount of light, and comparison of the relative response from multiple photomultiplier tubes allows localization of the scintillation event. Light quanta strike the photocathodes of the photomultiplier tubes, causing the release of electrons. The electrical signal is amplified by the photomultiplier tubes and transmitted to the energy discrimination and positioning circuitry of the camera.

capable of passing greater numbers of photons per unit of time, with somewhat poorer spatial resolution. "All-purpose" collimators have characteristics that are intermediate between these extremes.

Photons exiting the collimator strike a sodium iodide crystal that contains a trace amount of nonradioactive thallium. The crystal stops most of the photons and converts their energy into quanta of visible light. The more energetic the photons are, the more light quanta are produced. Light quanta are directed via a light pipe to adjacent photomultiplier tubes that convert the energy of the light quanta into an electrical current, and then amplify the strength of the current by several thousandfold. Special electronic circuitry is used to locate the $x$ and $y$ positions of the initial light impulse, and to analyze the energy of the incident photons.

Some of the photons that are emitted from the heart may be scattered before entering the collimator and striking the crystal. Scattered photons, because they have not traveled in a direct path, degrade the image. These scattered photons, however, lose energy in these collisions and scatter events. Setting an optimal "energy window" minimizes the contribution of scattered counts while preserving most of the desired nonscattered counts in the photopeak. The energy resolution of the camera determines the optimal setting for the energy window.

An image emerges as increasing numbers of photons (counts) are captured. State-of-the-art gamma cameras are capable of imaging about 200,000 counts per second, and some multiwire cameras are capable of even higher count rates. A camera with a high count rate capability is needed for high-quality first-pass imaging, (imaging that is performed while the radioactive tracer is being administered intravenously).

Images may be obtained using either *planar* or single-photon-emission computed tomographic (*SPECT*) acquisition techniques. Planar images are obtained with the gamma camera from several fixed views (usually anterior, left anterior oblique, and left lateral). Planar images may be acquired for a specific period of time, for a specific number of counts, or for a given number of cardiac cycles (radionuclide ventriculography).

## CARDIAC SPECT IMAGING

In SPECT imaging, pictures are obtained from multiple angles (projections) about the body. Current SPECT camera systems have between one and four camera heads that rotate about the patient. Images are typically acquired over 180- or 360-degree arcs, usually by "stepping and shooting" an image every 3 or 6 degrees. Information from the projection images is reconstructed using filtered back-projection or iterative reconstruction techniques and used to define the three-dimensional tracer distribution in space. Image sets orthogonal to the long axis of the heart (vertical long axis, horizontal long axis, and short axis) are then created.

SPECT images can be acquired with electrocardiogram (ECG) gating, and this permits assessment of ventricular function as well as perfusion. In gated imaging, the R–R interval of the ECG is usually divided into 8 or 16 equal time bins (frames) (Fig. 9–2). At each "step," the SPECT camera acquires 8 to 16 images gated to the patient's ECG, over

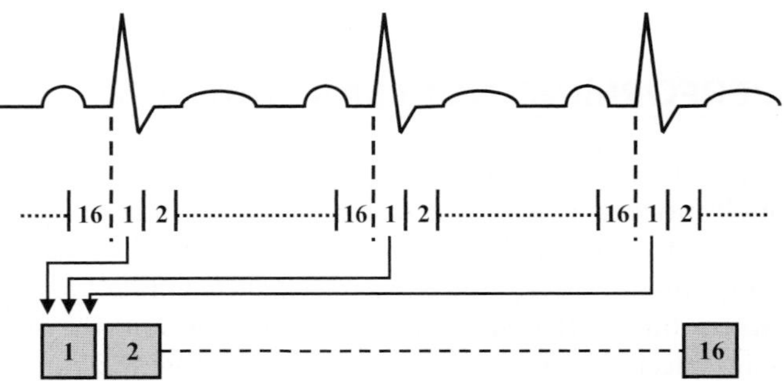


**Figure 9–2** Graphic representation of the process of ECG gating. Using the R wave of the patient's electrocardiogram as a timing signal, image count data from multiple cardiac cycles are added to the time bin corresponding to that portion of the R–R interval in which they were acquired. Counts in each bin increase with each succeeding cardiac cycle, improving the quality of the image represented by that time bin. Usually, 8 or 16 images are acquired per R–R interval, each representing a time-averaged look at that portion of the cardiac cycle. Once images are acquired, they can be displayed in a continuous ciné loop, depicting global and regional ventricular function.

multiple heart beats. Each of the frames depicts a different portion of the cardiac cycle. Gated image sets are reconstructed along the three major cardiac axes in the same fashion as the ungated images, providing functional information at each of the "slices" in these image sets. Currently available software packages can also display the gated information as a three-dimensional rendering, enabling the reviewer to visualize a graphical representation of the beating heart. Gated SPECT images provide information about regional wall motion and systolic thickening, as well as global left ventricular size and systolic function.

Because of the shorter 6-hour half-life of technetium-99m, higher doses of Tc-99m sestamibi or Tc-99m tetrofosmin can be administered with less radiation exposure to the patient than using thallium-201, which has a 73-hour half-life. Higher tracer doses provide a large enough number of counts to yield gated images that are of diagnostic quality. Although gated SPECT imaging with thallium has been used for ejection fraction measurements, clinical studies question whether there is sufficient count density on these images to enable reliable determination of regional wall motion and systolic thickening.

## CARDIAC PET IMAGING

Positron emission tomographic (PET) cardiac imaging is performed in some heart centers. PET imaging is a noninvasive, three-dimensional nuclear imaging technique that uses radioactive tracers to depict naturally occurring tissue processes in vivo. One of its uses is to assess perfusion, and it is more sensitive and specific for the detection of coronary artery disease than SPECT imaging. In addition, if it is performed with the metabolic tracer $^{18}$F-2-fluoro-2-deoxyglucose (FDG), PET imaging can provide important clinical information about regional myocardial viability.

As opposed to SPECT imaging tracers, tracers used for PET imaging decay by ejecting a positron (a $\beta^+$ particle) from a proton-rich nucleus. The positron interacts with atoms in the surrounding medium, producing excitations and ionizations that slow the positron. As the positron slows, it comes into close proximity with one of many electrons in the nearby surrounding medium. The electron and the positron mutually annihilate, releasing energy in the form of two 511-kiloelectron volt (keV) *annihilation photons,* which exit the site in opposite directions.

PET cameras employ circular banks of gamma-ray detectors connected by sophisticated electronic circuitry to identify paired scintillation events occurring about 180 degrees apart (*annihilation coincidence detection*). If two detectors opposite each other simultaneously register photons *in coincidence,* then an annihilation event is effectively localized to the volume between the two detectors (Fig. 9–3). If only a single photon is detected, the requirement for coincidence detection is not satisfied, and the scintillation event is not incorporated into the myocardial image. Employing

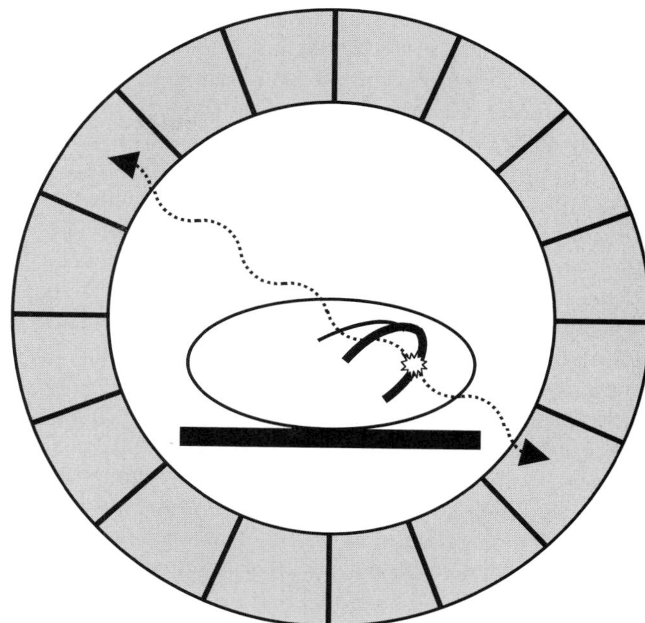

**Figure 9–3** Schematic representation of PET imaging. When a PET radiotracer decays, it emits a positron, the antiparticle of the electron. The positron travels a short distance before interacting with an electron, resulting in their mutual annihilation. The annihilation event produces two 511-keV photons traveling in diametrically opposed directions. PET imaging relies on the detection of two photons "in coincidence" (arriving at opposite detectors at about the same time) to identify true annihilation events and localize them to the volume between the two detectors.

data from millions of annihilation events, standard filtered back-projection or iterative reconstruction techniques are used to create an image of the tracer distribution within the plane of the ring of detectors (two dimensions). The three-dimensional spatial distribution of the tracer is achieved by the use of multiple rings of detectors adjacent to each other. A detector in one plane can be in the "line of sight" of some of the opposite detectors in the adjacent higher and lower ring planes. By using *interplane coincidences,* an additional set of interpolated images midway between the direct planes defined by the detector rings is generated.

PET images can be acquired at the moment of peak myocardial uptake of the tracer (*static image acquisition*), or a series of images can rapidly be acquired over time (*dynamic image acquisition*). The images acquired first, the *transverse images,* are orthogonal to the body. In most imaging centers, the transverse images are "resliced" into standard short-axis, and vertical and horizontal long-axis image sets analogous to those used in SPECT imaging. ECG-gated PET images can also be obtained to assess segmental wall motion and thickening, and ventricular volumes and ejection fractions.

PET has several advantages relative to SPECT for cardiac imaging, including better temporal and spatial image resolution and accurate correction for attenuation of emitted photons. Current PET tomographs can acquire multiple cross-sectional images of the heart as frequently as every 10 seconds, whereas SPECT imaging of the heart may take as long as 30 minutes. Unlike SPECT cameras, the spatial resolution of a PET tomograph depends mainly on the geometry of its detectors and is relatively insensitive to the depth of the scintillation event. PET tomographs have spatial resolutions on the order of 6 to 8 mm full-width, half-maximum (FWHM) in the center of the field of view, as compared to 12 to 15 mm FWHM for SPECT cameras.

Because PET images are corrected for tissue attenuation by use of measured attenuation coefficients, image counts accurately reflect true tissue activity concentrations. Measurements of rates of myocardial perfusion and/or metabolism can be obtained by examining the change in the tissue tracer concentration over time on dynamic PET images. Because the acquisition time of each image frame is operator-defined, it is possible to generate *time–activity curves* that depict tissue and vascular tracer activity concentrations as a function of time. Myocardial count data are fit using a mathematical model that describes the biologic behavior of the radioactive label. The parameter of interest (e.g., myocardial blood flow in milliliters per minute per gram of tissue or glucose consumption in micromoles per minute per gram of tissue) is then defined by the equation that fits the patient's myocardial time–activity data.

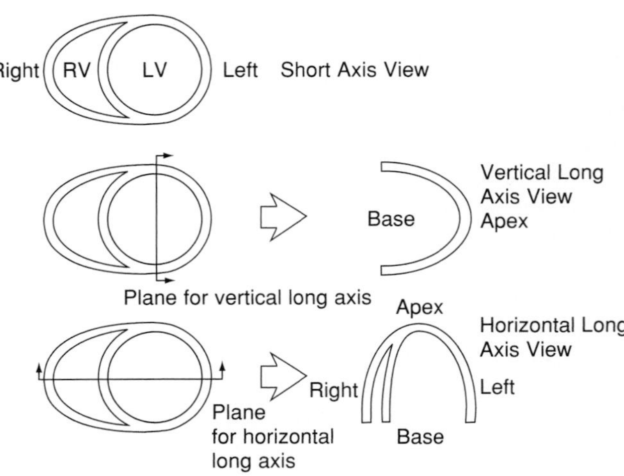


**Figure 9–4** Cardiac plane definition. (From American Heart Association, American College of Cardiology, and Society of Nuclear Medicine: Standardized Myocardial Segmentation and Nomenclature for Tomographic Imaging of the Heart. *Circulation* 1992;86:338–339, by permission.)

## INTERPRETATION OF NUCLEAR IMAGES

Planar and SPECT images are subjected to careful visual analysis by trained physicians. Care is taken to identify significant extracardiac activity (e.g., prominent pulmonary activity suggesting left ventricular dysfunction) that might affect image interpretation, to define cardiac chamber size, relative myocardial perfusion, and, where appropriate, regional and global function. As a quality-control measure for SPECT perfusion studies, the raw projection images are reviewed in a cinematic display. This enables the physician to look for motion and displacement of the heart during imaging, to identify interposed tissue that might attenuate the images, and to determine if the extracardiac distribution of the radioactive tracer is normal.

After the raw projection images are examined, the images are reviewed in each of the standard three orthogonal planes that are oriented orthogonal to the long axis of the left ventricle. Specifically, these are the short axis, vertical long axis, and horizontal long axis (Fig. 9–4). The ventricle is also divided into a standard 17-segment model in which each segment represents a near-equal proportion of the ventricular mass (6% for each segment except for the apical cap, which represents 4% of the left ventricular mass) (Fig. 9–5).

Segmental perfusion and function are scored semiquantitatively, based on visual interpretation of the images. One myocardial perfusion scoring system uses scores from 0 through 4; in this system, normal tracer uptake is scored as 0, a mild reduction in activity is scored as 1, a moderate reduction in activity is given a score of 2, a severe reduction in activity is considered a 3, and a complete absence of activity is given a 4. Indices of the severity of the observed perfusion abnormalities may be generated by summing the scores on stress and rest images separately. For example, if the stress images demonstrate a perfusion defect involving three segments, with visual scores of 4, 3, and 2, the *summed*

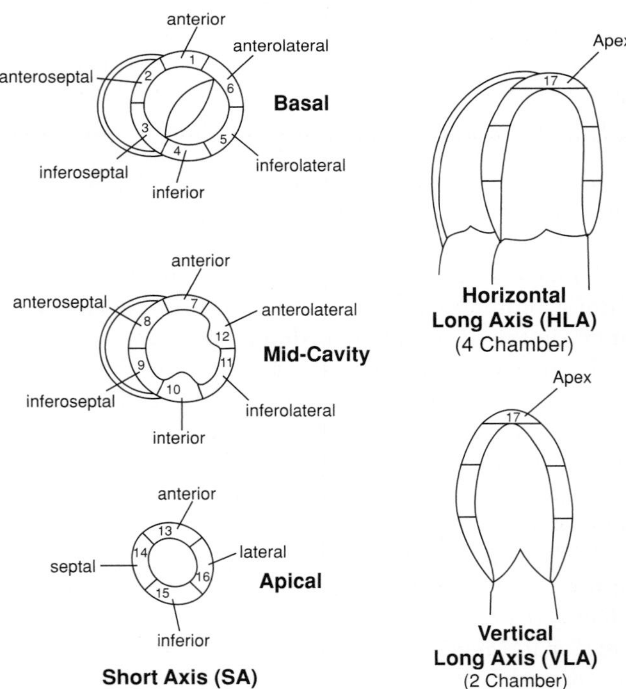


**Figure 9–5** Regional wall segments. This diagram demonstrates how the left ventricle can be divided into standardized segments for cardiac imaging. Short-axis, horizontal long-axis, and vertical long-axis views are depicted. (From Cerqueira, MD, et al. Standardized Myocardial Segmentation and Nomenclature for Tomographic Imaging of the Heart. *Circulation* 2002;105:529–542, by permission.)

*stress score* is 9 [ = (1 × 4) + (1 × 3) + (1 × 2)]. Defects on the rest images are scored in similar fashion and added together to calculate the *summed rest score*. Rest and stress summed scores are considered of low (0 to 4), intermediate (5 to 8) or high (>8) severity. The *summed difference score* is the sum of the differences between the stress and rest scores for each segment. The degree (or amount) of defect reversibility is considered low (summed difference score of 0 to 2), intermediate (summed difference score of 3 to 7) or high (summed difference score >7).

Augmenting the visual interpretation of the studies are computer-generated analyses of the nuclear images. *Circumferential profiles* of planar perfusion images display relative myocardial counts (counts expressed as a percent of the maximal counts in the tissue) as a function of the angle about the center of the image. Relative tracer concentrations in the patient's study are displayed along with those of gender-matched normals. For SPECT studies, quantitative analysis of the three-dimensional information is usually displayed in a two-dimensional "polar map." In the polar mapping technique, the ventricle is considered to be composed of a group of short-axis slices. The apical short-axis slice is smallest in diameter, and as the slices get closer and closer to the base of the heart the diameter of the slices gets larger and larger. Imagine that the smallest short-axis slice is put inside the center of the next larger slice. Both slices are oriented as if the observer is looking up the ventricle toward the base: the septum is on the observer's left, the anterior wall is above, the lateral wall is to the observer's right, and the inferior wall is below (Fig. 9–6). If those two slices are put inside the center of the third slice, and these three slices are put inside the center of the fourth slice, and so on, the process can be continued until all of the short-axis slices are stacked inside the largest basal short-axis slice, each having the same orientation. Basically, the image slices form a "target" with concentric rings and the three-dimensional information has been mapped into a two-dimensional display. The parameter of interest (e.g., relative technetium-99m sestamibi or thallium-201 activity) in each short-axis slice is then expressed as a percentage of the maximal value over the entire heart ("normalized" to peak myocardial values). The normalized activity in each picture element (voxel) can then be displayed using either a gray or color scale to provide the viewer a map of the activity distribution over the entire left ventricle in a single image. Normalized patient data are often referenced to gender-matched databases, and a second polar map is generated that displays the extent and the severity of the patient's abnormalities (e.g., two or three standard deviations from normal) on a voxel-by-voxel basis. A variety of parameters can be displayed using the polar mapping technique, including relative and absolute myocardial perfusion, relative systolic thickening (systolic change in counts on gated perfusion or metabolic images), segmental wall motion, thallium-201 redistribution, and PET perfusion–metabolism mismatches. These measurements provide an "independent observer" that assists the nuclear cardiologist in the interpretation of the images.

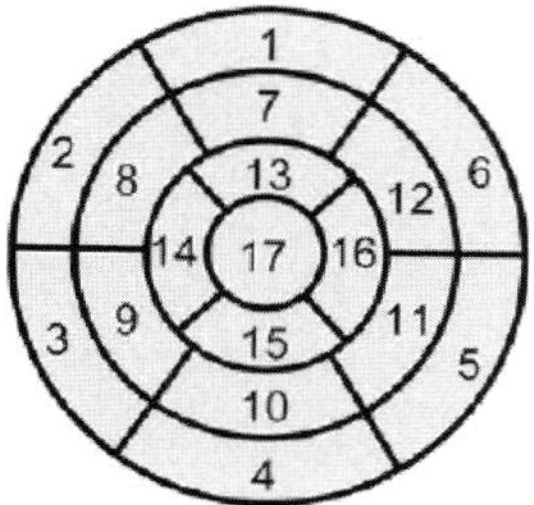


1) basal anterior
2) basal anteroseptal
3) basal inferoseptal
4) basal inferior
5) basal inferolateral
6) basal anterolateral
7) mid anterior
8) mid anteroseptal
9) mid inferoseptal
10) mid inferior
11) mid inferolateral
12) mid anterolateral
13) apical anterior
14) apical septal
15) apical inferior
16) apical lateral
17) apex

**Figure 9–6** Left ventricular segmentation. A polar plot demonstrating the 17 myocardial segments and the recommended nomenclature. (From Port SC. Imaging Guidelines for Nuclear Cardiology Procedures, Part 2. *J Nucl Cardiol* 1999;6:647–684, with permission of the American Society of Nuclear Cardiology.

## MYOCARDIAL PERFUSION IMAGING

Perfusion imaging is used to show relative regional myocardial blood flow during physiologic states of interest, usually during stress (exercise, pharmacologic) and at rest. The ideal perfusion tracer localizes to the myocardium in direct proportion to blood flow, such that tissue counts increase linearly as blood flow increases. In practice, only two perfusion tracers come close to exhibiting this linear relationship: technetium-99m teboroxime (SPECT imaging) and oxygen-15 water (PET imaging). The other tracers that are used for clinical SPECT and PET perfusion imaging exhibit progressively smaller increases in tissue uptake as blood flows increase above 2 mL/min per gram.

Perfusion imaging is used in clinical practice to detect coronary artery disease and to characterize its physiologic consequence. A summary of the various myocardial perfusion imaging protocols is given in Figure 9–7. In patients in whom exercise stress is not feasible, pharmacologic stress perfusion imaging is an acceptable alternative. As the severity of a coronary stenosis increases, the vessel loses its ability to increase blood flow in parallel with increases in tissue oxygen demand. In vascular territories supplied by a diseased artery, coronary flow reserve is impaired and a defect will be observed if images depicting myocardial perfusion during stress (exercise, hyperemia) are obtained. Unless the coronary stenosis is very severe, diseased vessels usually have a sufficient reserve to sustain blood flow during resting conditions, and perfusion images obtained in the basal state will not demonstrate a defect. *A reversible defect* (Table 9–1) is one that is present on stress images and not present on rest or redistribution images; it is the hallmark of stress-induced ischemia. Sometimes a coronary stenosis is severe enough to result in a perfusion defect if imaging is performed in a resting state. If a resting defect improves

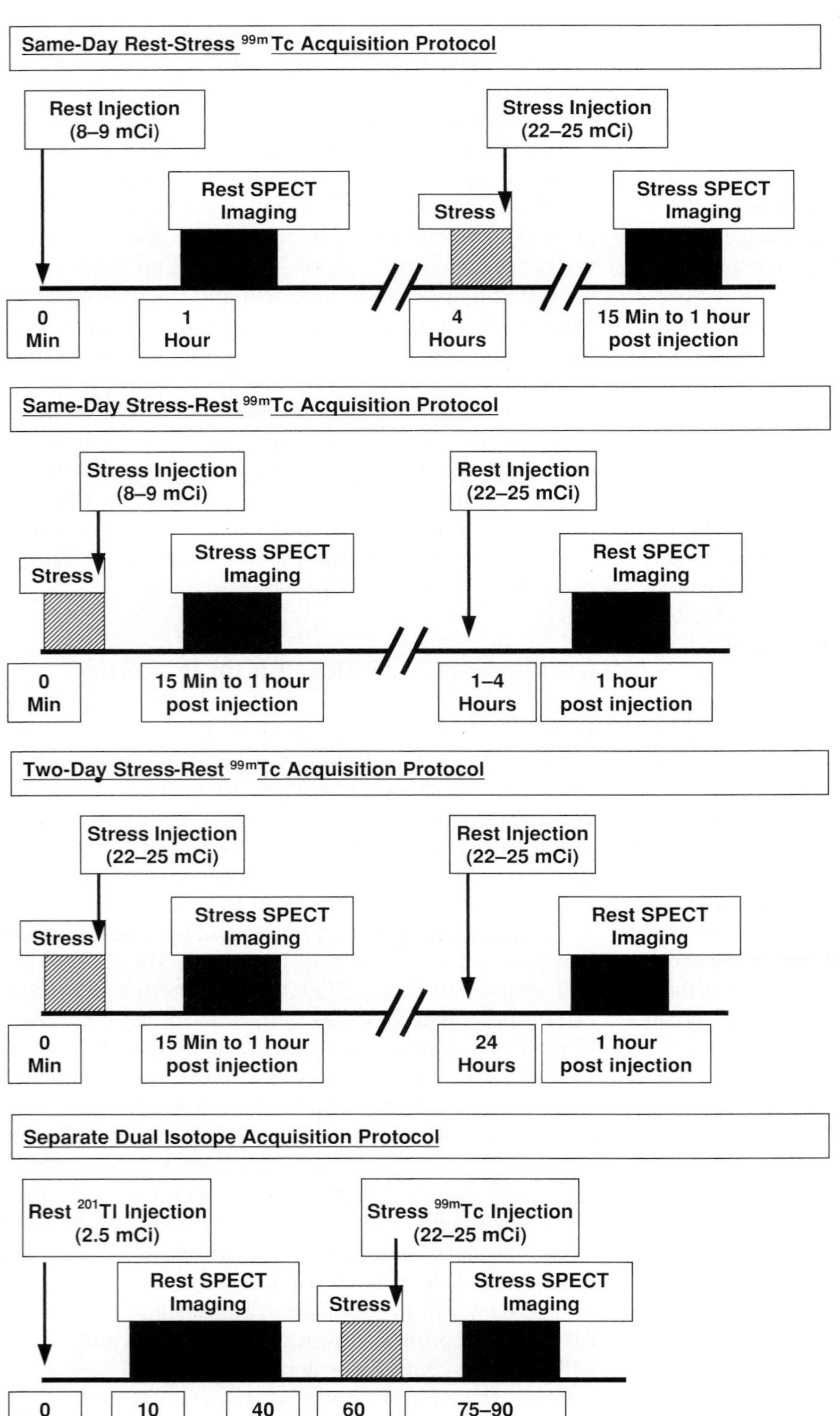


**Figure 9–7** Schematic summary of the various myocardial perfusion imaging protocols. (Adapted from DePuey EG. Updated Imaging Guidelines for Nuclear Cardiology Procedures, Part 1. *J Nucl Cardiology* 2001;8:641–646, with permission of the American Society of Nuclear Cardiology.)

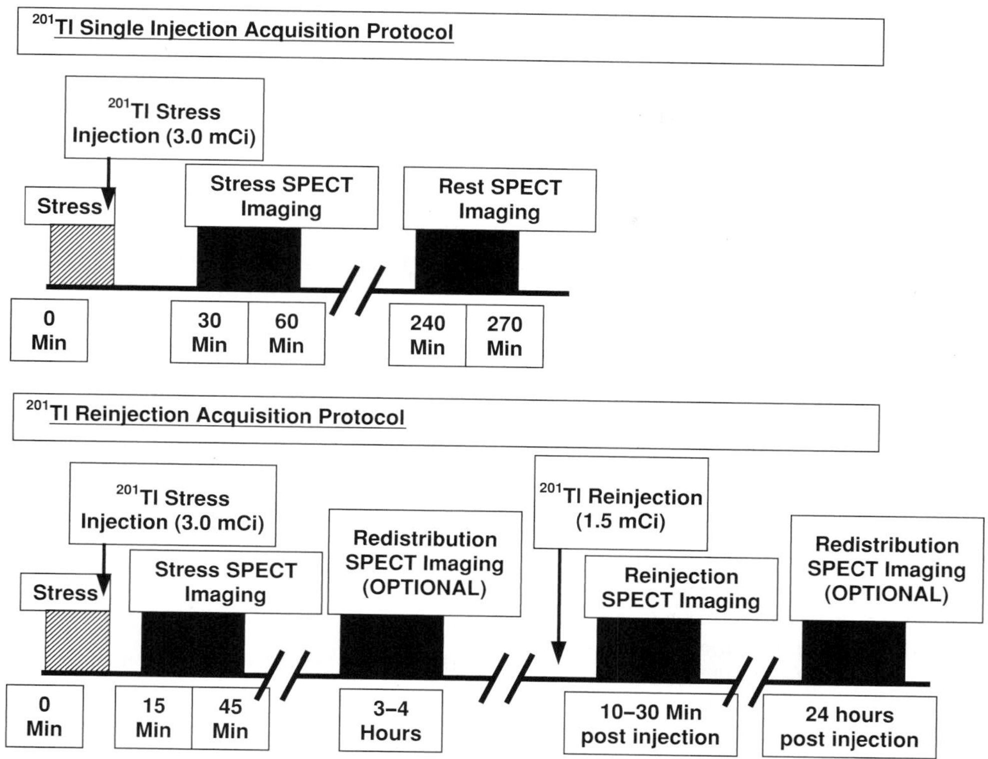


**Figure 9–7** *(continued)*

on redistribution or reinjection images, then the segment is viable and likely to benefit from revascularization.

In contrast, a perfusion defect that persists on both stress and rest or redistribution/reinjection images, *a fixed defect*, may reflect myocardial scar or myocardial hibernation. *Partially reversible defects* are stress defects that improve but do not normalize completely on rest or redistribution/reinjection images; these likely reflect nontransmural scar with superimposable ischemia. A defect is said to exhibit *reverse redistribution* if it is present on rest or redistribution images and is absent or much less prominent on stress images. Reverse redistribution has been identified in patients with multivessel coronary artery disease and in patients with acute myocardial infarction; it may reflect a differential wash-out of the perfusion tracer. Reverse redistribution may also reflect a technical artifact (oversubtraction of background activity on the rest/redistribution images).

**TABLE 9–1**
**DEFECT INTERPRETATION**

| Stress | Rest (or Early Redistribution) | Interpretation |
|---|---|---|
| Normal | Normal | Normal |
| Defect | Normal | Ischemia |
| Defect | Defect | Scar (or hibernation) |
| Normal | Defect | "Reverse redistribution" |

The specific coronary artery affected by a stenosis is inferred by the anatomic location of the perfusion defect. Typically, the left anterior descending artery supplies the anterior wall, anterior septum, and apex. When it is dominant, the right coronary artery usually supplies the inferior wall and the basal inferoseptum. The circumflex artery typically supplies the lateral wall when it is nondominant, and will additionally supply the inferior wall and basal inferoseptum when it is dominant (Fig. 9–8). Individual patient variations in the distribution of the coronary arteries do exist and may affect the patterns of myocardial perfusion identified on the nuclear images. In addition, observed perfusion patterns may be affected by the adequacy of coronary collaterals.

Myocardial perfusion imaging is utilized in clinical practice to identify coronary artery disease and to ascertain the physiologic significance of lesions of uncertain severity. It is used to stratify risk in patients following acute myocardial infarction and in patients with chronic coronary artery disease. The assessment of ventricular function from gated SPECT imaging provides incremental prognostic information beyond that provided by the pattern of myocardial perfusion alone. Myocardial perfusion imaging is also useful for risk stratification in patients prior to noncardiac surgical procedures, and in the follow-up of symptomatic patients

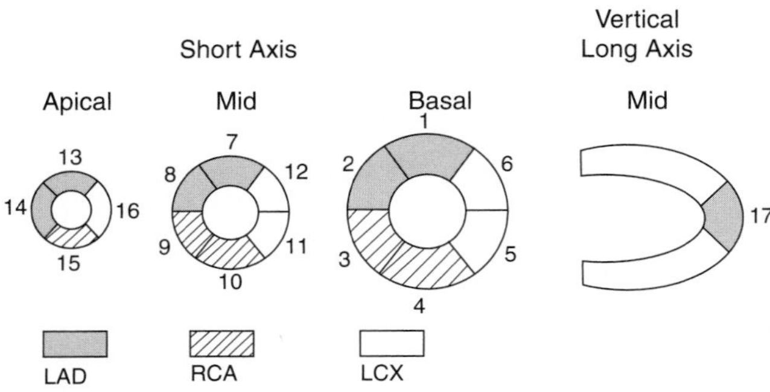


**Figure 9–8** Coronary artery territories. Assignment of the 17 myocardial segments to the territories of the left anterior descending (LAD), right coronary artery (RCA), and left circumflex coronary artery (LCX). (From Port SC. Imaging Guidelines for Nuclear Cardiology Procedures, Part 2. *J Nucl Cardiol* 1999;6:647–684, with permission of the American Society of Nuclear Cardiology.)

with prior percutaneous transluminal coronary angioplasty (PTCA) or coronary artery bypass grafts (CABG). It may also be useful for the differentiation of ischemic from nonischemic cardiomyopathies. In patients with ischemic cardiomyopathy, some have advocated late redistribution or reinjection imaging with thallium-201 to distinguish viable myocardium from scar.

## PET METABOLIC IMAGING FOR ASSESSING MYOCARDIAL VIABILITY

In patients with ischemic heart disease, the presence of tissue glucose metabolism in hypoperfused ventricular segments on PET metabolic imaging with FDG is a reliable marker of clinically important myocardial viability. This is manifest clinically by an improvement in regional contractile function in metabolically active myocardial segments following interventional restoration of blood flow. Ultimately, improvement in left ventricular ejection fraction and functional capacity are related to the anatomic extent and severity of the mismatch between perfusion and glucose metabolism on prerevascularization PET images. Individuals with the most extensive perfusion–metabolism mismatches derive the greatest functional benefit from revascularization. More simply, patients with evidence of FDG uptake in regions that have decreased uptake of perfusion tracers are more likely to regain myocardial function in the form of an improved ejection fraction.

## RADIONUCLIDE VENTRICULOGRAPHY

Two types of nuclear imaging are used to assess ventricular function. In *first-pass imaging*, high-temporal-resolution sequential (or *list mode*) images of the central circulation are obtained as the radioactive tracer is administered intravenously. A camera with a high count rate capability, (such as a multiwire camera) and a "tight" bolus of the radioactive tracer are required to achieve a high-quality study. Usually, first-pass images are acquired from either the anterior or the left anterior oblique projection. The images derived from a first-pass study depict the movement of the radioactivity through the heart's chambers with a sufficient temporal resolution to permit measurement of the left ventricular ejection fraction on a beat-to-beat basis. Measurements from 5 to 15 cardiac cycles are usually averaged to calculate the left ventricular ejection fraction (LVEF). The formula used to calculate the ejection fraction is

$$\text{LVEF} = \frac{(\text{end diastolic counts} - \text{end systolic counts})}{(\text{end diastolic counts})}$$

In this formula, end-diastolic and end-systolic counts represent the background-corrected counts in the left ventricle at end-diastole and end-systole, respectively.

First-pass studies may be used to assess the ventricular response to exercise stress. A tracer such as technetium-99m DTPA is employed, because the renal clearance of this radiopharmaceutical from the vascular space is rapid enough to permit sequential injections at baseline and during peak exercise stress. Counts in the right and left chambers of the heart are usually separated by a sufficiently long time interval so that it is possible to calculate both right and left ventricular ejection fractions at rest and with peak stress.

A second method of assessing ventricular performance is *gated radionuclide ventriculography* (multiple gated acquisition, or MUGA). In this technique, a radioactive tracer that remains in the vascular space, such as technetium-99m labeled red blood cells, is administered to the patient. Images over hundreds of cardiac cycles are then acquired, using the R wave of the patient's electrocardiogram as the timing marker for the computer's acquisition of the images. The nuclear medicine technologist first sets a "window," which instructs the computer on the length of the cardiac cycles that are to be accepted for imaging. Only cycles with the appropriate R–R intervals are incorporated into the imaging study, with rejection of shorter or longer cycles. Usually the R–R interval is divided into 16 to 24 frames of equal time duration. With each accepted cardiac cycle, counts from that portion of the cardiac cycle (each frame) are added to those of the corresponding frame from preceding cycles. Count data from about 400 to 600 cardiac cycles are allocated to 16 to 24 images representing different portions of the cardiac cycle. Once the acquisition is completed, the images are played in a continuous ciné loop to give a time-averaged estimate of ventricular function. The ejection fraction is calculated using background-corrected end-diastolic and end-systolic counts, employing the same formula as that for the first-pass studies. Unlike echocardiography, ejection fraction measurements made with this technique represent time-averaged values, and are not beat-to-beat measurements.

It is feasible to obtain gated images from differing projections (anterior, right anterior oblique, left anterior oblique, left lateral). In some centers, tomographic gated radionuclide ventriculography is performed. Visual estimates of chamber size and regional wall motion are obtained from the gated images. If there is a clinical need, gated images may also be obtained during intervention (stress, inotropic stimulation, sublingual nitroglycerin), to ascertain if there are regional or global differences in ventricular function elicited by the maneuver. A stable R–R interval is needed for gated radionuclide ventriculography. Patients with frequent ectopic beats, irregularly paced rhythms, and/or atrial fibrillation/flutter with an uncontrolled ventricular response rate benefit substantially by medical stabilization of the cardiac rhythm before referral for gated imaging.

Radionuclide ventriculography is used clinically to assess the severity of regional and global right and left ventricular dysfunction in both acute and chronic ischemic syndromes, and to determine the effect of medical or interventional treatments on cardiac function. In conjunction with exercise stress, radionuclide ventriculography can be utilized to determine the presence and extent of stress-induced ischemia. Both rest and stress ejection fraction measurements provide useful prognostic information to the clinician. Because ejection fraction measurements obtained with this imaging technique are count based and are not dependent on assumptions about the shape of the ventricle, they are highly reproducible if the imaging study is performed properly.

## RADIOACTIVE TRACERS FOR SPECT AND PET

Several different radioactive tracers are available to the nuclear cardiologist for clinical imaging. Each tracer has its own unique characteristics that may make it more or less suitable for a specific imaging task. Factors that influence the choice of tracer for the imaging study include: (a) whether SPECT or PET imaging is to be performed; (b) the physiologic property to be visualized (e.g., perfusion, metabolism, neuronal innervation); (c) the patient's body habitus; (d) the physical properties and the biologic behavior of the agent; and (e) the radiation dosimetry of the tracer. A brief overview of the radioactive tracers most frequently used for cardiac imaging in the United States is provided, to provide a basic understanding of the agents essential to the daily practice of nuclear cardiology.

### SPECT Perfusion Agents

The most commonly used SPECT tracers of myocardial perfusion are thallium-201, technetium-99m sestamibi, and technetium-99m tetrofosmin.

#### *Thallium-201*

Thallium-201 is a cationic, metallic element that is cyclotron produced. It has a relatively long physical half-life of 73 hours, compared to the 6-hour half-life of technetium-99m. It is administered intravenously as the chloride salt. Most of the photons emitted by thallium-201 are x-rays, with energies ranging from about 69 to 80 keV. Because the thallium-201 photons have lower energies than those of technetium-99m, they are more susceptible to scatter and attenuation by interposed tissue. Administered doses of thallium-201 are lower than those of the technetium-99m agents because of the radiation burden resulting from its longer half-life. Because of lower image counts, and lower photon energies, thallium-201 images may appear more "fuzzy" and less distinct than technetium-99m images.

Thallium-201 is a potassium analog. It enters the cardiac myocyte via the $Na^+/K^+$-ATPase pump in the cell membrane. Although thallium-201 uptake by the myocardium is directly proportional to blood flow at lower blood flows, the amount of the tracer that is retained in the tissue at higher flow rates underestimates actual tissue perfusion. This "roll-off" of the net tissue accumulation of the tracer at higher flows is common to all diffusible tracers; however, the "roll-off" begins at higher flow rates for thallium-201 than for technetium-99m-labeled agents, because of its greater first-pass extraction fraction.

One of the most important characteristics of thallium-201 is its property of redistribution. Following its intravenous administration, blood levels of thallium-201 peak very rapidly, and there is a concentration gradient of the tracer from the vascular space to inside the cell. Thallium-201 enters the cell, and then leaves the cell to go back into the circulation again as vascular tracer concentrations decline. For myocardial regions with lower flows at stress (a perfusion defect), the flux of the tracer into and out of the area is slower than in normally perfused tissue. As a consequence, initial images demonstrate a perfusion defect that appears to "fill in" or redistribute on delayed images. For areas with profound ischemia, there may be a defect even on the resting images, which fills in on delayed images or on images obtained following the reinjection of a "booster" dose of thallium-201. The implication of redistribution on delayed or reinjection images is that there is viable tissue in the myocardial region. This property is exploited for viability imaging with thallium-201 (described earlier).

#### *Technetium-99m-Labeled Agents*

The most commonly used technetium-99m-labeled agents are technetium-99m sestamibi and technetium-99m tetrofosmin. These agents may be prepared on site via kits using technetium-99m eluted from a molybdenum-99 generator, or are also generally available as prepared unit doses from commercial radiopharmacies.

Use of a technetium-99m-labeled tracer results in better image quality than use of thallium-201 because the higher-energy, monochromatic, 140-keV photons are less subject to scatter and attenuation than those of thallium-201. In addition, the short physical half-life of 6 hours permits the administration of significantly higher activity doses than thallium-201. The higher count rates achievable with the larger doses result in better image quality, and allow the acquisition of images gated to the patient's electrocardiogram. However, the extraction fractions of technetium-99m sestamibi and technetium-99m tetrofosmin (0.45 to 0.60) are lower than that of thallium-201. Therefore, net myocardial uptake of these tracers begins to plateau ("roll off") at lower flow rates than with thalium-201.

These lipid-soluble cationic compounds are retained within the myocardium predominantly by selective sequestration within the mitochondria of viable cells, because of the large negative transmembrane potential. Unlike thallium-201, technetium-99m sestamibi and technetium-99m tetrofosmin have minimal redistribution. As a result, these tracers are well suited for imaging of acute chest pain. Activity administered during chest pain can be imaged at a later time point and still accurately depict the pattern of perfusion at the time the tracer was administered.

## PET Tracers of Myocardial Perfusion

The most commonly used perfusion tracers for cardiac PET imaging are rubidium-82 chloride, nitrogen-13 ammonia, and oxygen-15 water. Important distinctions exist among these agents in their means of production, myocardial uptake, and physical half-lives.

### *Rubidium-82*

Rubidium-82 is an element with biologic properties similar to potassium. It is eluted directly off of a portable bedside strontium generator as the chloride salt. This obviates the need for an on-site cyclotron to do PET perfusion imaging. The physical half-life of rubidium-82 is 76 seconds. Uptake by the cardiac myocyte is predominantly via membrane-bound $Na^+/K^+$-ATPase. Clearance from the blood pool is prompt, and generally results in high-quality images. Like some other perfusion tracers, net myocardial uptake of rubidium-82 plateaus at higher myocardial blood flows.

### *Nitrogen-13 Ammonia*

Nitrogen-13 ammonia is a perfusion agent that is produced via a cyclotron, and because of its short half-life of 10 minutes, it must be produced on site. In the vascular space, there is a dynamic equilibrium between $^{13}NH_4^+$ and $^{13}NH_3$ and hydrogen ion. $^{13}NH_3$ diffuses across the membrane, and is trapped intracellularly via the glutamine synthetase reaction. Like rubidium-82, net myocardial uptake of nitrogen-13 ammonia also decreases at higher blood flows. It has a high single-pass extraction fraction and long tissue retention, which permits ECG-gated image acquisition.

### *Oxygen-15 Water*

Oxygen-15 is also cyclotron produced, and its short half-life of 2.1 minutes requires it to be produced on site. Unlike rubidium-82 and nitrogen-13 ammonia, it is freely diffusible. The fact that it is diffusible means that it is not rapidly cleared from the systemic circulation, image quality is lower because of relatively high background activity, and the images need to be corrected for vascular activity. However, the property of free diffusibility lends it a unique and important property. Net myocardial uptake of the tracer increases nearly linearly with increasing blood flow, and the tissue retention of the tracer is largely independent of tissue metabolism.

## PET Tracers of Myocardial Metabolism

Radiopharmaceuticals play an important role in distinguishing between viable and nonviable myocardium in patients with impaired left ventricular function. The most commonly used PET agent for this purpose is [$^{18}$F]-2-fluoro-2-deoxyglucose (FDG). (Other, less commonly used, metabolic PET agents include $^{11}$C-palmitate and $^{11}$C-acetate.) FDG is a glucose analog that enters the cardiac myocyte by facilitated transport. Once within the cell, it competes with glucose for the enzyme hexokinase. FDG is phosphorylated to FDG-6-phosphate, which is then trapped within the cardiac myocytes and not further metabolized. FDG imaging is utilized with perfusion imaging to identify myocardium that is normal (with normal uptake of both the FDG and the perfusion tracer), hibernating (defect on the perfusion images, with preserved uptake of FDG), or scarred (defect on the perfusion images with matching defect on the FDG metabolic images).

## BIBLIOGRAPHY

**Beller GA, Bergmann SR.** Myocardial perfusion imaging agents: SPECT and PET. *J Nucl Cardiol.*2004;11:71–86.

**Cerqueira MD, Weissman NJ, Dilsizian V, et al.** Standardized myocardial segmentation and nomenclature for tomographic imaging of the heart: a statement for healthcare professionals from the Cardiac Imaging Committee of the Council on Clinical Cardiology of the American Heart Association. *J Nucl Cardiol.* 2002;9:240–245.

**Chandra R.** *Nuclear Medicine Physics: The Basics.* Baltimore: Williams & Wilkins; 1998:xvi:182.

**Dilsizian V, Narula J.** *Atlas of Nuclear Cardiology.* Philadelphia: Current Medicine; 2003:ix:243.

**Heller GV, Hendel R.** *Nuclear Cardiology: Practical Applications.* New York: McGraw-Hill; 2004:xiii:369, [16] of plates.

Imaging guidelines for nuclear cardiology procedures, part 2. American Society of Nuclear Cardiology. *J Nucl Cardiol.* 1999;6: 647–648.

**Iskandrian AE, Verani MS.** *Nuclear Cardiac Imaging: Principles and Applications.*Oxford, New York: Oxford University Press; 2003:xiii:511, [16] of plates.

**Travin MI, Bergmann SR.** Assessment of myocardial viability. *Semin Nucl Med.* 2005;35:2–16.

Updated imaging guidelines for nuclear cardiology procedures, part 1. *J Nucl Cardiol.* 2001;8:G5–G58.

## QUESTIONS

1. Which of the following statements is *not* true?
   a. Collimator selection for a gamma camera reflects a trade-off between spatial resolution and efficiency.
   b. Photons that pass through the collimator and strike the imaging crystal produce visible light that is then converted to electrical current and amplified by photomultiplier tubes.
   c. By setting a more narrow energy window around the isotope's photopeak, one can increase the sensitivity of a camera to include more scattered photons.
   d. Planar images are typically obtained from several fixed views, whereas SPECT images are obtained from multiple projections that are then reconstructed.

Answer is c: The purpose for setting a narrow energy window around the photopeak of an isotope is to exclude lower-energy photons, which are more likely to be photons that have been scattered and thus lost some of their energy. In doing so, some of the true photons are also excluded, thus decreasing the sensitivity.

2. Assuming comparable biologic behavior, which of the following combinations of gamma-emitting isotopes and administered activity doses would result in the lowest absorbed dose of radiation to a patient?
   a. Short half-life, high dose
   b. Long half-life, high dose
   c. Short half-life, low dose
   d. Long half-life, low dose

Answer is c: Assuming comparable biologic behavior for the gamma-emitting isotopes, the lower the administered dose, the lower the exposure, thus excluding choices a and b. For the same dose, the isotope with the shorter half-life will result in a lower absorbed dose of radiation because of the shorter duration of exposure.

3. Assuming a "right dominant" coronary artery distribution, match each of the ventricular segments (from the standard 17-segment model) with its most likely corresponding coronary arterial distribution.
   (1) Basal anterior
   (2) Basal anteroseptal
   (3) Basal inferoseptal
   (4) Basal inferior
   (5) Basal inferolateral
   (6) Basal anterolateral
   (7) Mid anterior
   (8) Mid anterseptal
   (9) Mid inferoseptal
   (10) Mid inferior
   (11) Mid inferolateral
   (12) Mid anterolateral
   (13) Apical anterior
   (14) Apical septal
   (15) Apical inferior
   (16) Apical lateral
   (17) Apex
   a. Left anterior descending
   b. Right coronary artery
   c. Circumflex

Answers:
a. (1), (2), (7), (8), (13), (14), (17)
b. (3), (4), (9), (10), (15)
c. (5), (6), (11), (12), (16)

4. Given the following simplified count data obtained during radionuclide ventriculography, what is the ejection fraction?

   End-diastolic counts = 1,000
   End-systolic counts = 650

   a. 54%
   b. 65%
   c. 35%
   d. 30%

Answer is c: 35%, because LVEF = (end-diastolic counts – end-systolic counts)/(end-diastolic counts) = (1,000 – 650)/(1,000) = (350)/(1,000) = 0.35, or 35%.

5. Match the following combinations of stress and rest imaging findings with the appropriate interpretation:

| | Stress | Rest | Interpretation |
|---|---|---|---|
| a. | Defect | Normal | (i) Scar (or hibernation) |
| b. | Defect | Defect | (ii) Normal |
| c. | Normal | Defect | (iii) Ischemia |
| d. | Normal | Normal | (iv) Reverse redistribution |

Answers: a. (iii); b. (i); c. (iv); d. (ii)

# Coronary Artery Disease

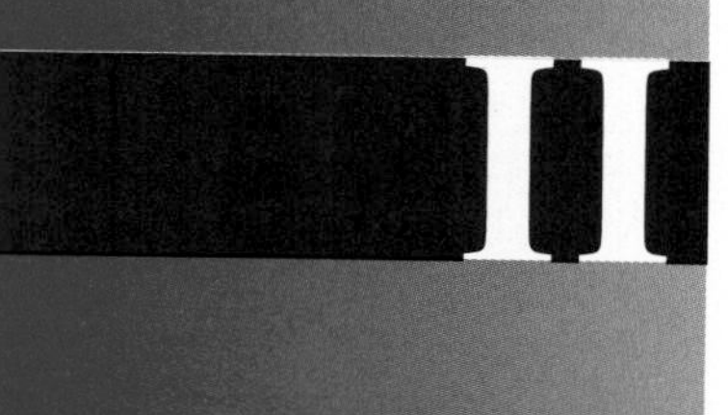

10

# Eval[illegible]on of Chest [illegible]nfort

[illegible]aib Donald A. Underwood

Chest pain or discomfort is a common complaint in the outpatient clinic, a common reason for admission from the Emergency Department, and a common occurrence on hospital floors and intensive care units (ICUs). The evaluation of chest discomfort, acute or chronic, is directed by the patient history, the physical examination, and the clinical scenario. The differential diagnosis should remain foremost in the clinician's mind during the evaluation, with the more life-threatening problems initially excluded and the underlying diagnosis ultimately clarified. What follows is an overview of the evaluation of chest discomfort.

## DIFFERENTIAL DIAGNOSIS

The differential diagnosis for chest discomfort can be divided into those diseases that cause acute chest discomfort and those that cause more subacute or chronic syndromes. Further, the causes of acute chest discomfort can be further subdivided into those syndromes that are urgent, life-threatening problems requiring immediate recognition and treatment, and those that warrant a more measured approach.

The acute, life-threatening problems in the differential diagnosis include acute myocardial infarction, acute aortic dissection, pulmonary embolism, spontaneous pneumothorax, and esophageal rupture. The acute coronary syndromes, including coronary spasm, should also be included in this differential, as those patients with non–ST-segment-elevation myocardial infarction are at high risk for ventricular dysrhythmias. Furthermore, hypertrophic obstructive cardiomyopathy with symptomatic obstruction, symptomatic aortic stenosis, and thoracic aortic aneurysm should also be considered in this group. These syndromes are each very different, and their successful recognition and treatment should likewise be individualized (Table 10–1).

Among the problems in the differential that may cause acute symptoms, but may not be life threatening in the near term, there are a variety of cardiac and noncardiac causes of chest discomfort. Acute pericarditis and myocarditis may cause oppressive symptoms with relatively acute onset. Pulmonary hypertension causing chronic cor pulmonale may be of more insidious onset, but can have acute symptoms superimposed. Pneumonia with pleuritis or pleuritis associated with other inflammatory illnesses can cause acute progressive chest discomfort, often exacerbated with inspiration or cough. Gastroesophageal disease such as reflux disease, peptic ulcer disease, and esophageal spasm may cause chest discomfort syndromes that may mimic angina pectoris. A variety of musculoskeletal injuries and inflammatory processes may cause chest wall pain syndromes of acute onset. All of these, while important causes of chest discomfort, are less critical in their clinical course and should therefore be pursued only after the acute, emergent diagnoses have been excluded.

Of the more chronic causes of chest discomfort, chronic stable angina may head the list of episodic discomfort, while more persistent symptoms may arise with chronic cor pulmonale due to chronic venous thromboembolic disease, severe underlying lung disease, and rheumatologic disease. These syndromes are typically addressed initially in the outpatient setting and may often be worked up on an outpatient basis. In any venue and across the range of symptom chronicity, in the majority of cases, the history and physical examination suggest the diagnosis.

**TABLE 10–1**
**CAUSES OF ACUTE CHEST DISCOMFORT**

| | | |
|---|---|---|
| Critical syndromes: | Acute myocardial infarction<br>Acute coronary syndromes<br>Acute aortic dissection<br>Thoracic aortic aneurysm<br>Critical aortic stenosis | HCM with obstruction<br>Pulmonary embolism<br>Spontaneous pneumothora<br>Boerhaave syndrome |
| Stable syndromes: | Pericarditis<br>Myocarditis<br>Mitral stenosis<br>Pulmonary hypertension<br>Pleuritis | Pneumonia<br>Gastroesophageal reflux disease<br>Esophageal spasm<br>Pancreatitis and biliary disease<br>Musculoskeletal syndromes |

## HISTORY

The evaluation should begin with a clinical history focusing on the characteristics of the discomfort. The location, quality, radiation, severity, timing, plaintive and palliative factors, context, and associated symptoms should be carefully and thoroughly documented. These syndrome attributes will form the basis of the physical examination, and inform the near-future decisions regarding further diagnostic studies. Further, the patient's background medical, social, and family histories, as well as medication history, are critical to an understanding of the patient's overall risk for acute and chronic disease processes under consideration.

## LOCATION

The location of the discomfort can suggest a specific diagnosis, or can help differentiate between chest wall and visceral organ pathology. Because the organs of the chest develop from the embryologic viscera, the innervation of the organ tissue can only loosely associate the inflamed tissue with a cutaneous distribution; as is the case with abdominal pain, inflammation or injury within the organs of the chest can cause diffuse or nonfocal discomfort. In fact, the term "chest pain" is often too specific a moniker for patients, and they will deny "chest pain" in favor of other, less specific sensations. Asking about chest "distress or disquiet" often leads to a story of typical angina pectoris when chest "pains" had been denied. In contrast, focal pains can be localized more consistently when they involve the parietal pleura or the chest wall itself. These structures have cutaneous dermatomal innervation, with inflammation or injury more commonly causing focal pain. Eliciting a careful description of the location of the pain or discomfort is critical to the overall assessment of the syndrome.

## QUALITY

The quality of the sensation is, as stated above, important in identifying the involvement of the viscera of the chest, or the chest wall. Is there pain or pressure? Heaviness o burning? These are typical complaints associated with visceral inflammation or injury. However, they are not specific to a particular organ tissue. The "squeezing" of myocardial ischemia may be perceived no differently than the "squeezing" sensation of esophageal spasm or pulmonary hypertension. Likewise, pleuritic pain, a sharp stabbing sensation often exacerbated by breathing or certain positioning, is no different than the perception of pericardial inflammation. Aortic dissection may cause a writhing, tearing, or stabbing sensation that is maximally intense at the onset and inescapable with different positioning, but has no variation with respiration. The quality of the discomfort contributes to the clinician's overall picture of the syndrome.

## RADIATION

Although chest discomfort is often localized to one single spot or generalized area, it may be described as "radiating" or migrating to another location. The discomfort of angina pectoris is often described as radiating to the arms or shoulders, the neck or jaw, or the back. In contrast, the pain of aortic dissection is classically described as tearing through to the back and migrating with the dissection. The pain of pulmonary embolism may cause diffuse, nonspecific tightness or heaviness (likely due to acute RV strain), evolving with time to include a focal pleural component representative of inflammation in the parietal pleura apposed to the infarcted lung tissue. This may felt to be "radiation" of pain or simply a separate component of the syndrome.

## SEVERITY

The severity of symptoms can provide the clinician an indication as to the severity of the underlying pathology. Likert pain scales are often used for patient self-assessment of pain severity and are helpful in following the patient's response to therapy, especially with acute coronary compared to the intensity and timing of their peak level of discomfort in acute chest discomfort syndromes. In more chronic syndromes, severity assessment may be helpful in following the progression of the disease.

## TIMING

The physician should make careful note of the symptom complex initial time of onset of, and the timing of the appearance of new symptoms as they occurred prior to presentation. The duration of symptoms may help differentiate acute ischemic injury or infarction with hours of persistent symptoms from an episode of unstable angina lasting 25 minutes. Furthermore, the duration of symptoms can be an important factor in the decision to administer certain therapies such as pharmacologic thrombolysis in acute myocardial infarction or pulmonary embolism.

## PLAINTIVE AND PALLIATIVE FACTORS

An assessment of the modifying factors of the primary complaint may in some cases help inform the diagnosis. Palliation of symptoms with medication such as nitroglycerin or resolution of symptoms with rest, discontinuation of strenuous activity, or changing position (sitting up, resulting in reduced preload and oxygen need) may suggest an anginal picture. Esophageal spasm is also thought to be palliated with nitroglycerin. Conversely, in acute coronary syndromes, pulmonary embolism, and chronic stable angina, exertion tends to be plaintive. So, while it is important to know what the patient has found to be palliative in his or her discomfort syndrome, it also helps to know what maneuvers may have exacerbated the symptoms.

## CONTEXT

The symptom context can assist in differentiating acute musculoskeletal injuries from unstable coronary syndromes. Sudden symptoms waking a patient from sleep at 4 A.M. may be more suggestive of an acute coronary syndrome than of a chest wall injury, whereas symptoms occurring while shoveling snow may be less clearly differentiated. Within the context of the occurrence of the symptoms should be an exploration of whether the patient has ever suffered a similar syndrome in the past. If the symptoms are recurrent, any previous studies performed to further evaluate the syndrome may be an invaluable resource. If the symptoms are novel, then more aggressive evaluation may be warranted.

## ASSOCIATED SYMPTOMS

A thorough exploration of associated symptoms with chest discomfort onset may help guide clinical decision making. Chest discomfort with associated dyspnea, nausea, vomiting, or diaphoresis may suggest significant autonomic and adrenergic activation, consistent with myocardial ischemia. Sudden presyncopal symptoms or frank syncope may be more concerning for ischemia-induced arrhythmias or critical aortic stenosis. Again, severity and duration of the symptoms as well as modifying factors may further clarify the picture of the larger syndrome.

## MEDICAL HISTORY

An exploration of the patient's prior medical history must be done and may help identify underlying risk factors for the various disease states under consideration. Risk factors for coronary artery disease, including patient age, presence of hypertension, hyperlipidemia, diabetes, peripheral vascular disease, history of prior myocardial infarction, cerebrovascular accident or transient ischemic attacks, all increase the likelihood of the presenting syndrome being attributable to coronary disease or acute aortic pathology. A history of estrogen use, hypercoagulable state, smoking, immobilization, or recent surgery may all point toward venous thromboembolic disease as an underlying cause of presenting symptoms.

## SOCIAL, FAMILY, AND MEDICATION HISTORY

Risk factors such as tobacco use, cocaine use, and even herbal supplement use, as in the case of ephedrine, may be helpful in further evaluating an acute chest discomfort syndrome. In addition, an assessment of the patient's family history may reveal a strong familial history of early coronary events, or aortic pathology as in the case of Marfan syndrome.

Medication history is important in assessing the new patient with chest discomfort. Medical compliance history in addition to the medications themselves and their dosing schedule may contribute to the clinical scenario, for example, a patient with chest discomfort and hypertension who was taking high-dose clonidine but ran out of medication. Rebound phenomena with $\alpha$- and $\beta$-antagonists may be active issues.

## PHYSICAL EXAMINATION

The physical examination should focus on findings supporting the diagnostic question and assess the suitability of any required invasive procedure. The head and neck examination should include assessment of the carotid pulses for their symmetry and quality of upstroke. The jugular veins should be observed for distention suggestive of volume overload, and normal a, c, and v waves. The cardiovascular exam should be sensitive to findings consistent with the differential diagnostic acute chest discomfort possibilities under consideration.

The pulmonary examination should assess for the presence of rales suggestive of fluid overload, but also for symmetric air movement in both lungs, tracheal shift from the midline, dullness to percussion suggestive of pleural effusion, or a cardiac border percussed lateral to the apex suggesting effusion. A complete (carotid, brachial, radial, femoral, popliteal, and dorsalis pedis/posterior tibialis pulsations) survey of the peripheral vasculature should be conducted to assess symmetry of the pulse. Any bruits should be documented, as the presence of bruits in the periphery may help inform the choice of vessel for arterial access if a left heart catheterization is needed. More important, bruits raise the likelihood of coronary insufficiency as the cause of the acute chest discomfort.

The extremities should be examined for edema, evidence of chronic venous stasis, cellulitis, vascular ulcerations, cords, or Homan's sign. Evidence of differential swelling or other signs hinting at the presence of deep venous thrombosis may give clues as to the etiology of the chest discomfort syndrome. Furthermore, an adequate neurologic examination is critical to establish baseline neurologic deficits that may be associated with the chest discomfort syndrome. The use of agents such as sedatives, opiate analgesics, and, more important, thrombolytics may be complicated by alterations in neurologic status.

## WORK-UP

The pace of the diagnostic evaluation is determined by the clinician's index of suspicion for critical acute chest disease. Chronic stable syndromes may be evaluated on an outpatient basis with diagnostic studies to rule out symptomatic obstructive coronary artery disease, gastroesophageal disease, peptic ulcer disease, and chronic lung, pericardial, or neuromuscular disease.

In the Emergency Department, patients presenting with acute chest discomfort are typically evaluated with an electrocardiogram (ECG) and chest x-ray. Critical evaluation of the ECG for evidence of myocardial ischemia, injury, or infarction should be conducted. A chest x-ray should be closely reviewed to assess for the presence of acute parenchymal or mediastinal changes. Serial cardiac markers and observation on telemetry may be performed in "chest pain" or clinical observation units in patients at low risk for acute coronary syndromes. After an appropriate observation period, if the biomarkers and ECG remain negative for evidence of coronary insufficiency, patients may undergo further risk stratification for coronary artery disease through exercise testing prior to discharge. Negative laboratory values and exercise stress testing during close observation is reassuring that the syndrome is unlikely to be attributable to coronary insufficiency, and an evaluation for other, less ominous causes of the chest discomfort syndrome can be pursued on an outpatient basis.

Patients at higher risk for acute coronary syndrome (ACS) should be treated more aggressively, with admission to the hospital and therapeutic anticoagulation, *if not contraindicated*. If suggested by the history and physical examination, ventilation/perfusion scan or helical computed tomography to rule out pulmonary embolism should be performed. Computed tomography or a transesophageal echocardiogram may be performed to assess for the presence of aortic aneurysm or dissection.

## SPECIAL CIRCUMSTANCES

"Atypical chest pain" is a term used to describe a syndrome of discomfort that does not follow the classically described pattern of discomfort attributable to coronary insufficiency. The pretest risk is uncertain based on symptoms, with the clinical risk-factor profile becoming important coupled with the physical examination.

Coronary disease with atypical symptoms occurs more commonly in women and in diabetics, and may be more difficult to recognize. Furthermore, the less common causes of chest discomfort, including the less common causes of myocardial ischemia, are more prevalent in women than in men. The presence of diabetes in women presenting with atypical chest discomfort appears to be the most predictive risk factor for angiographically evident coronary artery disease, arguing that these patients should be treated more aggressively and with a high clinical suspicion for ACS than the less typical symptoms might dictate.

## COCAINE-ASSOCIATED CHEST DISCOMFORT

Cocaine use is a commonly encountered comorbidity in patients presenting to the emergency department with acute chest discomfort. The initial evaluation of these patients proceeds in similar fashion to others presenting with similar complaints, save for the recognition that these patients have a higher risk for ACS and myocardial infarction. These patients are often younger and have fewer risk factors for coronary artery disease than those not using cocaine. They are at higher risk due to the increased incidence of accelerated atherosclerotic disease associated with cocaine use plus the increased incidence of coronary vasospasm. In the absence of ECG evidence of ongoing myocardial injury, cocaine-associated chest discomfort should be treated aggressively, similar to an ACS, with antianginals and antiplatelet and antithrombotic therapy until the discomfort is resolved and myocardial infarction has been excluded. One caveat in the treatment of cocaine-associated chest discomfort is that the use of $\beta$-antagonists without $\alpha$-antagonist activity is contraindicated because of the risk of a profound hypertensive response in the setting of unopposed $\alpha$-activity.

## VARIANT OR "PRINZMETAL" ANGINA

A small subset of patients with apparently ischemic chest discomfort and known angiographically normal coronaries suffer from transient vasospastic coronary obstruction. Patients who use tobacco, cocaine, or have other vasospastic syndromes such as Raynaud phenomenon or vascular headaches are at higher risk for variant angina. Patients present with typical anginal symptoms and ECG changes suggestive of acute injury, occurring at rest or with stress and resolving with nitrates and/or calcium antagonist therapy. Patients with recurrent episodes but without ECG changes often need provocative testing in the catheterization laboratory to confirm the diagnosis. Intracoronary *ergonovine* can reproduce the spasm and symptoms experienced by these patients. These patients frequently respond to therapy with long-acting nitrates and calcium antagonists, though higher than usual doses are often needed.

## SUMMARY

The evaluation of chest discomfort syndromes requires the performance of a careful history and physical examination with a focus on risk factors, signs, and symptoms indicative of critical pathology. Some basic laboratory studies and testing may guide the physician toward the diagnosis or help to rule out acute life-threatening syndromes. The pace of the evaluation is determined by the acuity of the clinical scenario and the clinical venue. In the absence of an acute syndrome, risk stratification for the presence of coronary artery disease is commonly undertaken, and further evaluation ensues.

## BIBLIOGRAPHY

**Bugiardini R, Bairey Merz CN.** Angina with "normal" coronary arteries: a changing philosophy. *JAMA.* 2005;293:477–484.

**Douglas PS, Ginsburg GS.** The evaluation of chest pain in women. *N Engl J Med.* 1996;334:1311–1315.

**Hollander JE.** The management of cocaine-associated myocardial ischemia. *N Engl J Med.* 1995;333:1267–1272.

**Lee TH, Goldman L.** Evaluation of the patient with acute chest pain. *N Engl J Med.* 2000;342:1187–1195.

# Coronary Artery Disease: Demographics and Incidence

11

***Taral N. Patel   Deepak L. Bhatt***

## GLOBAL BURDEN

It is widely acknowledged that cardiovascular diseases (CVDs) became the leading cause of mortality and a major cause of morbidity in adults worldwide over the course of the 20th century. Of these diseases, coronary artery or coronary heart disease (CAD) is the single most common cause, accounting for well over 40% of all CVD-related death. The World Health Organization (WHO) Global Burden of Disease (GBD) project estimates that >7 million deaths were attributable to CAD in 2002. More than 5.8 million new cases of CAD are added yearly. In order to further define the societal effects, the GBD designed a new measure to capture the effect of years of life lost as a result of both premature death and disability. This metric is termed the *disability-adjusted life-year* or DALY and reflects a year of healthy life lost to disease. In 2002, CAD accounted for the loss of nearly 59 million DALYs worldwide, making it the third leading cause overall, behind HIV/AIDs and depression (Table 11–1).

### Global Temporal Trends in Coronary Artery Disease

Great strides were made in the latter half of the 20th century in the identification and management of traditional risk factors and in the therapeutics and management of acute coronary events, to combat the rising tide of coronary disease. These efforts resulted in dramatic reductions in coronary event rates and CAD-related mortality, mostly in developed countries such as those of Northern Europe. Between the mid-1980s and the mid-1990s, coronary event rates decreased roughly 23% in women and 25% in men, while CAD-related mortality decreased 34% in women and 42% in men. One third of this reduction in CAD disease burden is attributable to improved therapeutics, whereas two-thirds is attributed to better identification and management of risk factors, leading to a decrease in acute coronary event rates.

Despite these improvements, the trend has been reversed and we are currently in the midst of a dramatic resurgence in CAD morbidity and mortality. Between 1990 and 2020, worldwide CAD mortality is expected to increase 100% in men and 80% in women. The majority of that increase is expected to occur in the developing world, where rates of CAD mortality are expected to increase 137% in men and 120% in women, whereas in developed countries the increases are a bit more modest, 48% in men and 29% in women. In terms of DALYs lost, the expected rise is nearly 40%, from 59 to 82 million. The reasons for this reversal are manifold. Reductions in mortality from infectious diseases and malnutrition paired with economic prosperity have lead to longer life spans. Along with these changes, modernization and industrialization have led to a decrease in physical activity and consumption of a high-fat, high-calorie diet. All of these factors have contributed to rising rates of obesity, diabetes, and lipid disorders and thus, along with cigarette smoking, to the inexorable rise of CAD.

**TABLE 11–1**
**WORLDWIDE BURDEN OF CAD AND CVD, 2000**

| | AFR | AMR | EUR | SEAR | WPR | EMR | World |
|---|---|---|---|---|---|---|---|
| | | | **Mortality in thousands** | | | | |
| CAD | 333 | 967 | 2,423 | 1,972 | 963 | 523 | 7,181 |
| Rheumatic | 29 | 111 | 34 | 132 | 108 | 24 | 338 |
| Other CVD | 227 | 352 | 845 | 407 | 380 | 152 | 2,363 |
| All CVDs | 985 | 1,980 | 5,042 | 3,797 | 3,745 | 1,037 | 16,585 |
| | | | **Societal Impact in millions of DALYs** | | | | |
| CAD | 3.26 | 6.51 | 16.00 | 20.24 | 7.37 | 5.35 | 58.72 |
| Rheumatic | 0.76 | 0.16 | 0.43 | 2.56 | 1.61 | 0.58 | 6.11 |
| Other CVD | 2.69 | 2.57 | 4.88 | 5.75 | 2.70 | 2.20 | 20.79 |
| All CVDs | 11.36 | 15.14 | 34.14 | 41.53 | 30.51 | 11.79 | 144.47 |

CAD, coronary artery disease; CVD, cardiovascular disease; AFR, Africa; AMR, America; EUR, Europe; SEAR, South East Asia region; WPR, Western Pacific region; EMR, Eastern Mediterranean region; DALY, disability = adjusted life-years.
Data obtained from the World Health Organization, with permission.

## BURDEN IN THE UNITED STATES

Coronary artery disease remains the most common manifestation of atherosclerotic CVD and the single most common cause of adult death in the United States, accounting for one of every five, and, in people over the age of 35 years, one of every three (Figs. 11–1 and 11–2, and Table 11–2). According to the American Heart Association, 494,382 people lost their lives to CAD in 2002, many at the peak of their productive lives. Currently, >13 million people are afflicted with this disease, with 1.2 million additional cases of myocardial infarction and/or fatal CAD in 2002. Of this number, 700,000 represent new cases, whereas 500,000 are recurrent. Approximately 865,000 people per year suffered a myocardial infarction (MI) from 1987 to 2000, 565,000 per year being new cases. Only 20% of MIs are accompanied by pre-existing stable angina. In 2002, 400,000 new cases of stable angina were added. Not included in these figures is the rate of silent MI, estimated at 175,000 new cases yearly. In terms of societal impact, CAD accounted for the loss of roughly 6.5 million DALYs in 2002, while the estimated average number of years of life lost due to MI is 11.5. It is the leading cause of premature permanent disability, accounting for 19% of Social Security disability outlays.

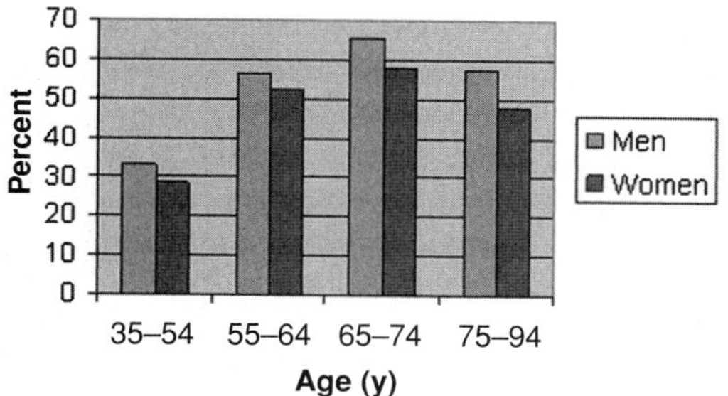


**Figure 11–1** Proportion of CVD as CAD by age and sex, from Framingham Study, 26-year follow-up. Lerner DJ, Kannel WB. Patterns of coronary heart disease mortality in the sexes: a 26-year follow-up of the Framingham population. *Am Heart J* 1986;111:383–390.

### Unrecognized and Silent Myocardial Ischemia and Infarction

The estimated prevalence of asymptomatic significant CAD that is detectable by stress testing or ambulatory ECG is 2% to 4% in the United States. Silent ischemia is actually the most common manifestation of clinically significant CAD, even more so than angina. The prevalence of silent myocardial ischemia in men with two or more traditional coronary risk factors (smoking, hyperlipidemia, family history, diabetes, age, hypertension, age >45 years, and obesity) is upwards of 10%. Of these patients, more than half will go on to develop overt clinical manifestations of CAD and come to medical attention. Further, often (75% in one study) these patients have multivessel disease when further investigated. In patients with known coronary disease and stable angina, the prevalence of silent ischemia is estimated to be between 25% and 50%. Additionally,

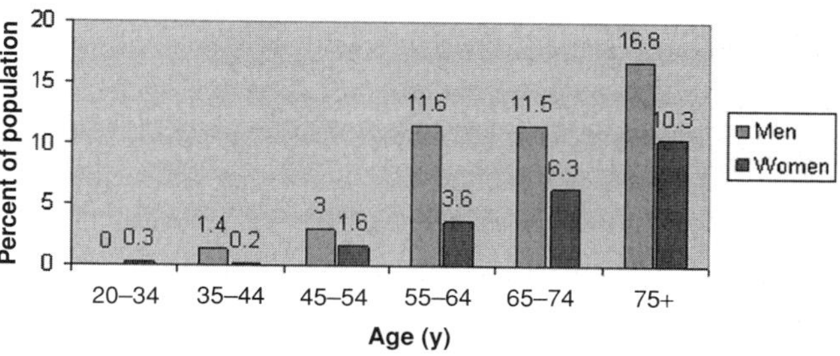


**Figure 11–2** Prevalence of coronary disease in the United States, by age and sex, from NHANES, 1999–2002. (From American Heart Association. *Heart Disease and Stroke Statistics—2005 Update*. Dallas, TX: American Heart Association; 2005.)

**TABLE 11–2**
**BURDEN OF CORONARY ARTERY DISEASE IN THE UNITED STATES, 2002**

| Population Group | Prevalence of CAD | Prevalence of MI | Prevalence of Angina | CAD Mortality Rate |
|---|---|---|---|---|
| Total population | 13 million | 7.1 million | 6.4 million | 171 |
| Men (%) | 8.4 | 5.0 | 4.2 | — |
| Women (%) | 5.6 | 2.3 | 3.6 | — |
| White men (%) | 8.9 | 5.1 | 4.5 | 221 |
| White women (%) | 5.4 | 2.4 | 3.5 | 131 |
| Black men (%) | 7.4 | 4.5 | 3.1 | 251 |
| Black women (%) | 7.5 | 2.7 | 4.7 | 170 |
| Mexican-American men (%) | 5.6 | 3.4 | 2.4 | — |
| Mexican-American women (%) | 4.3 | 1.6 | 2.2 | — |
| Hispanics (%)[a] | 4.8 | — | — | 138 |
| Asians (%)[a] | 5.0 | — | — | 116 |
| American Indians or Alaskan Natives (%)[a] | 3.6 | — | — | 124 |

CAD mortality rate is per 100,000 people. Data are for people age 20 years and older.
[a]Data are for people age 18 years and older.
*Source:* American Heart Association. *Heart Disease and Stroke Statistics—2005 Update*. Dallas, TX: American Heart Association; 2005.

70% to 80% of ischemic episodes in patients with stable angina are silent. Unrecognized MI has two components, asymptomatic or silent MI (~50%), and that which is associated with such atypical symptoms that infarction is not entertained as part of the differential (~50%). One in three MIs can actually be classified as unrecognized. The long-term morbidity and mortality of silent ischemia and unrecognized MI is similar to that of recognized MI (Figs. 11–3 and 11–4). Diabetic and hypertensive patients seem to be most susceptible to unrecognized MI.

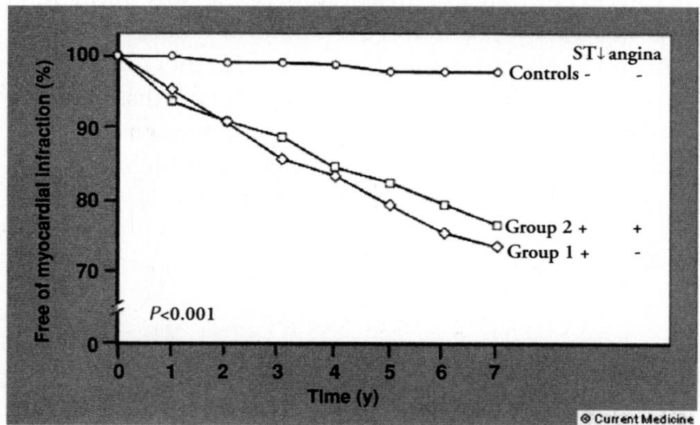


Figure 11–3 Outcome of patients with angina (Group 2) or silent ischemia (Group 2) and exercise-induced ST depression in the Coronary Artery Surgery Study (CASS) registry. Controls had no objective evidence of ischemia. Reprinted from Weiner DA, Ryan TJ, McCabe CH, et al. Risk of developing an acute myocardial infarction or sudden coronary death in patients with exercise induced silent myocardial ischemia: a report from the Coronary Artery Study (CASS) Registry. *Am J Cardiol.* 1988;62:1155–1158, with permission from Excerpta Medica Inc.

## Age and Gender Variation

The average age of a person presenting with a first MI in the United States is 66 years for men and 70 years for women. Figures 11–2 and 11–5 provide a sense of how strongly the prevalence and incidence of CAD is influenced by age and gender. The incidence of serious manifestations of CAD,

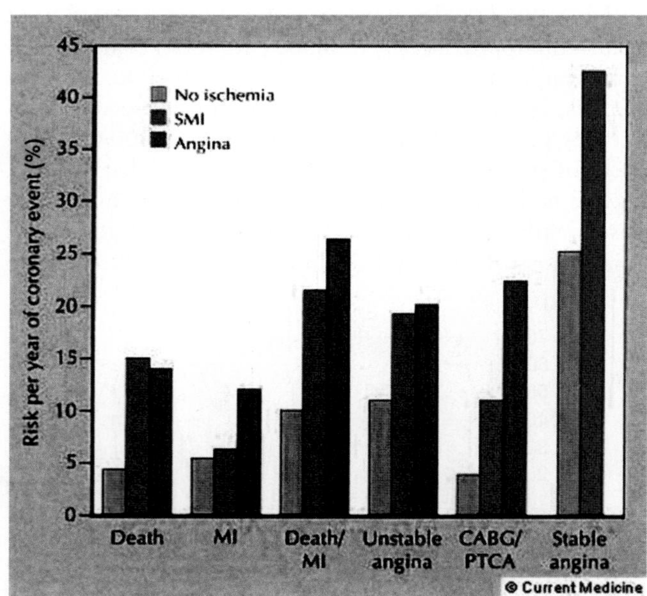


Figure 11–4 Long-term outcome of patients post–myocardial infarction with angina versus silent ischemia versus no objective ischemia. SMI, silent myocardial ischemia; CABG, coronary artery bypass grafting; PTCA, percutaneous coronary angioplasty; MI, myocardial infarction. (Data from Current Medicine: Braunwald *Atlas of Heart Diseases*, with permission.)

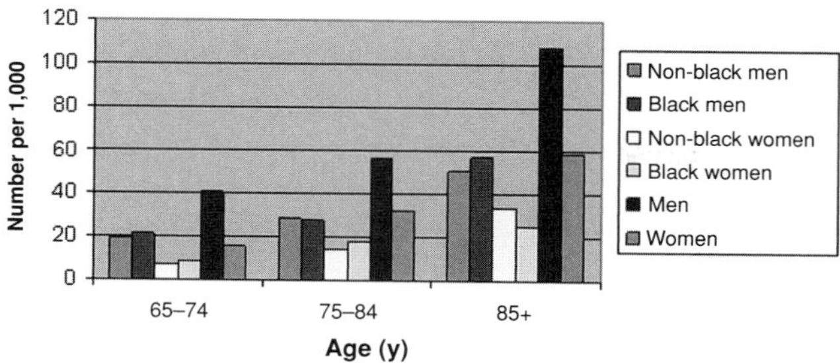


**Figure 11–5** Incidence of new MI or CAD death by age, sex, and race. (From American Heart Association. *Heart Disease and Stroke Statistics—2005 Update*. Dallas, TX: *American Heart Association;* 2005.)

such as MI or death, more than doubles between the age ranges of 65–74 and >85 for men and nearly quadruples for women. Further, data from the Centers for Disease Control (CDC) demonstrates that 83% of people who die from CAD are age 65 years or older. After age 40 years, men have a lifetime risk of developing CAD of 49%, while women have a risk of 32%. After age 70 years this risk decreases to 35% for men and 24% for women.

The incidence of any manifestation of CAD in women lags behind that in men by 10 years, whereas the incidence of myocardial infarction or sudden death lags by 20 years. In fact, excluding people >75 years of age, women are much more likely to present with angina as their first manifestation of CAD, whereas men more often present with MI (Fig. 11–6). In terms of CAD mortality, gender differences narrow significantly with age. Between the ages of 25 and 34 years the mortality related to CAD is three times higher in men than in women. This ratio decreases to 1.6 between the ages of 75 and 84 years.

Finally, menopause, whether natural or surgical, has a significant influence on the incidence and severity of CAD. Indeed, the incidence of serious manifestations of CAD is rare in premenopausal women but increases more than threefold in age-matched postmenopausal women. Of note, polycystic ovarian disease increases the likelihood of premature CAD in women.

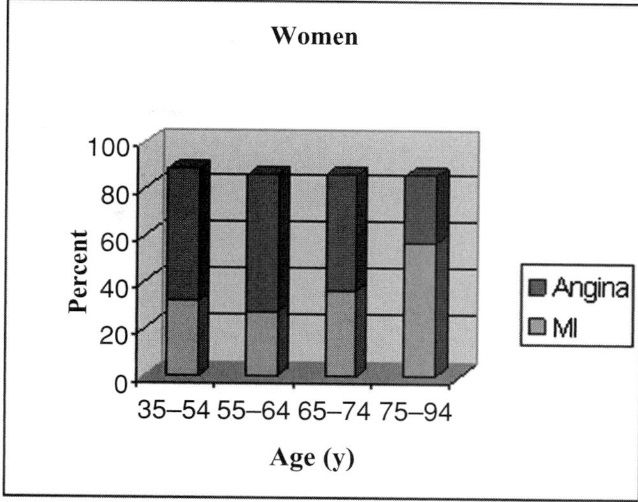


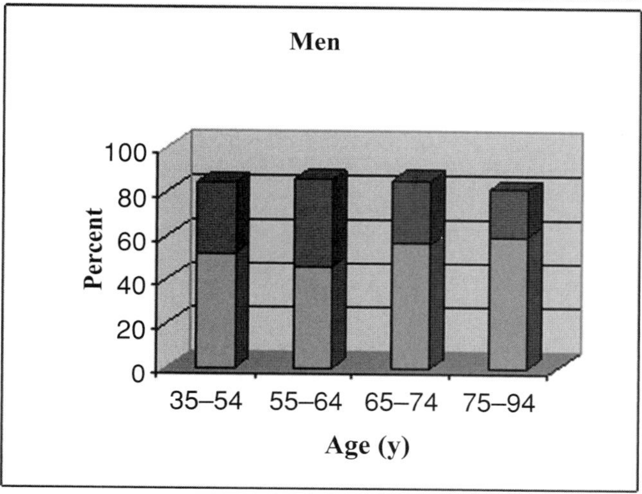


**Figure 11–6** First manifestation of CAD in men and women by age. MI, myocardial infarction. (Data from Lerner DJ and Kannel WB. Patterns of coronary heart disease morbidity and mortality in the sexes: a 26-year follow-up of the Framingham population. *Am Heart J* 1986;111:383–90.

## Racial and Socioeconomic Disparities

CAD as the leading cause of death in the United States holds for every major ethnic group, save East Asian-American women. The self-reported prevalence of CAD and MI and the CAD mortality rates in various racial and ethnic groups according to the latest AHA update are shown in Table 11–2. The most conspicuous feature of these data is that the CAD mortality rate is highest among blacks overall. This difference is particularly striking among younger people, aged 35 to 44 years, in whom the mortality among blacks is reported to be 50% higher than among whites. This difference disappears by age 75 years. Additionally, the incidence of CAD is particularly high among South Asians. The mortality rate among East Asians, Hispanics, and Native Americans or Alaskans is not nearly as high as that among whites or blacks. In terms of socioeconomic differences, numerous studies have linked lower income levels, lower educational levels, and other social factors to elevated CAD risk. One recent study showed a 2.5- to 3-fold increased risk in people living in poorer neighborhoods compared with those living in higher-income neighborhoods, even after adjusting for other socioeconomic and traditional risk factors.

## CAD in the Young

Symptomatic CAD in people under the age of 40 to 45 years is a fairly uncommon problem. In autopsy studies, however, the prevalence of anatomic CAD is roughly 20% in men and 8% in women aged 30 to 34 years. This is consistent with the finding of a delay in manifestations of CAD in

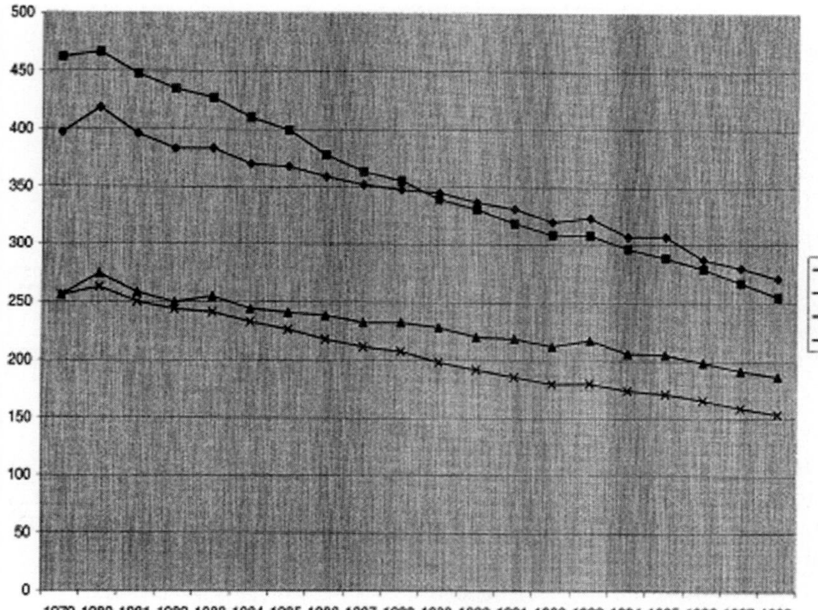


**Figure 11–7** U.S. CAD mortality rate by age and gender from 1979 to 1998. Rate is per 100,000 people. Reprinted from 33rd Bethesda. Conference: Preventive Cardiology: How can we do better? Task Force #1-Magnitude of the Prevention Problem: Opportunities and Challenges. *J Am Coll Cardiol* 2002;40:579–651. Copyright 2002 The American College of Cardiology Foundation and American Heart Association, Inc. Permission granted for one time use. Further reproduction is not permitted without permission from ACE/AHA.

women versus men and that atherosclerosis, despite its relative rarity in the young, is a process that begins at an early age. People presenting with CAD at a young age tend to have multiple risk factors as well as a significant family history of premature CAD. Tobacco use is very common among this population; however, the prevalence of dyslipidemia is similar to those presenting later in life. Often, this population tends to have some manifestations of the metabolic syndrome, such as low HDL, elevated triglycerides, and glucose intolerance. With the current epidemics of obesity and the metabolic syndrome in the United States, it seems likely that the incidence of symptomatic CAD in young people is either on the rise currently, or soon will be.

## Temporal Trends in CAD

Autopsy studies over the past few decades have shown a decreasing prevalence of anatomically significant CAD in people 59 years of age and younger in the United States. From the periods 1979 to 1983 and 1990 to 1994, the prevalence of CAD decreased from 42% to 32% among men and from 29% to 16% among women. There was no change in those >60 years of age. Similarly, the incidence of clinically manifested CAD decreased from the 1970s to the 1980s. The National Health and Nutrition Examination Survey (NHANES) tracked two cohorts of patients from 1971 to 1982 and from 1982 to 1992 and found that the prevalence of CAD over these time periods decreased from 133 to 114 cases per 10,000 persons per year of follow-up. Over a similar time period, the overall incidence of myocardial infarction has remained relatively stable. The incidence of ST-elevation myocardial infarction (STEMI) from 1975–1978 to 1997 decreased from 171 to 101 per 100,000 people, while the incidence of non-STEMI increased from 62 to 131 per 100,000 people.

In the United States, coronary heart disease mortality has declined steadily since it reached a peak in the mid-1960s (Fig. 11–7). The WHO estimated that between 1965–1969 and 1995–1997, overall CAD death rates declined 63% in men and 60% in women. Data from the Framingham study echo this, demonstrating a 59% reduction in CAD mortality and a 49% reduction in the rate of sudden cardiac death from 1950 to 1999. However, this trend is showing signs of slowing; the CDC found only a 27% reduction from 1992 to 2002. This is likely attributable to the epidemics of obesity, diabetes, and the metabolic syndrome in the United States at the end of the 20th century.

## Prognosis and Risk of Sudden Cardiac Death

Once an individual has been diagnosed with stable angina, prognosis shifts to a much higher risk stratum. The risk of future events, in particular subsequent MI, is increased, whereas survival is dramatically reduced with increasing age. The effect of age at presentation on risk of future events is more profound for women than for men. Overall, however, men remain at higher risk of subsequent MI and death at all age strata (Figs. 11–8 and 11–9).

Survivors of acute MI have 1.5 to 15 times the morbidity and mortality rate as the general population, depending on age, gender, and clinical outcome of the inciting event. In contrast to stable angina, the incidence of future adverse cardiovascular events in people after their initial recognized MI is, in general, higher in women than in men (Fig. 11–10). Following a recognized acute MI, the one-year mortality rate in men is 25%, whereas in women it is significantly higher, 38%. The majority of this risk occurs within the first 30 days after the event. The discrepancy between the male and female mortality and event rates can be explained

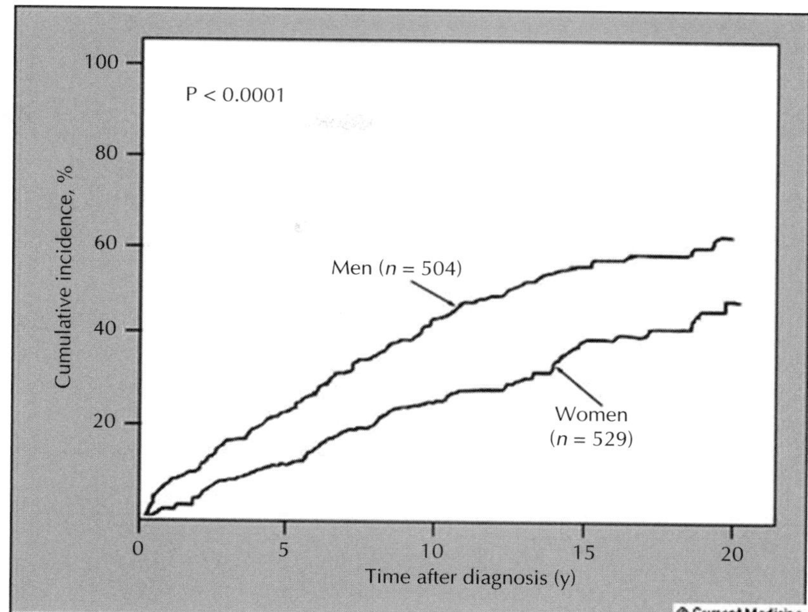


**Figure 11–8** Risk of subsequent MI or cardiac death after being diagnosed with angina, stratified by sex. Adapted from Orencia A, Baily K, Yaun P, et al. Effect of gender on long-term outcome of angina pectoris and myocardial infarction/sudden unexpected death. *JAMA* 1993;269:2392–2397.

by the later age and greater burden of risk factors on average at initial presentation in women.

Sudden cardiac death (SCD), mostly due to out-of-hospital ventricular fibrillation, accounts for >50% of total CAD-related mortality. The risk of SCD death in a person after the index MI is four to six times higher than for the age-matched general population. This risk also varies significantly as a function of age and sex. Overall, from 70% to 89% of all SCD cases occur in men, and the incidence of SCD is three to four times greater in men than in women. This disparity decreases as women age and their risk increases.

## Cost and Health Care Resource Utilization

Direct and indirect costs related to coronary heart disease are estimated to exceed $142 billion in the United States in 2005. This represents nearly half of the total cost related to

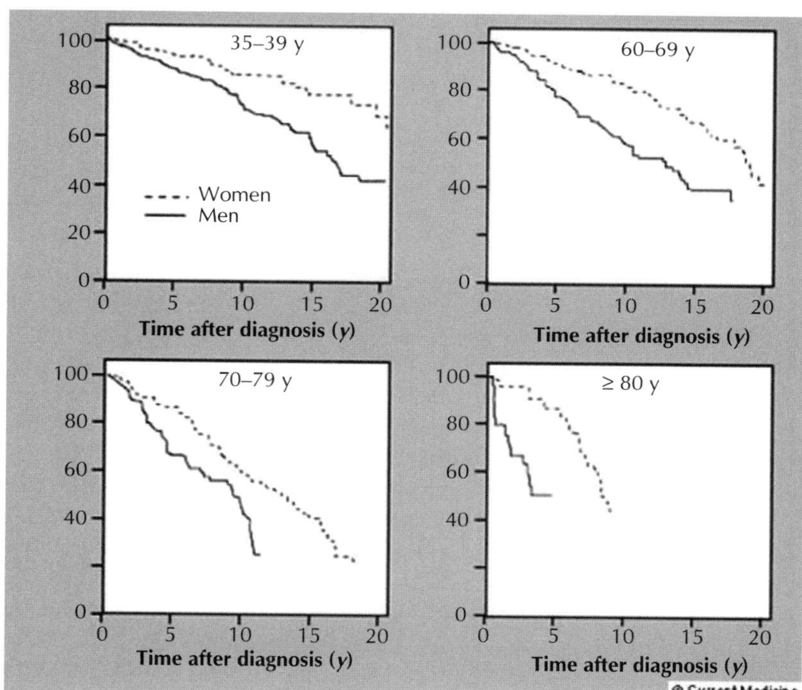


**Figure 11–9** Long-term survival after the diagnosis of uncomplicated angina, stratified by age and sex. Adapted from Orencia A, Baily K, Yaun P, et al. Effect of gender on long-term outcome of angina pectoris and myocardial infarction/sudden unexpected death. *JAMA* 1993;269:2392–2397.

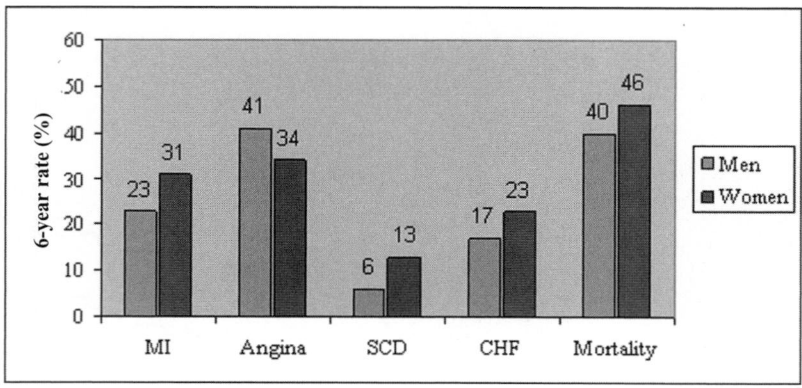


**Figure 11–10** Prognosis after myocardial infarction, from Framingham Study, 36-year follow-up. MI, myocardial infarction; SCD, sudden cardiac death; CHF, congestive heart failure. (From Prevalence, incidence, and mortality of coronary heart disease. In: *Atherosclerosis and Coronary Artery Disease*. Copyright Lippincott Williams & Wilkins, 1996, with permission.)

all cardiovascular diseases, including stroke, hypertension, and congestive heart failure (Table 11–3). In contrast, 2004 costs related to all forms of cancer were estimated to be $190 billion. Medicare estimates that the cost of CAD-related hospitalizations exceeded $10,000 for acute MI, $11,000 for coronary atherosclerosis, and $3,400 for "other" CAD diagnoses, per discharge, in 1999.

In terms of resource utilization, the median duration of hospital stay for acute MI decreased from 8.3 to 4.3 days from 1990 to 1999; however, overall CAD-related discharges from short-stay hospitals increased 22% from 1979 to 2002. In 2002, it was estimated that 1.4 million diagnostic cardiac catheterizations, 1.2 million percutaneous coronary interventions, and 515,000 bypass operations were performed in the United States.

## RISK FACTORS

### Traditional Modifiable Risk Factors

Epidemiologic studies undertaken in the latter half of the 20th century have firmly established links between certain demographic and clinical factors as well as social habits and the diagnosis of coronary heart disease. Among these, older age, dyslipidemia, hypertension, tobacco smoking, male sex, diabetes mellitus, and family history of premature coronary disease are among the more common and well recognized. Risk scores, most commonly the Framingham Risk Score, have been developed using these and other risks to predict accurately the long-term risk of CAD events. More than 90% of people carrying the diagnosis of

**TABLE 11–3**

**2005 ESTIMATED DIRECT AND INDIRECT COSTS (IN BILLIONS OF DOLLARS) OF CARDIOVASCULAR DISEASES IN THE UNITED STATES**

| Component | Heart Diseases[a] | Coronary Heart Disease | Total Cardiovascular Disease |
|---|---|---|---|
| *Direct costs* | | | |
| Hospital | $77.7 | $39.9 | $109.8 |
| Nursing home | 19.1 | 10.0 | 39.3 |
| Physicians/health professionals | 18.5 | 10.4 | 36 |
| Drugs/other medical durables | 19.4 | 9.0 | 45.9 |
| Home health care | 4.8 | 1.4 | 10.9 |
| Total expenditures[b] | $139.5 | $70.7 | $241.9 |
| *Indirect costs* | | | |
| Lost productivity/morbidity | $21.4 | $9.4 | $34.8 |
| Lost productivity/mortality[c] | 93.9 | 62.0 | 116.8 |
| Grand totals[b] | $254.8 | $142.1 | $393.5 |

[a]Includes coronary heart disease, congestive heart failure, part of hypertensive disease, cardiac dysrhythmias, rheumatic heart disease, cardiomyopathy, pulmonary heart disease, and other or ill-defined "heart" diseases.
[b]Totals do not add up secondary to rounding and overlap.
[c]Lost future earnings of persons who will die in 2005, discounted at 3%.
*Source:* American Heart Association. *Heart Disease and Stroke Statistics—2005 Update*. Dallas, TX: American Heart Association; 2005.

CAD have one of the following major risk factors: hypertension, hyperlipidemia, treatment for hypertension or hyperlipidemia, or diabetes. Further the INTERHEART study of >29,000 patients in 52 countries showed that >90% of the risk of an index MI is attributable to the following factors regardless of gender, ethnicity, or geography: tobacco, hyperlipidemia, hypertension, diabetes, obesity, sedentary lifestyle, alcoholism, low intake of fruits and vegetables, and psychosocial index.

### Tobacco

According to the AHA, >53 million Americans 18 years of age and older, including 1.4 million new smokers, used tobacco products in 2002. This constitutes 25% of all men and 20% of all women in the United States. From 1980 to 2002 the number of high school seniors who had smoked within the past month declined 12.5%, and since 1965, smoking among persons 18 years of age and older has decreased 47% overall. Smokers have a two- to fourfold higher risk of CAD than nonsmokers, and two- to threefold higher risk of CAD-related mortality. The INTERHEART study estimated that tobacco accounts for 36% of the population attributable risk of a first myocardial infarction.

Smoking cessation has proven benefits for CAD. According to the WHO, the risk of CAD decreases by 50% one year after abstention, and within 15 years the relative risk of death from CAD for an ex-smoker becomes equivalent to that of a lifetime nonsmoker.

### Lipids

The prevalence of lipid disorders in patients with CAD and in the general population is extraordinarily common. Of people with premature CAD, 75% to 85% have dyslipidemia. For further details on dyslipidemia and its effects on coronary disease, refer to Chapter 12.

### Hypertension

According to AHA figures, 65 million Americans carried the diagnosis of hypertension in 2002. An additional 59 million people are classified as having prehypertension (systolic blood pressure 120 to 139 mm Hg, or diastolic blood pressure 80 to 89 mm Hg) and are at risk for overt hypertension. Systolic blood pressure, diastolic blood pressure, and pulse pressure have all been separately identified as risk factors. According to the INTERHEART study, hypertension accounts for 18% of the population attributable risk of first MI. Further details on hypertension and its cardiovascular effects are included in the hypertension section.

### Diabetes Mellitus

The prevalence of diagnosed and undiagnosed diabetes mellitus among adults in the United States was 19.8 million in 2002. An additional 14.5 million are in the prediabetic phase of glucose intolerance. From 1990 to 2002, the prevalence of diabetes increased 61% in the United States. Mexican Americans and blacks currently have the highest rates of any ethnic group. Worldwide, the prevalence among all ages is 2.8%, and it is expected to nearly double to 4.4% by 2030. Diabetes increases the risk of MI or cerebrovascular accident by two- to threefold and doubles the risk of SCD. According to the INTERHEART study, diabetes accounts for 10% of the population attributable risk of first MI. In 2002 the National Cholesterol Education Program (NCEP) was compelled by these and additional statistics to elevate diabetes to the category of CAD equivalent.

### Obesity and the Metabolic Syndrome

According to the AHA, nearly 135 million perople could be classified as overweight or obese in 2002, 63 million being overtly obese. Further, the prevalence of overweight and obese children has quadrupled since the 1960s, to 9.1 million children in 2002. Obesity has reached epidemic proportions in the United States and shows no signs of slowing down. From 1988–1994 to 1999–2002 the prevalence of obesity % increased from 22.9 to 30% of the adult population. Mexican Americans constitute the ethnic group with the greatest prevalence. Obesity is now recognized as an independent risk factor for CAD, although it also mediates its effects through other factors that are highly associated with it, such as hypertension, insulin resistance, and hypertriglyceridemia. Obesity accounts for roughly 20% of the population attributable risk of a first MI.

The metabolic syndrome, as defined by the NCEP, consists of elevated triglycerides (>150 mg/dL), low high-density lipoprotein (HDL <40 mg/dL in men and <50 mg/dL in women), hypertension or prehypertension, impaired glucose tolerance, and overweight or obesity. The age-adjusted prevalence of the metabolic syndrome in U.S. adults is 23.7% or roughly 47 million. Among ethnic groups in the United States, Mexican Americans have the greatest prevalence. A diagnosis of metabolic syndrome carries with it an increased risk of overt diabetes mellitus, a twofold greater risk of CAD, an increased risk of CAD death.

## Novel Risk Factors

In addition to the classic modifiable risk factors newer measures are emerging that are leading to new insights and confirming the role of inflammation in atherosclerosis. Not all of these factors have obvious treatments or are modifiable, and some may prove to be risk markers rather than truly play a pathophysiologic role. Among these, high-sensitivity C-reactive protein (hs-CRP) has been at the forefront, although not without controversy. Levels of hs-CRP have been shown to predict the long-term risk of first myocardial infarction and improve risk stratification along with serum lipids in a primary prevention setting. Elevated serum homocysteine levels have similarly been shown to be linked with increased risk for CAD. Levels above the 95th percentile increase the risk of MI approximately threefold. Finally, elevated fibrinogen and brain natriuretic peptide levels (BNP) in otherwise asymptomatic healthy patients may predict increased risk for CAD, MI, and CVA.

Finally, peripheral vascular disease (PVD) as manifested by CVA, transient ischemic attack, or lower-extremity claudication significantly increases the risk of CAD and coronary events. This is somewhat intuitive, given that many of the risk factors are shared. CVA increases the risk of CAD or cardiac failure twofold, whereas intermittent claudication increases the risk two- to threefold. Carotid intimamedia thickness, a measure of carotid atherosclerotic disease as determined by ultrasound, has been shown to be predictive of future myocardial infarction, even after controlling for traditional risk factors. This lends further support to the role of systemic inflammation in the pathobiology of atherosclerotic vascular disease.

## BIBLIOGRAPHY


**American Heart Association.** Heart Disease and Stroke Statistics—2005 Update. Dallas, TX: American Heart Association; 2005.

**Azar RR, Waters DD.** Coronary heart disease and myocardial infarction in young men and women. In: Rose BD, Rush JM. *UpToDate Online 2005.*

**Bertolet BD, Pepine CJ.** Silent myocardial ischemia. In: Braunwald E. Atlas of Heart Diseases. Current Medicine Group; 2005.

**Gersh BJ.** Natural history of chronic coronary artery disease. In: Braunwald E. *Atlas of Heart Diseases.* Current Medicine Group; 2005.

**Kannel WB.** Epidemiologic relationship of disease among the different vascular territories. In: Fuster V, Ross R, Topol EJ. *Atherosclerosis and Coronary Artery Disease.* Vol 2. New York: McGraw-Hill Medical; 2001:13–21.

**Kannel WB.** Prevalence, incidence, and mortality of coronary heart disease. In: Fuster V, Ross R, Topol EJ. *Atherosclerosis and Coronary Artery Disease.* Vol 2. New York: McGraw-Hill Medical; 2001: 13–21.

**MacKay JMG.** *The Atlas of Heart Disease and Stroke.* 2005:46–49.

**Vasan RSBE, Sullivan LM, D'Agostino RB.** The burden of increasing worldwide cardiovascular disease. In: Fuster VAR, O'Rourke RA, eds. *Hurst's The Heart.* Vol. 7. New York: McGraw-Hill Medical; 2001:15–37.

**Wilson PWF.** Epidemiology and prognosis of coronary heart disease. In: Rose BD, Rush JM. *UpToDate Online 2005.*

**Wilson PWF, Culleton BF.** Overview of the risk factors for cardiovascular disease. In: Rose BD, Rush JM. *UpToDate Online 2005.*

# The Dyslipidemias

12

***Adam W. Grasso Michael B. Rocco***

Cardiovascular disease (CVD) is the leading cause of morbidity and mortality in the industrialized world, accounting for approximately 40% of all deaths in the United States. Coronary heart disease (CHD), a subcategory of CVD, kills one in every five Americans. Each year, 1.2 million people in the United States suffer a first or recurrent myocardial infarction (MI), and nearly 500,000 people experience sudden cardiac death (SCD). Stroke remains the third leading cause of mortality, with >700,000 strokes per year in the United States. More than half of the adult population in the United States (107 million people) has elevated total cholesterol, >200 mg/dL, and more than a quarter of adults (55 million) have low high-density lipoprotein (HDL) cholesterol, <40 mg/dL. Given the enormous burden of CVD, the high prevalence of lipid disorders, and effective evidence-based treatment strategies, recognition of and management of lipid disorders is an essential component of both primary and secondary prevention of CVD. In this chapter, we provide a clinically relevant discussion of dyslipidemias and their effective treatment to reduce CVD morbidity and mortality. In addition to defining lipoproteins and lipid disorders, the clinical trials and observational studies that form the cornerstone for modern treatment guidelines are reviewed.

## LIPIDS AND LIPOPROTEINS

*Lipids* are molecules with hydrocarbon skeletons, which play crucial roles in the storage, metabolism, and production of energy, the structure and behavior of cell membranes, and the transduction of signals both inside and between cells. Lipids are fat-soluble, or lipophilic, compounds, which are classified as either simple or complex. Simple lipids include free cholesterol (FC) and fatty acids (FA), and complex lipids, which are combinations of simple lipids, include cholesteryl esters (CE) and triglycerides (TG). The lipids with greatest pathologic significance appear to be CE, the predominant components of macrophage foam cell inclusions, and TG, which form the core of adipocyte inclusions. Packaged together with phospholipids and proteins known as *apolipoproteins*, lipids are transported between organs in the form of *lipoproteins*. Lipoproteins are classified according to their densities and electrophoretic mobilities and include, in decreasing density, high-density lipoproteins (HDL), low-density lipoproteins (LDL), intermediate-density lipoproteins (IDL), very-low-density lipoproteins (VLDL), and chylomicrons.

Lipid processing and transport can be envisioned as a bidirectional process. The first cycle begins with *triglyceride-rich lipoproteins (TGRL)*, namely, chylomicrons from the gut and VLDL from the liver (Fig. 12–1). These lipoproteins serve as substrates for lipoprotein lipase (LPL) and hepatic lipase (HL), two different enzymes bound to capillary endothelium. Free FA are released for the use of skeletal muscle, adipose tissue, and other organs, and FC and CE are delivered to distant tissues. Chylomicrons, VLDL, and their lipolysis products, such as chylomicron remnants, IDL, and LDL, bear apolipoprotein B (apoB) and apolipoprotein E (apoE) on their surfaces. ApoB has two isoforms: apoB100, which is present on lipoproteins secreted by the liver, and apoB48, which is present on gut-derived lipoproteins. LDL, IDL, and remnant particles can be taken up by hepatocytes via receptors that bind to apoB and apoE. Alternatively, they may migrate across the endothelium, undergo oxidation/modification, induce monocyte recruitment and foam cell formation, and initiate a cycle of inflammation, chemotaxis, and thrombotic activity leading to atherosclerosis and vascular events. IDL is the most atherogenic lipoprotein, but LDL (which carries 70% of plasma cholesterol) is the principal lipoprotein responsible for atherosclerosis. Cholesterol present in apoB-containing lipoproteins may be represented as *non–high-density lipoprotein cholesterol (non-HDL-C)*. *Small dense LDL (sdLDL)* is defined as LDL with a low ratio of LDL-C to LDL-apoB (<1.2), and represents a more atherogenic subclass of LDL.

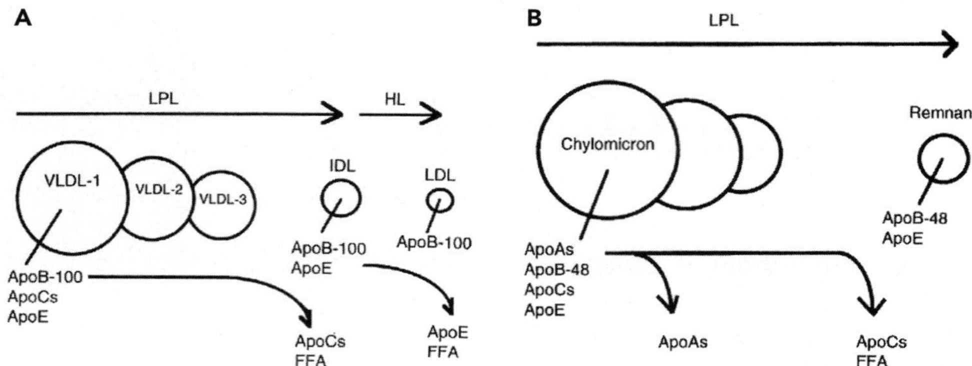


**Figure 12–1** Remodeling of triglyceride-rich lipoproteins. **A**: Stepwise lipolysis of VLDL subfractions 1, 2, and 3 by LPL. LPL catalyzes VLDL triglyceride hydrolysis with the concomitant transfer of the apoC proteins to HDL and the release of free fatty acids (FFA). Subsequently, HL catalyzes additional triglyceride hydrolysis that induces the transfer of apoE from IDL to HDL and the release of additional FFA. LDL contains apoB100 as its sole protein. **B:** Lipolysis of chylomicrons by LPL. Triglyceride hydrolysis is associated with the transfer of the apoC proteins to HDL and the release of FFA. The remnant contains apoB48, which is the major protein of chylomicrons, and apoE, which mediates the binding of remnants to hepatic receptors. (Reprinted from Betteridge DJ, Illingworth DR, and Shepherd J. *Lipoproteins in Health and Disease*. London: Edward Arnold; 1999:4, with permission.)

The other major transport cycle, sometimes termed reverse cholesterol transport (RCT), serves primarily to return cholesterol to the liver (Fig. 12–2). RCT involves HDL, the major structural protein of which is apolipoprotein A (apoA). Starting with a lipid-poor HDL known as pre-$\beta$ HDL, FC is progressively added from macrophages, and then esterified by the enzyme lecithin cholesterol acyltransferase (LCAT). These mature HDL-C particles can return to the liver by direct hepatic uptake of HDL, or CE can be transferred to apoB-containing lipoproteins, which then can be taken up by the liver. One clinically relevant reaction is catalyzed by the cholesteryl ester transfer protein (CETP), which transfers CE from HDL to LDL or VLDL in exchange for TG. Thus, CE and TG are rapidly equilibrated between HDL and the apoB-containing lipoproteins, a major reason why patients with hypertriglyceridemia tend to have low HDL cholesterol (HDL-C). The subsequent action of hepatic lipase (HL) on TG-rich HDL leads to the production of smaller, denser HDL in such individuals. Individuals with diminished or absent levels of serum CETP generally have elevated HDL-C, and lower rates of atherosclerosis. Pharmacologic inhibitors of CETP have been shown to significantly elevate HDL-C, and in the future may become important tools for the clinician. In addition to its role in lipid transport, HDL may mediate other antiatherosclerotic effects by inhibiting LDL oxidation, reducing endothelial dysfunction, reducing chemotaxis of inflammatory cells into plaques, and inhibiting thrombosis.

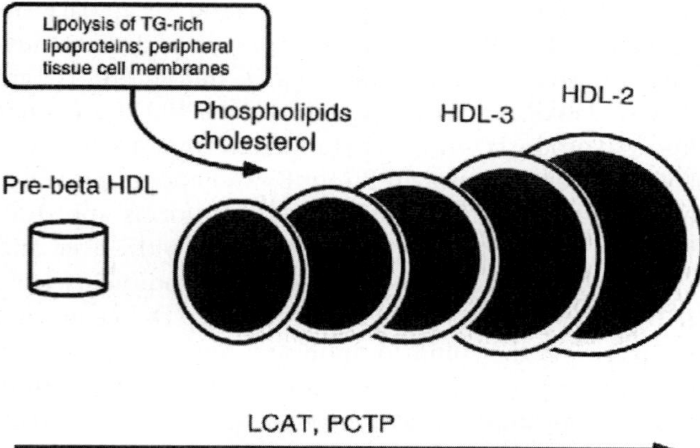


**Figure 12–2** Remodeling of HDL by LCAT and phosphatidylcholine transfer protein (PCTP, also known as phospholipid transfer protein or PLTP). Small, premigrating HDL composed of apoA-I, cholesterol, and lecithin is a substrate for LCAT, which forms cholesteryl esters within the core. Additional cholesterol and phospholipids from peripheral tissue cell membranes and lipolysis of triglyceride-rich lipoproteins are added to the HDL. Multiple cycles of lipid transfer to HDL and LCAT activity eventually produce large, mature HDL, which is a major carrier of cholesterol to the liver. (Reprinted from Betteridge DJ, Illingworth DR, and Shepherd J, eds. *Lipoproteins in Health and Disease*. London: Edward Arnold; 1999:4, with permission.)

Lipoprotein (a), or Lp(a), is an LDL-like particle of hepatic origin. Unlike LDL, apoB100 on the surface of Lp(a) is bound to a protein called apolipoprotein (a), or apo(a), which has strong homologies to plasminogen. Although apo(a) lacks enzymatic activity, Lp(a) can interfere with the binding of plasminogen to substrates such as fibrin, cell surfaces, and extracellular matrix, potentially promoting a prothrombotic state. Numerous retrospective and prospective studies have shown a clear association between high plasma Lp(a) levels and CHD, but evidence is still needed to test the hypothesis that pharmacologic reduction of Lp(a) levels will lower the incidence of coronary events.

## DIAGNOSIS OF DYSLIPIDEMIAS

Clinical interest is focused on dyslipidemias in which a causal or proposed causal relationship exists between abnormal serum lipid levels and atherosclerosis. Appropriate treatment of a particular dyslipidemia requires accurately characterizing a patient's lipid disorder. In order to classify a patient's dyslipidemia and exclude secondary causes and determine treatment strategies, the clinical practitioner should investigate the following.

- *Personal history*: abnormal serum lipid levels; CHD; manifestations of cerebrovascular disease, including transient ischemic attack (TIA) or cerebrovascular accident (CVA); peripheral vascular disease (PVD), including limb claudication, aortic aneurysm, or carotid atherosclerosis; diabetes mellitus (DM); hypothyroidism; renal insufficiency; nephrotic syndrome; hepatobiliary disease; pancreatitis; or pregnancy.
- *Medication history*: especially of thiazide diuretics, beta-blockers, oral contraceptives (OCP), hormone replacement therapy (HRT), isotretinoin, glucocorticoids, or highly active antiretroviral therapy (HAART) for HIV.
- *Family history*: dyslipidemias, CHD, TIA/CVA, PVD, sudden death, diabetes, hypertension, or central obesity. Suspicion of familial dyslipidemias should be followed up with lipid testing of family members.
- *Lifestyle history*: past and present tobacco use, excessive alcohol use (>40 g/day), sedentary lifestyle, or a diet rich in saturated fats or carbohydrates.
- *Physical exam findings*: body mass index (BMI), waist circumference, blood pressure, thyroid characteristics, xanthomas (cholesterol deposits of interdigital, tuberous, planar, or eruptive types), xanthelasmas (xanthomas of the palpebral fissures), arcus corneae, lipemia retinalis (pale-appearing retinal vessels), peripheral pulses, vascular bruits, or hepatosplenomegaly. See Figure 12–3 for representative examples of xanthomas.

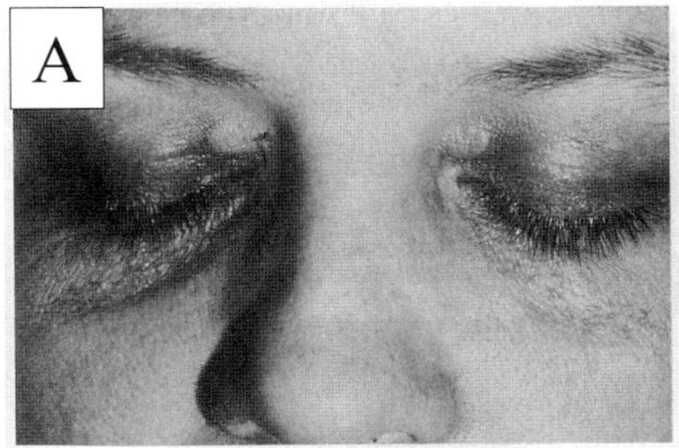


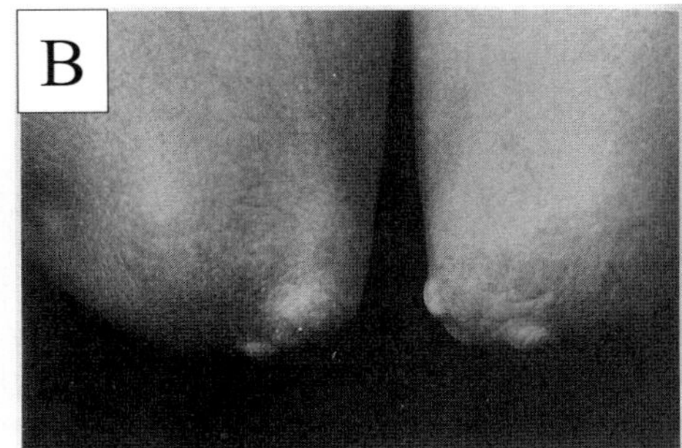


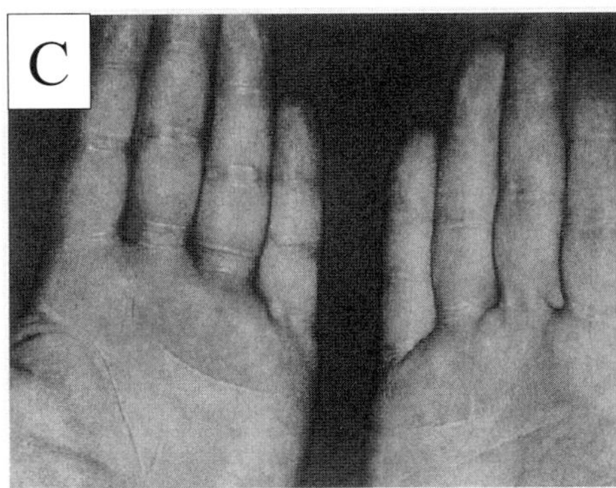


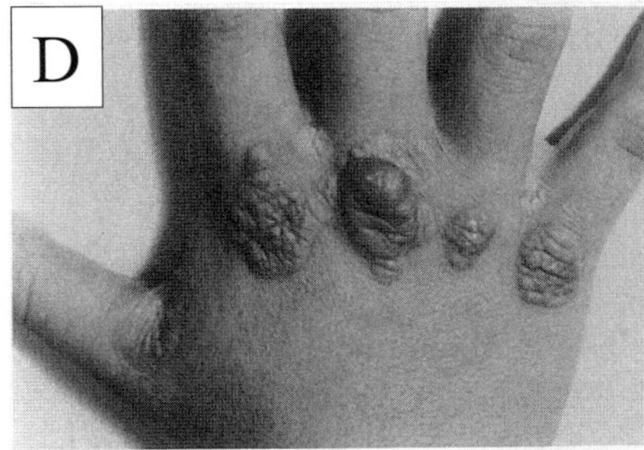


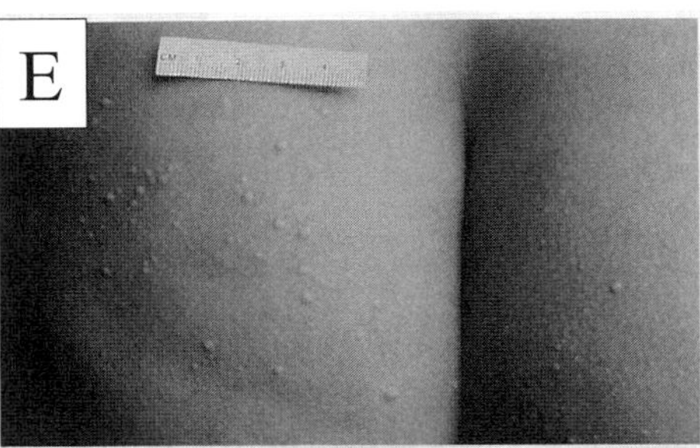


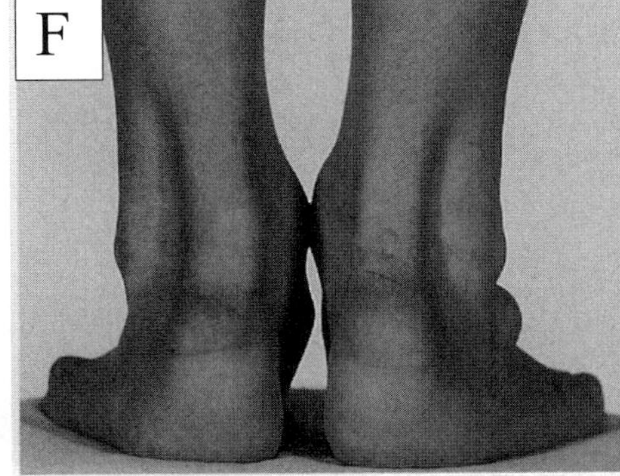


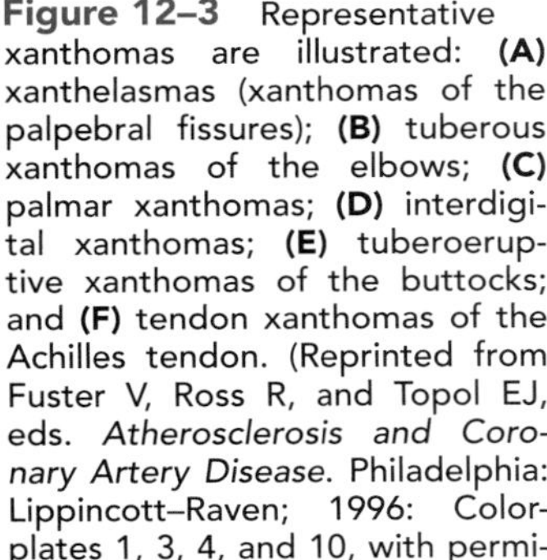

**Figure 12–3** Representative xanthomas are illustrated: **(A)** xanthelasmas (xanthomas of the palpebral fissures); **(B)** tuberous xanthomas of the elbows; **(C)** palmar xanthomas; **(D)** interdigital xanthomas; **(E)** tuberoeruptive xanthomas of the buttocks; and **(F)** tendon xanthomas of the Achilles tendon. (Reprinted from Fuster V, Ross R, and Topol EJ, eds. *Atherosclerosis and Coronary Artery Disease.* Philadelphia: Lippincott–Raven; 1996: Colorplates 1, 3, 4, and 10, with permission.)

- *Laboratory studies*: fasting serum lipid panel, fasting glucose, thyroid-stimulating hormone (TSH), high-sensitivity C-reactive protein (hsCRP), creatinine, hepatic function panel, urinalysis, and a screen for microalbuminuria. In most cases, it is not necessary to obtain lipoprotein subpopulation analysis, or levels of serum Lp(a).

## CLASSIFICATION OF DYSLIPIDEMIAS

In 1967, Fredrickson and colleagues (1) proposed a system to diagnose and classify lipid disorders based on the specific lipoprotein or lipoproteins elevated in the patient's serum. Although the Fredrickson classification system was useful shorthand for describing hyperlipidemias, it had two major shortcomings: its phenotypes did not provide or even imply etiology, and HDL was not included. In a more clinically relevant schema, lipid disorders can also be grouped into two broad categories. *Primary dyslipidemias* result from genetic variability in one or more loci controlling the expression of proteins involved in lipoprotein synthesis, metabolism, or clearance. *Secondary dyslipidemias* are the consequence of a separate pathologic process.

### Primary Dyslipidemias

The primary dyslipidemias of non-HDL-C are summarized in Table 12–1. *Familial hypercholesterolemia (FH)* is a common autosomal dominant disorder resulting from mutations in the LDL receptor (LDL-R), or apoB receptor, leading to impaired hepatic clearance of LDL from the circulation. *Heterozygous FH (HeFH)* occurs in one in 500 persons and is associated with serum LDL-C two to three times the average and a four- to sixfold increased risk for premature CHD. Without treatment, the average age for development of symptomatic CHD is 45 years in men and 55 years in women. By age 39, 90% of FH heterozygotes exhibit detectable xanthomas on the extensor tendons of the hands, or on the Achilles tendons (see Fig. 12–3). Several diagnostic criteria for FH exist, with that of the 15-year Simon Broome Register Group being the most commonly used.

*Definite FH* requires:

1. TC >290 mg/dL in adults or TC >260 mg/dL in children under 16
   *or* LDL-C >190 mg/dL in adults or >155 mg/dL in children
   PLUS
2. Tendon xanthomas in the patient, or in a first- or second-degree relative
   OR
3. DNA-based evidence of LDL-R mutation or familial defective apoB100

*Possible FH* is defined as 1 above plus one of 4 or 5 below:

4. MI before age 50 in 2nd degree relative, or before 60 in 1st degree
5. Elevated cholesterol in 1st degree relative, or >290 mg/dL in 2nd degree

*Homozygous FH (HoFH)* occurs in one in 1 million individuals. Patents with HoFH do not express any functional LDL receptors, and consequently exhibit a more severe phenotype. Total cholesterol (TC) levels are generally >600 mg/dL, with LDL-C levels six- to eightfold higher than average. Without treatment, death from MI occurs in the first or second decade of life. In addition to the xanthomas observed in heterozygotes, FH homozygotes are commonly affected by interdigital xanthomas, tuberous xanthomas on the hands, elbows, buttocks, and feet, and planar xanthomas on the posterior thighs, buttocks, and knees.

*Familial Defective Apolipoprotein B100* is associated with impaired LDL clearance due to reduced affinity of LDL for the LDL-R. The most common cause of this autosomal dominant condition is a single-base mutation in the apoB100 gene. Although the prevalence of familial defective apoB100 is unclear, and varies by ethnic background, it may be as common as one in 600. The lipoprotein concentrations, clinical features, and treatment are similar to those of FH heterozygotes.

*Polygenic hypercholesterolemia (PH)* is the most common cause of an isolated elevation in TC or LDL-C, with prevalence in the United States estimated at between one in 20 and one in 100. TG levels are generally normal. Alterations in the function or expression of several key proteins involved in LDL metabolism have been associated with PH, including mildly defective LDL-R and apoB100, increased synthesis of apoB, and the presence of the apoE4 allele, which has a higher affinity for the LDL-R than the other apoE isoforms, leading to downregulation of LDL-R synthesis and a secondary increase in serum LDL-C. Xanthomas are very rare or absent in patients with PH.

*Familial combined hyperlipidemia (FCH)* is the most common primary dyslipidemia in which multiple lipoprotein phenotypes exist, with a population prevalence of 1% to 3%. The three observed patterns of elevated VLDL, elevated LDL, or both can be seen within a family or within a single patient over time. Transmission is complex, with multiple genes likely to be involved. It is associated with an estimated two- to fivefold increased risk for CHD, accounting for one third to one half of familial CHD, and up to 20% of all premature CHD. Traditionally, diagnostic criteria include:

1. TC and/or TG levels >90th percentile for age- and sex-matched controls; TC of 250 to 350 mg/dL and TG >130 mg/dL (often higher, especially in diabetics)
2. At least one first-degree relative with elevated VLDL-C, LDL-C, or both
3. A strong family history of hyperlipidemia and premature CHD

## TABLE 12–1
## PRIMARY DYSLIPIDEMIAS OF NON-HDL-C

| Disorder | Molecular Basis | Inheritance/ Prevalence | Lipid Profile | Physical Findings | Symptomatic CHD Risk | Treatment (nondietary) |
|---|---|---|---|---|---|---|
| Familial hypercholesterolemia (FH) | LDL-R mutations<br>Dysfunctional receptor<br>↓ Hepatic LDL clearance | AD HeFH<br>1:500<br>HoFH<br>1:1 million | TC 300–400 mg/dL<br>LDL-C 200–300 mg/dL<br>TC >600 mg/dL<br>LDL-C >600 mg/dL | Xanthomas of extensor hand tendons, Achilles tendons<br>As in HeFH, plus interdigital, tuberous (hands, elbows, buttocks, feet), planar (thighs, buttocks, knees) xanthomas | 4–6 times average risk<br>Without treatment, fatal MI in nearly 100% by age 20 | Statins, resins, apheresis<br>Apheresis, statins, resins |
| Familial defective apoB100 | apoB100 mutation<br>↓ LDL affinity for LDL-R<br>↓ Hepatic LDL clearance | AD 1:600 | Similar to HeFH | Similar to HeFH | Similar to HeFH, often with slightly more benign course | Statins, resins, apheresis |
| Polygenic hypercholesterolemia (PH) | Presence of apoE4 allele, or<br>Mildly defective LDL-R, or<br>Mildly defective apoB100<br>↑ apoB synthesis | Complex<br>1:20 to 1:100 | TC 250–350 mg/dL<br>LDL-C 150–250 mg/dL<br>TG normal | No xanthomas | 1.5–2 times average risk | Statins, niacin, resins |
| Familial combined hyperlipidemia (FCH) | Multiple implicated genes | Complex<br>1:33 to 1:100 | TC 250–350 mg/dL<br>LDL-C 200–300 mg/dL and/or<br>TG >130 mg/dL (often much higher) | Arcus cornea<br>Xanthelasmas<br>No xanthomas | 2–5 times average risk | Statins (for phenotypes with ↑LDL)<br>Fibrates (for phenotypes with ↑VLDL) |
| Hyperapobetalipoproteinemia (Hyper-apoB) | ↑ Synthesis apoB | Inheritance and prevalence unclear | LDL-C <160 mg/dL (normal to borderline ↑)<br>LDL-apoB >130 mg/dL<br>TG normal or ↑ | Arcus cornea<br>Xanthelasmas<br>No xanthomas | If TG↑, >17 times average risk<br>If TG normal, 2–3 times average risk | Statins<br>Resins |
| Type III hyperlipidemia (familial dysbetalipoproteinemia) | Defective apoE<br>90% of patients are E2/E2 | Usually AR, but can be AD<br>1:1,000 to 1:5,000 | TC 300–600 mg/dL<br>TG 400–800 mg/dL and higher<br>VLDL-C:TG >0.3 | Planar xanthomas of the palmar creases<br>Tuberous xanthomas over knees and elbows, not attached to tendons | ↑↑ Compared to average (RR unknown) | Fibrates<br>Statins<br>Niacin |
| Familial endogenous and familial mixed hypertriglyceridemias | ↑ Hepatic VLDL, TG<br>↑ Hepatic VLDL, ↓ LPL activity | FEH: AD?<br>1:300<br>FMH: unclear<br>Rare | TG 200–500 mg/dL<br>TG >1,000 mg/dL | No xanthomas | CHD risk not consistently elevated; some kindreds at higher risk than others | Fibrates, niacin<br>Fibrates |
| Familial chylomicronemia | LPL or apoC-II mutations → serum accumulation of chylomicrons | AR 1 in 1 million | TG >1,000 mg/dL | Eruptive xanthomas on extensor limb surfaces, hepatosplenomegaly, pancreatitis, lipemia retinalis | Unclear association with CHD | Drug therapy ineffective |

AD, autosomal dominant; AR, autosomal recessive; HeFH, heterozygous FH; HoFH, homozygous FH; RR, relative risk.

Other major characteristics include elevated apoB (>120 mg/dL), a preponderance of sdLDL, and low HDL-C. FCH is usually diagnosed after age 20 years, and patients are often hypertensive, overweight, insulin resistant, or diabetic. Arcus cornea and xanthelasmas are commonly seen, but tendon xanthomas are unusual. Hence, the absence of tendon xanthomas in a hypercholesterolemic patient is a useful feature to differentiate FCH from FH.

Other, less common dyslipidemias of apoB metabolism are frequently characterized by elevations in TG, VLDL, or LDL-apoB concentrations. These include *hyperapobetalipoproteinemia (hyper-apoB)*, *type III hyperlipidemia* (also known as *familial dysbetalipoproteinemia* or *remnant disease*), *familial endogenous hypertriglyceridemia (FEH)*, *familial mixed hypertriglyceridemia (FMH)*, and *familial chylomicronemia* and are outlined in Table 12–1.

There exist a heterogeneous group of rare familial disorders of HDL-C, including *Tangier disease*, *familial LCAT deficiency*, and *partial LCAT deficiency* or *fish-eye disease*, which have not been consistently associated with premature CHD and are beyond the scope of this chapter. $ApoAI_{Milano}$ is a rare genetic variant of the apoAI protein that results in low HDL-C levels. However, individuals bearing the mutation display longevity and an exceptionally low risk of CHD. In a controlled trial of patients with a history of acute coronary syndrome (ACS), infusions of purified $\text{ApoAI}_{\text{Milano}}$ induced plaque regression, as assessed by intravascular ultrasound (IVUS). At present, such therapy is not available for clinical use, but these studies suggest a future role for HDL-C modification to reduce cardiovascular risk.

## Secondary Dyslipidemias

Evaluation of a dyslipidemia is not complete without a thorough search for secondary and contributing causes. A careful history and physical examination, accompanied by selected laboratory studies, including a fasting lipid panel, will frequently reveal the etiology of a patient's dyslipidemia. Breakdown by the abnormal lipid may simplify diagnosis of the dyslipidemia's cause:

- *Elevated TC and LDL-C:* a diet rich in saturated fat, drugs (oral contraceptives or OCP, HRT, HAART), hypothyroidism, nephrotic syndrome, chronic liver disease, and chronic biliary tract disease (classically, primary biliary cirrhosis)
- *Elevated TG:* a diet rich in carbohydrates, drugs (beta-blockers, thiazide diuretics, isotretinoin, glucocorticoids, HAART, OCP, HRT), excessive alcohol consumption, obesity, diabetes mellitus, hypothyroidism, CRI, chronic pancreatitis, and pregnancy.
- *Low HDL-C:* very-high-carbohydrate, very-low-fat diet, hypertriglyceridemia, obesity, sedentary lifestyle, smoking, diabetes mellitus.

Often, these dyslipidemias can be controlled by institution of lifestyle changes (including dietary improvement, weight loss, increased exercise, and smoking cessation), withdrawal and replacement on an implicated medication, or recognition and treatment of an underlying disorder. A typical example is the hyperlipidemic patient who is resistant to lipid-lowering therapy but is later found to be hypothyroid. Treatment with levothyroxine then corrects the secondary dyslipidemia.

# METABOLIC SYNDROME

Although it is not a distinct cause of dyslipidemia, because of the growing recognition of its prevalence and the association of this syndrome with a particularly dyslipidemic pattern, the metabolic syndrome (MetS) is reviewed here. During the late 1980s, Reaven observed that several CHD risk factors (namely, dyslipidemia, hypertension, and hyperglycemia) frequently cluster together (2). Originally referred to as *syndrome X* or *insulin resistance syndrome*, these descriptors have been supplanted by the more general term *metabolic syndrome*. The National Cholesterol Education Program's Adult Treatment Panel III report (ATP III, discussed later) identified six components of the MetS that relate to CHD: abdominal obesity, atherogenic dyslipidemia (high TG, low HDL-C, and sdLDL), HTN, insulin resistance, a prothrombotic state, and a proinflammatory state (3). Given the ongoing "epidemic of obesity," MetS is common and becoming more so, with approximately one quarter of American adults fulfilling ATP III criteria (4), as listed in Table 12–2. Observational data have shown that such persons

**TABLE 12–2**
**ATP III CLINICAL IDENTIFICATION OF METABOLIC SYNDROME (MetS)**

| Risk Factor (need 3) | Defining Level |
|---|---|
| Abdominal obesity[a] | Waist circumference[b] |
| Men | >102 cm (>40 in) |
| Women | >88 cm (>35 in) |
| Triglycerides | ≥150 mg/dL |
| HDL-C | |
| Men | <40 mg/dL |
| Women | <50 mg/dL |
| Blood pressure | ≥130/≥85 mm Hg |
| Fasting glucose | ≥110 mg/dL |

[a]Overweight and obesity are associated with insulin resistance and MetS. However, the presence of abdominal obesity is more highly correlated with the metabolic risk factors than is an elevated BMI. Therefore, the simple measure of waist circumference is recommended to identify the body-weight component of MetS.
[b]Some male patients can develop multiple metabolic risk factors when the waist circumference is only marginally increased, e.g., 37–39 in. (94–102 cm). Such patients may have a strong genetic contribution to insulin resistance. They should benefit from changes in life habits, similarly to men with categorical increases in waist circumference.
*Source:* Adapted from the Third Report of the National Cholesterol Education Program (NCEP) Expert Panel on the Detection, Evaluation, and Treatment of High Blood Cholesterol in Adults (ATP III), Final Report, 2002. A publication of the National Heart, Lung, and Blood Institute (NHLBI), a division of the National Institutes of Health (NIH), and the U.S. Department of Health and Human Services.

**TABLE 12–3**
**THERAPEUTIC LIFESTYLE CHANGES (TLC)**

| Component | Recommendation | Expected Change in Lipids |
|---|---|---|
| Diet | | |
| Saturated fat | <7% of total calories | ↓ LDL-C 8–10% |
| Dietary cholesterol | <200 mg/day | ↓ LDL-C 3–5% |
| Polyunsaturated fat | Up to 10% of total calories | |
| Monounsaturated fat | Up to 20% of total calories | |
| *n*-3 Fatty acids | "Higher" | |
| *trans*-Fatty acids | "Low" | |
| Total fat | 25–35% of total calories | |
| Carbohydrate | 50–60% of total calories | |
| Dietary fiber | 20–30 g/d | |
| Total protein | 15% of total calories | |
| Therapeutic options to ↓ LDL-C | | |
| Plant stanols/sterols | 2–3 g/d | ↓ LDL-C 6–15% |
| Increased viscous soluble fiber (from whole grains, fresh fruits, legumes, green leafy vegetables) | 5–10 g/d | ↓ LDL-C ~5% |
| Physical activity | Enough moderate activity to expend at least 200 kcal/d | ↓ TG 5–15%<br>↓ TC 0–5%<br>↓ LDL-C 0–3%<br>↑ HDL-C 3–5% (highly variable) |
| Weight loss | Goal BMI <25 kg/m$^2$ | ↓ TG ~7%<br>↓ LDL-C ~6%<br>↓ TC ~10%<br>↑ HDL-C ~8% (with 10 kg/22 lb weight loss)[a] |
| Smoking cessation | Immediate cessation of use of all tobacco products. Reasonable to use nicotine patch, gum, or bupropion for assistance in quitting. | ↑ HDL-C ~5% (highly variable) |

[a]Dattilo AM, Kris-Etherton PM. Effects of weight reduction on blood lipids and lipoproteins: a meta-analysis. *Am J Clin Nutr.* 1992;56:320–328.
*Source:* Adapted from the Third Report of the National Cholesterol Education Program (NCEP) Expert Panel on the Detection, Evaluation, and Treatment of High Blood Cholesterol in Adults (ATP III), Final Report, 2002. A publication of the National Heart, Lung, and Blood Institute (NHLBI), a division of the National Institutes of Health (NIH), and the U.S. Department of Health and Human Services.

have a three- to fivefold risk of CHD mortality, compared to those without MetS. A major health danger to persons with MetS appears to be a vastly increased risk of developing diabetes. MetS was highly predictive of new-onset diabetes in both men and women of the Framingham offspring cohort, as nearly half of the population-attributable risk of type 2 diabetes (DM2) could be explained by the presence of ATPIII-defined MetS (5). When overt diabetes develops, CHD risk increases sharply.

## TREATMENT STRATEGIES FOR DYSLIPIDEMIAS: THERAPEUTIC LIFESTYLE CHANGES

All dyslipidemic patients should be urged to adopt *therapeutic lifestyle changes (TLC)*, consisting of increased physical activity, ideal weight maintenance (often necessitating weight loss), smoking cessation, and the pursuance of a low-saturated-fat, low-cholesterol diet rich in fruits, vegetables, grains, and fiber (Table 12-3). In highly motivated individuals, TLC can result in an LDL-C reduction of nearly 30%, and should form the basis of all preventive treatment. Alcohol avoidance, smoking cessation, physical activity, and diet are essential in the management of dyslipidemias characterized by very high triglycerides. Most primary dyslipidemias other than HoFH, as well as the dyslipidemia associated with MetS, are very sensitive to changes in diet and adiposity, and thus should always be treated with a TLC diet and weight management, with a goal BMI <25 kg/m$^2$. Lifestyle changes are first-line therapy for the MetS, with obesity the primary target of intervention (6). The most critical goal of such modifications is to decrease the incidence of new-onset diabetes, which confers a similar risk of CHD events as known CHD. It may be challenging to implement such changes successfully, but every effort should be made to stress the clear health benefits of dietary modification, weight loss, and physical activity.

Whether TLC are sufficient alone, or should be accompanied by drug therapy, is determined by the dyslipidemic patient's CHD risk status, initial lipid levels, and treatment targets (to be discussed in later sections). Other nonpharmacologic approaches such as dietary intake of plant stanols/sterols (in certain labeled margarines and juices) and increased viscous soluble fiber (in oats, barley, psyllium, pectin-rich fruits, and legumes) may also aid in LDL-C reduction. Fish oil supplementation may aid in TG lowering. Consultation of a registered dietician or qualified nutritionist may be useful. If goal LDL-C has not been reached after 3 months, pharmacologic therapy should be considered.

## TREATMENT STRATEGIES FOR DYSLIPIDEMIAS: PHARMACOLOGIC THERAPY

Pharmacologic therapy should be initiated in patients whose lipids are inadequately lowered with TLC alone, those with lipids too high to be reasonably reduced with TLC alone, or those with CHD risk high enough to mandate drug initiation simultaneously with TLC. There are five major classes of drugs that can be used to regulate a patient's lipid profile, including (a) *HMG-CoA reductase inhibitors*, or "statins," (b) *bile acid sequestrants*, or "resins," (c) *fibric acid derivatives*, or fibrates, (d) *nicotinic acid*, or niacin, and (e) *cholesterol absorption inhibitors*, of which ezetimibe is the only clinically available member. Table 12–4 includes descriptions of these agents, their mechanisms of action, therapeutic indications and contraindications, effects on lipid levels, and adverse effects. The choice of a specific drug or combination of drugs is dependent on an understanding of each medication's mechanism of action, as well as the individual patient's lipid profile, cardiovascular risk, treatment goals, and contraindications. Medication choice should also be influenced by clinical outcome trials demonstrating reduction of cardiovascular events with specific treatments. Specific treatment guidelines are reviewed in a later section. Fasting lipid levels should be checked 6 weeks after drug initiation. Once the treatment goal has been achieved, fasting lipids should be redrawn every 4 to 6 months. Importantly, TLC should always be used concomitantly with drug therapy of dyslipidemias. Referral to a lipid specialist should be considered for complex combined lipid disorders or nonresponders.

Of the primary dyslipidemias, treatment of HeFH includes dietary approaches and aggressive pharmacologic therapy. Because the hepatocytes of these individuals still express the LDL-R, albeit at a lower concentration than normal, they are able to upregulate its level and thus increase clearance of LDL. Multiple studies involving adults with HeFH have shown high-dose statin therapy to be safe, well tolerated, and effective at reducing LDL-C levels, and CHD morbidity/mortality. Children and adolescents with HeFH are also treated effectively with statins. Despite concerns over possible interference with hormonal pathways, the growth parameters and sexual maturation in statin-treated children were similar to those given placebo (7). Often, combination drug therapy of a statin with ezetimibe and/or resins is necessary to lower LDL-C levels adequately. As for HoFH, dietary changes are not effective at reducing LDL-C. Given the complete absence of functional LDL receptors, one would not predict that FH homozygotes could be treated effectively with statins. However, multiple small studies have shown that statins reduce LDL-C by 15% to 35% in such persons, probably via decreased hepatic synthesis of VLDL and LDL.

Drug treatment of persons with other primary dyslipidemias is determined largely by their individual lipid profiles (Table 12–1). In general, elevated LDL-C should be treated with a statin unless contraindicated or not tolerated. Disorders of elevated TG are usually evaluated with a search for secondary causes, and treated with dietary modification, physical activity, and fibrates. The dyslipidemia associated with MetS should always be treated initially with lifestyle approaches, especially weight loss. However, failure to achieve full reversal of the MetS characteristics may necessitate pharmacologic therapy. Subgroup analyses of statin trials have shown that statins reduce risk for CVD events in MetS patients. A post-hoc analysis of recent fibrate trials strongly suggests that they reduce CVD endpoints in patients with atherogenic dyslipidemia and MetS. In some cases, drugs from multiple classes used in combination may be required for adequate LDL-C lowering and/or treatment of combined dyslipidemias. Studies have supported acceptable tolerance and improvement of the lipid profile with combination therapy in certain subgroups. Although lipoprotein improvements have been even more dramatic on combined statin–fibrate, statin–niacin, or stain–resin/ezetimibe therapy, no CVD endpoint data from large, controlled trials are available. Smaller trials and those employing surrogate vascular endpoints suggest clinical benefit of combination therapy. In the Familial Atherosclerosis Treatment Study (FATS), men with familial CHD and elevated apoB were treated with niacin and colestipol, lovastatin and colestipol, or colestipol alone (8). Compared to colestipol monotherapy, both combination therapies reduced the frequency of lesion progression and increased the frequency of lesion regression, as assessed by serial quantitative coronary angiography. Coronary events were significantly decreased in the niacin-based regimen. The HDL-Atherosclerosis Treatment Study (HATS) demonstrated similar benefits of combined simvastatin/niacin treatment for persons with CHD, low HDL-C, and average LDL-C (9). Despite these potential added benefits of combination therapy, it is important to be familiar with the adverse effects of lipid-regulating drugs (Table 12–4). Such adverse effects may occur more frequently with

**TABLE 12–4**
**LIPID-REGULATING DRUGS**

| Class | Specific Agents | Mechanism of Action | Indications/Contraindications | Changes in Lipid Levels | Adverse Effects |
|---|---|---|---|---|---|
| Statins | Lovastatin<br>Pravastatin<br>Fluvastatin<br>Simvastatin<br>Atorvastatin<br>Rosuvastatin | Inhibit HMG-CoA reductase, hepatic enzyme controlling rate-limiting step in cholesterol synthesis → upregulation of LDL-R and ↑ hepatic LDL clearance | High TC, high LDL-C, low HDL-C, high TG, high non-HDL-C, high apoB, mixed lipidemias, known CHD<br>AC: active or chronic liver disease, persistent ↑ transaminases, pregnancy, breast-feeding<br>RC: ↑ susceptibility to rhabdo-induced RF | ↓ TC 15–60%<br>↓ LDL-C 20–60%<br>↑ HDL-C 5–15%<br>↓ TG 10–25% | Major: myopathy, life-threatening rhabdomyolysis (rare)<br>Minor: ↑ hepatic transaminases, heartburn, abdominal pain, diarrhea, constipation, flatulence, headache, rash |
| Resins | Cholestyramine<br>Colestipol<br>Colesevelam | Bind intestinal bile acids, interrupt enterohepatic recycling, increase stool elimination of bile acids, leading to ↓ serum cholesterol | High TC, high LDL-C<br>Generally used only in familial disorders<br>AC: complete biliary obstruction, fasting TG >400 mg/dL<br>RC: fasting TG >200 mg/dL | ↓ TC 5–10%<br>↓ LDL-C 15–30%<br>↑ HDL-C 3–5%<br>TG may be ↑ | Major: bowel obstruction (rare)<br>Minor: constipation, diarrhea, flatulence, abdominal pain, bloating, heartburn, steatorrhea, hypertriglyceridemia |
| Fibrates | Clofibrate<br>Fenofibrate<br>Gemfibrozil<br>Bezafibrate[a]<br>Ciprofibrate[a] | Stimulate transcription factor PPAR-α →<br>↑ Catabolism of TGRL<br>↓ Formation of VLDL TG<br>↑ apoA synthesis<br>↓ TG lead to ↑ HDL-C | High TG, low HDL-C<br>AC: severe renal or hepatic dysfunction<br>RC: diabetic nephropathy, breast-feeding | ↓ TG 20–50%<br>↑ HDL-C 10–20%<br>↓ TC 15–20%<br>↓ LDL-C 5–20% | Major: myopathy (rare), but ↑ frequency with CRI, low albumin, or co-administration with statins<br>Minor: upper GI sx, HA, anxiety, fatigue, vertigo, sleep disorders, myalgia, ↓ libido, alopecia |
| Nicotinic acid | IR (crystalline)<br>ER (Niaspan)<br>SR (Slo-Niacin, enduracin) | ↓ Adipose tissue lipolysis<br>↓ Hepatic TG formation<br>↓ Hepatic HDL particle uptake and catabolism<br>↑ apoB100 catabolism<br>↓ Lp(a) synthesis | Low HDL-C, high TC, high LDL-C, high Lp(a)<br>AC: active or chronic liver disease, severe gout, peptic ulcer disease | ↑ HDL-C 5–35%<br>↓ LDL-C 5–25%<br>↓ TG 20–50%<br>↓ Lp(a) 20–30% | Major: hepatotoxicity (seen more in sustained-release), gout<br>Minor: Flushing, pruritis, upper GI distress, hyperuricemia, hyperglycemia |
| Cholesterol-absorption Inhibitors | Ezetimibe | ↓ Sterol transport across intestinal brush border | High TC, high LDL-C in patients with statin intolerance, or not at goal with statin<br>AC or RC: none | ↓ TC 10–15%<br>↓ LDL-C 15–20%<br>↓ TG 5–10% | Major: none<br>Minor: mild transaminase elevation |

AC, absolute contraindication; RC, relative contraindication; CRI, chronic renal insufficiency; HA, headache; IR, immediate-release; ER, extended release; SR, sustained release.
[a]not available in the United States.

combination therapy, including rhabdomyolysis (more common with statin + fibrate) and hepatic injury (statin + niacin, statin + ezetimibe).

## APHERESIS THERAPY

The mainstay of therapy for FH homozygotes is extracorporeal, namely, *LDL apheresis*. On average, LDL-C levels immediately after the procedure are decreased 50% to 80%. Because these values rebound fairly quickly, the process is performed every 2 weeks to keep intrapheresis LDL-C ≤120 mg/dL. U.S. Food and Drug Administration (FDA) indications since 1996 include: HoFH; HeFH in the absence of CHD when LDL-C ≥300 mg/dL despite maximal pharmacologic and dietary therapy; and HeFH in the presence of CHD when LDL-C ≥200 mg/dL despite maximal pharmacologic and dietary therapy. The benefits of apheresis to FH homozygotes, in terms of stabilization or regression of atherosclerotic lesions, and improvement in symptoms, have been clearly demonstrated. As for FH heterozygotes, combined apheresis and statin therapy have been shown to substantially reduce risk of coronary events, and to improve angiographic outcome.

## LIPID-REGULATING TRIALS FOR THE PREVENTION OF CHD

The rationale for aggressive management of lipid disorders for the purpose of reducing cardiovascular events is based on a large body of research spanning the past decade. A complete review of the research establishing an association between dyslipidemia and CHD is beyond the scope of this chapter, but it is important to highlight the observations and trials supporting recent cholesterol treatment recommendations. As early as the 1930s, associations were observed between cholesterol levels and atherosclerotic disease. Multiple, large observational and epidemiologic studies helped to form the basis of the *cholesterol hypothesis*, which posited that elevated serum cholesterol plays a causative role in the development of CHD, and that cholesterol reduction will reduce CHD risk (10). These studies included the Framingham Heart Study, the Seven Country Study, the Münster Heart Study (PROCAM), the Multiple Risk Factor Intervention Trial (MRFIT), and the Lipid Research Clinics (LRC) Prevalence Study. Data from these studies revealed a strong, graded, linear relationship between TC levels and risk of CHD, with an approximate 20% to 30% increase in CHD risk for each 10% increase in serum TC. An inverse correlation was observed for HDL-C, with every 1 mg/dL (0.026 mM) increase in HDL-C correlating with a 2% decrease in CHD risk for men, and a 3% decrease for women (11). Hypertriglyceridemia was long suspected to be an independent CHD risk factor, but this was difficult to prove given the tight inverse correlation between levels of TG and HDL-C. A meta-analysis of 17 population-based studies showed that each 1 mmol/L (88.5 mg/dL) increase in serum TG significantly increased the risk of a CHD event, by 32% in men and 76% in women. After multivariate analysis, including adjustment for HDL-C levels, a 1-mmol/L increase in TG continued to confer a significantly increased CHD risk, by 14% in men and 37% in women.

Once these relationships had been identified, clinical trials were designed to test the hypothesis that lipid-lowering therapy would slow or reverse the atherosclerotic process and decrease the incidence of CVD events. Despite the diversity in entry criteria and treatments, initial animal and human intervention studies demonstrated plaque regression or improvements in angiographic outcomes associated with improved lipid profiles. Although some of these trials did demonstrate decreased coronary events, the primary endpoints were typically surrogate outcomes, and the trials were not designed or powered to examine clinical outcomes. Subsequent intervention trials targeted "hard" clinical endpoints, including death and nonfatal MI. In *primary prevention* trials, individuals without known CVD underwent cholesterol reduction, with the goal of preventing a first CHD event. In *secondary prevention* trials, subjects with known CVD were treated to lower cholesterol, in an effort to prevent repeat events.

## EARLY TRIALS FOR PRIMARY AND SECONDARY CHD PREVENTION

A number of CVD endpoint trials, reviewed in detail in Table 12–5, were performed in the prestatin era, utilizing diet, bile acid sequestrants, fibrates, or niacin. These trials, in predominantly male populations both with and without CHD, using various treatments or combination of treatments, provided strong support for the cholesterol hypothesis, giving rise to the rule of thumb that a 1% lowering of TC decreases the incidence of CHD events by 2% to 3%. In several of these studies, noncardiovascular death was increased in the group treated with lipid-lowering therapy, raising concern over the safety of such treatment. However, a causal link was never established between lipid-lowering drugs and increased mortality. The early trials set the stage for the large statin trials of the 1990s.

These subsequent large, multicenter, randomized controlled trials irrefutably confirmed the cholesterol hypothesis, demonstrating conclusively that lowering LDL-C reduced the risk of coronary events, and in some cases, total mortality. The efficacy of statins was demonstrated in study populations with a wide range of risk factors and LDL-C levels, and in both primary and secondary CHD prevention. These trials also lay to rest concerns about the possible dangers of low cholesterol, the possibility of which had been raised by several of the prestatin trials. The major statin trials and their findings are summarized in Table 12–6.

## TABLE 12–5
## EARLY LIPID-REGULATING TRIALS

| Study | *N* | Sex, Age | Entry Criteria | Treatment, Control | *Y* | Lipid Change with Treatment | Clinical Outcome with Treatment[a] |
|---|---|---|---|---|---|---|---|
| | | | | **Primary CHD Prevention** | | | |
| LRC-CPPT | 3,806 | M, 35–59 y | TC ≥265 mg/dL<br>LDL-C ≥190 mg/dL<br>TG ≤300 mg/dL | Cholestyramine + diet<br>Placebo + diet | 7.4 | TC ↓ 13%<br>LDL-C ↓ 20% | 1° NFMI/CHDD ↓ 19%, new angina ↓ 20%, new + stress ↓ 25%<br>CABG ↓ 21% (NS), CHDD ↓ 24% (NS), TM ↓ 7% (NS) |
| WHO | >10K | M, 30–59 y | TC in upper tertile of those screened | Clofibrate<br>Placebo | 5.3 | TC ↓ 9% | NFMI/CHDD ↓ 20%<br>TM ↑ 47% but 13-y TM ↑ 11% (NS) |
| HHS | 4,081 | M, 40–55 y | Non-HDL-C >200 mg/dL | Gemfibrozil<br>Placebo | 5 | TC ↓ 10%<br>LDL-C ↓ 11%<br>HDL-C ↑ 11%<br>TG ↓ 35% | 1° NFMI/CHDD ↓ 34%<br>CHDD ↓ 26% (NS)<br>TM slightly ↑ (NS) |
| Oslo | 1,232 | M, 40–49 y | TC 290–380<br>SBP <150 mm Hg<br>Top quartile CHD risk (80% smokers) | Dietary and antismoking advice<br>Usual care | 5 | TC ↓ 13%<br>TG ↓ 20 | 1° NFMI/CHDD/SCD ↓ 47%<br>CHDD ↓ 55% (NS), TM ↓ 33% (NS) |
| | | | | **Secondary CHD Prevention** | | | |
| CDP | 8,341 | M, 30–64 y | MI | Niacin<br>Clofibrate<br>D-Thyroxine<br>E 2.5 mg/d<br>E 5.0 mg/d<br>Placebo | 5 | TC ↓ 10%<br>TG ↓ 22%<br>TC ↓ 6%<br>TG ↓ 22% | NFMI ↓ 27%, 15-y TM ↓ 11%<br>NFMI/CHDD ↓ 9% (NS), TM unchanged<br>↑ TM, arm stopped<br>↑ TE, CA, TM, arm stopped<br>↑ NFMI, lack of efficacy, arm stopped |
| Stockholm | 555 | M/F | MI | Clofibrate + Niacin<br>Placebo | 5 | TC ↓ 13%<br>TG ↓ 19% | CHDD ↓ 36%, TM ↓ 26% |
| BIP | 3,090 | M/F | MI, stable angina, or both | Bezafibrate | 6.2 | TC ↓ 4.5%<br>TG ↓ 21%<br>HDL-C ↑ 18% | MI or sudden death ↓ 7.3% (NS) |

*N*, number of patients in trial; *Y*, years of trial duration; 1°, primary endpoint; NFMI, nonfatal MI; CHDD, CHD death; SCD, sudden cardiac death; +stress, positive stress test; TM, total mortality; E, estrogen; NS, nonsignificant *p* value.
[a]All outcomes significant except as noted.

## TABLE 12–6
## LANDMARK STATIN TRIALS

| Trial[a] | N, Sex | Enrollment Lipids (mg/dL) | Drug, Dose (mg) | Y | Base LDL-C | Tx LDL-C | ΔLDL-C | Adverse Event, Relative Risk Reduction | Tx Rate | PC Rate | %ARR |
|---|---|---|---|---|---|---|---|---|---|---|---|
| **Primary Prevention** | | | | | | | | | | | |
| WOSCOPS | 6,595, M | LDL-C ≥155 | Prava 40 | 4.9 | 192 | 159 | −26% | NFMI or CHDD ↓ 31% | 5.3% | 7.5% | 2.2% |
| | | | | | | | | CABG or PTCA ↓ 37% | | | |
| | | | | | | | | All-cause mortality ↓ 22%* | 3.2% | 4.1% | 0.9% |
| | | | | | | | | CVA ↓ 11% (NS) | 1.4% | 1.5% | NS |
| AFCAPS/ TEXCAPS | 6,605, M/F | TC 180–264<br>LDL-C 130–190<br>HDL-C ≤45 M, ≤47 F | Lova 20–40 | 5.2 | 150 | 115 | −25% | NFMI, CHDD, USA, or SCD ↓ 37% | 3.5% | 5.5% | 2.0% |
| **High-Risk Primary and Secondary Prevention** | | | | | | | | | | | |
| HPS | 20,536, M/F | TC ≥135 | Simva 40 | 6 | 128 M<br>135 F | 89 | −40 mg/dL | All-cause mortality ↓ 12% | 12.9% | 14.6% | 1.7% |
| | | | | | | | | Vascular death ↓ 17% | 7.7% | 9.2% | 1.5% |
| | | | | | | | | Total CHD, CVA, or revasc ↓ 24% | 19.9% | 25.4% | 5.5% |
| | | | | | | | | CVA ↓ 25% | 4.3% | 5.7% | 1.4% |
| **Secondary Prevention** | | | | | | | | | | | |
| 4S | 4,444, M/F | TC 212–309 (mean 261) | Simva 20–40 | 5.4 | 188 | 122 | −35% | All-cause mortality ↓ 30% | 8.2% | 11.5% | 3.3% |
| | | | | | | | | NFMI, CHDD or resusc SCD ↓34% | 19.4% | 27.9% | 8.5% |
| | | | | | | | | CVA ↓ 30% | 3.2% | 4.4% | 1.2% |
| CARE | 4,159, M/F | TC <240<br>LDL-C 115–174 | Prava 40 | 5.0 | 139 | 98 | −32% | NFMI or CHDD ↓ 24% | 10.2% | 13.2% | 3.0% |
| | | | | | | | | CVA ↓ 31% | 2.6% | 3.8% | 1.2% |
| LIPID | 9,014, M/F | TC 155–270 | Prava 40 | 6.1 | 150 | 110 | −27% | CHDD ↓ 24% | 6.4% | 8.3% | 1.9% |
| | | | | | | | | All-cause mortality ↓ 22% | 11.0% | 14.1% | 3.1% |
| | | | | | | | | MI ↓ 29% | 7.4% | 10.3% | 2.9% |
| | | | | | | | | CVA ↓ 19%** | 3.7% | 4.5% | 0.8% |

*N*, number of subjects in trial; sex, sex of subjects in trial; *Y*, years of trial duration; base LDL-C, average baseline LDL-C; Tx LDL-C, average LDL-C with drug treatment; ΔLDL-C, change in average LDL-C with drug treatment compared to placebo, expressed in percent or mg/dL; Tx rate, adverse event occurrence rate in treatment group during study period; PC rate, adverse event occurrence rate in placebo control group during study period; %ARR, percent absolute risk reduction; Prava, pravastatin; Lova, lovastatin; Simva, simvastatin; Atorva, atorvastatin; NFMI, nonfatal MI; CHDD, CHD death; CVA, nonfatal and fatal stroke; USA, unstable angina; SCD, sudden cardiac death; revasc, coronary revascularization; resusc, resuscitated.
*$p = 0.051$; **$p = 0.048$; NS, not significant.
[a]Trials: WOSCOPS, West of Scotland Coronary Prevention Study; AFCAPS/TexCAPS, Air Force/Texas Coronary Atherosclerosis Prevention Study; 4S, Scandinavian Simvastatin Survival Study; CARE, Cholesterol And Recurrent Events trial; LIPID, Long-term Intervention with Pravastatin in Ischemic Disease trial.
*Source:* Adapted from Gotto AM, Pownall HJ. *Manual of Lipid Disorders.* 3rd ed. Philadelphia: Lippincott Williams & Wilkins; 2003:171–174, with permission.

## THE LANDMARK STATIN TRIALS—PRIMARY PREVENTION

The *West of Scotland Coronary Prevention Study (WOSCOPS)* (12) randomized 6,595 middle-aged men with high LDL-C (mean 192 mg/dL) to pravastatin 40 mg/day versus placebo, with dietary intervention in all subjects. The 26% reduction in LDL-C by pravastatin was double that seen in previous, nonstatin primary prevention trials. Over 4.9 years, pravastatin treatment significantly reduced coronary events (nonfatal MI or CHD death) by 31% and the need for coronary artery bypass grafting (CABG) or percutaneous translumenal coronary angioplasty (PTCA) by 37%. Total mortality was decreased 22%, with a $p$ value of borderline statistical significance ($p = 0.051$). Noncardiovascular deaths were not increased. A provocative post-hoc finding of WOSCOPS was that pravastatin treatment reduced the incidence of newly diagnosed diabetes by 30% ($p = 0.042$), by an as-yet undetermined mechanism. In summary, WOSCOPS demonstrated that LDL-C reduction with pravastatin was both safe and effective at preventing a first CHD event in hyperlipidemic men.

The *Air Force/Texas Coronary Atherosclerosis Prevention Study (AFCAPS/TexCAPS)* (13) was the first primary prevention trial of lipid regulation to include women, and subjects >65 years of age, but its most important feature was that it enrolled subjects with only average LDL-C (mean 150 mg/dL), and below-average HDL-C (mean 36 mg/dL in men, 40 mg/dL in women). At the time of the study, such therapy would have been considered aggressive in this population: only 17% would have qualified for lipid-lowering treatment by the existing 1993 NCEP guidelines, compared with 77% of the patients in WOSCOPS. Compared to placebo, lovastatin (20 to 40 mg/day over 5.2 years) reduced LDL-C 25% and increased HDL-C 6%. The rate of first major coronary event (unstable angina, MI, or sudden cardiac death) was reduced by 37%, fatal or nonfatal MI by 40%, unstable angina by 32%, and coronary revascularization by 33%. Total mortality and noncardiovascular deaths did not differ significantly between treatment groups. Benefit of statin therapy was observed for women, the elderly, smokers, and hypertensive persons. Equal benefit was seen in all quartiles of LDL-C level, without evidence for a threshold effect. Subjects with the lowest HDL-C (<35 mg/dL) enjoyed the greatest benefit of statin treatment, a 45% reduction in CHD events. AFCAPS/TexCAPS expanded the observations of WOSCOPS by demonstrating that statin therapy effectively prevented a first CHD event in both men and women with average LDL-C.

## THE LANDMARK STATIN TRIALS—SECONDARY PREVENTION

The *Scandinavian Simvastatin Survival Study (4S)* (14) enrolled 4,444 middle-aged men and women aged 35 to 60 years with mean LDL-C of 188 mg/dL and a history of angina pectoris or MI. Simvastatin (20 to 40 mg/day) for an average of 5.4 years lowered LDL-C by 35% (compared to a 1% increase in the randomized placebo group), and significantly decreased the primary endpoint of total (all-cause) mortality by 30% ($p = 0.0003$). Coronary mortality decreased 42%, without an increase in non-CVD death. Incidence of major coronary events (coronary death, nonfatal MI, and resuscitated cardiac arrest) was significantly reduced 34% by simvastatin. Interestingly, the reduction in risk for coronary events was similar in each quartile of baseline TC, LDL-C, or HDL-C. Pre-existing smoking, diabetes mellitus, impaired fasting glucose (IFG), and HTN did not mitigate these benefits. The risk of a major coronary event was significantly reduced by 35% in women, by 42% in diabetics, and by 38% in those with impaired fasting glucose. In summary, 4S provided robust evidence that LDL-C reduction with simvastatin safely reduced both CHD events and total mortality in men and women with known CHD.

The *Cholesterol and Recurrent Events (CARE)* trial (15) enrolled 4,200 post-MI men and postmenopausal women, aged 21 to 75 years, with average LDL-C (mean 139 mg/dL). LDL-C decreased by 28% with pravastatin 40 mg/day, relative to placebo. After 5 years, statin therapy yielded a 24% reduction in nonfatal MI or CHD death and decreased the need for CABG or PTCA by 27%. Women sustained better outcomes than men, with a 46% versus 20% reduction in combined coronary events, including CHD death, nonfatal MI, PTCA, and CABG (both with $p = 0.001$). Like the 4S trial, there was a greater than 30% reduction in CVA. The oldest patients (aged 65 to 75) enjoyed a decrease in combined coronary events of 32%, and those who had undergone previous CABG, PTCA, or both, experienced a 36% reduction in nonfatal MI or CHD. Treatment benefit was similar regardless of the presence or absence of HTN, diabetes, tobacco use, or left ventricular dysfunction. Therefore CARE demonstrated that both men and women (including the elderly) with a history of MI and only modest elevations in LDL-C levels experience fewer cardiovascular events when treated with pravastatin.

The *Long-term Intervention with Pravastatin in Ischemic Disease (LIPID)* trial (16) was designed to be applicable to as many patients with CHD as possible. LIPID enrolled 9,014 men and women with history of acute MI or hospitalization for unstable angina, with a broad range of serum lipids, as well as "average" LDL-C (mean 150 mg/dL). The 25% reduction in LDL-C with pravastatin 40 mg/day over 6.1 years was associated with reduction in the primary endpoint of CHD death by 24% ($p < 0.001$), the secondary endpoint of all-cause mortality by 22% ($p < 0.001$) and additional prespecified endpoints listed in Table 12–6. Effects of treatment were similar for all predefined subgroups, including women, the elderly, diabetics, and patients with TC <213 mg/dL. Importantly, a large percentage of subjects in both the placebo and treatment groups was on appropriate contemporary "background" therapy for CHD, including aspirin, beta-blockers, and antihypertensive medications. In summary, LIPID showed that a broad population of men and women with known CHD derived significant morbidity and mortality benefit from statin therapy, even in the context of average LDL-C levels and in addition to current non–lipid-lowering therapy for CHD.

## THE LANDMARK STATIN TRIALS—SECONDARY AND HIGH-RISK PRIMARY PREVENTION

The Medical Research Council/British Heart Foundation (MRC/BHF) *Heart Protection Study (HPS)* (17) was a "megastudy" of over 20,000 subjects, easily representing the largest trial of lipid-regulating therapy to date. Eligible patients included men and women between 40 and 80 years of age with fasting TC >135 mg/dL (>3.5 mM) at high risk for CHD death over the next 5 years. Subjects fell into one of three categories: (a) history of CHD, (b) PVD or cerebrovascular disease, or (c) diabetes mellitus or treated HTN in men ≥65 years of age. The HPS set out to test the hypothesis that treating the at-risk individual with a statin regardless of the level of pretreatment LDL-C would offer benefit. Simvastatin 40 mg/day reduced LDL-C by an average of 40 mg/dL in this placebo-controlled intent-to-treat analysis. Over an average of 5 years, the risk of a major vascular event (combination of total CHD, total CVA, or coronary and noncoronary revascularization) was significantly reduced by 24%, all-cause mortality by 12%, and CVA by 27% in the statin group compared to placebo. A 20% decreased risk for vascular events was seen in female subjects, the largest cohort reported to date. Significant reductions in vascular risk were observed both in patients younger than 70 years (24%), and in those 70 years or older (18%). Importantly, prior to HPS, evidence for a statin treatment benefit was lacking in large cohorts of patients with cerebrovascular disease, PVD, and diabetes, but without a history of MI or documented CHD ("high-risk primary prevention.") In HPS, effective reductions in vascular risk were provided by simvastatin to non-CHD subjects with history of CVA (15%), PVD (22%), or DM (24%).

Perhaps the most significant finding of HPS was that benefit occurred across all entry LDL-C concentrations, whether <116 mg/dL (21% reduction in vascular events), 116 to 135 mg/dL (26%), or >135 mg/dL (20%). This clear risk reduction in 6,973 patients with baseline LDL-C <116 mg/dL refutes the hypothesis (based largely on data from CARE) that cholesterol lowering below this level would not confer benefit. In fact, the investigators reported that, even in those subjects with LDL-C <100 mg/dL, there was a significant 21% reduction in vascular events. This finding prompted many to question whether the existing treatment LDL-C treatment goal of <100 mg/dL in high-risk patients was low enough, an issue that would be addressed in later trials. In conclusion, HPS demonstrated that men and women at high risk for a major vascular event (including those with DM, HTN, PVD, or cerebrovascular disease) benefit from statin therapy, regardless of baseline LDL-C. Data from HPS have helped shift our therapeutic paradigm from the treatment of elevated LDL-C to the treatment of elevated CVD risk.

In the preceding trials, statins were often started months to years after an acute coronary event and at moderate doses. Other studies addressed the safety and effectiveness of early high-dose statin therapy and set the stage for trials that would test the utility of more aggressive and early lipid lowering in the prevention of CHD.

The *Myocardial Ischemia Reduction with Aggressive Cholesterol Lowering (MIRACL)* trial tested the hypothesis that initiation of statin therapy in the acute post-ACS setting could be safe and provide clinical benefit. A cohort of 3,086 men and women with unstable angina or non–Q-wave MI were randomized to treatment with atorvastatin 80 mg/day or placebo within 24 to 96 hours of hospital admission. Mean LDL-C was reduced 40% in the atorvastatin group, versus a rise of 12% in the placebo group. After only 16 weeks, the primary endpoint of combined death, nonfatal MI, resuscitated cardiac arrest, or ischemia was reduced by 16% ($p = 0.048$) in the atorvastatin group. This benefit was due primarily to a reduction in symptomatic myocardial ischemia requiring rehospitalization, an endpoint that was reduced by 26% ($p = 0.02$). In summary, the MIRACL study showed that early initiation of high-dose atorvastatin was safe and possibly beneficial for immediate post-ACS patients.

The *Atorvastatin Versus Revascularization Treatments (AVERT)* trial was a small, short-term trial comparing high-dose atorvastatin therapy (80 mg/day) with angioplasty and usual care (73% of this group received some form of lipid-lowering therapy) in 341 angioplasty-eligible patients with stable CHD. LDL-C was reduced an average of 46% in the atorvastatin group, compared to 18% in the usual-care group. The rate of ischemic events was reduced by 36% in the atorvastatin group, compared to usual care/angioplasty, although the statistical significance was borderline ($p = 0.048$). AVERT contained the provocative result that, for patients with stable CHD, aggressive LDL-C reduction to levels well below 100 mg/dL with a high-dose statin was more effective at reducing coronary events than angioplasty.

## LESSONS FROM RECENT STATIN TRIALS

Since the NCEP ATP III guidelines appeared in 2001, a number of published trials in addition to the HPS have offered a rationale for modifications in these treatment recommendations (Table 12–7). Some have attempted to determine if more aggressive lipid lowering confers clinical benefit beyond moderate lipid lowering in patients after ACS (REVERSAL, PROVE-IT/TIMI-22, Phase Z of the A to Z Trial), and in those with stable CHD (TNT). Others have

## TABLE 12–7
## RECENT STATIN TRIALS

| Trial[a] | *N*, Sex | Drug, Dose (mg) | *Y* | Base LDL-C | Tx LDL-C | Adverse Event, Relative Risk Reduction | Tx Rate | PC Rate | %ARR |
|---|---|---|---|---|---|---|---|---|---|
| PROVE-IT TIMI-22 | 4,162, M/F | Atorva 80 vs. Prava 40 | 2 | 133 | 62 vs. 95 | 1° Death, MI, USA, revasc, or CVA: ↓ 16% | 22.4% | 26.3% | 3.9% |
| | | | | | | Death or MI ↓ 18% (NS) | 8.3% | 10.0% | 1.7% |
| | | | | | | Recurrent USA ↓ 29% | 3.8% | 5.1% | 1.3% |
| | | | | | | Revasc ↓ 14% | 16.3% | 18.8% | 2.5% |
| TNT | 10,001, M/F | Atorva 80 vs. Atorva 10 | 4.9 | 99 on Atorva 10 mg | 77 vs. 101 | NFMI ↓ 22% | 6.2% | 4.9% | 1.3% |
| | | | | | | Combined CV events ↓ 22% | 8.7% | 10.9% | 2.2% |
| | | | | | | CVA ↓ 25% | 3.1% | 2.3% | 0.8% |
| | | | | | | Fatal MI ↓ 20% NS | 2.5% | 2.0% | 0.5% |
| ASCOT-LLA | 10,305, M/F | Atorva 10 | 3.3 | 133 | 87 | NFMI or CHDD ↓ 36% | 5.2% | 8.3% | 3.1% |
| | | | | | | CV events/procedures ↓ 21% | 24.1% | 30.6% | 6.5% |
| | | | | | | Coronary events ↓ 29% | 10.8% | 15.2% | 4.4% |
| | | | | | | CVA ↓ 27% | 5.4% | 7.4% | 2.0% |
| | | | | | | Chronic stable angina ↓ 41% | 2.0% | 3.4% | 1.4% |
| CARDS | 2,838, M/F | Atorva 10 | 3.9 | 111 | 122 | Combined CV events ↓ 37% | 5.8% | 9.0% | 3.2% |
| | | | | | | USA, NFMI, CHDD ↓ 36% | 3.6% | 5.5% | 1.9% |
| | | | | | | CVA ↓ 48% | 1.5% | 2.8% | 1.3% |
| | | | | | | Total mortality ↓ 27%* | 4.3% | 5.8% | 1.5% |

*N*, number of subjects in trial; sex, sex of subjects in trial; *Y*, years of trial duration; Tx LDL-C, average LDL-C with drug treatment; Tx rate, adverse event occurrence rate in treatment group during study period; PC rate, adverse event occurrence rate in placebo control group or comparison group during study period; %ARR, percent absolute risk reduction; Prava, pravastatin; Atorva, atorvastatin; NFMI, nonfatal MI; CHDD, CHD death; CVA, nonfatal and fatal stroke; USA, unstable angina; SCD, sudden cardiac death; revasc, coronary revascularization; resusc, resuscitated.

[a]Trials: PROVE-IT/TIMI-22, Provastain or Atorvastain Evaluation and Infection Therapy-Thrombolysis in Myocardial Infarction 22; TNT, Treating to New Targets; ASCOT-LLA, Anglo-Scandinavian Cardiac Outcomes Trial—Lipid Lowering Arm; CARDS, Collaborative Atorvastatin Diabetes Study.

*$p = 0.059$; **$p = 0.048$; NS, not significant.

*Source:* Adapted in part from Gotto AM, Pownall HJ. *Manual of Lipid Disorders*. 3rd ed. Philadelphia: Lippincott Williams & Wilkins; 2003:171–174, with permission.

tested the hypothesis that initiation of statin therapy at levels of LDL-C previously not recommended for pharmacologic therapy would reduce CVD events in moderate risk individuals without known CHD (ASCOT-LLA in "primary care" hypertensive, nondyslipidemic patients with multiple risk factors and CARDS in patients with type 2 diabetes without significant elevation in LDL-C).

The *Reversal of Atherosclerosis with Aggressive Lipid Lowering (REVERSAL)* trial (18) compared the ability of moderate and intensive statin treatment to reduce progression of coronary atherosclerosis as assessed by intravascular ultrasound (IVUS). In this study, 502 patients with angiographically documented CHD were randomly assigned to receive pravastatin 40 mg/day or atorvastatin 80 mg/day, over a period of 18 months. The primary endpoint, percent change in total atheroma volume, did not change significantly in those subjects receiving atorvastatin, whereas it increased in those receiving pravastatin. Percentage changes in levels of LDL-C, hs-CRP, apoB100, and non-HDL-C correlated with the rate of progression of atherosclerosis. In summary, REVERSAL demonstrated that in patients with known CHD, there was a reduced rate of atherosclerotic progression associated with more aggressive statin treatment. Despite its use of a surrogate outcome (IVUS) and its lack of "hard" clinical endpoints, REVERSAL provided attractive biochemical and pathophysiologic data supporting intensive statin treatment to slow progression of CHD in high-risk groups.

The *Pravastatin or Atorvastatin Evaluation and Infection Therapy—Thrombolysis in Myocardial Infarction 22 (PROVE-IT/TIMI-22)* trial (19) enrolled 4,162 men and women who had been hospitalized for ACS within the previous 10 days, and randomized them to pravastatin 40 mg/day (standard therapy) or atorvastatin 80 mg/day (intensive therapy). Median LDL-C achieved during treatment was 95 mg/dL with pravastatin, and 62 mg/dL with atorvastatin. Over an average follow-up time of only 2 years, the primary endpoint (death from any cause, MI, documented unstable angina requiring rehospitalization, rehospitalization, revascularization performed $\geq$30 days after randomization, and stroke) occurred in 26% of the pravastatin group, and in 22% of the atorvastatin group, representing a 16% relative risk (RR) reduction for intensive therapy ($p = 0.005$). Prior to this trial, moderate-intensity statin treatment to a target LDL-C $<$100 mg/dL was felt to be adequate for patients with established CHD. However, PROVE-IT/TIMI-22 demonstrated that intensive statin therapy, with a goal LDL-C $<$70 mg/dL, provided greater protection against death or major cardiovascular events post ACS.

The *Treating to New Targets (TNT)* study (20) sought to determine if lowering LDL-C well below 100 mg/dL would provide additional benefit to patients with stable CHD. In this study, 10,001 patients with known CHD and LDL-C $<$130 mg/dL were randomized to either 10 mg or 80 mg of atorvastatin per day after documentation of at-goal response on a 10-mg dose. Over a median of 4.9 years, the mean LDL-C levels were 77 mg/dL during treatment with atorvastatin 80 mg/day, and 101 mg/dL during continued treatment with atorvastatin 10 mg/day. The primary endpoint (first major cardiovascular event, defined as CHD death, nonfatal non–procedure-related MI, rescuscitation after cardiac arrest, or CVA) occurred in 8.7% of patients receiving 80 mg/day of atorvastatin, compared to 10.9% of patients receiving 10 mg/day, representing a 22% RR reduction ($p < 0.001$). Total mortality was not different between the two groups. The TNT study showed that patients with stable CHD benefit from LDL-C reduction to levels considerably below 100 mg/dL.

The *Anglo-Scandinavian Cardiac Outcomes Trial—Lipid Lowering Arm (ASCOT-LLA)* (21) assessed the benefits of statin therapy for "the primary prevention of CHD in hypertensive patients not conventionally deemed dyslipidemic." In this study, 10,305 men and women with TC $\leq$250 mg/dL (mean LDL-C 133 mg/dL) were randomized to either atorvastatin 10 mg/day or placebo. At 1-year follow-up, LDL-C decreased 35% in the atorvastatin group, but was unchanged in the placebo group. The trial was stopped early (after 3.3 years, instead of the planned 5 years), because of a highly significant 36% reduction ($p = 0.0005$) in the primary endpoint of nonfatal MI and CHD death in the atorvastatin group. Hazard ratios for the primary endpoint were similar for subjects with baseline TC $\leq$217 mg/dL and those $>$217 mg/dL. Benefit was observed in most of the 18 prespecified subgroups, including women and diabetics. In conclusion, ASCOT-LLA demonstrated that men and women at moderately elevated risk for CHD should be considered for statin therapy, even if their LDL-C levels are only mildly elevated.

The *Collaborative Atorvastatin Diabetes Study (CARDS)* (22) tested the hypothesis that statin treatment could prevent primary CHD events in patients with DM2, serum creatinine $\leq$1.7 mg/dL, and fasting LDL-C $<$160 mg/dL (mean 111 mg/dL). In this study, 2,838 diabetic patients without known CHD, aged 40 to 75 years, with at least one other high-risk feature (retinopathy, albuminuria, current smoking, or HTN) were randomized to placebo or atorvastatin 10 mg/day. Over a median follow-up duration of 3.9 years, subjects treated with atorvastatin experienced a highly significant 37% reduction in the first occurrence of an acute CHD event, coronary revascularization, or CVA ($p = 0.001$). Assessed individually, CHD events, coronary revascularizations, and strokes were reduced significantly, by 36%, 31%, and 48%, respectively. Treatment also conferred a favorable trend toward reduced total mortality (RR reduction of 27%, $p = 0.059$). Therefore, CARDS demonstrated that atorvastatin 10 mg/day was safe and effective in reducing the risk of a first CVD event for patients with DM2 and average to low LDL-C, and that diabetic patients may benefit from statins, regardless of baseline LDL-C levels.

## TARGETING LIPIDS OTHER THAN LDL-C

As therapeutic target levels of LDL-C drop ever lower and the demographics of patients eligible for statin therapy grow ever wider, we may be soon approaching the limits of beneficial LDL-C treatment. In addition, with the increase in obesity, MetS, and DM2, more individuals are presenting with combined hyperlipidemias. Given the knowledge derived from epidemiologic and biochemical studies, it seems logical that altering concentrations of HDL-C and TG could reduce the incidence of CHD. A recent systematic review examining 19 prospective statin trials was unable to link changes in CHD mortality and morbidity to treatment-induced changes in HDL-C (23). Explanations for this negative result include the modest effect of statins on HDL-C levels, and the paucity of data on nonstatin therapies. Fibrates and niacin are the most potent agents available to decrease TG or increase HDL-C, with lesser effects on LDL-C. However, dissecting the relative contributions of changes in HDL-C and TG to decreasing CHD risk has been challenging. Earlier trials provided indirect data suggesting a benefit of such changes, but data from prospective studies testing this hypothesis directly have been only recently forthcoming. Monotherapy trials support a role for treatment with fibrates or niacin in select groups. An important clinical question is whether there is added benefit when other medications to modify HDL-C and TG are added to a background of statin therapy. However, long-term outcome trials examining combinations of these agents with statins are not yet available.

The Helsinki Heart Study (HHS) and the Bezafibrate Infarction Prevention (BIP) trial were primary and secondary prevention studies, respectively, using fibrates. Although both trials showed respectable increases in HDL-C and decreases in TG, nonfatal MI/CHD death was decreased 34% ($p < 0.02$) compared to placebo in HHS, while no such benefit was observed in BIP. Despite these conflicting results, post-hoc analysis of HHS provided tantalizing data suggesting the benefit of raising HDL-C. Application of a Cox proportional hazards model revealed that changes in both HDL-C and LDL-C were significantly associated with the reduction in CHD events, whereas the large reduction in TG had only a minimal contribution. Also, three groups of patients derived the greatest reduction in CHD event rate from gemfibrozil therapy: subjects with elevated VLDL and LDL, those in the lowest tertile of HDL-C, and those in the highest tertile of TG. The patients most likely to benefit from treatment were further defined as those with an LDL-C:HDL-C ratio >5 and TG >200 mg/dL. Together, these findings suggested that raising HDL-C could reduce the incidence of CHD events, especially in those with the atherogenic dyslipidemia of low HDL-C and high TG.

The Coronary Drug Project (CDP), initiated in the late 1960s, was a large secondary prevention study among men with several treatment arms, one of which utilized 3 g/day of niacin. Compared to placebo, niacin lowered TC by 10% and TG by 26% (LDL-C and HDL-C data not available), and after 6 years, significantly reduced nonfatal MI by 27%. Although all-cause mortality was not significantly different from placebo at the study's conclusion, a 15-year follow-up analysis (9 years after the interventions had ended) revealed a significant 11% decrease ($p < 0.004$) in total mortality. The investigators suggested that this reduction in mortality may have been due to the decrease in nonfatal MI during the period of niacin treatment.

The *Veterans Affairs Cooperative Studies Program High-Density Lipoprotein Cholesterol Intervention Trial (VA-HIT)* (24) assessed the benefit of gemfibrozil therapy for secondary CHD prevention in patients with low HDL-C and low LDL-C. A fibrate was chosen for treatment because of its minimal effects on LDL-C; the investigators hoped to evaluate the clinical benefit of raising HDL-C and lowering TG without the interference of changes in LDL-C. In this study, 2,531 men with mean HDL-C of 32 mg/dL, mean LDL-C of 112 mg/dL, and mean TG of 160 mg/dL, as well as CHD, defined as history of MI, angina with objective evidence of ischemia, coronary revascularization, or angiographic stenosis of >50% in one or more major coronary arteries, were randomized to gemfibrozil 1,200 mg/day or placebo, for an average period of 5.1 years. Gemfibrozil treatment was associated with 6% higher HDL-C and 31% lower TG and afforded a 22% reduction in nonfatal MI and CHD death over placebo ($p = 0.006$) and a 24% reduction in the combined primary outcome of nonfatal MI, CHD death, and stroke ($p < 0.001$). Decreased risk for CHD was predicted by increased HDL-C, but not by decreased TG. A multivariate Cox proportional hazards analysis published later showed a CHD event-rate reduction of 11% for every 5 mg/dL increase in HDL-C with therapy ($p = 0.02$). However, the HDL-C change seen in VA-HIT did not completely explain the treatment benefit of gemfibrozil.

The *Arterial Biology for the Investigation of the Treatment Effects of Reducing Cholesterol (ARBITER-2)* (25) study was a small secondary prevention trial of 167 persons (91% men) with known CHD and low HDL-C (<45 mg/dL, mean 40 mg/dL). Investigators sought to determine if the addition of an HDL-C–raising drug (niacin) to a background of statin treatment could slow the progression of atherosclerosis, the primary outcome measure being percent change in carotid intima-media thickness (CIMT). All subjects were at LDL-C treatment goals on a statin and then were randomized to additional treatment with once-daily extended-release niacin (1 g) or placebo. At 1 year, HDL-C increased an average of 21% in the niacin group. Mean CIMT increased significantly in the placebo group, but was not significantly changed in the niacin group. Although the overall difference in CIMT progression between niacin and placebo groups was not statistically significant ($p = 0.08$), niacin significantly reduced the CIMT progression rate in subjects without insulin resistance ($p = 0.026$). Coronary events occurred in three patients taking niacin (3.8%), and in seven patients taking placebo (9.6%, $p = 0.20$). Niacin treatment when added to statin therapy appeared to slow the rate of atherosclerotic progression in persons with CHD and low HDL-C. A large National Institutes of Health (NIH)-supported trial of statin and randomized addition of niacin has just begun recruitment. The benefit of the addition of a fibrate to statin in diabetics is being evaluated in the ACCORD trial. Future studies like these and others using drugs with more robust effects on HDL-C and TG should provide needed outcomes data.

## CURRENT TREATMENT GUIDELINES FOR DYSLIPIDEMIAS

The most recent full set of guidelines for the treatment of dyslipidemias is the National Cholesterol Education Program's Adult Treatment Panel III (NCEP ATP III), a 284-page document initially published in 2001 (26). ATP III highlighted early identification of lipid abnormalities, offered new recommendations for screening and detection, modified lipid and lipoprotein classifications, and re-emphasized the importance of nonpharmacologic management of lipid disorders. The main objective of ATP III was to promote more aggressive treatment of dyslipidemias in a broader spectrum of patients and over a wider range of cholesterol levels. LDL-C remained the primary target of therapy. This was based on knowledge of the linear relationship between serum cholesterol and coronary events (approximate 1% drop in CHD event risk for each 1% reduction in LDL-C), as well as knowledge gleaned from many of the large, prospective, randomized statin trials unavailable at the time of previous guidelines. For all patients, optimal LDL-C was redefined as <100 mg/dL (a lower threshold of LDL-C levels had not yet been established), threshold for low HDL-C increased from <35 mg/dL to <40 mg/dL, and TG classification cutpoints were reduced to bring more attention to moderate elevations (Table 12–8). Major CHD risk factors were once again identified (Table 12–9) and utilized as a basis for global risk assessment. Nonpharmacologic interventions such as TLC were intensified (see Table 12–3). One of the most important contributions of the newer guidelines was to highlight the importance of identifying the level of future cardiovascular risk and targeting therapeutic decisions to that risk level. In fact, applying the new risk assessment and treatment goals nearly tripled the number of adults suitable for initiation of simultaneous TLC and drug therapy to >36 million individuals. In August 2004, the NCEP generated a report proposing further modifications to the ATP III LDL-C treatment goals, based on studies published after its release, including HPS, ASCOT-LLA, and PROVE-IT/TIMI-22 (27). These suggested changes consist of optional lower goals for LDL-C targets, and a minimum 30% to 40% reduction in LDL-C from baseline, in high-risk and moderately high-risk patients.

The most recent cholesterol treatment guidelines and update identify four tiers of CHD risk with therapeutic lifestyle and pharmacologic recommendations for each risk level (Table 12–10). These tiers of risk are based largely on the known risk of clinically present cardiovascular disease or diabetes and epidemiologic data from the Framingham Heart Study. Individuals with known CHD, including a history of MI, unstable angina, PCI or CABG, or evidence of clinically significant myocardial ischemia, are at the highest risk for coronary events. Because noncoronary atherosclerotic disease confers a risk for coronary events comparable to that of known CHD, conditions such as symptomatic carotid artery disease, peripheral arterial disease, and abdominal aneurysm are referred to as "CHD risk equivalents." Starting with ATP III, diabetes also came to be regarded as a CHD risk equivalent based on

**TABLE 12–8**
**ATP III CLASSIFICATION OF LDL, TOTAL, AND HDL-CHOLESTEROL, AND TRIGLYCERIDES (mg/dL)**

| | |
|---|---|
| | **LDL Cholesterol—Primary Target of Therapy** |
| <100 | Optimal |
| 100–129 | Near-optimal/above optimal |
| 130–159 | Borderline high |
| 160–189 | High |
| ≥190 | Very high |
| | **Total Cholesterol** |
| <200 | Desirable |
| 200–239 | Borderline high |
| ≥240 | High |
| | **HDL Cholesterol** |
| <40 | Low |
| ≥60 | High |
| | **Triglycerides** |
| <150 | Normal |
| 150–199 | Borderline high |
| 200–499 | High |
| ≥500 | Very high |

*Source:* Adapted from the Third Report of the National Cholesterol Education Program (NCEP) Expert Panel on the Detection, Evaluation, and Treatment of High Blood Cholesterol in Adults (ATP III), Final Report, 2002. A publication of the National Heart, Lung, and Blood Institute (NHLBI), a division of the National Institutes of Health (NIH), and the U.S. Department of Health and Human Services.

**TABLE 12–9**
**MAJOR CHD RISK FACTORS (EXCLUSIVE OF LDL-C) THAT MODIFY LDL-C GOALS**

Cigarette smoking
HTN (BP ≥140/≥90 mm Hg or on antihypertensive medication)
Low HDL-C (<40 mg/dL)[a]
Family history of premature CHD (first-degree relative, male <55 y, female <65 y)
Age (men ≥45 y, women ≥55 y)

[a]HDL-C ≥60 mg/dL counts as a "negative" risk factor; its presence removes 1 risk factor from the total count.
*Source:* Adapted from the Third Report of the National Cholesterol Education Program (NCEP) Expert Panel on the Detection, Evaluation, and Treatment of High Blood Cholesterol in Adults (ATP III), Final Report, 2002. A publication of the National Heart, Lung, and Blood Institute (NHLBI), a division of the National Institutes of Health (NIH), and the U.S. Department of Health and Human Services.

TABLE 12–10

**ATP III LDL-C GOALS AND CUTPOINTS FOR THERAPEUTIC LIFESTYLE CHANGES (TLC) AND DRUG THERAPY IN DIFFERENT RISK CATEGORIES AND PROPOSED MODIFICATIONS BASED ON RECENT CLINICAL TRIAL EVIDENCE**

| Risk Category | LDL-C Goal | Initiate TLC | Consider Drug Therapy[a] |
|---|---|---|---|
| *High risk:* CHD[b] or CHD risk equivalents[d] (10-y risk >20%) | <100 mg/dL (optional goal: <70 mg/dL)[f] | ≥100 mg/dL[e] | ≥100 mg/dL[c] (<100 mg/dL: consider drug options)[a] |
| *Moderately high risk:* 2+ risk factors (10-year risk 10–20%)[g] | <130 mg/dL (optional goal: <100 mg/dL) | ≥130 mg/dL[c] | ≥130 mg/dL (100–129 mg/dL: consider drug options)[h] |
| *Moderate risk:* 2+ risk factors (10-year risk <10%)[g] | <130 mg/dL | ≥130 mg/dL | ≥160 mg/dL |
| *Lower risk:* 0–1 risk factor[i] | <160 mg/dL | ≥160 mg/dL | ≥190 mg/dL (160–189 mg/dL: LDL-lowering drug optional) |

[a]When LDL-lowering drug therapy is employed, it is advised that intensity of therapy be sufficient to achieve at least a 30–40% reduction in LDL-C levels.
[b]CHD includes history of MI, unstable angina, PCI or CABG, or evidence of clinically significant myocardial ischemia.
[c]If baseline LDL-C is <100 mg/dL, institution of an LDL-lowering drug is a therapeutic option on the basis of available clinical trial results. If a high-risk person has high TG or low HDL-C, combining a fibrate or nicotinic acid with an LDL-lowering drug can be considered.
[d]CHD risk equivalents include clinical manifestations of noncoronary forms of atherosclerotic disease (peripheral arterial disease, abdominal aortic aneurysm, and carotid artery disease [TIA or CVA of carotid origin or >50% obstruction of a carotid artery]), diabetes, and 2 + risk factors with 10-y risk for hard CHD >20%.
[e]Any person at high risk or moderately high risk who has lifestyle-related risk factors (e.g., obesity, physical inactivity, elevated triglyceride, low HDL-C, or metabolic syndrome) is a candidate for TLC to modify these risk factors regardless of LDL-C level.
[f]Very high risk favors the optional LDL-C goal of <70 mg/dL, and in patients with high triglycerides, non-HDL-C <100 mg/dL.
[g]Electronic 10-y risk calculators are available at www.nhlbi.nih.gov/guidelines/cholesterol.
[h]For moderately high-risk persons, when LDL-C is 100–129 mg/dL, at baseline or on lifestyle therapy, initiation of an LDL-lowering drug to achieve an LDL-C <100 mg/dL is a therapeutic option on the basis of available clinical trial results.
[i]Almost all people with zero or 1 risk factor have a 10-year risk <10%, and 10-year risk assessment in people with zero or 1 risk factor is thus not necessary.
*Source:* Adapted from Grundy SM, Cleeman JI, Merz CN, et al. Implications of recent clinical trials for the National Cholesterol Education Program Adult Treatment Panel III guidelines. *Circulation.* 2004;110: 227–239, with permission.

observational studies demonstrating a MI rate and mortality rate in diabetics without known CHD equivalent to that of nondiabetics with already-documented CHD (28). Patients with known CHD, or CHD risk equivalents, fall into the *high- risk* group for coronary events, and should thus receive the most aggressive lipid lowering. These are individuals with an estimated yearly risk of MI or death of 2% or greater. At the other end of the spectrum are those with 0–1 risk factors but no known CVD or diabetes. They are considered at *lower risk* for CHD events, with an estimated yearly MI or death rate of less than 0.5% to 1%, and require the least aggressive lipid control. Between these two extremes are individuals with 2 or more risk factors, but without known CVD or diabetes, for whom the 10-year risk of having a MI or dying from an MI can be estimated using the Framingham risk calculator. This is a point-based system (available online and in the "ATP III Guidelines At-A-Glance Quick Desk Reference," NIH Publication No. 01-3305) to assess risk in men and women, based on data from the Framingham Study, utilizing the parameters of age, TC, smoking status, HDL-C, and systolic BP. Those with 2+ risk factors and a 10-year risk >20% are grouped with the CHD and CHD risk equivalents (*high risk*), those with a 10-year risk of 10% to 20% are considered to be at *moderately high risk,* and those with a 10-year risk of <10% are said to be at *moderate risk.* Despite the utility of this calculator, important risk factors such as family history and obesity are not included, the calculation is heavily age and gender-weighted, and it may not apply equally to all ethnic groups. The guidelines have recommended the use of other novel risk markers [e.g., Lp(a)], measures of inflammation (e.g., hsCRP), and imaging for preclinical vascular disease (e.g., CT coronary calcification score, ankle-brachial index, carotid intima-medial thickness) to guide the intensity of therapy. These additional factors may be particularly useful in making more aggressive treatment decisions for intermediate-risk individuals with other compelling risk factors such as a strong family history of premature CHD.

The primary target of treatment is LDL-C. The LDL-C goal for therapy and LDL-C level for initiation of drug therapy are dependent on the individual's risk category. For example, the 2001 guidelines recommended that individuals falling into the CHD or CHD risk-equivalent category have a treatment goal of <100 mg/dL and have drug therapy initiated for an LDL-C of ≥130 mg/dL (between 100 and 129 mg/dL optional). After LDL-C goals have been met, non-HDL cholesterol (TC minus HDL-C) is a secondary target of therapy. The non–HDL-C target should be 30 mg/dL higher than the LDL-C goal. For example, in the high-risk group, if the LDL-C target is <100 mg/dL, the non-HDL-C target would be <130 mg/dL. This may be achieved by further reductions in LDL-C, lowering of TG, increase in HDL-C, or a combination. Specific recommendations for TG management have been outlined. If TG are borderline elevated at 150 to 199 mg/dL, weight reduction and increased physical activity should be prescribed. If TG are 200 to 499 mg/dL, this can be achieved by intensifying therapy with an LDL-lowering drug (i.e., increasing the statin dose), or by adding niacin or a fibrate to further lower VLDL-C. If TG are ≥500 mg/dL, TG should be lowered first to prevent pancreatitis. Treatment options include a very-low-fat diet (<15% of calories from fat), identification and treatment of secondary causes of elevated TG, weight reduction, and physical activity, and the addition of niacin or a fibrate. Once TG have been lowered to <500 mg/dL, LDL-C-lowering therapy should be initiated. Treatment of low-HDL-C remains a tertiary goal in lipid management, mainly because of the paucity of large outcome studies involving treatment of low HDL-C and less effective available medications. No specific target for ideal HDL-C has been proposed. Once LDL-C goal has been achieved, weight reduction and increased physical activity should be employed in an attempt to boost HDL-C. If TG are 200 to 499, the non–HDL-C goal should be achieved. If TG are <200 mg/dL (isolated low HDL-C) in high-risk individuals, one should consider initiating niacin or a fibrate. In the future, as better medications to raise HDL-C become available and more large trials address the utility of treating HDL-C to reduce CHD events, the priority of treating a low HDL-C may increase. Finally, ATP III recognized the MetS as a growing contributor to CHD risk, and stressed the importance of its identification and treatment. The ATP III definition of MetS and its treatment goals have already been discussed (see Table 12–2).

As noted earlier, newer studies since the 2001 publication of the ATP III guidelines confirm the benefit and safety of statins (particularly among high-risk patients), indicate that more intensive LDL-C–lowering therapy provides a greater benefit than less intensive LDL-C–lowering therapy, suggest that reducing LDL-C substantially below 100 mg/dL provides additional benefit, and support earlier initiation of therapy in moderately high-risk groups without known cardiovascular disease. These modifications published in 2004 offer the following recommendations and comments.

- LDL-C goal <70 mg/dL is a therapeutic option for very-high-risk patients.
- Option to reduce LDL-C to <70 mg/dL extends to patients at very high risk with baseline LDL-C <100 mg/dL.
- Factors favoring the optional goal of <70 mg/dL include CVD associated with multiple major risk factors (especially diabetes), severe and poorly-controlled other risk factors (especially smoking), MetS, or acute coronary syndrome.
- For moderately high-risk patients, LDL-C goal <100 mg/dL is a therapeutic option (e.g. hypertensive with multiple other risk factor).
- In patients with elevated LDL-C at baseline (≥160 mg/dL), standard statin doses may not be sufficient for optimal LDL-C reduction. Therefore, consider high-dose statins and/or combination therapy (e.g., statins + ezetimibe) to achieve aggressive LDL-C goals.
- Addition of fibrate or nicotinic acid should be considered for high-risk patients with high triglycerides (TG) or low high-density lipoprotein cholesterol (HDL-C).

Despite the enormous amount of information and widely disseminated treatment recommendations, a significant number of treatment-eligible patients are not identified or do not receive adequate treatment. ATP III suggests that all adults be screened with a full fasting lipid profile beginning at age 20. ATP III recommends screening the family members of individuals with genetic disorders such as familial hypercholesterolemia, familial defective apolipoprotein B-100, or polygenic hypercholesterolemia. The American Heart Association recommends that children of parents with premature CHD or significantly elevated cholesterol or children for whom a family history is unknown be screened after 2 years of age. The guidelines recommend early assessment of response and titration of nonpharmacologic and drug treatment strategies (every 6 weeks), and offer advice to help with patient, physician and health care provider adherence to the guidelines. Clearly we are faced with the challenge of finding better ways to implement cholesterol treatment recommendations.

See Tables 12–3 and 12–4 for detailed information on TLC and drug therapy, respectively, and Table 12–9 for an overview of the ATP III/Update treatment recommendations.

## FUTURE DIRECTIONS

In the past two decades, we have witnessed remarkable strides in the treatment of lipid disorders and coronary disease. These accomplishments can be attributed in large part to the development of statins, and their overwhelming success in multiple large-scale randomized trials of CHD prevention. Over the next two decades, we can expect to see continued progress in lipid and CHD therapies. Basic science findings will continue to further our understanding of atherosclerotic mechanisms. Lipid absorption and metabolism; lipoprotein structure, function, and transport;

inflammation, and the complex genetics of dyslipidemias and atherosclerosis, are just a few of the fertile research areas that will undergo further exploration. Clinical trials with agents with a capability to raise or modify HDL-C (such as the CETP inhibitors or ApoA1-Milano), long-term assessment of combination therapies along with statins, and better understanding of the role of hsCRP-directed therapy will likely further expand our treatment options for dyslipidemias and enhance our ability to reduce cardiovascular events.

## REFERENCES


1. Fredrickson DS, Levy RI, Lees RS. Fat transport in lipoproteins—an integrated approach to mechanisms and disorders. *N Engl J Med.* 1967;276:34–42, 94–103, 148–156, 215–225, 273–281.
2. Reaven GM. Banting lecture 1988. Role of insulin resistance in human disease. *Diabetes.* 1988;37:1595–1607.
3. Third report of the National Cholesterol Education Program (NCEP) Expert Panel on Detection, Evaluation, and Treatment of High Blood Cholesterol in Adults (Adult Treatment Panel III). Final Report. *Circulation.* 2002;106:3143–3421.
4. Ford ES, Giles WH, Dietz WH. Prevalence of the metabolic syndrome among US adults: findings from the third National Health and Nutrition Examination Survey. *JAMA.* 2002;287:356–359.
5. Grundy SM, Brewer HB, Cleeman JI, et al. Definition of metabolic syndrome: Report of the National Heart, Lung, and Blood Institute/American Heart Association Conference on Scientific Issues Related to Definition. *Circulation.* 2004;109:433–438.
6. Grundy SM, Hansen B, Smith SC Jr, et al. Clinical management of metabolic syndrome: report of the American Heart Association/National Heart, Lung, and Blood Institute/American Diabetes Association Conference on Scientific Issues Related to Management. *Circulation.* 2004;109:551–556.
7. Wiegman A, Hutten BA, de Groot E, et al. Efficacy and safety of statin therapy in children with familial hypercholesterolemia: a randomized controlled trial. *JAMA.* 2004;292:331–337.
8. Brown BG, Albers JJ, Fisher LD, et al. Regression of coronary artery disease as a result of intensive lipid-lowering therapy in men with high levels of apolipoprotein B. *N Engl J Med.* 1990;323:1289–1298.
9. Brown BG, Zhao XQ, Chait A, et al. Simvastatin and niacin, antioxidant vitamins, or the combination for the prevention of coronary disease. *N Engl J Med.* 2001;345:1583–1592.
10. Stamler J. Epidemiology, established major risk factors, and the primary prevention of coronary heart disease. In: Chatterjee K, Cheitlin MP, Karlines J, et al., eds. Cardiology: An illustrated text/reference. Philadelphia: JB Lippincott; 1991:1.
11. Gordon DJ, Probstfield JL, Garrison RJ, et al. High-density lipoprotein cholesterol and cardiovascular disease: four prospective American studies. *Circulation.* 1989;79:8–15.
12. Shepherd J, Cobbe SM, Ford I, et al. Prevention of coronary heart disease in men with hypercholesterolemia. *N Engl J Med.* 1995;333:1301–1307.
13. Downs JR, Clearfield M, Whitney E, et al. Primary prevention of acute coronary events with lovastatin in men and women with average cholesterol levels. *JAMA.* 1998;279:1615–1622.
14. The Scandinavian Simvastatin Survival Study Group. Randomised trial of cholesterol lowering in 4444 patients with coronary heart disease: the Scandinavian Simvastatin Survival Study (4S). *Lancet.* 1994;344:1383–1389.
15. Sacks FM, Pfeffer MA, Moye LA, et al. The effect of pravastatin on coronary events after myocardial infarction in patients with average cholesterol levels. *N Engl J Med.* 1996;335:1001–1009.
16. The Long-Term Intervention with Pravastatin in Ischaemic Disease (LIPID) Study Group. Prevention of cardiovascular events and death with pravastatin in patients with coronary heart disease and a broad range of initial cholesterol levels. *N Engl J Med.* 1998;339:1349–1357.
17. MRC/BHF Heart Protection Study of cholesterol lowering with simvastatin in 20,536 high-risk individuals: a randomised placebo-controlled trial. *Lancet.* 2002;360:7–22.
18. Nissen SE, Tuzcu EM, Schoenhagen P, et al. Effect of intensive compared with moderate lipid-lowering therapy on progression of coronary atherosclerosis: a randomized controlled trial. *JAMA.* 2004;291:1071–1080.
19. Cannon CP, Braunwald E, McCabe CH, et al. Intensive versus moderate lipid lowering with statins after acute coronary syndromes. *N Engl J Med.* 2004;350:1495–1504.
20. LaRosa JC, Grundy SM, Waters DD, et al. Intensive lipid lowering with atorvastatin in patients with stable coronary disease. *N Engl J Med.* 2005;352:1425–1435.
21. Sever PS, Dahlof B, Poulter NR, et al. Prevention of coronary and stroke events with atorvastatin in hypertensive patients who have average or lower-than-average cholesterol concentrations, in the Anglo-Scandinavian Cardiac Outcomes Trial—Lipid Lowering Arm (ASCOT-LLA): a multicentre randomised controlled trial. *Lancet.* 2003;361:1149–1158.
22. Colhoun HM, Betteridge DJ, Durrington PN, et al. Primary prevention of cardiovascular disease with atorvastatin in type 2 diabetes in the Collaborative Atorvastatin Diabetes Study (CARDS): multicentre randomised placebo-controlled trial. *Lancet.* 2004; 364:685–696.
23. Dean BB, Borenstein JE, Henning JM, et al. Can change in high-density lipoprotein cholesterol levels reduce cardiovascular risk?. *Am Heart J.* 2004;147:966–976.
24. Rubins HB, Robins SJ, Collins D, et al. Gemfibrozil for the secondary prevention of coronary heart disease in men with low levels of high-density lipoprotein cholesterol. Veterans Affairs High-Density Lipoprotein Cholesterol Intervention Trial Study Group. *N Engl J Med.* 1999;341:410–418.
25. Taylor AJ, Sullenberger LE, Lee HJ, et al. Arterial Biology for the Investigation of the Treatment Effects of Reducing Cholesterol (ARBITER) 2: a double-blind, placebo-controlled study of extended-release niacin on atherosclerosis progression in secondary prevention patients treated with statins. *Circulation.* 2004; 110:3512–3517.
26. National Cholesterol Education Program Expert Panel on Detection E, and Treatment of High Blood Cholesterol in Adults (Adult Treatment Panel III). Third Report of the National Cholesterol Education Program (NCEP) Expert Panel on Detection, Evaluation, and Treatment of High Blood Cholesterol in Adults (Adult Treatment Panel III): final report, NIH Publication 02-5215. September 2002.
27. Grundy SM, Cleeman JI, Bairey Merz CN, et al. Implications of recent clinical trials for the National Cholesterol Education Program Adult Treatment Panel III guidelines. *Circulation.* 2004;110:227–239.
28. Haffner SM, Lehto S, Ronnemaa T, et al. Mortality from coronary heart disease in subjects with type 2 diabetes and in nondiabetic subjects with and without prior myocardial infarction. *N Engl J Med.* 1998;339:229–234.


## QUESTIONS

1. Casey S. is an obese 54-year-old man (BMI = 35) with a history significant for obstructive sleep apnea and multiple joint complaints. A lower-extremity arterial duplex study, performed to work up the possibility of claudication, reveals noncritical peripheral arterial disease, with

bilateral ankle-brachial indices (ABIs) of 0.8. He denies ongoing exertional chest discomfort or dyspnea, but lives a fairly sedentary lifestyle. Physical exam reveals an obese man with normal blood pressure (BP), an unremarkable cardiac exam, and 1+ dorsalis pedis pulses. His fasting lipids are as follows: TC 240 mg/dL, TG 250 mg/dL, HDL-C 35 mg/dL, LDL-C (calculated) 155. Initial therapy should include:

a. TLC only
b. TLC plus a statin, with the goal of reducing LDL-C to <130 mg/dL
c. TLC plus niacin or a fibrate, with the goals of reducing LDL-C <100 mg/dL and TG < 150 mg/dL
d. TLC plus a statin, with the goal of reducing LDL-C to <100 mg/dL (<70 mg/dL optional)
e. TLC plus statin, as well as niacin or a fibrate, with the goals of reducing LDL-C <100 mg/dL and TG <150 mg/dL

Answer is d: Patients with a CHD equivalent (including clinically evident peripheral arterial disease) have an LDL-C goal of <100 mg/dL, with the optional goal of <70 mg/dL.

**2.** Donna O. is a 71-year-old retired executive whose father died at age 52 of a "massive MI." She is very worried about her own risk of a heart attack. She watches her weight (BMI = 23), does not smoke, and keeps physically fit, walking 3 miles on a treadmill three or four times a week. She denies angina or dyspnea on exertion, claudication, or history of TIA symptoms. Her BP is 120/80. Her fasting lipids are as follows: TC 250 mg/dL, TG 120 mg/dL, HDL-C 42 mg/dL, LDL-C (calculated) 151 mg/dL. Her calculated Framingham 10-year event risk is 5%. Initial therapy should include:

a. Nothing beyond her current lifestyle measures
b. Weight loss to bring BMI <20.
c. TLC plus a statin to reduce LDL-C to <130 mg/dL, or optionally <100 mg/dL
d. TLC to reduce LDL-C to <130 mg/dL
e. Statin and niacin to reduce LDL-C <130 mg/dL and increase HDL-C >50 mg/dL

Answer is d: The patient has two major risk factors: age (woman ≥55 years), and family history of CHD, with a 10-year CHD event risk of <10%. In such moderate-risk persons, TLC alone should be initiated if LDL-C is ≥130 mg/dL, and TLC plus drug therapy should be started for LDL-C ≥160 mg/dL. Because her LDL-C is ≥130 mg/dL, TLC measures should be initiated.

**3.** If Donna O. (Question 2) were found instead to have untreated HTN (systolic BP of 160), with all other data the same, what would be the preferred initial treatment, in addition to BP control? Her calculated 10-year Framingham risk score is now 11%.

a. Nothing beyond her current lifestyle measures
b. Weight loss to bring BMI <20
c. TLC plus a statin to reduce LDL-C to <130 mg/dL, or optionally <100 mg/dL
d. TLC to reduce LDL-C to <130 mg/dL
e. Statin and niacin to reduce LDL-C <130 mg/dL and increase HDL-C >50 mg/dL

Answer is c: Given her HTN, the patient now has three major risk factors and a 10-year risk of between 10% and 20%, placing her in the moderately high-risk category. By ATP III, her goal LDL-C is <130 mg/dL, with an optional goal of <100 mg/dL, per the 2004 updates. Since her LDL-C is ≥130 mg/dL, a statin should be started.

**4.** Richard D. is referred to you for lipid management. He denies any first-degree relatives with history of CHD, but reports that two uncles and a distant cousin have had heart attacks. He is currently asymptomatic. His BMI is 28. His physical exam reveals arcus cornea and xanthelasmas, but no xanthomas, and a BP of 150/80. His fasting lipid profile is as follows: TC 300 mg/dL, TG 430 mg/dL, HDL-C 50 mg/dL, LDL-C (direct) 200 mg/dL. Which primary dyslipidemia is this patient most likely to have?

a. Polygenic hypercholesterolemia
b. Heterozygous familial hypercholesterolemia
c. Familial combined hyperlipidemia
d. Hyperapobetalipoproteinemia
e. Familial endogenous hypertriglyceridemia

Answer is c: Familial combined hyperlipidemia is a common dyslipidemia (1:33 to 1:100 persons) characterized by complex inheritance. Xanthomas are rarely present (unlike in heterozygous FH), but xanthelasmas and arcus cornea can be seen. Affected individuals generally exhibit a TC of 250 to 350 mg/dL, LDL-C of 200 to −300 mg/dL, and TG >140 mg/dL (two thirds of patients with FCH have TG of 200 to 500 mg/dL. Patients with polygenic hypercholesterolemia have a similar lipid profile, except they do not generally have elevated TG.

**5.** What should the initial therapy be for Richard D. (Question 4)?

a. Statin
b. Fibrate
c. Statin and antihypertensive agent
d. Niacin
e. Apheresis

Answer is c: Because this patient's TG are <500, LDL-C reduction has first priority. A statin should be initiated, as well as an antihypertensive agent.

**6.** Which of the following statements is not correct?

a. 4S, CARE, LIPID, and HPS all involved secondary prevention of CHD.
b. Data from HPS, ASCOT-LLA, and PROVE-IT/TIMI-22 were influential in lowering the recommended treatment goals for LDL-C in the 2004 ATP III updates.
c. WOSCOPS and AFCAPS/TexCAPS were both primary CHD prevention studies that showed significant clinical benefits for statin therapy, with similar percentage reductions in LDL-C. The main difference between these trials was that subjects in AFCAPS/TexCAPS had considerably lower baseline LDL-C levels than those in WOSCOPS.
d. Early angiographic trials of lipid lowering showed significant reductions in coronary events, though they were not designed to show this.
e. ASCOT-LLA showed reductions in nonfatal MI, CHD death and all-cause mortality when patients with average lipids and HTN were treated with atorvastatin 10 mg daily for an average of 3.3 years.

Answer is e: Although ASCOT-LLA showed reductions in nonfatal MI and CHD death, coronary events or procedures, stroke, and chronic stable angina, it did not show a reduction in total mortality.

**7.** Gary P. is an obese, nonsmoking, gregarious 44-year-old talk show host with treated HTN and no family history of CHD. He has no personal history of known CHD. He has had elevated LDL-C in the past, and is taking atorvastatin 20 mg/day. His latest lipid panel is as follows: TC 220, HDL-C 40, direct LDL-C 120, and TG 450. His calculated 10-year risk of a CHD event is 5%. After recommending lifestyle modifications, what is your first goal of drug treatment?

a. Increase the HDL-C
b. Lower the LDL-C
c. Lower the non-HDL-C
d. Lower the TG
e. Lower the TG and increase the HDL-C

Answer is c: This man is currently at goal for his target LDL-C of <130 mg/dL. Given the fact that his TG are in the range 200 to 499, the next priority is to lower his non-HDL-C from its current level of 180 mg/dL to <160 mg/dL.

**8.** Which of the following would lower non-HDL-C?

a. Increase the dose of atorvastatin
b. Add a fibrate
c. Add niacin
d. Add ezetemibe
e. All of the above

Answer is e: Any of the therapeutic interventions would lower the non-HDL-C (TC minus HDL-C). However, risks of combination therapy and lack of long-term clinical trials assessing add-on therapy need to be considered. Emphasis on TLC with an increase in the statin dose would be an appropriate first step.

**9.** If the patient's TG were 600 mg/dL, what would be your next step in lipid management?

a. Increase the HDL-C
b. Lower the LDL-C
c. Lower the non-HDL-C
d. Lower the TG
e. Lower the TG and increase the HDL-C

Answer is d: When TG are ≥500 mg/dL, the priority is to reduce TG to <500 mg/dL, to avoid pancreatitis.

**10.** What would you prescribe for the patient in Question 9?

a. Raise the dose of atorvastatin to 40 mg/day
b. Add a fibrate
c. Add niacin
d. Add ezetemibe
e. Increase the statin dose and add a fibrate

Answer is b: This change could be most effectively achieved by adding a fibrate to his regimen.

# 13

# Stable Angina: Risk Stratification, Medical Therapy, and Revascularization Strategies

***Christian Simpfendorfer*** ***Conrad C. Simpfendorfer***

The syndrome of angina pectoris, first described in 1768 by William Heberden, is most commonly the symptomatic result of fixed coronary artery obstruction and impaired endothelial vasomotor activity in patients with advanced coronary atherosclerosis. In stable angina, symptoms occur in a predictable and reproducible fashion during periods of physical or emotional stress when increases in heart rate, cardiac contractility, and afterload increase myocardial oxygen requirements. Relief is usually brought on with rest or nitroglycerin. Symptom severity can be widely variable from patient to patient and is most commonly graded according to the Canadian Cardiovascular Scale (Table 13–1) (1).

The epidemiology of stable angina and coronary artery disease in the United States is changing because of continued advances in medical and revascularization therapies. From 1992 to 2002 the coronary heart disease death rate declined 26.5% and the in-hospital acute myocardial infarction survival rate improved by nearly 20% (2).

Despite these substantial improvements, coronary artery disease remains the number-one killer of both men and women in the United States and stable angina pectoris is among the most common initial clinical manifestations. Overall, an estimated 6.4 million of the nearly 14 million Americans with known coronary artery disease live with chronic angina, a number that is expected to increase as the population continues to age (2). The presence of symptomatic coronary artery disease affects quality of life negatively. It imparts significant morbidity and mortality, with a 3.5% annual risk of myocardial infarction and a 30% 10-year mortality risk, roughly twice that of age-matched controls (3,4). Pharmacologic and revascularization therapies aimed at reducing symptoms and improving survival in this broad population of patients are a fundamental aspect of modern clinical cardiology.

## DIAGNOSTIC TESTING/RISK STRATIFICATION

Evaluation of the patient with symptoms suspicious for coronary artery disease (CAD) begins with assessing for the presence of CAD historical predictors, such as pain character, age, sex, diabetes mellitus, smoking, and hyperlipidemia (5–7). In those with a significant suspicion for CAD, the spectrum of risk is broad and warrants different treatment strategies for different levels of risk. For patients determined to be at low-risk of adverse events, medical therapy alone is usually sufficient and may be superior to an invasive approach (8). For moderate- or high-risk subsets, there is evidence from randomized trials that medical therapy coupled with surgical revascularization improves long-term survival (8). The judicious use of noninvasive and invasive studies can help establish the diagnosis of CAD while simultaneously performing the critical risk stratification that is essential in determining the appropriate risk-reducing treatment strategies. More precisely, because all patients diagnosed with coronary disease should receive pharmacologic therapy, testing allows for the identification of individuals with high-risk features of coronary artery disease who may benefit from revascularization.

### Electrocardiography

Although the electrocardiograph (ECG) is normal in more than half of patients with chronic stable angina, an ECG is

**TABLE 13–1**
**CANADIAN CARDIOVASCULAR SOCIETY CLASSIFICATION OF ANGINA**

| | |
|---|---|
| Class I | No angina with ordinary physical activity. Strenuous activity may cause symptoms. |
| Class II | Angina causes slight limitation on ordinary physical activity. |
| Class III | Angina causes marked limitation on ordinary physical activity. |
| Class IV | Angina occurs with any physical activity and may be present at rest. |

**TABLE 13–2**
**DUKE TREADMILL SCORE**

| | |
|---|---|
| Calculation: | DTS = exercise time in minutes on the Bruce protocol − (5 × ST-segment deviation) − (4 × angina index [0 = none, 1 = nonlimiting, and 2 = exercise limiting]) |
| Risk stratification: | |
| Low risk, ≥5 | 0.25% annual mortality |
| Intermediate risk, −10 to +4 | 1.25% annual mortality |
| High risk, ≤−11 | 5.25% annual mortality |

a readily available first-line test that provides both diagnostic and prognostic information (Class I). A normal ECG at the time of diagnosis is associated with a favorable long-term prognosis, whereas abnormalities such as left ventricular hypertrophy, Q-waves suggestive of prior myocardial infarction, and persistent ST-segment depression identify patients at higher risk of future adverse events (9,10).

## Echocardiography

Most patients undergoing a diagnostic evaluation for stable angina do not require echocardiography. More specifically, in patients with a normal ECG, no history of prior myocardial infarction, and no clinical signs or symptoms of heart failure, valvular disease, or hypertrophic cardiomyopathy, it is currently contraindicated to obtain an echocardiogram (Class III). An exception to this rule is when the echocardiogram can be obtained during or within 30 minutes of chest pain to evaluate for regional wall motion abnormalities (Class I). In this setting, regional wall motion abnormalities have a positive predictive value for ischemia of 50% (11), whereas normal studies identify patients at low risk for an acute infarction (12).

## Exercise ECG Testing

In the largest published meta-analysis of exercise electrocardiography, the mean sensitivity and specificity for detecting angiographically significant disease was 68% and 77%, respectively (13). Although exercise electrocardiography is less sensitive than stress tests performed with imaging modalities, it remains the primary noninvasive tool for both diagnosis and risk stratification in patients with suspected CAD and interpretable ECGs. The American College of Cardiology/American Heart Association (ACC/AHA) Guidelines recommend that unless cardiac catheterization is more urgently indicated, symptomatic patients with suspected or known CAD should be considered for exercise testing to assess the risk of future cardiac events and the possible need for angiography (14). As a diagnostic tool, exercise testing is most useful in patients with stable chest pain syndromes and an intermediate risk of CAD (Class I indication). In those with a low or high pretest probability of coronary disease it has a Class IIb recommendation. As a prognostic tool, it can help identify patients with extensive atherosclerosis who would benefit from coronary angiography and possible revascularization.

The most important prognostic variables measured during exercise testing are exercise capacity, typically in metabolic equivalents tests (METs) and exercise-induced ischemic ST-segment changes. The Duke Treadmill Score integrates these two objective variables with the subjective presence or absence of anginal symptoms to generate a risk score that separates patients into high-, moderate-, and low-risk subsets (35%, 10%, and 3% 5-year mortality, respectively) (Table 13–2) (15,16). Patients with high-risk Duke Treadmill Scores frequently have left main or three-vessel disease that would benefit from revascularization, whereas low-risk patients have an excellent prognosis that is unlikely to improve with further evaluation or revascularization.

## Stress Testing with Nuclear and Echocardiography Imaging

Although stress imaging modalities have greater diagnostic accuracy than exercise electrocardiography, the increased cost of these tests precludes their routine use in all patients with suspected CAD. Most commonly, nuclear or echocardiographic stress imaging is reserved as first line testing in patients with abnormal baseline ECGs, an inability to exercise adequately, and in symptomatic patients with prior revascularization. As with exercise electrocardiography, stress imaging results can also separate patients who are appropriate for medical therapy (low-risk, ≤1% annual mortality) from those who may benefit from further angiographic evaluation and possible revascularization (intermediate risk, 1% to 3%; high risk, ≥3% annual mortality) (17) (Table 13–3).

## Coronary Angiography

Coronary angiography remains the "gold standard" diagnostic test for CAD. Additionally, anatomic estimation of disease extent and severity accurately identifies those patients with survival benefits as a result of surgical revascularization. Specifically, patients with severe left main trunk stenosis, three-vessel disease, and two-vessel disease

**TABLE 13–3**
**RECOMMENDATIONS FOR EXERCISE ECG TESTING AND STRESS IMAGING STUDIES IN STABLE ANGINA PECTORIS**

| | |
|---|---|
| | **Exercise ECG Testing without Imaging** |
| Class I | For diagnosis of obstructive CAD in patients with an intermediate pretest probability of CAD<br>For risk assessment and prognosis in patients undergoing initial evaluation |
| Class IIb | High pretest probability of CAD<br>Low pretest probability of CAD<br>Digoxin therapy with <1 mm ST-segment depression on baseline ECG<br>ECG criteria for LV hypertrophy and <1 mm of ST-segment depression |
| Class III | Pre-excitation (Wolff–Parkinson–White) syndrome<br>Electronically paced ventricular rhythm<br>More than 1 mm of rest ST depression<br>Complete left bundle-branch block (LBBB)<br>Risk stratification in patients with severe co-morbid conditions likely to limit life expectancy or prevent revascularization |
| | **Stress Imaging Studies** |
| Class I | Identify the extent, severity, location of ischemia in patients with normal ECGs<br>Patients with an intermediate pretest probability of CAD with abnormal baseline ECGs that preclude exercise ECG testing (dipyridamole or adenosine MPI preferred in patients with LBBB or electronically paced ventricular rhythm)<br>Exercise myocardial perfusion imaging or exercise echocardiography in patients with prior revascularization (either PCI or CABG) |
| Class IIb | Exercise or dobutamine echocardiography in patients with LBBB |
| Class III | Exercise myocardial perfusion imaging in patients with LBBB<br>Risk stratification in patients with severe comorbid conditions likely to limit life expectancy or prevent revascularization |

involving the proximal left anterior descending (LAD) are known to derive a survival benefit with bypass surgery (8). In general, coronary angiography is performed in patients with stable chest pain syndromes when noninvasive tests are inconclusive, when clinical or noninvasive testing suggests high-risk features, and when symptoms persist despite appropriate medical therapy. Less commonly, diagnostic coronary angiography is recommended for patients in whom coronary artery spasm is suspected, those with occupations that necessitate a definitive diagnosis, and survivors of sudden cardiac death (Table 13–4).

### Conclusion

Chest pain is the most common initial presenting symptom for patients diagnosed with coronary artery disease. Although coronary angiography provides powerful prognostic information and remains the gold standard for diagnosis, noninvasive tests are often more appropriate initial tools for patients with low or intermediate clinical predictors of coronary artery disease. Even for patients with a high pretest probability of coronary artery disease, noninvasive testing can be a useful prognostic tool that allows for selection of patients who warrant further invasive evaluation.

**TABLE 13–4**
**RECOMMENDATIONS FOR CORONARY ANGIOGRAPHY IN STABLE ANGINA PECTORIS**

| | |
|---|---|
| Class I | Disabling chronic stable angina despite medical therapy<br>High-risk criteria on clinical assessment or noninvasive testing regardless of anginal severity<br>Stable angina patients with sudden death or serious ventricular arrhythmia<br>Stable angina patients with congestive heart failure |
| Class IIa | Equivocal findings/uncertain diagnosis after noninvasive testing<br>Unable to undergo noninvasive testing due to disability, illness, or morbid obesity<br>Occupational requirement for a definitive diagnosis<br>Inadequate prognostic information after noninvasive testing |
| Class III | Risk of coronary angiography outweighs the benefits<br>Patients with CCS Class I or II angina who respond to medical therapy and have no evidence of ischemia on noninvasive testing<br>Patients who prefer to avoid revascularization |

## MEDICAL TREATMENT OF STABLE ANGINA

Percutaneous coronary interventions, although increasingly common and effective for symptom relief, do not reduce mortality or myocardial infarction incidence compared to medical therapy in patients with stable CAD (18). Coronary artery bypass surgery does have long-term survival benefits versus medical therapy, but only in a minority of patients with high-risk angiographic features (8). An initial trial of medical therapy, therefore, remains the mainstay of treatment for the majority of patients with chronic CAD. This is achieved through a combination of therapies that target both ischemic symptoms and modifiable risk factors known to aggravate angina and cardiovascular disease. Medications known to reduce the risk of myocardial infarction and death receive highest priority. Medications aimed at improving quality of life by reducing the frequency and severity of anginal episodes serve as important supplementary therapies.

### Symptomatic Medical Therapies: Antianginals

The currently available antianginal medications work to counteract the hemodynamic effects of flow-limiting stenosis by reducing myocardial oxygen requirements and/or by promoting coronary vasodilatation. They are all effective therapies for symptom relief but do not reduce death or myocardial infarction in patients with otherwise uncomplicated stable angina pectoris.

### *Beta-Blockers*

Beta-blockers function by competitively inhibiting the physiologic actions of catecholamines. The resulting decreases in heart rate, arterial blood pressure, and myocardial contractility substantially reduce myocardial oxygen demand. Their functional benefits in stable angina have been most clearly demonstrated by exercise studies in which beta-blocked patients experienced a delay or avoidance of ischemia onset with activity compared to baseline (19,20). In low-risk patients with otherwise uncomplicated stable angina, beta-blockers have not consistently reduced the incidence of major ischemic events. However, in high-risk subsets with a history of myocardial infarction or heart failure, the long-term benefit of beta-blockers in reducing death and recurrent myocardial infarction has been firmly established by multiple large-scale randomized trials. Studies comparing beta-blockers with calcium channel blockers have reported similar efficacy in controlling symptoms without a measurable difference in adverse events (21,22). The limited data directly comparing nitrates to beta-blockers as monotherapy for stable angina suggest superior symptomatic relief with beta-blockade (23). Given the benefits of beta-blockers in reducing death and adverse cardiovascular events in high-risk patients with stable angina, plus their equivalent efficacy in treating symptoms, these medications are first-line antianginal agents (Class I) in all patients with stable angina.

### *Calcium Channel Blockers*

All calcium channel blockers (CCBs) are vasodilators that act to reduce myocardial oxygen demand and increase myocardial oxygen supply. Although calcium channel antagonists do not improve survival or reduce myocardial infarctions in patients with stable angina pectoris, randomized trials have demonstrated that both dihydropyridine and nondihydropyridine agents are as effective as beta-blockers for symptom relief.

The safety of calcium channel antagonists in patients with hypertension and coronary atherosclerosis has generated significant debate following the publication of studies suggesting an increase in adverse outcomes among patients treated with short-acting formulations (24,25). Although further analysis of the published reports has failed to confirm an increased risk of adverse events (26), the safety of shorter-acting dihydropyridine calcium antagonists remains uncertain and they should be avoided in patients with coronary disease. In contrast, slow-release or long-acting vasoselective calcium antagonists are both safe and effective for symptom relief (27). The ACTION trial, a randomized study of long-acting nifedipine compared to placebo in >7,600 patients with stable angina, demonstrated a reduction in the need for coronary angiography and revascularization without an increase in mortality or adverse cardiovascular events (28). Based on these data, long-acting calcium channel antagonists have received a Class I indication as initial therapy for reduction of anginal symptoms when beta-blockers are contraindicated or not tolerated, and in combination with beta-blockers when initial treatment with beta-blockers alone is not successful. As initial monotherapy, long-acting nondihydropyridines, in lieu of beta-blockers, possess a Class IIa indication.

### *Nitrates*

Nitrates have been in clinical use for more than 100 years and have an excellent safety profile, well-recognized side effects, and few drug interactions. In patients with stable angina pectoris, nitrates reduce symptoms as both monotherapy and in combination with beta-blockers and calcium channel blockers (29,30). They do not improve survival or decrease the risk of myocardial infarction, regardless of estimated baseline risk (31). They are therefore recommended as combination agents in patients with persistent symptoms despite adequate doses of beta-blockers or calcium channel blockers (Class I) and as monotherapy only in patients who are intolerant of other medications (Class I).

### *Combination Therapy*

For many patients receiving treatment for angina pectoris, the symptoms persist despite monotherapy, illustrating the frequent need for combination pharmacotherapy. Although not all published trials of combination therapy have demonstrated greater efficacy over monotherapy, meta-analysis data suggest that the combination of a beta-blocker and calcium channel blocker allows for greater exercise tolerance when compared to either medication used alone (32). The combination of long-acting, second-generation, vasoselective dihydropyridine calcium antagonists with beta-blockers appears to be a particularly effective antianginal regimen as measured by indexes of angina, exercise tolerance, and nitroglycerin consumption (33). Nitrates also improve symptoms when used in combination with beta-blockers or calcium channel blockers (29,30). Both calcium antagonists and long-acting nitrates in combination with beta-blockers have a Class I indication when initial treatment with beta-blockers is not successful.

## Medical Therapy to Improve Survival

Although the symptoms of angina may be effectively reduced with the use of standard antianginal medications such a beta-blockers, nitrates, and calcium channel blockers, these therapies have not been shown to improve survival or reduce myocardial infarction incidence in patients with otherwise uncomplicated stable angina. Therefore, the management of patients with stable angina has evolved to include a set of standard therapies directed specifically at reducing adverse clinical outcomes.

### *Antiplatelet and Antithrombotic Therapy*

The benefit of aspirin in a broad spectrum of patients with both stable and unstable atherosclerotic syndromes has been well established for decades (34,35). Although it does not improve symptoms, clinical trials of aspirin in patients with chronic stable angina have demonstrated risk reductions for adverse cardiac events that are of a magnitude similar to that seen in patients with unstable coronary syndromes (35). In the Swedish Angina Pectoris Aspirin Trial (36), the largest randomized trial of aspirin therapy for chronic stable angina, the addition of 75 mg of aspirin to sotalol resulted in a 34% reduction in the primary composite endpoint of myocardial infarction and sudden death and a 22% to 32% decrease in the measured secondary vascular events (vascular death, all cause mortality, stroke). A similar 33% reduction in adverse cardiovascular events (vascular death, stroke, and myocardial infarction) was demonstrated among 2,920 patients with stable angina included in a meta-analysis performed by the Antithrombotic Trialists Collaboration (34). Aspirin, administered at 75 to 325 mg daily, is, therefore, first-line therapy in all chronic heart disease patients (Class I indication).

Thienopyridines are efficacious in acute coronary syndromes and post-percutaneous intervention, but have not been specifically studied in the subset of atherosclerotic patients with stable angina. In the CAPRIE trial, clopidogrel appeared to be slightly more effective than aspirin in decreasing the combined risk of myocardial infarction, vascular death, or ischemic stroke in patients with recent myocardial infarction, stroke, or symptomatic peripheral vascular disease (37). Combination antiplatelet therapy with aspirin and clopidogrel has only been studied in patients presenting with acute coronary syndromes (CURE trial) and is of unknown benefit in patients with stable angina pectoris (38). Given the limited data for clopidogrel in stable coronary syndromes, it is currently recommended only as replacement therapy for patients with a contraindication to aspirin (Class IIa).

### *Lipid-Lowering Therapy*

According to the most recent update from the National Cholesterol Education Program, cholesterol-lowering therapy is indicated for all patients with stable coronary syndromes and a low-density lipoprotein (LDL) value of $\geq$100 mg/dL (Class I) (39,40). The recommended LDL goal is $<$100 mg/dL, with the option of treating down to $<$70 mg/dL. If baseline LDL-C is already $<$100 mg/dL, institution of an LDL-lowering drug to achieve an LDL-C level $<$70 mg/dL is also a therapeutic option. The benefit of a more aggressive lipid-lowering strategy in patients with stable coronary syndromes was very recently established by the Treating to New Targets (TNT) trial (41). In this study, aggressive cholesterol reduction with 80 mg of atorvastatin daily (mean LDL = 77 mg/dL) produced an absolute 2.2% reduction in major adverse cardiovascular events (8.7% versus 10.9%, $p < 0.001$) compared to a more conventional 10 mg of atorvastatin daily (mean LDL = 101 mg/dL). These results are consistent with results from the PROVE-IT and REVERSAL trials, which showed similar benefits of very aggressive cholesterol reduction in patients with recent acute coronary syndromes (42,43).

In addition to improving outcomes, nuclear studies have demonstrated that statin therapy improves myocardial perfusion and reduces ischemia on ambulatory ECG monitoring in stable angina patients with both high or normal serum cholesterol levels (44). In patients with medically refractory angina that is not amenable to revascularization, aggressive lipid reduction with 80 mg daily of atorvastatin (LDL goal $<$77 mg/dL) has been shown to reduce symptoms of angina and decrease myocardial ischemic segments measured by dobutamine echocardiography when compared to more conventional therapy (LDL goal $<$116 mg/dL) (45).

### *Angiotensin-Converting Enzyme (ACE) Inhibitors*

The benefit of ACE inhibition in patients with diabetes and impaired left ventricular function has been firmly established by multiple large-scale clinical trials that have consistently demonstrated a reduction in adverse clinical events. ACE inhibitors are therefore recommended as first-line therapy (Class I) in all patients with coronary artery disease who also have diabetes or impaired left ventricular systolic function. In patients with stable coronary disease and preserved left ventricular function, the data are less consistent. Although both the HOPE and EUROPA trials demonstrated decreased mortality with ACE inhibition (ramipril and perindopril, respectively) in stable cardiovascular patients with preserved left ventricular function, a similar population of patients in the PEACE trial failed to benefit with trandolapril (46–48). In the most recent ACC/AHA Guidelines (2002), which predate publication of the EUROPA and PEACE trials, ACE inhibitors have a Class IIa recommendation for patients with coronary atherosclerosis or other vascular disease and preserved left ventricular function.

## Conclusion

Although no single class of medical therapy directed at symptom relief has proven to be prognostically superior in the treatment of uncomplicated stable angina pectoris, beta-blockers have been shown to reduce mortality in high-risk subsets of cardiovascular disease (prior myocardial infarction, heart failure, hypertension) and therefore serve as first-line agents for symptomatic treatment. Calcium channel blockers and nitrates are reserved for combination therapy in patients with persistent symptoms or as second-line agents in patients who are unable to tolerate beta-blockers (Table 13–5).

In addition to symptomatic treatment, it is essential that individual patient risk factors be identified and treated. The greatest emphasis should be placed on the treatment of modifiable factors that have the greatest potential for preventing disease progression and reducing the risk of future ischemic events. This includes antiplatelet therapy with

**TABLE 13–5**
**RECOMMENDED PHARMACOTHERAPY IN STABLE ANGINA PECTORIS**

Pharmacotherapy to prevent symptoms
- Beta-blockers
  - Class I: all patients without contraindications
- Calcium channel blockers
  - Class I: in combination with beta-blockers or in patients unable to tolerate beta-blockers
  - Class IIa: Long-acting nondihydropyridine calcium antagonists instead of beta-blockers as initial therapy
- Nitrates
  - Class I: in combination with beta-blockers or in patients unable to tolerate beta-blockers

Pharmacotherapy to prevent death or myocardial infarction
- Aspirin
  - Class I: all patients without contraindications
- Clopidogrel
  - Class IIa: when aspirin is absolutely contraindicated
- ACE inhibitors
  - Class I: patients with diabetes or left ventricular systolic dysfunction
  - Class IIa: patients with preserved left ventricular systolic dysfunction
- Statins
  - If LDL is ≥100 mg/dL, an LDL-lowering drug is indicated.
  - If LDL is ≤100 mg/dL, institution of an LDL-lowering drug to achieve an LDL level ≤70 mg/dL is a therapeutic option.

aspirin and aggressive treatment of hyperlipidemia, hypertension, and diabetes mellitus.

New pharmacologic agents targeting metabolic pathways (ranolazine, nicorandil) and sinus rate-lowering drugs (vidarabine) have unique mechanisms of action that may provide additive benefits when combined with traditional therapies, but further investigation is still required before these medications can receive FDA approval.

## REVASCULARIZATION IN STABLE ANGINA PECTORIS

In 2002 there were an estimated 515,000 coronary artery bypass surgeries and more than 1.2 million inpatient percutaneous interventions in the United States (2). The majority of these were performed electively in patients with stable ischemic syndromes. Despite the increasing prevalence of mechanical revascularization in the management of stable angina, evidence-based medicine dictates that patients with low-risk features are best managed medically, with revascularization reserved for those with refractory symptoms or high-risk clinical and angiographic features. As both medical and revascularization therapies continue to improve, identifying patients likely to derive sufficient symptomatic or survival benefit to warrant the immediate risk of an invasive procedure and selecting the most appropriate mode for revascularization remains an important challenge.

### CABG versus MEDS

The initial studies comparing medical therapy and coronary artery bypass surgery in stable coronary disease were performed prior to the advent of percutaneous therapies and before the routine use of antiplatelet and lipid-lowering pharmacotherapies. The three largest trials were the Veterans Administration Cooperative Study (VA Study), the Coronary Artery Surgery Study (CASS), and the European Coronary Surgery Study (ECSS) (49–51). In these trials, patients with significant coronary disease, defined angiographically as ≥70% stenosis of at least one major epicardial artery segment or ≥50% stenosis of the left main coronary artery, were randomized to medical therapy alone or with surgical revascularization. In all three trials, patients who underwent CABG had a marked improvement in anginal symptoms, exercise tolerance, and quality of life compared to medically treated patients. More than 90% were free of symptoms 1 year after surgery, 78% at 5 years, and 52% at 10 years (52). Accelerating vein graft attrition and progressive native vessel disease eventually reduce this number to 23% by 15 years (53). More important than symptom relief, these early trials identified high-risk angiographic features that predicted a survival benefit with CABG. Specifically, survival was improved for patients with severe left main stenosis (≥50%), two- or three-vessel disease that included >75% proximal LAD stenosis, and three-vessel disease with abnormal left ventricular systolic function regardless of proximal LAD involvement. These results were obtained across the range of the Canadian Classification System (CCS) of angina and were independent of other clinical variables. For low-risk patients, such as those with single-vessel disease, surgical revascularization provided better angina relief, but it did not improve survival. Myocardial infarctions were not significantly reduced in any subgroups, regardless of risk.

The data from individual trials are further bolstered by the CABG Trialists Collaboration meta-analysis, which included seven randomized trials comparing bypass surgery with medical treatment in 2,649 patients with stable coronary syndromes. Although the 5-year risk of myocardial infarction was not significantly reduced with bypass surgery (24.4% with bypass surgery versus 30.7% with medical therapy), a survival advantage was confirmed in patients with severe left main stenosis, three-vessel disease, or two-vessel disease with proximal LAD involvement (8). Within these subsets the presence of left ventricular dysfunction or a strongly positive exercise test predicted an even greater absolute benefit. The survival advantage of bypass surgery over medical therapy does not become apparent for 2 to 3 years because of early perioperative mortality. It remains statistically significant for up to 10 years and diminishes thereafter due to a combination of accelerating vein graft attrition and crossover of medically treated patients to bypass surgery (40% of medically assigned patients in the trials underwent CABG by 10 years). Long-term postoperative survival and symptoms have improved significantly with the routine use of internal mammary artery conduits, which have excellent long-term patency (85% at 10 years) and result in fewer reoperations compared to surgery with vein grafts alone (53,54).

A risk-stratification model performed as part of the CABG Trialists Collaboration meta-analysis, using clinical and angiographic variables (extent of CAD, left ventricular function, and severity of myocardial ischemia), demonstrated a significant survival benefit with bypass surgery among those deemed at high risk (5-year medical mortality 23%; relative risk 0.5, $p = 0.001$) and moderate risk (5-year medical mortality 11.5%; relative risk 0.63, $p = 0.05$). Patients in the lowest risk category (5-year medical mortality 5.5%) did not benefit from bypass surgery and showed a slight trend toward increased mortality with revascularization (relative risk 1.18, $p = 0.70$), further illustrating the need for careful patient selection.

## PTCA versus MEDS

The data comparing PTCA to medical therapy in stable coronary disease is limited to a few small trials that enrolled very low-risk patients, primarily with single-vessel disease, mild symptoms, and preserved left ventricular function. Although PTCA generally provided greater anginal relief than medical therapy, none of the individual trials suggested a reduction in mortality or myocardial infarction following percutaneous revascularization. The second Randomized Intervention Treatment of Angina (RITA-2) trial, the largest study comparing PTCA to medical therapy in stable coronary disease, actually noted that the composite primary endpoint of death or nonfatal myocardial infarction was increased in the revascularization arm (3.3% in the medical arm versus 6.3% in the PTCA arm; $p = 0.02$), due to an excess of myocardial infarctions (55). A meta-analysis of six randomized trials comparing PTCA to medical therapy in 1,904 patients with stable coronary disease demonstrated that while angioplasty significantly improves symptoms compared to medical therapy (RR 0.70; 95% CI 0.50–0.98), it does not decrease death (RR 1.32; 95% CI 0.65–2.70) or myocardial infarction (RR 1.42; 95% CI 0.90–2.25) (18). Additionally, initial treatment with PTCA resulted in significantly more bypass surgeries (RR 1.59; 95% CI 1.09–2.32) and a trend toward more repeat percutaneous interventions (RR 1.29; 95% CI 0.71–3.36).

Given the absence of evidence to suggest that percutaneous interventions improve long-term outcomes in low-risk patients with stable coronary syndromes, medical therapy is generally recommended as the initial strategy for the majority of patients with stable angina. For those with persistent lifestyle-limiting symptoms despite maximized medical therapy, percutaneous revascularization can provide symptomatic relief, but does increase the need for future revascularization procedures.

## PCI versus CABG in Single-Vessel CAD

Randomized trials of revascularization, surgical or percutaneous, in patients with stable single-vessel coronary artery disease have never demonstrated a survival benefit over medical therapy. Revascularization in this population is therefore generally reserved for patients with persistent symptoms despite optimal medical therapy. In this low-risk population, only three small trials have directly compared surgical and percutaneous revascularization. The MASS trial randomized 214 patients with stable angina, proximal LAD stenosis, and preserved left ventricular function to medical therapy, bypass surgery using an IMA graft, or PTCA (56). There was no difference in survival or myocardial infarction between the treatment arms at 3 years. Angina was improved compared to medical therapy following either form of revascularization, although initial bypass surgery provided greater relief and fewer repeat procedures than initial PTCA. The Lausanne Trial, which did not include a medical treatment arm, reported similar survival and symptomatic benefit at 5-year follow-up among 134 patients with a proximal LAD stenosis randomized to PTCA or bypass surgery (57). Lastly, a recent trial comparing the more contemporary approach of less invasive CABG versus stenting for a proximal LAD stenosis also failed to detect a difference in death or myocardial infarction, although recurrent symptoms and repeat interventions were more common following stenting (58).

## PCI versus CABG in Multivessel CAD

Multiple randomized trials comparing initial PCI versus CABG in multivessel coronary disease have shown that, except for the subset of patients with diabetes, the long-term risk of death or myocardial infarction is equivalent with both procedures. Percutaneous revascularization, however, is consistently associated with less anginal relief and the need for repeat revascularizations. The largest single study comparing these revascularization strategies for multivessel coronary disease was the Bypass Angioplasty Revascularization Investigation (BARI) (59). As initially noted in this trial and confirmed in subsequent publications, diabetic patients with multivessel disease have a significant survival benefit with surgery over PTCA. In BARI, this was apparent by 5 years (80.6% versus 65.5%; $p = 0.003$) and by 7 years (76.4% versus 55.7%) and was large enough to generate a significant difference in the overall population (84.4% versus 80.9%). The survival outcomes for nondiabetics were identical at 7 years (86.4% versus 86.8%). A meta-analysis combining results of eight randomized trials enrolling 3,371 patients with a mean follow-up of 2.7 years did not detect a difference in mortality (4.4% CABG versus 4.6% PTCA) or myocardial infarction (7.6% CABG versus 7.9% PTCA) (60), but did confirm that patients treated with angioplasty experienced less complete relief of anginal symptoms and required more repeat revascularizations (3.3% CABG versus 33.7% PTCA). In contrast, a more recently published meta-analysis of 13 trials on 7,964 patients with longer follow-up up to 8 years did demonstrate a significant 1.9% absolute survival advantage ($p = 0.02$) favoring CABG over PCI at 5 years that was no longer significant at 8 years (61). Subgroup analyses suggested that the mortality reduction was limited to diabetics, while nondiabetics again had equivalent outcomes. Anginal symptoms and repeat revascularizations were again significantly reduced following CABG, but the difference was markedly attenuated in patients receiving coronary stents.

### Coronary Stenting in Stable Angina Pectoris

Although stenting was initially introduced for the management of complications related to coronary angioplasty, it is now the dominant percutaneous coronary intervention modality because it significantly reduces restenosis compared with balloon angioplasty. A systematic review of 19 clinical trials comparing angioplasty to stenting in stable coronary disease demonstrated that while stenting does not reduce mortality or myocardial infarctions, it does dramatically reduce restenosis and the need for repeat revascularizations (62). When comparing conventional stenting to coronary bypass surgery, death and myocardial infarction are equivalent following both procedures, but surgery remains superior for repeat revascularizations, particularly in diabetics (63).

### Conclusion

Data from randomized trials and observational registries indicate that the benefits of revascularization in stable coronary syndromes are proportional to the patient's estimated long-term risk while on medical therapy (60,61). For low-risk patients with single-vessel coronary disease, medical therapy remains the initial treatment of choice, with revascularization reserved for symptom relief when medical treatment has failed. Patients with multivessel coronary disease are more complicated. Surgical revascularization provides the best long-term survival benefit for diabetics with multivessel disease and for all patients with high-risk angiographic features such as severe left main stenosis, three-vessel disease, or two-vessel disease involving the proximal LAD. For the remaining patients with moderate-risk multivessel disease, revascularization and medical therapy appear to provide similar outcomes (Table 13–6).

**TABLE 13–6**
**RECOMMENDATIONS FOR REVASCULARIZATION IN STABLE ANGINA PECTORIS**

Class I
- CABG for >50% left main trunk stenosis
- CABG for three-vessel disease and abnormal LV function or diabetes
- CABG for two-vessel disease with significant proximal left anterior descending CAD and abnormal LV function (ejection fraction <50)
- PCI or CABG for two- or three-vessel disease with significant proximal left anterior descending CAD, normal LV function, and no diabetes
- PCI or CABG for one- or two-vessel CAD without significant proximal left anterior descending CAD but with a large area of viable myocardium and high-risk criteria on noninvasive testing
- CABG or PCI for restenosis associated with a large area of viable myocardium and/or high-risk criteria on noninvasive testing
- PCI or CABG for persistent symptoms despite optimal medical therapy

Class IIa
- Repeat CABG for multiple saphenous vein graft stenosis. PCI may be appropriate in poor candidates for reoperation
- PCI or CABG for one- or two-vessel CAD without significant proximal LAD disease but with a moderate area of viable myocardium and ischemia on noninvasive testing
- PCI or CABG for one-vessel disease with significant proximal LAD disease

Class III
- PCI or CABG for one- or two-vessel CAD without significant proximal LAD CAD, who have mild symptoms that are unlikely due to myocardial ischemia, or who have not received an adequate trial of medical therapy and have only a small area of viable myocardium or have no ischemia on noninvasive testing
- PCI or CABG for borderline coronary stenoses (50% to 60% in locations other than the left main trunk) and no ischemia on noninvasive testing
- PCI or CABG for insignificant coronary stenosis (<50% diameter)
- PCI in patients with significant left main coronary artery disease who are candidates for CABG

## REFRACTORY ANGINA

Considerable progress has been made over the last 25 years in expanding the therapeutic options available in ischemic heart disease, including pharmacologic and revascularization therapies that improve both symptoms and prognosis. However, despite the efficacy of these treatments, there remains a subset of patients with severe symptoms who are refractory to conventional medical therapy and are deemed to be unsuitable for coronary revascularization. An estimated 300,000 to 900,000 patients in the United States suffer from refractory angina pectoris, with the prevalence expected to increase as the population ages and patients live longer with their coronary artery disease (64). For these patients with refractory angina there are adjunctive invasive and noninvasive therapies available that do not improve prognosis, but may serve to alleviate symptoms and improve quality of life.

### Enhanced External Counterpulsation

Although the mechanisms underlying the benefits observed with enhanced external counterpulsation (EECP) in patients with stable angina pectoris remain unclear, this is an effective noninvasive option in the management of patients with refractory angina pectoris. EECP utilizes three sets of pneumatic cuffs applied to the lower extremities that inflate sequentially during diastole to provide diastolic augmentation of coronary flow, reduced afterload, increased venous return, and increased cardiac output. A standard course of EECP involves 1 hour a day and a total of 35 hours of therapy performed over 7 weeks. Observational studies have demonstrated that EECP improves anginal class, exercise tolerance, and quality of life while reducing nitroglycerin use and the severity of ischemia measured with myocardial perfusion imaging. The data from these studies are further supported by a randomized, double-blind, sham-controlled study of EECP that demonstrated a reduction in angina, an increase in time to ST-segment depression during exercise, and an improvement in quality of life at 1 year (registry data suggest a benefit up to 2 years) (65). For those whose symptoms do eventually recur, a repeat course of EECP performed after 1 year may also be effective (66). EECP is FDA approved for treatment of refractory angina and has a Class IIb indication from the ACC/AHA.

## Transmyocardial Revascularization

Transmyocardial revascularization (TMR), another alternative treatment for patients with refractory angina, involves the formation of artificial channels in the subendocardium with either carbon dioxide or holmium:YAG lasers in an effort improve myocardial oxygen delivery. It is an invasive procedure that typically is performed from a left thoracotomy approach with a total of 25 to 40 conduits generated. The six small trials that have randomized patients with severe (Class III or IV) refractory angina to TMR plus medical therapy versus medical therapy alone have generally demonstrated an improvement of anginal symptoms and exercise tolerance without an improvement in mortality or myocardial perfusion (67). Based on the results of these trials, TMR has received a Class IIa indication for patients with medically refractory angina that is not amenable to revascularization.

Registry data from the Society of Thoracic Surgery examining the outcomes of TMR in clinical practice has demonstrated that the operative risks of TMR-only and TMR plus CABG in the community are significantly higher than those seen in the randomized trials with traditional revascularization procedures (6.4% 30-day mortality for TMR alone, 4.2% for TMR plus CABG) (67). The risk of death was particularly pronounced in the elderly, diabetics, and those with recent unstable coronary syndromes. These factors need to be carefully considered when selecting patients for this elective procedure.

## Spinal Cord Stimulation

Spinal cord stimulation (SCS) is an invasive procedure that involves the surgical placement of an epidural electrode at the level of C7 through T1 and a pulse generator in the left lower abdomen. Neuromodulation of the dorsal columns several times per day by the device is believed to inhibit the pain-conducting impulses originating from the spinothalamic tract. Several small observational studies have demonstrated improvements in anginal class and time to onset of ST-segment depression in up to 80% of patients treated with SCS. In a single randomized trial comparing SCS to CABG in 104 patients with stable angina, the two treatments provided equivalent symptom relief and an improved long-term quality of life (68). Mortality was improved at 6 months with SCS and similar between the two treatment arms at 5 years. Based on these results, SCS has a Class IIb indication for patients with refractory angina.

**TABLE 13–7**
**THERAPEUTIC TREATMENT OPTIONS FOR REFRACTORY ANGINA**

Transmyocardial revascularization (TMR)—Class IIa
Enhanced external counterpulsation (EECP)—Class IIb
Spinal cord stimulation (SCS)—Class IIb

## Transcutaneous Electrical Nerve Stimulation

Several small clinical trials have investigated the use of neuromodulation with transcutaneous electrical nerve stimulation (TENS) in patients with refractory angina. In these limited studies, patients treated with TENS demonstrated an increase in exercise tolerance, a decrease in anginal symptoms, and a reduction in ischemia noted on exercise electrocardiography (69). Because clinical trial data are so limited, the most recent (2002) ACC/AHA Guidelines do not specifically make recommendations on the utility of TENS in refractory angina (Table 13–7).

## REFERENCES

1. Campeau L. Grading of angina pectoris [letter]. *Circulation.* 1976; 54:522–523.
2. American Heart Association. *Heart Disease and Stroke Statistics—2005 Update.* Dallas, TX:American Heart Association; 2005.
3. Elveback LR, Connolly DC, Melton LJ III. Coronary heart disease in residents of Rochester, Minnesota 7. Incidence, 1950 through 1982. *Mayo Clin Proc.* 1986;61:896–900.
4. Kannel WB, Feinleib M. Natural history of angina pectoris in the Framingham study. Prognosis and survival. *Am J Cardiol.* 1972;29: 154–163.
5. Diamond GA, Forrester JS. Analysis of probability as an aid in the clinical diagnosis of coronary-artery disease. *N Engl J Med.* 1979;300:1350–1358.
6. Pryor DB, Harrell FE, Lee KL, et al. Estimating the likelihood of significant coronary artery disease. *Am J Med.* 1983;75:771–780.
7. Pryor DB, Shaw L, McCants CB, et al. Value of the history and physical in identifying patients at increased risk for coronary artery disease. *Ann Intern Med.* 1993;118:81–90.
8. Yusuf S, Zucker D, Peduzzi P, et al. Effect of coronary artery bypass graft surgery on survival: overview of 10-year results from randomised trials by the Coronary Artery Bypass Graft Surgery Trialists Collaboration. *Lancet.* 1994;344:563–570.
9. Connolly DC, Elveback LR, Oxman HA. Coronary heart disease in residents of Rochester, Minnesota, IV. Prognostic value of the resting electrocardiogram at the time of initial diagnosis of angina pectoris. *Mayo Clin Proc.* 1984;59:247–250.
10. Hammermeister KE, DeRouen TA, Dodge HT. Variables predictive of survival in patients with coronary disease. Selection by univariate and multivariate analyses from the clinical,

electrocardiographic, exercise, arteriographic, and quantitative angiographic evaluations. *Circulation.* 1979;59:421–430.

11. Cheitlin MD, Alpert JS, Armstrong WF, et al. ACC/AHA Guidelines for the Clinical Application of Echocardiography. A report of the American College of Cardiology/American Heart Association Task Force on Practice Guidelines (Committee on Clinical Application of Echocardiography). Developed in collaboration with the American Society of Echocardiography. *Circulation.* 1997;95: 1686–1744.
12. Peels CH, Visser CA, Kupper AJ, et al. Usefulness of two-dimensional echocardiography for immediate detection of myocardial ischemia in the emergency room. *Am J Cardiol.* 1990;65: 687–691.
13. Gibbons RJ, Balady GJ, Bricker JT, et al. ACC/AHA 2002 guideline update for exercise testing: a report of the American College of Cardiology/American Heart Association Task Force on Practice Guidelines (Committee on Exercise Testing). 2002. American College of Cardiology Web site. Available at: www.acc.org/clinical/guidelines/exercise/exercise_clean.pdf.
14. Gibbons RJ, Abrams J, Chatterjee K, et al. ACC/AHA 2002 guideline update for the management of patients with chronic stable angina—summary article: a report of the American College of Cardiology/American Heart Association Task Force on Practice Guidelines (Committee on the Management of Patients with Chronic Stable Angina). *J Am Coll Cardiol.* 2003;41(1):159–168.
15. Mark DB, Hlatky MA, Harrell FE, et al. Exercise treadmill score for predicting prognosis in coronary artery disease. *Ann Intern Med.* 1987;106:793–800.
16. Mark DB, Shaw L, Harrell FE, et al. Prognostic value of a treadmill exercise score in outpatients with suspected coronary artery disease. *N Engl J Med.* 1991;325:849–853.
17. Hachamovitch R, Berman DS, Shaw LJ, et al. Incremental prognostic value of myocardial perfusion SPECT for the prediction of cardiac death: differential stratification for risk of cardiac death and myocardial infarction. *Circulation.* 1998;97:533–543.
18. Bucher HC, Hengstler P, Schindler C, et al. Percutaneous transluminal coronary angioplasty medical treatment for non-acute coronary heart disease: meta-analysis of randomized controlled trials. *BMJ.* 2000;321:73–77.
19. Frishman WH, Heiman M, Soberman J, et al. Comparison of celiprolol and propranolol in stable angina pectoris. Celiprolol International Angina Study Group. *Am J Cardiol.* 1991;67:665–670.
20. Narahara KA. Double-blind comparison of once daily betaxolol versus propranolol four times daily in stable angina pectoris. Betaxolol Investigators Group. *Am J Cardiol.* 1990;65:577–582.
21. de Vries RJ, van den Heuvel AF, Lok DJ, et al. Nifedipine gastrointestinal therapeutic system versus atenolol in stable angina pectoris. The Netherlands Working Group on Cardiovascular Research (WCN). *Int J Cardiol.* 1996;57:143–150.
22. Fox KM, Mulcahy D, Findlay I, et al. The Total Ischaemic Burden European Trial (TIBET). Effects of atenolol, nifedipine SR and their combination on the exercise test and the total ischaemic burden in 608 patients with stable angina. The TIBET Study Group. *Eur Heart J.* 1996;17:96–103.
23. van de Ven LL, Vermeulen A, Tans JG, et al. Which drug to choose for stable angina pectoris: a comparative study between bisoprolol and nitrates. *Int J Cardiol.* 1995;47:217–223.
24. Psaty BM, Heckbert SR, Koepsell TD, et al. The risk of myocardial infarction associated with antihypertensive drug therapies. *JAMA.* 1995;274:620–625.
25. Furberg CD, Psaty BM, Meyer JV. Nifedipine: dose-related increase in mortality in patients with coronary heart disease. *Circulation.* 1995;92:1326–1331.
26. Ad Hoc Subcommittee of the Liaison Committee of the World Health Organization and the International Society of Hypertension. Effects of calcium antagonists on the risks of coronary heart disease, cancer and bleeding. *J Hypertens.* 1997;15:105–115.
27. Parmley WW, Nesto RW, Singh BN, et al. Attenuation of the circadian patterns of myocardial ischemia with nifedipine GITS in patients with chronic stable angina. *J Am Coll Cardiol.* 1992;19:1380–1389.
28. Lubsen J, Wagener G, Kirwan BA, et al. Effect of long-acting nifedipine on mortality and cardiovascular morbidity in patients with symptomatic stable angina and hypertension: the ACTION trial. *J Hypertens.* 2005;23(3):641–648.
29. Akhras F, Jackson G. Efficacy of nifedipine and isosorbide mononitrate in combination with atenolol in stable angina. *Lancet.* 1991;338:1036–1039.
30. Bassan MM, Weiler-Ravell D, Shalev O. Comparison of the antianginal effectiveness of nifedipine, verapamil, and isosorbide dinitrate in patients receiving propranolol: a double-blind study. *Circulation.* 1983;68:568–575.
31. Parker JD, Parker JO. Nitrate therapy for stable angina pectoris. *N Engl J Med.* 1998;338(8):520–531.
32. Heidenreich PA, McDonald KM, Hastie T, et al. Meta-analysis of trials comparing beta-blockers, calcium antagonists, and nitrates for stable angina. *JAMA.* 1999;281(20):1927–1936.
33. Ronnevik PK, Silke B, Ostergaard O. Felodipine in addition to beta-adrenergic blockade for angina pectoris. a multicentre, randomized, placebo-controlled trial. *Eur Heart J.* 1995;16:1535–1541.
34. Antithrombotic Trialists' Collaboration. Collaborative meta-analysis of randomised trials of antiplatelet therapy for prevention of death, myocardial infarction, and stroke in high-risk patients. *BMJ.* 2002;324:71–86.
35. Antiplatelet Trialists' Collaboration. Collaborative overview of randomised trials of antiplatelet therapy. I. Prevention of death, myocardial infarction, and stroke by prolonged antiplatelet therapy in various categories of patients. *BMJ.* 1994;308:81–106.
36. Juul-Moller S, Edvardsson N, Jahnmatz B, et al. Double-blind trial of aspirin in primary prevention of myocardial infarction in patients with stable chronic angina pectoris. The Swedish Angina Pectoris Aspirin Trial (SAPAT) Group. *Lancet.* 1992;340:1421–1425.
37. CAPRIE Investigators. A randomized, blinded trial of clopidogrel versus aspirin in patients at risk of ischemic events. *Lancet.* 1996;348:1329–1339.
38. Yusuf S, Zhao F, Mehta SR, et al. Effects of clopidogrel in addition to aspirin in patients with acute coronary syndromes without ST-segment elevation. *N Engl J Med.* 2001;345:494–502.
39. Gould KL, Martucci JP, Goldberg DI, et al. Atherosclerosis/coronary heart disease: short-term cholesterol lowering decreases size and severity of perfusion abnormalities by positron emission tomography after dipyridamole in patients with coronary artery disease: a potential noninvasive marker of healing coronary endothelium. *Circulation.* 1994;89:1530–1538.
40. Grundy SM, Cleeman JI, Merz CN, et al. Implications of recent clinical trials for the National Cholesterol Education Program Adult Treatment Panel III Guidelines. *J Am Coll Cardiol.* 2004; 44(3):720–732.
41. Larosa JC, Grundy SM, Waters DD, et al. Intensive lipid lowering with atorvastatin in patients with stable coronary disease. *N Engl J Med.* 2005;352:1425–1435.
42. Cannon CP, Braunwald E, McCabe CH, et al. Comparison of intensive and moderate lipid lowering with statins after acute coronary syndromes. *N Engl J Med.* 2004;350:1495–1504.
43. Nissen SE, Tuzcu EM, Shoenhagen P, et al. Statin therapy, LDL cholesterol, C-reactive protein, and coronary artery disease. *N Engl J Med.* 2005;352(1):29–38.
44. Huggins GS, Pasternak RC, Alpert NM, et al. Effects of short-term treatment of hyperlipidemia on coronary vasodilator function and myocardial perfusion in regions having substantial impairment of baseline dilator reverse. *Circulation.* 1998;98:1291–1296.
45. Fathi R, Haluska B, Short L, et al. A randomized trial of aggressive lipid reduction for improvement of myocardial ischemia, symptom status, and vascular function in patients with coronary artery disease not amenable to intervention. *Am J Med.* 2003;114:445–453.
46. The Heart Outcomes Prevention Evaluation Study Investigators. Effect of an angiotensin-converting–enzyme inhibitor, ramipril, on cardiovascular events in high-risk patients. *N Engl J Med.* 2000; 342:145–153.
47. Fox KM. Efficacy on perindopril in reduction of cardiovascular events among patients with stable coronary artery disease: randomised, double-blind, placebo-controlled, multicentre trial (the EUROPA study). *Lancet.* 2003;362:782–788.
48. The PEACE Trial Investigators. Angiotensin-converting–enzyme

inhibition in stable coronary artery disease. *N Engl J Med.* 2004; 351:2058–2068.
49. The Veterans Administration Coronary Artery Bypass Surgery Cooperative Study Group: Eleven-year survival in the Veterans Administration randomized trial of coronary bypass surgery for stable angina. *N Engl J Med.* 1984;311:1333–1339.
50. CASS Principal Investigators. Coronary Artery Surgery Study (CASS): a randomized trial of coronary artery bypass surgery. Survival data. *Circulation.* 1983;68:939–950.
51. European Coronary Surgery Study Group. Long-term results of prospective randomized study of coronary artery bypass surgery in stable angina pectoris. *Lancet.* 1982;2:1173–1180.
52. van Brussel BL, Plokker HW, Ernst SM, et al. Venous coronary artery bypass surgery: A 15-year follow-up study. *Circulation.* 1993;88:1187–1192.
53. ACC/AHA Guidelines for Coronary Artery Bypass Graft Surgery: A report of the ACC/AHA Task Force on Practice Guidelines. *J Am Coll Cardiol.* 2002;34:1262–1347, 1999.
54. Loop FD. Internal thoracic artery grafts: biologically better coronary arteries. *N Engl J Med.* 1996;334:263–265.
55. RITA-2 Trial Participants. Coronary angioplasty versus medical therapy forangina: the second Randomised Intervention Treatment of Angina (RITA-2) trial. *Lancet.* 1997;350:461–468.
56. Hueb WA, Bellotti G, de Oliveira SA, et al. The Medicine, Angioplasty or Surgery (MASS): A prospective randomized trial of medical therapy, balloon angioplasty or bypass surgery for single proximal left anterior descending artery stenosis. *J Am Coll Cardiol.* 1995;26:1600–1605.
57. Goy JJ, Eeckhout E, Burnand B, et al. Coronary angioplasty versus left internal mammary artery grafting for isolated left anterior descending artery stenosis. *Lancet.* 1994;343:1449–1453.
58. Diegeler A, Thiele H, Falk V, et al. Comparison of stenting with minimally invasive bypass surgery for stenosis of the left anterior descending coronary artery. *N Engl J Med.* 2002;347(8):561–566.
59. The Bypass Angioplasty Revascularization Investigation (BARI) Investigators. Comparison of coronary bypass surgery with angioplasty in patients with multivessel disease. *N Engl J Med.* 1996;335: 217–225.
60. Pocock SJ, Henderson RA, Rickards AF, et al. Meta-analysis of randomised trials comparing coronary angioplasty with bypass surgery. *Lancet.* 1995;346:1184–1189.
61. Hoffman SN, Ten Brook JA, Wolf MP, et al. A meta-analysis of randomized controlled trials comparing coronary artery bypass graft with percutaneous transluminal coronary angioplasty: one- to eight-year outcomes. *J Am Coll Cardiol.* 2003;41(8):1293–1304.
62. Nordmann AJ, Hengstler P, Leimenstoll BM, et al. Clinical outcomes of stents versus balloon angioplasty in non-acute coronary artery disease. A meta-analysis of randomized controlled trials. *Eur Heart J.* 2004;25(1):69–80.
63. Biondi-Zoccai GG, Abbate A, Agostoni P, et al. Stenting versus surgical bypass grafting for coronary artery disease: systematic overview and meta-analysis of randomized trials. *Ital Heart J.* 2003;4(4):271–280.
64. Yang EH, Barsness BW, Gersh BJ et al. Current and future treatment strategies for refractory angina. *Mayo Clin Proc.* 2004;79(10): 1284–1292.
65. Arora RR, Chou TM, Jain D, et al. The Multicenter Study of Enhanced External Counterpulsation (MUST-EECP): effect of EECP on exercise-induced myocardial ischemia and anginal episodes. *J Am Coll Cardiol.* 1999;33(7):1833–1840.
66. Michaels AD, Barsness BW, Soran O, et al. Frequency and efficacy of repeat enhanced external counterpulsation for stable angina pectoris (from the International EECP Patient Registry). *Am J Cardiol.* 2005;95(3):394–397.
67. Peterson ED, Kaul P, Kaczmarek RG, et al. From controlled trials to clinical practice: monitoring transmyocardial revascularization use and outcomes. *J Am Coll Cardiol.* 2003;42(9):1611–1616.
68. Mannheimer C, Eliasson T, Augustinsson LE, et al. Electrical stimulation versus coronary artery bypass surgery in severe angina pectoris: the ESBY study. *Circulation.* 1998;97(12):1157–1163.
69. Mannheimer C, Carlsson CA, Emanuelson H, et al. The effects of transcutaneous electrical stimulation in patients with severe angina pectoris. *Circulation.* 1985;71:308–316.

## QUESTIONS

**1.** An 85 year old hypertensive male referred to cardiology clinic with stable NYHA FC III angina for 3 months treated with aspirin, metoprolol succinate 150 mg daily, isosorbide mononitrate 120 mg daily, and simvastatin 40 mg daily. On exam, the heart rate is 57, the blood pressure is 98/60 mmHg, and the cardiopulmonary exam is unremarkable. Resting ECG is within normal limits. An exercise stress test is significant for 2 mm horizontal ST depression and exercise limiting chest discomfort at 6 METs.

The Duke Treadmill Score for this patient is:

a. −9, intermediate risk
b. −9, high risk
c. −10, intermediate risk
d. −14, intermediate risk
e. −14, high risk

Answer is e: This patient with exercise limiting angina has a DTS of −14 which predicts a high probability of severe angiographic coronary disease. The Duke treadmill score is calculated as follows:

DTS: Exercise time (minutes based on the Bruce protocol) − (5 × maximum ST segment deviation in mm) − (4 × exercise angina [0 = none, 1 = non-limiting, and 2 = exercise limiting]).

Patients are classified as low, moderate, or high risk according to their score: Low-risk ≥+5, Moderate-risk from −10 to +4, High-risk ≤−11. These patients have 3%, 10%, and 35% 5-year mortality, respectively. Patients with high risk Duke Treadmill Scores frequently have left main or three-vessel disease that would benefit from revascularization, while low risk patients have an excellent prognosis that is unlikely to improve with further evaluation or revascularization.

**2.** The most appropriate next step would be:

a. Increase nitrate dose
b. Increase beta blocker dose
c. Add calcium channel blocker
d. Cardiac catheterization
e. Echocardiography

Answer is d: This patient is maximized on medical therapy and unlikely to derive significant benefit from titration of his current medications or addition of further anti-anginals. Echocardiography is not warranted at this time in the absence of an abnormal ECG or clinical signs of heart failure or valvular disease. In patients with ischemic chest pain refractory to maximized medical therapy cardiac catheterization would be indicated.

# Unstable Coronary Syndromes

14

*Anthony A. Bavry*  *A. Michael Lincoff*

## TERMINOLOGY AND OVERVIEW

The current approach to unstable or acute coronary syndromes (ACS) recognizes a heterogeneous clinical spectrum that ranges from unstable angina (UA) and non-ST-elevation myocardial infarction (NSTEMI) to ST-elevation myocardial infarction (STEMI). ACS is one manifestation of atherothrombotic disease. Other clinical manifestations of vascular disease include ischemic/embolic stroke, transient ischemic attack, renal insufficiency/failure, and limb ischemia/claudication. There is considerable overlap in the burden of vascular disease, so the presence of atherothrombosis in one vascular bed should raise the suspicion for disease in another vascular bed. As an example, an individual who has limb claudication is also likely to have coronary artery disease and should undergo equally aggressive atherothrombotic risk factor modification.

Various classifications have been used to describe the syndrome of unstable angina. The Braunwald Classification of Unstable Angina is a widely used mechanism for providing diagnostic and prognostic information about the patient. In this system, angina is divided into acute rest (class III), subacute rest (class II), or exertional angina (class I). Acute rest angina is chest pain that occurred at rest within 48 hours of presentation, while subacute rest angina is chest pain that occurred at rest within the previous month, although more than 48 hours prior to presentation. Exertional angina is chest pain that has been present for <2 months' duration that is described as new onset, severe, or accelerating in nature. This type of angina occurs with any exertion or less exertion than would normally bring about chest pain, with no rest angina for the previous 2 months. The Braunwald classification system also describes the clinical circumstances in which the angina is occurring. For example, secondary UA is caused by a clinical process that causes demand ischemia, such as gastrointestinal bleeding resulting in tachycardia. This process is in contrast to primary UA, in which supply ischemia results from plaque rupture with partial or total coronary occlusion. Postinfarction angina is a special clinical circumstance to consider, as these patients are at higher risk for adverse cardiac outcomes.

The classification for an ACS focuses on electrocardiographic (ECG) findings in the first minutes to hours of an event. This approach ensures that the most appropriate management (i.e., early invasive therapy with appropriate coronary revascularization versus a more conservative approach) occurs as rapidly as possible. Older ACS terminology is inefficient, as it focused on the ECG findings after the completion of the coronary event. Historical terms such as Q-wave and non-Q-wave myocardial infarction should therefore be avoided.

This chapter discusses the spectrum that encompasses UA and NSTEMI, while another chapter focuses on STEMI. Other causes of chest pain syndromes such as aortic dissection, acute pericarditis, or pulmonary embolus will not be discussed here. These chapters follow the American College of Cardiology/American Heart Association (ACC/AHA) guidelines (Table 14–1).

## EPIDEMIOLOGY AND PROGNOSIS

There are over 5 million annual visits to emergency departments in this country for the evaluation of chest pain, with approximately 1.5 million hospitalizations for UA/NSTEMI. This number is expected to increase over the next decade. Atherothrombotic disease and especially ACS significantly shortens an individual's life span. A survived

**TABLE 14–1**
**ACC/AHA CLASSIFICATION FOR RECOMMENDATIONS**

| | |
|---|---|
| Class I | Conditions for which there is evidence and/or general agreement that a given procedure/treatment is useful and effective |
| Class II | Conditions for which there is conflicting evidence and/or a divergence of opinion about the usefulness/efficacy of a procedure/treatment |
| Class IIa | Weight of evidence/opinion is in favor of usefulness/efficacy |
| Class IIb | Usefulness/efficacy is less well established by evidence/opinion |
| Class III | Conditions for which there is evidence and/or general agreement that the procedure/treatment is not useful/effective and in some cases may be harmful |

*Source:* From Braunwald E, Antman EM, Beasley JW, et al. ACC/AHA guidelines for the management of patients with unstable angina and non-ST-segment elevation myocardial infarction. A report of the American College of Cardiology/American Heart Association Task Force on Practice Guidelines (Committee on the Management of Patients with Unstable Angina). *J Am Coll Cardiol.* 2000;36:970–1062.

acute myocardial infarction shortens the expected life expectancy for a 60-year-old individual by approximately 9 years, whereas a cerebrovascular accident shortens an individual's expected life span by about 12 years. Coronary disease is the single largest cause of mortality worldwide and the second largest cause for mortality in the United States (cancer is now responsible for more deaths). This translates into approximately one of every five deaths in the United States being attributable to atherothrombotic disease. The shift in the epidemiology of coronary disease in this country, with improved overall mortality, is due to effective prevention and treatment of cardiovascular disease over the last several decades.

Most acute coronary syndromes occur in individuals >65 years old, and nearly 50% occur in women. When women present with chest pain, the etiology is less likely to be secondary to obstructive coronary disease, and when coronary disease is present, it tends to be less severe than in men. In-hospital mortality of UA and NSTEMI patients is less than for STEMI patients, although because the former are at risk for recurrent events, their long-term risk is equivalent or worse compared to STEMI patients.

## CLINICAL PRESENTATION

UA and NSTEMI patients typically present with substernal chest discomfort, described as a pressure or a heavy sensation. This more accurately describes angina than terminology such as "pain". Symptoms typically last <30 minutes, although they may recur frequently throughout the day or evening upon minimal exertion. Symptoms may occur at rest. Angina that occurs with minimal exertion is usually relieved promptly with rest or nitroglycerin. Anginal equivalents include neck and jaw discomfort, although the most common anginal equivalent is worsening dyspnea upon exertion. Atypical findings such as nausea, vomiting, and fatigue are easily overlooked, although these symptoms should be considered as angina in diabetics, women, and the elderly. Findings that are typically not characteristic of myocardial ischemia include sharp/pleuritic pain, pain that has been present for several hours, or brief pain that lasts only a few seconds. Up to 20% of myocardial infarctions are "silent" and occur without any appreciable symptoms.

ECG findings include transient ST elevations, ST depressions (horizontal or down-sloping), T-wave inversions, or nonspecific changes. The ECG may also appear normal. Deep symmetric T-wave inversions predict higher risk than small T-wave inversions. Ischemic T waves may also have a biphasic appearance. Dynamic ECG changes that are obtained during an episode of chest pain are particularly valuable, especially if the changes resolve in the absence of symptoms. It is important to repeat the ECG frequently, as a non–ST-elevation ACS may progress to a STEMI. Conversely, initial ST elevations may resolve quickly, thus changing the focus of early management.

## PATHOPHYSIOLOGY FOR PRIMARY AND SECONDARY CAUSES OF ANGINA

The above discussion assumes a primary coronary etiology for an unstable coronary syndrome. The corresponding pathophysiology for a primary ACS is felt to be rupture of a vulnerable plaque. Vulnerable plaques overlie lipid-rich cores that are surrounded by thin fibrous caps. Exposure of the underlying plaque to blood is a potent activator of platelets and thrombus formation. This subsequently results in microembolization of platelet aggregates and intermittent coronary vasoconstriction. The fibrous cap can become unstable as a result of fissures caused by proteinases secreted by neighboring macrophages. As a plaque matures, the fibrous cap becomes thicker and more stable. An important observation has been that acute myocardial infarctions do not occur at sites of severe coronary narrowing. Two thirds of events that are caused by an acutely occluded coronary vessel are in the location of a previous mild stenosis (i.e., stenosis <50%).

Secondary causes of ACS that are responsible for demand ischemia should be screened for and corrected if present before proceeding down the appropriate ACS management algorithm. Secondary causes include hypertensive crises, anemia/hypovolemia, worsened chronic obstructive pulmonary disease/hypoxia, hyperthyroidism, arteriovenous fistula in dialysis patients, and systemic infection. Aortic stenosis and hypertrophic obstructive cardiomyopathy are cardiac diseases that may cause demand myocardial ischemia. Cocaine use is a special condition to consider, as it can produce both demand ischemia (increased heart rate and blood pressure) as well a supply ischemia (coronary vasospasm and thrombus formation).

## RISK STRATIFICATION

### ECG

Risk stratification is a necessary component in the initial management of coronary disease patients. The ECG is a first-line test that provides not only diagnostic but also prognostic information. Data from the GUSTO IIb trial revealed a lower 6-month survival among patients with ST depressions treated conservatively compared to STEMI patients treated with fibrinolysis. The lowest-risk ACS patients (among those with any ECG changes) were those with T-wave inversions. Patients with a completely normal ECG had the lowest overall risk. A similar analysis from the RISC Study Group found the highest risk to be among those with ST elevations and reciprocal changes (ST depressions). The lowest risk was among those with no ST changes or nonspecific ST-T changes.

### Biomarkers

While the ECG is being performed and interpreted, blood work should be sent for analysis of complete blood count (CBC), chemistry, cardiac biomarkers, markers of inflammation and volume overload, and a lipid profile. Although it is not usually thought of for this purpose, information available from the CBC can be helpful in providing a crude measure of risk stratification. An elevated white blood cell (WBC) count has been shown to predict worse cardiac outcomes in ACS patients.

The role of high-sensitivity C-reactive protein (hs-CRP) as a marker of inflammation is continually expanding, as it provides prognostic information in unstable coronary syndromes. An elevated hs-CRP predicts a three- to fourfold increased risk for future cardiac events. This increased risk for myocardial infarction can be attenuated by the use of aspirin. An hs-CRP level >3 mg/L is considered high risk, while a level >10 mg/L is considered an acute-phase response and should be repeated in 3 weeks. An elevated CRP predicts future cardiac events better than elevated cholesterol or presence of the metabolic syndrome.

An elevated troponin I or T also carries independent prognostic information. A recent meta-analysis showed that troponin positive ACS patients have a fourfold increased risk for death compared to troponin-negative patients. Similarly, an analysis of the TIMI IIIb trial documented an eightfold increased risk of death at 42 days for patients with an elevated troponin I (>9 ng/mL) compared to troponin-negative patients. The 42-day mortality in patients with an elevated troponin was 7.5%, compared to 1% in those with a negative troponin.

An elevated brain natriuretic peptide (BNP) predicts increased risk for adverse cardiac events across the spectrum of ACS, although the predictive effect is greatest for UA and NSTEMI. The combination of multiple biomarkers has incremental value. An hs-CRP combined with cardiac biomarkers (i.e., troponin I or T) and markers of pressure/volume overload (i.e., BNP) predict an increased risk for major cardiac events. In the OPUS-TIMI 16 trial there was a sixfold increased risk for 30-day cardiac events when all three markers were elevated. Similarly, in the TACTICS-TIMI 18 trial there was a 13-fold increased risk in 30-day cardiac events. So hs-CRP, troponin I or T, and BNP provide prognostic information in ACS patients. Other inflammatory markers such as CD-40 ligand are experimental, although they may have a role in the future in predicting the overall risk for cardiac events in ACS.

### TIMI Risk Score

The TIMI Risk Score incorporates data derived from the TIMI 11B trial and has been validated by three additional trials. The TIMI risk score is an easily used model that has important prognostic and therapeutic implications. It incorporates seven variables that are readily available from the history, ECG, and cardiac biomarkers (Fig. 14–1). The presence of six or seven risk factors predicts a 40% incidence of death, myocardial infarction, or ischemia requiring repeat revascularization by 30 days. This is in contrast to zero or one risk factors, where the 30-day cardiac event rate is less than 5%. The seven variables used to calculate the TIMI risk score are age ≥65 years, ≥3 coronary disease risk factors (defined as diabetes, hypertension, hyperlipidemia, use of tobacco, and family history of premature coronary disease), a known coronary stenosis of >50%, ST deviation (transient ST elevations, ST depressions, or T-wave inversions), ≥2 anginal events in the past 24 hours, aspirin use in the last 7 days, and elevated cardiac biomarkers (i.e., elevated CK-MB or troponin).

Data from the PURSUIT trial has also been used to predict future adverse cardiac outcomes. This model additionally incorporates findings from the physical exam into the global risk assessment. In this model, the following variables were most predictive for death in patients presenting with an unstable coronary syndrome: advanced age, elevated heart rate, hypotension, signs of heart failure, ST depression, and elevated cardiac biomarkers.

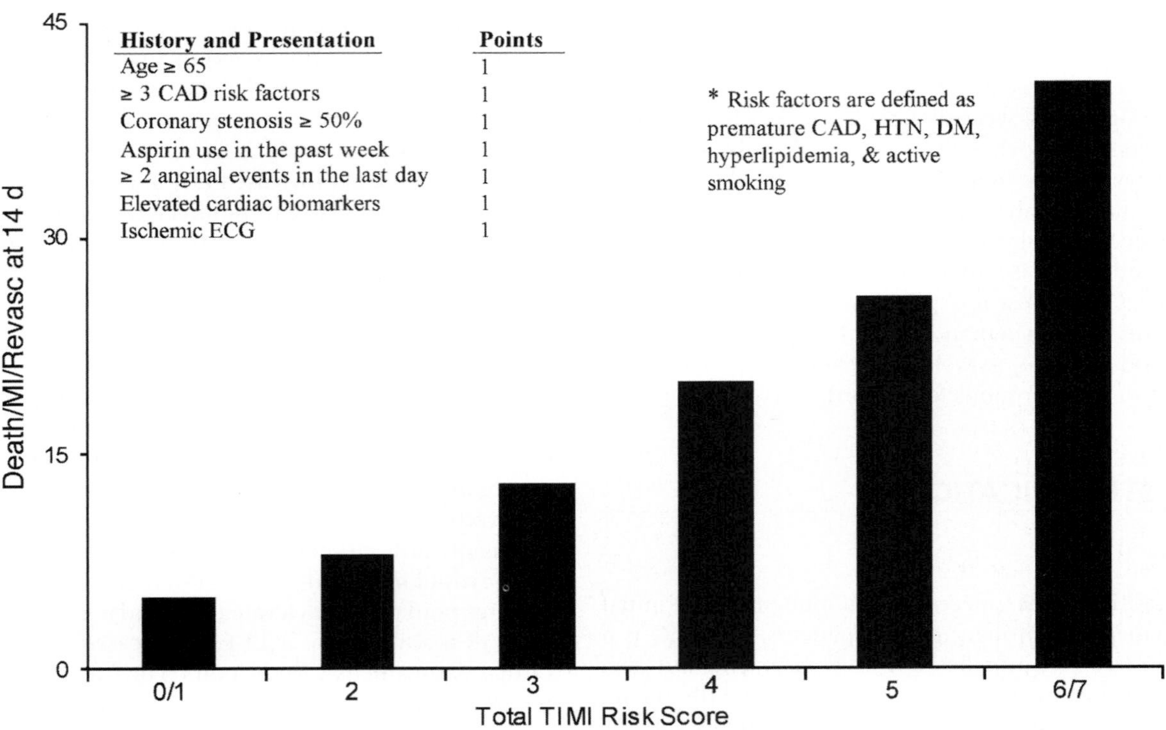


**Figure 14–1** TIMI risk model for prediction of short-term adverse cardiac events in UA/NSTEMI patients. (From Antman EM, Cohen M, Bernink PJ, et al. The TIMI risk score for unstable angina/non-ST elevation MI: a method for prognostication and therapeutic decision making. *JAMA.* 2000;284:835–842.)

## MANAGEMENT

### Initial Approach

The initial assessment of UA/NSTEMI coronary syndromes includes establishing intravenous access and starting supplemental oxygen in patients who are hypoxic or who show signs of respiratory distress. Simultaneously, an ECG must be interpreted, a targeted history and physical exam taken, and cardiac biomarkers measured. Preferred cardiac biomarkers include troponin I or T and CK-MB. Total CK (without MB) should not be used to evaluate an ACS (class III recommendation).

The primary management focus during an ACS, while antithrombotic and anti-ischemic medicines are administered, is to determine a patient's suitability for early invasive therapy versus conservative therapy (Fig. 14–2). While fibrinolytic therapy plays an invaluable role in STEMI patients, it should not be used for the management of UA/NSTEMI unstable coronary syndromes (class III recommendation).

### Invasive Therapy

Early trials failed to show a benefit from an invasive approach in UA/NSTEMI patients. A meta-analysis performed in the current percutaneous coronary intervention (PCI) era analyzed all available studies that randomized patients to early invasive therapy versus conservative management. In those studies, patients who were treated conservatively could have an angiogram performed if they had recurrent chest pain, ischemic ECG changes, a large reversible defect with noninvasive stress testing, or elevated cardiac biomarkers. Only contemporary trials that used GP IIb/IIIa inhibitors and intracoronary stents were included. Five studies, involving nearly 7,000 UA/NSTEMI patients, were analyzed. This analysis revealed a 6- to 12-month survival advantage from early invasive therapy compared to conservative management (RR = 0.80, 95% CI 0.63 to 1.03). In contrast, studies that enrolled patients before the routine use of stents and GP IIb/IIIa inhibitors revealed a harmful association from early invasive therapy (RR 1.31, 95% CI 0.98 to 1.75).

One of the larger studies that contributed to this meta-analysis was the TACTICS-TIMI 18 trial. In this trial, ACS patients were randomized to early invasive therapy versus conservative management. Both groups were treated with aspirin, unfractionated heparin (5,000-U bolus, followed by 1,000 U/h for 48 hours), and tirofiban (0.4 $\mu$g/kg, followed by 0.1 $\mu$g/kg/min for 48 hours or until revascularization and for 12 hours after revascularization). Other medicines such as beta-blockers, nitrates, and lipid-lowering agents were encouraged and used according to physician preference. Patients in the invasive arm

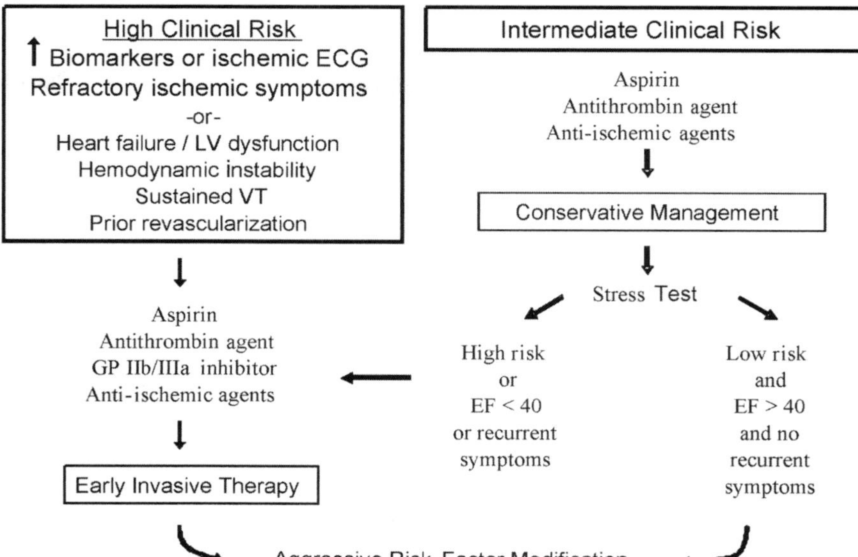


**Figure 14–2** Unstable coronary syndrome pathway for intermediate- and high-risk patients. Low-risk patients can be evaluated with serial cardiac enzymes in a chest pain unit or short hospital stay. All patients should undergo aggressive risk-factor modification. (From Braunwald E, Antman EM, Beasley JW, et al. ACC/AHA guidelines for the management of patients with unstable angina and non-ST-segment elevation myocardial infarction. A report of the American College of Cardiology/American Heart Association Task Force on Practice Guidelines (Committee on the Management of Patients with Unstable Angina). *J Am Coll Cardiol.* 2000;36:970–1062.)

underwent angiography a median of 22 hours after randomization, while for conservatively treated patients who eventually underwent angiography, the median time was 79 hours. Invasive therapy reduced the primary endpoint of death, myocardial infarction, or rehospitalization for an ACS at 6 months by approximately 20% (OR = 0.78, 95% CI 0.62 to 0.97, $p = 0.025$). Additionally, the benefit of invasive therapy was clustered in high-risk individuals who had a TIMI risk score of $\geq 3$.

The ACC/AHA guidelines recommend (class I) an early invasive approach to patients with angina in the presence of heart failure symptoms (pulmonary edema, an $S_3$ gallop, or new mitral regurgitation), known left ventricular dysfunction, hemodynamic instability, positive noninvasive stress test (large area of ischemia), sustained ventricular tachycardia or prior revascularization [prior coronary artery bypass grafting (CABG), or PCI within the last 6 months (see Fig. 14–1). The updated guidelines additionally recommend that individuals with rest angina despite intensive anti-ischemic therapy or with new ST depressions or elevated cardiac biomarkers be directed to early invasive therapy. Invasive therapy is discouraged in low-risk patients and those with extensive co-morbidities (class III recommendation).

Intermediate-risk patients can initially be treated by either an early invasive or a conservative approach with careful monitoring for the development of high-risk features. High-risk features include refractory pain, angina with dynamic ECG changes, or elevated cardiac biomarkers. Such a change in clinical status should advance therapy to a more invasive approach along with adjunctive GP IIb/IIIa inhibitor use.

Low-risk patients can often be treated as outpatients or screened for myocardial infarction with serial cardiac enzymes in a chest pain unit with a goal of early discharge. Invasive therapy is discouraged in these patients. Risk-factor modification is emphasized to all patients regardless of their risk at presentation.

Once the decision is made to perform coronary angiography, the patient's suitability for coronary revascularization is determined. Two options for revascularization are PCI (i.e., percutaneous transluminal coronary angioplasty [PTCA] and intracoronary stents) or CABG. The choice of which revascularization to perform is beyond the scope of this chapter, although several general guidelines exist. Severe left main trunk disease is usually an indication for CABG, although left main PCI can be performed in select cases (i.e., the patient is not a candidate for open heart surgery). Severe three-vessel disease or severe two-vessel disease involving the left anterior descending artery, along with left ventricular dysfunction or diabetes, also favor CABG (Fig. 14–3).

## Antiplatelet Agents

### *Aspirin*

Aspirin is the cornerstone of treatment for all unstable coronary syndromes unless there is a serious contraindication to its use (class I recommendation). Aspirin blocks the conversion of arachidonic acid to thromboxane $A_2$ by irreversibly acetylating cyclooxygenase (Fig. 14–4). Full-dose aspirin exerts maximal antiplatelet effects within 30 minutes of absorption; therefore an initial 325 mg of aspirin orally (or by rectal suppository if necessary) is given during an ACS (Table 14–2). Low-dose aspirin (75 to 150 mg daily) is effective in primary prevention by reducing the incidence of myocardial infarction. In secondary prevention, aspirin improves survival. Bleeding complications increase

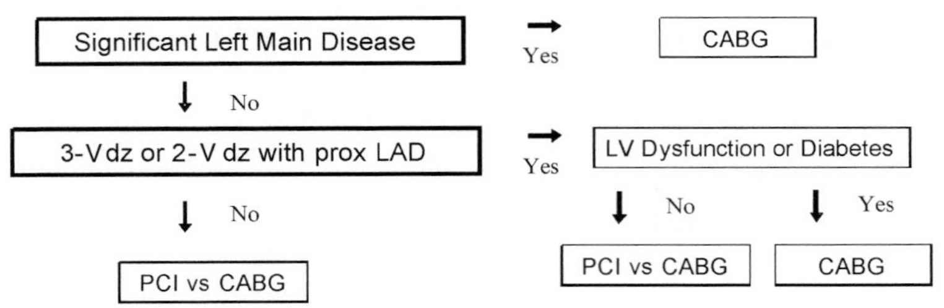


**Figure 14–3** Recommendations for PCI versus CABG once coronary anatomy is defined. (From Braunwald E, Antman EM, Beasley JW, et al. ACC/AHA guidelines for the management of patients with unstable angina and non-ST-segment elevation myocardial infarction. A report of the American College of Cardiology/American Heart Association Task Force on Practice Guidelines (Committee on the Management of Patients with Unstable Angina). *J Am Coll Cardiol.* 2000;36:970–1062.)

with increasing dosage; therefore ongoing aspirin therapy is typically an 81-mg tablet daily unless there is a compelling reason for using a higher dosage, such as mitigating the cutaneous side effects of niacin. Dipyridamole is not indicated in the care of UA/NSTEMI patients (class III recommendation). Despite aspirin's proven benefit in reducing myocardial infarction and death, it does not fully block platelet aggregation, especially when aggregation is induced by adenosine diphosphate. Other agents such as thienopyridines play a valuable role in the management of UA/NSTEMI patients because they complement the actions of aspirin.

### *Thienopyridines*

Thienopyridines are represented by ticlopidine and clopidogrel. These agents act by inhibiting adenosine diphosphate receptor-mediated platelet activation. These agents may be used alone if a patient has a hypersensitivy to aspirin, but they are ideally used adjunctively with aspirin. Clopidogrel is preferred over ticlopidine, given its lower incidence of neutropenia and thrombocytopenia and its rapid onset of action. A loading dose of 300 to 600 mg of clopidogrel produces maximal antiplatelet effects in 4 to 6 hours. The important studies that document the benefit of clopidogrel in unstable coronary syndromes are the CAPRIE, CURE, and CREDO trials.

The CAPRIE trial randomized over 19,000 vascular disease patients to receive aspirin or clopidogrel. Vascular disease was manifested as a history of ischemic stroke, myocardial infarction, or symptomatic peripheral arterial disease. After nearly 2 years of follow-up, clopidogrel reduced a composite endpoint of ischemic stroke, myocardial infarction, or death from vascular causes (5.3% versus 5.8%, $p =$ 0.04).

Patients with vascular disease that is manifested by an ACS are at increased risk for both short- and long-term recurrence of cardiac events. The CURE trial sought to provide protection from these events beyond that of aspirin by the addition of clopidogrel to aspirin and standard medical therapy. This trial randomized over 12,000 non–ST-elevation acute coronary syndrome patients within 24 hours of their onset of chest pain to clopidogrel versus placebo. Patients were eligible if they had ischemic ECG changes or elevated cardiac biomarkers. Individuals who were randomized to clopidogrel received a loading dose of 300 mg, followed by 75 mg/day for 3 to 12 months.

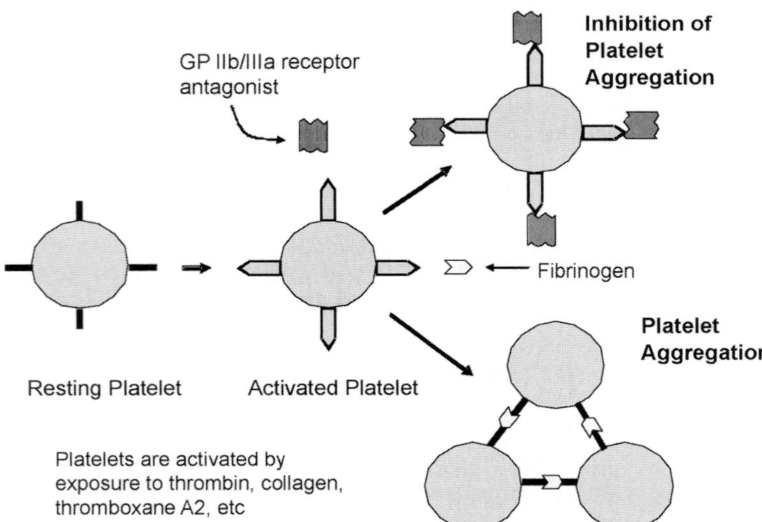


**Figure 14–4** Schema for platelet aggregation and inhibition of platelet aggregation by GP Iib/IIIa inhibitors. Platelets are activated by adenosine diphosphate, thrombin, epinephrine, collagen, and thromboxane A2. Aspirin blocks the conversion of arachidonic acid to thromboxane A2. Clopidogrel blocks adenosine diphosphate-mediated platelet activation. GP IIb/IIIa inhibitors cause a conformational change in the GP Iib/IIIa receptor that prevents fibrinogen-mediated platelet aggregation. (From Yeghiazarians Y, Braunstein JB, Askari A, Stone PH. Unstable angina pectoris. *N Engl J Med.* 2000;342:101–114.)

**TABLE 14–2**
**CLASS I ANTIPLATELET AND ANTITHROMBOTIC RECOMMENDATIONS**

| High Risk—Invasive Strategy | Intermediate Risk—Conservative Strategy | Low Risk |
|---|---|---|
| Aspirin<br>Antithrombin agent[a]<br>GP IIb/IIIa inhibitor | Aspirin<br>Antithrombin agent[b] | Aspirin |

Clopidogrel is indicated for high-risk patients who are managed conservatively, for invasively managed patients when PCI is planned, or for aspirin hypersensitivity.
[a]There is no benefit of low-molecular-weight heparin over unfractionated heparin.
[b]There may be a marginal benefit of low-molecular-weight heparin over unfractionated heparin as long as there is no renal insufficiency and patients are <75 years of age.
*Source:* From Braunwald E, Antman EM, Beasley JW, et al. ACC/AHA guidelines for the management of patients with unstable angina and non-ST-segment elevation myocardial infarction. A report of the American College of Cardiology/American Heart Association Task Force on Practice Guidelines (Committee on the Management of Patients with Unstable Angina). *J Am Coll Cardiol.* 2000;36:970–1062.

Aspirin could be given at a dose of 75 to 325 mg/day. This was largely a conservatively treated population, as <50% of the patients underwent angiography. Among enrolled patients, <20% underwent CABG, and <25% had percutaneous coronary revascularization. Also, <10% of individuals were treated with a GP IIb/IIIa inhibitor in addition to the other antithrombotic agents. The mean treatment of clopidogrel was 9 months. A composite of cardiac outcomes was significantly reduced at 30 days (RR = 0.79, 95% CI 0.67 to 0.92) and 1 year by the regimen of clopidogrel plus aspirin versus aspirin alone (RR = 0.8, 95% CI 0.72 to 0.9, $p$ <0.001). The incidence of myocardial infarction was significantly reduced by clopidogrel, while other individual components of the composite cardiac outcome were not. The primary outcome was reduced across a range of patients regardless of whether or not they were revascularized.

Important safety data also came from the CURE trial. Major bleeding was significantly increased by the use of clopidogrel, although this did not include hemorrhagic strokes. Patients who had clopidogrel discontinued more than 5 days before CABG did not have an increase in major postoperative bleeding, while individuals whose clopidogrel was stopped within 5 days of CABG appeared to have an increase in major bleeding (9.6% in clopidogrel versus 6.3% in placebo, RR 1.53, $p = 0.06$). Additionally, patients on clopidogrel who were treated with high-dose aspirin (325 mg/day) suffered more bleeding than individuals on approximately 81 mg/day.

The CREDO trial was designed to explore two questions. The first was whether a loading dose of clopidogrel reduces composite cardiac outcomes over the short term, and the second was whether long-term use of clopidogrel after PCI reduces composite cardiac outcomes at 1 year. This trial enrolled >2,000 patients who were either scheduled to undergo elective PCI or were felt to be at high risk of undergoing PCI. Patients were eligible if they had anginal symptoms, a positive stress test, or dynamic ECG changes. Participants were randomized to a loading dose of clopidogrel (300 mg, at least 3 hours and up to 24 hours before the procedure) versus placebo in addition to aspirin and standard medical therapy. Both groups received clopidogrel (75 mg/day) after the procedure until day 28, at which time clopidogrel was continued in the arm receiving the loading dose and replaced by placebo in the arm without a loading dose. A loading dose of clopidogrel did not significantly reduce 28-day events, although when the analysis was restricted to individuals who received clopidogrel 6 hours or more prior to the procedure, there was a marginally significant reduction in 28-day events (RR = 0.61, 95% CI 0.37 to 0.98, $p = 0.051$). There was a significant reduction in all-cause mortality, myocardial infarction, or stroke at 1 year from the long-term use of clopidogrel (RR = 0.73, 95% CI 0.56 to 0.96). Major bleeding that occurred from the use of clopidogrel was usually in the setting of CABG or PCI.

Clopidogrel should be considered in addition to aspirin (or alone when there is hypersensitivity to aspirin) for all UA/NSTEMI patients when PCI is planned or for those managed conservatively (class I recommendation) (see Table 14–2). Duration of therapy is at least 1 month and possibly longer. An important caveat with clopidogrel is that it likely increases the risk for major bleeding during surgery and so it should be held for at least 5 days before cardiac surgery is performed. For this reason, clopidogrel is often given on the catheterization table (loading dose) after coronary anatomy is defined and it is clear that cardiac surgery will not be required. A loading dose of clopidogrel is 300 to 600 mg. When a significant aspirin allergy exists, clopidogrel should be used in its place (class I recommendation).

### *Glycoprotein IIb/IIIa Inhibitors*

Glycoprotein (GP) IIb/IIIa inhibitors are effective in the management of high-risk UA/NSTEMI patients managed by early invasive therapy. GP IIb/IIIa inhibitors further complement the actions of aspirin and clopidogrel by blocking the final pathway involved in platelet activation and aggregation (see Fig. 14–4). In individuals for whom an invasive strategy is planned, the use of a GP IIb/IIIa inhibitor reduces mortality and myocardial infarction rates. Accordingly, the use of a GP IIb/IIIa inhibitor in high-risk UA/NSTEMI patients managed by early invasive therapy is a class I recommendation. This information comes principally from a meta-analysis that analyzed 19 trials involving >20,000 patients undergoing PCI. These individuals were randomized to a GP IIb/IIIa inhibitor versus placebo in addition to standard medial therapy including aspirin and heparin. Most of these trials used abciximab. Fewer trials used eptifibatide, and only two trials used tirofiban. This was a contemporary analysis as the use of stents was well

**TABLE 14–3**
**GP IIb/IIIa INHIBITOR DOSAGES**

| GP IIb/IIIa Inhibitor | Dose for Normal CrCl | Dose for Reduced CrCl |
|---|---|---|
| Abciximab (ReoPro) | 0.25 mg/kg bolus, followed by 0.125 mg/kg/min for 12 to 24 hours | No reduced dose for renal insufficiency |
| Eptifibatide (Integrilin) | 180 μg/kg bolus, followed by 2 μg/kg/min for 72 to 96 hours | 180 μg/kg bolus, followed by 1 μg/kg/min for 72 to 96 hours |
| Tirofiban (Aggrastat) | 0.4 μg/kg/min for 30 min followed by 0.1 μg/kg/min for 72 to 96 hours | 0.2 μg/kg/min for 30 min followed by 0.05 μg/kg/min for 72 to 96 hours |

*Source:* From Braunwald E, Antman EM, Beasley JW, et al. ACC/AHA guidelines for the management of patients with unstable angina and non-ST-segment elevation myocardial infarction. A report of the American College of Cardiology/American Heart Association Task Force on Practice Guidelines (Committee on the Management of Patients with Unstable Angina). *J Am Coll Cardiol.* 2000;36:970–1062.

represented in the trials. The use of a GP IIb/IIIa inhibitor reduced mortality by approximately 30% at 30 days (RR = 0.69, 95% CI 0.53 to 0.90), 20% at 6 months (RR = 0.79, 95% CI 0.64 to 0.97), and 20% during longer follow-up (RR = 0.79, 95% CI 0.66 to 0.94). This translates into the number of patients needed to treat to save one life as 320, 220, and 170, respectively, for 30-day, 6-month, and longer follow-up. There was a modest increase in bleeding from the use of a GP IIb/IIIa inhibitor (0.68%, 95% CI −0.05% to 1.40%). There was an increase in major bleeding among studies that continued heparin after the procedure (RR = 1.70, 95% CI 1.36 to 2.14) in contrast to studies that discontinued heparin after the procedure (RR = 1.02, 95% CI 0.85 to 1.24). Cardiac outcomes were the same regardless of whether heparin was continued or discontinued after the procedure.

When invasive therapy is planned and the patient is already on aspirin, clopidogrel, and an antithrombin agent, the need for a GP IIb/IIIa inhibitor is downgraded to a class IIa recommendation. This is a result of insufficient evidence for using "quadruple therapy" during PCI. The choice of which GP IIb/IIIa inhibitor to use as an adjunct to invasive therapy is further influenced by the Do TARGET trial and the GUSTO IV–ACS trial.

The TARGET trial showed a reduction in composite cardiac outcomes at 30 days in patients undergoing PCI who were randomized to abciximab instead of tirofiban ($p$ = 0.038). This complements the findings from the GP IIb/IIIa in PCI meta-analysis, in which mortality was reduced by abciximab (RR = 0.69, 95% CI 0.51 to 0.94) but not tirofiban (RR = 1.05, 95% CI 0.42 to 2.61).

In GUSTO IV–ACS, however, the use of continuous abciximab in patients who were not intended to undergo revascularization resulted in worsened mortality at 48 hours ($p$ = 0.008). Therefore, if invasive therapy is anticipated to occur quickly, abciximab should be used. More than several hours' delay in performing invasive therapy should probably necessitate the use of eptifibatide or tirofiban (Table 14–3). Such a scenario might be expected in a patient being transferred from a community hospital to a tertiary-care center for PCI. Abciximab should not be used for conservative therapy, as was highlighted in GUSTO IV–ACS (class III recommendation).

When invasive therapy is not planned as part of the management of unstable coronary syndromes, the use of a GP IIb/IIIa inhibitor is less clear. In this setting, using a GP IIb/IIIa inhibitor is a class II recommendation. A large meta-analysis was performed on six trials with >31,000 patients with acute coronary syndromes who were not routinely scheduled to undergo early invasive therapy. This analysis revealed a small reduction in the composite outcome of mortality and myocardial infarction (OR = 0.91, 95% CI 0.84 to 0.98, $p$ = 0.015), but mortality was not significantly reduced (OR = 0.91, 95% CI 0.81 to 1.03, $p$ = 0.14) at 30 days. According to the ACC/AHA guidelines, for patients who are managed conservatively and who continue to have ischemia, the use of a GP IIb/IIIa inhibitor is considered a class IIa recommendation. This is in contrast to conservatively treated individuals who do not have continued ischemia (class IIb recommendation). The dosages for GP IIb/IIIa inhibitors are listed in the table.

Multiple trials have reported unfavorable results for the use of oral GP IIb/IIIa inhibitors in patients with coronary disease. The most recent study in this context was the BRAVO trial. This trial was terminated early after 30% increased mortality was detected in the oral GP IIb/IIIa inhibitor group. As such, oral GPIIb/IIIa inhibitors do not have a role in the management of coronary disease patients.

## AntiThrombin Therapy

### *Unfractionated Heparin and Low-Molecular-Weight Heparin*

Heparins have been used in the management of coronary syndromes and during PCI for the last several decades.

Unfractionated heparin is a glycosaminoglycan composed of polysaccharide chains that range in weight from 3,000 to 30,000. Heparin causes a conformational change in antithrombin III that inhibits the activity of thrombin (factor IIa) and factor Xa. This results in the inhibition of platelet aggregation and fibrin formation. In contrast to unfractionated heparin, low-molecular-weight heparins have high bioavailability and a more predictable pharmacokinetic effect. Low-molecular-weight heparins are also easy to administer and do not require monitoring. The various low-molecular-weight heparins have different ratios of anti-Xa to IIa. For example, the ratios of anti-Xa to IIa for enoxaparin and dalteparin are 3.8 and 2.7, respectively. Higher ratios appear to be associated with improved outcomes, although more research is need to define the most optimal agents, dosage, and duration of therapy.

Heparin and aspirin reduce death and myocardial infarction in non–ST-elevation acute coronary syndromes compared to treatment with aspirin alone. Therapy with unfractionated heparin is a class I recommendation in the care of intermediate- or higher-risk ACS patients (see Fig. 14–2). Low-molecular-weight heparin may have marginal benefit over unfractionated heparin in conservatively treated patients, and can be considered in patients who do not have renal insufficiency or when surgical revascularization is not planned within 24 hours (class IIa recommendation). For invasively treated patients, there is no clear advantage of low-molecular-weight heparin over unfractionated heparin, and institutional preference should govern the choice of a particular agent.

The SYNERGY trial was a contemporary analysis that randomized nearly 10,000 patients to subcutaneous enoxaparin or intravenous unfractionated heparin in addition to standard medical therapy. More than half of the participants received a GP IIb/IIIa inhibitor, and >90% were managed by an invasive approach. Mortality at 30 days was equivalent (3.2% for enoxaparin versus 3.1% for unfractionated heparin), although major bleeding was increased by low-molecular-weight heparin (9.1% for enoxaparin versus 7.6% for unfractionated heparin).

The dose of unfractionated heparin in conservatively treated patients is 80 U/kg bolus followed by 18 U/kg/h infusion. Heparin dosage is lowered if a patient will be managed invasively with a GP IIb/IIIa inhibitor and will be at higher risk for bleeding. The heparin dose in this case is 60 U/kg bolus (maximum 5,000 U) followed by 12 U/kg/h infusion (maximum 1,000 U/h) for a goal pTT of 45 to 65. Conservative dosing for enoxaparin is 1 mg/kg subcutaneously twice a day, while the dose used in conjunction with invasive therapy is 0.75 mg/kg subcutaneously twice a day.

The large meta-analysis on GPIIb/IIIa inhibition in the setting of PCI revealed an increase in major bleeding when heparin was continued after PCI, although major adverse cardiac outcomes (myocardial infarction, stroke, urgent revascularization) were not increased by stopping heparin at the time of completion of PCI. Accordingly, heparin or coumadin should not be continued post-PCI, unless there is a specific indication for their use. The routine use of coumadin in stabilized UA/NSTEMI patients is a class IIb recommendation. An indication for continuing antithrombin therapy after PCI would be a patient with atrial fibrillation or a mechanical valve. The optimal duration of heparin in conservatively treated patients is unknown, although if patients are asymptomatic, the duration of heparin therapy usually should not exceed 48 hours. If conservatively treated patients continue to have signs of ischemia, then longer duration of heparin therapy may be indicated.

### *Direct Thrombin Inhibitors*

In contrast to heparins, direct thrombin inhibitors (DTI) block factor only IIa via a mechanism that does not require the action of antithrombin III. These agents overcome important limitations of heparin, including unpredictable pharmacokinetics, increased bleeding, and the potential to cause heparin-induced thrombocytopenia (HIT). Representative agents in this class of medicines include hirudin, argatroban, and bivalirudin.

The Bivalirudin Angioplasty Study examined cardiac outcomes in >4,000 UA patients undergoing coronary angioplasty who were randomized to bivalirudin or unfractionated heparin. The combined endpoint occurred in 16% of the bivalirudin group, versus 19% of the heparin group (OR = 0.82, 95% CI 0.70 to 0.96, $p = 0.012$) at 90 days, while bleeding was significantly reduced in the bivalirudin group (3.5% versus 9.3% for the heparin group, $p < 0.001$).

A 2002 meta-analysis analyzed available trials that randomized over 35,000 ACS and PCI patients to DTI versus heparin. This was a heterogeneous population, as it included STEMI and UA/NSTEMI patients. At 30 days of follow-up, death or myocardial infarction was significantly reduced (OR = 0.91, 95% CI 0.84 to 0.99). This finding was preserved when the analysis was restricted to studies that enrolled >20,000 patients with non–ST-elevation unstable coronary syndromes (OR = 0.80, 95% CI 0.70 to 0.92). This outcome was driven entirely by a reduction in myocardial infarctions (OR = 0.87, 95% CI 0.79 to 0.95). Death or myocardial infarction was reduced in studies that used hirudin and bivalirudin, whereas no benefit was seen with univalent agents. Major bleeding was increased by the use of hirudin (OR = 1.28, 95% CI 1.06 to 1.55), although it was reduced by bivalirudin (OR = 0.44, 95% CI 0.34 to 0.56).

The previously mentioned studies revealed that bivalirudin was comparable to heparin in clinical efficacy, although it was associated with less bleeding. The REPLACE-2 trial expanded on these findings by specifically studying this agent during contemporary PCI. Although the patients in this trial were relatively stable, some lower-risk UA patients were enrolled. This trial documented the noninferiority of bivalirudin and a provisional GP IIb/IIIa inhibitor compared to unfractionated heparin and a planned GP IIb/IIIa

**TABLE 14–4**
**CLASS I ANTI-ISCHEMIC RECOMMENDATIONS**

| Therapy |
|---|
| Bed rest with continuous ECG monitoring |
| Supplemental oxygen to keep $SaO_2 > 90\%$ |
| Intravenous NTG |
| Intravenous or oral beta-blockers[a,b] |
| Intravenous morphine for anxiety, pulmonary congestion, and pain[c] |
| IABP for refractory ischemia or hemodynamic instability |
| ACE-I for control of hypertension or LV dysfunction after MI[d] |

The listed therapies are indicated for ongoing ischemia.
[a]Intravenous beta-blockers should be converted to oral dosing when ischemia is controlled.
[b]Calcium channel blockers may be used when beta-blockers are not successful, or there is a contraindication to their use.
[c]Care must be taken, however, not to obscure symptoms and confound treatment of ongoing myocardial ischemia with excessive morphine doses.
[d]ACE-I are continued when ischemia is controlled, especially for LV dysfunction or diabetes.
*Source:* From Braunwald E, Antman EM, Beasley JW, et al. ACC/AHA guidelines for the management of patients with unstable angina and non-ST-segment elevation myocardial infarction. A report of the American College of Cardiology/American Heart Association Task Force on Practice Guidelines (Committee on the Management of Patients with Unstable Angina). *J Am Coll Cardiol.* 2000;36:970–1062.

inhibitor. Additionally, bivalirudin was shown to significantly reduce the risk for major bleeding (2.4% in the bivalirudin group versus 4.1% in the heparin group, $p < 0.001$). The ACUITY trial of 13,000 patients is comparing bivalirudin to heparin-based regimens in invasively managed unstable coronary syndromes and will help to clarify the use of this agent in ACS.

## Anti-ischemic Agents

Regardless of whether a patient will be directed to an early invasive approach versus a conservative approach, anti-ischemic medications are a priority. Nitroglycerin and beta-blockers are the first-line agents to consider (Table 14–4). Nitroglycerin is initiated by a 0.4-mg sublingual tablet (repeated several times every 5 minutes if symptoms persist and hypotension does not develop), followed by intravenous infusion started at 10 to 20 5 $\mu$g/min (titrated up until resolution of symptoms or hypotension develops). An intravenous dose of 200 $\mu$g/min is considered a ceiling, although doses as high as 400 $\mu$g/min are occasionally used if needed. Sildenafil use within 24 hours of presentation is a class III recommendation to the use of nitroglycerin.

Beta-blockers are administered along with nitroglycerin and help to blunt the reflex tachycardia that may occur from its use. Beta-blockade is initiated intravenously (i.e., 5 mg metoprolol intravenously, repeated several times every 5 minutes), followed by oral administration (i.e., 25 mg metoprolol orally twice to three times per day and titrated up to effect) if there are no contraindications to its use. Contraindications include significant conduction abnormalities (marked first-degree AV block, or second/third-degree block), asthma, or decompensated heart failure. If beta-blockers are used at maximal dose or there are contraindications to their use, a nondihydropyridine (i.e., diltiazem or verapamil) may be considered to control symptoms. Morphine (1 to 5 mg intravenously) is also considered a class I anti-ischemic medication and is particularly helpful for anxious patients. Care must be taken, however, not to obscure symptoms and confound treatment of ongoing myocardial ischemia with excessive morphine doses.

If hemodynamics are well controlled with anti-ischemic medications (i.e., heart rate is 50 to 60 beats/minute and systolic blood pressure is 90 to 100 mm Hg but ischemia persists, an intra-aortic balloon pump (IABP) should be considered (class IIa recommendation). Hemodynamic instability is another class IIa indication for using an IABP in the management of UA/NSTEMI. In either scenario, the device is used as a bridge to coronary angiography or until stabilization occurs after invasive therapy has been performed.

## Miscellaneous Agents

Angiotensin-converting enzyme inhibitors (ACE-I) should be considered in patients after an unstable coronary syndrome (class IIa recommendation) (Table 14–5). An ACE-I is usually not given in the first hours of an ACS, to ensure that the patient is hemodynamically stable. The presence of diabetes or left ventricular dysfunction strengthens the recommendation for an ACE-I after UA/NSTEMI (class I recommendation).

**TABLE 14–5**
**MEDICAL RECOMMENDATIONS FOR STABILIZED UA/NSTEMI PATIENTS**

| Therapy | Class of Recommendation |
|---|---|
| Aspirin | I |
| Clopidogrel[a] | I |
| Nitrates | I |
| Beta-blockers | I |
| Calcium channel blockers[b] | I |
| ACE-I[c] | I or IIa |
| Warfarin | IIb |
| Dipyridamole | III |

[a]The duration of clopidogrel is 1 month and possibly up to 9 months. Patients with drug-eluting stents will require longer duration of clopidogrel than bare-metal stent recipients.
[b]Calcium channel blockers are class I when beta-blockers are not successful, or there is a contraindication to their use.
[c]ACE-I are class I when there is heart failure/LV dysfunction and class IIa otherwise.
*Source:* From Braunwald E, Antman EM, Beasley JW, et al. ACC/AHA guidelines for the management of patients with unstable angina and non-ST-segment elevation myocardial infarction. A report of the American College of Cardiology/American Heart Association Task Force on Practice Guidelines (Committee on the Management of Patients with Unstable Angina). *J Am Coll Cardiol.* 2000;36:970–1062.

Early statin trials excluded ACS patients, although more recent studies have addressed this high-risk population. The PROVE IT-TIMI 22 trial randomized >4,000 patients within 10 days of an ACS to intensive lipid lowering (80 mg/day atorvastatin) versus moderate lipid lowering (40 mg/day pravastatin). The outcome was a composite of death, myocardial infarction, ACS requiring rehospitalization, revascularization, and stroke. Follow-up was 18 to 36 months, with a mean follow-up of 24 months. Atorvastatin was more effective in lowering cholesterol (median LDL 62 mg/dL) than pravastatin (median LDL 95 mg/dL). The primary outcome was reached in 22% of the atorvastatin group and 26% of the pravastatin group, representing a 16% reduction in the hazard ratio (95% CI 5 to 26%, $p = 0.005$). Intensive lipid-lowering therapy appeared to beneficially lower the primary outcome as early as 30 days after enrollment. Both medications were well tolerated, with 23% of the atorvastatin group discontinuing therapy at 1 year because of an adverse event, compared to 21% for pravastatin ($p = 0.3$). Atorvastatin was associated with more elevations in liver enzymes (defined as alanine aminotransferase more than three times the upper limit of normal) (3.3% of the atorvastatin group, 1.1% of the pravastatin group).

**TABLE 14–6**
**NONINVASIVE RISK STRATIFICATION**

| |
|---|
| High risk (>3% annual mortality): |
| Severe resting or exercise LV dysfunction (<35%) |
| High-risk treadmill score (≤−11) |
| Large stress perfusion defect (especially anterior) |
| Multiple moderate stress perfusion defects |
| Large fixed defect or moderate perfusion defect with LV dilitation or increased lung uptake |
| Wall motion abnormalities (>2 segments) at low-dose dobutamine or low heart rate |
| Extensive ischemia by stress echo |
| Intermediate risk (1% to 3% annual mortality): |
| Mild/moderate resting LV dysfunction |
| Intermediat- risk treadmill score (−11 to 5) |
| Moderate perfusion defect without LV dilitation or increased lung uptake |
| Limited stress echo wall motion (≤2 segments) only at high-dose dobutamine |
| Low risk (<1% annual mortality): |
| Low-risk treadmill score (≥5) |
| Normal to small rest or stress perfusion defect |
| Normal stress echo wall motion |

*Source:* From Braunwald E, Antman EM, Beasley JW, et al. ACC/AHA guidelines for the management of patients with unstable angina and non-ST-segment elevation myocardial infarction. A report of the American College of Cardiology/American Heart Association Task Force on Practice Guidelines (Committee on the Management of Patients with Unstable Angina). *J Am Coll Cardiol.* 2000;36:970-1062.

## DISCHARGE PLANNING AND NONINVASIVE STRESS TESTING

All stabilized UA/NSTEMI patients need aggressive risk-factor modification (including smoking cessation) and must have their discharge medicines reviewed. For intermediate- and low-risk patients managed conservatively (either hospitalized or observed in a chest pain unit), a noninvasive stress test provides important additional risk stratification (Table 14–6). A noninvasive stress test should be performed in intermediate-risk patients who have been free of chest pain and without heart failure symptoms for 2 to 3 days and in low-risk patients who have been free of chest pain and without heart failure symptoms for 12 to 24 hours. Patients who have an interpretable baseline ECG and are able to exercise should have an exercise ECG performed. Radionuclide or echocardiographic imaging should be used if there is a noninterpretable ECG (i.e., the presence of a left bundle branch block or left ventricular hypertrophy with repolarization changes). Patients who are unable to exercise should have a pharmacologic stress test.

## SUMMARY

Patients with unstable coronary syndromes are a heterogeneous group that includes UA and NSTEMI. These patients have a high burden of atherothrombotic disease in other vascular beds and are at high risk for future adverse cardiac events. Risk stratification helps to guide therapy and should take place by one of several mechanisms during the initial assessment of the patient. The ECG is one simple and readily available diagnostic test that should be performed in all ACS patients that provides important prognostic information.

High-risk patients benefit from early invasive therapy with adjunctive use of a GP IIb/IIIa inhibitor in addition to aspirin and an antithrombin agent (i.e., unfractionated heparin). Clopidogrel is beneficial, in either invasively or conservatively managed patients. Lower-risk patients can be managed without a GP IIb/IIIa inhibitor unless high-risk features develop during the hospital course. Lowest-risk patients can be treated with aspirin and managed expeditiously in a chest pain unit or discharged home with noninvasive stress testing performed on an outpatient basis. In addition to antiplatelet and antithrombin agents, anti-ischemic agents should be used judiciously, with the goal of relieving ischemic symptoms and improving hemodynamics. Nitroglycerin and beta-blockers are first-line anti-ischemic medications, unless there is a contraindication to their use. Calcium channel blockers are considered second-line anti-ischemic agents. Intensive statin therapy and possibly an ACE-inhibitor (especially if the patient is diabetic or there is left ventricular dysfunction) should be part of the discharge regimen. Once ACS patients are risk stratified, stabilized, and possibly revascularized, discharge planning goals are centered on aggressive risk-factor modification. Lower-risk patients who were not revascularized should have plans made for a future noninvasive stress test.

## BIBLIOGRAPHY


**Antiplatelet Trialists'Collaboration**. Collaborative overview of randomized trials of antiplatelet therapy, I: prevention of death, myocardial infarction, and stroke by prolonged antiplatelet therapy in various categories of patients. *Br Med J.* 1994;308:81–106.

**Antman EM, Cohen M, Bernink PJ, et al**. The TIMI risk score for unstable angina/non-ST elevation MI: a method for prognostication and therapeutic decision making. *JAMA.* 2000;284:835–842.

**Bavry AA, Kumbhani DJ, Quiroz R, Ramchandani SR, Kenchaiah S, Antman EM**. Invasive therapy along with glycoprotein IIb/IIIa inhibitors and intracoronary stents improves survival in non-ST-segment elevation acute coronary syndromes: a meta-analysis and review of the literature. *Am J Cardiol.* 2004;93:830–5.

**Bittl JA, Chaitman BR, Feit F, et al**. Bivalirudin versus heparin during coronary angioplasty for unstable or postinfarction angina: final report reanalysis of the Bivalirudin Angioplasty Study. *Am Heart J.* 2001;142:952–959.

**Blazing MA, de Lemos JA, White HD, et al**. Safety and efficacy of enoxaparin vs unfractionated heparin in patients with non-ST-segment elevation acute coronary syndromes who receive tirofiban and aspirin: a randomized controlled trial. *JAMA.* 2004;292:55–64.

**Boersma E, Harrington RA, Moliterno DJ, et al**. Platelet glycoprotein IIb/IIIa inhibitors in acute coronary syndromes: a meta-analysis of all major randomised clinical trials. *Lancet.* 2002;359:189–198.

**Braunwald E, Antman EM, Beasley JW, et al**. ACC/AHA guidelines for the management of patients with unstable angina and non-ST-segment elevation myocardial infarction. A report of the American College of Cardiology/American Heart Association Task Force on Practice Guidelines (Committee on the Management of Patients with Unstable Angina). *J Am Coll Cardiol.* 2000;36:970–1062.

**Cannon CP, Braunwald E, McCabe CH, et al**. Intensive versus moderate lipid lowering with statins after acute coronary syndromes. *N Engl J Med.* 2004;350:1495–1504.

**Cannon CP, Weintraub WS, Demopoulos LA, et al**. Comparison of early invasive and conservative strategies in patients with unstable coronary syndromes treated with the glycoprotein IIb/IIIa inhibitor tirofiban. *N Engl J Med.* 2001;344:1879–1887.

**Eikelboom JW, Anand SS, Malmberg K, et al**. Unfractionated heparin and low-molecular-weight heparin in acute coronary syndrome without ST elevation: a meta-analysis. *Lancet.* 2000;355:1936–1942.

**Ferguson JJ, Califf RM, Antman EM, et al**. Enoxaparin vs unfractionated heparin in high-risk patients with non-ST-segment elevation acute coronary syndromes managed with an intended early invasive strategy: primary results of the SYNERGY randomized trial. *JAMA.* 2004;292:45–54.

**Karvouni E, Katritsis DG, Ioannidis JP**. Intravenous glycoprotein IIb/IIIa receptor antagonists reduce mortality after percutaneous coronary interventions. *J Am Coll Cardiol.* 2003;41:26–32.

**Lincoff AM, Bittl JA, Harrington RA, et al**. Bivalirudin and provisional glycoprotein IIb/IIIa blockade compared with heparin and planned glycoprotein IIb/IIIa blockade during percutaneous coronary intervention: REPLACE-2 randomized trial. *JAMA.* 2003;289:853–863.

**Ottervanger JP, Armstrong P, Barnathan ES, et al**. Long-term results after the glycoprotein IIb/IIIa inhibitor abciximab in unstable angina: one-year survival in the GUSTO IV-ACS (Global Use of Strategies to Open Occluded Coronary Arteries IV—Acute Coronary Syndrome) Trial. *Circulation.* 2003;107:437–442.

**Petersen JL, Mahaffey KW, Hasselblad V, et al**. Efficacy and bleeding complications among patients randomized to enoxaparin or unfractionated heparin for antithrombin therapy in non-ST-segment elevation acute coronary syndromes: a systematic overview. *JAMA.* 2004;292:89–96.

**Ridker PM, Cushman M, Stampfer MJ, et al**. Inflammation, aspirin, and the risk of cardiovascular disease in apparently healthy men. *N Engl J Med.* 1997;336:973–979.

**Sabatine MS, Morrow DA, de Lemos JA, et al**. Multimarker approach to risk stratification in non-ST elevation acute coronary syndromes: simultaneous assessment of troponin I, C-reactive protein, and B-type natriuretic peptide. *Circulation.* 2002;105:1760–1763.

**Steinhubl SR, Berger PB, Mann JT 3rd, et al**. Early and sustained dual oral antiplatelet therapy following percutaneous coronary intervention: a randomized controlled trial. *JAMA.* 2002;288:2411–2420.

**Topol EJ, Moliterno DJ, Herrmann HC, et al**. Comparison of two platelet glycoprotein IIb/IIIa inhibitors, tirofiban and abciximab, for the prevention of ischemic events with percutaneous coronary revascularization. *N Engl J Med.* 2001;344:1888–1894.

**Yeghiazarians Y, Braunstein JB, Askari A, Stone PH**. Unstable angina pectoris. *N Engl J Med.* 2000;342:101–114.

**Yusuf S, Zhao F, Mehta SR, et al**. Effects of clopidogrel in addition to aspirin in patients with acute coronary syndromes without ST-segment elevation. *N Engl J Med.* 2001;345:494–502.


## QUESTIONS

**1.** All of the following are recommended mechanisms to decrease bleeding complications in the management of unstable coronary syndromes, except:

a. Decreasing the maintenance dose of aspirin from 325 to 81 mg daily
b. Stopping clopidogrel a minimum of 5 days prior to a major surgical procedure
c. Stopping the routine use of heparin after percutaneous coronary intervention
d. Withholding the loading dose of clopidogrel
e. Reducing the dose of heparin for patients who are also on aspirin and a glycoprotein IIb/IIIa inhibitor

Answer is d: When clopidogrel is used for either invasively or conservatively managed unstable coronary syndromes, a loading dose of 300 to 600 mg should be used. Giving 75 mg of clopidogrel daily without a loading dose would require up to 7 days to reach full antiplatelet effect. All of the other listed strategies may be effective in reducing bleeding complications.

**2.** All of the following are high-risk features of the TIMI risk score for stratifying patients with unstable coronary syndromes, except:

a. Elevated cardiac biomarkers
b. Age >65 years
c. Tachycardia
d. Ischemic electrocardiographic changes
e. A known coronary stenosis of more than 50%

Answer is c: Although tachycardia (and hypotension) have been identified through the PURSUIT trial to be markers of high risk, they are not part of the formal TIMI risk model. All the other variables are components of the TIMI risk score.

**3.** All of the following therapies are class I recommendations for conservatively treated patients with unstable coronary syndromes, except:

a. ACE inhibitor therapy
b. Nitrate therapy
c. Aspirin therapy
d. Beta-blocker therapy
e. Clopidogrel therapy

Answer is a: All of the listed therapies are class I recommendations for stabilized patients with unstable coronary syndromes except ACE inhibitors, which are a class IIa recommendation. ACE inhibitors are strengthened to a class I recommendation if patients have diabetes or left ventricular dysfunction. Clopidogrel is a class I recommendation for both invasive and conservatively managed patients with unstable coronary syndromes.

**4.** All of the following are class III recommendations in the treatment of unstable coronary syndromes, except:

a. Use of fibrinolytic therapy for non–ST-elevation acute coronary syndromes
b. Use of abciximab for conservatively managed high-risk patients who continue to have ischemic symptoms
c. The use of a low-molecular-weight heparin instead of unfractionated heparin for conservatively managed unstable coronary syndromes
d. Use of nitroglycerin within 24 hours of sildenafil (Viagra)
e. Invasive therapy in low-risk patients who present with a chest pain syndrome

Answer is c: There may be a marginal benefit of low-molecular-weight heparin over unfractionated heparin for conservatively managed patients, and this strategy is a class IIa recommendation. Nitroglycerin should not be used within 24 hours from the last dose of sildenafil. Fibrinolytics should only be used for ST-elevation myocardial infarctions. Ideally, high-risk patients should be managed invasively, but for high-risk individuals who defer invasive therapy or who have extensive co-morbidities and continue to have ischemic symptoms, the use of a glycoprotein IIb/IIIa inhibitor is a class IIa recommdation. However, eptifibitide or tirofiban should be used in this setting, while abciximab should be used only during invasive management.

**5.** Which of the following are causes of secondary angina?

a. An anemic patient from a gastrointestinal bleed
b. A dialysis patient with an arterio-venous fistula
c. A dyspneic patient with underlying emphysema
d. a and c
e. a, b, and c

Answer is e: Anemia, anterior-venous shunting, and hypoxemia can all cause demand ischemia. Note that a left-arm arterio-venous fistula can produce shunting as well as subclavian steal in patients with a previous left internal mammary artery graft.

# Acute Myocardial Infarction

15

***Anthony A. Bavry    A. Michael Lincoff***

## INTRODUCTION AND EPIDEMIOLOGY OF ST-ELEVATION MYOCARDIAL INFARCTION

This chapter focuses on the diagnosis and management of ST-elevation myocardial infarction (STEMI). STEMI represents the most urgent acute coronary syndrome (ACS). This condition mobilizes a health care network with the aim of promptly restoring coronary perfusion in order to improve myocardial salvage and patient survival. This is a distinct clinical entity from unstable angina (UA) and non–ST-elevation myocardial infarction (NSTEMI), which were discussed in the previous chapter. In contrast to UA, which is characterized by ST depressions or T-wave inversions without elevated cardiac biomarkers, and NSTEMI, which is characterized by elevated cardiac biomarkers without ST-segment elevations, STEMI presents with ST elevations in the territory of the infarcted myocardium.

Acute myocardial infarction or angina is the usual initial presentation for coronary disease, although about 20% of individuals with a coronary event do not even present to the hospital. For these individuals, sudden cardiac death is their initial manifestation of coronary disease. Unless defibrillation occurs within minutes, death ensues quickly. Fortunately, automated external defibrillators have become more available and are now found in many public places.

More than half a million hospital presentations per year are attributable to STEMI. This condition is responsible for higher in-hospital mortality than UA or NSTEMI. Whereas the early management decision in UA/NSTEMI is deciding whether a patient should be directed to an early invasive approach versus conservative management, in STEMI the focus is on rapid pharmacologic or mechanical reperfusion.

Issues such as risk stratification, fibrinolysis, primary percutaneous coronary intervention (PCI), adjunctive medical therapy, and discharge planning are discussed in the following text. A controversial issue is whether patients with suspected acute myocardial infarction should be directed to the nearest hospital or to a facility with cardiac catheterization and surgical capabilities. Important patient characteristics and logistical considerations will be reviewed that may favor one approach over another. This chapter follows the American College of Cardiology/American Heart Association (ACC/AHA) guidelines.

## CLINICAL PRESENTATION

STEMI typically presents with substernal chest discomfort that is described as a pressure or heavy sensation that lasts more than 30 minutes. Symptoms are often described as "vicelike" or "an elephant sitting on my chest." Patients may display the Levine sign by clutching their fist over their chest. STEMI is often accompanied by dyspnea, nausea, vomiting, and diaphoresis. Atypical symptoms are more common in diabetics, women, and the elderly (similar to UA/NSTEMI patients). There is a small subset (approximately 20%) of patients who have myocardial infarctions in the absence of symptoms.

## DIAGNOSIS

The *sine qua non* for the diagnosis of STEMI is recognizing ST elevations in a typical coronary distribution or a new left bundle branch block in the setting of typical (or atypical) symptoms. Waiting for cardiac biomarkers to return before

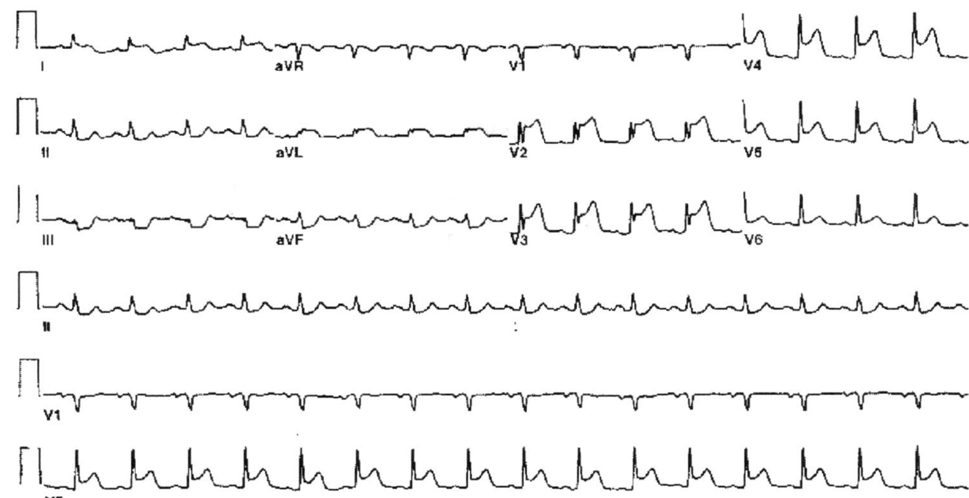


**Figure 15–1** Anterior ST-elevation acute myocardial infarction. There is also ST elevation in leads I and aVL, suggesting a left anterior descending artery occlusion proximal to a major diagonal branch.

making a diagnosis of acute myocardial infarction and initiating emergency therapy is inappropriate (class III recommendation). A brief phase before ST-elevations appear is often unrecognized. This phase is characterized by hyperacute T waves in the infarct related territory. The hyperacute electrocardiogram (ECG) findings rapidly progress to typical ST elevations. ST elevations are usually convex or "tombstone" in appearance, although they can be concave. STEMI is diagnosed when at least 1-mm ST elevations are recognized in two or more contiguous leads. Figures 15–1 through 15–4 show various ECG examples of STEMI.

The ECG can also help to localize the location of the coronary occlusion. For example, high lateral (i.e., I and aVL) ST elevations that accompany an anterior myocardial infarction indicate a left anterior descending artery occlusion proximal to a major diagonal branch. An anterior STEMI with ST segment elevation in lead V1 and QRS complex prolongation indicates a left anterior descending artery occlusion proximal to a major septal perforator. ST elevations resolve later (hours to days) in the course of an acute myocardial infarction, at which time the T waves become inverted. Most ST-elevation myocardial infarctions (70% to 80%) eventually progress into Q waves in the region of the infarcted myocardium.

Although the ECG is absolutely essential for the diagnosis of STEMI, there are other conditions that cause ST-elevations and must be simultaneously screened and evaluated. These include acute pericarditis, hyperkalemia, left ventricular hypertrophy, early repolarization, and ventricular aneurysm (Table 15–1).

A posterior myocardial infarction is an important STEMI equivalent. This is often seen in the setting of an inferior or inferolateral myocardial infarction. The ECG findings

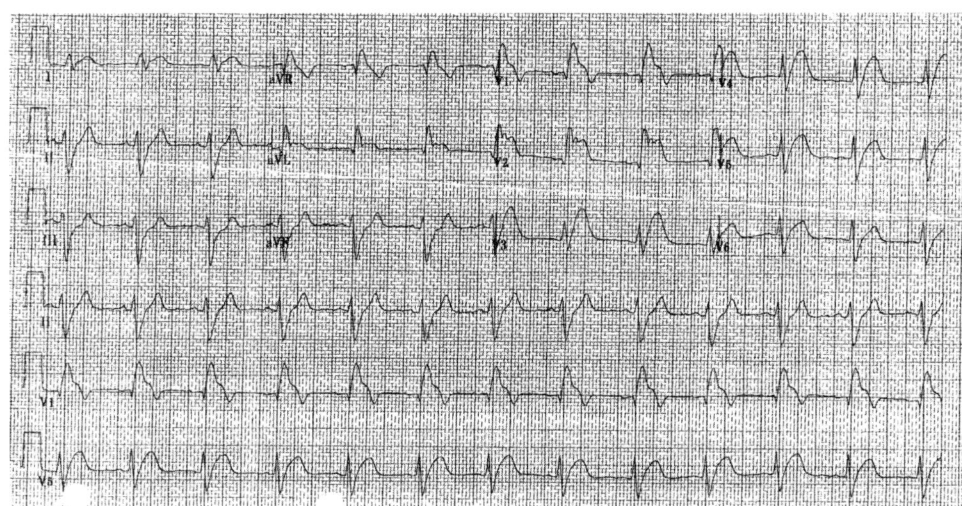

**Figure 15–2** Anterior ST-elevation acute myocardial infarction. In addition to ST elevation in leads I and aVL, there is also QRS prolongation, suggesting a left anterior descending artery occlusion proximal to a major diagonal branch and a major septal perforator.

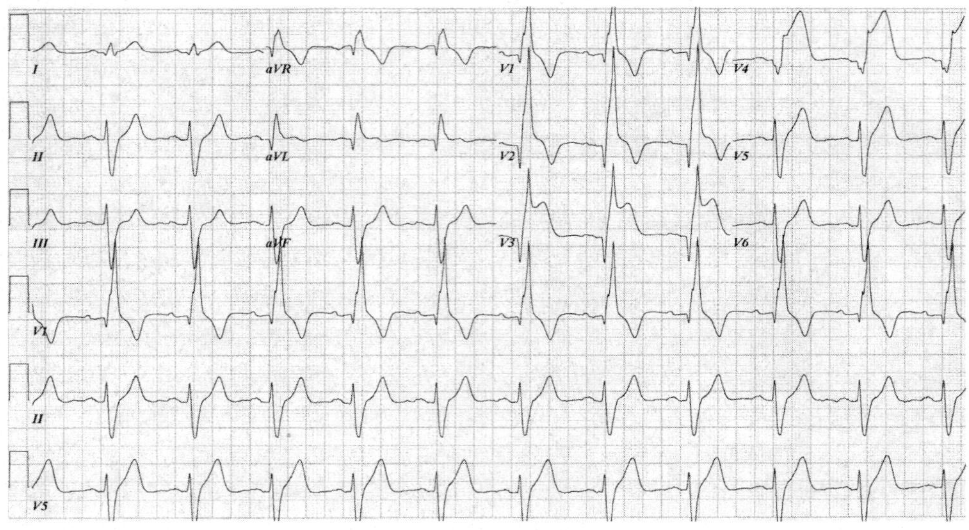


**Figure 15–3** Anterior ST-elevation acute myocardial infarction in the setting of a pre-existing RBBB. ST elevation is noted in leads V3–V6.

are a tall R wave in V1 with ST depressions in V1–V2. It is critical to recognize an isolated posterior infarction as a STEMI, because patient prognosis hinges on the prompt restoration of coronary flow.

The other STEMI equivalent to consider is a new or presumably new complete left bundle branch block (LBBB). Not surprisingly, patients who present with a complete LBBB have high in-hospital mortality rates (up to 25%), in part due to the fact that they are nearly 80% less likely to receive reperfusion therapy than patients who present with recognizable ST elevations. However, even with reperfusion therapy, mortality rates are higher in patients with new complete LBBB than with ST elevation, attesting to the high-risk nature of this population. Although ischemic changes are interpretable in the context of a right bundle branch block (RBBB), this task becomes more difficult with a complete LBBB. There are criteria that can help diagnose a LBBB as an acute myocardial infarction with good specificity (Table 15–2), which look at the degree of ST elevation or depression and the concordance or discordance of the ST segment with the QRS.

## RISK STRATIFICATION

### Killip Class and TIMI Risk Score

Since all patients with STEMI are initially eligible for reperfusion therapy, risk models are used primarily to determine prognosis and not to direct therapy as in UA/NSTEMI risk models. Initial information for risk stratification comes from the physical exam. Assessing for signs of heart failure is a useful tool for risk stratification. Patients who present with cardiogenic shock have a 30-day mortality rate of approximately 60% (Table 15–3). Cardiac biomarkers

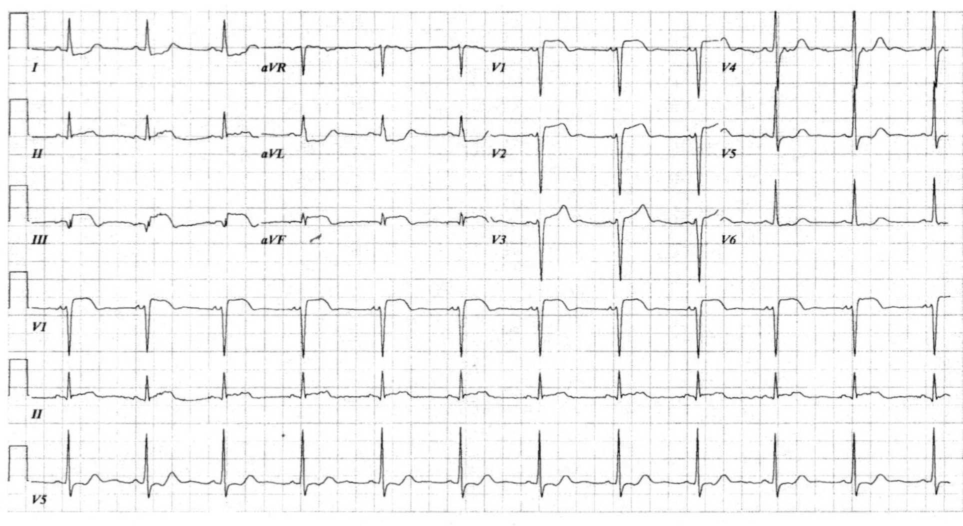


**Figure 15–4** Inferior ST-elevation acute myocardial infarction. There is also ST elevation in leads V1–V3, suggesting right ventricular (RV) involvement. RV leads should also be done to confirm RV involvement (i.e., occlusion proximal to acute marginal branch).

**TABLE 15–1**
**DIFFERENTIAL FOR ST-SEGMENT ELEVATION**

| Condition | Features |
|---|---|
| Male pattern | 90% of healthy young men, most pronounced in V2 |
| Early repolarization | J point notching most pronounced in V4, upright T |
| LVH | Concave, other criteria for left ventricular hypertrophy |
| LBBB | Concave |
| Acute pericarditis | Diffuse ST↑, ST↓ Avr and PR↓ |
| Hyperkalemia | Wide QRS, peaked T, low-amplitude P, down-sloping ST |
| Brugada syndrome | rSR′ in V1 and V2, down-sloping ST↑ in V1 and V2 |
| Pulmonary embolism | Can simulate inferior and anteroseptal AMI |
| Cardioversion | Pronounced transient ST↑ after DCC |

*Source:* From Wang K, Asinger RW, Marriott HJ. ST-segment elevation in conditions other than acute myocardial infarction. *N Engl J Med.* 2003;349:2128–2135.

(troponin I or T and total CK and CK-MB isoenzyme) supplement the physical exam by gauging infarct size and providing additional prognostic information.

Risk models have been created that provide a more accurate prediction of risk. These models combine multiple variables that are most predictive for future adverse cardiac outcomes. The TIMI risk score is an easily used and validated model that has important prognostic implications. It incorporates eight variables that are readily available from the history, physical exam, ECG, and cardiac biomarkers (Fig. 15–5). The presence of more than eight risk factors predicts an approximately 35% incidence of death at 30 days. This is in contrast to zero or one risk factor, for which the 30-day mortality rate is less than 2%. The strongest variable that predicts an adverse prognosis is advanced age (where age ≥75 years receives 3 points and age 65 to 74 years receives 2 points). Other variables include hypotension, tachycardia, or Killip class II–IV at presentation, history of diabetes or hypertension, low body weight, anterior ST elevation (also complete LBBB), and a time to treatment of >4 hours.

**TABLE 15–2**
**ECG CRITERIA FOR THE PRESENCE OF AMI IN THE SETTING OF LBBB**

| Criterion | Score |
|---|---|
| ST elevation ≥1 mm, concordant with QRS | 5 |
| ST depression ≥1 mm, in lead V1, V2, or V3 | 3 |
| ST elevation ≥5 mm, discordant with QRS | 2 |

*Source:* From Sgarbossa EB, Pinski SL, Barbagelata A, et al. Electrocardiographic diagnosis of evolving acute myocardial infarction in the presence of left bundle-branch block. GUSTO-1 (Global Utilization of Streptokinase and Tissue Plasminogen Activator for Occluded Coronary Arteries) Investigators. *N Engl J Med.* 1996;334:481–487.

**TABLE 15–3**
**KILLIP CLASS—30-DAY MORTALITY**

| Killip Class | Characteristics | Patients (%) | Mortality (%) |
|---|---|---|---|
| I | No evidence for CHF | 85 | 5 |
| II | Rales, ↑ JVD, S3 | 13 | 14 |
| III | Pulmonary edema | 1 | 32 |
| IV | Cardiogenic shock | 1 | 58 |

*Source:* From Lee KL, Woodlief LH, Topol EJ, et al. Predictors of 30-day mortality in the era of reperfusion for acute myocardial infarction. Results from an international trial of 41,021 patients. GUSTO-I Investigators. *Circulation.* 1995;91:1659–1668.

## MANAGEMENT

### Initial Approach

The initial assessment of a patient suspected of having an acute myocardial infarction is to establish intravenous access and start supplemental oxygen for individuals who are hypoxic or who show signs or respiratory distress. Simultaneously, a targeted history and physical exam should be obtained. The history and physical exam provide prognostic information, but also can suggest an alternative diagnosis and help identify mechanical complications of STEMI. An important alternative diagnosis to screen for in any patient with a chest pain syndrome is aortic dissection.

If fibrinolysis is considered, the history and physical exam should screen for contraindications to its use. Because the most feared complication with the use of fibrinolytics is intracranial hemorrhage, patients with an increased risk for this complication must be identified. Risk factors for intracranial hemorrhage are advanced age, female gender, uncontrolled hypertension, and low body weight. Patients with coagulopathies (e.g., patients on Coumadin therapy) are also at increased risk for bleeding. Absolute contraindications to fibrinolytics include previous hemorrhagic stroke, known intracranial neoplasm, active bleeding, or suspected aortic dissection. Relative contraindications include severe hypertension (any reliable measurement of blood pressure >180/110 mm Hg during the current hospitalization), use of anticoagulation, recent head trauma or other serious trauma, recent internal bleeding, or pregnancy.

### Reperfusion Therapy

Time is of paramount importance in reinstituting coronary flow. The greatest improvement on mortality comes from

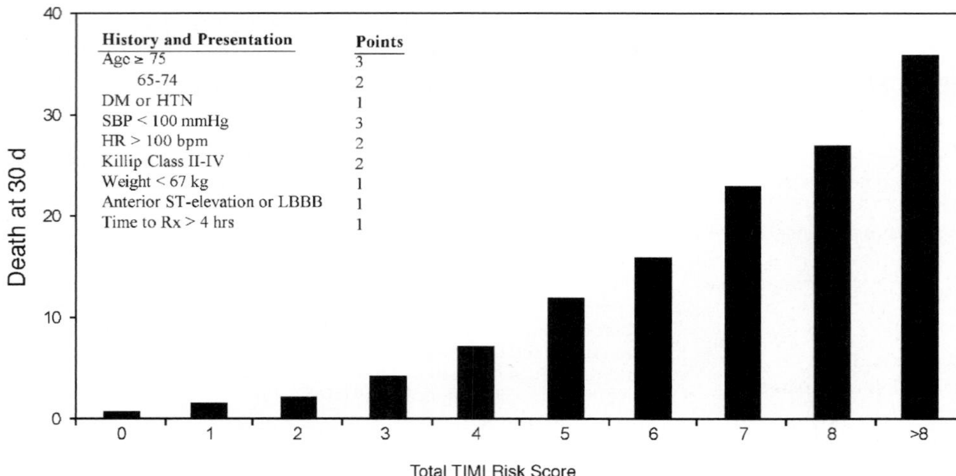


**Figure 15–5** TIMI risk model for prediction of short term mortality in STEMI patients. (From Morrow DA, Antman EM, Charlesworth A, et al. TIMI risk score for ST-elevation myocardial infarction: a convenient, bedside, clinical score for risk assessment at presentation: an intravenous nPA for treatment of infarcting myocardium early II trial substudy. *Circulation.* 2000;102: 2031–2037.)

reperfusion within the first hour, the so-called "golden hour." Reperfusion therapy can be considered up to 12 hours from the onset of chest pain and even longer in select cases. In order to facilitate rapid coronary reperfusion, a pharmacologic or mechanical approach should be decided on quickly. The current goal for door-to-lytic time is 30 minutes, whereas the goal for door-to-balloon time is 90 minutes.

In general, if primary PCI can be performed immediately (i.e., the patient presents to a center capable of performing PCI), this is the preferred choice for reperfusion. This information comes from a meta-analysis of 23 trials that randomized nearly 8,000 STEMI patients to fibrinolytic therapy versus primary PCI. The hospitals included in the analysis were largely experienced providers of coronary intervention and were able to deliver mechanical reperfusion in a timely fashion, although some studies enrolled patients who were transferred for primary PCI versus given immediate fibrinolysis. This study was a contemporary analysis, as stents were used in 12 of the trials and glycoprotein (GP) IIb/IIIa inhibitors were used in eight. General inclusion criteria required that patients have ischemic symptoms within the previous 6 to 12 hours and at least 1-mm ST elevations in contiguous leads or a new/presumable new complete LBBB. Patients also needed to be candidates for fibrinolysis to be eligible for enrollment. A notable exception was the SHOCK trial, as this study enrolled patients in cardiogenic shock and chest pain within the preceding 36 hours. Since the SHOCK trial was the outlier to the overall analysis, the analysis was performed with and without this study. Most patients (76%) received fibrin-specific (i.e., t-PA) lytic agents, whereas the remainder received streptokinase. This analysis revealed a short-term survival advantage as well as a reduction in recurrent myocardial infarction and hemorrhagic stroke in those who received primary PCI. Short-term mortality was 7% in the primary PCI group, compared to 9% in the fibrinolytic group ($p = 0.0002$). Long-term mortality was also significantly reduced ($p = 0.0019$). Thus, among patients who present within 12 hours of the onset of chest pain to a tertiary care center that is capable of performing primary PCI expeditiously, the data support the use of mechanical reperfusion.

In reality, though, only a minority of acute myocardial infarction patients present to a center that is capable of performing coronary intervention. Most individuals present to a community hospital, at which time the question becomes whether to transfer the patient to a primary PCI center or to administer immediate fibrinolysis.

Fibrinolysis is limited by postlysis TIMI 3 flow of less than 50% at 90 minutes which results in recurrent ischemia and reinfarction. There is also a definite risk for intracranial hemorrhage (up to 0.9% in many trials and even greater in high-risk patients). There are also numerous contraindications to consider. These limitations have led to trials that specifically addressed if delaying immediate reperfusion to allow transfer for primary PCI may be beneficial.

A subanalysis from the previously mentioned meta-analysis examined the studies that transferred patients for primary PCI versus giving immediate fibrinolytics. The mean time that was required for transfer to a primary PCI center was 39 minutes. Mortality was similar between the two groups ($p = 0.057$), although a composite outcome that included death, reinfarction, or stroke was reduced by transfer for primary PCI ($p < 0.001$).

Another meta-analysis specifically addressed this issue using available clinical trial information. This study examined only trials that randomized patients to immediate fibrinolysis or transfer to a center capable of performing primary PCI. The inclusion criteria were similar to the previous study: acute ST-elevation myocardial infarction within 6 to 12 hours from the onset of chest pain and eligibility to receive a fibrinolytic agent. Six trials were available for analysis, involving nearly 4,000 patients. The following individual trials deserve special comment. The AIR-PAMI study randomized patients who were high risk to one of these reperfusion strategies. High risk was defined as age

>70 years of age, heart rate >100 beats/min, systolic blood pressure <100 mm Hg, Killip class II/III, complete LBBB, or anterior myocardial infarction. This was the smallest study that was included in the analysis, although there was no noticeable harm in transferring patients for PCI. The CAPTIM trial was unique in that patients were randomized before arrival to the hospital, which enabled fibrinolytics to be given in an even more timely fashion. This was the only trial that showed a nonsignificant trend in mortality favoring fibrinolysis. The PRAGUE-2 trial examined the effect of time from the onset of chest pain on transferring a patient for PCI. The study was stopped prematurely, as mortality was increased 2.5-fold among patients who presented more than 3 hours from the onset of chest pain who received fibrinolysis. Patients who presented within 3 hours from the onset of chest pain had similar mortality (7.4% with fibrinolysis and 7.3% with primary PCI), in contrast to increased mortality for patients who presented from 3 to 12 hours from the onset of chest pain (15% with fibrinolysis and 6% with primary PCI, $p < 0.02$).

So, while transferring a STEMI patient for primary PCI versus immediately administering fibrinolysis is controversial, some patient characteristics and logistical considerations favor one approach over another. Fibrinolytics are more successful if administered early after the onset of chest pain. Accordingly, this strategy may be preferred over PCI in patients who present within 3 hours of chest pain and who are at low risk of bleeding, especially if a catheterization laboratory capable of performing PCI is not available by transfer in a timely fashion (i.e., transport time more than 2 hours). Conversely, for patients who are at high risk for bleeding or who present more than 3 hours after the onset of chest pain, transfer for primary PCI may be favored. Additionally, patients who are in cardiogenic shock benefit from mechanical revascularization, but have not been shown to have a mortality reduction with fibrinolysis. Lastly, if there are contraindications to fibrinolytics or the diagnosis of STEMI is in doubt, PCI should be considered.

## Fibrinolytic Therapy

A large body of research involving tens of thousands of patients documented the benefit of fibrinolytic therapy in reducing infarct size, preserving left ventricular function, and improving survival in acute myocardial infarction patients. For every 1,000 patients treated with fibrinolytics within 1 hour of onset of symptoms, the number of lives saved is 26, while treatment within 3 to 6 hours from the onset of chest pain saves 18 lives. There is still a survival advantage from 6 to 12 hours, although it is smaller in magnitude than giving lytics closer to the onset of chest pain. Accordingly, fibrinolysis is indicated for 1 mm or more of ST elevations in contiguous leads, or a new complete LBBB within 12 hours from the onset of chest pain. Patients with stuttering infarcts may benefit from lytics up to 24 hours after the onset of chest pain. Asymptomatic patients more than 24 hours out from the onset of chest pain should not receive lytic therapy (class III recommendation). Patients who undergo lysis and continue to have recurrent ischemia, persistent ST elevation, or labile hemodynamics should be referred for rescue PCI.

If lytic therapy is selected, it is important to know about the different agents used for fibrinolysis and which are available at a given institution. Additionally, contraindications to the use of fibrinolytics should be reviewed in every eligible patient. The choice of one agent over another is made according to hospital availability and physician experience with a given agent.

The following discussion explores the four commercially available fibrinolytic agents. All the lytic agents are similar in terms of 3-hour patency, although 90-minute patency rates may differ.

Streptokinase was the first-generation fibrinolytic agent. It is capable of lysing circulating and clot-bound fibrin. Allergic reactions are common, and re-exposure to streptokinase should be avoided. This is the least expensive lytic agent, at around $500 per dose. Streptokinase may not require adjunctive heparin therapy unless the patient is at high risk for emboli (i.e., atrial fibrillation or known left ventricular thrombus). Accordingly, lysis with streptokinase is associated with a slightly less intracranial hemorrhage risk (0.5% compared to 0.7% for fibrin-specific agents). This property makes streptokinase attractive if an individual is not a candidate for PCI, and is at high risk for bleeding. An example would be a small elderly hypertensive female who refuses or is not a candidate for PCI.

Fibrin-specific agents activate plasminogen directly and are relatively selective against clot-bound fibrin rather than circulating fibrinogen. Allergic reactions do not occur with these agents, as can occur with streptokinase. Fibrin-specific agents include alteplase (tPA), reteplase (rPA), and tenecteplase (TNK-tPA). Because these fibrin-specific agents do not produce a systemically lytic state and because they activate platelets, the use of heparin therapy appears to improve and maintain vessel patency.

The GUSTO-1 trial was a landmark study published in 1993 that compared streptokinase to various fibrin-specific strategies. Up until this trial there was no known advantage of one agent over another. This trial studied >40,000 patients with acute myocardial infarction and revealed the superiority of accelerated tPA over streptokinase. Accelerated tPA with intravenous heparin resulted in a 14% reduction in mortality and higher rates of TIMI 3 flow at 90 minutes (54% versus 31%) compared to streptokinase-based regimens. The accelerated tPA dose is a 15-mg bolus, then 0.75 mg/kg (up to 50 mg) over 30 minutes, followed by 0.5 mg/kg over 60 minutes (up to 35 mg).

Reteplase is less fibrin-specific than alteplase. This agent is equivalent to alteplase in terms of efficacy, although it is easier to administer (two 10-mg boluses administered 30 minutes apart). Tenecteplase is the easiest lytic to administer, because it is given as a single bolus (dose ranges from

**TABLE 15–4**
**WEIGHT-BASED DOSING OF TENECTAPLASE**

| Weight | Dose |
|---|---|
| <60 kg | 30 mg |
| 60 to 69 kg | 35 mg |
| 70 to 79 kg | 40 mg |
| 80 to 89 kg | 45 mg |
| ≥90 kg | 50 mg |

*Source:* From Antman EM, Anbe DT, Armstrong PW, et al. ACC/AHA guidelines for the management of patients with ST-elevation myocardial infarction—executive summary. A report of the American College of Cardiology/American Heart Association Task Force on Practice Guidelines (Writing Committee to revise the 1999 guidelines for the management of patients with acute myocardial infarction). *J Am Coll Cardiol.* 2004;44:671–719.

30 to 50 mg, adjusted for body weight). See Table 15–4 for dosing. This agent is more fibrin-specific and has a slower plasma clearance than the other fibrin-specific agents. The ASSENT 2 trials showed the noninferiority of tenecteplase compared to alteplase. In this trial, there was also less major bleeding with tenecteplase, and a trend toward less intracranial hemorrhage in elderly women. Equivalent efficacy, enhanced safety, and ease of administration make tenecteplase an attractive fibrinolytic agent.

## Percutaneous Coronary Intervention

When PCI is selected for reperfusion, eligibility criteria are the same as those used for fibrinolytics: 1 mm or more of ST elevations in contiguous leads or a new/presumably new complete LBBB within 12 hours of the onset of chest pain. A posterior myocardial infarction should be treated as a STEMI equivalent. The goal of PCI is to achieve revascularization of the infarct related artery. Multivessel revascularization at the time of primary PCI is usually not indicated (class III recommendation), except in patients with cardiogenic shock.

Several approaches to PCI exist in the setting of STEMI. Most data support the use of primary PCI. In primary PCI, fibrinolytics are not given prior to intervention. Patients either present directly to a PCI center, or they are transferred (without fibrinolysis) from a community hospital to a center capable of performing PCI. As mentioned previously, the downside in transferring a patient for primary PCI is the delay in time that is required until mechanical reperfusion can occur.

In contrast to primary PCI, facilitated or rescue PCI combines lysis with PCI. In facilitated PCI, patients are routinely transferred for PCI after lysis, a strategy that has intuitive appeal but has not yet been shown to improve clinical outcome in randomized trials. In the approach of rescue PCI, patients undergo PCI only for persistent ST elevation, recurrent ischemia, or hemodynamic instability. The REACT trial enrolled patients who had persistent STelevation 90 minutes after lysis. Eligible patients were randomized to repeat lysis, conservative management, or rescue PCI. At 6 months a composite endpoint of death, myocardial infarction, stroke, or heart failure was reduced by rescue PCI (30% conservative management versus 15% rescue PCI, $p = 0.002$). The role of late or delayed PCI more than 12 to 24 hours after the initial event is not clear, but some evidence supports the open-artery hypothesis. This approach may be selected if a large area of viable myocardium in the territory of the infarct-related artery exists.

Historically, STEMI patients who were selected for mechanical reperfusion underwent percutaneous transluminal coronary angioplasty (PTCA). With the advent of intracoronary stents, randomized trials were designed to determine if PCI using intracoronary stents would improve outcomes. A meta-analysis that involved nearly 3,000 patients with STEMI who were randomized to PTCA versus PCI with intracoronary stents revealed an advantage to the use of stents. This analysis documented a reduction in the composite endpoint of death, myocardial infarction, or target vessel revascularization at 6 months by the use of stents (14% versus 26%, $p < 0.0001$), a difference that was driven by a reduction in the need for target vessel revascularization. The largest trial in this analysis was the CADILLAC trial. This study showed no reduction in death or myocardial infarction from the use of stents, although there was less clinical and angiographic restenosis at follow-up. Drug-eluting stents dramatically reduce restenosis, although they have not been fully evaluated in acute myocardial infarction trials.

With the success of intracoronary stents and adjunctive GP IIb/IIIa inhibitors, PCI is usually successful in achieving TIMI 3 flow in the infarct-related artery. Coronary artery bypass grafting is still indicated for left main disease, failed PCI, or mechanical complications of infarction (e.g., myocardial rupture). Additionally, patients with three-vessel disease (or two-vessel disease that includes the proximal left anterior descending artery) in the setting of left ventricular dysfunction or diabetes may have a better clinical outcome with surgery, although logistic difficulties in performing bypass grafting within a rapid time frame may favor initial reperfusion by percutaneous techniques followed by later elective surgical revascularization.

## Antiplatelet Agents

### *Aspirin and Thienopyridines*

Just as aspirin is the cornerstone of treatment for all UA/NSTEMI patients, it is also a class I recommendation for STEMI patients (see Fig. 15–4). Aspirin is associated with a mortality benefit similar to that achieved by streptokinase. Unless there is a serious contraindication to its use, full-dose aspirin should be given to all STEMI patients. If there is any question as to whether the patient received aspirin prior to arrival in the emergency department, another dose should be given. If the patient is vomiting, aspirin can be given by rectal suppository if necessary (at the same dose). An 81-mg aspirin daily is sufficient for ongoing therapy.

When significant hypersensitivity to aspirin exists, clopidogrel should be given in its place. An important caveat with clopidogrel is that it increases the risk for major bleeding during surgery, and so it should be withheld for at least 5 days before cardiac surgery is performed. If there is any suspicion of an early mechanical complication requiring the need for open-heart surgery, clopidogrel should be withheld. Similarly, coronary angiography may define coronary disease that requires CABG. For this reason, clopidogrel is usually withheld until coronary anatomy is defined and the decision is made to perform PCI using stents. In STEMI patients who undergo lysis, the recent CLARITY trial revealed a reduction in the composite endpoint of occluded infarct-related artery, death, or recurrent myocardial infarction before angiography by the addition of clopidogrel to aspirin, heparin, and standard medical therapy. The COMMIT trial randomized nearly 46,000 STEMI patients to clopidogrel or placebo in addition to standard medical therapy that included aspirin. This trial had sufficient power to detect a survival advantage from the use of clopidogrel. Rates of bleeding were similar in the two trials. Therefore, if STEMI patients will be managed by fibrinolysis, the addition of clopidogrel to standard therapy that includes aspirin and heparin should be considered.

### *GP IIb/IIIa Inhibitors*

The role of a GP IIb/IIIa inhibitor with full or half-dose lytics remains investigational. In contrast, there is much more experience with GP IIb/IIIa inhibition during PCI. An analysis that included ADMIRAL, CADILLAC, ISAR-2, and the RAPPORT trials revealed a reduction in rates of the composite endpoint of death, recurrent myocardial infarction, or target revascularization by 6 months with the adjunctive use of abciximab during PCI compared to placebo (OR = 80, 95% CI 0.67 to 0.97). The dose of abciximab is a 0.25-mg/kg intravenous bolus, followed by an infusion of 0.125 mg/kg for 12 hours. Most experience with GP IIb/IIIa inhibitors during PCI in the setting of acute myocardial infarction is with abciximab. Accordingly, the use of abciximab during PCI is a class IIa recommendation, while the use of eptifibatide or tirofiban is a class IIb recommendation.

## Antithrombotic Agents

Most STEMI patients should receive heparin therapy, although the dose will vary depending on the reperfusion strategy selected. The dose of unfractionated heparin is 60 U/kg as a bolus (maximum 5,000 U), followed by 12-U/kg/h infusion (maximum 1,000 U/h) to achieve a pTT of 45 to 65 seconds in patients undergoing fibrinolysis or patients undergoing PCI with an adjunctive GP IIb/IIIa inhibitor. The goal of intraprocedural ACT in this case is 200 to 250 seconds. For patients undergoing PCI without adjunctive GP IIb/IIIa inhibitor, the dose of unfractionated heparin is 80 U/kg as a bolus, followed by 18-U/kg/h infusion to achieve a pTT of 50 to 75 seconds and an ACT of 300 to 350 seconds during the PCI. In general, heparin should not be continued after PCI, because there is increased risk for major bleeding and no incremental benefit. Exceptions to this rule include patients at high risk for systemic emboli, such as with large anterior infarction/left ventricular thrombus and atrial fibrillation. Deep venous thrombosis should be prevented during periods of immobilization by unfractionated heparin, 5,000 to 7,000 U, twice to three times per day when therapeutic doses of heparin are not being used.

Low-molecular-weight heparin may be considered as an alternative to unfractionated heparin in patients undergoing fibrinolysis (class IIb recommendation). The ASSENT-3 trial tested various antithrombotic regimens with weight-based tenecteplase. Low-molecular-weight heparin was represented by enoxaparin initiated by 30-mg intravenous bolus, followed by 1.0 mg/kg subcutaneously every 12 hours up to discharge or revascularization, for a maximum of 7 days. Tenecteplase plus enoxaparin reduced a composite endpoint of death, in-hospital reinfarction, or in-hospital refractory ischemia compared to unfractionated heparin. For patients who are >75 years old or who have renal insufficiency (creatinine >2.5 mg/dL for men and >2.0 mg/dL for women) the use of a low-molecular-weight heparin is not recommended (class III).

Direct thrombin inhibitors (DTI) are considered an alternative to heparin-based regimens if there is an allergy to heparin (i.e., heparin-induced thrombocytopenia). The DTI used in the HERO-2 trial was bivalirudin. In this trial, 17,073 STEMI patients were randomized to streptokinase and bivalirudin or streptokinase and unfractionated heparin. The primary endpoint of mortality was not reduced by bivalirudin, although reinfarction was reduced by 30% within 96 hours. There was a small increase in mild to moderate bleeding with bivalirudin. If this agent is selected, the dose is 0.25 mg/kg bolus, followed by 0.5 mg/kg/h for 12 hours and 0.25 mg/kg/h for 36 hours with a pTT not to exceed 75 seconds. There is no recommendation for a DTI over unfractionated heparin in the setting of lysis, although bivalirudin or enoxaparin are considered acceptable alternatives.

## Anti-ischemic Agents

Nitroglycerin and beta-blockers are first-line anti-ischemic agents (class I recommendation). Nitroglycerin is initiated by a 0.4-mg sublingual tablet (repeated several times every 5 minutes if symptoms persist and hypotension does not develop), followed by intravenous infusion of 10 to 20 $\mu$g/min (titrated up until resolution of symptoms or until hypotension develops). An intravenous dose of 200 $\mu$g/min is considered a ceiling, although the dose is occasionally increased to 400 μg/min if needed. Notably, large-scale randomized trials have failed to observe any reduction in mortality with nitroglycerin, and indications for this agent in the setting of STEMI are thus to relieve ischemia, hypertension, or congestive heart failure. Sildenafil use within 24 hours of presentation is a class III recommendation against the use of nitroglycerin.

Beta-blockers are administered along with nitroglycerin and help to blunt the reflex tachycardia that may occur from their use. A large body of evidence supports the use of beta-blockers (class I recommendation). A pooled analysis from the prefibrinolytic era in >24,000 patients (dominated by the ISIS-1 trial) documented a 14% reduction in 7-day mortality (23% long-term reduction) among patients who received beta-blockade. Interestingly, in the reperfusion era, only the CAPRICORN trial with carvedilol has shown a mortality reduction with a beta-blocker. Other trials in the reperfusion era have only shown reduced reinfarction or recurrent ischemia.

Beta-blockade is initiated intravenously (i.e., 5 mg metoprolol intravenously, repeated several times every 5 minutes), followed by oral administration (i.e., 25 mg metoprolol orally twice to three times per day and titrated up). Contraindications to beta-blockers include significant conduction abnormalities (marked first-degree AV block, or second/third-degree block), asthma, or decompensated heart failure. If beta-blockers are used at maximal dose or there are contraindications to their use, a nondihydropyridine (i.e., diltiazem or verapamil) may be considered to control symptoms. Morphine (1 to 5 mg intravenously) is also considered a class I anti-ischemic medication and is particularly helpful for anxious patients.

## Miscellaneous Agents

### *Angiotensin-Converting Enzyme Inhibitors*

Angiotensin-converting enzyme inhibitors (ACE-I) are indicated in all STEMI patients (class IIa recommendation) as soon as patients are felt to be hemodynamically stable. For this reason, an oral ACE-I is usually not used sooner than 6 hours into the hospital course. The presence of an anterior infarction, left ventricular dysfunction (ejection fraction <40%), or diabetes strengthens the use of an ACE-I to a class I recommendation. Intravenous ACE-I should not be used within 24 hours (class III recommendation). Patients with a class I recommendation for an ACE-I should continue it indefinitely, in contrast to all others, for whom 4 to 6 weeks may be appropriate. For patients who are intolerant of an ACE-I, an angiotensin-receptor blocker should be considered unless there is history of angioedema.

### *Vasopressors, Inotropes, and Anti-arrhythmics*

Inotropic or vasopressor agents (i.e., dopamine, dobutamine, norepinephrine) are not used routinely except for cardiogenic shock that does not respond to an intra-aortic balloon pump (IABP). Dobutamine may also be used for right ventricular infarction that does not respond to intravenous fluids. Anti-arrhythmics are indicated for significant arrhythmias. Amiodarone, lidocaine, and procainamide are used for ventricular arrhythmias. For ventricular fibrillation or pulseless ventricular tachycardia, the dose of amiodarone is a 300-mg intravenous bolus, repeated in 150-mg boluses up to 2.1 g in a 24-hour period. For unstable ventricular tachycardia the dose is a 150-mg intravenous bolus, then 1 mg/min for 6 hours, then 0.5 mg/min until oral amiodarone is started. The dose of lidocaine varies depending on left ventricular function (Table 15–5). Procainamide is an alternative to amiodarone and lidocaine for ventricular fibrillation/ventricular tachycardia. The dose of procainamide is 20 mg/min intravenously until the arrhythmia is suppressed, hypotension develops, or the QRS widens by 50%. Atropine (0.5 to 1 mg intravenously every 5 minutes to a total of 3 mg) is used for bradyarrhythmias and magnesium for torsades de pointes (1 to 2 g intravenous).

**TABLE 15–5**
**LEFT VENTRICULAR-BASED DOSING OF LICOCAINE**

| Left Ventricular Function | Dose |
|---|---|
| Normal function | 75-mg IV bolus, then 50 mg IV q5 min × 3 (total 225 mg), then 2 mg/min |
| Moderate dysfunction | 75-mg IV bolus, then 50 mg IV q5 min × 1 (total 125 mg), then 1 mg/min |
| Severe dysfunction | 50- to 75-mg IV bolus, then 0.5 mg/min |

*Source:* From Antman EM, Anbe DT, Armstrong PW, et al. ACC/AHA guidelines for the management of patients with ST-elevation myocardial infarction—executive summary. A report of the American College of Cardiology/American Heart Association Task Force on Practice Guidelines (Writing Committee to revise the 1999 guidelines for the management of patients with acute myocardial infarction). *J Am Coll Cardiol.* 2004;44:671–719.

### *Miscellaneous*

As with UA/NSTEMI patients, HMG-CoA reductase inhibitors (statins) should be considered for all STEMI patients regardless of their presenting lipid profile. Gemfibrozil, niacin, and fish oil should be considered for patients with a low HDL. Based on clinical trial data, atorvastatin has been studied most extensively at a dose of 80 mg daily. Magnesium is not routinely indicated in STEMI patients unless there is hypomagnesemia or torsades de pointes.

## Mechanical Devices

### *Intra-aortic Balloon Pump*

The use of an intra-aortic balloon pump (IABP) is recommended for patients in cardiogenic shock. A pulmonary artery catheter should be used during the management of cardiogenic shock. Shock can result from early pump failure that may respond to multivessel revascularization. Hemodynamic instability may remain after revascularization for a period of time. The differential for hemodynamic instability after revascularization includes hypovolemia, anemia, right ventricular infarction, and mechanical complications. Mechanical complications to consider in every acute myocardial infarction patient with hemodynamic instability/cardiogenic shock include papillary muscle dysfunction/rupture, ventricular septal defect, and myocardial free wall rupture with tamponade. Electrical complications may occur during the course of the acute myocardial infarction, either before or after reperfusion, and an IABP may be considered for unstable ventricular arrhythmias. Moreover, an IABP is indicated for patients with recurrent myocardial ischemia that is refractory to pharmacologic therapy until revascularization may be performed. Therefore the IABP is used for stabilization until revascularization, as a bridge to CABG or repair of a mechanical complication, or for continued hemodynamic instability after revascularization.

#### *Temporary Right Ventricular Pacing*

Right ventricular pacing may be indicated in the management of conduction disturbances. Bradyarrhythmias are common in the setting of inferior myocardial infarctions, especially with right ventricular involvement. If such a patient exists who does not respond to chronotropic agents such as dobutamine or dopamine, temporary right ventricular pacing may be needed until electrical and hemodynamic stability returns. Complete heart block can be seen with anterior myocardial infarctions that involve a large septal perforator branch.

### Pericarditis

Acute pericarditis develops in 10% to 15% of acute myocardial infarction patients within 2 to 4 days. Pain that occurs within the first 24 hours of a STEMI is unlikely to be secondary to pericarditis. Pericardial effusion is common, although frank tamponade is infrequent. Unlike ischemic pain, pericarditic pain is more often sharp, worse with deep inspiration and recumbancy. A pericardial friction rub is helpful in making the diagnosis, although it is not always present. The ECG may show diffuse ST elevation with PR depression. The treatment consists of aspirin (650 mg, three to four times per day). Alternatively, 600 to 800 mg of ibuprofen four times per day may be used. Indomethacin is effective, although it should be avoided given its reduction in coronary blood flow and gastrointestinal toxicity. Colchicine, 0.6 mg twice a day, may be added to aspirin or ibuprofen for refractory cases. Steroids should be avoided if possible, because of the concern for increased risk of myocardial rupture.

Dressler's syndrome is the finding of pleuropericarditis 1 to 2 weeks after the infarct. This inflammatory reaction occurs in 1% to 2% of acute myocardial infarction patients. The clinical course is usually benign, although constrictive pericarditis may result. The treatment is generally the same as for acute pericarditis.

## PREDISCHARGE RISK STRATIFICATION

Stress testing is a widely used mechanism for risk stratification after coronary reperfusion. There are several options for postreperfusion stress testing. One approach is a submaximal stress test at 4 to 7 days, followed by symptom-limited stress test at 6 weeks. An alternative approach is to defer the submaximal stress test and perform a symptom-limited stress test in 10 to 14 days. Every patient after an acute myocardial infarction should have an assessment of his or her left ventricular function. Patients with moderate to severe left ventricular dysfunction are at higher risk for adverse events. For these individuals, the use of beta-blockers and ACE-inhibitors is especially important. Additionally, the implantation of an intracardiac defibrillator (ICD) may be indicated, after a period of convalescence from an acute myocardial infarction.

## SUMMARY

STEMI is a distinctly different clinical entity than UA/NSTEMI, with a higher early mortality. Risk models such as the TIMI risk score are used to determine prognosis, not to guide therapy. In STEMI there is a limited window of opportunity (generally less than 12 hours and preferably less than 3 to 6 hours) for revascularization to preserve left ventricular function and improve survival. Primary PCI is preferred over lytic therapy if it can be performed rapidly, and potentially even if there is a delay in transport to a PCI center. Certain patient characteristics and logistical considerations favor one approach over another. Fibrinolysis is a viable option if primary PCI is not available in a timely fashion. Rescue PCI should be undertaken if fibrinolysis was unsuccessful. Failed fibrinolysis is characterized by continued ischemia, hemodynamic instability, or incomplete ST-segment resolution.

All STEMI patients should receive aspirin and an antithrombin agent (the dose of heparin varies depending on the use of adjunctive medicines). Clopidogrel should be given if there is a hypersensitivity to aspirin, and may be beneficial in all patients receiving thrombolysis. GP IIb/IIIa inhibitors (represented by abciximab) are indicated during PCI, although their role during fibrinolysis is less clear. Beta-blockers and nitrates are first-line anti-ischemic agents and should be used judiciously. Calcium channel blockers may be used if the patient has a significant intolerance to beta-blockers. Statins are important across the spectrum of acute coronary syndromes, including STEMI. ACE-inhibitors are indicated when the patient becomes hemodynamically stable (usually not before 6 hours), and are especially useful for anterior myocardial infarctions, in the presence of left ventricular dysfunction, and in diabetics.

Acute myocardial infarction patients should be monitored for the development of mechanical and electrical complications. Mechanical complications are life-threatening conditions that necessitate the use of an IABP and urgent surgical repair. Electrical complications may necessitate the use of anti-arrhythmics and potentially right ventricular pacing for bradyarrhythmias. Once patients are revascularized, they should be risk stratified in order to identify residual ischemia and determine the need for future ICD implantation.

## BIBLIOGRAPHY

**Andersen HR, Nielsen TT, Rasmussen K, et al**. A comparison of coronary angioplasty with fibrinolytic therapy in acute myocardial infarction. *N Engl J Med.* 2003;349:733–742.

**Antman EM, Anbe DT, Armstrong PW, et al**. ACC/AHA guidelines for the management of patients with ST-elevation myocardial infarction—executive summary. A report of the American College of Cardiology/American Heart Association Task Force on Practice Guidelines (Writing Committee to revise the 1999 guidelines for the management of patients with acute myocardial infarction). *J Am Coll Cardiol.* 2004;44:671–719.

**Bonnefoy E, Lapostolle F, Leizorovicz A, et al**. Primary angioplasty versus prehospital fibrinolysis in acute myocardial infarction: a randomised study. *Lancet.* 2002;360:825–829.

**Dalby M, Bouzamondo A, Lechat P, Montalescot G.** Transfer for primary angioplasty versus immediate thrombolysis in acute myocardial infarction: a meta-analysis. *Circulation.* 2003;108:1809–1814.

**Dargie HJ.** Effect of carvedilol on outcome after myocardial infarction in patients with left-ventricular dysfunction: the CAPRICORN randomised trial. *Lancet.* 2001;357:1385–1390.

**ASSENT-3 Investigators.** Efficacy and safety of tenecteplase in combination with enoxaparin, abciximab, or unfractionated heparin: the ASSENT-3 randomised trial in acute myocardial infarction. *Lancet.* 2001;358:605–613.

**Grines CL, Westerhausen DR Jr, Grines LL, et al**. A randomized trial of transfer for primary angioplasty versus on-site thrombolysis in patients with high-risk myocardial infarction: the Air Primary Angioplasty in Myocardial Infarction study. *J Am Coll Cardiol.* 2002;39:1713–1719.

**Keeley EC, Boura JA, Grines CL.** Primary angioplasty versus intravenous thrombolytic therapy for acute myocardial infarction: a quantitative review of 23 randomised trials. *Lancet.* 2003;361: 13–20.

**Lee KL, Woodlief LH, Topol EJ, et al**. Predictors of 30-day mortality in the era of reperfusion for acute myocardial infarction. Results from an international trial of 41,021 patients. GUSTO-I Investigators. *Circulation.* 1995;91:1659–1668.

**Morrow DA, Antman EM, Charlesworth A, et al**. TIMI risk score for ST-elevation myocardial infarction: a convenient, bedside, clinical score for risk assessment at presentation: an intravenous nPA for treatment of infarcting myocardium early II trial substudy. *Circulation.* 2000;102:2031–2037.

**Sabatine MS, Cannon CP, Gibson CM, et al**. Addition of clopidogrel to aspirin and fibrinolytic therapy for myocardial infarction with ST-segment elevation. *N Engl J Med.* 2005;352:1179–1189.

**Sgarbossa EB, Pinski SL, Barbagelata A, et al**. Electrocardiographic diagnosis of evolving acute myocardial infarction in the presence of left bundle-branch block. GUSTO-1 (Global Utilization of Streptokinase and Tissue Plasminogen Activator for Occluded Coronary Arteries) Investigators. *N Engl J Med.* 1996;334:481–487.

**Wang K, Asinger RW, Marriott HJ.** ST-segment elevation in conditions other than acute myocardial infarction. *N Engl J Med.* 2003;349:2128–2135.

**White H.** Thrombin-specific anticoagulation with bivalirudin versus heparin in patients receiving fibrinolytic therapy for acute myocardial infarction: the HERO-2 randomised trial. *Lancet.* 2001;358:1855–1863.

**Widimsky P, Budesinsky T, Vorac D, et al**. Long distance transport for primary angioplasty vs immediate thrombolysis in acute myocardial infarction. Final results of the randomized national multicentre trial—PRAGUE-2. *Eur Heart J.* 2003;24:94–104.

## QUESTIONS

**1.** In the TIMI risk score model, the variable that has the strongest prediction for subsequent 30-day mortality is:

a. Low body weight (i.e., <67 kg)
b. Tachycardia
c. Advanced age (i.e., >75 years)
d. Killip class II–IV at presentation
e. Left bundle branch block at presentation

Answer is c: Advanced age (>75 years) predicts the worst outcome for 30-day mortality and receives 3 points in the risk model. The other variables receive 1 to 2 points each. Hypotension (i.e., systolic blood pressure <90 mmHg) at presentation is also a high-risk variable and receives 3 points in the risk model.

**2.** Which of the following is not included in the differential diagnosis for electrocardiographic ST elevations?

a. ST-elevation myocardial infarction
b. Left ventricular aneurysm
c. Hypokalemia
d. Pericarditis
e. Left ventricular hypertrophy

Answer is c: Among the electrolyte abnormalities, hyperkalemia, not hypokalemia can cause ST elevations that mimic ST-elevation myocardial infarctions.

**3.** Risk factors for intracranial hemorrhage during administration of fibrinolytics include all of the following except:

a. Uncontrolled hypertension
b. Advanced age
c. Female gender
d. Preexisting coagulopathy
e. Morbid obesity

Answer is e: Low body weight, not morbid obesity, is a risk factor for intracranial hemorrhage.

**4.** All of the following are class III recommendations except:

a. Performing revascularization of non–infarct-related arteries at the time of primary PCI
b. Waiting for cardiac biomarkers to return before making the diagnosis of an ST-elevation myocardial infarction
c. Administering fibrinolytics to asymptomatic patients more than 24 hours from the onset of chest pain
d. The use of a low-molecular-weight heparin along with fibrinolytics in elderly patients (i.e., >75 years old) or those with renal insufficiency
e. The use of an oral ACE-inhibitor within 24 hours of an anterior ST-elevation myocardial infarction

Answer is e: The use of an oral ACE inhibitor is generally recommended early in the hospital course as long as the patient is hemodynamically stable (usually at least 6 hours after presentation). In contrast, the use of an intravenous ACE inhibitor during the first 24 hours is not recommended. Non–infarct-related coronaries should not be revascularized except in the setting of cardiogenic shock. Fibrinolytics are recommended for ST-elevation myocardial infarction within 12 hours from the onset of chest pain. Administering fibrinolytics 12 to 24 hours from the onset of chest pain is generally not recommended, however individuals with stuttering chest pain during this time period may still be eligible to receive fibrinolytics. In elderly individuals (i.e., >75 years old) and/or those with renal insufficiency who also receive fibrinolytics, the use of unfractionated heparin is preferred over low-molecular- weight heparin.

5. The fibrinolytic agent associated with the least intracranial hemorrhage is
   a. Alteplase (tPA)
   b. Streptokinase
   c. Reteplase (rPA)
   d. Tenecteplase (TNK-tPA)

Answer is b: Among the various fibrinolytic agents, streptokinase does not necessitate the use of heparin. This may help to explain the smaller incidence of intracranial hemorrhage seen with this agent.

# 16

# Fibrinolytic Therapy for Acute Myocardial Infarction

***Juhana Karha Sorin J. Brener***

Acute ST-segment-elevation myocardial infarction (STEMI) remains a common and lethal illness in the United States. The management of STEMI is predicated on the open artery hypothesis, which links the early restoration of antegrade blood flow in the infarct-related artery (IRA) to improved survival. In practice, this means the immediate recanalization of the culprit epicardial coronary artery, preferably within 12 hours of symptom onset. The two ways to restore blood flow to the affected myocardium are fibrinolytic therapy and primary percutaneous coronary intervention (PCI), each with its own set of benefits and limitations. Whereas head-to-head randomized trials have demonstrated that primary PCI is superior to fibrinolytic therapy, many logistical considerations often make fibrinolytic therapy the preferred strategy. In fact, the administration of fibrinolytic agents is the most commonly used therapy to achieve reperfusion in STEMI, mainly due to wide availability and ease of application. Additional advantages of fibrinolytic therapy are its initial lower cost and easier learning curve for the personnel providing the therapy. Persistent challenges are the incompleteness and lack of durability of reperfusion and the higher incidence of intracranial hemorrhage.

## INDICATIONS AND CONTRAINDICATIONS

The American College of Cardiology (ACC) and the American Heart Association (AHA) have issued guidelines regarding the use of fibrinolytic therapy for the treatment of acute STEMI (Table 16–1). The indications for reperfusion therapy (fibrinolytic therapy or primary PCI) center around making the diagnosis of acute STEMI (ischemic symptoms and ST-segment elevation of greater than 0.1 mV in at least two contiguous leads, or a new left bundle branch block, or an electrocardiogram (ECG) consistent with a true posterior STEMI) in a patient who presents within 12 hours of symptom onset.

The contraindications for fibrinolytic therapy focus on the increased bleeding risk associated with it. The most worrisome complication is intracranial hemorrhage (ICH), which may be fatal in up to two thirds of cases. Contraindications therefore include patient characteristics that increase the risk of ICH, such as prior ICH, recent (within 3 months) ischemic stroke or head trauma, intracranial neoplasm, and any elevated blood pressure measurement (exceeding 180/110 mm Hg). Other variables that increase the bleeding risk associated with fibrinolytic therapy are older age, female gender, African American race, lower weight, excessive anticoagulation, and the use of tissue plasminogen activator (t-PA) versus streptokinase. Other co-morbid conditions that preclude the use of fibrinolytic therapy are aortic dissection, active bleeding, and major surgery within the last 4 weeks. Relative contraindications that require consideration on an individual basis are prolonged cardiopulmonary resuscitation, diabetic retinopathy, chronic anticoagulation, bleeding diatheses, and pregnancy. Streptokinase should be avoided if the patient has been exposed to it in the past. If ICH is suspected during or following

**TABLE 16–1**
**SUMMARY OF GUIDELINES FOR ADMINISTRATION OF FIBRINOLYTIC AGENTS IN PATIENTS WITH STEMI**

| | |
|---|---|
| Class I | 1. In the absence of contraindications, fibrinolytic therapy should be administered to STEMI patients with symptom onset within the prior 12 hours and ST elevation greater than 0.1 mV in at least two contiguous precordial leads or at least two adjacent limb leads. (Level of Evidence: A)<br>2. In the absence of contraindications, fibrinolytic therapy should be administered to STEMI patients with symptom onset within the prior 12 hours and new or presumably new LBBB. (Level of Evidence: A) |
| Class IIa | 1. In the absence of contraindications, it is reasonable to administer fibrinolytic therapy to STEMI patients with symptom onset within the prior 12 hours and 12-lead ECG findings consistent with true posterior MI. (Level of Evidence: C)<br>2. In the absence of contraindications, it is reasonable to administer fibrinolytic therapy to patients with symptoms of STEMI beginning within the prior 12 to 24 hours who have continuing ischemic symptoms and ST elevation greater than 0.1 mV in at least two contiguous precordial leads or at least two adjacent limb leads. (Level of Evidence: B) |
| Class III | 1. Fibrinolytic therapy should not be administered to asymptomatic patients whose initial symptoms of STEMI began more than 24 hours earlier. (Level of Evidence: C)<br>2. Fibrinolytic therapy should not be administered to patients whose 12-lead ECG shows only ST-segment depression except if a true posterior MI is suspected. (Level of Evidence: A) |

fibrinolytic therapy, fibrinolytic, antiplatelet, and anticoagulant therapies should be suspended immediately. Neurologic evaluation with brain imaging should be undertaken with consideration given to administration of cryoprecipitate, fresh-frozen plasma, protamine, and platelets. Other measures in the treatment of ICH include elevation of the head of the bed (30 degrees), blood pressure optimization, intubation with hyperventilation, administration of mannitol, as well as neurosurgical evacuation of ICH.

## THE FIBRINOLYTIC AGENTS

The use of fibrinolytic therapy in acute STEMI is associated with an approximately 20% lower short-term risk of death compared to standard therapy without reperfusion. The STEMI patients who are at the highest risk of death derive the most benefit from fibrinolytic therapy. These include patients with anterior myocardial infarction (MI) and those with greater total ST-segment deviation or new left bundle branch block. Moreover, the benefit with fibrinolytic therapy is greatest when administered early on after symptom onset, especially in the first 1 to 2 hours.

A number of fibrinolytic agents are available in the United States. They all work by activating plasminogen. Their characteristics are summarized in Table 16–2. Streptokinase (SK), the first agent to be evaluated, binds plasminogen relatively nonspecifically, even in the absence of fibrin. Tissue plasminogen activator (t-PA, alteplase), a second-generation fibrinolytic agent, is more fibrin specific than SK. The accelerated infusion regimen of t-PA (over 90 minutes) demonstrated a survival benefit compared to SK, saving one life for each 100 patients treated and thus becoming the benchmark fibrinolytic agent. It is also the most commonly used agent in the United States. Reteplase (r-PA), a third-generation agent, is a nonglycosylated deletion mutant of wild-type t-PA. The GUSTO-III trial randomized nearly 15,000 acute STEMI patients to rPA

**TABLE 16–2**
**SUMMARY OF PROPERTIES OF FIBRINOLYTIC AGENTS USED IN CLINICAL PRACTICE**

| | Streptokinase | t-PA | r-PA | TNK-t-PA |
|---|---|---|---|---|
| Source | Group C Streptococci | Recombinant | Recombinant | Recombinant |
| Fibrin specificity | None | ++ | + | +++ |
| Half-life, min | 18–23 | 3–4 | 14 | 20–24 |
| Dose | 1.5 MU | 15-mg bolus, 0.75 mg/kg for 30 min, then 0.5 mg/kg for 60 min for up to 100 mg total dose | 10 MU × 2, 30 min apart | 30–50 mg according to 5 weight categories |
| Cost | $300 | $2,200 | $2,200 | $2,200 |
| Advantages | Cost, no need for heparin co-therapy | More effective than SK, short half-life | Bolus administration | Bolus administration, may be more effective with late presentation |

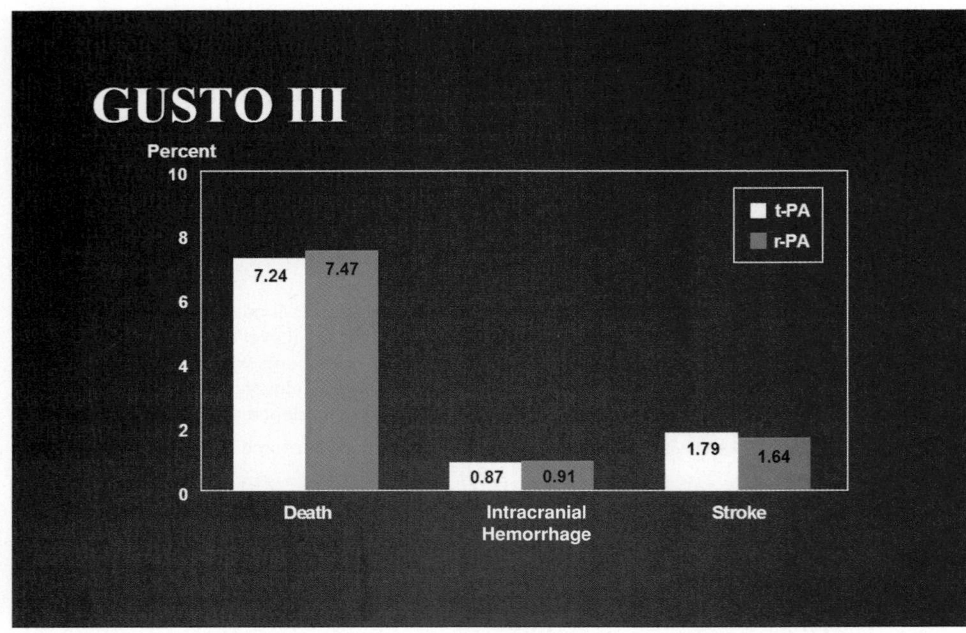


**Figure 16–1** GUSTO III: Comparison between t-PA and r-PA. (Adapted from A comparison of reteplase with alteplase for acute myocardial infarction. The Global Use of Strategies to Open Occluded Coronary Arteries (GUSTO III) Investigators. *N Engl J Med* Oct 16 1997;337(16):1118–1123.)

versus t-PA and documented similar mortality (Figure 16–1). The 30-day mortality was 7.24% and 7.47% for t-PA and r-PA, respectively. The rate of ICH at 30 days was 0.87% and 0.91% for t-PA and r-PA, respectively. Tenecteplase (TNK-t-PA) is a triple mutant of t-PA with greater fibrin specificity and greater resistance to plasminogen activator inhibitor (PAI)-1. In the ASSENT-2 trial, 16,949 acute STEMI patients were randomized to receive weight-adjusted TNK-t-PA versus t-PA. There was no difference in the incidence of 30-day mortality (6.15% for t-PA versus 6.18% for TNK) or ICH (0.93% for t-PA vrsus 0.94% for TNK) between the treatment arms, but fewer patients receiving tenecteplase required a blood transfusion, thus suggesting modest improvement in the safety profile (Figure 16–2). Patients presenting later than 4 hours from symptom onset seemed to derive greater benefit from TNK than from t-PA, presumably because of its greater resistance to PAI-1.

The administration of fibrinolytic therapy prior to the arrival in the hospital emergency room is recommended (ACC/AHA Guideline Class IIa indication), provided that a physician is present in the ambulance or that the emergency medical services (EMS) system is well developed and can transmit 12-lead ECGs. Prehospital fibrinolytic

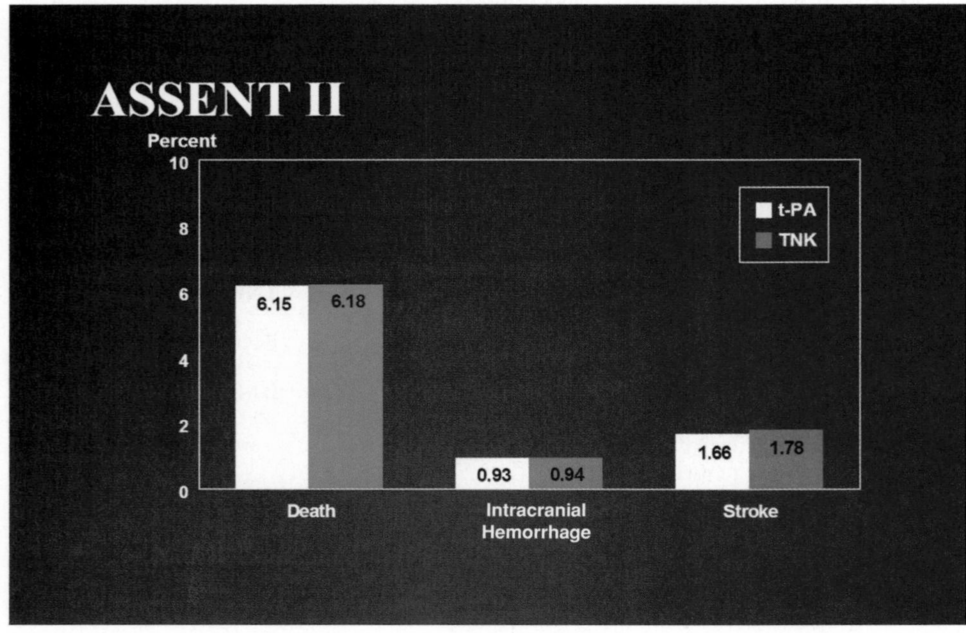


**Figure 16–2** ASSENT II: Comparison between t-PA and TNK-t-PA. (Adapted from Single-bolus tenecteplase compared with front-loaded alteplase in acute myocardial infarction: the ASSENT-2 double-blind randomised trial. Assessment of the Safety and Efficacy of a New Thrombolytic Investigators. *Lancet* 1999;354(9180):716–722.)

therapy may have especially pronounced benefits within those EMS systems that have longer transport times to hospitals.

## COMPARISON WITH PRIMARY PERCUTANEOUS CORONARY INTERVENTION (PCI)

Several randomized trials have compared primary PCI with fibrinolytic therapy in the management of acute STEMI. A meta-analysis of these trials ($n = 7{,}739$) by Keeley et al. revealed that primary PCI is associated with improved clinical outcomes compared to fibrinolytic therapy (Table 16–3). Short-term mortality was lower in the angioplasty group (7.0% versus 9.3%, $p = 0.0002$), corresponding to a 27% relative risk reduction. Stroke and nonfatal reinfarction were also reduced in the angioplasty group. The mortality benefit of PCI persisted over 6 to 12 months of follow-up. Thus, for patients with acute STEMI who present to medical centers with available interventional cardiology facilities, the preferred strategy is primary PCI. However, this recommendation comes with a number of requirements. The operators and the catheterization laboratory personnel must be experienced, and the procedure must be performed without excessive delay. The ACC/AHA Guideline recommended maximum door-to-balloon time is 90 minutes. The same time applies to patients who may need to be transferred to another facility to undergo primary PCI. The corresponding benchmark time for fibrinolytic therapy is the door-to-needle time of 30 minutes, referring to the interval between presentation and the initiation of fibrinolytic therapy. In practice, however, the 90-minute door-to-balloon time is often not achieved, and if this is foreseen, fibrinolytic therapy should be administered immediately.

The key issue in choosing between the two reperfusion strategies is how much of a PCI-related relative delay is acceptable. The ACC/AHA Guideline committee has set this time interval at 60 minutes (that is, the difference between the door-to-balloon and the door-to-needle times). A number of variables influence the threshold "needle–balloon" interval. For patients with elevated (>4%) estimated risks of ICH or other major bleeding, longer PCI-related delays are clearly acceptable. Likewise, one would favor primary PCI despite a longer needle–balloon interval for patients who present late (perhaps in the 3- to 12-hour window after symptom onset, and particularly if later than 12 hours but have persistent angina). The same would be the case for older patients, and for patients with features of larger MIs (e.g., anterior MI). Every effort should be made to offer primary PCI to patients who present in or develop cardiogenic shock. Finally, in cases of failed fibrinolytic therapy (evident by persistent chest discomfort and ST-segment elevation signifying ongoing ischemia), performance of rescue PCI is indicated.

## SUBGROUPS

Fibrinolytic therapy maintains its mortality benefit over placebo across a broad range of subgroups. These include elderly patients, women, and diabetics (in fact, diabetics have greater mortality benefit than do nondiabetics). In general, the larger the MI, the greater the benefit offered by fibrinolytic therapy. Accordingly, this is true for cardiogenic shock and for anterior MI location. In addition, those patients with inferior MI who also have right ventricular involvement or anterior ST depression signifying a larger territory have greater benefit with fibrinolytic therapy. The other major variable is the time of presentation, and patients who present within 3 hours of symptom onset derive the greatest benefit from fibrinolytic therapy.

## COMBINATION THERAPY WITH REDUCED-DOSE FIBRINOLYTIC PLUS IIb/IIIa INHIBITOR

The strategy of reduced-dose fibrinolytic agent plus platelet glycoprotein IIb/IIIa inhibitor in the treatment of acute STEMI has been evaluated in two large randomized trials, namely, GUSTO-V and ASSENT-3. Neither trial documented a survival benefit when compared with full-dose fibrinolytic regimen. However, the incidence of recurrent in-hospital MI was reduced (but notably, without leading to long-term survival benefit), but at the expense of increased incidence of bleeding complications. The combination therapy–associated increase in bleeding risk was magnified among patients over the age of 75 years. The only subgroup that appeared to derive some survival benefit from the combination therapy in a retrospective analysis was comprised of younger patients with anterior MI.

A summary of the results of important clinical trials of reperfusion therapy in STEMI patients is provided in Table 16–4.

## OTHER ADJUNCTIVE PHARMACOTHERAPIES

Unfractionated intravenous heparin has traditionally been a mainstay adjunctive pharmacologic agent in the treatment of acute ischemic syndromes. Given that streptokinase itself is a systemic anticoagulant due to fibrinogen depletion, the utility of adding heparin is unclear, but almost universally done. However, the more fibrin-specific agents (alteplase, reteplase, and tenecteplase) do not have a systemic anticoagulant effect, and thus need adjunctive antithrombin therapy, traditionally in the form of intravenous unfractionated heparin (with a target activated partial thromboplastin time of 50 to 70 seconds).

The ASSENT-3 trial compared unfractionated intravenous heparin with enoxaparin, a low-molecular-weight heparin (LMWH), as an adjunct to tenecteplase. Therapy

## TABLE 16–3
## MAJOR TRIALS COMPARING FIBRINOLYSIS WITH PRIMARY PCI

| | Patients' Characteristics | Symptom Duration (h) | Number Randomized to PTCA ($n = 3,872$) | Number Randomized to Thrombolysis ($n = 3,872$) | Stents Used | Glycoprotein IIb/IIIa Antagonists Used | Thrombolytic Agent Used, Administration Time | Time to Treatment (min) PTCA | Time to Treatment (min) Thrombolytic Theraphy |
|---|---|---|---|---|---|---|---|---|---|
| **Streptokinase Trials ($n = 1,837$)** | | | | | | | | | |
| Zijlstra[8] | Age ≤75 y, ST↑ | <6 | 152 | 149 | No | No | 1.5 million U SK, 1 h | 62* | 30* |
| Riberio[9] | Age <75 y, ST↑ | <6 | 50 | 50 | No | No | 1.2 million U SK, 1 h | 238 | 179 |
| Grinfeld[10] | ST↑ | <12 | 54 | 58 | No | No | 1.5 million U SK, 1 h | 63† | 18† |
| Zijlstra[11] | ST↑, low risk | <6 | 47 | 53 | No | No | 1.5 million U SK, 1 h | 68* | 30* |
| Akhras[12] | ST↑ | <12 | 42 | 45 | No | No | 1.5 million U SK, 1 h | NA | NA |
| Widimsky[13]** | ST↑, LBBB | <6 | 101 | 99 | Yes | No | 1.5 million U SK, 1 h | 80† | 70† |
| de Boer[14] | Age ≥76 y; ST↑ | <6 | 46 | 41 | Yes | No | 1.5 million U SK, 1 h | 59* | 31* |
| Widimsky[15] | ST↑ | <12 | 429 | 421 | Yes | Yes | 1.5 million U SK, 1 h | 277‡,§ | 277‡,§ |
| **Fibrin-Specific Trials ($n = 5,902$)** | | | | | | | | | |
| DeWood[16] | Age ≤76 y; ST↑ | <12 | 46 | 44 | No | No | Duteplase, 4 h | 126* | 84* |
| Grines[17] | ST↑ | <12 | 195 | 200 | No | No | t-PA, 3 h | 60† | 32† |
| Gibbons[18] | Age <80 y; ST↑ | <12 | 47 | 56 | No | No | Duteplase, 4 h | 45† | 20† |
| Ribichini[19,20] | Age <80 y; inferior MI, anterior ST↓ | <6 | 55 | 55 | No | No | Accelerated t-PA | 40† | 33† |
| Garcia[21,22] | anterior MI | 5 | 95 | 94 | No | No | Accelerated t-PA | 84* | 69* |
| GUSTO IIb[23] | ST↑, LBBB | <12 | 565 | 573 | No | No | Accelerated t-PA | 114† | 72† |
| Le May[24] | ST↑, LBBB | <12 | 62 | 61 | Yes | Yes | Accelerated t-PA | 77‡,¶ | 15† |
| Bonnefoy[25] | ST↑ | <6 | 421 | 419 | Yes | Yes | Accelerated t-PA | 190† | 130† |
| Schomig[26] | ST↑ | <12 | 71 | 69 | Yes | Yes | Accelerated t-PA | 65*,¶ | 30*,¶ |
| Vermeer[27]** | Age <80 y; ST↑ | <6 | 75 | 75 | Yes | No | Accelerated t-PA | 100† | 85† |
| Andersen[28] | ST↑ | <12 | 790 | 782 | Yes | NA | Accelerated t-PA | NA | NA |
| Kastrati[29] | ST↑, LBBB | <12 | 81 | 81 | Yes | Yes | Accelerated t-PA | 75*,¶ | 35*,¶ |
| Aversano[30] | ST↑ | <12 | 225 | 226 | Yes | Yes | Accelerated t-PA | 102*,¶ | 46*,¶ |
| Grines[31] | ST↑ | <12 | 71 | 66 | Yes | Yes | Accelerated t-PA | 155* | 51* |
| Hochman[7] | Cardiogenic shock | <36 | 152 | 150 | Yes | Yes | Accelerated t-PA | 75*,¶ | 6,168†,¶,‖ |

PCI, percutaneous coronary intervention; ST↑, St-segment elevation; y, years; h, hours; u, units; min, minutes; PTCA, percutaneous transluminal coronary angioplasty; SK, streptokinase; t-PA, tissue plasminogen activator; LBBB, left bundle branch block; GUSTO IIB, the Global Use of Strategies to Open Occluded Coronary Arteries in Acute Coronary Syndromes.

Reproduced with permission from Keeley EC, Boura JA, Grines CL. Primary angioplasty versus intravenous thrombolytic therapy for acute myocardial infarction: a quantitative review of 23 randomized trials. *Lancet.* 2003;361:13–20.

**TABLE 16–4**
**PRIMARY RESULTS OF MAJOR TRIALS AND ANALYSES OF REPERFUSION THERAPY IN STEMI**

| Trial | Year | Design | Primary Endpoint | Relative Reduction in EP |
|---|---|---|---|---|
| ISIS-2 | 1988 | SK vs ASA vs both vs neither | 30-d mortality | SK or ASA: ~20%<br>Both: 40% |
| ISIS-3 | 1992 | SK vs APSAK vs t-PA | 35-d mortality | None |
| GUSTO I | 1993 | t-PA vs SK vs both | 30-d mortality | t-PA : 14%<br>Both : none |
| GUSTO III | 1997 | r-PA vs t-PA | 30-d mortality | None |
| ASSENT II | 1999 | TNK vs t-PA | 30-d mortality | None |
| GUSTO V | 2001 | r-PA + abciximab vs r-PA | 30-d mortality | None |
| Meta-analysis of PCI vs lytics | 2003 | PCI vs lytics | 30-d mortality | PCI: 27% |

with enoxaparin was associated with a lower incidence of a 30-day major adverse cardiac event endpoint, although among patients older than 75 years it also was associated with more bleeding. The ASSENT-3 PLUS trial noted that both major bleeding and the incidence of ICH were increased among older patients receiving enoxaparin. It is important to recognize that the ASSENT-3 trial excluded patients with severe chronic renal insufficiency, in whom the effects of LMWH may be more long lasting.

Aspirin at doses of 162 to 325 mg is indicated for all patients with acute STEMI. Recently, the CLARITY TIMI 28 study evaluated the utility of adding clopidogrel (300-mg loading dose, followed by a daily dose of 75 mg) to the regimen of aspirin, heparin, and a fibrinolytic agent among 3,491 patients with acute STEMI. Patients receiving clopidogrel had a lower incidence of the 30-day combined endpoint of cardiovascular death, recurrent MI, or recurrent ischemia requiring urgent revascularization. It is notable that patients older than 75 years were excluded. Thus, both aspirin and clopidogrel should be administered to patients receiving fibrinolytic therapy who are younger than 75 years old, and who are not at increased risk of bleeding.

## BIBLIOGRAPHY


**Antman EM, Anbe DT, Armstrong PW, et al.** ACC/AHA guidelines for the management of patients with ST-elevation myocardial infarction—executive summary: a report of the American College of Cardiology/American Heart Association Task Force on Practice Guidelines (Writing Committee to Revise the 1999 Guidelines for the Management of Patients with Acute Myocardial Infarction). *Circulation.* 2004;110:588–636.

**Boersma E, Maas AC, Deckers JW, Simoons ML.** Early thrombolytic treatment in acute myocardial infarction: reappraisal of the golden hour. *Lancet.* 1996;348:771–775.

**Keeley EC, Boura JA, Grines CL.** Primary angioplasty versus intravenous thrombolytic therapy for acute myocardial infarction: a quantitative review of 23 randomized trials. *Lancet.* 2003;361:13–20.

**Morrison LJ, Verbeek PR, McDonald AC, et al.** Mortality and prehospital thrombolysis for acute myocardial infarction: A meta-analysis. *JAMA.* 2000;283:2686–2692.


## QUESTIONS

1. A 54-year-old man with a history of hypertension presents with chest pain that started 2 hours ago and is diagnosed in the Emergency Department with anterior STEMI. His blood pressure is 205/100 mm Hg. He receives intravenous metoprolol and the blood pressure falls to 170/85 mm Hg. What is the most appropriate reperfusion strategy?
   a. Fibrinolytic therapy
   b. Angiography and PCI
   c. Medical therapy alone and PCI at a later date

Answer is b: The patient's admission systolic blood pressure is quite elevated and represents a relative contraindication for fibrinolytic therapy. Therefore, primary PCI is the preferred reperfusion strategy in this case.

2. A 75-year-old woman presents to a community hospital (without invasive capabilities) with 6 hours of chest pain and is diagnosed with inferior STEMI. The anticipated transfer to a medical center with primary PCI capability will take 2 hours. What is the preferred reperfusion therapy?
   a. Fibrinolytic therapy at the presentation hospital
   b. Transfer for angiography and PCI
   c. Half-dose fibrinolysis and GP IIb/IIIa inhibition at the presentation hospital and

transfer for rescue PCI, if it fails to produce reperfusion

Answer is a: The transfer-related delay of 2 hours tips the balance in favor of fibrinolytic therapy, according to the 2004 ACC/AHA Guidelines.

3. A 48-year-old man with an anterior STEMI receives fibrinolytic therapy with reteplase. 30 minutes after the second bolus he continues to have chest pain and his ECG demonstrates mild (estimated 30%) resolution of the ST segment elevations. What is the next correct step in his management?
   a. Readministration of a different fibrinolytic agent
   b. Administration of GP IIB/IIIA inhibitor
   c. Immediate coronary angiography and rescue PCI
   d. Symptomatic relief of angina and heart failure

Answer is c: The patient has failed fibrinolytic therapy as evidenced by ongoing ischemic symptoms and insufficient ST resolution (<50%). Coronary angiography and consideration for rescue PCI are advisable.

4. An 80-year-old woman with chest discomfort for the last 15 hours and progressively worsening dyspnea over the last few hours presents to the Emergency Department and is diagnosed with anterior STEMI. What, if any, reperfusion measures should be undertaken?
   a. Fibrinolysis
   b. Immediate coronary angiography and PCI
   c. Symptomatic relief of angina and heart failure

Answer is b: The benefit of fibrinolytic therapy after 15 hours of ischemic symptoms is unclear. Moreover, it sounds as if the patient's MI may be complicated by heart failure, and she is best managed with medical therapy. An invasive strategy should be considered if she develops cardiogenic shock.

5. A 77-year-old thin woman with a history of gastroesophageal reflux disease presents in the first hour of an acute inferior STEMI. The blood pressure is normal. Invasive facilities are not readily available. What is the preferred strategy for reperfusion therapy?
   a. Fibrinolytic therapy
   b. Transfer for immediate coronary angiography and PCI
   c. Half-dose fibrinolysis and GP IIb/IIIa inhibition
   d. Symptomatic relief of angina only

Answer is a: Even though advanced age, female gender, and low body mass index (BMI) are all risk factors for bleeding complications, the patient will have a mortality benefit with fibrinolytic therapy and should receive it.

## HOW TO PREPARE FOR THE BOARDS

Thoroughly review the indications and contraindications of administering fibrinolytic therapy. Also, familiarize yourself with available adjunctive pharmacotherapy and its indications. The continued evaluation of the patient who has just received fibrinolytic therapy is important in terms of both ischemic symptoms and possible bleeding complications. When taking the examination, keep in mind that administering fibrinolytic therapy for acute STEMI is appropriate when significant delays are expected with primary PCI.

# Percutaneous Coronary Intervention

17

*Soundos Moualla* *Brendan Duffy* *Stephen Ellis*

It was 1977 when Gruntzig first attempted to manage flow-limiting coronary atherosclerosis with percutaneous transluminal coronary angioplasty (PTCA). Since then, numerous advances involving stent design, equipment, techniques, strategies, and adjunct therapeutics have been achieved. The procedure is now referred to as percutaneous coronary intervention (PCI), to encompass not only angioplasty and stenting, but also all percutaneous techniques capable of relieving coronary narrowing, including rotational atherectomy, directional atherectomy (DCA), extraction atherectomy (TEC), laser angiography (ELCA), and brachytherapy. The field of PCI has been the focus of some of the most important clinical trials in cardiology. These studies have shaped clinical practice and defined the algorithms established in the 2001 American College of Cardiology/American Heart Association (ACC/AHA) guidelines. In this chapter, we will cover the ACC/AHA guidelines, summarize the major clinical trials comparing and contrasting PCI to other modes of revascularization therapy, and discuss patient risk stratification, complications, technical aspects of PCI, and adjunct anticoagulation and antiplatelet therapy. It is important to keep in mind that PCI is constantly evolving, with versatile changes in therapy and indications. This makes it challenging to present from the perspective of the Cardiology Board exam, which is based mostly on the most current ACC/AHA guidelines and thus lags current practice by a few years.

The goals of revascularization therapy are to extend survival, prevent myocardial infarction (MI), improve anginal symptoms, and improve exercise capacity. Assessing the effect of PCI on these goals is essential, as PCI is increasingly being used, and is now attempted in patients with previous MI, older patients, and those with multivessel and complex coronary artery disease (CAD) lesions. It is estimated that more than a million PCI procedures are performed yearly in the United States.

## INDICATIONS

The ACC/AHA classify indications as Class I, II, or III, and classify the weight of evidence in support of indications as level A, B, or C. Refer to the 2001 ACC/AHA guidelines for percutaneous coronary intervention (revision of the 1993 PTCA guidelines) for precise definitions. The guidelines incorporate risk stratification of patients (low, moderate, high risk) and predictors of success/complications based on multiple factors, including anatomic and clinical factors, risk of death, gender, age, and presence of diabetes mellitus (DM) or coronary artery bypass graft (CABG). Patients with a wide range of clinical presentations can be candidates for PCI, ranging from asymptomatic to those with a variable severity of symptoms. The major guidelines are summarized as follows.

### Asymptomatic or Mild Angina Patients

Before the ACIP study (see later description), the consensus for management of the majority of asymptomatic or mildly symptomatic patients was medical therapy. The ACIP study, though not definitive, increased concern about a medical therapy approach in high-risk patients with a similar symptom profile. The stratification system for low versus high risk is discussed in a later section. The recommendations for PCI in high-risk but asymptomatic or mildly symptomatic patients are shown in Table 17–1 and are adapted from the ACC/AHA practice guidelines.

**TABLE 17–1**
**ACC/AHA GUIDELINES FOR PCI IN ASYMPTOMATIC OR MILDLY SYMPTOMATIC PATIENTS**

| Class | | Level of Evidence |
|---|---|---|
| Class I | Patients with<br>■ No diabetes<br>■ One or more significant lesions in one or two coronary arteries, with high likelihood of procedure success<br>■ High-risk anatomy: vessels to be intervened on should supply a large area of viable myocardium based on stress testing | B |
| Class IIa | Patients with<br>■ Similar clinical and anatomic requirements as for Class I<br>■ Except patients treated for diabetes<br>■ Or the vessel to be intervened on supplies a moderate area of viable myocardium | B |
| Class IIb | Patients with<br>■ Three or more coronary arteries suitable for PCI with a high likelihood of procedural success—vessels to be intervened on should supply at least a moderate area of viable myocardium<br>■ Myocardial ischemia based on stress testing (ECG, nuclear, or echo) or intracoronary anatomic or physiologic assessment of severity of stenosis, such as fractional flow reserve or intravascular ultrasound | B |
| Class III | Patients who do not meet the criteria for Class I or II and who have<br>■ Left main trunk disease<br>■ Small area of viable myocardium at risk<br>■ Lesions <50% in severity<br>■ No ischemia based on stress tests | C |

*Source:* Adapted from the ACC/AHA 2001 JACC 2001;37(8):2339i

## Patients with Angina Class II–IV, or Unstable Angina, or Non–ST-Elevation Myocardial Infarction

This group of patients has been the center of multiple trials, including TIMI-IIIB, VANQWISH, FRISC II, and TACTICS, with inconsistent results. TACTICS was the only study evaluating what is contemporary therapy, particularly in the use of glycoprotein IIb/IIIa inhibitors. The ACC/AHA guidelines assume that these patients are already on intensive medical therapy, either with an inadequate symptom response or with significant disease that merits intervention. Intensive medical therapy includes aspirin, heparin, beta-blockers, statins, and glycoprotein IIb/IIIa antagonists. A summary of these guidelines is given in Table 17–2.

## Patients with Acute ST-Elevation Myocardial Infarction (STEMI)

The role of fibrinolytics in improving survival of acute MI compared to conservative management has long been established (GUSTO, GISSI, ISIS-2, FTT trials). Subsequent trials established the importance of the 90-minute patency profile on improved left ventricular (LV) function postthrombolysis (TIMI-1, ECSG). This time profile was extrapolated to PCI. Primary PTCA (before stents) demonstrated reduction in recurrent ischemia, reinfarction, reocclusion, and strokes compared to patients treated with fibrinolysis. The long-term mortality benefit was not consistent amongt various studies (GUSTO-2B, PAMI, Zwolle, and other studies), but meta-analysis by Weaver et al. showed a 34% relative reduction in mortality for PTCA compared to thrombolysis. Subsequent studies showed that stenting in acute ST-elevation MI is more effective than PTCA alone, in terms of postintervention lumen size, reclosure risk, risk of subsequent ischemic events, and risk of redo target vessels revascularization (GRAMI, FRESCO, STENTIM, PASTA, PSAAMI, stent-PAMI). However, there is no survival benefit for stents compared to PTCA alone. Indications for PCI in STEMI are based on the timing of PCI relative to the MI and/or relative to fibrinolytics if used (Tables 17–3 and 17–4).

**TABLE 17–2**

**ACC/AHA RECOMMENDATION FOR PCI IN PATIENTS WITH CLASS II–IV ANGINA, UNSTABLE ANGINA, OR NON–ST-ELEVATION MYOCARDIAL INFARCTION ALREADY ON MEDICAL THERAPY**

| Class | | Level of Evidence |
|---|---|---|
| Class I | Low-risk patients<br>■ With one or more lesions in one or more vessels and high likelihood of procedural success<br>■ Vessels to be intervened on should supply at least a moderate to a large area of viable myocardium | B |
| Class IIa | Patients with<br>■ SVG with focal lesions or multiple lesions, but not total occlusions<br>■ Patients who are poor candidates for redo CABG | C |
| Class IIb | Patients with<br>■ One or more high-risk lesions<br>■ Or moderate area of viable myocardium supplied by the vessel to be intervened on<br>■ Or two- or three-vessel disease, or significant proximal LAD disease or abnormal LV<br>■ Or diabetic | B |
| Class III | Patients with<br>■ No evidence of ischemia or injury with no trial of medical therapy, or small area of affected myocardium, or high-risk lesions<br>■ Insignificant stenosis (<50%)<br>■ Significant LMT disease and candidate for CABG | C<br>C<br>B |

SVG, or CABG, coronary artery bypass graft; LAD, left arteries descending; LV, left ventricular; LMT, left main trunk. *Source:* Adapted from the ACC/AHA 2001 JACC 2001;37(8):2339i.

*Immediate PCI* is intervention done immediately after successful fibrinolysis. In patients with successful fibrinolysis who are asymptomatic, earlier trials showed no evidence that immediate PCI of the infarct-related artery provided any added benefit in death rate reduction, reinfarction, or myocardial salvage (SWIFT and TIMI II). It is important to note that in these trials, clopidogrel or glycoprotein IIb/IIIa inhibitors were not used. In these studies, interventions were associated with increased incidence of events including death, recurrent ischemia, emergency CABG, recurrent ischemia, and higher transfusion rates (SWIFT and TIMI II). However, immediate PCIs show mortality benefit when performed on patients with a history of MI compared to a conservative approach. This benefit was not evident in patients with a first MI (TIMI-II reanalysis). More recent but smaller trials showed contradictory results; SIAM III showed significant reduction in mortality and ischemic events in those who underwent immediate PCI after successful fibrinolysis.

Numerous advances have been made since many of these trials were conducted. A recent trial that addressed this controversy is CAPITAL AMI (Combined Angioplasty and Pharmacological Interventions versus Thrombolytics Alone in Acute MI). Patients with ST-elevation MI were randomized to TNK followed by immediate PCI versus TNK alone. The combined invasive approach group had reduced major adverse cardiac events (MACE) at 30 days and 6 months; there was no increased risk of bleeding with the invasive approach. Another trial, GARCIA-1, addressed the issue of immediate PCI after thrombolysis. Patients with acute ST-elevation MI treated with tPA were randomized to an invasive approach (PCI and stenting within 24 hours) versus a conservative approach (intervention guided by evidence of ischemia). The invasive-approach group had a lower risk of death, reinfarction, and revascularization at 1 year as a composite endpoint. Furthermore, the patients experienced no increase in bleeding and shorter hospital stays.

*Facilitated PCI* refers to early PCI done with a reduced dose of fibrinolytics with or without IIb/IIIa antagonist therapy prior to the PCI. The idea originated from the observation of an improved prognosis of acute MI patients referred to primary PCI when TIMI-3 flow was seen on baseline angiography, as compared to TIMI-0-2. Facilitated PCI without IIb/IIIa antagonists did not demonstrate a difference in the rate of TIMI 3 flow after the intervention (PACT). However, the combination of reduced-dose fibrinolysis with IIb/IIIa antagonist prior to PCI demonstrated

**TABLE 17–3**
**ACC/AHA RECOMMENDATIONS FOR PCI IN ACUTE MYOCARDIAL INFARCTION AS AN ALTERNATIVE TO FIBRINOLYSIS**

| Class | | Level of Evidence |
|---|---|---|
| Class I | Patients with | |
| | ■ Acute MI with STEMI or new/presumed new LBBB + PCI <12 h from symptoms onset or >12 h of presistent symptoms, + PCI to be done 90 ± 30 min from hospital admission; procedure to be done by skilled operators in experienced Cath labs[a] | A |
| | ■ STEMI within 36 h of ST elevation or LBBB + cardiogenic shock + <75 y of age + PCI to be done within 18 h of onset of shock by skilled operators in experienced Cath lab | A |
| Class IIa | Patients with acute MI who have contraindications to thrombolytics | C |
| Class IIb | No recommendation | |
| Class III | Patients with | |
| | ■ Acute MI and PCI to a non–infarct-related artery at the time of acute MI (except patients with shock) | C |
| | ■ PCIs on patients with acute MI who received thrombolytics with successful results/no symptoms | C |
| | ■ PCIs by inexperienced operators on patients with acute MI; candidates for thrombolytics | |
| | ■ PCI 12 h after onset of initial symptoms with no evidence of ongoing ischemia or symptoms | |

[a]Though current guidelines do not recommend reperfusion treatment in STEMI patients who present more than 12 h after the onset of symptoms, a multicenter European trial showed that there is an increased degree of myocardial salvage in patients who had later reperfusion (12–48 h after symptom onset and without persistent symptoms).
STEMI, ST-elevation myocardial infarction; Cath lab, cardiac catheterization lab; LBBB, left bundle branch block; MI, myocardial infarction.
*Source:* Adapted from the ACC/AHA 2001 JACC 2001;37(8):2339i.

higher rates of TIMI 3 flow compared to PCI alone, with no increased risk of hemorrhagic complications (SPEED and TIMI 14). Recently, in the BRAVE trial, patients with STEMI were randomized to facilitated PCI with half-dose reteplase with abciximab, or abciximab alone. There was no difference in infarct size or MACE between the two groups.

Patients who fail fibrinolysis (continuing or recurrent ischemia) benefit from rescue PCI (within 12 hours

**TABLE 17–4**
**ACC/AHA RECOMMENDATIONS FOR PCI AFTER THROMBOLYSIS**

| Class | | Level of Evidence |
|---|---|---|
| Class I | Patients who received thrombolysis with objective evidence of recurrent infarction or ischemia (rescue PCI) | B |
| Class IIa | Patients who received thrombolytics with cardiogenic shock or hemodynamic instability | B |
| Class IIb | Patients who received thrombolytics with recurrent angina but no objective evidence of ischemia | C |
| | ■ PCI of infarct-related vessel within 48 h of successful thrombolytics and no evidence of ischemia or symptoms | B |
| Class III | ■ PCI within 48 h post-failed thrombolytics | B |
| | ■ PCI of infarct-related artery immediately after successful fibrinolytics | A |

*Source:* Adapted from the ACC/AHA 2001 JACC 2001;37(8):2339i.

of lytics) in terms of mortality, congestive heart failure (CHF), and improved LV function as well fewer adverse in-hospital events (Gusto-I, Rescue I, TAMI-5, MERLIN, REACT, STOPAMI). MERLIN (Middlesbrough Early Revascularization to Limit Infarction study) studied patients who received streptokinase but had no resolution of ST segments. Patients were randomized to either left heart catheterization (LHC)/PCI or medical therapy. There was no mortality difference between the two groups; major adverse cardiac events were lower in the invasive group, except strokes and transfusions, which were increased in the invasive treatment group. REACT (the larger REscue Angioplasty versus Conservative Therapy or repeat thrombolysis trial) randomized patients who failed thrombolysis to either rescue PCI, repeat thrombolysis, or a conservative approach. Patients who had rescue angioplasty experienced a lower rate of death, reinfarction, and heart failure (composite endpoint) than either of the other groups. STOPAMI (Stent Or Percutaneous transluminal coronary Angioplasty for occluded coronary arteries with acute MI) found rescue PCI with stenting was associated with better myocardial salvage than PCI without stenting. In conclusion, the current recommendations are that patients who fail thrombolysis should proceed to rescue PCI.

*Delayed PCI*, performed electively 1 to 7 days after successful fibrinolysis without recurrent ischemia, was not shown to have added survival benefit, reduction of reinfarction, or LV preservation compared to conservative therapy (TIMI-2B).

Patients with acute MI complicated by cardiogenic shock have usually been excluded from major clinical trials. The only large study to address this issue (SHOCK) found that early revascularization (by PCI or CABG) for acute MI complicated by cardiogenic shock (not secondary to mechanical complications of acute MI) had improved long-term mortality benefit (after 6 months) compared to patients managed by medical therapy among patients 75 years of age and younger. Patients who were younger than 75 had reduced mortality at 30 days, and after 6 months, with PCI compared to medical therapy.

## Patients Who Are Undergoing PCI Post-CABG

Patients who undergo CABG are still at risk of ischemia, as a result of graft occlusion or progression of disease in the native vessels. Considering that repeat CABG carries a higher risk, a post-CABG patient with recurrent ischemia may require PCI procedures to the grafts or the native vessels. Timing of ischemia following CABG has been divided into very early (<30 days after CABG), early (30 days to 1 year after CABG), and late (>1 year after CABG). Ischemia within 30 days is usually secondary to graft failure from thrombosis. It can also be secondary to unbypassed native vessel disease. Ischemia occurring 30 days to 1 year following CABG is usually secondary to perianastomotic graft stenosis. Ischemia occurring >1 year after CABG is usually secondary to disease progression in the grafts and/or native coronary vessels. The role of PCI after CABG varies based on the timing of ischemia relative to the CABG procedure. PCI may be used to recanalize thrombosed vessels, dilate anastomotic points, or balloon or stent native vessels or grafts.

It is important to keep in mind that the choice of PCI versus redo CABG in patients with recurrent ischemia after CABG depends on graft conduits (arterial versus venous), the number of grafts and how many are occluded, the location of recurrent disease (in native vessels versus grafts), LV function, and associated co-morbidities. The ACC/AHA guidelines for PCI following CABG are shown in Table 17–5.

**TABLE 17–5**
**ACC/AHA RECOMMENDATIONS FOR PCI AFTER CABG**

| Class | | Level of Evidence |
|---|---|---|
| Class I | Patients with early ischemia within 30 d after CABG | B |
| Class IIa | Patients with ischemia 1–3 y after CABG with normal LV and focal lesions in the grafts | B |
| | Patients with ischemia from new disease in the native vessels | B |
| | Patients <3 y from CABG with diseased vein grafts | B |
| Class IIb | None | |
| Class III | Patients with chronic total vein graft occlusion | B |
| | Patients with multivessel disease, multiple SVG occlusion, and impaired LV | B |

CABG, coronary artery bypass graft, LV, left ventricular, SVG.
*Source:* Adapted from the ACC/AHA 2001 JACC 2001;37(8):2339i.

**TABLE 17–6**
**ACC/AHA CORONARY LESION CLASSIFICATION FOR PREDICTION OF PROCEDURAL SUCCESS AND COMPLICATIONS**

| | |
|---|---|
| Low risk/Type A lesion | Discrete (<1 cm in length), accessible to intervention, concentric, nonangulated (<45 degree), smooth contour, noncalcified, nonostial, no major side branch involvement, nonthrombotic lesions |
| Moderate risk/Type B lesion | Longer tubular lesions (1–2 cm in length), eccentric, angulated (45 degree), tortuous, irregular in contour, moderately or heavily calcified, subacute total occlusion (<3 mo), ostial lesions, bifurcating lesions, thrombotic lesions |
| High risk/Type C lesion | Diffuse (>2 cm in length), highly tortuous, extremely angulated (>90 degrees), chronic total occlusion (>3 mo), unprotected major side branch, degenerated vein grafts |

## PATIENT SELECTION AND PREDICTORS OF OUTCOME

Factors that can help predict the likelihood of procedural success or complications can be divided into two major categories: clinical predictors and angiographic predictors.

Clinical predictors include age, gender, heart failure, cardiogenic shock, unstable angina, evolving MI, other comorbidities such as diabetes mellitus, and chronic renal insufficiency (CRI). Patients older than 75 years of age are at increased risk of PCI complications, mainly because they have increased incidence of prior MIs, CHF, and associated morbidities. Diabetic patients are three times more likely to have complications from PCI, and have three times higher mortality rates than nondiabetics. Women presenting for PCI have similar procedural success rates as men with similar anatomy, similar in-hospital mortality, MI, emergency CABG, and 5-year mortality. However, women have a higher incidence of CHF and pulmonary edema compared to men with similar disease burden. This is postulated to be secondary to small vessel size in women, a greater incidence of diastolic dysfunction, and hypertension with older age when women present with coronary artery disease. Patients with chronic renal insufficiency have increased risk of post-PCI contrast nephropathy, particularly if they are diabetics and particularly if their creatinine is more greater than 2.0 mg/dL.

Angiographic predictors of outcomes involve focality of the lesion, total versus subtotal versus partial occlusions, degenerated SVG, restenosis after PTCA (increased long-term risk, but not acute risk), in-stent restenosis, small vessels, bifurcating lesions, ostial lesions, left main trunk disease (LMT) lesions, decreased LV function, multivessel CAD, amount of myocardium supplied by the vessel to be intervened upon, severity of calcification, length of the lesion, and angulation of the vessel. The classification systems that have been used for lesion description and risk stratification are the ACC/AHA classification with its modification and the Society for Cardiovascular Angiography and Interventions (SCAI) classification.

The current ACC/AHA lesion classification, issued in 1990, modified from the original issued in 1986, utilizes 26 lesion features, some of which were mentioned above. There are three major categories of lesion classification: low risk, moderate risk, and high risk (Table 17–6). The initial ACC/AHA classification, developed in the PTCA era, is not as useful in the stent and glycoprotein IIb/IIIa inhibitor era. Also, the procedural success rates are not applicable in the stent era. The outcomes of Type B lesions have improved with the use of coronary stents. In addition, the various features of Type B lesions as described in the initial guidelines are not equal in terms of risk. Bifurcating lesions, for example, are higher risk than eccentric lesions or moderate-length lesions. Thus, in 1990, Ellis et al. proposed to further subdivide the B lesions into B1 and B2 types. Lesion Type B1 has one Type B characteristic, whereas a Type B2 lesion has two or more Type B characteristics. In their evaluation, Ellis et al. found that the modified B1/B2 lesion classification system and the presence of diabetes were the only variables that were independently predictive of procedural success. Analysis of success and complications according to this scheme showed 92% success and 2% complication rate for Type A lesions; for Type B1 lesions, an 84% success and 4% complication rate was seen; for Type B2 lesions, a 76% success and a 10% complication rate; for Type C lesions, a 61% success rate and a 21% complication rate. It is important to keep in mind that these rates are reflective of the prestent and pre–glycoprotein IIb/IIIa era.

The SCAI has proposed another system for lesion classification. This system uses vessel patency in addition to the ACC/AHA classification to predict procedure complication and success. Class B and C lesions are further subdivided into patent and occluded lesions. There are four classes in the SCAI system (Table 17–7). Basically, the SCAI system emphasizes the importance of Type C lesion and occluded vessels in predicting success and complications.

**TABLE 17–7**
**SOCIETY FOR CARDIAC ANGIOGRAPHY AND INTERVENTIONS (SCAI) LESION CLASSIFICATION**

| | | |
|---|---|---|
| Type I lesion | Non-C and patent lesion | 96.8% success rate |
| Type II lesion | Patent C lesion | 90% success rate |
| Type III lesion | Non-C and occluded lesion | 87.6% success rate |
| Type IV lesion | Occluded C lesion | 75% success rate |

With the advent of stents and the wide use of glycoprotein IIb/IIIa inhibitors during PCI, there were dramatic changes in the approach to PCI, allowing treatment of more complex lesions with lower overall risk. The new approach to PCI needed a more updated classification system concordant with the current use of stents and IIb/IIIa inhibitors. Ellis et al. proposed such a new classification system in 1999. The risk factors were divided into:

- Strongest correlates (nonchronic total occlusion and degenerated SVG)
- Moderately strong correlates ($\geq$10-mm lesion length, lumen irregularity, large filling defect, calcium and angle >45°, eccentric lesion, severe calcification, or SVG $\geq$10 years)

The lesions were classified into:

- Class I/low risk (no risk factors)
- Class II/moderate risk (1 to 2 moderate correlates and the absence of strong correlates)
- Class III/high risk ($\geq$3 moderate correlates and the absence of strong correlates)
- Class IV/highest risk (either of the strongest correlates)

These classes (I to IV) had risks of death, MI, or emergency CABG of 2.1%, 3.4%, 8.2%, and 12.7%, respectively. In the same analysis, the scheme was validated against the ACC/AHA classification. Class A lesions had 2.5% risk of death, MI, or emergency CABG. Class B1 had 3% risk, B2 had 5.2% risk, and class C had 6.6% risk. The proposed classification scheme is more predictive than the ACC/AHA lesion scheme. It reflects current practice with use of IIb/IIIa inhibitors (41% of patients in the study) and stenting (64% of patients in the study). The study utilizes fewer specific correlates (nine) and risk factors, making it easier to use and more applicable in clinical practice.

## CLINICAL TRIALS

In this section, we review in more detail the major clinical trials in separate categories, comparing and contrasting the various revascularization strategies as divided in Table 17–8. Keep in mind that this approach is somewhat historic; many advances in techniques, devices (particularly stents), and pharmacotherapy (e.g., glycoprotein IIb/IIIa inhibitors, statins, angiotensin-converting enzyme [ACE] inhibitors bivalirudin) were not available during most of these trials. However, it is important to see the progression of available data into the stent era, which defined evidence-based practice and formed the basis for most of the PCI ACC/AHA guidelines.

**TABLE 17–8**
**SUMMARY OF MAJOR CLINICAL TRIALS COMPARING VARIOUS THERAPEUTIC MODALITIES AND REVASCULARIZATION STRATEGIES**

| Medical Therapy vs. PCI in Stable Angina | Conservative vs. Invasive Therapy in ACS | Medical Therapy vs. CABG | PCI vs. CABG | |
|---|---|---|---|---|
| | | | Isolated disease | Multivessel LAD disease |
| ACME | TIMI IIB | VA Cooperative | BARI | MASS |
| ACME 2 | VANQUISH | CASS | CABRI | SIMA |
| RITA II | FRISC II | European Cooperative | EAST | |
| AVERT | TACTICS-TIMI 18 | | GABI | |
| TIME | RITA III | | RITA I | |
| ACIP | | | ERACI-I | |
| | | | ERACI-II (stent) | |
| | | | ARTS (stent) | |
| | | | ARTS II (stent) | |
| | | | SOS (stent) | |

ACS, acute coronary syndrome; CABG, coronary artery bypass grant.

## Medical Therapy versus PCI

*ACME.* The Veterans Affairs ACME trial was a randomized trial comparing medical therapy versus plain old balloon angioplasty (POBA) in 212 patients with single- and double-vessel coronary artery disease. In the single-vessel group, there was no difference in death or MI between the two groups; however, PCI offered earlier and more complete relief of angina and was associated with better exercise tolerance and less ischemia during exercise testing at 6 months. Among the patients with double-vessel disease, no difference was found between the treatment groups in relief from angina or exercise duration.

*ACME-2.* The ACME-2 trial was a randomized comparison of PTCA versus medical therapy in 101 patients with stable angina and evidence of ischemia on stress testing. At 6 months there was no difference in exercise duration, freedom from angina, or overall quality-of-life score.

*RITA-II.* The RITA-II trial was a randomized trial comparing the long-term effects of PTCA versus conservative care in 1,018 patients considered suitable for either treatment option. After 2.7 years, death or definite MI occurred in 6.3% of patients treated with PCI, whereas these endpoints occurred in 3.3% of patients with medical care ($p = 0.02$). Adverse events included one death and seven periprocedural nonfatal MIs. At 7 years the incidence of death or MI was comparable in both groups. PCI was associated with greater symptomatic improvement. This study lags behind contemporary practice, however, because only 7.6% of the patients received stents, and the antiplatelet regimens used were not mentioned.

*AVERT.* The AVERT trial compared statin therapy to PCI in 341 stable patients with mild or no symptoms. After 18 months, 13% of patents who received aggressive statin therapy had experienced ischemic events, compared with 21% of patients who underwent PCI ($p = 0.048$). This result was not statistically significant when adjusted for interim analysis. A limitation of the study was that restenosis requiring reintervention was more likely to occur in the PCI group than the conservatively treated group, and only 30% of the PCI group received stents. In addition, the PCI group did not receive aggressive contemporary statin therapy. Statins did not show an anti-ischemic effect, but the study suggested they might prevent coronary events.

*ACIP.* The ACIP trial compared strategies of angina-guided medical therapy, ischemia-guided medical therapy, revascularization with CABG, or PTCA in 558 patients with documented CAD and severe symptoms who had both stress-induced ischemia and at least one episode of silent ischemia on 48-hour Holter monitoring. After 2 years, the total mortality was 6.6% in the angina-guided group, 4.4% in the ischemia-guided group, and 1.1% in those receiving revascularization. These data suggested a benefit from initial revascularization compared to medical therapy for relief of ischemia.

*TIME.* The TIME trial compared revascularization versus medical therapy in 301 patients >75 years old with Canadian Cardiac Society (CCS) Class II chronic angina despite taking at least two antiangina drugs. Patients had relief from angina and improvement in quality of life regardless of their assignment to invasive or medical therapy. At 6 months, however, a major adverse event (death, nonfatal MI, or repeat hospitalization) had occurred more frequently in the medical treatment group (49% versus 19%). Survival rates were better if patients were revascularized within the first year.

A meta-analysis of the above six studies indicated that PTCA is more effective than medical therapy in relieving angina (risk ratio 0.70, 95% CI). However, there was no difference between the two modalities in terms of the risk of MI, death, or need for PTCA and/or CABG in the future.

Overall, PCI is more effective than medical therapy in relieving angina and improving exercise capacity in patients with chronic stable angina. Although PCI alone has not been shown to prevent MI or lower mortality, a strategy of initial medical management in this population is safe.

## Conservative Therapy versus Invasive Therapy in Acute Coronary Syndrome

According to the CRUSDADE registry, a group of 30,295 high-risk non–ST-elevation acute coronary syndrome (NSTEACS) patients who were treated at 248 U.S. hospitals between March 2000 and September 2002, <50% of those eligible underwent an invasive procedure. Proponents of a conservative strategy cite the following studies.

*TIMI IIIB.* The Thrombolysis In Myocardial Ischemia (TIMI) IIIB trial compared 1,473 patients with unstable angina to alteplase or placebo, and to a conservative or early invasive approach. In the conservative arm, patients underwent catheterization only if they developed evidence of recurrent ischemia. In the invasive arm, cardiac catheterization was performed within 18 to 24 hours, followed by POBA or CABG as indicated. At 1 year there was no difference in death or nonfatal MI between the groups, although the invasive treatment group had shorter hospital stays and fewer rehospitalizations.

*VANQWISH.* The Veterans Affairs Non-Q Wave Infarction Strategies In-Hospital (VANQUISH) trial compared 920 patients with NSTEMI to an early invasive strategy (coronary angiography followed by revascularization as dictated by anatomic findings) 72 hours after the last episode of chest pain or an early conservative strategy with angiography and revascularization only if spontaneous ischemia was associated with ST-segment changes or if a thallium stress test suggested the presence of residual ischemia. Revascularization was performed on 44% of the patients randomized to the invasive approach. At the time of hospital discharge, death and nonfatal MI had occurred more frequently in this group (7.8% versus 3.2%, $p = 0.004$).

Proponents for an early invasive approach in acute coronary syndrome (ACS) cite the following studies.

*FRISC II.* The second Fragmin and Fast Revascularization during Instability in Coronary artery Disease (FRISC) trial examined 2,457 patients with unstable angina who were randomly assigned after 48 hours to an invasive approach (catheterization followed by intervention within 7 days) or a noninvasive approach (angiography only if there was objective evidence of ischemia). The rate of death or MI was lower in the invasive approach group at 1 year (10.4% versus 14.1%, $p = 0.005$). Additionally, there was a 50% reduction in angina and need for readmission in the invasive group.

*TACTICS-TIMI 18.* In the Treat Angina with aggrastat and determine Cost of Therapy with an Invasive or Conservative Strategy–Thrombolysis In Myocardial Infarction (TACTICS-TIMI 18) trial, 2,220 unstable angina and NSTEMI patients were randomized to an invasive (catheterization within 4 to 48 hours followed by PCI or CABG) approach or conservative medical therapy. All patients received aspirin, beta-blockers, heparin, and tirofiban for 48 to 108 hours. At 6 months, death, MI, and revascularization occurred less frequently with an invasive strategy (15.8% versus 19.4% OR 0.78, $p = 0.025$).

*RITA-III.* In the RITA-III trial, 1,810 patients with NSTEMI were randomized to early angiography (within 2 days) and revascularization (primary POBA) compared to conservative therapy. At 4 months, the combined endpoint of death, MI, and refractory angina was lower in the invasive group (9.6% versus 14.5%, $P = 0.001$).

*ISAR-COOL.* The ISAR-COOL trial compared a medical "cooling off" strategy versus immediate PCI in NSTEMI patients. All patients received aspirin, clopidogrel, heparin, and tirofiban. Median time to catheterization was 86 hours in the "cooling off" strategy and 2.4 hours in the immediate PCI group. The primary endpoint of death or nonfatal MI at 30 days occurred in 11.6% of patients in the "cooling off" group and in 5.9% in the immediate PCI group ($p = 0.04$).

Many lessons were learned during these various trials, not the least of which is the importance of patient selection and risk stratification, which allow the cardiologist to tailor treatment strategies on a patient-to-patient basis. Higher-risk patients are likely to benefit from an earlier, more invasive approach, whereas low- to intermediate-risk patients may be initially treated successfully with medical therapy.

## Medical Therapy versus CABG

*VA Cooperative Study.* This study was designed to compare the effects of CABG to standard medical therapy on survival, incidence of MI, and relief of symptoms. Multiple reports including 10-year, 17–year, and 22-year follow-up were published subsequently. The VA Cooperative Study represents the longest and most complete follow-up of any randomized trial of bypass surgery versus medical therapy. It is important to note that the study was done between 1972 and 1974, when medical therapy was limited to aspirin and beta-blockers; statins and ACE inhibitors were not yet available. Furthermore, internal mammary arteries (IMA) were not used in CABG. In the study, 686 patients with stable angina were randomized to medical therapy or CABG. Survival was superior in the CABG group up to 7 years only, despite high operative mortality at that time (5.8%). A significant survival benefit in CABG patients was observed in high-risk subgroups, including patients with prior MI during follow-up. This survival benefit was attributed to duration of graft patency (7 to 10 years). Patients with significant left main disease (LMT) had better survival when treated with CABG.

*CASS.* The National Heart, Lung, and Blood Institute (NHLB) Coronary Artery Surgery Study was a multicenter patient registry and a randomized controlled clinical trial. Between 1975 and 1979, 780 patients with stable coronary artery disease were randomized to CABG or medical therapy (nitrates and beta-blockers). There was no significant difference in survival rates between the two treatment groups, or for most of the subgroups (patients with single-, double-, or triple-vessel disease). Patients with three vessel disease and LVEF $< 50\%$ had better survival with surgery. The limitation of the study, as in the VA Cooperative Study, is that medical therapy in the 1970s was limited to aspirin, beta-blockers, and nitrates.

*European Coronary Surgery Study Group.* This multicenter study randomized 768 patients with at least two-vessel disease between medical therapy and CABG.

Survival was significantly better in patients randomized to CABG compared to those given medical therapy. This survival advantage was increased if patients had significant LMT disease, three-vessel disease, or two-vessel disease with proximal LAD disease. No significant difference between the two groups in patients with two-vessel disease was seen. Patients who had CABG received significantly less beta-blockers compared to patients in the medical therapy group. Furthermore, patients who had CABG had significantly more symptomatic relief of angina compared to those on medical therapy. Exercise performance increased in both treatment subgroups, but was significantly increased in the surgical groups compared with the medical group. This difference tended to diminish with time. The study cannot be compared to the VA study because of significant population differences. In the VA study, patients had lower ejection fractions, some patients had single-vessel disease, and the study population was older. Furthermore, operative mortality in the VA study was higher than in this study.

A meta-analysis of the above trials, as well as other smaller studies comparing medical treatment to CABG, was completed. The overall population from all studies combined was 2,649 patients. There was a clear survival benefit in the CABG group over the medical therapy group. This was mainly for patients with three-vessel disease, and LMT disease. It took nearly 2 years for the survival benefit to appear, mostly because of the increased up-front risk of operative mortality during CABG and that benefit had begun to narrow by year ten.

## PCI versus CABG

PCI, on the one hand, is a relatively easy procedure that avoids general anesthesia, thoracotomy, extracorporeal circulation with secondary CNS complications, and a prolonged recovery period. On the other hand, PCI has its own limitations, including risk of early restenosis and inability to revascularize many totally occluded arteries or arteries with extensive atherosclerotic lesions. CABG has greater durability, with >90% graft patency at 10 years using arterial conduits. CABG can be used to completely revascularize complex lesions. The major finding in many of these trials was that survival was similar with CABG and PTCA; although patients with diffuse CAD were excluded from randomization. However, repeat intervention was much more common with PTCA. Comparison between PCI and CABG should be divided into two subsets, isolated LAD disease and multivessel disease, with and without drug-eluting stents (DES). Studies comparing treatment modalities for multivessel disease include the following.

*BARI*. The Bypass Angioplasty Revascularization Investigation was a multicenter study completed between 1988 and 1991. The study compared the effectiveness of POBA to CABG in 1,829 symptomatic patients with multivessel disease undergoing a first revascularization procedure. The initial mean follow-up was 5.4 years. There was no significant difference in 5-year survival between POBA and CABG. However, patients who had CABG instead of PTCA had fewer hospitalizations, fewer subsequent revascularization procedures, and a greater improvement of angina. However, they had higher rates of in-hospital Q-wave MI compared to the PTCA group. Furthermore, treatment with CABG was associated with higher survival rates among diabetic patients compared to PTCA. The benefit of CABG in diabetic patients was more evident in patients requiring insulin, those who received internal mammary grafts, and those who had four or more lesions.

*CABRI*. The Coronary Angioplasty versus Bypass Revascularization Investigation trial was a European multinational, multicenter (26-center) study that looked at 1,054 patients with follow-up at 1 year and 5 years. Similar to BARI, the patients were symptomatic with multivessel disease. As in BARI, there was no difference in mortality rates between the two revascularization modalities at 1 year. Patients who received PTCA required significantly more reinterventions, had more clinically significant angina (particularly among women), and required more medications at 1 year compared to CABG patients. This was secondary to increased restenosis and a higher likelihood of residual disease following PTCA compared to CABG.

*EAST*. The Emory Angioplasty versus Surgery Trial was a smaller (392 patients) single-center study with follow-up at 1 year and 3 years. Patients had multivessel disease, 60% two-vessel disease, 40% three-vessel disease, and had not had prior revascularization procedures. The combined endpoint of mortality, Q-wave MI, and thallium perfusion defect were similar between the PTCA and CABG groups. Similar to the above two studies, more patients treated with PTCA required additional revascularization procedures at 3 years (70% versus 87%, $p < 0.001$).

*GABI*. The German Angioplasty Surgery Investigation was a multicenter study. The patients had complete revascularization of at least two major vessels supplying different myocardial segments by either PTCA or CABG. The primary endpoint was freedom of angina at 1 year. Secondary endpoints included death, MI, and the need for revascularization. The results showed that both CABG and PTCA were equally effective in relieving angina at 1 year. In addition, in-hospital deaths were similar between the two groups. However, more patients in the CABG groups sustained Q-wave MI and had periprocedure morbidity during hospitalization, as among the BARI. Patients in the PTCA group required more interventions, as in BARI and CABRI.

*RITA-I.* The Randomized Intervention Treatment of Angina trial followed 1,011 patients in the United Kingdom over 5 years. The trial compared the long-term effects of PTCA and CABG in patients with one, two, or three diseased vessels, with lesions deemed equivalent in terms of revascularization achieved by either procedure. Of these patients, 55% had two or more diseased coronary arteries, leaving 45% with single-vessel disease. The inclusion of single-vessel disease patients in this study was interesting, because this is usually not an indication for CABG (unless LAD). There was no difference in death rate between the PTCA and CABG groups (3.1% versus 3.6%). Similarly, there was no difference in the rates of nonfatal MI. As in the above studies, patients who received PTCA had higher rates of repeat coronary angiography (31% versus 7%), revascularization procedures (32% versus 5%), and increased frequency of angina compared to the CABG group.

*ERACI-I.* This Argentine randomized trial similarly compared PTCA to CABG in 127 patients with multivessel disease. As in RITA-I, the lesions were equally amenable to PTCA and CABG. There was no difference in death rates and freedom from MI between the two groups. However, freedom from angina, repeat revascularization, and from combined events was higher in the CABG group compared to the PTCA group. More complete anatomic revascularizations were achieved by CABG compared to PTCA (88% versus 51%, $p < 0.001$). There was no difference in terms of in-hospital complications. The in-hospital cost and added cost at 1 year (despite the need for more revascularization procedures) were still lower in the PTCA group compared to the CABG group.

Pocock et al. completed a meta-analysis of the above trials (BARI was not included). There was no difference in cardiac death or MI at 1 year between CABG and PCI. However, as shown above, CABG was better at relieving angina pectoris than PTCA. Patients who had CABG required fewer revascularization procedures compared to the PTCA group. Keep in mind that in the above analysis, patients were a relatively low-risk population: <10% had LV dysfunction, and 70% had one- or two-vessel disease.

Since the above studies were performed, stents have been shown to decrease acute complications, late stenosis, and the need for repeat revascularization. Hence, since their introduction, several trials have compared PCI (with stenting) to CABG in symptomatic patients with multivessel disease. These trials include ERACI-II, ARTS, and SOS. However, the data on the need for repeat target vessel revascularization in these trials are probably not applicable to current practice, given the availability of drug-eluting stents that markedly reduce restenosis.

*ERACI-II.* This Argentine randomized study was larger than ERACI-I: 450 patients were randomized to PCI with stenting or to CABG. Significant differences were seen in hospital and 30-day outcomes between the two strategies of revascularization. Mortality was lower in the stenting group (0.9% versus 5.7% in the CABG group, $p < 0.013$). Similarly, the rate of Q-wave MI was lower in the stenting group versus the CABG group (0.9% versus 5.7%, $p < 0.013$). These advantages were maintained at 1-year follow-up. Like the previous studies, freedom from repeat revascularization was significantly improved with the CABG patients compared to stenting (95.2% versus. 83.2%, $p < 0.001$). Unlike in ERACI-I, the short-term and long-term cost of either technique was similar. This is partly secondary to the cost of stents, glycoprotein IIb/IIIa inhibitors, in-hospital complications, and repeat revascularization procedures. It is important to point out that despite the increased need for repeat revascularization procedures with stenting compared to CABG, the rate of repeat procedures was lower than that observed in PTCA without stenting (16.8% versus a range of 30% to 40%).

*ARTS-I.* The Arterial Revascularization Study was a multicenter study that randomized 1,205 patients with multivessel disease to PCI with stenting (bare-metal stents [BMS]) or CABG. The study population included 17% who were diabetic. At 1 year, there was no difference in death, stroke, or MI between the two groups. Event-free survival was lower with stenting compared to CABG, due primarily to an increase in repeat revascularization in the stenting group. Event-free survival was significantly lower in diabetic patients undergoing stenting compared to those treated with CABG (63% versus 84%). PCI with stenting was more cost effective than CABG during the initial hospitalization. The net difference remained in favor of stenting, but it decreased by 1 year. Throughout the 1-year period of observation, more patients were free of angina after bypass surgery than after stenting.

*ARTS II.* ARTS II was a multicenter, prospective registry of patients with multivessel disease who had sirolimus-eluting stents placed. This was a single-arm study with similar entry criteria to ARTS-I. The main goal was to demonstrate noninferiority in clinical effectiveness and cost effectiveness of sirolimus-eluting stents compared to the data from ARTS-I. The primary endpoint was freedom from major cardiac and cerebrovascular events (MACCE). Patients who received sirolimus-DES had less MACCE than either ARTS-I (CABG) patients or ARTS-I (PCI with BMS) patients. Furthermore, patients who received sirolimus-DES had lower composite endpoints of death/CVA/MI than ARTS-I (CABG) and ARTS-I (PCI). With regard to revascularization, ARTS-II patients had higher rates of CABG or repeat revascularization than ARTS-I (CABG) patients, but lower rates than ARTS-I (PCI with BMS) patients. Though this was a registry and not a randomized trial, the data are reassuring regarding the use of sirolimus stents as a strategy for patients with multivessel disease who are suitable for stenting.

*SOS*. The Stent Or Surgery trial randomized 988 symptomatic patients with multivessel disease to PCI with stenting or CABG with an arterial graft. PCI with stenting was associated with a significantly higher incidence of repeat revascularization, as in ARTS and ERACI-II (21% versus 6%). There were significantly more deaths with PCI compared to CABG (5% versus 2%, hazard ratio 2.9), due to a large number of cancer deaths in the stenting group. The incidence of cardiac, vascular, and noncardiovascular mortality was higher in the PCI group than in the CABG group. As observed in prior studies, patients were more angina free at 1 year in the CABG group. Of note, SOS reported only a very limited use of glycoprotein IIb/IIIa inhibitors.

*MASS*. The Medicine, Angioplasty or Surgery Study was a prospective randomized trial of medical therapy, PTCA, or CABG for single proximal LAD disease. It was a single-center study of 214 patients with stable angina and normal LV function, and a proximal LAD stenosis of >80%. There was no difference in mortality or MI rates among the three groups at 3 years follow-up. All three strategies resulted in controlling angina, though CABG and PTCA resulted in greater symptomatic relief. There was less need for revascularization in the CABG group. The study recommended a more aggressive therapeutic approach, with initial CABG for patients with severe proximal LAD disease, despite no added mortality or MI benefit.

*SIMA*. The objective of the Stenting versus Internal Mammary Artery study was to compare CABG with stenting in patients with proximal isolated LAD disease. The patients had ejection fraction (EF) >45%. SIMA was a multicenter study in which 123 patients were randomized to CABG or stenting. The primary composite endpoint was event-free survival, with no death, MI, or need for revascularization. Secondary endpoints were functional class, antianginal therapy, and quality of life. The primary endpoint occurred in 31% of patients in the stenting group versus 7% of patients in the CABG group ($p < 0.001$). The significant difference in clinical outcome was due to a higher incidence of additional revascularization in the stent group. The incidence of death and MI were similar between the two groups. The functional class, need for antianginal therapy, and quality-of-life assessment showed no significant difference between stenting and CABG.

Recently, Hannan et al. published a report on long-term outcomes of CABG versus stent implantation. They used observation data obtained from New York registries that identified 37,212 patients with multivessel disease who underwent CABG, and 22,102 patients with multivessel disease who underwent PCI. Survival rates in all anatomic subgroups, particularly if the patients had more than two diseased coronary arteries, were significantly higher among patients who had CABG than among those who received a stent. Need for revascularization was considerably higher in the stent groups than in the CABG group. However, patients who underwent CABG were significantly older, had lower ejection fractions, had more coexisting conditions, and were more likely to have three-vessel CAD compared to the stent group. Note that this was not a randomized, controlled trial, and observational studies may fail to identify all confounders. Furthermore, since most of the above studies (CABG versus stenting) were completed, drug-eluting stents have been introduced and "off-pump" CABG has become more common. Certainly, future studies will be needed to compare long-term outcomes for DES with CABG in patients with various anatomies and co-morbidities. For now, there are many considerations when a physician is deciding on CABG versus percutaneous intervention, such as age, life expectancy, co-morbidities, and expertise in available services.

## COMPLICATIONS

Complications following PCI vary according to the baseline clinical severity of the patient, operator skill, and technologic capability. It is important to remember that techniques of PCI, competing technologies (DES, etc.) and adjunctive pharmacotherapeutic regimens are evolving and will continue to affect the incidence of complications associated with PCI and possibly precipitating as yet unrecognized complications. With the recent dramatic advances in technology, PCI success rates are higher and patient clinical factors play a dominant role in predicting outcomes.

### Patient Risk Assessment

Decisions on access site (femoral versus brachial versus radial), guide catheters and guidewires, whether to balloon or primary stent, the type, length, and size of the stent, and whether to use adjunctive devices such as filter devices or brachytherapy should be left to the acumen of the interventional cardiologist based on current data. The introduction of glycoprotein IIb/IIIa inhibitors and stents in the 1990s has decreased the incidence of emergency CABG and STEMI to <1%. Also, the incidence of NSTEMI was approximately 5% in most trials and the need for blood transfusion 3%, while stroke is a complication in 0.07% to 0.4% of procedures. Mortality after PCI varies between 1.1% to 1.7% and several multivariable risk models exist, mostly validated within the institution at which they were developed, but others created by the American College of Cardiology National Cardiovascular Data Registry (ACC/NCDR).

Understanding of clinical and anatomic risk factors is essential to enable the cardiologist to gauge potential risk and have been discussed under risk stratification. Clinical and anatomic risk factors for major complications (death, MI, urgent CABG) with an odds ratio >2.0 are given here.

Clinical risk factors with an overall risk of major complications of 5% are

- Acute MI/ACS
- Age >80 years
- IABP pre-PCI
- Creatinine >2.0 mg/dL
- Female sex

Anatomic risk factors with an overall risk of a major complication of 2% to 13% are

- Older severely diseased SVG
- Nonchronic total occlusions
- Lesion length >10 mm
- Presence of thrombus
- Calcified and angulated vessels >45 degrees

Factors such as anemia, prior beta-blocker use, left ventricular ejection fraction, same-vessel intervention, and prior bypass also affect risk.

The Mayo Clinic derived a risk score to identify contemporary patients at increased risk for major complications after PCI. The score was derived from >5,600 first PCI procedures performed between 1996 and 1999 and then validated in almost 1,800 procedures performed in 2000. The score is relevant to current clinical practice because it was performed after stenting became routine, plus patients were usually treated with thienopyridine and intravenous glycoprotein IIb/IIIa inhibitors (Tables 17–9 and 17–10). A predictive point score was based on eight clinical and angiographic variables; the usual score ranged from 0 to 25. Major complications include in-hospital mortality, ST-elevation MI, urgent or emergency CABG, and stroke.

Hypotension is a common complication during PCI and has a variety of causes:

- Ischemia/acute vessel closure
- Coronary perforation/tamponade
- Hypovolemia/bleeding
- Vagal reaction
- Drug reaction
- Dissection of coronary arteries

**TABLE 17–9**
**MAYO CLINIC COMPLICATION RISK SCORING SYSTEM**

| Predictors of Complications | Score |
|---|---|
| Age (1 point for each decade above 40) | 40–49 = 1 point, 50–59 = 2 points, etc. |
| Periprocedural shock | 5 |
| Left main disease | 5 |
| Creatinine >3 mg/dL | 3 |
| Multivessel disease | 2 |
| NYHA Class III/IV congestive heart failure | 2 |
| Urgent or emergent PCI | 2 |
| Presence of thrombus | 2 |

*Source:* Modified from Singh et al. JACC 2002;40:387.

Acute vessel closure manifests by acute ischemia and hypotension during the PCI and can be caused by coronary dissection, intracoronary thrombus formation, and guide catheter damping and coronary spasm. The incidence of coronary perforation and tamponade is approximately 0.1% to 0.3%. These patients usually present with hypotension, and this complication is fatal in 25% of cases.

Risk factors associated with coronary perforation are

- Old age
- Female sex
- Use of devices (atheroablative or intravascular ultrasound)
- Distal migration of hydrophilic wires in the presence of antiplatelet therapy
- High-pressure stent implantation

Management of hypotension that is refractory to fluid resuscitation should include assessment of LMT dissection or occult perforation. If the occlusion cannot be readily reversed, IABP placement should be performed along with hemodynamic stabilization with inotropic support if necessary, followed by emergency CABG.

**TABLE 17–10**
**RISK OF MAJOR COMPLICATIONS BASED ON MAYO CLINIC SCORING SYSTEM**

| Risk Score | Risk of Complications (%) |
|---|---|
| Very low risk (0–5) | 0–2% |
| Low risk (6–8) | 2–5% |
| Moderate risk (9–11) | 5–20% |
| High risk (12–14) | 10–25% |
| Very high risk (15–25) | >25% |

### Other Complications of PCI

PCI may be followed by several more minor complications, many of which are similar to those following diagnostic catheterization. Those more specific to PCI include:

- Hypotension, discussed above
- Retained guidewire: A rare complication caused by entrapment of the distal end of a guidewire in a high-grade stenosis. These can be removed by a commercially available snare or bioptome if in the proximal vessel. If this is unsuccessful, surgical removal of the retained fragment should be considered, unless fragments are confined to branch vessels.
- Ventricular arrhythmias: Occur in 1.5% to 2% of patients undergoing PCI. Etiologies include forceful injection into the right coronary artery if dye is allowed to remain static in the coronary vessel. Correction of electrolyte disturbance and treatment of the arrhythmia according to the ACLS standard is recommended.
- New conduction defects: New defects are noted in 0.9% of PCI cases but almost always disappear by hospital discharge.
- Dissection: Dissection may occur secondary to trauma from the guidewire as well as during balloon inflation. It appears as slow flow of contrast through the dissection and the distal portion. Usually, the area requires PTCA and stenting to restore flow.
- Intramural hematoma: Coronary artery intramural hematoma is defined as an accumulation of blood within the medial space displacing the internal elastic membrane inward and the external elastic membrane outward, with or without identifiable entry and exit points. It can occur in 6.7% of procedures; the incidence is lower with stenting compared to PTCA. Patients may have a higher incidence of TVR at 30 days.
- Side-branch occlusion: Occlusion of side branches has been reported in up to 19% of cases in the bare-metal stent era. However, by 6 to 9 months, the majority of these branches are patent. Stent-induced occlusion of a branch may result in significant ischemia, leaving the branch in "stent jail." It is often possible to place a guidewire into this jailed branch and dilate it through the stent struts.
- Vascular access site complications are among the most common complications and occur in up to 5% of patients. These include need for blood transfusion (3%), arteriovenous fistula (2%), pseudo-aneurysm (up to 5%), acute occlusion (3%), and infections (<0.1%).
- Contrast-induced nephropathy (CIN) can occur in up to 20% of patients. Renal failure is manifest as an increase in serum creatinine of ≥25% and/or ≥0.5 mg/dL. The risk factors and predictive scores for developing renal failure after PCI are shown in Tables 17–11 and 17–12.

**TABLE 17–11**
**RISK FACTORS FOR CIN FOLLOWING PCI**

| Independent Predictors of CIN | Score |
|---|---|
| Hypotension SP <80 mm Hg for at least 1 h requiring inotropic support | 5 |
| IABP within 24 h periprocedurally | 5 |
| CHF | 5 |
| Chronic kidney disease baseline Cr >1.5 mg/dL | 4 |
| Diabetes | 3 |
| Age >75 y | 4 |
| Anemia, HCT<39% men, HCT<36% women | 3 |
| Volume of contrast (for each 100 cc used) | 1 |

CIN, contrast-induced nephropathy; SP, systolic pressure; IABP, intra-aortic balloon pump; CHF, congestive heart failure; HCT, hematocrit.

## ADJUNCT THERAPY FOR PCI

Pharmacotherapy has played an integral role since the first clinical application of PCI. The demand for improved clinical outcomes has led to more aggressive medical regimens and more efficacious therapies.

Pretreatment with an intracoronary (IC) bolus of nitroglycerine is recommended to unmask vasospasm, to assess true vessel size, and to reduce the risk of vasospastic reactions. Boluses may be repeated during the procedure. No or slow reflow (reduction in coronary flow without an obstructive lesion), most commonly caused by microvascular spasm and distal embolization, can be treated with intracoronary vasodilators. Powerful microvascular vasodilators include verapamil (200 $\mu$g), adenosine (36 to 72 $\mu$g), nitroprusside (50 to 200 $\mu$g), and nicardipine (100 to 200 $\mu$g). Lower-osmolar ionic contrast causes fewer arrhythmias and less nausea during angiography.

### Antiplatelet Therapies

Three classes of antiplatelet agents (aspirin, thienopyridines, and glycoprotein (GP) IIb/IIIa inhibitors) are currently used regularly in catheterization laboratories. Platelet activation and aggregation play a central role in

**TABLE 17–12**
**PREDICTIVE SCORES FOR CIN AND DIALYSIS POST-PCI BASED ON RISK FACTORS**

| Risk Score | Risk of CIN | Risk if Dialysis |
|---|---|---|
| ≤5 | 7.5% | 0.04% |
| 6–10 | 14% | 0.12% |
| 11–16 | 26.1% | 1.09% |
| ≥16 | 57.3% | 12.6% |

CIN, contrast-induced nephropathy.
*Source:* Modified from Mehran et al. JACC Vol. 44, No. 7, 2004.

the propagation of intracoronary thrombi after atherosclerotic plaque disruption that results in myocardial ischemia or infarction in the acute coronary syndromes (ACS), or the mechanical disruption that results from PCI.

### *Aspirin*

Aspirin inhibits cyclo-oxygenase (COX), thus blocking the conversion of arachidonic acid to thromboxane A2 in the platelets. Because it inhibits only one pathway by which platelet activation and aggregation occur, it is a relatively weak antiplatelet agent. Despite this, it is the cornerstone of treatment for ischemic syndromes, secondary prevention, and primary prevention in high-risk subgroups. The Antithrombotic Trialists' Collaboration meta-analysis showed that there is no greater benefit in reduction of events using chronic aspirin doses of >75 mg. M-HEART was the only placebo-controlled RCT, and it showed a significant improvement in clinical outcomes compared to placebo (30% versus 41%). Additionally, in the ISIS-2 trial, aspirin was shown to be almost as effective as streptokinase in the treatment of STEMI. Recently, the concept of aspirin resistance has been observed in up to 20% of patients and is linked to worse outcome. Aspirin sensitivity can manifest as a respiratory illness in up to 10% of patients and as an urticarial rash in 0.2% of patients. Desensitization can be performed by a rapid challenge procedure and may allow aspirin reintroduction within a few hours.

### *Glycoprotein IIb/IIIa Inhibitors*

Abciximab, eptifibatide, and tirofiban are the three GP-IIb/IIIa inhibitors that are commercially available. They block fibrinogen binding to the receptor that is critical to the process of platelet thrombus formation and serve as the final common pathway for platelet aggregation. However, they differ in their modes of action, costs, and the specific circumstances in which they should be used.

Abciximab is a chimeric monoclonal antibody that binds nonspecifically to the GPIIb/IIIa receptor. Additionally, abciximab inhibits Mac 1 and vitronectin receptors, potentially inhibiting white blood cell diapedesis and smooth muscle proliferation, respectively. In the EPILOG trial abciximab was given as a 0.25-mg/kg dose followed by a 0.125-μg/kg/min infusion (to a maximum dose of 10 μg/min) for 12 hours postprocedure. In this trial, heparin was weight adjusted at 70 IU/kg, which decreased the amount of bleeding that had been seen in previous trials.

Eptifibatide is a cyclic heptapeptide with a lysine–glycine–aspartic acid (KGD) sequence that binds selectively to the GP-IIb/IIIa receptor. The ESPRIT trial established the recommended dose of eptifibatide as two IV boluses of 180 μg/kg 10 minutes apart, followed by a 2-μg/kg/min infusion for 18 to 24 hours.

Tirofiban hydrochloride is a nonpeptide derivative of tyrosine that binds selectively to the GP-IIb/IIIa receptor. The optimal dosage regimen for Tirofiban has been the subject of recent trials. The ADVANCE trial used a dosage regimen of 25 μg/kg for 3 minutes, followed by 0.15 μg/kg/min for 24 to 48 hours.

For stable CAD, recent data from ISAR REACT suggest that there is no benefit to adding abciximab for patients undergoing PCI if they have been loaded with 600 mg of clopidogrel at least 2 hours before the procedure. Additionally, in the higher-risk diabetic group, results from the ISAR SWEET trial again suggest a lack of benefit if patients are similarly loaded with clopidogrel. However, these trials have been critiqued as underpowered, and larger studies will be needed to confirm these results. GP-IIb/IIIa inhibitors remain useful in unstable lesions, as bailout herapy (for the direct treatment of abrupt closure, no reflow, coronary thrombosis, or other similar PCI complicatons). In ACS, the TACTICS-TIMI 18 study used tirofiban to show the benefit of an early invasive strategy. The IMPACT II trial and the CAPTURE trials also confirm the benefit of using eptifibatide or abciximab in this setting. However abciximab has the most robust evidence for use during STEMI. A meta-analysis by Topol et al. shows an overall reduction in the composite endpoint of death, reinfarction, and TVR of 46% at 30 days.

## Antithrombin Therapies

The use of unfractionated heparin (UFH) to prevent thrombus formation has been standard since the first clinical application of PCI. Currently, UFH is given as an IV bolus of 100 IU/kg to maintain an activated clotting time (ACT) of 250 to 350 seconds, or 50 to 60 IU/kg to maintain an ACT of 200 to 250 seconds if a GP-IIb/IIIa inhibitor is used. The sheath can be removed when the ACT is <180 seconds if a closure device is not used. ACT-guided dosing is recommended because of the variable bioavailability of UFH. The antithrombotic effects of heparin are variable because of its strong binding to plasma proteins, leading to unpredictable levels of heparin. Low-molecular-weight heparin (LMWH) inhibits factor Xa, and because of its more consistent plasma levels, is considered more predictable. Although its use as a sole agent in PCI is scant, recent data suggest that both approaches appear to be safe and efficacious in patients with ACS, although a concern remains about increased bleeding rates with LMWH use. Additionally, UFH is effectively reversed with protamine, whereas LMWH is only partially reversed. Currently there is no evidence to support a preference for LMWH over UFH.

Bivalirudin is a direct thrombin inhibitor and has been suggested as a replacement for UFH because it causes significantly less bleeding when compared with heparin alone in stable patients undergoing PCI. The REPLACE-2 trial established that bivalirudin monotherapy in a dose of 0.75 mg/kg bolus prior to the start of PCI plus provisional

GPIIb/IIIa inhibition, followed by infusion of 1.75 mg/kg per hour for the procedure duration, is comparable to heparin plus GP-IIb/IIIa inhibition in patients undergoing elective and urgent PCI. The half-life of bivalirudin is 25 minutes in patients with normal renal function, and the sheath can be removed in 1 to 2 hours after completion of the procedure. The reduction in hemorrhagic complications, cost savings, and ease of administration establish bivalirudin plus provisional GPIIb/IIIa inhibition as an attractive antithrombotic strategy for patients undergoing elective or urgent PCI. Unfortunately, the effects of bivalirudin cannot be reversed.

### Thienopyridines

Both ticlopidine and clopidogrel inhibit adenosine diphosphate (ADP)-receptor-mediated platelet activation and have been shown to reduce the incidence of acute and subacute thrombosis after PCI following stent implantation. Clopidogrel is considered safer and more efficacious. Aspirin and clopidogrel are synergistic in their antiplatelet effects. At present, the majority of PCI procedures conclude with stent implantation, and patients should be considered for pretreatment with clopidogrel and aspirin. The CREDO and TARGET propensity analyses suggest that 300 mg of clopidogrel should be given at least 2 hours before PCI. The ISAR REACT study and the recently published ARMYADA-2 study suggest that if a 600-mg loading dose of clopidogrel is used in a stable patient, then GP-IIb/IIIa inhibitors may be unnecessary. The duration of clopidogrel treatment after PCI is subject to debate. If a bare-metal stent is used, treatment for 4 weeks may suffice; however, if a drug-eluting stent is used, clopidogrel should be continued for at least 6 and possibly 12 months or longer after stent implantation.

## TECHNICAL ASPECTS OF ANGIOGRAPHY AND PCI

Covering all the technical aspects of angiography and PCI in detail is beyond the scope of this book. We will attempt to cover the topics that may be seen on the boards.

### Stents

The concept of implanting intravascular stents to support the arterial wall was proposed in 1964 by Dotter and Judkins. Today, more than 1 million stents are implanted each year in the United States. There are a variety of different types of intracoronary stents. They vary in

- Metallic composition: stainless steel (BX-Velocity, MultiLink), nitinol (Radius), tantalum, and platinum (Wallstent). Gold coating has been added to improve radiographic opacity.
- Strut design: different numbers of cells, thick versus thin struts.
- Delivery and deployment systems.
- Luminal surface coverage: closed-cell and open-cell designs. The former cover more of the luminal surface and as a result are less flexible. The latter cover less of the luminal surface and as a result are more flexible so it is easier to reach side branches.

These characteristics affect the flexibility and ease of delivery of the stent into the coronary artery.

Stents can be classified into various categories:

- Balloon expandable (BX-Velocity, Express, Multi-Link Tetra and Ultra) versus self-expandable (Radius, Magic Wallstent).
- Tubular (Bx-Velocity, Express, Multi-Link) versus coil (Flexstent, Wiktor) versus hybrid (AVE GFX, S7).
- Short (8 to 18 mm) versus medium length (23 to 28 mm) versus long (>30 mm).
- Bifurcating stents.
- Coated stents: Heparin-coated stents and silicon carbide-coated have been used in an attempt to reduce thrombogenic potential of stents.
- Covered stents: The JoStent balloon-expandable stent with SVG covering has been used mainly in coronary perforation.
- Drug-eluting stents: These stents are designed to provide local and sustained delivery of antiproliferative agents such as sirolimus/rapamycin (Cypher stent) and paclitaxel/taxol (Taxus stent). Sirolimus is a naturally occurring antibiotic produced by *Streptomyces* fungus. It is an immunosuppressant that inhibits cell proliferation (cytostatic) in the G1 phase of the cell cycle. Paclitaxel is derived from the pacific yew tree, *Taxus brevifolia*, and is an inhibitor of microtubules that prevent cell division (cytotoxic) in the M phase of the cell cycle.

The two DES stents were compared in terms of safety and efficacy in the SIRTAX trial. Major adverse cardiac events (MACE) occurred less frequently in the Cypher stent versus the Taxus stent. Target lesion revascularization (TLR) was the only component of the composite endpoint that was statistically lower with Cypher compared to Taxus stents. Furthermore, in-segment late loss was significantly lower in Cypher stents compared to Taxus stents. The REALITY trial was another study that compared the two types of DES. The primary endpoint was in-lesion binary restenosis by quantitative coronary angiography at 8 months. There was no statistically significant difference between the two stents in terms of the primary outcome. No difference in mortality, risk of MI, TLR, or MACE was seen between the two stents. Cypher stents showed a significantly lower in-stent late loss, and a significantly lower risk of stent thrombosis, compared to Taxus stents. The ISAR-Diabetes trial compared the two types of DES in diabetic patients. The study was designed to show noninferiority of Taxus stents

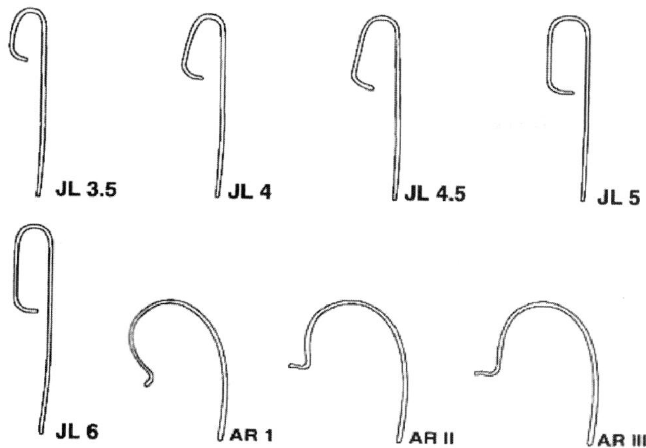


Figure 17–1 Illustration of the various sizes of Judkins left catheters and Amplatz left catheters. (Courtesy of Deepak Bhatt and LWW. From Griffing BP, Topol EJ, eds. *Manual of Cardiovascular Medicine.* 2nd ed. Philadelphia: Lippincott Williams & Wilkins; 2004.)

compared to Cypher stents in diabetics. Late lumen loss, which was the primary endpoint, was more frequent with Taxus stents compared to Cypher (it failed to show noninferiority). Taxus stents showed more angiographic restenosis and TLR compared to Cypher stents. There was no difference in terms of death or risk of MI between the two stents.

## Catheters

Catheters are usually made of polyethylene or polyurethane. Catheters commonly used to enter the left coronary circulation are Judkins left (JL) catheters and Amplatz left (AL) catheters (Fig. 17–1). The Judkins left catheter has a double curve. The length of the segment (in centimeters) between the first and second curves determines the size of the catheter (JL 3.5, 4, 5, or 6 cm). The aortic length and width and the overall habitus of the patient affect the choice of size, longer and dilated ascending aortas requiring larger-size catheters such as JL 5 or JL 6. The left Amplatz (AL) catheter has a preshaped half-circle with a tip extending out of the curve and perpendicular to it, giving the catheter three curves. AL catheters come in three sizes, 0.5, 0.75, and 1 cm. The size indicates the diameter of the half-circle/secondary curve. Larger sizes are used for a dilated ascending aorta. An LMT that is located superiorly may require a smaller JL catheter (JL-3.5), or and AL catheter. LMT that is located inferiorly may require a multipurpose catheter instead of the JL. When the LMT is short or there are separate ostia for the LAD and CX, AL catheters may cannulate the vessels better.

Catheters that are used to enter the right circulation are Judkins right (JR) catheters and Amplatz right (AR) and modified AR catheters (Fig. 17–2). The various sizes are JR 3.5, 4, 5, and 6 cm. The JR catheter can also used to cannulate SVG and subclavian arteries. Similar to the JL, the size reflects the size of the segment between the first and second curves. The AR and modified AR have three curves, as in AL catheters. The AR and modified AR sizes are 1, 2, and 3 cm; the size represents the width of the secondary curve. AR are very useful when the RCA origin is inferior. A high anterior RCA origin may be better accessed by using an AL catheter. Another, less often used form of right-side catheters is the 3DRC, which is a no-torque right coronary artery catheter (it has multiple curves leading to a three-dimensional configuration, hence the name 3D, and consequently does not require manipulation to cannulate the right coronary artery as is normally done with the JR).

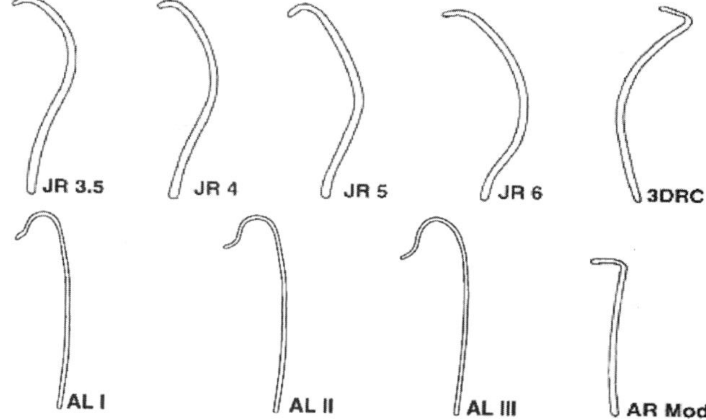


Figure 17–2 Illustrations of catheters used to cannulate the right coronary circulation. (Courtesy of Deepak Bhatt and LWW. From Griffing BP, Topol EJ, eds. *Manual of Cardiovascular Medicine.* 2nd ed. Philadelphia: Lippincott Williams & Wilkins; 2004.)

Other catheters used are multipurpose (MP) catheters, internal mammary (IM) and special IM catheters, left coronary bypass (LCB) and right coronary bypass (RCB) catheters, and the PIG, which is a pigtail catheter (Fig. 17–3). The names suggest the uses of these catheters. PIG catheters are used for ventriculograms and aortograms.

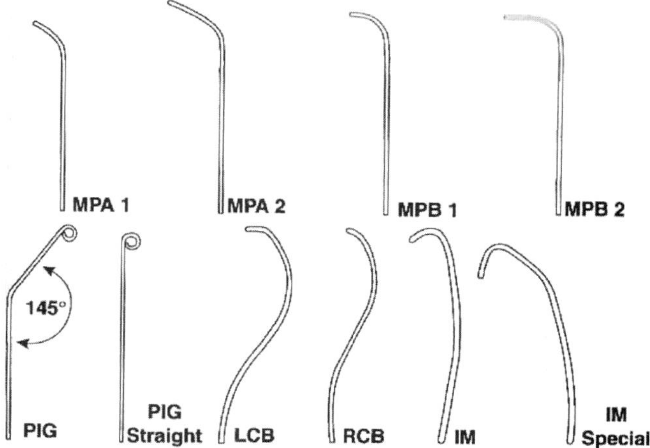


Figure 17–3 Illustrations of various other catheters used in coronary angiography. (Courtesy of Deepak Bhatt and LWW. From Griffing BP, Topol EJ, eds. *Manual of Cardiovascular Medicine.* 2nd ed. Philadelphia: Lippincott Williams & Wilkins; 2004.)

TABLE 17–13
**SUMMARY OF THE VARIOUS TYPES OF CONTRAST AGENTS USED IN CORONARY ANGIOGRAPHY**

| Class | Trade Name | Generic Name | Iodine (mg/mL) | Osmolality (mOsm/kg)[a] | Sodium (mEq/L) |
|---|---|---|---|---|---|
| **Ionic:** | | | | | |
| High osmolar | MD 76 R | Sodium diatrizoate | 370 | 2,140 | 190 |
| | Angiovist 370 | Sodium diatrizoate | 370 | 2,076 | 150 |
| | Hypaque | Sodium diatrizoate | 370 | 2,076 | 160 |
| Low osmolar | Hexabrix | Ioxaglate | 320 | 600 | 157 |
| **Nonionic:** | | | | | |
| Low osmolar | Omnipaque | Iohexol | 350 | 844 | Trace |
| | Optiray 320 | Ioversol | 320 | 702 | Trace |
| | Oxilan 350 | Ioxilan | 350 | 695 | Trace |
| Isosmolar | Visipaque 320 | Iodixanol | 320 | 290 | Trace |

[a]Blood osmolality is 275 mOsmol/L.
*Source:* Adapted from Introduction guide to cardiac catheterization, LWW.

Coronary guide catheters used during PTCA and stenting are generally stiffer than diagnostic catheters. Their role is to provide support in addition to cannulating the coronary artery. There are various shapes of guiding catheters, more than there are diagnostic catheters. Some are designed specifically for use with adjunct devices such as in directional atherectomy.

## Contrast Material

All contrast agents used in coronary angiography contain iodine, which absorbs X-rays more than the surrounding tissue, which in turn gives the contrast its radio-opacity. Contrast dye is a derivative of benzoic acid with a variable number of iodine molecules. Contrast agents are commonly classified based on their osmolality (high, low, or isosmolar), and their ionicity/sodium content (ionic or nonionic) (Table 17–13). High-osmolar agents are ionic and are differentiated by their possession of calcium-binding properties. Low-osmolar agents are classified by their ionicity. Ionic agents have six iodine atoms associated with each osmotically active particle, whereas nonionic agents have three iodine atoms for each isomotically active particle. This difference leads to an osmolality seven times that of serum for ionic agents, versus twice that of serum for nonionic agents.

Contrast agents affect myocardial physiologic and electrical functions, as well as coagulation and renal function. Higher-osmolar agents and hypertonic agents are more likely to cause peripheral vasodilatation/hypotension, myocardial stiffening/elevation of LV filling pressure, and depression of myocardial function. This is particularly important in patients who have low cardiac reserve (LMT disease, severe LV dysfunction, or severe aortic stenosis). Furthermore, high-osmolar and ionic agents could precipitate heart failure because of fluid shifting into the vasculature. Higher-osmolar and ionic agents are more likely to cause bradycardia, QRS complex, and QT-interval prolongation. However, there is no evidence that these electrical changes lead to an increased risk of ventricular arrhythmias. With regard to coagulation, in vitro and in vivo studies have suggested that nonionic contrasts agents are more thrombogenic than ionic agents. Some have even recommended avoiding nonionic contrast in acute MI. The clinical importance of this potential effect is usually buffered by the use of heparin and thrombin inhibitors during catheterization and/or interventions.

The effect of contrast agents on renal function is well established. Pre-existing renal impairment, diabetes mellitus, CHF, multiple myeloma, age (>70 years), dehydration, hypotension, IABP use, cardiogenic shock, renal transplant, and other nephrotoxic drugs are known risk factors for contrast-induced nephropathy. Contrast amount, osmolality of contrast, and repeat exposure within 72 hours are procedural risk factors for increased contrast-induced nephropathy. The mechanism of injury is not well understood; vasoconstriction or glomerular and tubular injuries have been proposed as possible culprits. Renal function deterioration is usually seen within 48 hours after catheterization, peaks at 5 days postcatheterization, and normalizes by 7 to 10 days postexposure. Fewer than 1% of patient progress to requiring chronic dialysis. Hydration, low-osmotic contrast agents, and bicarbonate have been shown to reduce contrast nephropathy. N-acetylcysteine (NAC) (Mucomyst) is commonly used in patients with renal insufficiency prior to contrast exposure. Two large meta-analyses showed a borderline significant ($p = 0.05$) protective effect of NAC. Mannitol, furosemide, dopamine, theophylline, fenoldopam, and L-arginine have not been shown to prevent nephropathy. With regard to statins, two nonrandomized retrospective studies demonstrated a reduction in contrast nephropathy with statin use.

Contrast allergy is another potential side effect of contrast agents. Mortality is 4 to 23 deaths/million. Some reactions are anaphylactoid (IgG mediated) and anaphylactic (IgE mediated). Patients who are asthmatic with nasal polyps have six to nine times increased incidence of contrast allergic reactions. Reactions vary from mild (nausea, flushing, or urticaria) to moderate (angioedema) to severe (anaphylaxis). Repeat allergic reactions occur in 15% to 40% of patients, on average. Hence, preparation of patients with prior reactions using prednisone and antihistamine is the standard of care. Furthermore, nonionic contrast is recommended in these cases. In the VIP trial, iodixanol (Visipaque) was associated with lower hypersensitivity reactions than ioxaglate (an ionic, low-osmolar contrast agent).

## ADJUNCTIVE DEVICES FOR PCI

### Intracoronary Brachytherapy for in-Stent Restenosis (ISR)

This procedure is no longer used, but it is described briefly here because the pathophysiologic concept of brachytherapy can be considered the platform for drug-eluting stents. There are several established clinical outcomes and angiographic risk factors for the development of ISR:

- Lesion length >30 mm
- Longer stent length
- Vessel diameter <2.5 mm
- Smaller posttreatment lumen diameter
- Reopened chronic total occlusion
- Location of ostial bifurcation
- Presence of diabetes mellitus
- Aorto-ostial location

Brachytherapy utilizes radiation to damage cellular DNA and thereby prevent neointimal hyperplasia. Balloon angioplasty for ISR is associated with high recurrence rates. Several retrospective clinical trials have demonstrated that brachytherapy results in improvement in angiographic and clinical status in native coronary arteries and in SVGs compared to balloon angioplasty. However, it can only be used once in each vessel, and if inadequate radiation is given to an injured segment, neointimal proliferation and restenosis can occur and clinical benefit is lost after 4 years. Recent studies looked at brachytherapy for treatment of de novo lesions to prevent restenosis. There appears to be a significant reduction in in-stent neointimal proliferation, but this benefit is offset by an edge effect (stenosis on angiographic follow-up occurring after VBT <5 mm proximal or distal to the tip of the radiation source) in the treated vessels. The edge effect occurs as a result of inadequate radiation coverage of the edges. Furthermore, there is a higher rate of late thrombosis in patients treated with brachytherapy.

### Cutting Balloon

The cutting balloon (CB) device is fitted with three or four metal razors that make longitudinal plaque incisions at dilatation. Based on data from retrospective studies, the cutting balloon has been used primarily to treat ISR. These trials did not support a benefit to CB in the treatment of ISR compared with angioplasty. The RESCUT trial compared this device with balloon angioplasty in 428 patients with ISR, and although less slippage was noted with the cutting balloon, there was no difference in restenosis at 7 months ($p = 0.82$). However, there may still be a place for the cutting balloon in ISR to avoid slipping-induced vessel trauma during the intervention.

### Rotablation

High-speed diamond-burr rotablation ablates atheroma and can remove calcium and plaque from coronary arteries. The procedure may be complicated by spasm and no/slow-flow phenomenon, which is characterized by inadequate flow at the tissue level despite a fully dilated epicardial coronary artery. The technique compares favorably to balloon angioplasty in the treatment of de novo lesions but does not show any long-term benefit. Data on the treatment of ISR are largely equivocal when compared to angioplasty. The dramatic increase in the use of DES that require optimal stent apposition and the practical ability of being able to dilate heavily calcified vessels may herald the reintroduction of rotablation into clinical practice.

### Directional Coronary Atherectomy

Directional coronary atherectomy is an over-the-wire cutting and retrieval technique that attempts to remove obstructive coronary plaque with directional control to obtain a large vessel lumen rather than compressing plaque with stents. However, compared to angioplasty it results in higher costs, higher rates of early complications, and no clear clinical benefit.

### Embolic Protection Devices

In most interventions, but particularly SVG interventions, there is exposure to distal embolization of particles. The use of GP-IIb/IIIa inhibitors and polytetrafluoroethylene (PTFE) stents during PCI has failed to reduce event rates in SVG PCIs. Areas of no/reflow are caused by microvascular disruption secondary to embolized particles. Current devices are aimed at filtering or aspirating such particles.

#### *Filter Devices*

The use of an obstructing balloon placed distally and an aspiration catheter (FilterWire) significantly improved myocardial perfusion grade and decreased major adverse cardiac events (MACE) in SVG PCI. Distal protection with a catheter-based filter offers the advantage of maintained antegrade perfusion. Data on the best protection device for SVG PCI are mixed. The PRIDE trial showed equal efficacy at the 30-day MACE endpoint when the TriActiv distal balloon occlusion system was compared to either the GuardWire or FilterWire device. The CAPTIVE trial compared the MedNOVA EmboShield filter with the Medtronic GuardWire, and at 30 days the incidence of MACE (a composite of death, MI, TVR, and emergency CABG) was 11.4% in the EmboShield group versus 9.1% in the GuardWire group ($p = 0.057$). However, the benefits of this technique in SVG graft interventions are not duplicated in the setting of primary PCI of the native vessels in STEMI.

#### *Proximal Suction Devices*

The main difficulties in using a distal protection device are the need to cross the stenotic lesion without trauma and the need for a suitable landing zone for the device. The Angiojet is essentially a guide catheter with a suction device. It failed to show a difference in reducing infarct size in acute MI patients in the AiMI trial, and similarly, in the VeGAS-2 trial, it failed to reduce MACE in patients with visible thrombus during SVG interventions when compared to Urokinase.

## ADJUNCTIVE DIAGNOSTIC TECHNOLOGY

### Intravascular Ultrasound

Intravascular ultrasound (IVUS) allows tomographic assessment of luminal area, plaque size, distribution, and composition. It is a valuable adjunct to angiography and provides extended insights into the diagnosis and therapy, including stent implantation and apposition. It is very useful as a clinical tool when the angiogram is ambiguous or when a complicated situation arises during the intervention and the interventionalist needs more detailed information in order to proceed.

### Fractional Flow Reserve (FFR)

Diffuse coronary lesions are often complex, with distorted luminal shapes, and are difficult to assess using planar angiography. The fractional flow reserve (FFR) wire has a pressure transducer that is placed distal to the stenosis, allowing a translesional gradient to be measured. Hyperemia is induced by an intracoronary or intravenous bolus of adenosine, and the ratio of the distal coronary pressure to the aortic pressure is known as the FFR. A ratio of $<0.75$ is very specific and represents inducible ischemia. An FFR $>0.8$ excludes ischemia in 90% of patients, making it ideal for interrogating intermediate lesions.

## PERSPECTIVE

Because this book was written with the Cardiology Boards in mind, we strove to emphasize the guidelines as well as the trials (even if outdated) that shaped most of these guidelines. This approach may have falsely given a rigid impression of the discipline, which is very dynamic, with great potential advances. It is important to keep in mind that by the time this book is published, the anticipated 2006 ACC/AHA guidelines will have been published, and many trials will have been concluded, which may contradict some of the data presented.

From a restenosis point of view, numerous trials have demonstrated that drug-eluting stents are superior to bare-metal stents in reducing the risk of in-stent restenosis and target lesion revascularization. Multiple studies have looked at other DES (besides sirolimus and paclitaxel). These stents include everolimus-coated stents, actinomycin D-coated stents, and high-dose dexamethasone loaded on phosphorylchlorine-coated stents. Other trials have looked at the role of adjunct oral therapy to the DES to reduce or limit in-stent restenosis. Verapamil was used versus placebo after DES placement. There was a significant reduction in target vessel revascularization, but no difference in in-stent restenosis. Oral sirolimus as an adjunct therapy to bare-metal stenting was also studied. High-dose sirolimus given before the PCI and continued for a total of 10 days was associated with a reduction in in-stent restenosis compared to placebo or low-dose sirolimus. Other trials are evaluating interventions that may modulate metabolism during acute MI to improve myocardial salvage. Some of these therapies are hyperoxemic reperfusion with aqueous oxygen during acute MI (no difference in infarct size, or ST resolution), and intravascular cooling (no difference in mortality or infarct size). Other studies have looked at the possibility of a myoblast transplant into an infarcted myocardium, showing improved viability by PET imaging, but with increased malignant arrhythmias. Other trials are assessing the potential use of stem cells in myocardial regeneration.

## BIBLIOGRAPHY

**Antman, et al.** Management of patients with STEMI: executive summary. ACC/AHA guidelines for the management of patients with ST-elevation myocardial infarction. *J Am Coll Cardiol.* 2004;44:671–719.

**Braunwald E, et al.** ACC/AHA 2002 guideline update for the management of patients with unstable angina and non-ST-segment elevation myocardial infarction—summary article. *J Am Coll Cardiol.* 2002;40:1366–1374.

**Douglas JS.** Intervnetional cardiology. *J Am Coll Cardiol.* 2005;45: 4B–8B.

**Eagle KA, Guyton RA, et al.** ACC/AHA 2004 guideline update for coronary artery bypass graft surgery. *Circulation.* 2004;110:1–104.

**Ellis SG, Guetta V, Miller D, et al.** Relationship between lesion characteristics and risk with percutaneous intervention in the stent and glycoprotein IIb/IIIa era. *Circulation.* 1999;100:1971–1976.

**Ellis SG, Vandormael MG, Cowley MJ, et al.** Coronary morphologic and clinical determinants of procedural outcome with angioplasty for multivessel coronary disease. *Circulation.* 1990;82:1193–1202.

**Flaherty JD, Davidson CJ, Crouse JR III, et al.** Coronary artery bypass grafting versus stent implantation. *N Engl J Med.* 2005;353:735–737.

**Gibbons RJ, et al.** ACC/AHA 2002 Guideline update for the management of patients with chronic stable angina—summary article. *J Am Coll Cardiol.* 2003;41:159–168.

**Griffin BP, Topol EJ, eds.** *Manual of Cardiovascular Medicine.* 2nd ed. Philadelphia: Lippincott Williams & Wilkins; 2004.

**Hannan EL, Racz MJ, Walford G, et al.** Long term outcomes of coronary-artery bypass grafting versus stent implantation. *N Engl J Med.* 2005;352:2174–2183.

**Holmes DR, et al.** Modeling and risk prediction in the current era of interventional cardiology a report from the National Heart, Lung, and Blood Institute Dynamic Registry. *Circulation.* 2003;107:1871–1876.

**Kim HS, Waksman R, Cottin Y, et al.** Edge stenosis and geographical miss following intracoronary gamma radiation therapy for in-stent restenosis. *J Am Coll Cardiol.* 2001;37:1026–1304.

**Manson JE, Buring JE, Ridker PM, Gaziano JM.** *Clinical Trials in Heart Disease, A Companion to Braunwald's Heart Disease.* 2nd ed. Elsevier Saunders; 2004.

**Mehran R, et al.** A simple risk score for prediction of contrast-induced nephropathy after percutaneous coronary intervention. *J Am Coll Cardiol.* 2004;44:1393–1399.

**Merten GJ, et al.** Prevention of contrast-induced nephropathy with sodium bicarbonate. *JAMA.* 2004;291:2328–2334.

**Mohan NB, Lawrence J, Patrick B, et al.** A hierarchical Bayesian meta-analysis of randomized clinical trials of drug-eluting stents. *Lancet.* 2004;364:583–591.

**O'Neill WW, Dixon SR, Grines CL.** The year in interventional cardiology. *J Am Coll Cardiol.* 2005;45:1117–1133.

**Popma JJ, Berger P, Ohman EM, et al.** The Seventh ACCP Conference on Antithrombotic and Thrombolytic Therapy: Antithrombotic Therapy during Percutaneous Intervention. *Chest.* 2004;126:576S–599S.

**Rihal CS, et al.** Indications for coronary artery bypass surgery and percutaneous coronary intervention in chronic stable angina: review of the evidence and methodological considerations. *Circulation.* 2003;108:2439–2445.

**Schomig A, Ndrepepa G, Mehilli J, et al.** A randomized trial of coronary stenting versus balloon angioplasty as a rescue interventional after failed thrombolysis in patients with acute myocardial infarction. *J Am Coll Cardiol.* 2004;44:2073–2079.

**Singh M, et al.** Correlates of procedural complications and a simple integer risk score for percutaneous coronary intervention. *J Am Coll Cardiol.* 2002;40:387–393.

**Smith SC Jr, Feldman TE, et al.** ACC/AHA/SCAI 2005 guideline update for percutaneous intervention—summary article. *Circulation.* 2006;113:1–20.

**Smith SC Jr.** ACC/AHA guidelines for percutaneous coronary intervention (revision of the 1993 PTCA guidelines). *J Am Coll Cardiol.* 2001;37(8):2239i–2239lxvi.

**Stadius ML.** Diminishing returns. . . too many choices. . . the saga of pharmacologic therapy to reduce the complications of percutaneous coronary interventions. *J Am Coll Cardiol.* 2004;44:25–27.

**Sutton AG, Campbell PG, Graham R, et al.** A randomized trial of rescue angioplasty versus a conservative approach for failed thrombolysis in ST-segment elevation myocardial infarction. The Middlesbrough Early Revascularization to Limit Infarction trial (MERLIN). *J Am Coll Cardiol.* 2004;44:287–296.

**Topol EJ, ed.** Califf RM, Isner JM, et al., assoc eds. *Textbook of Cardiovascular Medicine.* 2nd ed. Philadelphia: Lippincott Williams & Wilkins; 2002.

**Topol EJ, Neumann FJ, Montalescot G.** Referred reperfusion strategies for acute myocardial infarction. *J Am Coll Cardiol.* 2003;42:1886–1889.

## QUESTIONS

**1.** A 73-year-old man underwent PCI after a non–ST-elevation myocardial infarction. He was pretreated with 325 mg of aspirin and 600 mg of clopidogrel, plus unfractionated heparin and weight-adjusted abciximab were administered during the intervention. A drug-eluting stent is deployed into the mid-LAD. Following the procedure, which of the following statements is correct?

a. Both heparin and abciximab infusions should be stopped. The arterial sheath should be removed when the ACT <150 seconds, and 4 hours later an abciximab infusion should be restarted and continued for 12 hours.

b. Heparin should be stopped, the abciximab infusion should be continued for 12 hours, the arterial sheath should be removed when the ACT is <150 seconds, and 75 mg of clopidogrel should be continued for up to 1 year.

c. The heparin should be stopped, the abciximab infusion should be continued until the time of sheath removal; the arterial sheath should be removed when the ACT is <150 seconds.

d. Heparin infusion at 700 U/h should be started, the abciximab infusion should be continued for 12 hours, the arterial sheath should be removed when the ACT is <150 seconds, and 75 mg of clopidogrel should be continued for 4 weeks.

Answer is b: Heparin should be stopped, the abciximab infusion should be continued for 12 hours, the arterial sheath should be removed when the ACT is less than <150 seconds, and 75 mg of clopidogrel should be continued for up to 1 year. In the EPIC trial, prolonged sheath dwells and high heparin dose resulted in more major bleeding complications with abciximab than with placebo (14% versus 7%). However, reduction in heparin dose and early sheath removal resulted in fewer major bleeding complications with abciximab than with heparin alone in both the EPILOG (2.0% versus 3.1%) and the EPISTENT (1.5% versus 2.2% major bleeding) trials. Recently, concern has arisen regarding late thrombosis with drug-eluting stents. Theoretically, complete healing of the stent may take up to 2 years. Currently, continuing clopidogrel for 6 to 12 months is recommended.

**2.** A 62-year-old woman with crescendo angina has presented for elective PCI to a known focal stenosis in a moderate-sized first diagonal branch. She is not taking medications and has a severe allergy to shellfish (hives), and she also reports an allergy to aspirin although she cannot specify the reaction. Which of the following statements regarding patient management is correct?

a. Administer 100 mg hydrocortisone IV, 50 mg diphenhydramine (Benadryl) IV, and 600 mg clopidogrel orally before the procedure, then proceed with the scheduled intervention.
b. Administer 40 mg methylprednisolone IV, 50 mg diphenhydramine (Benadryl) IV, 600 mg clopidogrel orally, and standard-dose abciximab before the procedure, then proceed with the scheduled intervention.
c. Administer 100 mg hydrocortisone IV, 50 mg diphenhydramine (Benadryl) IV, 325 mg aspirin, and 300 mg clopidogrel orally before the procedure, then proceed with the scheduled intervention.
d. Administer 100 mg hydrocortisone IV, 50 mg diphenhydramine (Benadryl) IV, 300 mg clopidogrel orally, and standard-dose abciximab before the procedure, then proceed with the scheduled intervention.
e. Consult an allergy specialist and postpone the intervention.

Answer is e: Consult an allergy specialist and postpone the intervention. Manifestations of aspirin sensitivity such as exacerbations of respiratory tract disease and urticaria can occur in up to 10% and 0.2% of the general population, respectively An urgent intervention could be undertaken with the pharmacologic therapy described in the second option. However, an elective intervention should be postponed, awaiting appropriate workup and desensitization. There is little or no experience with aspirin desensitization in patients with aspirin-induced anaphylaxis. Potent platelet inhibitors, such as ticlopidine and clopidogrel, have demonstrated value in unstable angina and may have value in patients with aspirin allergy; pretreatment for 2 to 4 days prior to intervention is recommended to achieve optimal platelet inhibition. Abciximab has been shown to reduce ischemic complications following high-risk (EPIC and CAPTURE trials) and elective coronary interventions (EPILOG trial) in patients receiving aspirin; its role in the aspirin-allergic patient has not been defined but is theoretically appealing. Investigational oral platelet receptor antagonists may be useful.

**3.** A 50-year-old man presents to the emergency room (ER) about 100 minutes after the onset of chest pain. The pain is substernal, radiates to the left arm, and is associated with vomiting and diaphoresis. On examination, the patient is tachycardic with a heart rate of 104, hypertensive with blood pressure of 150/88. An electrocardiogram showed 3 mm ST elevation in the anterior and lateral leads. Symptoms were not relieved with sublingual nitroglycerin or beta-blocker therapy. An IV nitroglycerin drip was titrated to control the patient's symptoms. The closest interventional cardiology center is 120 minutes away. The patient has asked about the therapeutic options at this point. What can you tell him about the various therapeutic modalities?

a. Primary PCI is recommended over thrombolytics because PCI has short-term mortality benefit, reduced reinfarction risk, and reduced risk of stroke, regardless of duration of symptoms and time required to PTCA.
b. Thrombolysis is recommended over PCI because door-to-balloon time is ≥90 minutes.
c. Half-dose thrombolysis should be recommended; then the patient should be transferred for PCI.
d. The patient should be referred for emergency CABG for better survival advantage.

Answer is b: Current ACC/AHA guidelines for management of patients with ST-elevation MI are dependent on the duration of symptoms, mortality risk of the STEMI, the risk of bleeding, and the difference between time to PCI and time thrombolytics. PCI is recommended over thrombolysis when experienced operators restore blood flow in ≤90 minutes. The patient in this question is relatively young, with a large STEMI that has a high mortality risk. He has been having symptoms for 80 minutes and requires 120 minutes or more to have perfusion established with PCI. He is hemodynamically stable. Delayed treatment affects outcome negatively, whether treatment is PCI or thrombolytics. Thrombolysis is highly effective in restoring coronary flow in STEMI, particularly when the patient has presented within 3 hours of symptoms. Data from the National Registry of MI showed increased mortality when PCI is delayed beyond 2 hours. Hence, this patient will likely have better outcome if he receives thrombolysis.

**4.** A 62-year-old woman, current smoker, diabetic, hypertensive and hyperlipidemic, presented to the ER with a 2-day history of intermittent chest pain. On examination, she was tachycardic with a heart rate of 101 beats/min, and hypertensive with a blood pressure of 160/100 mm Hg. The patient does not have any signs of heart failure. An electrocardiogram showed 2-mm depression in V2–V6. The patient was started on heparin and given IV metoprolol for rate control, as well as nitroglycerin. In addition, she was started on an eptifibatide infusion. The patient remained asymptomatic until her coronary angiogram. The left heart catheterization showed 90% stenosis in the proximal third of the LAD, 80% stenosis in the proximal RCA, with 30% disease in the middle circumflex artery. The best plan of treatment for this patient is

a. PCI to both the LAD and RCA now
b. Referral for two-vessel CABG
c. PCI to the LAD with staged intervention to the RCA
d. Medical management with no PCI or CABG

Answer is b: The patient is diabetic with multivessel coronary artery disease. CABG has been shown to provide a survival benefit over PTCA according to the BARI trial. However, in the stenting era, one could recommend PCI with stenting, because there is no survival benefit of CABG over stenting according to ERACI-II, ARTS, and SOS. The patient is more likely to require further revascularization and more antianginal medication. Hence the recommendation according to the pre–drug-eluting stents ACC/AHA guidelines is to refer this patient to CABG.

# Risk Stratification and Post–Myocardial Infarction Therapy

18

**Ryan D. Christofferson    Samir R. Kapadia**

Unstable angina, non–ST-segment-elevation myocardial infarction, and ST-segment-elevation myocardial infarction represent a spectrum of ischemic coronary disease of similar etiology—atherosclerotic plaque instability and rupture—termed acute coronary syndrome (ACS). The role of risk stratification in ACS is to identify which patients have increased risk for adverse events and are therefore more likely to benefit from the array of mechanical and pharmacologic therapies available. Risk stratification after myocardial infarction (MI) begins during the initial clinical encounter, continues throughout the index hospitalization, and remains important after discharge. Although modern advances have had a significant impact on outcomes of MI, post-ACS morbidity (and mortality) remain a challenging problem, most notably recurrent ischemia and infarction, congestive heart failure, and sudden cardiac death.

The use of noninvasive risk stratification versus invasive assessment for postinfarction ischemia remains controversial, although recent data favor an early invasive approach. Early aggressive lipid-lowering therapy post-MI is clearly beneficial, with lower targets for low-density lipoprotein (LDL) levels. The importance of neurohormonal blockade has become apparent, particularly in patients with left-ventricular systolic dysfunction. Antiplatelet therapies have become essential, both during and after ACS, but in particular following percutaneous coronary intervention (PCI). The role of the implantable cardioverter-defibrillator (ICD) after MI has become clearer, with recent trials indicating no benefit to ICD early in the course post-MI, but demonstrable subsequent benefit in patients with significant left ventricular dysfunction. The recognition of the role of inflammation in ACS has led to the development of clinical assays measuring inflammatory markers such as C-reactive protein (CRP), augmenting the clinical risk assessment. Lifestyle modification and risk-factor reduction remain important, including smoking cessation, diabetes and hypertension management.

## RISK STRATIFICATION FOR ST-ELEVATION MI (STEMI)

Identification of high-risk characteristics early after myocardial infarction is important because 25% of deaths during the first postinfarction year occur within the first 48 hours of hospitalization, and more than one half of deaths occur within the first month after STEMI (Figs. 18–1 and 18–2). Demographic and clinical data, electrocardiogram (ECG), serum markers, and various diagnostic tests assist in the risk assessment.

### Initial Presentation

#### *Clinical and Demographic Factors*

The most important predictors of death within 30 days are age, systolic blood pressure and heart rate at presentation, evidence of congestive heart failure (CHF) on physical

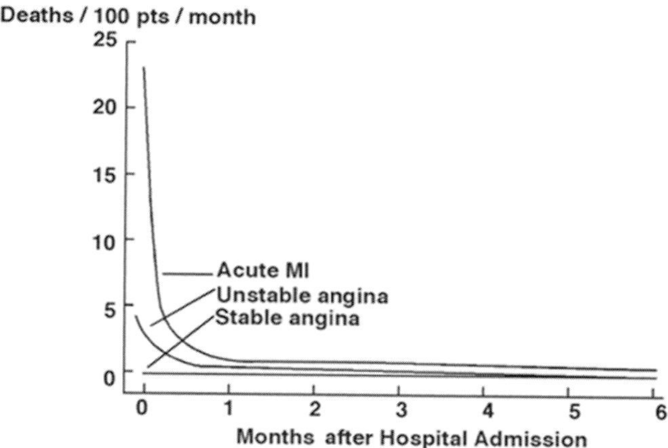


**Figure 18–1** Mortality rate according to patient characteristics at time of presentation. (From *Circulation.*1994;90:613–622.)

**TABLE 18–1**

**PREDICTORS OF MORTALITY IN ST-ELEVATION MYOCARDIAL INFARCTION**

| Variable | TIMI-II ($n = 3{,}339$) | GISSI-2 ($n = 10{,}219$) | GUSTO-I ($n = 41{,}021$) |
|---|---|---|---|
| Age | ++ | ++ | ++ |
| Prior MI | ++ | ++ | ++ |
| Diabetes | ++ | + | ++ |
| Smoking | ++ | — | ++ |
| Hypertension | + | + | ++ |
| Female gender | ++ | + | + |
| Vascular disease | — | — | ++ |

+, univariate predictor; ++, multivariate predictor.

examination, location of infarction, and previous infarction. In the GUSTO-1 study these predictors accounted for >90% of the total prognostic information. Additional important prognostic factors include female gender, history of diabetes, hypertension, smoking, and vascular disease (Table 18–1).

Advanced age has been recognized as an important predictor of mortality in several studies. In the NRMI (National Registry of Myocardial Infarction) registry, a community-based database with information on >350,000 patients with acute MI at U.S. hospitals, in-hospital mortality ranged from 3% for patients younger than 55 years of age to 28% for individuals more than 84 years of age. Older patients are more likely to possess a history of a prior MI, have more severe coronary disease, and consequently are more likely to develop CHF and cardiogenic shock after MI. Additionally, several reports have shown that older patients are also less likely to receive life-saving therapies such as immediate reperfusion therapy, beta-blockers, and aspirin, which may contribute to the worsened prognosis.

In several studies, women have been shown to have higher mortality after STEMI. In the GUSTO-1 (Global Utilization of Streptokinase and TPA for Occluded Arteries—I) trial, women had higher 30-day mortality (11.3% versus 5.5%), occurrence of shock (9% versus 5%), and reinfarction (5.1% versus 3.6%) compared to men. Part of this increased risk can be explained by the advanced age and increased prevalence of pre-existing diabetes and hypertension. Additionally, women are more likely to present late during an infarction.

Paradoxically, smokers possess a lower risk for early mortality, most likely because of their younger age. Diabetes mellitus has been associated with a 1.5 to 3.0 times higher mortality after STEMI. Whether this is due to a higher atherosclerotic burden, or some other characteristic induced by the diabetic state, such as silent ischemia or a larger infarct size, remains unclear. Further, the nonfatal complications are also higher in diabetic patients, including a greater incidence of postinfarction angina, reinfarction, and heart failure.

### *Physical Examination*

The clues to right ventricular (RV) and left ventricular (LV) dysfunction on physical examination provide the most important prognostic information. Accordingly, variables

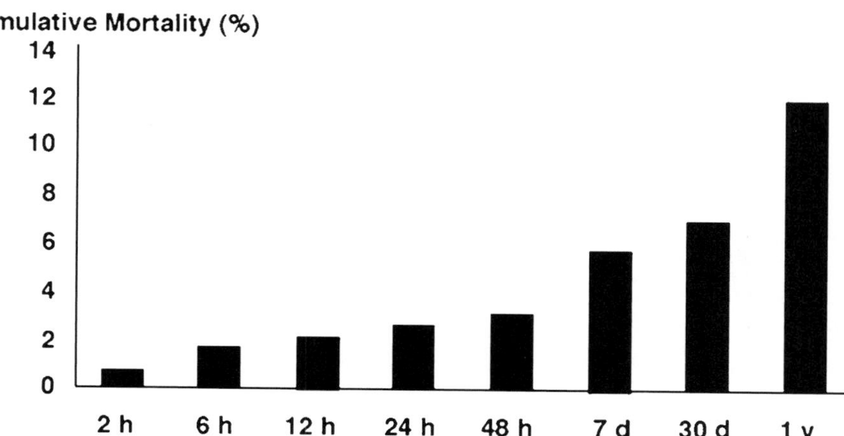


**Figure 18–2** Mortality rate according to duration of time after presentation with acute myocardial infarction. (From *N Engl J Med.* 1993;329:673–682.)

**TABLE 18–2**
**KILLIP CLASSIFICATION AND MORTALITY FROM GUSTO-I TRIAL**

| Killip Class | Features | Patients on Entry (%) | 30-Day Mortality (%) |
|---|---|---|---|
| I | No CHF | 70 | 2 |
| II | Early CHF (crackles, S3) | 20 | 20 |
| III | Pulmonary edema (1/2 lung fields) | 5 | 33 |
| IV | Cardiogenic shock | 5 | 66 |

CHF, congestive heart failure.

predictive of a worsened outcome include hypotension, tachycardia, jugular venous distension, an S3 gallop, pulmonary edema, and evidence of peripheral hypoperfusion, many of which are captured by the Killip classification (Table 18–2). The physical examination can also help to identify mechanical complications of MI, such as acute mitral regurgitation, ventricular septal defect, and free wall rupture, all of which have been associated with significant mortality.

### Electrocardiogram

The ECG provides useful information about the location and size of infarction, likelihood of tissue reperfusion after treatment, presence of ongoing ischemia, and conduction system dysfunction. The finding of ST elevation or depression has similar prognostic implications (Fig. 18–3). Mortality is greater in patients experiencing anterior wall MI compared to after inferior MI, even when corrected for infarct size. Patients with RV infarction complicating inferior infarction have a higher mortality rate than patients sustaining an inferior infarction without RV involvement. Patients with multiple leads showing ST-segment elevation and those with a high degree of ST-segment elevation have increased mortality, especially if their infarct is anterior. Patients with persistent or advanced heart block (e.g., Mobitz type II, second-degree, or third-degree AV block) or new intraventricular conduction abnormalities (bifascicular or trifascicular) in the course of an acute MI have a worse prognosis than do patients without these abnormalities. The influence of high-grade conduction block is particularly important in patients with RV infarction, for such patients have a markedly increased mortality. Other ECG findings suggesting a worse outcome are persistent horizontal or down-sloping ST-segment depression, Q-waves in multiple leads, evidence of RV infarction accompanying an inferior infarction, ST-segment depressions in anterior leads in patients with an inferior infarction, and atrial arrhythmias (especially atrial fibrillation).

Other than these well-established predictors on ECG, ST-segment resolution has generated renewed interest in determining effectiveness of reperfusion therapy. Resolution of ST elevation predicts successful perfusion at the myocardial level, which is the most important predictor of LV function and survival. Continuous ST-segment monitoring has been shown to yield important prognostic information after 60 min of observation. In the ASSENT 2 (Assessment of Safety and Efficacy of a New Thrombolytic) and ASSENT-PLUS studies, the optimal cutoff for ST-segment resolution analyses was found to be 50%, measured at 60 min. Patients with ST resolution (40%) by this criterion had a 30-day mortality of only 1.4%.

### Biomarker Assessment

Two separate groups of biomarkers have been used to predict outcome after MI. One group includes the myocardial enzymes that predict infarct size and another group assesses

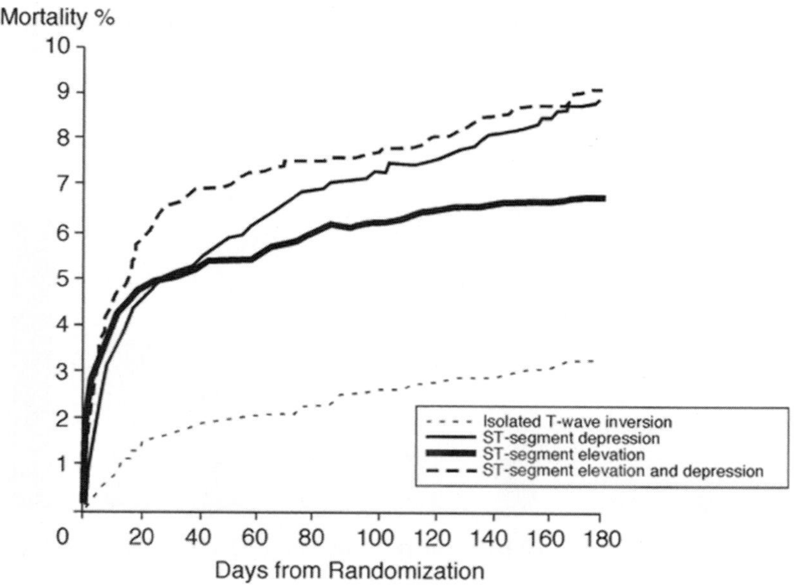


**Figure 18–3** Mortality rate according to electrocardiographic findings on presentation with acute myocardial infarction in the GUSTO IIb trial. (From *JAMA*.1999;281:707–713.)

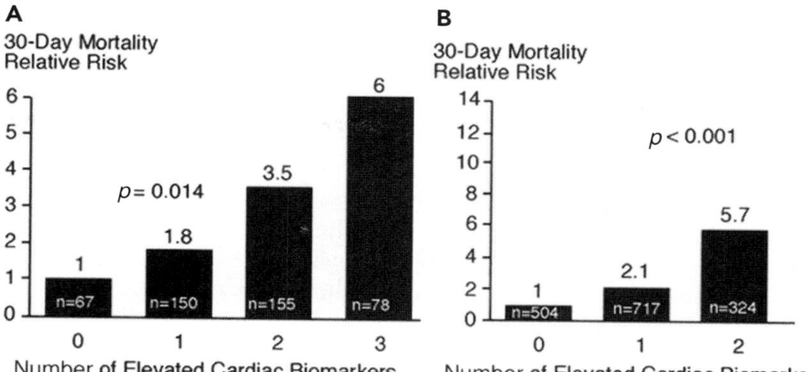


**Figure 18–4** Relative risk for mortality at 30 days according to cardiac biomarker elevation. (From *N Engl J Med.* 1996;335:1333–1341.)

the degree of systemic vascular inflammation. The prognostic value of CRP, endothelin, brain natriuretic peptide (BNP), CD40, and CD40 ligand has recently been investigated extensively. These markers of inflammation seem to predict active atherosclerotic disease process. Aggressive risk-factor modification may be more important when the levels of these markers are high.

More conventional markers of myocardial damage include troponin-I or -T, creatine kinase (CK), CK-MB 1 and 2 isoforms, CK-MB isoenzyme mass, and occasionally myoglobin. The presence and degree of troponin, CK, and CK-MB isoenzyme elevation on admission and thereafter have been associated with poorer outcome in the setting of both ST-elevation and non–ST-elevation MI. However, there is less information on troponin levels in STEMI. In the GUSTO IIa study, 30-day mortality was substantially higher among patients who were troponin-T positive (Fig. 18–4). Given their more rapid return to baseline, CK and CK-MB isoenzymes are also helpful for identifying high-risk individuals by facilitating the diagnosis of reinfarction shortly after an ST- or non–ST-elevation MI. Currently, infarct size is determined by CK-MB mass; the role of troponin-I or -T in this matter has been less well established.

### *Imaging*

Imaging at the time of acute infarction is used to determine the amount of jeopardized myocardium. Contrast echocardiography and technetium-based imaging can be used to quantify perfusion noninvasively. Nuclear scanning is superior for quantifying perfusion, whereas echocardiography is better for assessing function. Acute imaging has been used principally in clinical trials to determine the degree of myocardial salvage, which is the percent of ischemic myocardium at presentation that has adequate perfusion on follow-up.

## During Hospitalization

Recurrent angina is an important predictor of a worsened outcome and the need for revascularization. Recurrent chest pain frequently signifies ischemic myocardium; either in the peri-infarct territory supplied by the infarct-related artery, or ischemia at a distance secondary to a non–infarct-related artery. Early revascularization is required in many patients who have postinfarct angina. Other important predictors include LV or RV dysfunction and mechanical complications of MI. Cardiogenic shock possesses a very high mortality in which medical management is not effective. Early revascularization in patients who develop cardiogenic shock within 36 hours of an MI is recommended, based on the findings of the SHOCK (Should We Emergently Revascularize Occluded Coronary Arteries for Cardiogenic Shock) trial, which showed reduced mortality with early revascularization compared to medical stabilization (33.3 versus 51.6%). Arrhythmias, including high-grade AV block, atrial fibrillation, or ventricular tachycardia, also predict poor outcome.

### *Predischarge Assessment*

Although significant emphasis is placed on predischarge risk stratification, many high-risk patients will declare themselves clinically during their hospital stay. The challenge for the clinician during the predischarge phase is to distinguish the few patients who remain at higher risk from the many relatively lower-risk patients. Although multiple testing technologies have been developed to aid in this process, the low event rate in these patients (1-year mortality rates of 2% to 5%) mandates that these tests must be highly sensitive and specific if they are to have clinical value. What tests should be routinely performed for predischarge risk stratification is highly debated. Risk stratification at discharge can be accomplished by determining three factors: (a) resting LV function, (b) residual potentially ischemic myocardium, and (c) susceptibility to serious ventricular arrhythmias. More sophisticated testing may provide additional data but may not be as useful in changing patient outcomes.

### *LV Function Assessment*

Assessment of LV function is typically performed by echocardiography or by ventriculography at the time of cardiac catheterization. However, imaging of the left ventricle at rest may not distinguish between infarcted, irreversibly damaged myocardium and hibernating myocardium.

Therefore, many different techniques have been used to determine viable myocardium, including dobutamine echocardiography, rest-redistribution thallium, positron emission tomography (PET) scanning, and magnetic resonance imaging (MRI). Dobutamine echocardiography can provide functional assessment along with information on viability and ischemia. However, the results are directly dependent on the expertise and experience of the interpreter. Radionucleotide imaging provides higher sensitivity to detect ischemia, but specificity can be compromised by the size of the patient, diaphragmatic or breast attenuation. Further, regional wall motion assessment is not as precise as with echocardiography. Regardless of the imaging modality chosen, the prognosis is worse if there is significant LV dysfunction, or if there is a large amount of ischemic myocardium.

#### *Stress Testing*

Patients who do not have high-risk features after successful thrombolysis should be considered for exercise stress testing. Although the predictive accuracy of exercise stress testing has diminished in the reperfusion era as a result of the lower incidence of adverse outcomes, it is still given a Class I indication under current American College of Cardiology/American Heart Association (ACC/AHA) Guidelines. In addition, although it is not known whether exercise testing can effectively risk-stratify patients who have not received acute reperfusion therapy, it is also assumed to be effective in this setting. Low-level exercise appears to be safe in patients who have been free of angina or heart failure and who possess a stable baseline ECG during the previous 2 to 3 days. Patients who are unable to exercise or who have baseline ECG abnormalities that would preclude interpretation should undergo an exercise test with imaging. Patients who cannot achieve a 3 or 4 MET workload, those who develop ischemia at a low level of exercise, or those in whom blood pressure drops during exercise should undergo coronary angiography. No further testing should be necessary in patients without these high-risk findings.

#### *Assessment for Risk of Sudden Cardiac Death*

Determination of risk for sudden cardiac death (SCD) after MI is important because it is highest in the first 1 to 2 years after the index event. The most important predictor for SCD is LV dysfunction. Provocative electrophysiology studies are not necessary for risk stratification. Signal-averaged ECG, heart-rate variability, QT dispersion, and baroreflex sensitivity have been investigated to select specific patients with LV dysfunction who might benefit from an ICD. The presence of a filtered QRS complex duration > 120 milliseconds and abnormal late potentials recorded on a signal-averaged ECG after acute MI signifies somewhat higher risk for SCD. However, the signal-averaged ECG suffers from a high false-positive rate, which makes the test clinically less useful. Depressed heart-rate variability is an independent predictor of mortality and arrhythmic complications after acute MI. A depressed baroreflex sensitivity value (3.0 ms/mm Hg) is associated with about a threefold increase in the risk of mortality. These tests may provide useful prognostic information, but at present, only assessment of ejection fraction is necessary to determine eligibility for a device, where significant LV dysfunction qualifies a patient for ICD placement. Recent data indicate, however, that ICD therapy is not beneficial in the early post–MI period, and most likely should be delayed for several months after an infarction.

### Predischarge Management

An outline for predischarge management is presented in Figure 18–5. It is important to note that routine angiography is not recommended for all patients with an acute ST-segment-elevation MI. Initially, a judgment is made as to the presence of clinical variables indicative of high risk for future cardiac events. Patients with spontaneous episodes of ischemia or depressed left ventricular function who are considered suitable candidates for revascularization based on their overall medical condition should be referred for cardiac catheterization. These patients are at increased risk of recurrent infarction (and subsequent increased mortality), and may benefit from revascularization if severe coronary artery disease is identified at catheterization.

## NON–ST-ELEVATION ACS

Many patients with acute coronary syndrome present without ST elevation on ECG. It is important to note that although the risk of mortality during the index hospitalization is less than in those with ST-elevation ACS, the prognosis at 1 year is similar (see Fig. 18–3). Typically, the underlying pathophysiology is a high-grade stenosis with plaque rupture, but unlike ST-elevation MI, the vessel is not totally occluded. Indeed, fibrinolysis has been shown to be of no benefit and may actually be harmful in this patient cohort. Multiple trials have investigated the role of early angiography and PCI versus conservative management in these patients. (Fig. 18–6) It appears that early invasive strategy in the high-risk population provides the best outcome and may even be more cost effective than a conservative strategy.

### Non–ST-Elevation MI Risk Stratification

#### *Initial Presentation*

A number of historical features predictive of a worse prognosis following non–ST-elevation ACS have been derived from existing trial data. These features are summarized in Table 18–3. The most important are older age, greater number of cardiac risk factors, known coronary artery disease, peripheral vascular or cerebrovascular disease, prior MI, previous PCI or coronary artery bypass graft surgery, history of congestive heart failure (CHF), a more severe

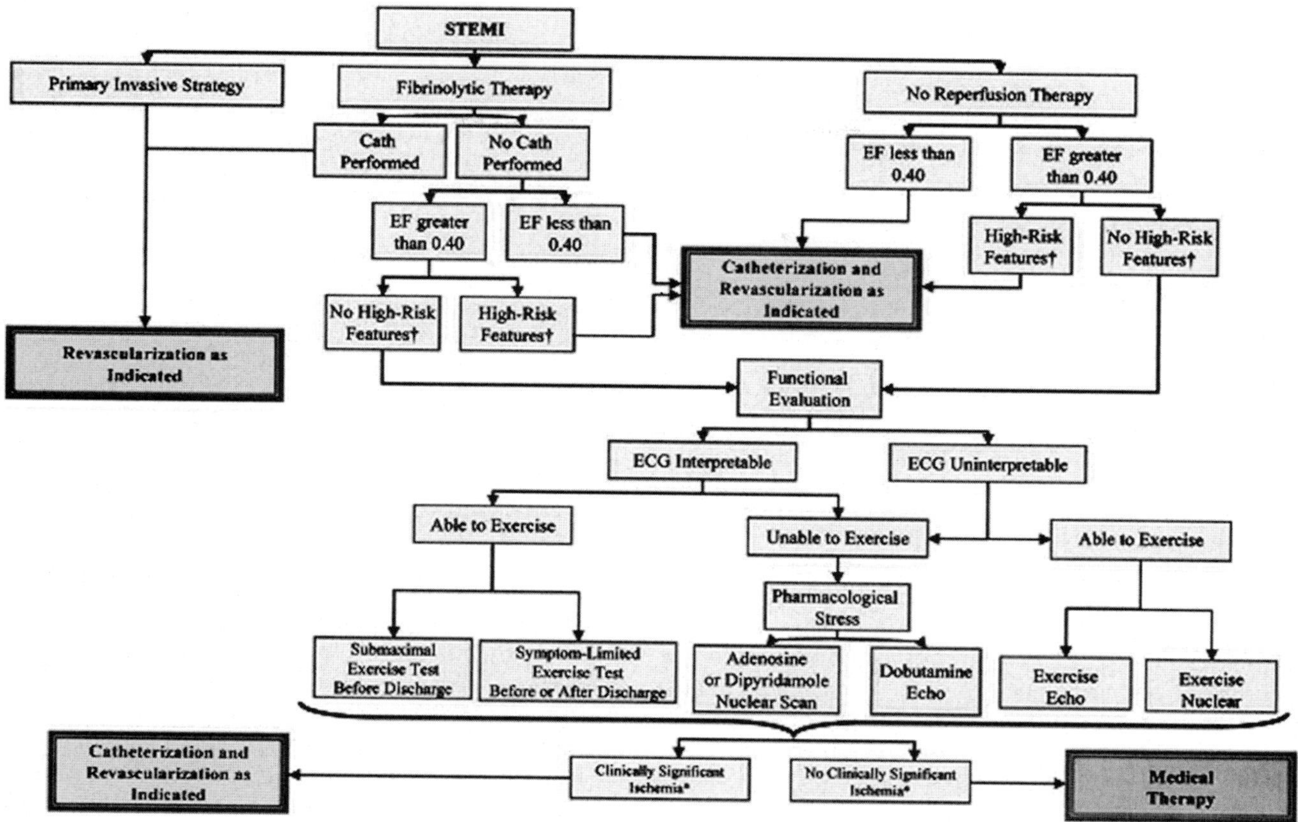


**Figure 18–5** An algorithm for management of ST-elevation myocardial infarction from the ACC/AHA guidelines. (From Antman EM, Anbe DT, Armstrong PW, et al. ACC/AHA guidelines for the management of patients with ST-elevation myocardial infarction; a report of the American College of Cardiology/American Heart Association Task Force on Practice Guidelines (Committee to Revise the 1999 Guidelines for the Management of Patients with Acute Myocardial Infarction). *J Am Coll Cardiol*. 2004;44:E1–E211.)

anginal pattern, and the use of aspirin within a week of presentation.

### *Electrocardiogram*

Among patients with non–ST-elevation ACS, the presence of Q-waves, ST changes associated with angina or at presentation (in particular, ST-segment depression), T-wave inversions of significant amplitude (i.e., >0.2 mV), or the absence of ECG changes during angina are important predictors of future events (see Fig. 18–3). When clinical variables are also considered, heart rate and the presence of ST depression on admission ECG are the most important multivariable predictors.

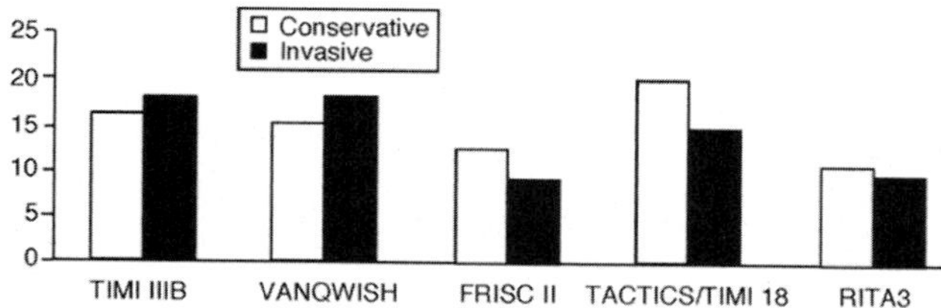


**Figure 18–6** Invasive versus conservative strategy in acute non–ST-elevation myocardial infarction.

### *Biomarkers*

The presence and degree of troponin elevation on admission and thereafter can identify patients who are at increased risk of experiencing adverse outcomes. Cardiac troponin-I and troponin-T are particularly useful

**TABLE 18–3**

**PREDICTORS OF A WORSE PROGNOSIS IN NON-ST-ELEVATION MYOCARDIAL INFARCTION**

| Variable | PURSUIT ($n = 9,461$) | TIMI-IIB ($n = 1,957$) | ESSENCE ($n = 3,171$) |
|---|---|---|---|
| Age | ++ | ++ | ++ |
| Coronary artery disease | — | ++ | ++ |
| Diabetes | ++ | — | ++ |
| Vascular disease | ++ | — | — |
| Congestive heart failure history | ++ | — | — |
| Anginal severity | ++ | ++ | ++ |
| Aspirin within 7 days | — | ++ | — |

Other study predictors include female gender, number risk factors, previous MI, prior PCI/CABG.

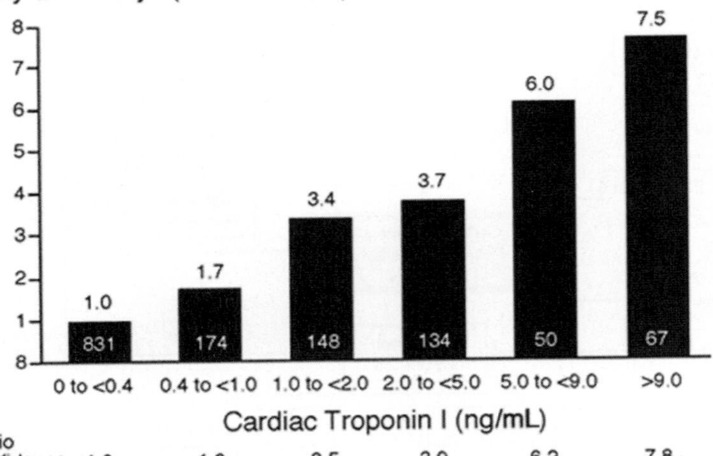


**Figure 18–7** Mortality and troponin-I levels.

in identifying high-risk patients with non–ST-elevation ACS (Fig. 18–7). Other markers of inflammation, such as C-reactive protein (CRP), CD-40, CD-40 ligand, fibrinogen levels, or B-type natriuretic peptide (BNP) can add to the prognostic information in ACS. Adding multiple markers to assess a patient may add important prognostic information, as illustrated in the OPUS-TIMI 16 (Oral Glycoprotein IIb/IIIa Inhibition with Orbofiban in Patients with Unstable Coronary Syndromes) trial and the TACTICS-TIMI 18 (Treat Angina with Aggrastat and Determine Cost of Therapy with an Invasive or Conservative Strategy) analyses (Fig. 18–8). However, at the present time, there is no clear consensus on how to incorporate these markers in patient management.

### *Risk Scores*

An essential element of risk stratification following an ACS is the quantification of short-term and long-term risk. Although there are many historical, physical exam, ECG, and biomarker variables that are significantly and independently associated with worse short-term outcome, the integration of these into an accurate estimation of risk is complex and has traditionally required the use of sophisticated multivariable modeling (Figs. 18–9, 19–10, and 19–11). Nevertheless, simplified nomograms and risk scores incorporating the most important variables have been derived from a number of these analyses and allow for a reasonably accurate categorization of patients into low-risk, intermediate-risk, and high-risk groups. In the analysis by Boersma et al. (see Fig. 18–11), patient age, heart rate, systolic blood pressure, ST-segment depression, signs of heart failure, and elevation of cardiac markers were the most important predictors of death or MI at 30 days. In the analysis by Antman et al. (TIMI risk score, see Fig. 18–9), age >65 years, >3 coronary risk factors, prior CAD, ST deviation, >2 angina episodes in last 24 hours, use of aspirin within 7 days, and elevated cardiac markers were important in determining death, reinfarction, or recurrent severe ischemia requiring revascularization (termed TIMI risk score).

## During-Hospitalization and Predischarge Risk Stratification

Patients who develop recurrent ischemia or reinfarction, CHF, hemodynamic compromise, or life-threatening arrhythmias are candidates for early angiography. Additionally, ACC/AHA Guidelines recommend angiography in

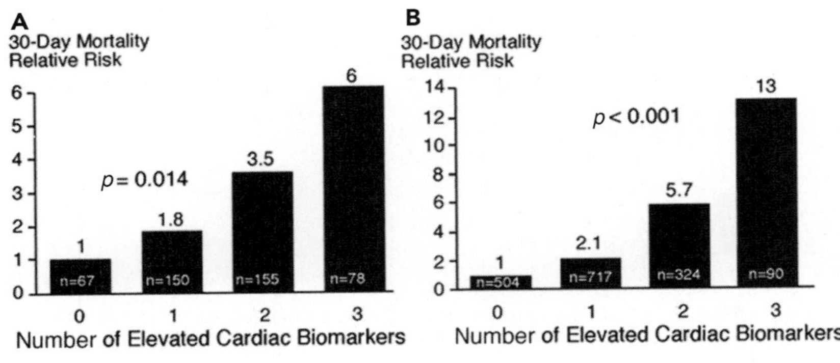


**Figure 18–8** Relative 30-day mortality risks in OPUS-TIMI 16 **(A)** and TACTICS-TIMI 18 **(B)** in patients stratified by the number of elevated cardiac biomarkers (TnI, CRP, and BNP). (From *Circulation*. 2002;105:1760.)

1) Age >65 years
2) ≥3 CAD risk factors
3) Coronary stenosis >50%
4) ST deviation
5) Severe anginal symptoms
6) ASA use in last 7 days
7) Elevated cardiac markers

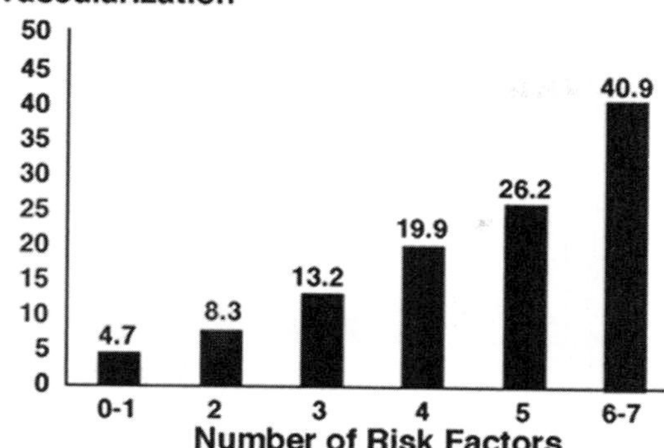


**Figure 18–9** TIMI risk score (TIMI IIB and ESSENCE): 14-day outcome after non–ST-elevation ACS (From *JAMA*. 2000;284:835–842.)

those who have had prior PCI or CABG. There is considerable controversy over the nonacute risk stratification of patients with unstable angina and non–ST-elevation MI who have stabilized on medical therapy. The TIMI IIIb (Thrombolysis in Myocardial Ischemia) and VANQUISH (Veterans Affairs Non-Q-Wave Infarction Strategies in Hospital) trials suggest a more conservative approach with catheterization only in those who develop high-risk features, spontaneously or during provocation (i.e., selective approach). In contrast, the FRISC II (Fast Revascularization during Instability in Coronary Artery Disease) and TACTICS-TIMI 18 studies reported significant decreases in the rate of death or MI at 6 months among patients randomized to early angiography with revascularization as needed (i.e., early invasive approach). Both the early invasive and conservative strategies are given Class I indications in the ACC/AHA Guidelines. In the absence of high-risk clinical features or post–ACS complications, patients who have not undergone coronary angiography should be considered at low or intermediate risk pending the results of further risk stratification. Noninvasive testing provides useful supplementary information beyond that available from clinically based assessments of risk in this cohort.

The purpose of noninvasive testing is to identify ischemia and estimate prognosis. Accordingly, noninvasive evaluation should include an assessment of LV function and/or ischemia in order to identify patients who are at increased risk of adverse outcomes who are likely to benefit from coronary angiography and revascularization. High-risk findings on noninvasive testing should direct patients to coronary angiography if they are eligible for revascularization (Table 18–4). It is not clear whether LV function assessment or myocardial perfusion imaging (with rest and during exercise or pharmacologic stress) is superior in assessing prognosis. The ability of most noninvasive tests to dichotomize patients into low-risk and high-risk groups appears similar (Table 18–5). Selection of the appropriate test should be based on patient characteristics, availability of the test, and institutional expertise in performance and interpretation.

The ACC/AHA Guidelines recommend exercise ECG as the primary mode of noninvasive stress testing. Patients with baseline ECG abnormalities that preclude accurate interpretation (Table 18–6) should undergo an exercise test with imaging. Those who are unable to exercise (the cohort at highest risk of future adverse outcomes) should undergo pharmacologic stress testing with imaging. According to the ACC/AHA Guidelines, stress testing is safe in low-risk patients who have been free of ischemia or CHF for 12 to 24 hours and for 2 to 3 days in intermediate-risk patients. Patients who do not have any high-risk findings on noninvasive evaluation require no further testing.

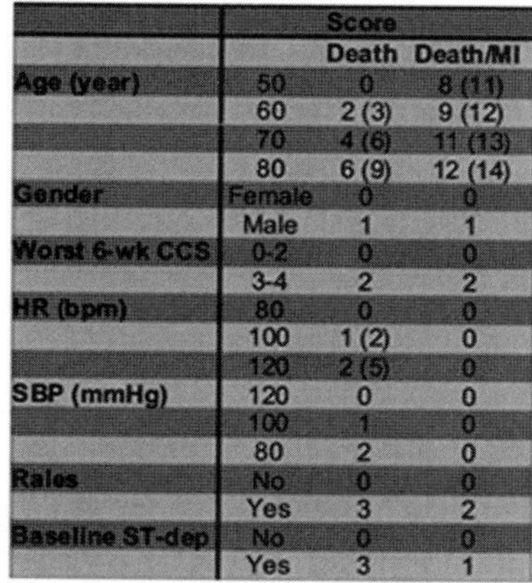

| | Score | | |
|---|---|---|---|
| | | Death | Death/MI |
| Age (year) | 50 | 0 | 8 (11) |
| | 60 | 2 (3) | 9 (12) |
| | 70 | 4 (6) | 11 (13) |
| | 80 | 6 (9) | 12 (14) |
| Gender | Female | 0 | 0 |
| | Male | 1 | 1 |
| Worst 6-wk CCS | 0-2 | 0 | 0 |
| | 3-4 | 2 | 2 |
| HR (bpm) | 80 | 0 | 0 |
| | 100 | 1 (2) | 0 |
| | 120 | 2 (5) | 0 |
| SBP (mmHg) | 120 | 0 | 0 |
| | 100 | 1 | 0 |
| | 80 | 2 | 0 |
| Rales | No | 0 | 0 |
| | Yes | 3 | 2 |
| Baseline ST-dep | No | 0 | 0 |
| | Yes | 3 | 1 |

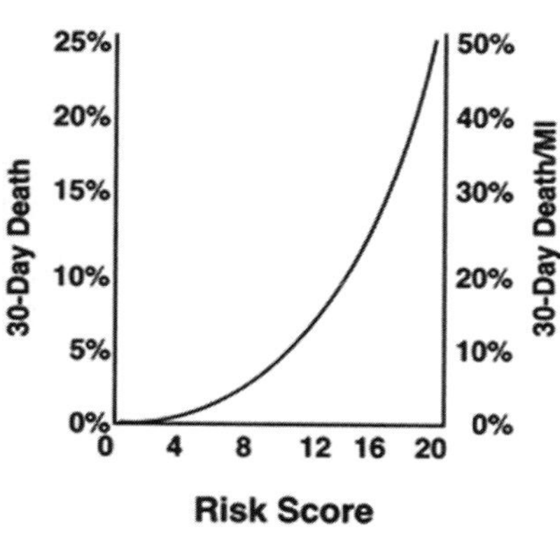


**Figure 18–10** PURSUIT risk score 30-day outcome after non– ST-elevation ACS. (From *Circulation*. 2000;101:2557–2567.)

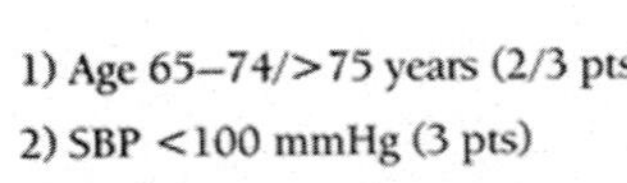
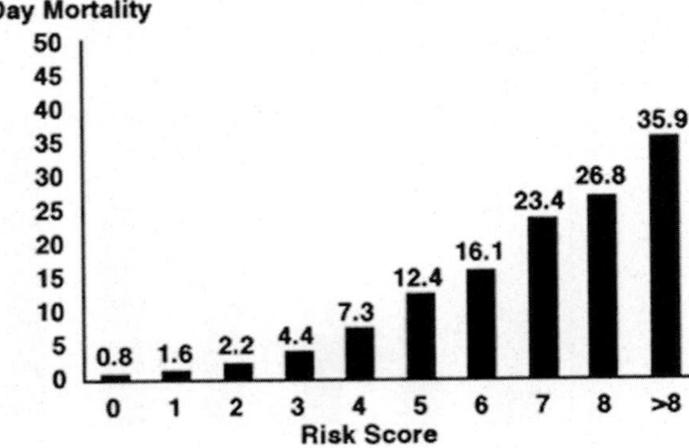


**Figure 18–11** Mortality at 30 days according to clinical characteristics.

## POST–MYOCARDIAL INFARCTION THERAPY

After myocardial infarction, secondary prevention of cardiovascular events depends on prompt institution of appropriate pharmacotherapy, lifestyle changes, and co-morbid disease management. In this area, recent advances have revealed the significant benefits of antiplatelet therapy, neurohormonal blockade, and lipid-lowering therapy. The importance of diet and exercise, as well as smoking cessation, cannot be overemphasized. In addition, optimal management of diabetes and hypertension are paramount to preventing further events. As demonstrated in Figure 18–12, residual LV function after MI is a strong determinant of the proper approach to post–MI pharmacotherapy. This section outlines the role of these therapies as well as lifestyle changes in the post–MI patient.

### Antiplatelet Therapy

A large number of randomized, controlled trials, summarized in meta-analysis by the Antiplatelet Trialists' Collaboration, have documented the benefit of daily aspirin therapy after myocardial infarction. The recommended daily dose of aspirin is 75 to 325 mg orally, to be given indefinitely, based on a 25% reduction in recurrent infarction, stroke, or vascular death. Although the universal application of aspirin therapy among patients without contraindications is accepted, a subset of patients can be shown to exhibit either biochemical or clinical resistance to aspirin. Such patients may potentially benefit from dual antiplatelet therapy, with the addition of a thienopyridine (clopidogrel) or ticlopidine, although there is no current consensus on the assessment of aspirin resistance, or its treatment. Regardless of aspirin resistance status, clopidogrel has also been shown to be beneficial when added to aspirin among patients with UA/NSTEMI. The CURE (Clopidogrel in Unstable Angina to Prevent Recurrent Events) study demonstrated a 20% reduction in composite endpoint of nonfatal myocardial infarction, stroke, and cardiovascular death after 9 months' follow-up. Clopidogrel therapy after myocardial infarction is also indicated for reduction in recurrent events in the setting of coronary stent implantation, based on analysis of the CREDO (Clopidogrel for the Reduction of Events during Observation) trial. The optimal duration of therapy with combined clopidogrel and aspirin after intracoronary stent implantation is currently debated, especially with use of drug-eluting stents, however, evidence indicates that up to 1 year of therapy may be beneficial. Among patients with a true aspirin allergy or gastrointestinal intolerance, it is currently recommended that clopidogrel be used as monotherapy in a dose of 75 mg orally daily.

Of note, ibuprofen may attenuate the beneficial effects of aspirin in patients with cardiovascular disease, and its regular use should be discouraged for patients taking aspirin after myocardial infarction.

### Anticoagulation

The primary use of oral anticoagulation (warfarin) in the post-MI patient has been shown to be at least as effective as aspirin in terms of risk reduction for recurrent myocardial infarction. Its use as a substitute for aspirin is only recommended among aspirin-allergic patients, however, as the difficulty of administering oral anticoagulation and risk for major bleeding makes this a less than optimal

**TABLE 18–4**
**HIGH RISK FINDINGS ON NON-INVASIVE TESTING LEADING TO CORONARY ANGIOGRAPHY EKG-ABNORMALITIES THAT PRECLUDE ACCURATE INTERPRETATION OF AN EXERCISE STRESS TEST**

1. Severe resting LV dysfunction (LVEF <0.35)
2. High-risk treadmill score (score≤ −11)
3. Severe exercise LV dysfunction (exercise LVEF <0.35)
4. Stress-induced large perfusion defect (particularly if anterior)
5. Stress-induced multiple perfusion defects of moderate size
6. Large, fixed perfusion defect with LV dilation or increased lung uptake (thallium-210)
7. Stress-induced moderate perfusion defect with LV dilation or increased lung uptake (thallium-201)
8. Echocardiographic wall motion abnormality (involving >2 segments) developing at a low dose of dobutamine (≤10 mg/kg min$^{-1}$) or at a low heart rate (<120 bpm)
9. Stress echocardiographic evidence of extensive ischemia

**TABLE 18–5**
**STRESS TEST PREDICTORS OF CARDIAC DEATH AND MYOCARDIAL INFARCTION**

| | Sensitivity | | Specificity | | PPV | | NPV | |
|---|---|---|---|---|---|---|---|---|
| | CD | CD/MI | CD | CD/MI | CD | CD/MI | CD | CD/MI |
| Exercise ECG | | | | | | | | |
| ST-depression | 0.42 | 0.44 | 0.75 | 0.70 | 0.04 | 0.16 | 0.98 | 0.91 |
| Impaired SBP | 0.44 | 0.23 | 0.79 | 0.87 | 0.11 | 0.21 | 0.96 | 0.88 |
| Time of exercise | 0.56 | 0.53 | 0.62 | 0.65 | 0.10 | 0.18 | 0.95 | 0.91 |
| Exercise perfusion | | | | | | | | |
| Reversible defect | 0.89 | 0.80 | 0.38 | 0.48 | 0.07 | 0.16 | 0.98 | 0.95 |
| Multiple defects | 0.64 | 0.75 | 0.71 | 0.76 | 0.07 | 0.17 | 0.98 | 0.97 |
| Exercise ventricular function | | | | | | | | |
| Exercise RVG | | | | | | | | |
| Peak EF <40% | 0.63 | 0.60 | 0.77 | 0.75 | 0.27 | 0.31 | 0.94 | 0.91 |
| Change in EF <5% | 0.80 | 0.55 | 0.67 | 0.74 | 0.15 | 0.18 | 0.98 | 0.94 |
| New wall motion defect | | 0.78 | | 0.50 | | 0.17 | | 0.94 |
| Exercise echocardiography | | | | | | | | |
| Change in EF <5% | | 0.56 | | 0.60 | | 0.14 | | 0.92 |
| New wall motion defect | 1.00 | 0.62 | 0.62 | 0.79 | 0.18 | 0.48 | 1.00 | 0.86 |
| Pharmacologic stress myocardial perfusion | | | | | | | | |
| Reversible defect | 0.56 | 0.71 | 0.46 | 0.49 | 0.10 | 0.19 | 0.90 | 0.91 |
| Multiple defects | | 0.50 | | 0.64 | | 0.17 | | 0.90 |

PPV, positive predictive value; NPV, negative predictive value; SBP, systolic blood pressure; RVG, radionuclide ventriculography; EF, ejection fraction.

alternative. In fact, the use of a thienopyridine (clopidogrel) appears more practical in aspirin-allergic patients. Combination therapy with aspirin and low-intensity warfarin (INR <2.0) has not been shown to be superior to aspirin alone. Moderate and high-intensity oral anticoagulation plus aspirin has been shown to reduce subsequent cardiac events over aspirin alone, with increased bleeding risk only among the high-intensity patients. The use of oral anticoagulation with dual antiplatelet therapy has not been extensively studied. Current guidelines specifically recommend the use of warfarin in post-STEMI patients with atrial fibrillation, left ventricular thrombus, or other indication for anticoagulation. It may also be used for secondary prevention, in combination with aspirin, among patients with left ventricular dysfunction, with or without congestive heart failure, and/or extensive regional wall motion abnormalities. The current recommendations for long-term antithrombotic therapy at hospital discharge after STEMI as shown in Figure 18–13. These guidelines can be generalized to NSTEMI patients as well.

**TABLE 18–6**
**EKG ABNORMALITIES THAT PRECLUDE ACCURATE INTERPRETATION OF AN EXERCISE STRESS TEST**

Left bundle branch block
Left ventricular hypertrophy
Interventricular conduction deficit
Ventricular pacing
Ventricular pre-excitation
Digoxin effect

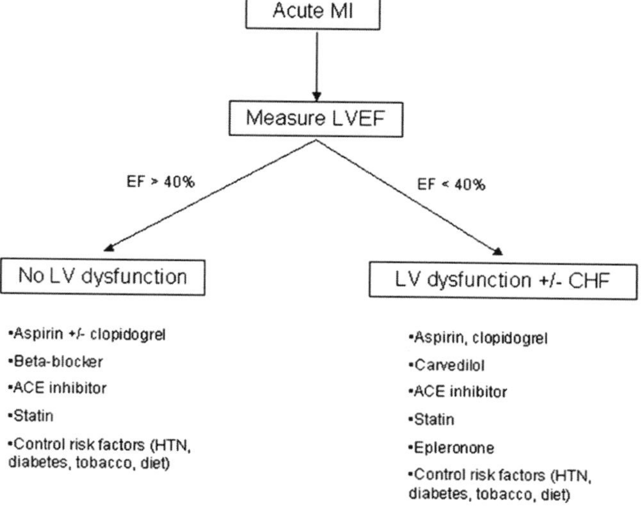


**Figure 18–12** Pharmacologic therapy post-MI in patients with and without significant LV dysfunction.

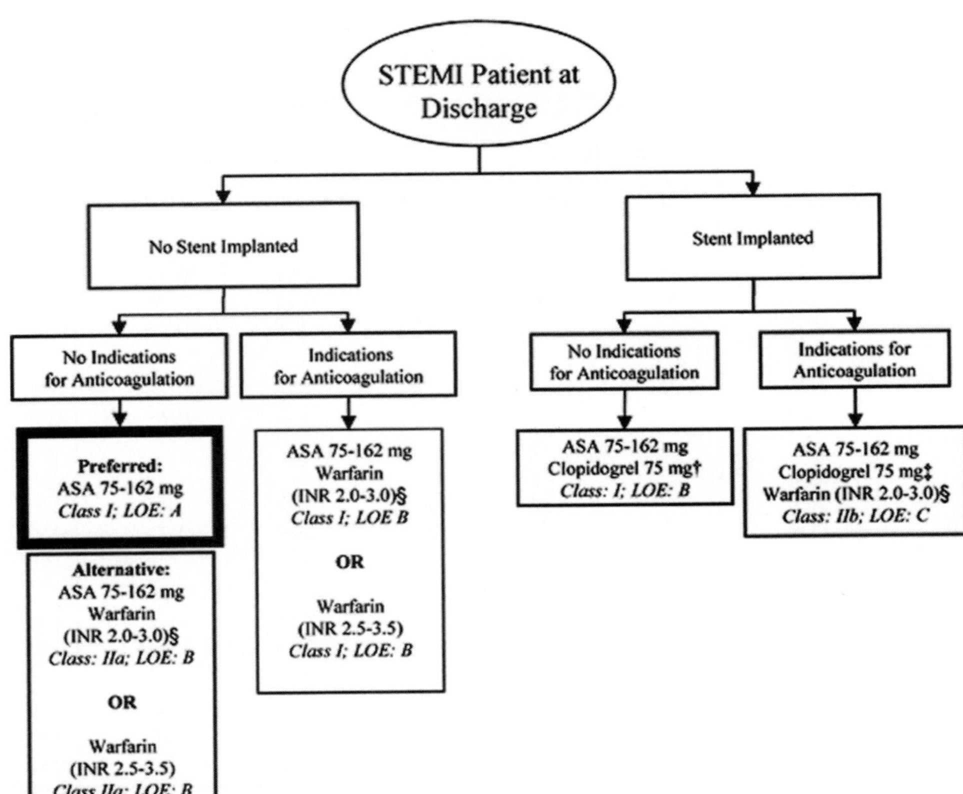


**Figure 18–13** Current ACC/AHA guidelines for anticoagulation and antithrombotic therapy at time of discharge in patients with STEMI. (Adapted from Antman EM, Anbe DT, Armstrong PW, et al. ACC/AHA guidelines for the management of patients with ST-elevation myocardial infarction; a report of the American College of Cardiology/American Heart Association Task Force on Practice Guidelines (Committee to Revise the 1999 Guidelines for the Management of Patients with Acute Myocardial Infarction). *J Am Coll Cardiol.* 2004; 44:E1–E211.)

## Neurohormonal Blockade

### *Renin–Angiotensin–Aldosterone System Inhibition*

The finding of left ventricular dysfunction after myocardial infarction is a strong predictor of subsequent mortality. The renin-angiotensin-aldosterone system is pivotal in modulating the extent of post-MI remodeling and LV dysfunction. Pharmacologic agents have been developed to block this critical pathway at various levels. Many well-designed trials have indicated that angiotensin-converting enzyme inhibitor (ACE inhibitor) use can improve long-term survival and attenuate the progression of LV failure and LV dilatation among post-MI patients with LV dysfunction. This is particularly true for patients with large, anterior STEMI. Current ACC/AHA Guidelines for UA/NSTEMI extend their use only to patients with CHF, LV dysfunction, hypertension, or diabetes. More recently developed ACC/AHA Guidelines for STEMI recommend the use of ACE inhibitors in all post-STEMI patients, based on presumed benefit, even in patients without apparent LV dysfunction. This recommendation was founded on the results of the HOPE (Heart Outcomes Prevention Evaluation) trial, which evaluated the effect of long-term ACE inhibitors among high-risk patients, many of whom (52%) had a prior MI. This trial found a highly significant reduction in MI, stroke, and cardiovascular mortality among such patients. In addition, subsequent secondary analysis of the initial trials confirmed the extension of benefit to all post-MI patients. Many different ACE inhibitors have been studied, and it does appear that ACE inhibitors demonstrate a "class effect," leading to no specific recommendation on the brand of ACE inhibitor.

Similar to ACE inhibitors, positive results have been found for the use of angiotensin-receptor blockers (ARBs) in post-MI patients. This class of medications can provide an alternative to ACE inhibitors among patients with intolerance or allergy to ACE inhibitors, when LV dysfunction or CHF is present. However, given the extensive clinical experience with ACE inhibitors, and the potential positive effects of ACE inhibitors on the vascular endothelium through the bradykinin pathway, ACE inhibitors remain the first line of therapy in patients without contraindication. The combination of ACE inhibitor (captopril) and ARB (valsartan) has been evaluated in immediately post-MI patients in the VALIANT trial (Valsartan in Acute Myocardial Infarction Trial). In this population, combination ACE inhibitor and ARB did not show any benefit over ACE inhibitor alone or ARB alone, although the combination did have increased adverse effects. Of note, valsartan was roughly equivalent to captopril in outcomes. The CHARM trial (Candesartan in Heart Failure Assessment in Reduction of Mortality) focused on patients with chronic congestive heart failure, although 60% of the patients studied had an ischemic etiology. This trial found a small absolute risk reduction with the addition of candesartan to an ACE inhibitor. Based on the findings of these two trials, the combination of ACE inhibitor and ARB can be considered in the long-term management of STEMI patients with persistent symptomatic heart failure and LVEF less than 0.40 (CHARM), but should be avoided in the acute setting (VALIANT).

Finally, aldosterone blockade has been shown to be beneficial in post–MI patients. The RALES trial (Randomized Aldactone Evaluation Study) evaluated patients with New York Heart Association Class III or IV heart failure (55% of patients had ischemic cardiomyopathy) and found a reduction a 24% relative risk reduction in all-cause mortality with 25 to 50 mg of spironolactone daily. More recently, the EPHESUS trial (Eplerenone Post–Acute Myocardial

Infarction Heart Failure Efficacy and Survival Study) evaluated the use of an aldosterone-receptor blocker, eplerenone, in acute MI patients with LV dysfunction (EF ≤0.40). The patients in this trial received optimal therapy, with reperfusion, aspirin, ACEI, beta-blockers, and statins. A significant relative risk reduction for all-cause mortality of 15% was seen among patients receiving eplerenone. It is important to note that patients with severe renal impairment (serum creatinine >2.5 mg/dL) or hyperkalemia (serum potassium >5.0 mmol/L) were excluded from this trial. These findings led to the inclusion of eplerenone in the current STEMI guidelines as a Class I(A) indication.

### *Beta-Receptor Blockade*

Beta-receptor blockade (beta-blockers) has long been considered important in patients with acute myocardial infarction to reduce myocardial ischemia by decreasing oxygen demand. However, long-term beta-blocker therapy in the convalescent phase of MI has also been demonstrated to be beneficial in numerous trials, as demonstrated in Figure 18–14.

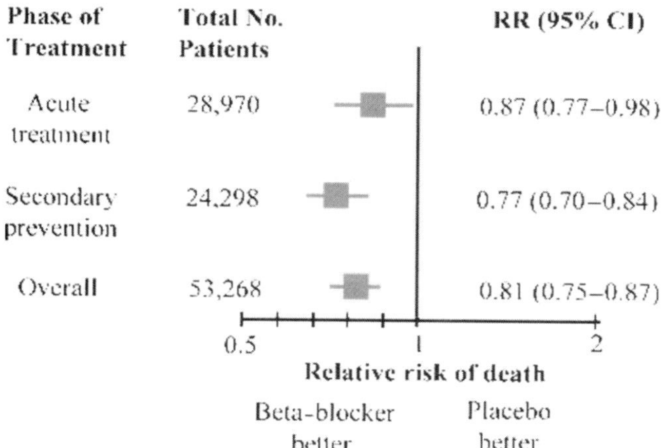


**Figure 18–14** Summary of data from a meta-analysis of trials of beta-blockers for acute MI. (From Antman EM, Anbe DT, Armstrong PW, et al. ACC/AHA guidelines for the management of patients with ST-elevation myocardial infarction; a report of the American College of Cardiology/American Heart Association Task Force on Practice Guidelines (Committee to Revise the 1999 Guidelines for the Management of Patients with Acute Myocardial Infarction). *J Am Coll Cardiol.* 2004;44:E1–E211).

The postulated mechanism of benefit is similar to that seen with the renin–angiotensin–aldosterone system, which is modulation of LV remodeling and LV dysfunction post–MI. After MI, the sympathetic nervous system has been found to increase infarct size, activate the RAAS, and promote myocyte injury. The initiation of beta-blockade, if not begun in the acute treatment phase, is reasonable to begin 24 to 48 hours after freedom from a relative contraindication, such as bradycardia or heart failure. The BHAT trial (Beta-Blocker Heat Attack Trial), a prethrombolytic study, compared 180 to 240 mg of propranolol daily to placebo in post-MI patients, finding a 26% relative risk reduction for all-cause mortality, and a 28% reduction in sudden death. Although metoprolol and atenolol are frequently prescribed to post–MI patients, these agents have not been demonstrated to reduce mortality during long-term therapy. The MERIT-HF (Metoprolol CR/XL Randomised Intervention Trial in Congestive Heart Failure) trial evaluated the use of metoprolol in chronic CHF with EF <40% and found a 33% reduction in mortality. This trial included 66% of patients with ischemic cardiomyopathy. The COMET (Carvedilol or Metoprolol European Trial) compared carvedilol, a nonselective beta-blocker with alpha-blocking capability, with metoprolol in patients with chronic CHF, and found a 17% reduction in the risk of death from carvedilol, relative to metoprolol. More recently, the CAPRICORN trial (Carvedilol Post-Infarct Survival Control in Left Ventricular Dysfunction) tested carvedilol in post-MI patients with significant LV dysfunction (EF ≤0.40). This trial found similar reductions in all-cause mortality and sudden death to the BHAT trial. Current ACC/AHA Guidelines support the use of beta-blockers in all post-MI patients without contraindication, and recommend reassessment of candidacy in the convalescent phase, after resolution of contraindications.

## Lipid Management

Pharmacologic lipid management after myocardial infarction is crucial for secondary prevention of cardiac events. The National Cholesterol Education Program (NCEP) published guidelines in 2001 (ATP III) for lipid-lowering therapy that encourage the use of "therapeutic lifestyle changes" including weight reduction, increased physical activity, increased fiber intake, and reduced intake of saturated fats and cholesterol. The recommended drug therapy for lipid lowering includes statins, bile acid sequestrants, nicotinic acid (niacin), or fibric acids, depending on the patient's lipid profile and potential side effects.

The ATP III guidelines also established a low-density lipoprotein (LDL) goal of <100 mg/dL among patients with known cardiovascular disease. However, since publication of that document, several trials have demonstrated that there is added benefit to additional LDL lowering in very-high-risk patients. This finding has led the ACC/AHA Guidelines writers to recommend targeting an LDL goal of

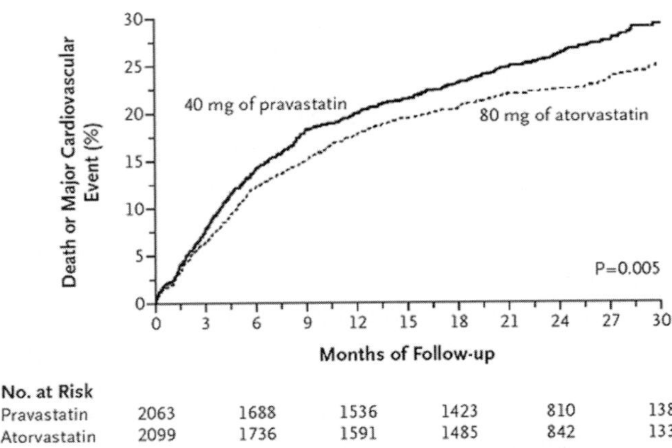


**Figure 18–15** Kaplan-Meier estimates of the incidence of all-cause mortality in the PROVE-IT TIMI 22 study. (*N Engl J Med.* 2004;350(15):1495–1504.)

"substantially less than 100 mg/dL" among STEMI patients. The PROVE-IT TIMI 22 (Pravastatin or Atorvastatin Evaluation and Infection Therapy-Thrombolysis in Myocardial Infarction 22) study was pivotal in the change in recommendation. This trial compared moderate lipid lowering (40 mg of pravastatin) to aggressive lipid lowering (80 mg of atorvastatin) among patients with ACS. The LDL level attained with 40 mg of pravastatin was 95 mg/dL, while 80 mg of atorvastatin resulted in an LDL of 62 mg/dL, representing a 35% difference. The composite cardiovascular endpoint at 2 years was reduced by 16% with atorvastatin (Fig. 18–15).

This trial, as well as other recent trials such as MIRACL (Myocardial Ischemia Reduction with Acute Cholesterol Lowering), and Phase Z of the A to Z trial, demonstrates that more intensive LDL lowering does result in additional benefit in high-risk patients. It may be that the additional benefit to aggressive lipid lowering relates to reduction in inflammation, as evidenced by recent data from the REVERSAL (Reversal of Atherosclerosis with Aggressive Lipid Lowering) trial, showing a relationship between progression of atherosclerosis and CRP levels.

## Risk-Factor Management

Diabetic patients represent a high-risk subset because of macrovascular and microvascular complications including severe coronary artery disease, hypertension, peripheral vascular disease, and renal dysfunction. Tight glucose control during admission for STEMI has been shown to be beneficial in terms of mortality. Continued control of glucose after discharge, with a target HbA1C of <7.0%, reduces microvascular disease and may reduce macrovascular events. Clinical trials have shown that combined neurohormonal blockade with ACE inhibitors, aldosterone antagonists, and beta-blockers are essential in treatment of diabetic patients with prior MI. There is some concern about beta-blockers masking the symptoms of hypoglycemia in diabetic patients, but they have been shown to be beneficial and should be used with appropriate caution in this high-risk subset.

Hypertension management post-MI is important in risk reduction for subsequent MI. In addition to important lifestyle changes such as weight control, exercise, and sodium restriction, current guidelines state that treatment of blood pressure with drug therapy post-MI should be initiated to reach a target blood pressure of 140/80 for all patients, and 130/80 for diabetics and patients with renal insufficiency. However, it is reasonable to treat all patients post-MI to a target blood pressure of 120/80, considering the high-risk population represented by post-MI patients. These recommendations are based on the Seventh Report of the Joint National Committee on Prevention, Detection, Evaluation, and Treatment of High Blood Pressure (JNC-7). The same committee recommends the initiation of two agents if the blood pressure is more than 20/10 mm Hg above goal. From a practical perspective, the post-MI patient should already be receiving a beta-blocker and ACE inhibitor for reasons detailed above, especially among patients with LV dysfunction (EF <40%). Although achieving maximal doses of these medications is essential, the optimal method of reaching target dose is a matter of conjecture. In addition to beta-blockers and ACE inhibitors, thiazide diuretics and long-acting calcium channel antagonists are excellent antihypertensive therapy choices with excellent supporting data from large, multicenter randomized trials, in particular the ALLHAT results (Antihypertensive and Lipid-Lowering Treatment to Prevent Heart Attack Trial).

Obesity is a major risk factor for coronary disease and should be carefully addressed in the post-MI patient as part of a comprehensive secondary risk-reduction strategy. In particular, body mass index and waist circumference have been shown to be important in risk assessment. The desirable body mass index range is 18.5 to 24.9 kg/m$^2$, and the desired waist circumference is less than 40 inches in men and 35 inches in women. Overweight patients should be advised regarding weight-management strategies and appropriate levels of physical activity. An initial weight loss of 10% of body weight over 6 months is the recommended target, at 1 to 2 pounds per week. Patients with an elevated waist circumference should be screened for the metabolic syndrome, a significant risk factor for coronary disease.

Smoking cessation is a must for every post-MI patient. It is imperative that the treating physician provides adequate counseling and pharmacologic therapy to achieve this goal. Smoking has been shown to trigger coronary spasm, reduce effectiveness of beta-blockers, and increase mortality after STEMI. Patients recovering from MI should be provided with counseling and appropriate pharmacologic therapy. Of note, routine use of nicotine-replacement therapy during hospitalization with acute MI is not recommended because of the potential sympathomimetic effects of nicotine.

## CONCLUSIONS

Risk stratification in myocardial infarction is essential to determine appropriate therapy, and for allocation of limited health care resources to high-risk patients. In STEMI, the most important predictors of death include age, systolic blood pressure and heart rate at presentation, congestive heart failure, and location of infarction. Early revascularization is critical to reducing the mortality rate. In NSTEMI, high-risk features, such as biomarker elevation or elevated TIMI risk score, can be used to determine which patients should be eligible for an early invasive strategy. Patients who develop evidence of recurrent ischemia or LV dysfunction after myocardial infarction have a worse prognosis, so the identification of these features is important to guiding predischarge management.

The appropriate use of pharmacotherapy after myocardial infarction also depends on identification of high-risk features. Under most circumstances, post-MI therapy should include daily aspirin, a statin, and a beta-blocker, and may also include clopidogrel (especially if a stent is placed). If significant LV dysfunction is present, an ACE inhibitor and/or ARB, potentially with aldosterone blockade, are needed. Lifestyle modification remains essential to post-MI management, including smoking cessation and control of risk factors such as diabetes and hypertension.

## BIBLIOGRAPHY

**Antman EM, Anbe DT, Armstrong PW, et al.** ACC/AHA guidelines for the management of patients with ST-elevation myocardial infarction; a report of the American College of Cardiology/American Heart Association Task Force on Practice Guidelines (Committee to Revise the 1999 Guidelines for the Management of Patients with Acute Myocardial Infarction). *J Am Coll Cardiol.* 2004;44: E1–E211.

**Braunwald E, Antman EM, Beasley JW, et al.** ACC/AHA 2002 guideline update for the management of patients with unstable angina and non-ST-segment elevation myocardial infarction—summary article: a report of the American College of Cardiology/American Heart Association Task Force on Practice Guidelines (Committee on the Management of Patients with Unstable Angina). *J Am Coll Cardiol.* 2002;40:1366–1374.

**Griffin BP, Topol EJ.** *Manual of Cardiovascular Medicine.* Philadelphia: Lippincott Williams & Wilkins; 2004.

**Topol EJ, Califf RM.** *Textbook of Cardiovascular Medicine.* Philadelphia: Lippincott Williams & Wilkins; 2002.

**Zipes DP, Braunwald E.** *Braunwald's Heart Disease:* A Textbook Of Cardiovascular Medicine. Philadelphia: Elsevier Saunders; 2005.

## QUESTIONS

**1.** A 52-year-old man presented to the Emergency Department with an acute anterior wall myocardial infarction and received successful lytic therapy. Physical exam findings were notable for a systolic blood pressure of 90 mm Hg, a heart rate of 120 beats/min, and rales at both lung bases. The most important determinant of 30-day mortality in this patient is

a. Age
b. Infarct location
c. Killip class
d. Systolic blood pressure
e. Heart rate

Answer is a: An analysis of 41,021 patients with acute MI enrolled in GUSTO-I, a trial of lytic therapy, found that age was the most significant predictor of 30-day mortality in a multivariable analysis. In addition, anterior infarct location, higher Killip class, elevated heart rate, and lower systolic blood pressure were predictors, although they were not as significant as age. Together, these five characteristics included 90% of the prognostic information in the baseline clinical data (Lee et al., *Circulation.* 1995;91:1659–1668).

**2.** The patient in Question 1 had an uncomplicated in-hospital course. All of the following are acceptable risk-factor stratification strategies except:

a. Assessment of LV function
b. Predischarge cardiac catheterization
c. Submaximal stress on days 4 to 6
d. Symptom-limited stress on days 10 to 14

Answer is e: The current ACC/AHA Guidelines for STEMI recommend assessment of LV function as part of a risk-stratification algorithm. It is acceptable to proceed to cardiac catheterization, particularly in patients with EF <0.40 or with high-risk features. In patients who do not undergo cardiac catheterization, it is recommended that those with an interpretable ECG, and who can exercise, undergo exercise stress testing, either as a submaximal stress test on days 4 to 6 or a symptom-limited test on days 10 to 14. EP testing is not part of the recommended algorithm for risk stratification.

**3.** The patient in Question 1 has a brief episode of chest pain (less than 1 minute) with transient ST depression on the morning of his scheduled submaximal stress test. The pain was relieved with one sublingual nitroglycerin tablet. You should:

a. Proceed with submaximal stress as planned
b. Wait two or three additional days and proceed with stress testing if he remains asymptomatic
c. Order echocardiography to see if there have been any additional wall motion abnormalities
d. Schedule for coronary catheterization prior to discharge

Answer is d: Recurrent ischemia after myocardial infarction is a high-risk predictor, and patients with recurrent ischemia should undergo cardiac catheterization and revascularization as indicated.

4. BF is a 48-year-old man who presents for a submaximal stress test prior to discharge after successful thrombolysis for an inferior wall myocardial infarction. His baseline ECG demonstrated a complete LBBB but was unchanged during stress testing. He achieved 5.5 METs and the stress test was stopped because of general fatigue. You are asked to review his stress test and decide to:

   a. Discharge the patient home and schedule him for a symptom-limited stress test in 10 to 14 days
   b. Schedule a symptom-limited stress test in 2 to 3 weeks
   c. Perform cardiac catheterization because of the low METs achieved
   d. Repeat the stress test with perfusion imaging secondary to baseline LBBB

Answer is d: Left bundle branch block precludes interpretation of a stress ECG and is a contraindication to exercise ECG testing, in the absence of nuclear perfusion imaging.

5. JT is a 65-year-old woman who developed cardiogenic shock 10 hours after presenting with an anterior wall myocardial infarction. The most appropriate management strategy is

   a. Administration of thrombolytics
   b. Watchful waiting after initiation of inotropic support and insertion of an intra-aortic balloon pump
   c. Coronary angiography with revascularization within 18 hours of shock onset

Answer is d: Baseline ECG abnormalities can preclude ECG stress test interpretation. LVH with strain, WPW, ventricular pacemaker, and baseline ST depression fall into this category. However, the ECG in RBBB is interpretable, as ST segments are generally normal in this condition.

# Complications of Myocardial Infarction

19

**Amy L. Seidel** **E. Murat Tuzcu**

Despite advances in technology and therapeutics, in-hospital mortality following acute myocardial infarction (AMI) remains high. The leading cause of death in these patients is cardiogenic shock, which has an incidence of approximately 7% (1). Cardiogenic shock (CGS) in the AMI setting can result from severe left or right ventricular systolic dysfunction, dynamic left ventricular outflow tract (LVOT) obstruction, or mechanical complications. These include acute mitral regurgitation (MR) from papillary muscle rupture, tamponade from cardiac free wall rupture, and left-to-right shunting from a ventricular septal defect (VSD). Arrhythmias and inflammatory sequelae are most often less deleterious unless they occur in an unmonitored setting or in a patient who is already in shock or hemodynamically tenuous.

## LEFT VENTRICULAR DYSFUNCTION COMPLICATED BY CARDIOGENIC SHOCK

Isolated left ventricular (LV) failure accounts for the majority of shock cases following AMI. In the Should We Emergently Revascularize Occluded Coronaries for Cardiogenic Shock (SHOCK) Trial and concurrent SHOCK Trial registry, predominant LV failure was the cause of CGS in 78.5% of the patients, and in hospital mortality was 59.2% (2). Autopsy studies have shown that those patients who develop this complication have lost approximately 40% of their myocardial mass to necrosis (3). This generally occurs after a large transmural myocardial infarction or following a relatively small, nontransmural event in someone with prior ischemic damage. In the Global Utilization of Streptokinase and Tissue Plasminogen Activator for Occluded Coronary Arteries (GUSTO-I) Trial that examined outcomes associated with thrombolytic therapy in 41,021 patients with acute ST-elevation myocardial infarction (STEMI), risk factors for the development of shock were advanced age, female gender, prior infarction, anterior infarction location, and diabetes mellitus (4).

### Symptoms and Signs

Patients typically experience chest pain and shortness of breath. Despite this, symptoms usually do not clarify the diagnosis. The physical examination on presentation is more helpful. One of the most popular systems to categorize these patients is the Killip classification (Table 19–1). Shock is present if there are signs of inadequate tissue perfusion with or without hypotension, which is defined as a systolic blood pressure less than 90 mm Hg. Signs of inadequate tissue perfusion include altered mental status, oliguria, and chemical evidence of end-organ damage such as a rise in serum creatinine, lactate, and/or liver transaminases. Patients are often tachycardic, hypothermic, and have cool extremities. Neck vein distention can be seen and an $S_3$ gallop is sometimes heard on physical examination. Peripheral edema and displacement of the point of maximal impulse is less likely unless it existed prior to the AMI.

### Diagnosis

In addition to the symptoms and physical findings mentioned above, the electrocardiogram (ECG) is critical in diagnosis. Anterior STEMI is the most common cause of shock in the AMI setting (2,4). Chest x-ray (CXR) can demonstrate an enlarged cardiac silhouette, although this is rare in the acute phase if prior myocardial damage has not

**TABLE 19–1**
**KILLIP CLASSIFICATION**

| Killip Class | Exam Findings |
|---|---|
| I | No CHF |
| II | Mild to moderate CHF: $S_3$, rales <½ posterior thorax, JVD |
| III | Overt pulmonary edema |
| IV | Cardiogenic shock |

occurred, plus varying degrees of pulmonary venous congestion and edema can be seen. Transthoracic echocardiography (TTE), though not necessary for diagnosis, should be performed urgently in patients with shock or signs of congestive heart failure (CHF) in order to assess the extent of LV and/or RV dysfunction and exclude mechanical complications. Right heart catheterization can also be used to confirm the diagnosis and to monitor therapy. In cardiogenic shock, the cardiac index is typically <2.2 L/min/m$^2$ body surface area, the mixed venous oxygen saturation is low, typically <65%, and the pulmonary capillary wedge pressure (PCWP) is elevated, typically >18 mm Hg.

### Treatment

Treatment involves a combination of revascularization, medication, and mechanical therapy. It is important to remember that mechanical complications other than isolated left ventricular dysfunction must be ruled out in the initial phases of management. Although this can be done with TTE, transport to the catheterization laboratory and implementation of aggressive supportive measures such as placement of an intra-aortic balloon pump (IABP) should not be delayed for this purpose. Patients should be monitored closely in the intensive care unit (ICU), and it is an American College of Cardiology/American Heart Association (ACC/AHA) Class I recommendation that both intra-arterial blood pressure monitoring and right heart catheterization be used to monitor patients in cardiogenic shock (5).

## REVASCULARIZATION

Thrombolytic therapy has a limited effect on the high mortality rate associated with AMI complicated by cardiogenic shock (2,4). Data to support this comes from the Italian Group for the Study of Streptokinase in Myocardial Infarction (GISSI), which randomized >11,000 patients with AMI to thrombolytic therapy versus no thrombolytic therapy. In both groups, the subset of patients with cardiogenic shock had a 70% mortality rate (6). Fortunately, with the advent of more aggressive and invasive strategies for the management of AMI, survival of patients with AMI complicated by cardiogenic shock has improved. Although the SHOCK Trial did not show a significant reduction in 30-day mortality between patients undergoing early revascularization and those receiving initial medical stabilization, 6-month and 1-year survival were both significantly improved in those who underwent early revascularization, defined as within 18 hours of the diagnosis of shock (2,7). Only one subgroup in this study, those 75 years of age or older, did not benefit from early revascularization at 6 months and 1 year. It is therefore an ACC/AHA Class I recommendation that patients younger than 75 years of age with an acute STEMI (including new-onset left bundle branch block) complicated by cardiogenic shock undergo early revascularization with either percutaneous coronary intervention (PCI) or coronary artery bypass grafting (CABG) (5). This recommendation applies only to patients who present within 36 hours of MI onset and who can be revascularized within 18 hours of shock development. This recommendation is Class IIa for patients who are 75 years of age or older. Therefore, treatment must be individualized in this group of patients. Whether shock is present upon arrival or manifests during the course of hospitalization, patients should be transferred to a tertiary care facility capable of performing emergency revascularization and skilled in the management of critically ill patients.

Although the use of thrombolytic therapy has limited efficacy on the high mortality rate associated with this condition, it is acceptable in two circumstances. The first is when the patient is not a candidate for either surgical intervention or PCI. The second is when PCI or CABG is expected to be delayed. For specific recommendations regarding thrombolytic, interventional, and surgical strategies following AMI, see Chapters 16, 17, and 18.

## MEDICAL AND MECHANICAL THERAPIES

Although prompt cardiac catheterization and percutaneous or surgical revascularization are the primary goals in patients with AMI complicated by cardiogenic shock, measures to stabilize the blood pressure and achieve adequate tissue perfusion must begin immediately. If the patient does not possess signs of volume overload, therapy can begin with rapid volume expansion. If this is not corrective, or the patient has volume overload, vasopressor therapy becomes necessary. Dopamine is the drug of first choice, and if the patient remains hypotensive or has signs of inadequate tissue perfusion on maximum doses, norepinephrine should be added. It is acceptable to start with norepinephrine if the patient's blood pressure is very low, with an attempt to transition to dopamine once the patient's systolic blood pressure reaches 80 mm Hg (5). Epinephrine and phenylephrine are not first choices in cardiogenic shock because of their significant $\alpha$-agonist activity, which can lead to an increase in afterload and subsequent decrease in cardiac output. They may become necessary, however, if dopamine and norepinephrine fail to stabilize the patient. It is recommended that inotropic agents such as dobutamine and milrinone not be started until the patient has a systolic blood pressure of 90 mm Hg. For dosing guidelines, see Chapter 60.

## Intra-Aortic Balloon Counterpulsation

In the reperfusion era, a large randomized trial and two large registries have shown benefit of IABP use in patients with AMI complicated by cardiogenic shock. In GUSTO-I, early insertion of an IABP in conjunction with thrombolytic therapy demonstrated a trend toward lower 30-day and 1-year mortality, though the bleeding risk was higher (8). This trial also demonstrated that patients who received no or late IABP therapy had a much higher mortality within the first 8 hours of hospitalization than those receiving IABP therapy early. In the SHOCK Trial Registry and the second National Registry of Myocardial Infarction, patients who received both IABP therapy and thrombolytic therapy had a significant mortality benefit over patients who received thrombolytic therapy alone (9,10). In addition, those who received early IABP and thrombolytic therapy in the SHOCK Trial Registry had a higher likelihood of receiving revascularization. Early IABP therapy, therefore, appears to have a mortality benefit in patients with cardiogenic shock complicating AMI. This is why insertion under these circumstances remains an ACC/AHA Class I recommendation, provided no contraindications exist. These contraindications are aortic dissection, more than moderate aortic regurgitation, sepsis, bleeding diatheses, iliac or aortic atherosclerosis that impairs lower extremity blood flow, patent ductus arteriosis, and an anatomic abnormality of the femoral artery, iliac artery, or aorta that prevents insertion (11). IABP insertion should be performed concomitant with the early stabilization efforts discussed previously. Once in place, it may allow for weaning of both vasopressor and inotropic agents, which increase myocardial workload and are therefore not ideal in the AMI setting.

## Inotropes

Although inotropic agents are not ideal in the setting of active ischemia, in the setting of AMI complicated by shock, they sometimes become necessary. The two most common agents used are dobutamine, which acts primarily by stimulating $\beta_1$-adrenergic receptors, and milrinone, which works through phosphodiesterase inhibition. Dobutamine causes less hypotension and is preferred in the AMI setting.

## Circulatory-Assist Devices

Decisions regarding placement of circulatory-assist devices in the AMI setting, other than an IABP, should involve collaboration with a cardiothoracic surgeon skilled in their placement and follow-up. In addition, the medical and surgical cardiac transplantation teams should be consulted. Decisions regarding their placement are complex and involve multiple considerations in addition to the hemodynamic status of the patient. Mechanical cardiac support devices in AMI complicated by isolated LV dysfunction should be considered when patients remain hemodynamically unstable and have evidence of end-organ hypoperfusion despite IABP therapy and maximal inotropic support. In addition, surgically correctable, mechanical complications of myocardial infarction must be ruled out. Specific hemodynamic criteria include a systolic blood pressure $<$80 mm Hg, with a cardiac index $<$2 L/min/m$^2$ or a PCWP $>$20 mm Hg. Other issues such as transplant candidacy, potential reversibility of cardiac dysfunction, bleeding risks, expected duration of support, and the absence or presence of biventricular dysfunction are also important. In addition, the patient's age, body habitus, and co-morbid conditions must be considered.

There are a number of different circulatory-assist devices, grouped best into two categories. The first category consists of devices used in cardiogenic shock patients who are felt to have stunned myocardium with potential for recovery or those who require immediate hemodynamic stabilization before decisions about long-term treatment can be made. The devices in the first category consist of extracorporeal membrane oxygenation (ECMO), centrifugal ventricular assist devices, the Abiomed ventricular assist device (VAD), and the Thoratec VAD. These do not require ventricular cannulation. If a patient is subsequently refused for transplantation, he or she can be weaned from the device and removal can occur without reinstitution of cardiopulmonary bypass. These devices are useful because they allow for observation of myocardial recovery after a period of rest and provide decision time concerning transplant candidacy. The second category of devices consists of VADs that are suitable for long-term support. Two common devices in this category are the Novacor and HeartMate VADs. If a patient is deemed a transplant candidate in the acute setting, some centers will immediately place this type of device. If a short-term device was used initially, switching to a long-term device can be done, although the Thoratec and Abiomed devices can likewise serve as bridges to transplantation.

## Vasodilators

Vasodilator therapy is ideal in patients with a low cardiac output who are not hypotensive. The two drugs most frequently used in the ICU setting are nitroprusside and nitroglycerin. Nitroprusside is a direct intravenous vasodilator that produces a balanced effect on both arteries and veins. It is initiated at low doses and titrated to a mean arterial blood pressure (MAP) of 65 to 70 mm Hg. Thiocyanate and cyanide toxicity have been reported but are uncommon unless patients receive a prolonged infusion. Patients with renal dysfunction are more prone to the former, and those with liver dysfunction, the latter. Thus, nitroprusside must be used cautiously in patients with these co-morbidities. Intravenous nitroglycerin is the drug of first choice in the setting of AMI and CHF. In addition to its vasodilatory effect, it has anti-ischemic properties, plus, when compared to nitroprusside, is less likely to cause coronary steal. Both of these drugs should be avoided in hypotensive patients.

### Cardiac Glycosides

Because of their narrow therapeutic index and potential for cardiotoxicity, cardiac glycosides should not be used in the treatment of cardiogenic shock associated with AMI.

### Beta-Blockers

Both intravenous and oral beta-blockers should be avoided in patients with AMI complicated by cardiogenic shock. Once the patient is hemodynamically stable and has been weaned from inotrope and IABP support, it is safe to institute low doses of beta-blocker. For recommendations regarding upward titration in stable patients, see Chapter 30.

### Diuretics

Intravenous diuretics are frequently necessary in the setting of AMI complicated by cardiogenic shock, for the treatment of pulmonary edema and volume overload. These can cause hypotension and therefore measures to stabilize the blood pressure should be instituted before diuretics are administered to a hypotensive patient. If the patient is in extremis from a respiratory standpoint, intubation should be considered.

### Angiotensin-Converting Enzyme Inhibitors and Angiotensin-II Receptor Blockers

Multiple trials studying the administration of oral angiotensin-converting enzyme inhibitors (ACE-I) during the first few days following AMI complicated by congestive heart failure (CHF) have shown a decrease in both mortality and adverse cardiovascular events (12–14). Angiotensin-II receptor blockers (ARBs) have also been shown to lower mortality and adverse cardiovascular events when instituted early in patients with AMI complicated by CHF (15,16). Importantly, these trials did not include patients in cardiogenic shock. Once shock has resolved, ACE-I and/or ARBs can be initiated at low doses, provided no contraindications to these drugs exist. See Chapter 30 for further recommendations regarding medical management of the stable heart failure patient.

## MECHANICAL COMPLICATIONS

### Ventricular Septal Defect

Ventricular septal defect is a serious complication of AMI that increases the risk of mortality substantially, even in patients who have undergone urgent surgical correction. In the prethrombolytic era, its occurrence was between 1% and 2%, and it accounted for approximately 5% of AMI-related deaths. The incidence has decreased with the use of thrombolytic agents, as demonstrated in the GUSTO-I Trial,in which the incidence was 0.2% (17). Also noteworthy in GUSTO-I was that the most important predictors of VSD were advanced age, female sex, anterior infarct location, and no current smoking (17). In addition, a history of hypertension was common among patients. Angiographically, >50% of the patients had two- and three-vessel coronary disease and those patients with a VSD were more likely to have had total occlusion of the infarct-related artery (17).

VSD typically presents in the first week after myocardial infarction and usually within 3 to 5 days of symptom onset. It was noted to occur earlier in the GUSTO-I and SHOCK Trials, with a median time of 1 day and 16 hours from MI symptom onset, respectively (17,18). Many of the patients in both of these trials received thrombolytic therapy, which has led investigators to hypothesize that timely administration of thrombolytic therapy restores patency of the infarct-related artery, thereby preventing or limiting the extensive transmural necrosis required for ventricular septal rupture. If it does occur, myocardial hemorrhage is increased and therefore VSD will present earlier (17).

VSD occurs with equal frequency in anterior, inferior, or posterior myocardial infarctions. When it occurs in the setting of a right coronary artery (RCA) or dominant left circumflex artery (LCx) occlusion, the location of the defect is typically in the posterobasal region of the septum as opposed to the apical-septal region, seen with anterior infarctions. Posterobasal ruptures are often complex, with serpiginous courses and/or containing multiple small defects. This differs from the direct, through-and-through communications common with apical-septal defects. These two anatomic differences make surgical and percutaneous closure of posterobasal ruptures more difficult. Additionally, patients with inferior or posterobasal infarctions often present with varying degrees of right ventricular (RV) infarction, which adds to management complexity.

#### *Symptoms and Signs*

VSD results in a left-to-right shunt that leads to RV volume overload, increased pulmonary blood flow, and reduced systemic blood flow. These hemodynamic alterations often lead to shock (see above). Patients demonstrate signs of biventricular failure that include elevated neck veins and pulmonary edema. Peripheral edema is uncommon in the acute setting, as is displacement of the point of maximal impulse. There is often a loud, holosystolic, precordial murmur that has widespread radiation. A palpable, precordial thrill is present in >50% of these patients (19).

#### *Diagnosis*

The physical examination is diagnostic in most patients with a VSD. The test of first choice to confirm its presence

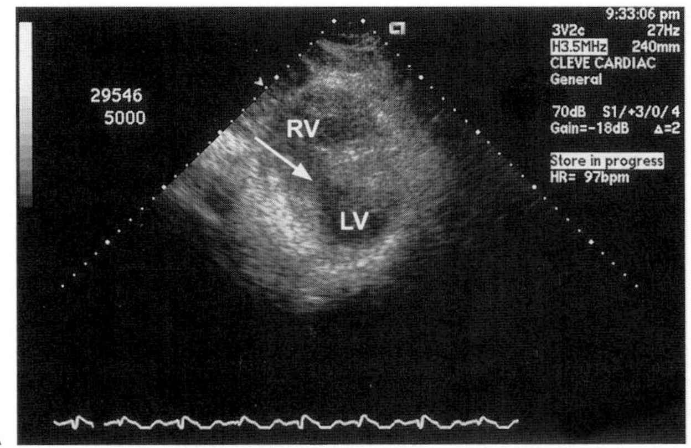


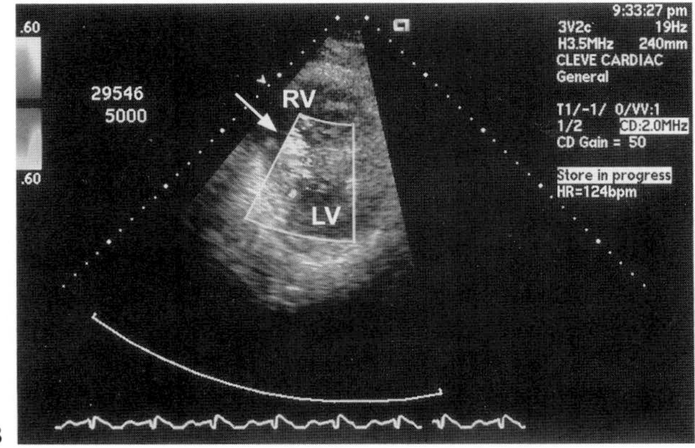


**Figure 19–1** **A.** Subcostal short-axis view demonstrating an inferobasal VSD (arrow). **B.** Same view with color Doppler across the defect, demonstrating a left-to-right shunt. RV, right ventricle; LV, left ventricle.

is TTE with color Doppler imaging. A basal VSD can be visualized in multiple views, including the parasternal long-axis view with medial angulation, the apical long-axis view, the subcostal long-axis view, and the parasternal short-axis view (Fig. 19–1). An apical VSD is best visualized in the apical four-chamber view, although it too can be appreciated in multiple views.

Diagnosis can be confirmed by right heart catheterization with a saturation run. This is performed by sequentially sampling blood from the pulmonary artery (PA), RV, right atrium (RA), superior vena cava (SVC), and inferior vena cava (IVC). It is important to discard several milliliters of blood prior to sampling in each chamber, so that blood from the prior chamber is not admixed within the catheter. In the case of a VSD, there will be a 7% step-up in the RV and PA saturations relative to the saturation in the RA; which normally ranges between 64% and 67%. Subsequently, by using the saturation obtained in the right atrium and the arterial oxygen saturation, one can calculate the degree of shunting, which is expressed as the ratio of pulmonary to systemic blood flow (Qp:Qs) (Fig. 19–2).

Lastly, VSD can be diagnosed by ventriculography. Typically, the best view for this is the LAO projection with cranial angulation, such as LAO 60 degrees with 20 degrees of cranial angulation. This nicely demonstrates the full length of the septum and, with contrast injection, passage of the material will be seen crossing into the RV (Fig. 19–3).

### *Treatment*

Emergency cardiac surgery with concomitant CABG is recommended for patients who present with VSD following AMI. This applies to both stable and unstable patients because stability can change rapidly if the necrotic edges of the defect expand abruptly. While surgical consultation is being obtained, patients should be placed in the ICU for invasive hemodynamic monitoring, initial treatment of shock, and consideration of IABP insertion (see above). If the patient is not hypotensive, a short-acting vasodilator such as nitroprusside can be used to optimize hemodynamics. Percutaneous closure for a VSD complicating AMI has been reported in several case series. It remains investigational,

**Fick Method for Calculating Intracardiac Shunts**

**Qp/Qs**

$$\text{Qp (pulmonary flow, L/min)} = \frac{\text{Oxygen consumption (mL/min)}}{\text{10 (pulmonary AvO}_2\text{ difference)}}$$

$$\text{Qs (systemic flow, L/min)} = \frac{\text{Oxygen consumption (mL/min)}}{\text{10 (systemic AvO}_2\text{ difference)}}$$

Oxygen consumption is estimated from the patient's body surface area (125 mL/min/$m^2$)
$AvO_2$ difference = arterial – venous $O_2$ content
$O_2$ content = (oxygen saturation/100) × 1.36 × hemoglobin concentration (g/dL)

**Simplified Formula**

$$\text{Qp/Qs} = \frac{SaO_2 - MvO_2}{PvO_2 - PaO_2}$$

$SaO_2$ = arterial oxygen saturation
$MvO_2$ = mixed venous oxygen saturation
$PvO_2$ = pulmonary vein saturation
$PaO_2$ = pulmonary artery saturation

**Figure 19–2** Calculation of left-to-right intracardiac shunts. When no shunt exists, $MvO_2$ = pulmonary artery saturation. When a left-to-right shunt is present, $MvO_2$ = the saturation in the chamber prior to the oxygen step-up. If there is no right-to-left shunt, and $PvO_2$ is not collected, it is assumed to be 95%.

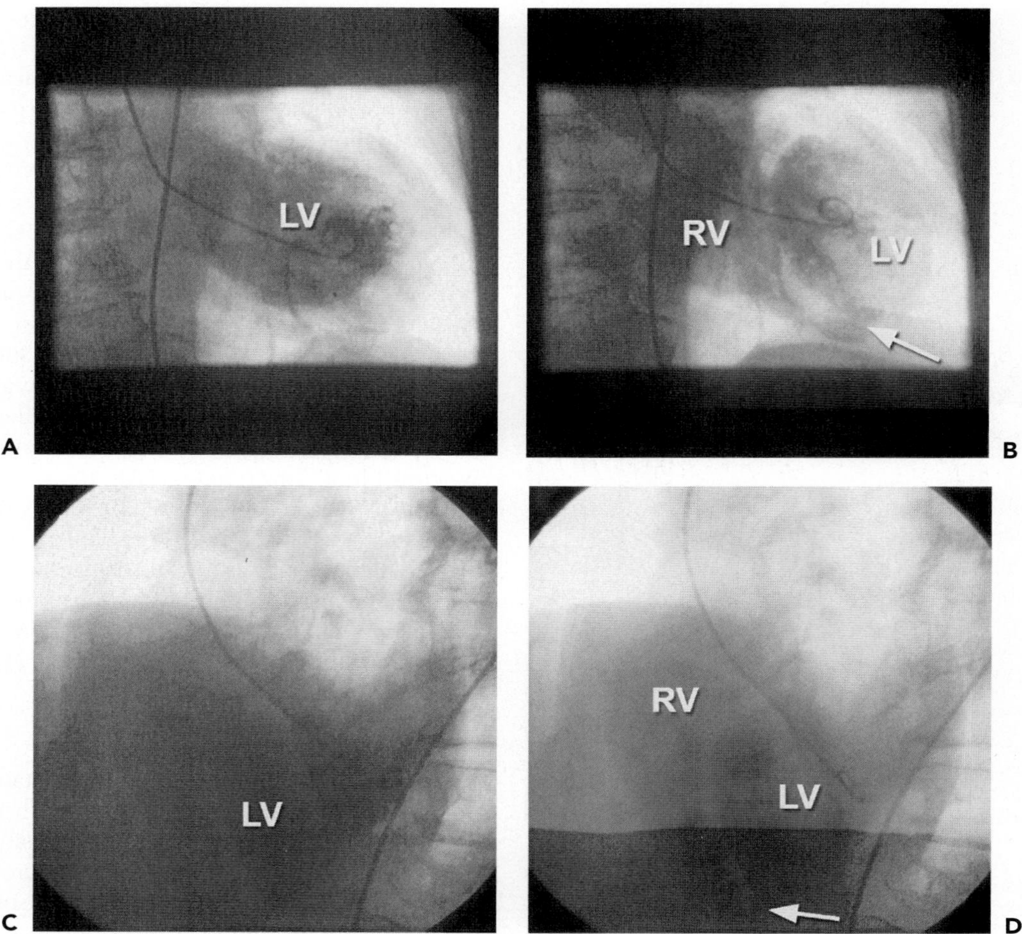


**Figure 19–3** **A.** RAO 20-degree projection demonstrating filling of the left ventricle (LV). **B.** Same view demonstrating filling of the right ventricle (RV) from the LV through an inferoapical VSD (arrow). **C.** LAO 40-degree, cranial 25-degree projection demonstrating filling of the LV. **D.** Same view demonstrating filling of the RV from the LV through and inferoapical VSD (arrow).

as patient numbers were small, follow-up was short, different devices were used, and most patients underwent closure several weeks following the acute event.

Even in patients who undergo emergency surgical repair, mortality at 30 days in the thrombolytic era is estimated to be approximately 50%. This is in comparison to a 94% 30-day mortality in patients managed medically (17). This underscores the importance of prompt recognition, early placement of an IABP, and expeditious triage to the operating room for surgical repair.

## Acute Mitral Regurgitation from Papillary Muscle Rupture or Functional Mitral Regurgitation

Mitral regurgitation in the setting of AMI can occur for various reasons. It can result from papillary muscle rupture, which complicates 1% of AMIs and results in approximately 5% of AMI-related deaths. It can also result from abnormal coaptation of the mitral valve leaflets during systole, secondary to mitral annular dilation or dyssynchronous contraction of the left ventricular walls. The latter is more commonly referred to as functional MR in the setting of ischemic left ventricular damage, and in its mild to moderate form is quite common following AMI.

Although any degree of MR following AMI has been associated with an increase in mortality, severe functional MR and papillary muscle rupture carry the gravest prognosis. In patients who develop severe, functional MR, the infarct is often extensive. In contrast, papillary muscle rupture is more often the result of a small infarction affecting the papillary muscle itself, and typically occurs between the second and seventh days following AMI (19). Rupture of the posteromedial papillary muscle in the setting of an inferior infarction is more common because it has a single vessel blood supply from the posterior descending branch of the dominant coronary artery. The anterolateral papillary muscle receives a dual blood supply from the left anterior descending (LAD) and LCx arteries, making it more resistant to necrosis.

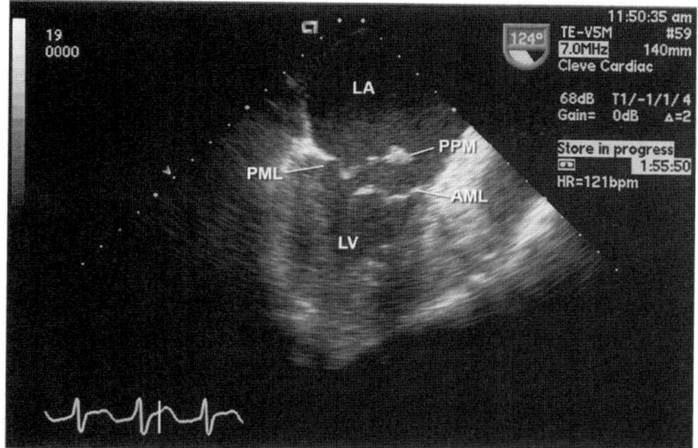


**Figure 19–4** TEE at 124 degrees at the mid-esophageal level demonstrating papillary muscle rupture and a flail posterior mitral leaflet. LV, left ventricle; LA, left atrium; PML, posterior mitral leaflet; AML, anterior mitral leaflet; PPM, posterior papillary muscle.

### *Symptoms and Signs*

Severe MR caused by papillary muscle rupture or functional (ischemic) MR manifests as sudden shortness of breath followed by rapid hemodynamic deterioration. The median time to its development in the SHOCK Trial registry was 12.8 hours (20). Also noteworthy in the SHOCK Trial Registry was that ST elevation was less frequent in those patients with cardiogenic shock and severe MR in comparison to patients with cardiogenic shock caused by severe left ventricular dysfunction without MR (20). This important observation shows that an ECG with a relatively benign appearance in the setting of abrupt and severe hemodynamic deterioration should raise the suspicion of acute MR. Signs of shock are typically present (see above), and patients frequently have pulmonary rales. A precordial, systolic murmur may be heard, and its quality varies significantly from patient to patient. In some cases there is no appreciable murmur due to the rapid equilibration of pressures between the left ventricle and left atrium.

### *Diagnosis*

Although physical examination is quite helpful, accurate diagnosis can be made by TTE or transesophageal echocardiography (TEE) with color Doppler imaging. The left ventricular ejection fraction (LVEF) may be normal or even supranormal in the case of papillary muscle rupture, as the infarcts occurring in this setting are often less extensive, plus the MR possesses an unloading effect on the left ventricle. If rupture has occurred, one will see the head of the papillary muscle attached to a flail mitral leaflet (Fig. 19–4).

RHC, though important for hemodynamic monitoring and therapy in MR complicating AMI, should not be used as a diagnostic modality. It can, however, help to confirm the diagnosis. In addition to an elevated PCWP, there will often be giant V-waves in the PCWP tracing (Fig. 19–5). Left ventriculography can also confirm the diagnosis, but it is often unnecessary because echocardiography is sufficient to make both diagnostic and treatment decisions.

### *Treatment*

Stabilization efforts for papillary muscle rupture and severe, functional MR are the same as those discussed for patients with cardiogenic shock related to isolated LV dysfunction. With regard to medical therapy, patients who are not hypotensive can be managed with an intravenous vasodilator such as sodium nitroprusside. This will reduce left ventricular afterload, improve cardiac output, and subsequently reduce the degree of mitral regurgitation and pulmonary edema. An IABP should be placed if the patient is in shock or has overt pulmonary edema. In patients with papillary muscle rupture, even if these two signs are not present, IABP therapy should be considered because stability can change rapidly. Stabilization efforts should begin immediately, but not prevent rapid transport to the catheterization laboratory. Patients should be cared for in the ICU, and there is general agreement that a RHC is warranted for short-term guidance of pharmacologic and/or

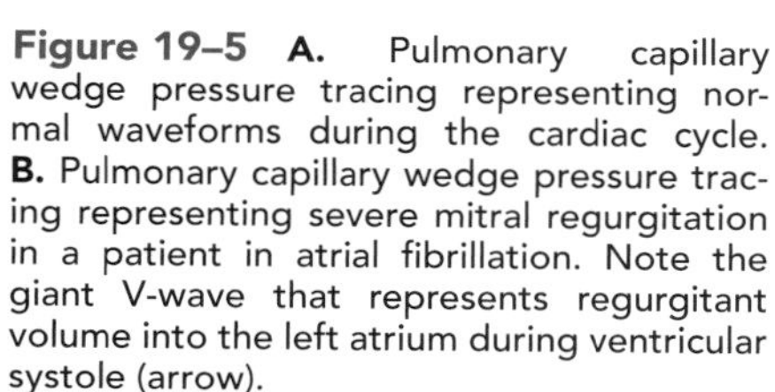

**Figure 19–5 A.** Pulmonary capillary wedge pressure tracing representing normal waveforms during the cardiac cycle. **B.** Pulmonary capillary wedge pressure tracing representing severe mitral regurgitation in a patient in atrial fibrillation. Note the giant V-wave that represents regurgitant volume into the left atrium during ventricular systole (arrow).

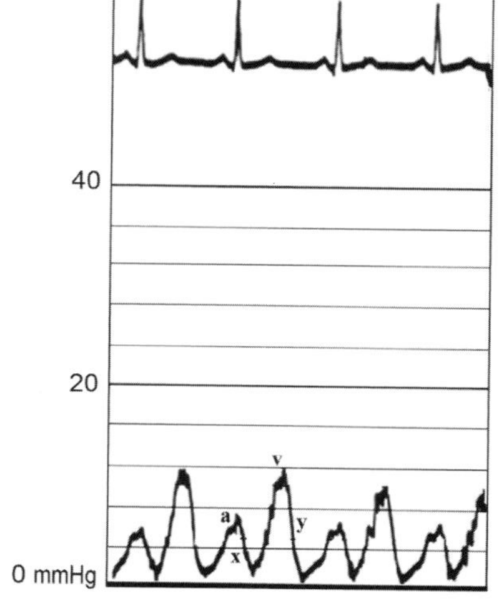


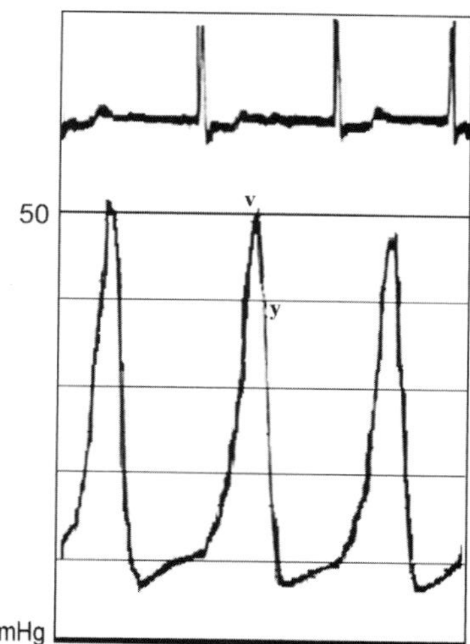

mechanical management of severe MR complicating AMI (21). Diuretics should be used judiciously for relief of pulmonary edema.

Emergency cardiac surgery with concomitant CABG is indicated in all cases of AMI complicated by papillary muscle rupture. Stability can change rapidly, so stabilization and triage to the operating room must be swift. In-hospital mortality in surgically treated patients is approximately 40%, substantially lower than for those treated medically (20). In patients who survive to hospital discharge, short- and long-term survival remain excellent. Although a patient with severe functional MR may ultimately require CABG and mitral valve repair or replacement, emergency surgery is not necessary for the MR alone. This is because the degree of regurgitation often improves with revascularization and aggressive medical and/or mechanical therapies. If the patient's coronary anatomy is felt to require surgical revascularization, the degree of mitral regurgitation should be reassessed and valve repair or replacement considered if it is moderate or greater (5).

## Cardiac Free Wall Rupture

Cardiac free wall rupture, though an infrequent complication of AMI, is the second leading cause of in-hospital mortality in AMI patients. Approximately half of cardiac ruptures occur within the first 5 days of AMI, and approximately 90% within the first 2 weeks. It can present in an acute or subacute fashion. The acute presentation is typically not compatible with life. Subacute rupture presents more subtly, and if diagnosis is made early, prognosis with surgery is favorable.

Rupture most commonly involves the LV, but on occasion may involve the RV. Although the incidence of cardiac rupture has decreased recently, there has been an increase in the incidence of in-hospital mortality following rupture. This is particularly more common in the first 2 days following AMI, in those patients who have received thrombolytic therapy (22,23). Risk factors associated with free wall rupture have been variable across studies, but those commonly seen include: age >70 years, female gender, no history of prior myocardial infarction or angina, transmural myocardial involvement, poor coronary collateral blood flow, and hypertension (24–27).

### *Signs and Symptoms*

The acute presentation of free wall rupture is typically one of cardiovascular collapse and electromechanical dissociation. This is commonly associated with transmural, through-and-through tears that cause abrupt tamponade. The subacute presentation is less severe, and patients slowly begin to manifest signs of cardiogenic shock (see above) from tamponade. This is due to the slow egress of blood into the pericardial space from gradual or incomplete rupture of the infarcted myocardium. It can also occur when thrombus or pericardium incompletely seals off the rupture site, also known as a pseudoaneurysm, or contained rupture. Patients may experience persistent or recurrent chest pain with ST- and T-wave abnormalities. Additionally, they may experience episodes of transient hypotension, nausea, a feeling of doom, and/or have a fleeting pericardial friction rub prior to decompensation. Signs of tamponade, such as hypotension, tachycardia, and neck vein distention, may be present.

### *Diagnosis*

In addition to the above symptoms and signs, the ECG often demonstrates persistent ST elevation and evidence of infarct extension or expansion (27). Hemodynamics by RHC will demonstrate elevation of intracardiac pressures, along with equalization of diastolic filling pressures and a reduced cardiac output. Pulsus paradoxus can be appreciated on the intra-arterial waveform, along with blunting of the Y decent on the right atrial and pulmonary arterial pressure waveforms (Fig. 19–6). TTE will demonstrate a large pericardial effusion and signs of tamponade, including right atrial collapse during ventricular systole (Fig. 19–7), right ventricular collapse during ventricular diastole (Fig. 19–8), respiratory variation of the tricuspid and mitral valve inflow velocities, and a plethoric inferior vena cava (IVC) (see Fig. 19–7) that fails to collapse by 50% of its diameter with inspiration. It is important to note that pericardial effusion is a common finding following uncomplicated myocardial infarction. Its presence should heighten one's suspicion for the possibility of subacute rupture. Serial echocardiography and close clinical observation can then be performed in order to exclude further accumulation of pericardial fluid.

### *Treatment*

Patients with acute or subacute rupture should be supported with intravenous fluids and, if hypotensive, with vasopressors while emergency cardiothoracic surgical consultation is obtained. Pericardiocentesis should be performed only in the operating room, as decompression of the pericardial space will result in further bleeding. If a patient is hemodynamically unstable despite treatment with fluids and vasopressors, pericardiocentesis can be performed as a last resort because decompression is the only chance for survival.

## Pseudoaneurysm

Although it is an infrequent complication of AMI, it is important to recognize a pseudoaneurysm because it is prone to complete rupture. It occurs when pericardial adhesions and thrombus seal off an area of myocardial rupture. Although this can happen at any location, a recent review found that the posterior wall was the most common area of involvement. This was followed by the lateral, apical, and finally inferior regions of the myocardium (28). In comparison to a true aneurysm, there is no myocardium

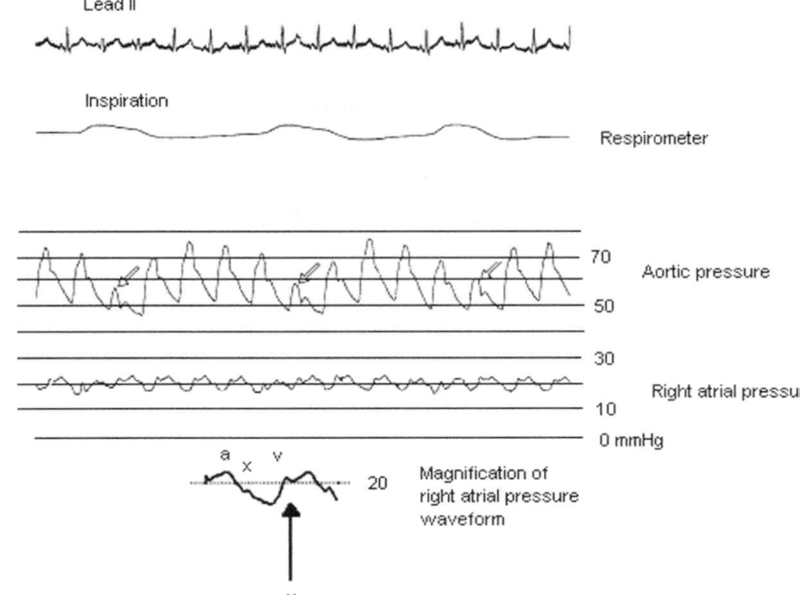


**Figure 19–6** Hemodynamic findings in tamponade. Note that the aortic pressure tracing demonstrates hypotension and pulsus paradoxus (drop in systolic blood pressure by greater than 10 mm Hg upon inspiration). In addition, the right atrial pressure is elevated and the y-descent is extremely blunted (arrow). a, atrial contraction; x, atrial relaxation; v, atrial filling (ventricular systole); y, atrial emptying (ventricular diastole). (Modified from Wu LA, Nishimura RA. Pulsus paradoxus. *N Engl J Med.* 2003;349(7):666.)

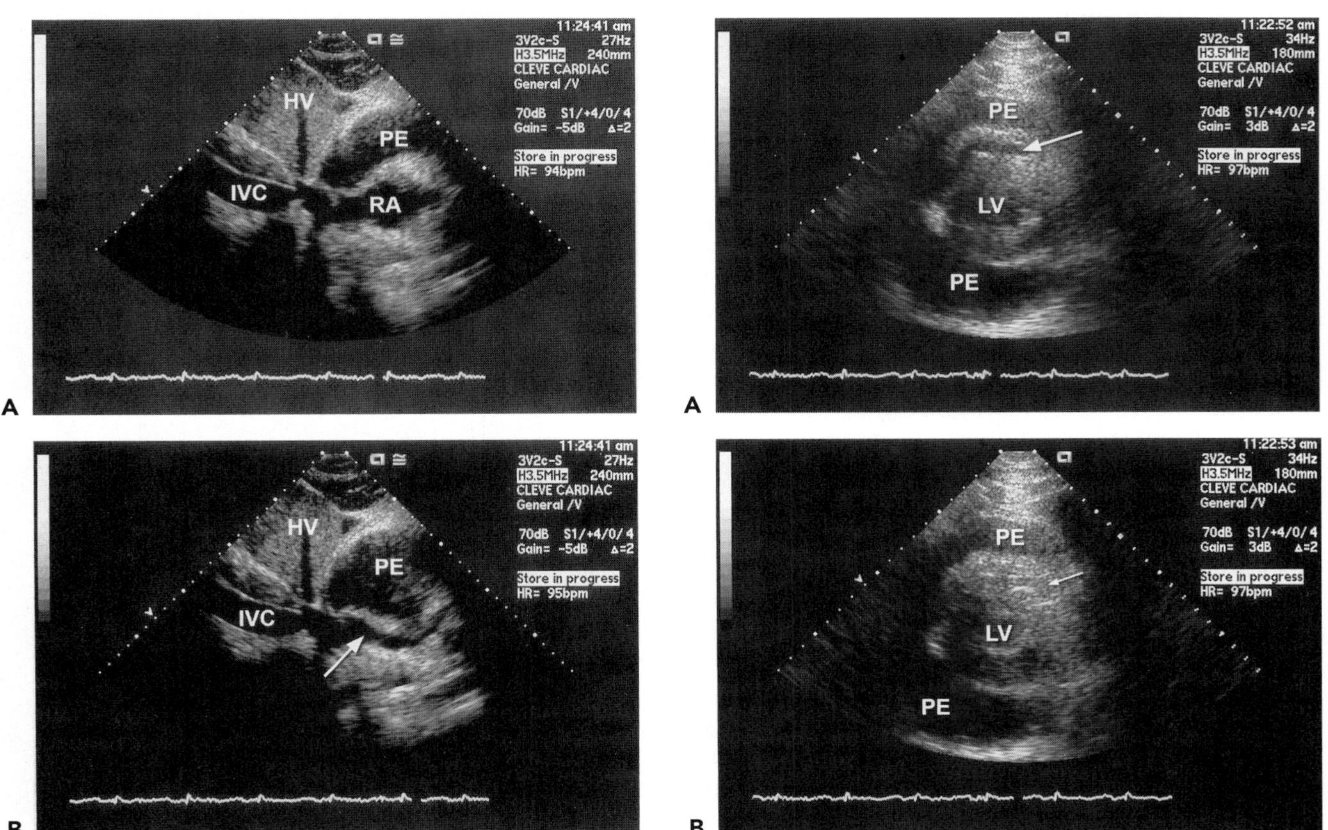


**Figure 19–7** **A.** Subcostal long-axis view demonstrating a large pericardial effusion adjacent to the right atrium. **B.** Same view demonstrating right atrial wall inversion (arrow) during systole. Note that inferior vena cava (IVC) plethora is present in both images. HV, hepatic vein; PE, pericardial effusion; RA, right atrium.

**Figure 19–8** **A.** Parasternal short-axis view demonstrating that the right ventricle, while small and underfilled, remains open during systole (arrow). **B.** Same view demonstrating right ventricular diastolic collapse (smaller arrow). LV, left ventricle; PE, pericardial effusion.

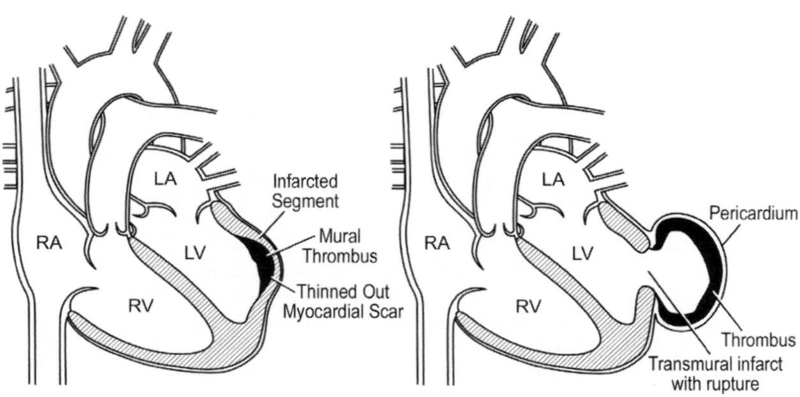


**Figure 19–9** Pseudoaneurysm versus aneurysm. (Modified from Cercek B, Shah PK. Complicated acute myocardial infarction: heart failure, shock, mechanical complications. *Cardiolo Clin.* 1991;9(4): 569–593.)

between the left ventricular cavity and the pericardial space (Fig. 19–9), hence the propensity for complete rupture. Risk factors for the development of postinfarction pseudoaneurysm are similar to those for myocardial free wall rupture (see above).

### *Symptoms and Signs*

Pseudoaneurysms are often silent and are discovered on follow-up imaging or postmortem. Gradual enlargement of the aneurysmal cavity can lead to progressive heart failure symptoms, although this is rare. The diagnosis should be considered if a patient develops dyspnea on exertion, lower-extremity edema, orthopnea, paroxysmal nocturnal dyspnea, and fatigue following AMI. Some present with arrhythmias, most commonly ventricular. Others develop signs and symptoms of systemic arterial embolization due to egress of thrombus from the aneurysmal cavity. The physical examination can be normal or consistent with CHF. Some patients will have a new murmur on auscultation, although 30% will have no murmur (28). Rarely, a patient will present in cardiogenic shock (see above).

### *Diagnosis*

The ECG may show persistent ST elevation or regional pericarditis, although it most often demonstrates nonspecific ST changes (28). CXr can demonstrate an abnormal bulge around the site of involved myocardium but more frequently shows cardiomegaly. There are several imaging modalities available for diagnosis, including contrast ventriculography, TTE, TEE, magnetic resonance imaging (MRI), and computed tomography (CT). None of these tests has been 100% accurate, and no adequate comparisons between modalities have been made. Contrast ventriculography is the "gold standard" and has been associated with a high degree of diagnostic accuracy. One will see a narrow orifice leading to a saccular cavity. If concomitant coronary arteriography is performed, there will be a lack of vessels at the site of the pseudoaneurysm. Because this is an invasive modality, TTE with color Doppler is a reasonable test to perform first, although its diagnostic accuracy was found to be 26% for this condition (28) (Fig. 19–10). Although TEE and MRI have shown a higher

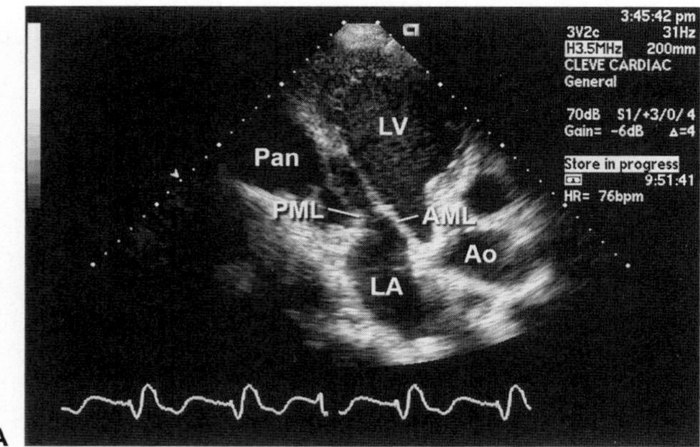


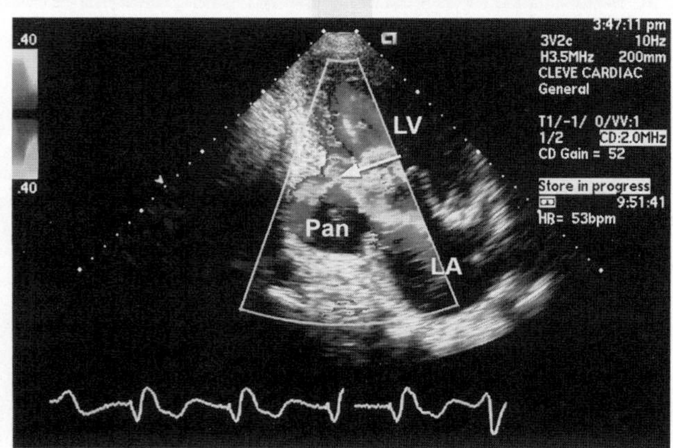


**Figure 19–10** **A.** Apical long-axis view demonstrating a pseudoaneurysm of the posterior left ventricular (LV) wall. **B.** Same view with color Doppler demonstrating the rupture site (arrow) with turbulence of blood flow in and surrounding the cavity. LA, left atrium; AML, anterior mitral leaflet; PML, posterior mitral leaflet; Pan, pseudoaneurysm; Ao, aorta.

degree of diagnostic accuracy, only small numbers have been studied and a definitive conclusion regarding superiority cannot be made. If MRI is used, cine will increase diagnostic sensitivity with its ability to highlight abnormal blood flow patterns and turbulence in and around the cavity of a pseudoaneurysm. In addition, it will often demonstrate loss of epicardial fat at the site of rupture.

### *Treatment*

Once a pseudoaneurysm is diagnosed, urgent surgery is indicated because of a 30% to 45% risk of rupture (28). If the pseudoaneurysm is incidentally diagnosed or the patient is asymptomatic, the patient should be monitored until surgical evaluation has occurred.

## Left Ventricular Aneurysm

A true ventricular aneurysm differs anatomically from a pseudoaneurysm in that myocardium is present in its wall and there is no communication between the ventricular cavity and pericardial space (see Fig. 19–9). Its incidence following AMI has been reported as high as 38%. With the advent of reperfusion therapy, its frequency has decreased to between 8% and 15% (19,29). Ventricular aneurysms most commonly complicate transmural anterior wall myocardial infarctions and are thought to be the result of infarct expansion. In contrast to post-MI pseudoaneurysms, true ventricular aneurysms rarely rupture because the walls become fibrotic and calcified with time. True aneurysms have a wide base and are frequently associated with mural thrombus (19).

### *Signs and Symptoms*

Aneurysms place the entire ventricle, including the noninfarcted portion, at a mechanical disadvantage. Contractile energy is expended during passive outward expansion of the aneurysmal wall, and cardiac output decreases. This functional decline is more significant with acute aneurysms because the aneurysmal wall is more compliant and therefore expands to a greater degree during systole. Additionally, the distorted geometry can lead to misalignment of the mitral valve apparatus and result in mitral regurgitation.

Patients can present early or several weeks following AMI. They can be asymptomatic, or develop congestive heart failure, cardiogenic shock, or recurrent ventricular arrhythmias. The index event is less often systemic embolization. The physical examination may demonstrate signs of congestive heart failure and/or cardiogenic shock. In addition, patients may have a diffuse, dyskinetic apical impulse that is shifted leftward. Auscultation may reveal a murmur suggestive of mitral regurgitation or a third heart sound.

### *Diagnosis*

In addition to the above physical findings, as with pseudoaneurysms, the chest x-ray may demonstrate cardiomegaly and a bulge representing the aneurysmal area. The ECG will often show evidence of a transmural anterior myocardial infarction and persistent ST-segment elevation. TTE is the diagnostic test of choice and will show thinning of the myocardium and dyskinetic wall motion at the site of infarction. Thrombus should always be excluded, as it is found in more than half of the surgical and autopsy cases that have been studied. If there is inability to exclude thrombus with a standard surface echocardiogram, contrast can be given simultaneously to improve distinction between the ventricular cavity and endocardial lining. Other imaging modalities such as cardiac MRI or CT scanning can be useful in this regard.

### *Treatment*

Diagnosis of a ventricular aneurysm in itself does not change the treatment algorithm for a post–myocardial infarction patient with comparable degrees of heart failure and/or cardiogenic shock (see above). It is important to note that administration of an ACE-I within 24 hours of infarction is especially crucial in this situation, because of the drug's inhibitory effect on infarct expansion and beneficial effect on ventricular remodeling. If a patient is stable off mechanical and vasopressor support, an ACE-I should be started.

Surgery, which should include an LV aneurysmectomy and concomitant CABG, is indicated when there are symptoms and signs related to the aneurysm (5). This includes refractory heart failure, ventricular arrhythmias, angina, plus systemic embolization despite therapeutic levels of anticoagulation. Patients with small or moderate-sized, asymptomatic aneurysms should not undergo surgery. They do require medical management for heart failure when it is present. Management of large, asymptomatic aneurysms is controversial, and decisions to proceed with surgery are often individualized.

Anticoagulation with warfarin for at least 3 months is indicated for all post-STEMI patients who develop a mural thrombus in the acute setting. This applies to diagnoses made within 1 month of the event. Anticoagulation is indicated because systemic embolization can occur in as many as 10% with documented mural thrombi, and the risk of late thromboembolism appears to be decreased with oral anticoagulant therapy (30,31). Although the risk of embolization decreases dramatically in the subsequent months following the infarction, therapy should be continued indefinitely for those patients who are not at an increased risk of bleeding (5). Anticoagulation in these patients consists of the early administration of intravenous, unfractionated heparin or subcutaneous low-molecular-weight heparin, along with Coumadin therapy until the international normalized ratio is between two and three. Once this has been achieved, heparin may be discontinued. Patients who develop a LV aneurysm but no identifiable thrombus in the acute setting should similarly be anticoagulated because the incidence of thrombus in these patients, postmortem and intraoperatively, is at least 50% (30). There is limited evidence to support long-term anticoagulation in these patients, and practice patterns often differ.

## ADDITIONAL COMPLICATIONS

### Right Ventricular Infarction with Hemodynamic Compromise

RV infarction rarely happens in isolation and more commonly occurs during an inferior or infero-posterior left ventricular myocardial infarction. Patients present with various degrees of RV dysfunction, but only 10% to 15% develop hemodynamically significant RV impairment. This typically occurs when there is an ostial or proximal right coronary artery occlusion prior to take-off of the RV marginal branches.

#### *Symptoms and Signs*

If one understands the hemodynamic relationship between the LV, RV, and pericardium, the symptoms and signs of RV infarction become clear. It is important to realize that many of the hemodynamic changes overlap with tamponade, constrictive pericarditis, and restrictive cardiomyopathy. This makes clinical context and echocardiographic examination very important.

When RV infarction occurs, the right ventricular filling pressure becomes elevated due to systolic and diastolic dysfunction, which in turn causes elevation of right atrial filling pressures. Simultaneously, a decrease in right ventricular output leads to a reduced left ventricular end diastolic volume and the PCWP will be low. This is not always the case when there is concomitant LV dysfunction from a previous infarction or the current event. Left ventricular preload becomes further reduced when intrapericardial pressure is increased by abrupt dilation of the RV. Similar to tamponade, the LV and RV become interdependent (32). This combination of events leads to the triad of hypotension, elevated neck veins, and clear lung fields (33). Neck vein distention may not be seen if the patient is hypovolemic but may become apparent following aggressive fluid resuscitation, one of the key aspects of treatment.

#### *Diagnosis*

This diagnosis should be considered in any patient who presents with inferior ST-segment elevation on ECG. In fact, it is an ACC/AHA Class I indication to obtain a tracing of lead $V_4R$ and a TTE to look for RV infarction in patients with inferior STEMI and hemodynamic compromise (5). RV infarction should also be considered in patients with ST depression in leads $V_1$ and $V_2$, as this may represent acute infarction of the posterior myocardium as opposed to septal, subendocardial ischemia. Again, TTE can confirm the diagnosis by demonstrating hypokinesis and dilatation of the RV. Right heart catheterization can help confirm the diagnosis, but findings are nonspecific and may overlap with those of tamponade, constriction, and restriction. One will see elevated RV filling pressures that are equal to or greater than LV filling pressures, normal or low pulmonary arterial and PCWP, and a reduced cardiac index. Another clue to significant RV involvement in patients with inferior or posterior myocardial infarction is hypotension following the administration of preload reducing agents such as diuretics and nitrates.

#### *Treatment*

Similar to patients with AMI and cardiogenic shock secondary to LV dysfunction, patients with AMI complicated by severe RV dysfunction should undergo emergency diagnostic angiography and revascularization. If CABG is indicated, then the ACC/AHA feels that it is reasonable (IIa) to delay it in patients with clinically significant RV dysfunction, because right ventricular function frequently improves following several weeks of medical therapy (5).

Patients should be monitored in the ICU with both intra-arterial blood pressure monitoring and a RHC. If shock is present, the first line of therapy is aggressive fluid resuscitation. This is done with isotonic saline until the PCWP is between 15 and 18 mm Hg. If shock remains after this is achieved, an inotropic agent should be added. Dobutamine is the preferred drug in this situation because it causes less hypotension than milrinone. If vasopressors are required, a pure $\alpha$-agonist should be avoided, as it will lead to pulmonary arterial vasoconstriction and further decrease forward flow into the left ventricle. If severe LV dysfunction and an elevated pulmonary capillary wedge pressure exist, unlike the situation of isolated LV systolic dysfunction complicating AMI, sodium nitroprusside should be avoided. These patients should be considered for IABP counterpulsation. It is important to avoid factors that increase RV afterload, such as hypoxemia, $\alpha$-agonists, and elevations in PCWP, which includes positive end expiratory pressure (PEEP). In addition, one should avoid anything that decreases RV preload. This includes medications such as nitrates, morphine, and diuretics; but also dysrhythmias that lead to disruption of atrioventricular (AV) synchrony, such as atrial fibrillation and high degree AV block.

Atrial fibrillation must be dealt with emergently in the hemodynamically unstable patient following RV infarction, with immediate direct-current cardioversion (DCCV). If the patient is not hemodynamically compromised, a trial of antiarrhythmic therapy can be attempted; however, if sinus rhythm is not restored promptly, general anesthesia followed by DCCV should be performed. When general anesthesia is performed, it is advisable to have an anesthesiologist available, should prompt intubation be required.

Bradyarrhythmias, a frequent complication of inferior myocardial infarction (IMI) with RV involvement, can be quite dangerous even when the atrium and ventricle contract synchronously. This is because the dilated right ventricle has a relatively fixed stroke volume and depends largely on heart rate to increase its output. Management of bradycardia in AMI will be discussed in a subsequent section. It is important to know that if a patient with RV infarction requires temporary pacing; both atrial and ventricular leads should be placed, in order to maintain AV synchrony.

## Dynamic Left Ventricular Outflow Tract Obstruction

Although development of dynamic LVOT obstruction is a rare complication of myocardial infarction, it is important to recognize because many of the traditional therapies used in the treatment of AMI complicated by cardiogenic shock should be avoided. These include nitrates, afterload reduction, diuretics, IABPs, and inotropic agents.

Dynamic LVOT obstruction most often occurs in the setting of an anteroapical myocardial infarction with compensatory basal hyperkinesis. This combination of segmental wall motion abnormalities causes a decrease in the cross-sectional area of the LVOT and acceleration of blood flow across this region. The acceleration of blood flow decreases pressure above the mitral valve, causing systolic anterior motion (SAM) of the anterior mitral leaflet against the interventricular septum, which worsens the LVOT obstruction (34). These patients often have a single, significant stenosis in the left anterior descending (LAD) coronary artery, in addition to mild concentric left ventricular hypertrophy or asymmetric septal hypertrophy.

### *Symptoms and Signs*

Patients with dynamic LVOT obstruction usually have chest pain and evidence of an anterior or anteroapical ST-elevation myocardial infarction. This complication has also been seen in non–ST-elevation myocardial infarction (NSTEMI), but much less frequently. Symptoms and signs of CHF and cardiogenic shock are often present (see above). Patients can have a holosystolic murmur at the left lateral sternal border that radiates to the apex and represents MR in addition to a harsh crescendo-decrescendo systolic murmur in the left second intercostal space, representing LVOT obstruction.

### *Diagnosis*

The possibility of LVOT obstruction should be considered in patients who have progressive hemodynamic deterioration in the setting of standard medical and mechanical therapies used to treat patients with AMI and CGS. The diagnosis is made by TTE. LV ejection fraction may be normal or depressed. Apical hypo or akinesis along with hyperkinesis of the basal segments of the heart will be seen, in addition to SAM and regurgitation of the mitral valve. The left ventricular outflow tract, best interrogated with continuous-wave Doppler in the apical five- and three-chamber views, will demonstrate a gradient greater than 30 mm Hg.

### *Treatment*

Standard revascularization and anticoagulant therapy for AMI must be instituted in these patients. What is different are the supportive measures used during the peri-infarction period. This consists of beta-blockers and fluids. If shock is present, an $\alpha$-agonist should be used. All of these therapies decrease the degree of LVOT obstruction. Phenylephrine, the most commonly used $\alpha$-agonist, is started at 20 to 40 $\mu$g/min and titrated upward, until there is clinical improvement or the maximum dose has been reached.

## Pericarditis

There are two forms of pericarditis that occur in the setting of myocardial infarction. The first, typically occurring within 24 to 96 hours of transmural MI, is a form of localized inflammation in the pericardial region above the necrotic myocardium, which tends to run a benign course. The second, a form of post–cardiac injury syndrome also referred to as Dressler syndrome, can manifest 1 to 8 weeks following MI. Although the exact mechanism is unclear, it is felt to be the result of an autoimmune reaction involving myocardial antigen and antibody complexes. This form of pericarditis tends to be a more systemic inflammatory process, is often refractory to first-line therapies, and frequently recurs.

### *Symptoms and Signs*

Patients with pericarditis often develop positional chest pain. This tends to be sharp, pleuritic, exacerbated by recumbency, and commonly radiates to the trapezius ridge. If the patient has Dressler syndrome, he or she may also complain of arthralgias and myalgias. Dressler syndrome can also be associated with pleuritis and pleural effusions. Although these effusions are typically small, they may enlarge and cause dyspnea. Patients may be febrile in both forms of pericarditis, and those with Dressler syndrome can run fevers as high as 40°C. All patients with pericarditis may have leukocytosis and elevation of inflammatory markers such as the erythrocyte sedimentation rate and C-reactive protein. Physical examination may demonstrate a pericardial friction rub. The rub classically has three components, representing atrial systole, ventricular systole, and ventricular diastole. All three are not always appreciated at the same time.

### *Diagnosis*

Symptoms and the presence of a pericardial friction rub are quite specific for pericarditis. ECG can be helpful but is less sensitive, especially in the acute situation, as the evolutionary changes seen following myocardial infarction can mask the typical ECG features of pericarditis (Table 19–2). Although TTE is not diagnostic in situations of post-MI pericarditis, it must be obtained to rule out a significant pericardial effusion, seen more commonly in patients with Dressler syndrome. It is important to realize that the

**TABLE 19–2**
**ECG CHANGES IN PERICARDITIS VERSUS STEMI**

| Stage | ECG Changes Typically Associated with Pericarditis[a] |
|---|---|
| I | Diffuse, concave-up ST elevation; ST depression in aVR and V1; PR depression in the limb leads and left chest leads; PR elevation in aVR |
| IIa | ST and PR segments return to baseline, while T-waves remain upright |
| IIb | T-waves begin to flatten and invert, largely in the leads that had ST elevation |
| III | Diffuse T-wave inversion |
| IV | Prepericarditis ECG, however, T-wave inversions may persist |
| **Stage** | **Evolutionary ECG Changes Typically Associated with STEMI** |
| I | Convex-upward ST segment elevation and upright T-waves overlying area of infarct; ST-segment depression in opposite leads; Q-waves begin to develop |
| II | Gradual T-wave inversion followed by deep, symmetrically inverted T-waves; Q-waves continue to evolve |
| III | Resolution of ST elevation,[b] T-waves begin to normalize |

[a]In pericarditis, the evolution of repolarization abnormalities does not always occur simultaneously as they typically do in MI. In addition, the distribution of repolarization abnormalities in myocardial infarction remains constant, whereas in pericarditis, multiple areas on the electrocardiogram can demonstrate different repolarization patterns.
[b]If ST-segment elevation does not resolve by 6 weeks, consider the possibility of ventricular aneurysm or a large area of dyskinetic myocardium.

presence of an effusion is not diagnostic, as it is commonly seen following uncomplicated AMIs. Likewise, absence of a pericardial effusion does not exclude the diagnosis.

#### *Treatment*

There are two issues to consider and balance when treating patients with post-MI pericarditis. One is the need for anti-inflammatory agents and the need to avoid anticoagulation. In terms of anti-inflammatory agents, aspirin is the first line of therapy. If patients are refractory to standard doses, as much as 650 mg every 4 to 6 hours may be used. When high doses are needed, it is advisable to place the patient on a proton pump inhibitor. Some patients will be refractory to or unable to take high-dose aspirin therapy. In these patients, 0.6 mg of colchicine every 12 hours and/or 650 mg of acetaminophen every 4 to 6 hours can be tried. Nonsteroidal anti-inflammatory drugs (NSAIDs) and corticosteroids should be used only as a last resort. Corticosteroids and NSAIDs adversely affect myocardial scar formation, which can lead to thinning of the scar and, in some circumstances, infarct expansion. There are reports suggesting that both drug classes put the patient at increased risk for myocardial rupture following AMI.

Clinical judgment is necessary if anticoagulation is required for a patient with post-MI pericarditis. It is an ACC/AHA Class I indication to discontinue anticoagulant therapy if an effusion develops or enlarges. This decision must be individualized and based on the risk-to-benefit ratio. If a decision is made to continue anticoagulation, the patient must be observed diligently for effusion enlargement and impending tamponade.

## ARRHYTHMIC COMPLICATIONS

### Bradyarrhythmias

In the setting of AMI, management of bradyarrhythmias is complex because decisions regarding temporary and permanent pacing must be made and require multiple considerations. In the acute setting, if a patient is hemodynamically stable despite a bradyarrhythmia, a decision must be made regarding the need for prophylactic, back-up pacing. This requires one to predict which patients are likely to progress to a life-threatening rhythm abnormality such as third-degree AV block. The route by which pacing is performed must involve considerations regarding patient stability, the need for AV synchrony, and the bleeding risks associated with the use of thrombolytic and postinterventional therapies.

Sinus bradycardia occurs in approximately 30% to 40% of AMIs, most commonly with inferior MI and reperfusion of the RCA (5). Although multiple mechanisms can be responsible, the most common is hyperactivity of parasympathetics due to stimulation of vagal afferents. This is termed the Bezold-Jarisch reflex and causes both bradycardia and hypotension. When patients become symptomatic from sinus bradycardia or from sinus pauses greater than 3 seconds in duration, intravenous atropine is the first line of therapy (5). This should be administered in doses of 0.5 mg to 1 mg every 3 minutes until the patient is no longer symptomatic or a total dose of 0.4 mg/kg has been reached. If symptomatic bradycardia persists, transcutaneous or transvenous pacing must be initiated.

The development of atrioventricular conduction block (AVB), intraventricular conduction delay (IVCD), and/or bundle branch block (BBB) in the setting of AMI is associated with an increased risk of in-hospital mortality. Decisions regarding prophylactic or therapeutic temporary pacing depend on the infarction location, the type of block and its presumed relationship to the AV node, the extent of pre-existing conduction system disease, and the presence or absence of symptoms.

An important factor to consider when dealing with any form of heart block is its relationship to the AV node. This is important because blocks proximal to or within the AV node, often referred to as intranodal block, are generally benign, with prophylactic and eventual permanent pacing typically not required. This is in contradistinction to infranodal blocks, which tend to be more dangerous, often

**TABLE 19–3**

**CLASS I RECOMMENDATIONS FOR PROPHYLACTIC, TEMPORARY PACING IN AMI**

| Intraventricular Conduction | Atrioventricular Conduction: First-Degree AVB, Anterior MI | First-Degree AVB, Other MI | Second-Degree AVB Type I, Anterior MI | Second-Degree AVB Type I, Other MI | Second-Degree AVB Type II, Anterior MI | Second-Degree AVB Type II, Other MI |
|---|---|---|---|---|---|---|
| Normal | Observe | Observe | TC | TC | TC | TC |
| New or old fascicular block | TC | TC (IIa) | TC | TC | TC | TC |
| Old BBB | TC | TC | TC | TC | TC | TC |
| New BBB | TC | TC | TC | TC | *TV* | *TV* |
| Fascicular block + RBBB | TC | TC | TC | TC | *TV* | *TV* |
| Alternating left and right BBB | *TV* | *TV* | *TV* | *TV* | *TV* | *TV* |

The actions listed—transcutaneous (TC) pacing, transvenous (TV) pacing, or observation—are based on the patient's atrioventricular and intraventricular conduction patterns as well as the location of the MI. To determine the Class I indication, follow the row containing the patient's intraventricular conduction pattern to the column containing the patient's atrioventricular conduction pattern and MI location. Class I recommendations are those for which there is evidence and/or general agreement that the treatment is beneficial, useful, and effective. Class IIa recommendations are those for which there is conflicting evidence and/or a divergence of opinion regarding the usefulness/effectiveness of the treatment; however, the weight of evidence or opinion is in favor of usefulness/efficacy. Class IIa included only when a Class I recommendation does not exist. AVB, atrioventricular block; BBB, bundle branch block; RBBB, right bundle branch block.
Modified from Antman EM, Anbe DT, Armstrong PW, et al. ACC/AHA guidelines for the management of patients with ST-elevation myocardial infarction—executive summary. *J Am Coll Cardiol.* 2004:44(3): 671–719.

require prophylactic and therapeutic temporary pacing, and frequently result in permanent pacemaker insertion prior to hospital discharge (5). Typical intranodal blocks are first-degree and second-degree, Mobitz type I AVB. These are usually seen in inferior or inferoposterior AMIs, and the RCA is usually the culprit artery, although the LCx can be involved. If third-degree AVB develops in the intranodal region, the QRS width is typically less than 0.12 seconds, the escape rate tends to be between 45 to 60 beats per minute (bpm), and asystole is uncommon. Common infranodal blocks are second-degree, Mobitz type II AVB and third-degree AVB. When infranodal blocks are present, the LAD is typically the culprit lesion. When third-degree AVB of the infranodal variety is present, the QRS width tends to be wider than 0.12 seconds, escape rates are often less than 30 bpm, and asystole is common. Hence, the majority of these patients require either prophylactic or therapeutic temporary pacing during the AMI setting. It is important to remember that whereas atropine is commonly the first line of treatment in patients with symptomatic, presumed intranodal AVB and sinus bradycardia, it can be dangerous in the presence of infranodal AVB. This is due to an increase in the sinus rate without an increase in the escape rate, leading to a decrease in the effective ratio of conduction and a decrease in ventricular rate (5). Atropine is administered in intravenous doses of 0.5 to 1 mg and repeated if no response, to a total dose of 0.04 mg/kg. If the patient is hemodynamically unstable and not responsive to atropine, temporary pacing is indicated. For a summary of the Class I recommendations regarding prophylactic, temporary pacing in AMI complicated by AV and intraventricular conduction abnormalities, see Table 19–3. Third-degree AVB in the AMI setting should be treated with transvenous temporary pacing. Ventricular asystole should be treated as per the Advanced Cardiac Life Support guidelines. For indications regarding permanent pacemaker insertion following AMI, see Chapter 52.

## Tachyarrhythmias

Tachyarrhythmias are common in the setting of AMI. The most deadly, primary ventricular fibrillation (VF), occurs in 3% to 5% of patients within the first few hours of STEMI. This high frequency and early occurrence underscores the importance of early hospitalization and rapid triage to an area where continuous monitoring and rapid defibrillation can occur. Treatment of supraventricular and ventricular rhythm disturbances is reviewed in Chapters 50, 51, and 52. In addition, current guidelines for implantation of implantable cardiac defibrillators (ICD) following myocardial infarction can be found in Chapter 51.

In the setting of AMI, especially when complicated by cardiogenic shock, tachyarrhythmias must be dealt with emergently. They increase myocardial oxygen consumption, exacerbate ischemia, and can lead to or worsen CHF and cardiogenic shock. Beta-blockers and calcium channel blockers must be avoided if shock or significant heart failure is present, as they can contribute to hemodynamic decompensation. Often cardioversion becomes the treatment of first choice. Heightened vigilance is appropriate when sinus tachycardia is present in the AMI setting, as this may be compensatory for a severely depressed myocardium. Although beta-blocker administration has been proven beneficial in the AMI setting, it can be deadly if used to treat sinus tachycardia that is compensatory for a severely depressed myocardium. Lastly, accelerated idioventricular rhythm occurs in approximately 30% of AMI patients, often in those with involvement of the inferior wall and following reperfusion therapy (32). It is characterized by a wide complex QRS with regular rates between 60 and 120 bpm, atrioventricular dissociation (AV) with the V-rate surpassing the A-rate, with fusion and capture beats. It occurs because an ectopic ventricular focus assumes the role of the predominant pacemaker. Accelerating the sinus rhythm or atrial pacing can cause suppression of this rhythm if treatment becomes necessary. Treatment is indicated only when there is hemodynamic compromise, symptoms as a result of the rhythm, or the R-wave consistently falls on the T-wave, predisposing to more serious ventricular arrhythmias.

## CONCLUSION

Although short- and long-term mortality following AMI has improved with the use of thrombolytic therapy and early coronary reperfusion strategies, both remain high. The greatest fraction of deaths comes from cardiogenic shock, which results from isolated left ventricular systolic dysfunction or mechanical disruption of the myocardium. It is imperative that these patients be identified early for the institution of appropriate therapeutic measures in a prompt manner. These include immediate efforts to achieve hemodynamic stability, rapid transport to the cardiac catheterization laboratory, and emergency percutaneous coronary intervention or surgical consultation when indicated. These patients should be monitored closely in an ICU setting, where arrhythmias and other potentially catastrophic complications can be dealt with expediently.

## REFERENCES


1. Goldberg RJ, Samad NA, Yarzebski J, et al. Temporal trends in cardiogenic shock complicating acute myocardial infarction. *N Engl J Med.* 1999;340(15):1162–1168.
2. Hochman JS, Buller CE, Sleeper LA, et al. Cardiogenic shock complicating acute myocardial infarction—etiologies, management and outcome: a report from the SHOCK Trial Registry. Should we emergently revascularize Occluded Coronaries for cardiogenic shock? *J Am Coll Cardiol.* 2000;36(3 suppl A):1063–1070.
3. Domanski MJ, Topol EJ. Cardiogenic shock: current understandings and future research directions. *Am J Cardiol.* 1994;74(7):724–726.
4. Holmes DR Jr, Bates ER, Kleiman NS, et al. Contemporary reperfusion therapy for cardiogenic shock: the GUSTO-I trial experience. The GUSTO-I Investigators. Global Utilization of Streptokinase and Tissue Plasminogen Activator for Occluded Coronary Arteries. *J Am Coll Cardiol.* 1995;26(3):668–674.
5. Antman EM, Anbe DT, Armstrong PW, et al. ACC/AHA guidelines for the management of patients with ST-elevation myocardial infarction—executive summary. A report of the American College of Cardiology/American Heart Association Task Force on Practice Guidelines (Writing Committee to Revise the 1999 Guidelines for the Management of Patients with Acute Myocardial Infarction). *J Am Coll Cardiol.* 2004;44(3):671–719.
6. Effectiveness of intravenous thrombolytic treatment in acute myocardial infarction. Gruppo Italiano per lo Studio della Streptochinasi nell'Infarto Miocardico (GISSI). *Lancet.* 1986;1(8478):397–402.
7. Hochman JS, Sleeper LA, Webb JG, et al. Early revascularization in acute myocardial infarction complicated by cardiogenic shock. SHOCK Investigators. Should We Emergently Revascularize Occluded Coronaries for Cardiogenic Shock. *N Engl J Med.* 1999; 341(9):625–634.
8. Anderson RD, Ohman EM, Holmes DR Jr, et al. Use of intraaortic balloon counterpulsation in patients presenting with cardiogenic shock: observations from the GUSTO-I Study. Global Utilization of Streptokinase and TPA for Occluded Coronary Arteries. *J Am Coll Cardiol.* 1997;30(3):708–715.
9. Sanborn TA, Sleeper LA, Bates ER, et al. Impact of thrombolysis, intra-aortic balloon pump counterpulsation, and their combination in cardiogenic shock complicating acute myocardial infarction: a report from the SHOCK Trial Registry. Should we emergently revascularize Occluded Coronaries for cardiogenic shock? *J Am Coll Cardiol.* 2000;36(3 suppl A):1123–1129.
10. Barron HV, Every NR, Parsons LS, et al. The use of intra-aortic balloon counterpulsation in patients with cardiogenic shock complicating acute myocardial infarction: data from the National Registry of Myocardial Infarction 2. *Am Heart J.* 2001;141(6):933–939.
11. Caracciolo EA, Donohue TJ, Kern MJ, et al. High risk cardiac catheterization. In: Kern MJ, ed. *The Cardiac Catheterization Handbook.* 3rd ed. St. Louis, MO: Mosby; 1999:461–500.
12. Pfeffer MA, Braunwald E, Moye LA, et al. Effect of captopril on mortality and morbidity in patients with left ventricular dysfunction after myocardial infarction. Results of the Survival and Ventricular Enlargement trial. The SAVE Investigators. *N Engl J Med.* 1992;327(10):669–677.
13. Kober L, Torp-Pedersen C, Carlsen JE, et al. A clinical trial of the angiotensin-converting-enzyme inhibitor trandolapril in patients with left ventricular dysfunction after myocardial infarction. Trandolapril Cardiac Evaluation (TRACE) Study Group. *N Engl J Med.* 1995;333(25):1670–1676.
14. Effect of ramipril on mortality and morbidity of survivors of acute myocardial infarction with clinical evidence of heart failure. The Acute Infarction Ramipril Efficacy (AIRE) Study Investigators. *Lancet.* 1993;342(8875):821–828.
15. Pfeffer MA, McMurray JJ, Velazquez EJ, et al. Valsartan, captopril, or both in myocardial infarction complicated by heart failure, left ventricular dysfunction, or both. *N Engl J Med.* 2003; 349(20):1893–1906.
16. Dickstein K, Kjekshus J. Effects of losartan and captopril on mortality and morbidity in high-risk patients after acute myocardial infarction: the OPTIMAAL randomised trial. Optimal Trial in Myocardial Infarction with Angiotensin II Antagonist Losartan. *Lancet.* 2002;360(9335):752–760.
17. Crenshaw BS, Granger CB, Birnbaum Y, et al. Risk factors, angiographic patterns, and outcomes in patients with ventricular septal defect complicating acute myocardial infarction. GUSTO-I (Global Utilization of Streptokinase and TPA for Occluded Coronary Arteries) Trial Investigators. *Circulation.* 2000;101(1):27–32.
18. Menon V, Webb JG, Hillis LD, et al. Outcome and profile of ventricular septal rupture with cardiogenic shock after myocardial

infarction: a report from the SHOCK Trial Registry. Should we emergently revascularize Occluded Coronaries in cardiogenic shock? *J Am Coll Cardiol.* 2000;36(3 suppl A):1110–1116.
19. Cercek B, Shah PK. Complicated acute myocardial infarction. Heart failure, shock, mechanical complications. *Cardiol Clin.* 1991;9(4):569–593.
20. Thompson CR, Buller CE, Sleeper LA, et al. Cardiogenic shock due to acute severe mitral regurgitation complicating acute myocardial infarction: a report from the SHOCK Trial Registry. Should we use emergently revascularize Occluded Coronaries in cardiogenic shock? *J Am Coll Cardiol.* 2000;36(3 suppl A):1104–1109.
21. Mueller HS, Chatterjee K, Davis KB, et al. ACC expert consensus document. Present use of bedside right heart catheterization in patients with cardiac disease. American College of Cardiology. *J Am Coll Cardiol.* 1998;32(3):840–864.
22. Becker RC, Hochman JS, Cannon CP, et al. Fatal cardiac rupture among patients treated with thrombolytic agents and adjunctive thrombin antagonists: observations from the Thrombolysis and Thrombin Inhibition in Myocardial Infarction 9 Study. *J Am Coll Cardiol.* 1999;33(2):479–487.
23. Becker RC, Gore JM, Lambrew C, et al. A composite view of cardiac rupture in the United States National Registry of Myocardial Infarction. *J Am Coll Cardiol.* 1996;27(6):1321–1326.
24. Alexander RW, Pratt CM, Ryan TJ, Roberts R. ST Segment myocardial infarction: clinical presentation, diagnostic evaluation, and medical management. In: Fuster V, Alexander RW, O'Rourke RA, et al., eds. *Hurst's The Heart.* 11th ed. New York: McGraw-Hill; 2004:1277–1349.
25. Moreno R, Lopez-Sendon J, Garcia E, et al. Primary angioplasty reduces the risk of left ventricular free wall rupture compared with thrombolysis in patients with acute myocardial infarction. *J Am Coll Cardiol.* 2002;39(4):598–603.
26. Pohjola-Sintonen S, Muller JE, Stone PH, et al. Ventricular septal and free wall rupture complicating acute myocardial infarction: experience in the Multicenter Investigation of Limitation of Infarct Size. *Am Heart J.* 1989;117(4):809–818.
27. Figueras J, Cortadellas J, Soler-Soler J. Left ventricular free wall rupture: clinical presentation and management. *Heart.* 2000; 83(5):499–504.
28. Frances C, Romero A, Grady D. Left ventricular pseudoaneurysm. *J Am Coll Cardiol.* 1998;32(3):557–561.
29. Glower DG, Lowe JE. Left ventricular aneurysm. In: Cohn LH, Edmunds LH, eds. *Cardiac Surgery in the Adult.* New York: McGraw-Hill; 2003:771–788.
30. Keeley EC, Hillis LD. Left ventricular mural thrombus after acute myocardial infarction. *Clin Cardiol.* 1996;19(2):83–86.
31. Sherman DG, Dyken ML, Fisher M, et al. Antithrombotic therapy for cerebrovascular disorders. *Chest.* 1989;95(2 suppl):140S–155S.
32. Lavie CJ, Gersh BJ. Mechanical and electrical complications of acute myocardial infarction. *Mayo Clin Proc.* 1990;65(5):709–730.
33. Reeder GS. Identification and treatment of complications of myocardial infarction. *Mayo Clin Proc.* 1995;70(9):880–884.
34. Haley JH, Sinak LJ, Tajik AJ, et al. Dynamic left ventricular outflow tract obstruction in acute coronary syndromes: an important cause of new systolic murmur and cardiogenic shock. *Mayo Clin Proc.* 1999;74(9):901–906.

## QUESTIONS

**1.** All of the following should raise suspicion of subacute free wall rupture, *except*:

a. Intermittent chest pain, hypotension, and electromechanical dissociation
b. Agitation and apprehension
c. Intermittent, nonspecific, ST–T-wave abnormalities
d. Pericardial effusion and echodensities in the pericardium
e. Nonsustained ventricular tachycardia

Answer is e: A high index of suspicion is needed to diagnose subacute free wall rupture. Accurate and timely diagnosis provides valuable time for surgical treatment before acute rupture and pericardial tamponade lead to death. Intermittent chest pain, nausea, electromechanical dissociation, and hypotension along with dynamic ST–T-wave changes and agitation can all be present in cases of subacute rupture.

**2.** Which of the following statements regarding ventricular septal rupture complicating acute myocardial infarction is true?

a. It is usually seen in elderly, hypertensive patients with a history of multiple prior infarctions.
b. It is more common in anterior than inferior infarctions.
c. A 4/6 holosystolic murmur indicates a large defect.
d. Either echocardiography or right heart catheterization can be used as the initial diagnostic tool.
e. Surgery should be delayed several weeks until infarct healing occurs.

Answer is d: In most series, the frequency of ventricular septal rupture was equal in anterior and inferior myocardial infarctions. Although it is usually seen in elderly hypertensive patients, many times it occurs in the setting of a first myocardial infarction. The intensity of the murmur is usually inversely proportional to the size of the defect. Both echocardiography and right heart catheterization can be used as initial diagnostic modalities. Surgery should be performed emergently.

**3.** Which of the following statements regarding papillary muscle rupture complicating acute myocardial infarction is true?

a. Papillary muscle rupture is most frequently seen in large, anterolateral infarctions.
b. Patients should be referred for emergency catheterization and percutaneous intervention.
c. A harsh holosystolic murmur and systolic thrill are very common.
d. Despite pulmonary edema or shock, overall left ventricular systolic function may be normal.

e. Right heart catheterization is the diagnostic modality of choice.

Answer is d: Many times a relatively small myocardial infarction may be the culprit in papillary muscle rupture. Hyperdynamic left ventricular function in the setting of a relatively small myocardial infarction may appear puzzling in a patient with severe pulmonary edema and cardiogenic shock. Papillary muscle rupture is most frequently seen in inferior and posterior myocardial infarctions because of the single blood supply of the posteromedial papillary muscle. Although coronary angiography may be needed before surgery, definitive treatment requires emergency surgery, not percutaneous intervention. In many patients a systolic murmur may be audible, but the absence of a murmur does not rule out presence of papillary muscle rupture. A systolic thrill is very uncommon in papillary muscle rupture, as opposed to ventricular septal rupture. The diagnostic modality of choice is echocardiography.

**4.** *Case:* A 75-year-old woman with a history of hypertension and hyperlipidemia presents to the Emergency Department with dyspnea and fatigue. Thirty-six hours prior to presentation, she experienced substernal chest pressure that was severe, sudden in onset, and persisted for "a few hours." She provides a history of exertional chest discomfort for the past 2 months.

Exam: Blood pressure 95/60, heart rate 110, respiratory rate 28, pulse oximetry 88%, room air temperature 37°C
Neck: Elevated neck veins
Lungs: Bibasilar inspiratory crackles halfway up posterior thorax
Heart: PMI displaced laterally, palpable thrill over the left, fourth intercostal space, tachycardic, regular, S1 and S2 normal, 3/6 holosystolic murmur heard best at left, lateral sternal border
Extremities: Trace edema, somewhat cool, 2+ distal pulses throughout
ECG: sinus tachycardia, Q-waves and T-wave inversion in leads $V_1$–$V_5$.
CXR: Cardiomegaly, pulmonary edema
Labs: CK 500 U/L, CKMB 50 ng/ml, troponin-T 12 ng/mL, creatinine 1.5 mg/dL

A. In addition to ordering oxygen therapy, lasix, aspirin, and nitroglycerin, what should be performed next?

(1) Arterial blood gas
(2) Left heart catheterization
(3) Transthoracic echocardiogram
(4) Placement of a right heart catheter
(5) Cardiac CT scan

Answer is (3): The clinical picture is consistent with an anterior myocardial infarction that occurred more than 24 hours ago and the patient now presents in Killip Class III heart failure. Although the CHF may very well be secondary to a large anterior MI, her exam creates concern of a mechanical complication. In addition to oxygen therapy and initial measures to treat her pulmonary edema, she should have an emergency TTE. An arterial blood gas is not essential in this situation because the clinical picture is clear and $CO_2$ retention is not a concern at the moment. One can follow her oxygenation status by pulse oximetry. Although urgent left heart catheterization is indicated in patients with AMI complicated by CHF and CGS, this patient is several hours out of her acute event and the route of revascularization will be dictated by the presence or absence of a mechanical complication. A ventriculogram can diagnose a VSD as well, but there is time to obtain a transthoracic echocardiogram in the present situation. A right heart catheterization is also indicated in this situation, but this can be performed in the catheterization laboratory or the coronary intensive care unit and does not need to be done immediately. A cardiac CT has no place in this situation.

B. The above study demonstrated that the patient had an apical VSD, an akinetic anterior wall, and RV dilation. What should be the next step?

(1) Cardiothoracic surgery consultation
(2) Left heart catheterization
(3) Placement of an intra-aortic balloon pump
(4) Placement of a right heart catheter

Answer is (1): The next step should be a consultation to cardiothoracic surgery. Make the page, and while you are waiting for a response, make arrangements for the patient to go to the catheterization laboratory and subsequently the coronary intensive care unit until surgery can be performed. In the catheterization laboratory, in addition to obtaining the coronary anatomy, an IABP and RHC can be placed. Further medical management can occur in the coronary care unit while plans for surgery are being made.

# The Science of Hemodynamic Measurements

20

***Frederick A. Heupler, Jr.***

## PHYSICS OF PRESSURE MEASUREMENT

The most common method of measuring pressures in the cardiac catheterization laboratory is to use fluid-filled catheter systems that convey the pressure wave from the site of interest through a catheter, manifold, and a pressure transducer that converts the pressure waveform to an electrical signal. A catheter with a pressure transducer at the tip provides a more accurate pressure recording, but these catheters are too expensive for routine clinical use.

Fluid-filled catheters commonly produce several types of artifacts in recorded waveforms:

1. Low-frequency response
2. Overshoot
3. Zero level

Low-frequency response and overshoot are common to all types of fluid-filled pressure-transmitting devices. The natural resonant frequency of a catheter–manometer system is the frequency at which the system oscillates when stimulated. The desirable frequency response for a catheter system is about 20 Hz or more. When the natural resonant frequency response of a catheter system is below about 12 Hz, low-frequency catheter oscillation waves will obscure high-frequency cardiac waveforms. The angiographer should try to minimize the following factors that lower the frequency response of a catheter–manometer system:

1. Air bubbles in the catheter system
2. High-viscosity fluid in the catheter (e.g., contrast material instead of saline)
3. Long fluid-filled tubing between the catheter and the pressure transducer
4. A long catheter
5. A narrow-bore catheter
6. A catheter made of soft, compliant material

Overshoot is produced by reflected waves within the catheter–manometer system. The magnitude of overshoot can be reduced by mechanical or electrical damping. Overdamping eliminates overshoot, but it reduces frequency response. Optimal damping reduces overshoot without producing a major drop in frequency response (Fig. 20–1).

The pressure transducer in a fluid-filled catheter system must be placed at a level equal to the mid-height atrial level to achieve the "zero level." This is approximately one half the distance between the front and back of the chest. If the transducer is placed on the anterior chest surface of a supine patient, the recorded pressures will be falsely low.

The ultimate goal of setting up a fluid-filled catheter pressure measurement system is to achieve the highest frequency response possible, optimally damp the system to eliminate overshoot, and locate the pressure transducer at the zero level.

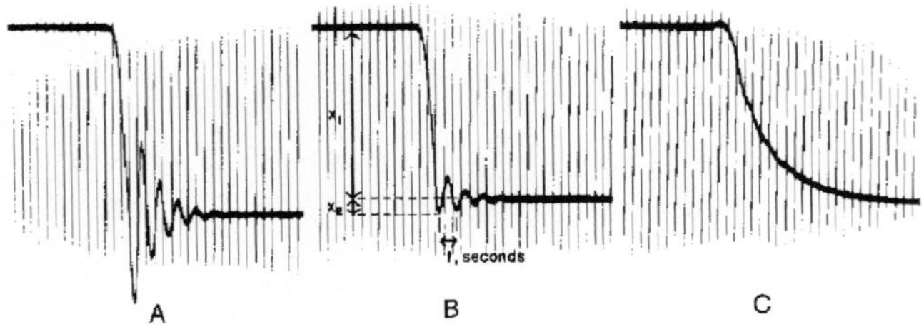


**Figure 20–1** A, Underdamped; B, Optimally damped; C, Overdamped.

## BASIC INTRACARDIAC WAVEFORMS

The basic configuration of waveforms is similar for the right and left atria. The V-wave amplitude is generally greater than the A wave in the left atrium, whereas the A-wave predominates in the right atrium. Electromechanical delay is about 40 to 80 milliseconds. The basic intra-atrial waveforms and the events to which they correspond are listed below:

A: atrial contraction
C: ventricular contraction
V: rising atrial pressures during ventricular systole; occurs during the T wave
C-V, or systolic: severe atrioventricular valve regurgitation
X descent: atrial relaxation; occurs after the A wave peak, before the C wave
X′ descent: atrial relaxation; occurs after the C wave and before the V wave
Y descent: opening of the atrioventricular valve; occurs after the V wave (Fig. 20–2).

Arrhythmias may produce a variety of changes in intracardiac pressures:

1. Atrial fibrillation will eliminate A waves.
2. Junctional rhythm will displace A waves closer to the C wave (or systolic upstroke in the ventricle).
3. PVCs and ventricular pacemaker rhythm may produce cannon A waves in the atrium as a result of atrial contraction against a closed atrioventricular valve.

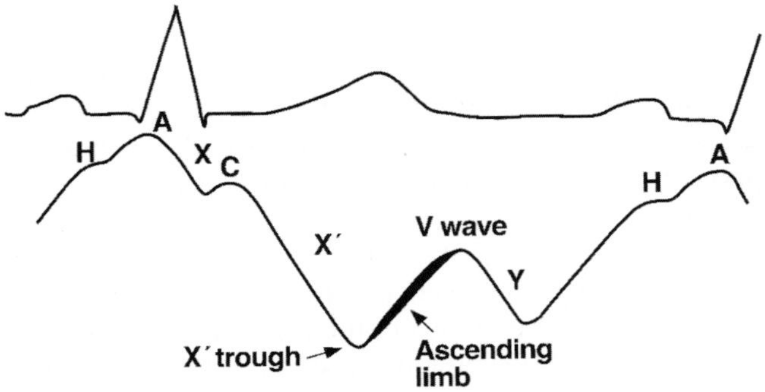


**Figure 20–2**

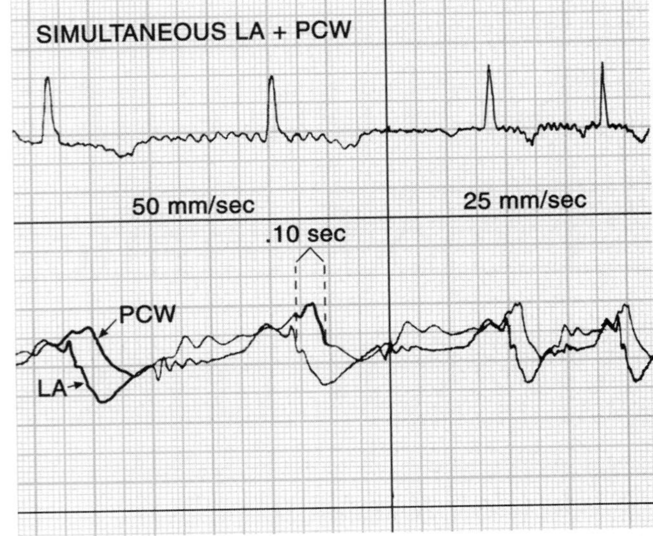


**Figure 20–3**

Pulmonary capillary wedge (PCW) pressures indirectly reflect left atrial pressures. PCW waveforms demonstrate a mechanical time delay, decreased amplitude, and decreased frequency response compared to left atrial waveforms (Fig. 20–3). The reason for these changes is the retrograde transmission of pressure waves from the left atrium through the pulmonary veins, capillaries, and arterioles to the wedged catheter in the pulmonary artery. The mechanical time delay is determined in part by the location of the wedged catheter in the pulmonary arterial circuit and in part by the catheter–manometer–tubing assembly. A stiff 7-French end-hole catheter (e.g., Cournand), will wedge farther out in the pulmonary artery, with a mechanical time delay of about 70 to 80 milliseconds. A balloon-tipped catheter will wedge farther from the terminal pulmonary artery branches, with a mechanical time delay of 150 to 160 milliseconds.

Normal values for intracardiac pressures are listed in Table 20–1.

### Pressure Wave Artifacts

In addition to the artifacts that may be produced by low-frequency response and overshoot, catheter structure or placement may introduce artifacts in pressure recordings.

**TABLE 20–1**
**NORMAL VALUES FOR INTRACARDIAC PRESSURE**

| Chamber | Normal Pressure (mm Hg) |
|---|---|
| Right atrium | 5 (±2) |
| Right ventricle | 25 (±5)/5 (±2) |
| Pulmonary artery | 25 (±5)/10 (±2) |
| Left atrium | 10 |

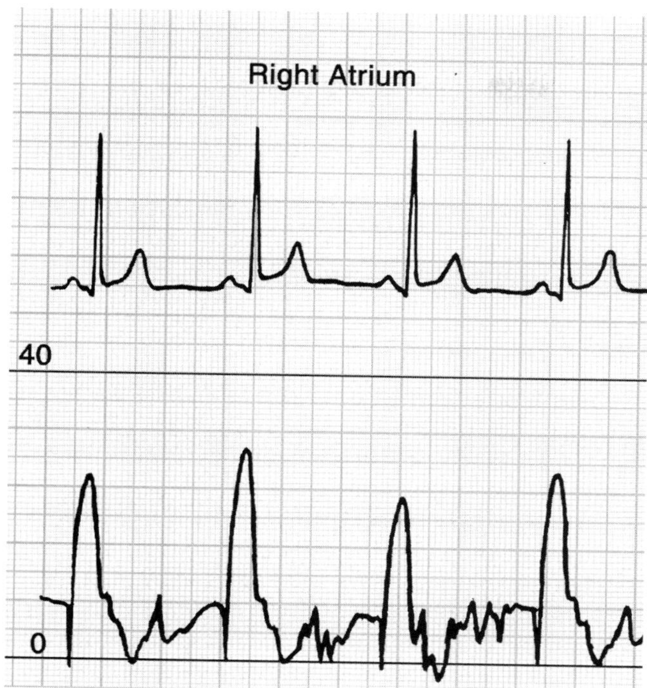


**Figure 20–4**

End-hole artifacts may occur when the tip of an end-hole catheter becomes occluded during contraction of an atrial or ventricular wall. If this occurs during atrial systole with a catheter in the atrium, the A wave will appear greatly magnified (Fig. 20–4).

Simultaneous recording of ventricular and aortic pressures may occur when the tip of a pigtail catheter is located in the ventricle and the side port in the aorta. This may produce a bizarre-looking pressure wave with an apparently elevated diastolic left ventricular pressure.

Catheter-whip artifact is a high-frequency oscillation that results from rapid movement of the catheter by blood flow. This is particularly likely to occur in the pulmonary artery and above a stenotic aortic valve.

## Cardiac Output Measurement

The fundamental function of the heart is to deliver enough blood to the systemic circulation to meet the oxygen demands of tissues. The normal resting cardiac output (C.O.) increases with body size and exercise and decreases with age. Numerous other factors may affect resting cardiac output. In order to account for body size, the cardiac output is normalized to body surface area in square meters ($m^2$), and the result is the cardiac index. Body surface area (BSA) may be obtained from a nomogram or calculated by the following formula:

$$\text{BSA}\,(\text{m}^2) = \sqrt{\frac{\text{Ht (cm)} \times \text{Wt (kg)}}{3{,}600}}$$

The normal resting cardiac index falls from about 4.5 $L/min/m^2$ at age 7 years to 3 $L/min/m^2$ in middle age, and to 2.5 $L/min/m^2$ at age 70.

The two major methods for measurement of cardiac output in the cardiac cath lab are the Fick oxygen technique and the indicator dilution technique.

### The Fick Technique

The Fick principle states that the total uptake or release of any substance (such as oxygen) by an organ (such as the lungs) is the product of blood flow to the organ and the arteriovenous (A-V) concentration difference of the substance. If pulmonary blood flow equals systemic blood flow, then:

$$\text{C.O.} = \frac{\text{O}_2\text{ consumption}}{\text{A-V O}_2\text{ difference}}$$

Oxygen consumption by the lungs can be estimated by measuring the oxygen uptake from room air by use of a Douglas bag or metabolic hood. In order to conserve time and expense, many laboratories estimate oxygen consumption using an assumed oxygen consumption based on the formula 125 $mL/min/m^2$ for younger patients (110 $mL/min/m^2$ for older patients) or 3 mL/min/kg. However, assumed oxygen consumption values may produce discrepancies of $\pm 10\%$ to 25% in about half of patients.

A-V oxygen difference is obtained by subtracting the oxygen content of pulmonary arterial from pulmonary venous blood. Oxygen content may be calculated using the formula

$$\text{O}_2\text{ content} = \text{O}_2\text{ saturation} \times 1.36\,(\text{mL O}_2/\text{g Hb}) \times (\text{g Hb}/100\,\text{mL blood})$$

where Hb is hemoglobin.

The final formula for calculation of cardiac output then becomes

$$\text{C.O.} = \frac{\text{O}_2\text{ consumption (mL/min)}}{(\text{arterial O}_2 - \text{mixed venous O}_2\text{ saturation}) \times 1.36\,\text{Hb} \times 10}$$

Estimation of pulmonary arterial oxygen content by using "mixed venous" blood from the venae cavae is less accurate. Mixed venous blood oxygen saturation is an estimation of what the pulmonary artery saturation would be if no shunt were present. This can be approximated by the following formula:

$$\text{Mixed venous blood} = \frac{3\,\text{SVC} + \text{IVC}}{4}$$

where SVC and IVC are the respective $O_2$ saturations.

Use of arterial blood to estimate pulmonary venous blood oxygen content is acceptable, because, in the absence of shunts, only a small amount of venous blood enters the arterial circuit within the heart via the Thebesian veins. Narrow A-V oxygen differences (as seen with high cardiac output) are more likely to introduce error than wide differences (as seen with low cardiac output). Thus, the

Fick method is most accurate in patients with low cardiac output.

Assume that a patient has the following measured values:

Oxygen consumption = 250 mL/min
Femoral artery oxygen saturation = 97%
SVC oxygen saturation = 70%
IVC oxygen saturation = 78%
Hb concentration = 14.0 g%

The mixed venous blood saturation will be

$$\frac{3\,(0.7) + (0.78)}{4} = 0.72$$

In this case, the cardiac output (C.O.) can be calculated as

$$\text{C.O.} = \frac{250\ \text{mL/min}}{(0.97 - 0.72) \times 1.36 \times 14 \times 10} = 5.25\ \text{L/min/m}^2$$

## Indicator Dilution Methods

The most commonly used indicator dilution method today is the thermodilution technique. This method utilizes a bolus injection of chilled saline, followed by continuous measurement of the temperature of the blood by a thermistor in the pulmonary artery. The resulting curve is analyzed by computer to derive the cardiac output using the basic indicator dilution equation. With this method, the temperature of the injectate (measured in the injectate fluid container before injection) is assumed to increase by a predictable amount during injection.

Accurate measurement of both blood and injectate temperatures immediately before injection is important for measuring thermodilution cardiac outputs. According to the formula for calculating thermodilution cardiac output, the temperature difference between blood and injectate (typically 16°C when room-temperature injectate is used) is directly proportional to cardiac output. Small errors in either of these measurements can produce errors in calculated cardiac output.

Thermodilution cardiac output will be overestimated if the injectate temperature is inappropriately increased by permitting the injectate to remain in the syringe or by holding the syringe in the hand before and during injection. Use of cooled injectate, as opposed to room-temperature injectate, may produce an even greater mean error, probably because warming of the cooled injectate in the tubing and syringe produces an even greater increase in temperature than use of room-temperature injectate. Even though there is a theoretical advantage to iced injectate because of its greater signal-to-noise ratio, most studies have shown no advantage to iced over room-temperature injectate. A dual-thermistor catheter appears to minimize these problems with injectate temperature, resulting in more consistent and accurate cardiac output measurements, but at increased expense.

The thermodilution technique will overestimate cardiac output in low-flow states because of warming of blood by the cardiac chambers. The thermodilution method is most accurate in high-flow states. It is unreliable in the presence of significant tricuspid regurgitation. Overall, the thermodilution method should have an error of no more than 5% to 10% when performed correctly.

## Shunt Calculation

A shunt is an abnormal communication between the left and right heart chambers. A left-to-right shunt increases pulmonary blood flow in relation to systemic flow, and a right-to-left shunt does the opposite.

Oximetry is the most common method for calculating intracardiac shunts in the catheterization laboratory, although dye dilution curves and angiography may also be used. Oximetry is not as sensitive as dye dilution curves for detecting small shunts, but it should be capable of detecting any shunt that is large enough to merit surgical correction. Detailed oximetric analysis requires sampling in the right atrium (three sites), superior vena cava (high and low), inferior vena cava (at renal artery level and below the diaphragm), right ventricle (three sites), pulmonary artery, and aorta.

When a left-to-right shunt exists at the atrial level, it is necessary to use the SVC and IVC oxygen saturations to calculate the mixed venous blood saturation, as described above. A significant increase in oxygen saturation in the right side of the heart is considered to exist when there is a > 7% increase from the SVC/IVC to the right atrium (RA), >5% from the RA to the right ventricle (RV), and >5% from the RV to the PA.

Left-to-right shunts are commonly expressed as $Q_p/Q_s$. $Q_p$, or pulmonary flow, and $Q_s$, or systemic flow, are calculated using the formula given above for calculating cardiac output. The A-V $O_2$ difference for $Q_p$ requires pulmonary arterial and pulmonary venous samples (or assumption of a pulmonary venous saturation of 95%). The A-V $O_2$ difference for $Q_s$ requires arterial and mixed venous samples. A $Q_p/Q_s$ <1.5 signifies a small left-to-right shunt, 1.5 to 2.0 an intermediate size, and >2.0 a large shunt. A $Q_p/Q_s$ <1.0 indicates a net right-to-left shunt.

When $Q_p/Q_s$ is calculated, all the components of the cardiac output formula factor out, leaving only the oxygen saturations. Therefore, $Q_p/Q_s$ can be calculated by the following formula:

$$Q_P/Q_S = \frac{\text{systemic arterial oxygen saturation} - \text{mixed venous oxygen saturation}}{\text{pulmonary venous oxygen saturation} - \text{pulmonary artery oxygen saturation}}$$

Assume that a patient with an ostium secundum interatrial septal defect has the following measured values:

LV oxygen saturation = 96%
SVC oxygen saturation = 67.5%
IVC oxygen saturation = 73%
PA oxygen saturation = 80%

The mixed venous blood saturation is

$$\frac{3(0.675) + (0.73)}{4} = 0.69$$

In this case, $Q_P/Q_S$ is calculated as follows:

$$Q_P/Q_S = \frac{0.96 - 0.69}{0.96 - 0.80} = 1.69$$

### Vascular Resistance

Vascular resistance is defined by the ratio of pressure gradient across a vascular circuit divided by the flow. In a rigid tube with steady laminar flow of a homogeneous fluid, the relationship between pressure and flow is described by Poiseuille's law, which states that the pressure drop across a circuit with fluid flowing at a constant rate (and therefore its resistance) is directly proportional to the length of the tube and the viscosity of the fluid and indirectly proportional to the fourth power of the radius of the tube. Within the bloodstream, Poiseuille's law is inaccurate because blood flow is pulsatile and nonlaminar, blood is not homogeneous, and blood vessels are nonlinear and elastic. However, the basic principles of this law still apply in clinical measurements of resistance.

For clinical purposes, two important vascular resistance concepts are commonly derived from pressure and flow data:

$$\text{Systemic vascular resistance (SVR)} = \frac{\overline{Ao} - \overline{RA}}{Q_S}$$

$$\text{Pulmonary vascular resistance (PVR)} = \frac{\overline{PA} - \overline{LA}}{Q_P}$$

where $\overline{Ao}$ = mean systemic arterial pressure; $\overline{RA}$ = mean right atrial pressure; $\overline{PA}$ = mean pulmonary arterial pressure; $\overline{LA}$ = mean left atrial pressure; $Q_S$ = systemic blood flow; and $Q_P$ = pulmonary blood flow. The mean pulmonary capillary wedge pressure is often used as an approximation of the left atrial pressure.

These calculations yield vascular resistance in Wood units, named after Dr. Paul Wood. To convert to metric resistance units, expressed in dynes-sec-cm$^{-5}$, multiply by 80. Vascular resistance index (VRI) is obtained by multiplying vascular resistance by body surface area.

Normal values for vascular resistance (in dynes-sec-cm$^{-5}$) are

SVR: 1,150 ± 300
SVRI: 2,100 ± 500
PVR: 70 ± 40
PVRI: 125 ± 70

Clinically, SVR calculations are commonly used to diagnose and treat patients with hypotension or heart failure, and PVR to evaluate suitability of patients with congenital heart disease for cardiac surgery. Because the length of the vascular bed is likely to be constant in any adult patient, changes in SVR and PVR reflect either altered viscosity of blood or a change in the cross-sectional area of the vascular bed. Severe chronic anemia lowers the values for measured vascular resistance. If the hematocrit remains stable, changes in SVR are produced primarily by altered arteriolar tone. Thus, measurement of SVR becomes the basis for hemodynamic evaluation of shock.

In congenital heart disease, the ratio of PVR to SVR is commonly used as a criterion for operability. Normal is $<0.25$. Moderate pulmonary vascular disease is 0.25 to 0.75, severe is 0.75 to 1.0, and $\geq 1.0$ is generally considered inoperable. Administration of oxygen or vasodilator drugs permits differentiation of reversible vasoconstriction versus permanent obliterative changes in the pulmonary vasculature.

## CALCULATION OF VALVE ORIFICE AREA

Proper calculation of stenotic valve orifice area (VOA) is critically important for proper timing of valve surgery and valvuloplasty. The "gold standard" for calculating VOA is the Gorlin formula, which was developed by Richard Gorlin.

### Gorlin Formula

The Gorlin formula relies on measurement of three variables: cardiac output; mean pressure gradient; and flow period, which is the portion of the cardiac cycle during which pulsatile flow actually occurs. The diastolic filling period (DFP) is used for the mitral and tricuspid valves, because flow occurs through these valves only during diastole; the systolic ejection period (SEP) is used for the aortic and pulmonic valves. The final formula for the calculation of VOA is

$$\text{VOA} = \frac{\text{C.O.}/(\text{HR})(\text{DFP or SEP})}{44.3C\sqrt{\Delta P}}$$

where VOA = valve orifice area in cm$^2$, C.O. = cardiac output (cm$^3$/min), DFP = diastolic filling period (s/beat), SEP = systolic ejection period (s/beat), HR = heart rate (beats/min), $C$ = empiric constant, and $\Delta P$ = pressure gradient. An empiric constant of 0.85 is used for mitral valve calculations, and 1.0 for all other valves.

### Hakki Formula

A simplified formula for calculating VOA was introduced by Hakki, and it is

$$\text{VOA} = \frac{\text{C.O. (L/min)}}{\sqrt{\Delta P}}$$

This simplification is based on the fact that, at normal heart rates, the product of heart rate, SEP or DFP, and the Gorlin constant is approximately 1.0 for all patients.

However, in the presence of tachycardia, the simplified formula may be less useful because the percentage of time/min spent in systole or diastole changes markedly at higher heart rates. Therefore, Angel introduced a correction for heart rate: the Hakki equation should be divided by 1.35 when the heart rate is <75 beats/min with mitral stenosis and >90 beats/min with aortic stenosis.

## Aortic Valve Resistance

Aortic valve resistance (AVR) is another method of estimating severity of aortic stenosis. The simplified method of AVR calculation is

$$AVR = \frac{(LV\text{-}Ao) \times 80}{C.O. \times 2.5}$$

where (LV-Ao) = mean aortic valve gradient, 80 = conversion factor to dynes-s-cm$^{-5}$, C.O. = cardiac output, and 2.5 assumes that the systolic ejection period comprises 40% of the R-R cycle. Severe aortic stenosis (aortic VOA <0.7 cm$^2$) corresponds to AVR ≥300 dynes-s-cm$^{-5}$.

# SPECIFIC HEMODYNAMIC EXAMPLES

## Mitral Valve Disease

The typical atrial waveform configuration of mitral or tricuspid stenosis depends on its severity and the pliability of the valve. The characteristic features are elevation of the mean pressure, a diastolic gradient that is higher in early diastole, and a slow Y descent (Fig. 20–5). The A and C waves are increased in amplitude when the valve is pliable.

The characteristic atrial pressure waveform in mitral or tricuspid regurgitation consists of an earlier V-wave upstroke, increased amplitude, and a steep Y descent. In severe mitral regurgitation, the V wave may fuse with the C wave, producing a systolic wave (Fig. 20–6). The amplitude of the systolic wave in mitral regurgitation is determined by the severity and acuity of the regurgitation and the size of the atrium. Acute severe mitral regurgitation is often as-

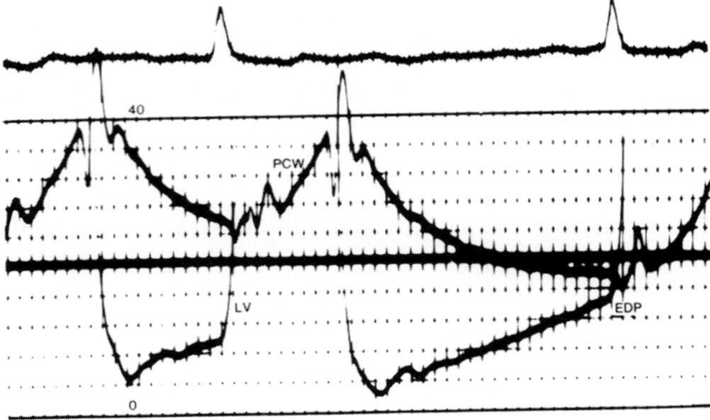


Figure 20–5

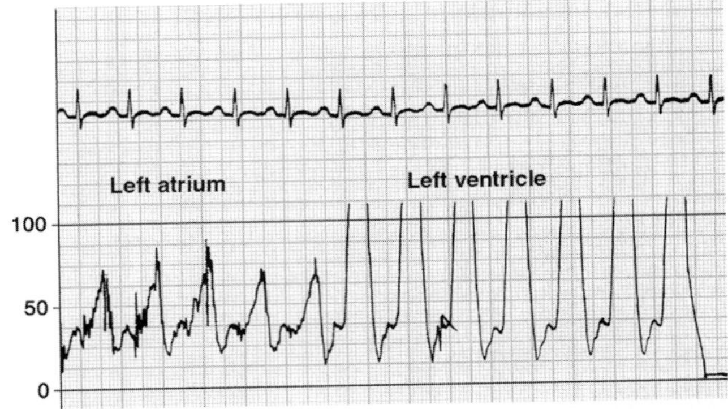


Figure 1–6

sociated with normal atrial size, in which case the atrium is noncompliant and the systolic wave is very high. When the atrium is quite dilated and compliant, as with chronic rheumatic mitral regurgitation, the systolic wave is likely to be much lower in amplitude.

The normal mitral valve area is 4.0 to 5.0 cm$^2$. A normal cardiac output of about 5 L/min can be maintained across a mitral valve with only a minimal diastolic gradient until the valve area falls to about 2.0 cm$^2$. When the valve area falls to about 1.0 cm$^2$, the resting gradient increases to about 10 mm Hg with this cardiac ouput, and substantial increases in the diastolic gradient, and therefore in left atrial and PCW pressures, will occur as the pulse rate rises. Therefore, a mitral valve area of 1.0 cm$^2$ is generally the "critical" area at which intervention may be required. For a large patient, an area of 1.2 may be critical.

Several factors may interfere with accurate determination of mitral valve area, including cardiac output measurements, presence of mitral regurgitation, and the phase delays and amplitude of PCW pressures compared to left atrial pressures.

Cardiac output measurements should ideally be made simultaneously with the measurement of pressure gradients. When mitral regurgitation coexists with mitral stenosis, calculations of valve area using only net forward flow will underestimate the actual valve orifice area because they fail to take into account the additional diastolic flow across the valve due to the regurgitation.

PCW pressure is commonly used as a substitute for left atrial pressures to calculate mitral VOA. Some authors suggest that, especially in prosthetic mitral valve stenosis, use of the PCW results in overestimation of transvalvular gradients. Others claim that the PCW pressure is adequate for this purpose, as long as the right heart catheter is properly wedged, which can be demonstrated by:

1. A mean PCW pressure about 10 mm Hg lower than mean PA pressure
2. Blood withdrawn from the wedged catheter has an oxygen saturation at least equal to arterial saturation

The following is an example of measurements made in a patient with mitral stenosis:

Cardiac output = 4,700 mL/min
Heart rate = 80 beats/min
Diastolic filling period = 0.4 s/beat
Mean mitral diastolic gradient = 20 mm Hg

From these values, the mitral valve orifice area can be calculated by the Gorlin formula as follows:

$$\text{Mitral orifice area} = \frac{(4{,}700\ \text{mL/min})/(80\ \text{beats/min})(0.4\ \text{s/beat})}{(44.3)(0.85)(\sqrt{20\ \text{mm Hg}})} = 0.9\ \text{cm}^2$$

The mitral valve orifice area can be calculated by the Hakki formula as follows:

$$\text{Mitral orifice area} = \frac{4.7\ \text{L/min}}{\sqrt{20\ \text{mm Hg}}} = 1.0\ \text{cm}^2$$

## Aortic Valve Disease

The aortic waveform in aortic stenosis is generally characterized by a slow upstroke, but the upstroke may be brisk in elderly patients with stiff, noncompliant vessels.

The aortic waveform in chronic severe aortic regurgitation is characterized by a wide pulse pressure, commonly >100 mm Hg, and a low diastolic pressure, often <50 mm Hg. When the pulse is fast, the aortic diastolic pressure tends to be higher and the left ventricular diastolic pressure lower. When the pulse rate is slow, the aortic diastolic pressure falls, and it may become equal to the left ventricular diastolic pressure. Patients with severe aortic insufficiency tolerate bradycardia poorly because of the resulting increase in LV end-diastolic pressure.

The aortic transvalvular gradient may be expressed as:

1. Peak-to-peak gradient, which uses the maximum left ventricular and maximum aortic pressures. This measurement has no physiologic meaning because the two peaks occur at different times. This gradient approximates the mean gradient in severe aortic stenosis.
2. Peak instantaneous gradient, which is usually derived from Doppler flow velocity.
3. Mean gradient, which represents the planimetered area under the simultaneous aortic–left ventricular curves.

Normal aortic valve area is about 3.0 to 4.0 cm$^2$. Aortic stenosis is generally considered severe enough to produce symptoms when the aortic VOA is reduced to <0.8 cm$^2$. In a very large person—for example, someone with a body surface area of >2.2 m$^2$—an orifice area of 0.9 to 1.0 cm$^2$ may be considered severe. Unlike mitral stenosis, in which the transvalvular gradient increases with increasing heart rate, the gradient in aortic stenosis increases with decreasing heart rate.

Several factors may interfere with accurate determination of aortic VOA, including use of simultaneous left ventricular and peripheral arterial pressures, catheter position in the left ventricular outflow tract, low-flow states, and pullback pressures, especially in the presence of arrhythmias. In addition, aortic VOA calculations in patients with associated severe aortic regurgitation will underestimate the aortic flow, and therefore the VOA.

Ideally, the aortic valve gradient should be measured simultaneously in the left ventricle and ascending aorta, either with a double-lumen catheter or with separate catheters. Compared to the ascending aorta pressure, the femoral artery pressure wave is delayed and widened, and the peak systolic pressure is amplified. If the femoral artery and ventricular waveforms are aligned, the mean gradient is overestimated by nearly 10 mm Hg. With alignment, the gradient is underestimated by about 10 mm Hg. These errors are of particular significance when the gradient is <50 mm Hg.

Patients with aortic stenosis who have low cardiac output and a small gradient present a special problem. For instance, a 0.7-cm$^2$ aortic VOA combined with a cardiac output of 3 L/min will produce a gradient of only 20 mm Hg. The Gorlin formula becomes very flow dependent at cardiac outputs of <3–4 L/min. Maneuvers such as exercise or infusion of an inotropic agent or sodium nitroprusside may produce a higher cardiac output, which allows calculation of a more reliable VOA. In mild aortic valve disease, the calculated valve area increases, indicating that surgery may not be necessary. In severe aortic stenosis, the valve area remains small.

Pullback pressures across the aortic valve may introduce errors in calculation of the VOA as a result of respiratory variation or to transient changes that occur in the systolic pressure during sinus beats that follow a PVC during pullback. In addition, when the VOA is less then 0.6 cm$^2$, a 7 or 8 French catheter may occupy a significant amount of the remaining valve orifice area, in which case the catheter temporarily increases the severity of the stenosis.

The following is an example of measurements obtained in a patient with aortic stenosis:

Cardiac output = 4,500 mL/min
Heart rate = 72 beats/min
Systolic ejection period = 0.33 s/beat
Mean aortic systolic gradient = 50 mm Hg

From these values, the aortic valve orifice area can be calculated as follows:

$$\text{Aortic orifice area} = \frac{(4{,}500\ \text{mL/min})/(72\ \text{beats/min})(0.33\ \text{s/beat})}{(44.3)\sqrt{50\ \text{mm Hg}}} = 0.6\ \text{cm}^2$$

The aortic valve orifice area can be calculated by the Hakki formula as follows:

$$\text{Aortic orifice area} = \frac{4.5\ \text{L/min}}{\sqrt{50\ \text{mm Hg}}} = 0.6\ \text{cm}^2$$

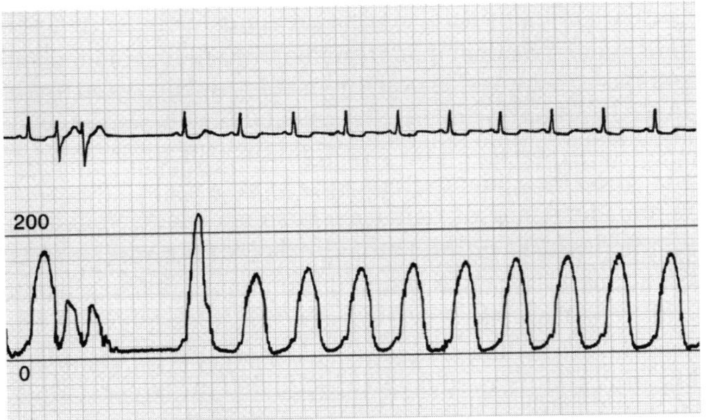


Figure 20–7

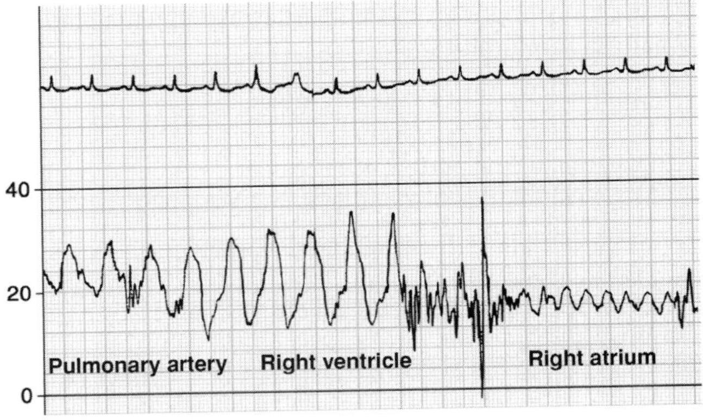


Figure 20–8

The aortic valve resistance (AVR) in this patient can be calculated by the following formula:

$$\text{AVR} = \frac{50\ \text{mm Hg} \times 80}{4.5\ \text{L/min} \times 2.5} = 356\ \text{dynes-s-cm}^{-5}$$

## Hypertrophic Obstructive Cardiomyopathy

Hypertrophic obstructive cardiomyopathy (HOCM) produces characteristic hemodynamic changes that may vary greatly with physiologic maneuvers. It is important to understand the underlying physiology of HOCM because there may be no gradient at rest, and therefore it is necessary to provoke the gradient during the catheterization procedure. The three principal mechanisms that may provoke an intraventricular gradient in HOCM are

1. Decreased LV end-diastolic volume (e.g., Valsalva maneuver, nitroglycerin, dehydration, upward tilt, phlebotomy)
2. Increased force or duration of ventricular contraction (e.g., following a PVC, intravenous isoproterenol infusion)
3. Decreased aortic outflow resistance (e.g., amyl nitrite inhalation)

PVCs produce characteristic changes in LV pressure and gradient in HOCM (Fig. 20–7). The peak LV systolic pressure of the sinus beat that follows a PVC is

- Lower in the normal heart
- Higher with left ventricular outflow tract obstruction (HOCM, valvular aortic stenosis), severe mitral stenosis, and severe dilated cardiomyopathy

A characteristic feature of HOCM that differentiates it from valvular aortic stenosis is the Brockenbrough sign: with HOCM, the arterial pulse pressure of the sinus beat that follows a PVC, is lower than the sinus beat that precedes the PVC; with valvular aortic stenosis, it is higher. In addition, both the Valsalva maneuver and nitroglycerin increase the gradient in HOCM, but decrease the gradient in valvular aortic stenosis.

## Constrictive Physiology

Pericardial tamponade and chronic constrictive pericarditis are the two classic syndromes of constrictive physiology. A third syndrome, effusive-constrictive pericarditis, has intermediate hemodynamic features. All three are characterized by diastolic dysfunction, with impaired atrial and ventricular filling patterns. Clinically, the differentiation of pericardial tamponade and constrictive pericarditis is simple. However, the differentiation of constrictive pericarditis and restrictive cardiomyopathy may be much more difficult, even with the use of modern diagnostic tools.

### *Pericardial Tamponade*

The classic features of pericardial tamponade include:

- Elevation and equalization of right and left ventricular diastolic pressures and right and left atrial pressures
- Pulsus paradoxus, that is, exaggerated (>10 mm Hg) inspiratory fall in arterial pressures
- Prominent X descent with blunted Y descent
- Arterial hypotension, as a late event (Fig. 20–8)

Pulsus paradoxus is a characteristic finding in pericardial tamponade, but it may be found in chronic obstructive pulmonary disease and rarely in pulmonary embolus and in constrictive pericarditis. Pulsus paradoxus in tamponade is associated with narrowing of the pulse pressure during inspiration, but the pulse pressure is normal in chronic pulmonary disease (Fig. 20–9). Pulsus paradoxus may be impossible to detect in a patient with an irregular rhythm, such as atrial fibrillation.

Three phases of cardiac tamponade have been described:

*Phase 1.* Only intrapericardial and right atrial pressures are elevated.

*Phase 2.* Elevated intrapericardial pressure produces equilibration of right atrial and right ventricular diastolic pressures, but not pulmonary capillary wedge (or left ventricular filling) pressure. It is also

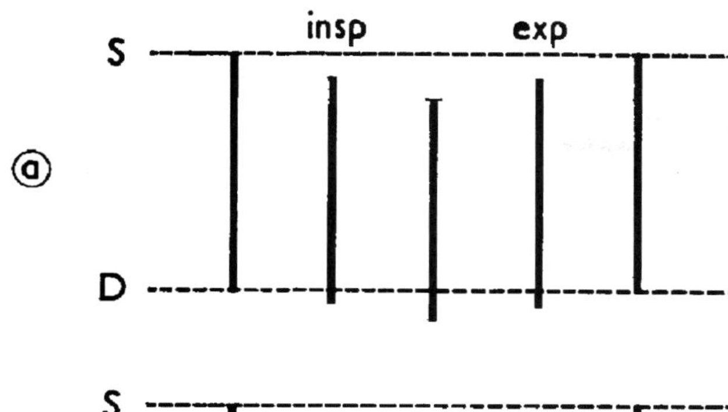


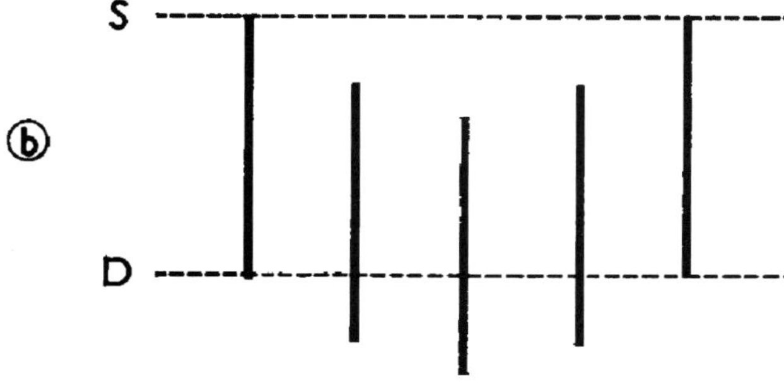


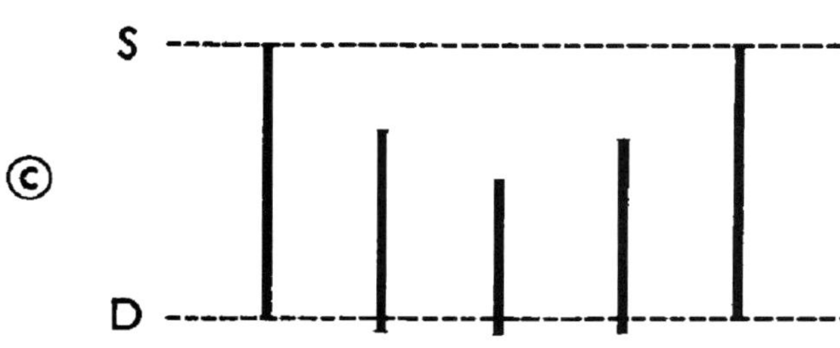


Figure 20–9

associated with pulsus paradoxus and a modest decrease in cardiac output.

*Phase 3.* Elevated intrapericardial pressure results in equilibration of right and left ventricular filling pressures; marked pulsus paradoxus; decreased cardiac output; and hypotension.

Echocardiography is sensitive for the detection of phases 2 and 3 of cardiac tamponade, characterized by right heart chamber collapse during diastole in the presence of pericardial effusion.

### *Constrictive Pericarditis and Restrictive Cardiomyopathy*

The classic features of constrictive pericarditis include:

- Elevation and equalization of diastolic pressures in all four cardiac chambers
- Deep, rapid Y descent (corresponding clinically to Friedrich sign)
- Attenuation of the X descent, which, in conjunction with the deep Y descent, produces an M or W configuration in the atrial tracing
- Elevation of the right atrial mean pressure during inspiration (corresponding clinically to Kussmaul sign)
- "Dip and plateau" pattern in right and left ventricular pressures
- RVEDP > one third the RVSP
- PA systolic pressure <55 mm Hg
- Pulsus paradoxus when pericardial pressures are equilibrated with right, but not left, ventricular filling pressures (Fig. 20–10)

None of these features is diagnostic of constrictive pericarditis. Pulsus paradoxus without a Kussmaul sign is characteristic of cardiac tamponade, whereas Kussmaul sign

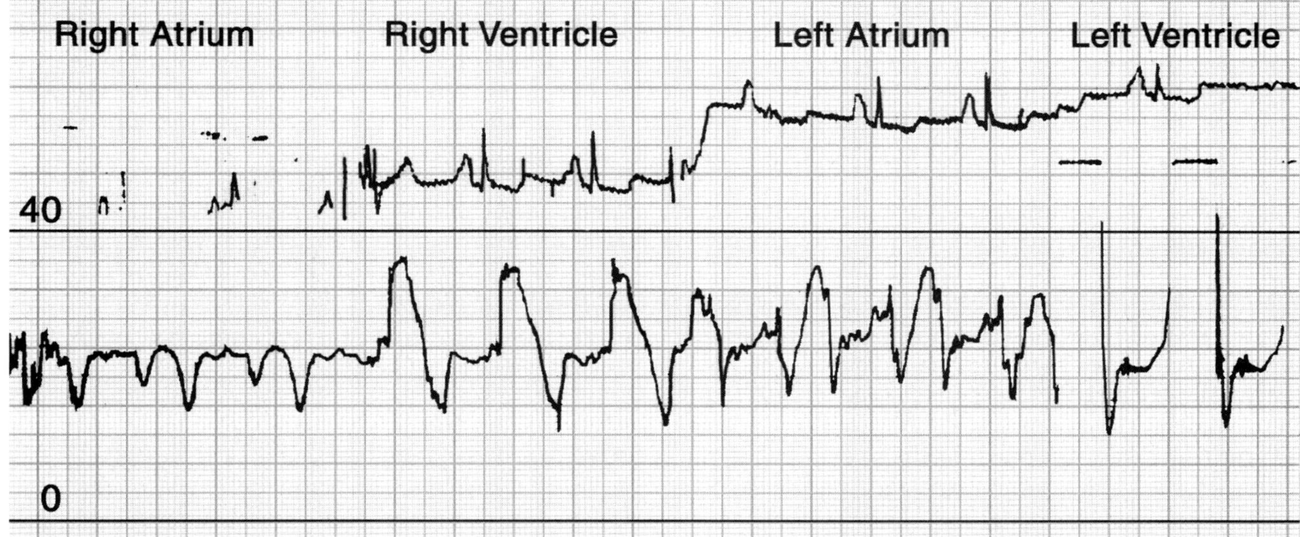


Figure 20–10

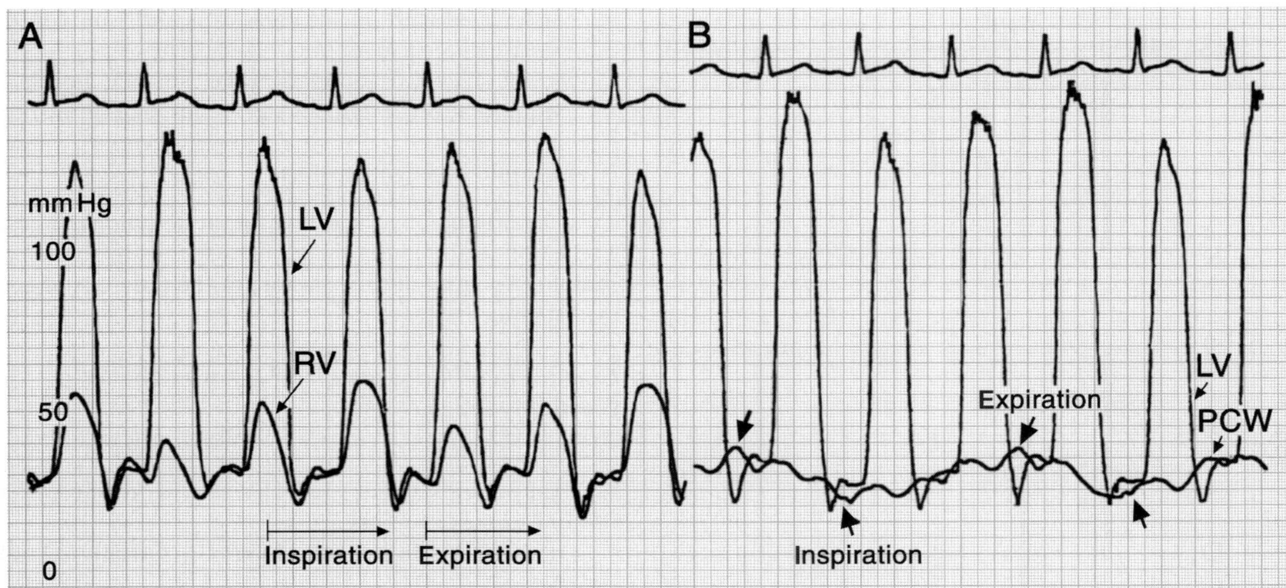


**Figure 20–11**

without pulsus paradoxus is characteristic of pericardial constriction. However, Kussmaul sign and a rapid Y descent in the right atrial pressure tracing may be seen in right ventricular dysfunction of any cause, such as right ventricular infarction and restrictive cardiomyopathy. Kussmaul sign may also occur in respiratory failure, when the systolic and diastolic pressures fall equally with no change in pulse pressure, whereas tamponade produces a fall in systolic pressure and pulse pressure. A dip-and-plateau pattern is not diagnostic of constrictive pericarditis, and it may be absent in constrictive pericarditis if the pulse rate is rapid.

### *Hemodynamic Criteria*

Two hemodynamic criteria, based on respiratory dynamics, have been introduced recently, and they improve accuracy in differentiating constrictive pericarditis from restrictive cardiomyopathy. They are

- Respiratory discordance in early diastolic PCW-LV pressure gradient
- Respiratory discordance in left and right ventricular systolic pressures

In the normal heart and in restrictive cardiomyopathy, the drop in intrathoracic pressure that occurs with inspiration is transmitted to both the pericardial sac (and therefore the heart) and the pulmonary veins. The effective filling gradient (EFG) between the PCW pressure and the left ventricular diastolic pressure remains nearly constant.

However, in cardiac tamponade and constrictive pericarditis, inspiration decreases both the intrathoracic pressure and the pulmonary venous pressure (and PCW pressure), but does not affect the pressures in the pericardial sac or left ventricular diastolic pressure. This produces a discordance in the EFG: with inspiration, the PCW falls but the LV diastolic pressure does not, resulting in a marked decrease in EFG, which corresponds to the decrease in diastolic flow across the mitral valve seen on the echocardiogram. With expiration, the PCW and the EFG rise and the diastolic flow across the mitral valve increases.

Discordance in the right and left ventricular systolic pressures with inspiration may occur because the relatively fixed intracardiac volume imposed by constrictive pericarditis produces ventricular "interdependence" (Fig. 20–11). Because the ventricles in constrictive pericarditis cannot fill independently of one another, the filling of one ventricle impairs the filling of the other. Inspiration augments the diastolic filling of the right ventricle at the expense of the left ventricle, with a shift of the interventricular septum to the left. During inspiration, the RV systolic pressure increases due to the increased RV volume, whereas, the LV systolic pressure decreases.

The presence of an irregular rhythm, especially atrial fibrillation, may obscure the respiratory variations that occur in the hemodynamics of constrictive pericarditis. In this case, the varying R-R intervals may be regularized with a temporary pacemaker.

Diagnosis of constrictive pericarditis may be problematic in a variety of circumstances:

- Severe lung disease with marked respiratory changes
- Right ventricular infarction
- Severe tricuspid regurgitation
- Low filling pressures, e.g., due to diuresis. If the filling pressure is <15 mm Hg, constrictive pericarditis can be "unmasked" by infusion of 500 to 1,000 mL of saline.

## BIBLIOGRAPHY


**Angel J, Soler-Soler J, Anivarro I, Domingo E.** Hemodynamic evaluation of stenotic cardiac valves: II. Modification of the simplified valve formula for mitral and aortic valve area calculation. *Cathet Cardiov Diagn.* 1985;11:127–138.

**Assey ME, Zile MR, Usher BW, et al.** Effect of catheter positioning on the variability of measured gradient in aortic stenosis. *Cathet Cardiovasc Diagn.* 1993;30:287–292.

**Baim DS, Grossman W,** eds, *Cardiac Catheterization, Angiography and Intervention.* 5th ed. Philadelphia: Williams & Wilkins; 1996.

**Blitz LR, Kolansky DM, Hirshfeld JW.** Valve function: stenosis and insufficiency. In: Pepine C, Hill J, Lambert CR, eds. *Diagnostic and Therapeutic Cardiac Catheterization.* 3rd ed. Baltimore: Williams & Wilkins; 1998:516–540.

**Bonow RO, Carabello B, deLeon AC, et al.** ACC/AHA guidelines for the management of patients with valvular heart disease. *J Am Coll Cardiol.* 1998;32:1486–1588.

**Hakki AH, Iskandrian AS, Bemis CE, et al.** A simplified valve formula for the calculation of stenotic cardiac valve areas. *Circulation* 1981;63:1050–1055.

**Hurrell DG, Nishimura RA, Higano ST, et al.** Value of respiratory changes in left and right ventricular pressures for the diagnosis of constrictive pericarditis. *Circulation* 1996;93:2007–2013.

**Kegel JG, Schalet BD, Corin WJ, Iskandrian AS.** Simplified method for calculating aortic valve resistance: correlation with valve area and standard formula. *Cathet Cardiovasc Diagn.* 1993;30:15–21.

**Kern MJ,** ed. *Hemodynamic Rounds.* New York: Wiley-Liss; 1999.

**Lange RA, Hillis LD.** Cardiac catheterization and hemodynamic assessment. In: Topol EJ, ed. *Textbook of Cardiovascular Medicine.* Philadelphia: Lippincott-Raven, 1998:1957–1976.

**Lehmann KG, Platt MS.** Improved accuracy and precision of thermodilution cardiac output measurement using a dual thermistor catheter system. *J Am Coll Cardiol.* 1999;33:883–891.

**Sigwart U.** *Automation in Cardiac Diagnosis. The Computer-Assisted Acquisition of Cardiac Catheterization Data.* Basel; Schwabe, 1978.

# 21

# Electrocardiographic Stress Testing

*Julie C. Huang   Michael S. Lauer*

## ESSENTIAL FACTS

1. With few exceptions, exercise stress testing is the test of choice for initial evaluation of suspected coronary artery disease.
2. Diagnosis of coronary artery disease using exercise stress testing is limited by verification bias and an uncertain "gold standard."
3. Exercise capacity is the most important prognostic factor derived from exercise stress testing; Duke treadmill score, heart rate recovery, chronotropic response, and ventricular ectopy during recovery also provide important prognostic information.
4. Exercise stress testing is most useful for intermediate-risk patients.

## ESSENTIAL EVIDENCE/CURRENT GUIDELINES

The exercise electrocardiographic (ECG) stress test is one of the most commonly performed diagnostic tests in modern medicine and is the test of choice for the initial evaluation of suspected coronary artery disease. Its advantages include its low cost, general safety and noninvasive nature, and its usefulness in providing information regarding functional capacity. Despite excitement over new imaging techniques, it has recently become realized that the "plain old treadmill test" is vastly underappreciated, particularly for its ability to predict short- and long-term risk.

Traditionally, the primary goal of exercise stress testing is the diagnosis of obstructive coronary artery disease (CAD) and myocardial ischemia in patients with symptoms of angina or risk factors for heart disease. This goal, however, is hampered by verification bias; because the majority of patients who undergo coronary angiography to confirm the diagnosis of CAD have had a positive stress test, it cannot be known for certain how sensitive or specific the stress test is—those who had a negative stress test are not evaluated similarly with angiography. Furthermore, the use of coronary angiography as the gold standard for the diagnosis of CAD is increasingly questioned, as more recent studies have suggested that, because of arterial remodeling, an angiographically normal-appearing artery can actually have a significant amount of atherosclerotic disease upon evaluation by other methods such as intravascular ultrasound. For these reasons, some cardiologists discourage the notion of exercise stress testing as a "diagnostic" tool, but instead consider it a "prognostic" tool.

### Safety

Exercise treadmill testing is generally considered to be very safe, but can rarely be associated with serious complications. These may include myocardial infarction (3.5/10,000 tests), serious arrhythmias (4.8/10,000), and death (0.5/10,000). Exercise testing after myocardial infarction is also safe at as early as 3 to 5 days, though is usually limited to submaximal testing using endpoints of 70% age-predicted maximal heart rate or a peak work level of 5 METs.

### Indications and Contraindications to Exercise ECG Stress Testing

Most commonly, exercise stress testing is ordered for the diagnosis of obstructive or flow-limiting coronary artery disease; it is most useful in patients with an intermediate pretest probability based on age, gender, and symptoms of having CAD. In a patient with a high pretest probability of CAD (e.g., a middle-aged male with typical anginal symptoms and multiple cardiac risk factors), a negative stress test does not sufficiently preclude a diagnosis of CAD and is more likely to be a false negative result. In contrast, in a patient with a low pretest probability of CAD (e.g., a young woman with unusual symptoms and no significant risk factors), a positive stress test is more likely to be a false positive result. The sensitivity and specificity of testing is therefore highest in patients with intermediate pretest probability. Patients must also have a baseline ECG in which ST segments and subsequent changes are interpretable. Patients with left bundle branch block, paced rhythms, >1 mm of resting ST depression (e.g., digoxin therapy or left ventricular hypertrophy), and Wolff–Parkinson–White syndrome are therefore not recommended for exercise ECG testing without adjunctive imaging.

Stress testing can be used to assess prognosis in patients with known or suspected CAD. It is indicated after myocardial infarction for activity or exercise prescription, entrance into cardiac rehabilitation, and evaluation of medical therapy; after revascularization to evaluate symptoms and as periodic monitoring of high-risk, asymptomatic patients. In patients with valvular heart disease, stress testing is used for evaluation of exercise capacity and may be very useful in determining the appropriate timing of surgery. Use of stress testing is also indicated for adjustment of pacemaker settings, assessment of suspected exercise-induced arrhythmias, and evaluation of therapy in patients with suspected exercise-induced arrhythmias. Before a patient returns to work, testing may provide a comparison of peak workload achieved to that required in employment.

There are no Class I indications for testing of asymptomatic patients, and routine screening is classified as a Class III indication. However, patients who are asymptomatic but have multiple risk factors, those planning to start vigorous exercise or engaged in occupations that may affect public safety (e.g., pilots, bus drivers), and those who are at high risk of cardiovascular disease because of comorbidities such as diabetes mellitus can still be referred for exercise stress testing though these are listed as Class II indications.

Contraindications to exercise stress testing are listed in Table 21–1 and include testing of extremely low-risk patients and those with recent myocardial infarction, unstable angina, or dynamic ECG changes; active or unstable arrhythmias or congestive heart failure; aortic dissection; or other acute cardiac or systemic processes. Relative contraindications are at the discretion of the physician: testing may proceed if the benefit outweighs the risk.

**TABLE 21–1**
**CONTRAINDICATIONS TO EXERCISE TESTING**

| |
|---|
| Absolute contraindications |
| Recent significant change in resting ECG |
| Recent MI (2 days) |
| Unstable angina not medically controlled |
| Uncontrolled arrhythmias causing hemodynamic compromise |
| Uncontrolled heart failure |
| Acute pulmonary embolism/infarction |
| Acute myocarditis or pericarditis |
| Suspected or known aortic dissection |
| Acute infection |
| Relative contraindications |
| Left main coronary stenosis |
| Moderate stenotic valve disease |
| Electrolyte abnormalities ($K^+$, $Mg^{2+}$) |
| SBP >200 mm Hg, DBP >110 mm Hg |
| Symptomatic tachy- or bradyarrhythmias |
| Hypertrophic cardiomyopathy |
| Neuromuscular, musculoskeletal, or rheumatoid disorders that are exacerbated by exercise |
| High-degree AV block |
| Ventricular aneurysm |
| Uncontrolled metabolic diseases |
| Chronic infections (e.g., hepatitis, HIV) |

MI, myocardial infarction; SBP, systolic blood pressure; DBP, diastolic blood pressure; AV, atrioventricular.
*Source:* Gibbons RJ, et al. ACC/AHA 2002 guideline update for exercise testing, 2002.

## Methods of Testing

Ideally, the exercise stress test should last 8 to 12 minutes; this provides a reasonable compromise for assessment of functional capacity without fatigue and attainment of anaerobic threshold. It is therefore important to choose the appropriate exercise protocol to suit the patient's projected ability to perform the test. For instance, the widely used Bruce protocol may be an appropriate test for most average patients, but is likely too difficult for an elderly patient undergoing risk stratification before hospital discharge. A truncated test provides a less accurate assessment of functional capacity.

Although bicycle protocols allow for a more precise measurement of work capacity, most patients in the United States have more familiarity with treadmill methods and treadmill is therefore more commonly used. The disadvantage of treadmill is that work is only estimated and tends to be overestimated, depending on the degree of reliance (leaning) on handrails.

Placement of electrodes for ECG measurement differs in exercise testing compared to standard 12-lead ECG and may result in rightward axis shift and false positive or negative inferior Q waves. Lead V5 is often the best for assessment of ST changes. ECGs are obtained at rest, during each stage of exercise, at peak exercise, and every 1 to 2 minutes for at least 5 minutes of recovery. Other data obtained during testing include rhythm, heart rate, blood pressure, symptoms, and the patient's rating of perceived exertion. The test is completed when the patient attains 85% of the age-predicted maximum heart rate or cannot proceed because of symptoms. The age-predicted maximum heart rate is calculated as 220–age in years.

Indications for termination of stress testing are listed in Table 21–2, and include symptoms, drop in systolic

**TABLE 21–2**
**INDICATIONS FOR TERMINATION OF ECG STRESS TESTING**

Absolute indications for terminating testing
- SBP drop of ≥10 mm Hg in the presence of other signs of ischemia
- Moderate to severe angina
- Increasing ataxia, dizziness, near-syncope
- Pallor or cyanosis
- Technical difficulties with ECG or blood pressure monitoring
- Subject request
- Sustained VT
- ST elevation ≥1 mm in leads without pathologic Q waves

Relative indications for terminating testing
- SBP drop of ≥10 mm Hg in the absence of other signs of ischemia
- ST depression >2 mm
- Arrhythmias other than sustained VT
- Fatigue, dyspnea, wheezing, leg discomfort, claudication
- Development of bundle branch block or IVCD that cannot be distinguished from VT
- Increasing chest pain
- SBP >250 mm Hg or DBP >115 mm Hg

SBP, systolic blood pressure; VT, ventricular tachycardia; IVCD, intraventricular conduction defect; DBP, diastolic blood pressure.
*Source:* Gibbons RJ, et al. ACC/AHA 2002 guideline update for exercise testing.

blood pressure, sustained ventricular arrhythmias, and the development of ST elevation. Relative indications for termination of testing are also listed.

## Diagnostic Interpretation

Interpretation of the ECG stress test primarily involves evaluation of the ST segment. The classic positive finding is ≥1 mm of horizontal or down-sloping ST-segment depression 80 ms after the J point, though many labs also consider up-sloping ST-segment depression ≥1.5 mm a positive finding. Ischemic changes tend to occur in leads I and V4–V6; the more widespread the ECG changes, usually the more severe the disease. ST-segment depression does *not* localize ischemia; however, ST-segment elevation in leads without Q waves *does* localize the distribution of ischemia and is an indication for termination of the test. Markers of severe CAD during testing include a drop in systolic blood pressure below resting value, exercise-limiting angina, poor exercise capacity <5 METs, down-sloping ST depression in recovery, and ST depression at low work load.

## Prognostic Interpretation

Of as much importance as evaluation of ST segments during stress testing is the contribution of other markers of risk to overall prognosis. Exercise capacity is the most important prognostic variable; it is widely accepted that patients able to perform >10 METs are in general at low risk for cardiovascular events (Table 21–3). The heart rate recovery (HRR)(difference in heart rate from peak exercise to 1 minute recovery) is known to be a very strong prognostic indicator, and patients with HRR of 12 beats or less have a significantly elevated mortality compared with those whose HRR is >12 beats. The Duke treadmill score (DTS), a composite of exercise capacity and angina, also provides important information. It is calculated as

$$\text{DTS} = \text{minutes of Bruce protocol} - 5 \times \text{ST deviation} - 4 \times \text{angina index}$$

where the angina index is 0 = no angina, 1 = angina, but not test limiting, and 2 = test-limiting angina. DTS interpretation is as follows:

Low (≥+5): mortality risk <1% per year
Intermediate (−10 to +4): mortality risk 1% to 3% per year
High (<−10): mortality risk >3% per year

**TABLE 21–3**
**AGE AND GENDER ESTIMATED FUNCTIONAL CAPACITY**

| | Estimated Functional Capacity (METs) | | | | |
|---|---|---|---|---|---|
| **Age (y)** | **Poor** | **Fair** | **Average** | **Good** | **High** |
| | | | **Women** | | |
| ≤29 | <7.5 | 8–10 | 10–13 | 13–16 | >16 |
| 30–39 | <7 | 7–9 | 9–11 | 11–15 | >15 |
| 40–49 | <6 | 6–8 | 8–10 | 10–14 | >14 |
| 50–59 | <5 | 5–7 | 7–9 | 9–13 | >13 |
| ≥60 | <4.5 | 4.5–6 | 6–8 | 8–11.5 | >11.5 |
| | | | **Men** | | |
| ≤29 | <8 | 8–11 | 11–14 | 14–17 | >17 |
| 30–29 | <7.5 | 7.5–10 | 10–12.5 | 12.5–16 | >16 |
| 40–49 | <7 | 7–8.5 | 8.5–11.5 | 11.5–15 | >15 |
| 50–59 | <6 | 6–8 | 8–11 | 11–14 | >14 |
| ≥60 | <5.5 | 5.5–7 | 7–9.5 | 9.5–13 | >13 |

The use of beta-blockers during stress testing may affect certain variables such as chronotropic incompetence and peak heart rate; but has little if any effect on the Duke treadmill score and its prognostic implications. Presence of ventricular ectopy during exercise recovery is a significant negative prognostic indicator.

### Metabolic Gas-Exchange Analyses

Metabolic stress testing is indicated for the evaluation of exercise capacity and response to therapy in patients with heart failure being considered for heart transplantation as well as for differentiation of cardiac from pulmonary causes of exercise intolerance. It may also be used for the evaluation of exercise capacity when subjective measurement is unreliable; for the assessment of responses to specific therapeutic interventions, and for the determination of exercise intensity for a cardiac rehabilitation program. It is not indicated for routine evaluation of exercise capacity.

Several standard measurements are made in metabolic stress testing in addition to the above-mentioned variables used in routine ECG testing. The peak $Vo_2$ (oxygen uptake) defines the patient's aerobic capacity and is proportional to the cardiac output; a peak $Vo_2$ of $<14$ mL/kg/min identifies hig- risk patients who are reasonable candidates for cardiac transplant despite ambulatory status. The respiratory exchange ratio (RER), calculated as $Vco_2/Vo_2$, where $Vco_2$ is the production of carbon dioxide, identifies the adequacy of the test, with RER $>1.09$ suggesting adequate effort for reliable analysis of the test. Other important variable measurements include $Vo_2$ at anaerobic threshold; the VE/MVV (proportion of breathing reserve used); and $Vo_2$ pulse or $Vo_2$/HR (measure of stroke volume).

## SUMMARY

In modern medical practice with its large array of available diagnostic testing, there is still a role for exercise ECG testing in the evaluation of suspected ischemic heart disease. It should be used primarily for evaluation of symptoms, but it is also important for risk stratification in patients with risk factors, as well as in evaluation of the effectiveness of therapy. In its use as a tool for diagnosis of CAD, it is best used in patients with an intermediate pretest probability based on patient characteristics and symptomatology. In this situation the sensitivity and specificity of the test are highest, generally reported as 68% and 77%, though these values are hampered by verification bias.

The prognostic information gained from stress testing is just as important, and includes exercise capacity, heart rate recovery, chronotropic competence, and the Duke treadmill score.

## BIBLIOGRAPHY

**Cole CR, Blackstone EH, Pashkow FJ, et al.** Heart-rate recovery immediately after exercise as a predictor of mortality. *N Engl J Med.* 1999;341:1351–1357.

**Diaz LA, Brunken RC, Blackstone EH, et al.** Independent contribution of myocardial perfusion defects to exercise capacity and heart rate recovery for prediction of all-cause mortality in patients with known or suspected coronary heart disease. *J Am Coll Cardiol.* 2001;37(6):1558–1564.

**Froelicher VF, Lehmann KG, Thomas R, et al.** The electrocardiographic exercise test in a population with reduced workup bias: diagnostic performance, computerized interpretation, and multivariable prediction. Veterans Affairs Cooperative Study in Health Services #016 (QUEXTA) Study Group. Quantitative Exercise Testing and Angiography. *Ann Intern Med.* 1998;128:965–974.

**Frolkis JP, Pothier CE, Blackstone EH, Lauer MS.** Frequent ventricular ectopy after exercise as a predictor of death. *N Engl J Med.* 2003;348(9):781–790.

**Gibbons RJ, Balady GJ, Beasley JW, et al.** ACC/AHA guidelines for exercise testing. A report of the American College of Cardiology/American Heart Association Task Force on Practice Guidelines (Committee on Exercise Testing). *J Am Coll Cardiol.* 1997;30(1):260–311.

**Gibbons RJ, Balady GJ, Bricker JT, et al.** ACC/AHA 2002 guideline update for exercise testing: summary article. A report of the American College of Cardiology/American Heart Association Task Force on Practice Guidelines (Committee to Update the 1997 Exercise Testing Guidelines). *J Am Coll Cardiol.* 2002;40(8):1531–1540.

**Gibbons RJ, Chatterjee K, Daley J, et al.** ACC/AHA/ACP-ASIM guidelines for the management of patients with chronic stable angina: a report of the American College of Cardiology/American Heart Association Task Force on Practice Guidelines (Committee on Management of Patients with Chronic Stable Angina). *J Am Coll Cardiol.* 1999;33(7):2092–2197.

**Lauer MS.** Exercise electrocardiogram testing and prognosis. Novel markers and predictive instruments. *Cardiol Clin.* 2001;19(3):401–414.

**Mark DB, Shaw L, Harrell FE Jr, et al.** Prognostic value of a treadmill exercise score in outpatients with suspected coronary artery disease. *N Engl J Med.* 1991;325:849–853.

**Nishime EO, Cole CR, Blackstone EH, et al.** Heart rate recovery and treadmill exercise score as predictors of mortality in patients referred for exercise ECG. *JAMA.* 2000;284(11):1392–1398.

**Patterson RE, Horowitz SF.** Importance of epidemiology and biostatistics in deciding clinical strategies for using diagnostic tests: a simplified approach using examples from coronary artery disease. *J Am Coll Cardiol.* 1989;13:1653–1665.

**Wei M, Kampert JB, Barlow CE, et al.** Relationship between low cardiorespiratory fitness and mortality in normal-weight, overweight, and obese men. *JAMA.* 1999;282(16):1547–1553.

## QUESTIONS

1. A 40-year-old asymptomatic man with no risk factors undergoes stress testing as part of an "Executive Physical" program. His resting ECG is normal and he is taking no medications. He has an exercise capacity of 14 METs (13.5 minutes on the Bruce protocol), no angina, a peak heart rate

of 180, and 1 mm of down-sloping ST-segment depression noted in lead V5. His Duke treadmill score is

a. 9
b. 8.5
c. 7.5
d. 3.5
e. 2

Answer is b: DTS = 13.5 minutes − 5 × 1 mm of ST depression − 4 × 0 angina = 8.5.

2. Given these test results, the next most appropriate step is

a. No further cardiac testing
b. A stress imaging study
c. A repeat stress test in 1 year
d. Coronary angiography

Answer is a: A DTS ≥5.5 implies low risk of death (≤1% per year) and therefore no further testing is needed.

3. A 55-year-old woman presents with intermittent substernal chest pain that radiates to the left arm. The pain is not clearly exertional and is not clearly relieved with rest. There is no history of gastrointestinal problems; her symptoms are not related to meals or body position. Her resting ECG is normal and she is taking no medications. She is referred for an exercise test and is found to have ST-segment depression. Assuming that the true, unbiased sensitivity of exercise ST-segment changes is 45% and the specificity is 85%, the likelihood that she has at least one 50% coronary artery stenosis is

a. 0.25
b. 0.50
c. 0.75
d. 0.80
e. 0.90

Answer is c: This is the positive predictive value, where PPV = (Sens)(Prev)/[(Sens)(Prev) + (1 − Spec)(1 − Prev)]. The patients has atypical angina, and given her age and gender therefore has an intermediate-risk (0.50) pretest likelihood. Substituting values, the PPV is 0.75.

4. A 60-year-old man with chronic obstructive pulmonary disease (COPD) (FEV1 1.25) and chronic ischemic cardiomyopathy (EF 30%) is referred for metabolic stress testing, which shows the following: peak $VO_2$ 15 mL/kg/min, peak $VCO_2$ 18 mL/kg/min, $VO_2$ at anaerobic threshold 10 mL/kg/min, peak VE 45 L/min. Which of the following is true?

a. The test was submaximal.
b. The primary limitation to exercise is cardiac.
c. The primary limitation to exercise is pulmonary.
d. The patient should be referred for cardiac transplantation.
e. It is not possible to differentiate cardiac from pulmonary limitations to exercise in this patient.

Answer is c: The MVV is 40 × 1.25 = 50. Given his VE of 45, he used up 90% of his breathing reserve.

5. A 60-year-old man presents with exertional pressure-like chest discomfort that is relieved with rest and that often radiates to the left arm and jaw. His resting ECG is normal. He is taking no medications. Which of the following is true?

a. The patient should be referred for coronary angiography.
b. The patient should have an exercise test to determine whether obstructive coronary artery disease is present.
c. The patient should be referred for an exercise imaging study.
d. The patient should have an exercise test to determine his short- and long-term prognosis.
e. The patient need not have any test; he should be started on a beta-blocker, aspirin, and a lipid-lowering agent and then followed.

Answers is d: The patient has typical angina and a very high pretest likelihood of disease. Exercise testing is appropriate to assess prognosis. If he is found to be at low risk, medical management will be appropriate.

# Nuclear Stress Testing 22

**Richard C. Brunken** **Omosalewa O. Lalude**

Nuclear cardiac imaging has become an integral component of the clinical practice of cardiology over the last several decades. Myocardial perfusion imaging facilitates the detection of coronary artery disease, permits assessment of the physiologic effects of equivocal coronary artery stenoses, and assists in the identification of patients who are likely to benefit from coronary revascularization. In individuals with known or suspected coronary artery disease, myocardial perfusion imaging provides incremental prognostic information beyond that afforded by stress electrocardiography alone, and can be used for individual risk stratification for future cardiac events. The fundamentals of nuclear cardiac imaging and image interpretation are discussed in Chapter 9. This chapter focuses primarily on the clinical utility of myocardial perfusion imaging for patients with suspected or established coronary artery disease, and how the information derived from these nuclear imaging studies can be used to assist in the care of the patient. The contribution of nuclear imaging to the management of patients with congestive heart failure will also be briefly discussed.

## MYOCARDIAL PERFUSION IMAGING

### Principles of Cardiac Nuclear Stress Testing

The usual goal of myocardial perfusion imaging is to compare the pattern of tissue perfusion in the resting state to that under stress conditions, in order to detect flow-limiting coronary artery stenoses. To understand how myocardial perfusion imaging is used for this purpose, it is helpful to recall certain aspects of cardiovascular physiology. In the basal resting state, oxygen extraction from myocardial capillary blood approaches 70% and is near maximal. Thus, there is little capacity to augment tissue oxygen delivery by increasing the myocardial extraction of oxygen from the blood when the ventricular workload increases. As a result, increases in the left ventricular workload must be accompanied by nearly proportional increases in myocardial perfusion, in order to meet the oxygen demands of the tissue. Healthy coronary vessels have *flow reserves* between 3 and 6, meaning that they can increase blood flows about three to six times above rest values during periods of stress (1).

In most patients with coronary artery disease, autoregulatory changes in arteriolar vascular resistance are capable of maintaining normal tissue perfusion in the resting state. The left ventricular workload is low in the resting state and the coronary circulation is usually capable of meeting basal myocardial oxygen demands. Thus, images of rest myocardial perfusion are typically normal in patients with coronary artery disease who have not had a prior infarction or an acute ischemic event. To detect an obstructive coronary stenosis, it is frequently necessary to use maneuvers that increase tissue perfusion, in order to distinguish between vessels with and without an *impaired coronary flow reserve*.

### Detection of Coronary Stenoses

In an artery with an atherosclerotic lesion, coronary flow reserve decreases nonlinearly as the luminal narrowing increases. The ability of the coronary vessel to increase tissue perfusion during periods of stress becomes increasingly and progressively limited as the luminal stenosis becomes more pronounced (1). During stress, perfusion in the myocardium supplied by a coronary vessel with a limited flow reserve will be less than that in regions subtended by healthy arteries. Measurements of stress perfusion in affected areas (in milliliters of blood flow per minute per gram of tissue) typically will exceed resting values, but remain less than the values in normal myocardium. Stenoses of 50% to 60% luminal cross-sectional area or greater are usually of sufficient magnitude to impair coronary flow reserve. However, other factors, such as the presence or absence of nonlaminar flow in the vessel, the presence or absence of collateral vessels, the presence of several stenoses in series, stenosis length, eccentricity of the lumen, absolute luminal cross-sectional area, heart rate, and the pressure gradient across the stenosis, may influence the physiologic effects of a coronary stenosis on tissue perfusion.

Images depicting myocardial perfusion during stress conditions show a reduction in the relative tracer concentration, or a *stress perfusion defect*, in the vascular territories supplied by the arteries with flow-limiting stenoses. The hallmark of stress-induced ischemia is a *reversible* perfusion defect, one that is present on stress perfusion images but absent on rest perfusion images. In studies in which measurements of coronary flow reserve made with intracoronary Doppler catheters have been compared to SPECT myocardial perfusion images, a strong correlation has been noted between stenosis flow reserves less than 2.0 and the presence of a reversible perfusion defect. Similarly, noninvasive measurements of myocardial perfusion reserve obtained with positron emission tomography (PET) in patients with coronary artery disease suggest that reversible SPECT defects are usually associated with perfusion reserves of 1.8 or less. In general, the more severe the luminal stenosis, the greater is the likelihood that it will be associated with a stress perfusion defect.

The anatomic extent of the stress perfusion defect and the magnitude of the reduction in the relative tracer activity within the defect provide objective information about the effects of a coronary stenosis on tissue perfusion during conditions of high oxygen demand. Commercially available computer programs can be used to compare the count data from a specific patient's images to those of a normal sex-matched population, to assist in the identification and quantification of myocardial perfusion defects (see Chapter 9). The relative tracer activity concentration within the stress defect provides an indication of the severity of the ischemia. Defect extent, or the amount of the left ventricle that is affected by the perfusion abnormality, can be expressed as the number of myocardial segments with an abnormal tracer concentration, or as the proportion (percent) of all myocardial voxels that have an abnormal tracer concentration. A proximal stenosis in a major epicardial artery will generally produce a stress defect that is larger and more readily detected than one resulting from a stenosis in a distal vessel or a smaller branch artery. The anatomic location of the perfusion defect can be used to infer which of the three major coronary vessels is (are) diseased (see Chapter 9). It may also be possible to deduce whether the stenosis is proximal, mid, or distal, based on the location and anatomic extent of the defect on the stress perfusion images.

## Assessment of Relative versus Absolute Myocardial Perfusion

The SPECT or PET myocardial perfusion images used in routine clinical practice for coronary artery disease (CAD) detection depict *relative* tissue perfusion. It is assumed that at least one area of the visualized myocardium is supplied by a vessel with a normal or near-normal coronary flow reserve. However, in some patients with multivessel coronary artery disease, there may be "balanced ischemia," a situation in which the coronary flow reserve of each of the three major coronary arteries is equally or nearly equally impaired. In balanced ischemia, the pattern of perfusion on the stress images appears relatively homogenous. A regional perfusion defect is not identified because the stress defect involves essentially all of the visualized left ventricular myocardium. PET measurements of absolute myocardial perfusion and perfusion reserve in such a situation can be expected to show reduced hyperemic perfusion (relative to a control population) and a global reduction in myocardial perfusion reserve. The prevalence of balanced ischemia in CAD patients is not well defined, and is likely to depend on each nuclear laboratory's specific referral pattern. In large cardiac referral centers, the prevalence of balanced ischemia is probably less than 5% of patients referred for nuclear stress testing, and it may be smaller in an office-based practice. Other observations from the stress test can alert the nuclear cardiologist to the possibility of balanced ischemia. These include the onset of anginal symptoms with stress, a significant drop in systolic blood pressure with exercise, electrocardiographic ST-segment changes in response to stress, and acute ventricular dilatation and/or new systolic dysfunction on the gated stress perfusion images. When incorporating the results of SPECT perfusion imaging study into the management of the patient, the possibility of balanced ischemia should be considered, especially if there are other clinical observations that suggest this possibility.

## Resting Perfusion Defects

Perfusion defects on images acquired in the resting state may arise in several different situations. When a coronary stenosis is very severe (>90% to 95% area stenosis) or there is an unstable lesion with intermittent dynamic obstruction of the lumen, a defect can sometimes be identified on resting perfusion images. In this situation, the diseased vessel may be incapable of maintaining perfusion commensurate with the tissue's oxygen demands. A second set of perfusion images acquired at a later time may show *redistribution*, or "fill in" of the resting perfusion defect, as the tissue tracer concentration in this area equilibrates with that in adjacent normal myocardium. Sometimes, a supplemental dose of the perfusion tracer may be given prior to obtaining the late set of images, to assist in the "fill in" of the defect. The clinical implication of the filling in of a resting perfusion defect on *redistribution or reinjection perfusion images* is that the tissue is viable, and supplied by a vessel with a severe coronary stenosis.

A resting perfusion defect that persists on redistribution or reinjection images sometimes indicates a myocardial scar. In a scar there is replacement of cardiac myocytes by relatively avascular fibrous tissue. Residual tissue perfusion in the segment with the scar is lower than in normal myocardium, resulting in a reduction in the relative tracer concentration on both the resting and redistribution/reinjection perfusion images. Because of the limited spatial resolution of current gamma cameras and PET tomographs, reductions in perfusion due to a nontransmural scar will be averaged over the minimum resolvable volume of the instrument (the *partial volume effect*). Thus, it is not possible to attribute an observed reduction in myocardial tracer activity to a scar specifically in the subendocardial, mid-myocardial or epicardial portion of the ventricular wall, as counts will be averaged over the entire thickness of the tissue. In studies of subjects with clinical myocardial infarction (MI), the extent and severity of persistent resting perfusion defects have generally paralleled the loss of viable myocytes, as measured by the size of the leak of cardiac enzymes or by the amount of tissue fibrosis on ventricular specimens (2).

If a resting perfusion defect persists on redistribution or reinjection images, an alternative diagnostic possibility is *myocardial hibernation*, a state in which there is a sustained downregulation of tissue perfusion, metabolism, and function. Although the mechanism by which human myocardium enters into a state of "hibernation" is not well defined, accumulating evidence suggests that multiple repetitive episodes of ischemia (repetitive stunning) may eventually result in myocardial hibernation (3). Histopathologic studies of hibernating myocardium have identified structural and ultrastructural alterations in the tissue. These include a loss of myofibrillar protein, myocyte hypertrophy, accumulation of glycogen within the cytosol of the cardiac myocyte, and alterations in myocyte mitochondrial size and appearance. Modest increases in tissue collagen content have also been reported. As the name suggests, the clinical implication of hibernating myocardium is that the dysfunctional tissue is viable, and that it can be "awakened" by restoration of blood flow and benefit functionally by coronary revascularization.

In both hibernating tissue and myocardial scar, there is a persistent reduction in tissue perfusion. Because there is little or no capacity to increase tissue perfusion with stress in either situation, reductions in relative tracer concentration on resting perfusion images will also be present on stress perfusion images, and therefore appear as a *fixed perfusion defect*. Myocardial scar and hibernating tissue both exhibit systolic dysfunction, and may be indistinguishable from each other on conventional gated myocardial perfusion scintigraphy. Additional imaging studies are frequently needed in order to distinguish between hibernating (viable) tissue and myocardial scar. Low-dose dobutamine echocardiography, contrast magnetic resonance imaging, and glucose metabolic imaging with positron emission tomography (below) are some of the methods that have been used to distinguish myocardial hibernation from scar (4).

## Stress Options for Myocardial Perfusion Imaging

Exercise is generally the preferred stress modality because it permits the simultaneous assessment of other parameters of clinical interest including patient symptoms, functional capacity, vital signs, and the rate–pressure product as an indirect index of myocardial oxygen consumption. Graded exercise is most commonly performed on a treadmill, using one of several standard stress protocols (see Chapter 24). In order to optimize the examination for the detection of coronary stenoses, it is important to increase the ventricular workload high enough to elicit a significant increase in myocardial perfusion. In clinical practice, the usual goal is for the patient to achieve at least 85% of the maximum predicted heart rate (MPHR) for age. The radioactive perfusion tracer is administered intravenously about 1 to 2 minutes prior to the end of stress, to allow a long enough period of time for myocardial uptake of the imaging agent prior to the termination of exercise.

In some patients, an adequate level of exercise cannot be achieved because of orthopedic limitations, peripheral vascular disease, complicating medical illnesses, or the use of medications such as beta-blockers. Stress perfusion imaging is still feasible if a pharmacologic agent can be used to increase myocardial blood flow. About 40% of the myocardial perfusion imaging tests in the United States are performed using pharmacologic stress (5). The two most commonly used pharmacologic stress agents, adenosine and dipyridamole, are potent coronary vasodilators. These agents increase myocardial perfusion by directly dilating the coronary vasculature, thereby "uncoupling" myocardial perfusion from ventricular work. The third agent used for myocardial perfusion imaging is a synthetic catecholamine, dobutamine, which increases tissue perfusion primarily by increasing tissue oxygen demand through its positive inotropic and chronotropic effects. The pharmacologic agents used for stress perfusion imaging are summarized in Table 22–1.

*Adenosine* is a small molecule that is produced by vascular smooth muscle and endothelial cells. Adenosine can also be generated by the extracellular dephosphorylation of adenosine triphosphate (ATP) and adenosine diphosphate (ADP). Free adenosine within the vascular space can re-enter endothelial, vascular smooth muscle, or red blood cells by facilitated transport, or it can bind to specific receptors on the cell membrane. Adenosine induces coronary vasodilation when it binds to specific $A_{2A}$ receptors on the surface of the cell. Binding to the receptor causes an increase in intracellular cyclic AMP (cAMP) concentration via a coupled G-protein system that in turn results in coronary artery dilatation. Adenosine has a very short half-life (2 to 10 seconds), because it is rapidly cleared from the vascular space by uptake into endothelial and red blood cells. In normal coronary arteries, adenosine leads to increases in

**TABLE 22–1**
**AGENTS FOR PHARMACOLOGIC STRESS TESTING**

| Drug | Mechanism | Dose | Risks | Comments |
|---|---|---|---|---|
| Adenosine | Coronary vasodilatation (binds to $A_{2A}$ receptor, which results in arteriolar dilatation) | 140 $\mu$g/kg/min by continuous IV infusion over 6 min | Bronchospasm, ischemia/MI AV block | Caffeine blocks. Short half-life of 2–10 s Aminophylline reverses. Perfusion tracer injected midway during adenosine infusion. |
| Dipyridamole | Coronary vasodilatation (blocks cellular uptake of adenosine, increasing binding of adenosine to $A_{2A}$ receptors) | 0.142 mg/kg/min, by continuous IV infusion over 4 min | Bronchospasm, ischemia/MI, rarely AV block | Caffeine blocks. Reversed by aminophylline. Tracer injected 4 min after end of dipyridamole infusion. |
| Dobutamine | Increases myocardial perfusion by increasing tissue oxygen demand | Incremental steps, beginning at 5–10 up to a maximum of 40 $\mu$g/kg/min. Can add isometric hand-rip or up to 1 mg of atropine if target heart rate not achieved | Ischemia/MI, arrhythmias, hypotension, hypertension | Useful for patients with asthma or other bronchospastic pulmonary disease who are unable to exercise. Unlike echocardiography, online monitoring of ventricular function is not possible during the period of stress. Beta-blockers are useful for treating side effects such as arrhythmias. |

blood flows that are generally three to six times those in the resting state. Adenosine is usually administered as a continuous intravenous infusion at a rate of 140 $\mu$g/kg/min over a period of 6 minutes. The radioactive perfusion radiotracer is injected at 3 minutes, midway through the adenosine infusion.

*Dipyridamole* blocks the cellular reuptake of adenosine. This causes more of the endogenous adenosine within the vascular space to bind to the $A_{2A}$ receptors on the cell surface. Greater receptor binding by adenosine, in turn, promotes coronary vasodilatation. Dipyridamole has a significantly longer half-life than adenosine, inducing coronary vasodilatation that may persist for as long as 30 minutes following its administration. Dipyridamole is given by continuous intravenous infusion over 4 minutes, at a rate of 0.142 mg/kg/min. The radioactive perfusion tracer is injected about 4 minutes after the end of the dipyridamole infusion, to allow achievement of maximal myocardial hyperemia.

The side effects of adenosine and dipyridamole are similar and include flushing, chest pain, dyspnea, headache, nausea, hypotension, bronchospasm, and AV block. Side effects, especially AV block, are more commonly seen with adenosine but tend to be shorter-lived with this agent. Usually, simply turning off the adenosine infusion is all that is necessary to abate its side effects. With dipyridamole, the side effects tend to persist longer, and treatment with aminophylline (50 to 100 mg IV), a nonselective competitive antagonist, may be required. Clinical studies suggest that the side effects of dipyridamole and adenosine may be attenuated if the patient is capable of performing exercise in conjunction with the pharmacologic stress. Image quality may also benefit from the performance of adjunctive exercise. Contraindications to the administration of the vasodilator agents include asthma or a history of bronchospastic pulmonary disease, hypotension, unstable angina or acute myocardial infarction within 2 days, high-degree AV block without a pacemaker, uncontrolled arrhythmias, and critical aortic or mitral valve stenosis. Unlike stress with exercise or IV dobutamine (below), the adequacy of the myocardial hyperemia induced by IV adenosine or dipyridamole cannot be inferred from the changes in heart rate or systemic blood pressure induced by the administration of these agents.

For both adenosine and dipyridamole stress, it is important that the patient refrain from the use of drugs such as aminophylline and theophylline prior to the test, as these medications are competitive antagonists of the adenosine membrane receptor (6). These medications effectively blunt the hyperemia induced by adenosine or dipyridamole and may cause a falsely negative imaging study. Caffeine and caffeinelike substances such as theobromine, whose effects are similar to those of aminophylline, should also be avoided prior to pharmacologic stress testing with vasodilators. Current joint guidelines issued by the American Heart Association (AHA), the American College of Cardiology (ACC), and the American Society of Nuclear Cardiology (ASNC) recommend that patients refrain from the use of caffeine for at least 24 hours prior to vasodilator stress testing (7).

*Dobutamine* is a short-lived (half-life of about 2 minutes) $\beta_1$-adrenergic receptor agonist which is widely used for stress echocardiography. Unlike stress echocardiography, when dobutamine is used as the stress for nuclear perfusion imaging it is not possible to monitor ventricular function "online." Dobutamine stress should therefore be used with caution for nuclear imaging in patients with reduced left ventricular ejection fraction, as new regional contractile abnormalities incited by ischemia could precipitate further deterioration in ventricular function. Dobutamine can be used in patients with bronchospastic pulmonary disease, in whom there is a relative contraindication to the use of dipyridamole or adenosine. Dobutamine increases cardiac contractility and heart rate, and is contraindicated in patients with recent myocardial infarction, uncontrolled hypertension, or significant cardiac arrhythmias.

Dobutamine is administered as a continuous intravenous infusion, typically starting at 5 to 10 $\mu$g/kg/min for 3 minutes and then increasing by 10 $\mu$g/kg/min every 3 minutes to a maximum dose of 40 $\mu$g/kg/min. If the patient does not achieve 85% of his or her age-related maximal predicted heart rate, he or she can be instructed to perform handgrip exercise and/or be given up to 1 mg of atropine IV to increase the heart rate. The perfusion tracer is administered intravenously 1 to 2 minutes before the end of the dobutamine infusion, to allow enough time for myocardial uptake of the imaging agent. Side effects of dobutamine include palpitations, chest pain, hypertension, hypotension, atrial fibrillation, and ventricular tachycardia. The side effects usually respond to stopping the infusion, or to the intravenous administration of a beta-blocker.

## Indications for Myocardial Perfusion Imaging

The Class I indications for myocardial perfusion imaging, as listed by the ACC/AHA/ASNC guidelines (7), are summarized in Table 22–2.

### *Acute Chest Pain Syndromes*

Prompt identification of individuals with acute coronary syndromes provides the best opportunity to salvage viable myocardial tissue and save lives. In some who present to the Emergency Department with chest pain, elevated cardiac enzyme levels and an abnormal electrocardiogram provide definitive evidence of an acute myocardial infarction, and there is no need for imaging to establish the diagnosis. On the other hand, in those with chest pain that is clearly noncardiac in origin, there is little utility in pursuing an aggressive (and expensive) diagnostic imaging strategy to exclude coronary disease. There are, however, about 6 million patients who present to Emergency Departments each year in the United States with chest pain of uncertain etiology, who have normal enzyme levels and a nondiagnostic electrocardiogram. It is these patients, in whom an acute coronary syndrome remains a diagnostic possibility, that myocardial perfusion imaging has the highest clinical benefit (8). Although the relative proportion of individuals with an acute coronary syndrome in this patient group is not large, the probability of an adverse outcome in those with a true coronary event is high if the diagnosis is missed. Reported mortality in Emergency Department patients with an acute coronary syndrome who are mistakenly sent home is as high as 5% to 6%. On the other hand, for those without an acute coronary syndrome who are admitted to the hospital for observation, there are substantial costs associated with the unnecessary utilization of health care services.

Rest SPECT myocardial perfusion imaging is useful for the evaluation of patients with suspected acute coronary syndromes. Rest myocardial perfusion imaging can detect a regional perfusion abnormality in the absence of acute necrosis, especially if the radioactive tracer is injected during or shortly after an episode of chest pain. Reported negative predictive values of a normal rest myocardial perfusion scan in patients with suspected acute coronary syndromes are as high as 99% to 100%, and up to 97% of patients who have a negative perfusion study in this setting will remain free of cardiac events over a short-term follow-up. Two randomized, prospective studies have shown that access to acute myocardial perfusion imaging has a beneficial effect on length of stay and hospital costs. It is the position of the American Society of Nuclear Cardiology that the evidence supports the use of acute rest myocardial perfusion imaging for the triage of selected Emergency Department patients with suspected acute coronary syndromes (8). However, rest perfusion imaging is less helpful in those with a history of prior myocardial infarction because it is not possible to distinguish a resting perfusion defect due to an acute ischemic event from that of a preexisting scar.

Both thallium-201– and technetium-99m–labeled tracers have been used for rest myocardial imaging in Emergency Department patients. Thallium-201 begins redistributing shortly after its uptake by the myocardium, and images obtained later than 10 to 15 minutes following tracer injection may miss a regional perfusion abnormality. The technetium-99m–labeled tracers are preferred for imaging because they are rapidly trapped in the myocardium and permit imaging of tissue perfusion *at the time of tracer injection* up to 4 hours later. The sensitivity of acute rest myocardial perfusion imaging is highest if the radioactive tracer is injected during chest pain, or shortly thereafter. Ideally, the tracer should be administered within 2 hours of the episode of chest pain. In those without prior infarction, identification of a perfusion defect and/or a segmental wall motion abnormality on the rest gated SPECT perfusion images will ordinarily prompt hospital admission and an aggressive work up for an acute coronary syndrome. By contrast, those who have normal scans can be discharged home with a low probability of sustaining an ischemic event in the immediate future.

Current imaging guidelines indicate that rest myocardial perfusion imaging is not appropriate for patients with obvious acute myocardial infarction (7). However, some who have imaging because of an uncertain clinical picture at presentation will subsequently rule in for acute infarction, and the perfusion images can provide useful information

**TABLE 22–2**
**INDICATIONS FOR MYOCARDIAL PERFUSION IMAGING**

| Patient Group | Condition | Imaging Technique |
|---|---|---|
| ER patient with chest pain | For risk stratification in pt with possible ACS. Initial serum markers and enzymes, ECG are nondiagnostic. | Rest perfusion imaging (with ECG gating, if possible). |
| | For CAD diagnosis in pt with possible ACS and nondiagnostic ECG. Negative serum markers and enzymes or normal rest perfusion scan. | Same-day rest/stress (ECG gated) myocardial perfusion imaging. |
| Acute MI/unstable angina | Assessment of LV function. | Rest myocardial perfusion imaging with ECG gating (rest gated radionuclide angiography is alternative option). |
| ST-elevation MI | Measurement of infarct size and residual viable myocardium. | Rest myocardial perfusion imaging with ECG gating, or with stress perfusion imaging with ECG gating |
| | Thrombolysis without coronary angiogram, to identify inducible ischemia and myocardium at risk. | Rest and stress myocardial perfusion imaging, with ECG gating whenever possible. |
| Non–ST-elevation MI/unstable angina | In those at intermediate or low risk for major adverse cardiac events, to determine the extent and severity of inducible ischemia, either in the distribution of the "culprit"vessel or in remote myocardium. | Rest and stress myocardial perfusion imaging, with ECG gating whenever possible. |
| | In individuals whose angina is stabilized on medical therapy, or in whom the diagnosis is uncertain, to identify the extent and severity of inducible ischemia. | Rest and stress myocardial perfusion imaging, with ECG gating whenever possible. |
| | To assess the hemodynamic significance of a coronary stenosis on angiography. | Rest and stress myocardial perfusion imaging. |
| CAD diagnosis in an individual with an intermediate probability of disease, and/or risk stratification in someone with an intermediate or high likelihood of disease *and* able to exercise to 85% MPHR or more | Those with pre-excitation, LVH, on digoxin, or more than 1-mm ST-segment depression on resting ECG. | Rest and exercise stress myocardial perfusion imaging, with ECG gating whenever possible. |
| | Individuals with left bundle branch block or ventricularly paced rhythm. | Rest and vasodilator stress myocardial perfusion imaging, with ECG gating whenever possible. |
| | Patients with an intermediate Duke treadmill score. | Rest and exercise stress myocardial perfusion imaging, with ECG gating whenever possible. |
| | In an individual with a prior rest and stress myocardial perfusion scan, but in whom a change in symptoms suggests a different risk for a cardiac event. | Repeat rest and exercise stress myocardial perfusion imaging, with ECG gating whenever possible. |
| CAD diagnosis in an individual with an intermediate probability of disease, and/or risk stratification in someone with an intermediate or high likelihood of disease *and* not able to exercise | To identify the extent, severity, and location of inducible ischemia. | Rest and vasodilator stress myocardial perfusion imaging, with ECG gating whenever possible. |
| | In an individual with a prior rest and stress myocardial perfusion scan, but in whom a change in symptoms suggests a different risk for a cardiac event. | Rest and vasodilator stress myocardial perfusion imaging, with ECG gating whenever possible. |
| Individuals with lesions of intermediate severity (25–75%) on coronary angiography | To determine the physiologic consequence of the coronary stenosis. | In those able to exercise, rest and exercise stress myocardial perfusion imaging, with ECG gating whenever possible. *or* In those unable to exercise, rest and vasodilator stress myocardial perfusion imaging, with ECG gating whenever possible. |

(*continued*)

**TABLE 22–2**
**(continued)**

| Patient Group | Condition | Imaging Technique |
|---|---|---|
| Prior to noncardiac surgery | Initial diagnosis of CAD in those with intermediate probability of disease and abnormal ECG or inability to exercise. | In those able to exercise, rest and exercise stress myocardial perfusion imaging, with ECG gating whenever possible.<br>*or*<br>In those unable to exercise, rest and vasodilator stress myocardial perfusion imaging, with ECG gating whenever possible. |
| | In individuals with established or suspected CAD with abnormal ECG or inability to exercise. | In those able to exercise, rest and exercise stress myocardial perfusion imaging, with ECG gating whenever possible.<br>*or*<br>In those unable to exercise, rest and vasodilator stress myocardial perfusion imaging, with ECG gating whenever possible. |
| | Diagnosis of CAD in patients with left bundle branch block and intermediate pretest probability of disease. | Rest and vasodilator stress myocardial perfusion imaging, with ECG gating whenever possible. |
| | In suspected or established CAD, prognostic assessment of those with left bundle branch block on rest ECG. | Rest and vasodilator stress myocardial perfusion imaging, with ECG gating whenever possible. |
| | Individuals with poor functional capacity (less than 4 METs) and intermediate (mild angina, prior MI, compensated or prior CHF, diabetes, renal insufficiency) or minor (advanced age, abnormal ECG, rhythm other than sinus, low functional capacity, prior CVA, uncontrolled hypertension) clinical risk predictors prior to high-risk noncardiac surgery. | Rest and vasodilator stress myocardial perfusion imaging, with ECG gating whenever possible. |
| | Patients with intermediate clinical risk predictors, abnormal rest ECG and moderate or excellent functional capacity (>4 METs) who require high-risk noncardiac surgery. | Rest and exercise stress myocardial perfusion imaging, with ECG gating whenever possible. |
| Equivocal SPECT myocardial perfusion scan | Clinically indicated SPECT perfusion study is equivocal for CAD diagnosis or risk stratification purposes. | Rest and adenosine or dipyridamole stress PET myocardial perfusion study. |
| CAD patient with systolic dysfunction and CHF, with little or no angina | Prediction of improvement in regional/global LV function following revascularization. | Stress/redistribution/reinjection thallium-201 SPECT perfusion imaging<br>*or*<br>Rest/redistribution SPECT perfusion imaging<br>*or*<br>Myocardial perfusion plus FDG PET metabolic imaging<br>*or*<br>Resting sestamibi SPECT perfusion imaging. |
| | Prediction of improvement in natural history following revascularization. | Stress/redistribution/reinjection thallium-201 SPECT perfusion imaging<br>*or*<br>Rest/redistribution thallium-201 SPECT perfusion imaging<br>*or*<br>Myocardial perfusion plus FDG PET metabolic imaging. |

about the anatomic site of injury. If the rest perfusion images are repeated prior to hospital discharge, a measure of the degree of myocardial salvage afforded by treatment can be achieved by subtracting the perfusion defect size on the resting images at discharge (final infarct size) from that on the early images (region at risk).

### *Risk Assessment after ST-Elevation Myocardial Infarction*

Patients with acute ST-elevation myocardial infarction (STEMI) who are suitable for primary percutaneous intervention are usually referred directly for angiography and coronary revascularization. However, current practice guidelines indicate that noninvasive risk stratification is appropriate for stable, low-risk patients (ejection fractions >40%) who have not received reperfusion therapy or who have been treated with fibrinolytic agents (9). Final infarct size, the extent of inducible ischemia, and left ventricular ejection fraction are the key elements of risk stratification for stable patients following ST-segment elevation myocardial infarction, and gated myocardial perfusion imaging is well suited for measurement of these parameters (10).

*Infarct size* can be determined by measuring the amount of the left ventricle with a resting perfusion defect prior to hospital discharge. Clinical studies of patients with acute infarction suggest that resting perfusion defect size is a variable that contributes independently to cardiac risk. Patients with only small fixed perfusion defects generally have a good prognosis, whereas those with resting perfusion defects involving 20% or more of the left ventricle are at higher risk for cardiac events over the ensuing 24 months. The extent of *inducible ischemia* can be derived from the images by careful subtraction of the size of the rest perfusion defect from that of the stress defect. Inducible ischemia, whether in the clinical infarct zone or in other vascular territories, also contributes to cardiac risk. Patient risk increases as the percent of the left ventricle with stress-induced ischemia increases, with involvement of 10% or more of the ventricle by a reversible perfusion defect placing the patient into a high-risk group. Measurements of *left ventricular ejection fraction* and ventricular volumes can also readily be obtained from the gated perfusion images. In general, as the left ventricular ejection fraction declines to <40% there is a progressive and nonlinear increase in the risk of cardiac events. Other scintigraphic observations that have been associated with increased clinical risk in the post–MI patient include transient ischemic dilatation (TID) of the left ventricle on the stress images, and increased pulmonary tracer uptake (especially with thallium scintigraphy) on the stress images.

Stress perfusion imaging with adenosine or dipyridamole can safely be performed as early as 2 days following an acute infarction (11), while present guidelines suggest that submaximal exercise stress testing not be performed before 5 days after an acute event. Myocardial perfusion imaging with vasodilator stress provides incremental prognostic information beyond that afforded by conventional clinical and stress electrocardiographic variables. Vasodilator stress perfusion imaging is more sensitive for the identification of ischemia than submaximal exercise stress testing and is more useful for risk stratification, probably because it is possible to safely achieve a greater degree of hyperemia without inducing frank ischemia using vasodilator stress (Fig. 22–1). Early risk stratification facilitates identification of the high-risk patient and appropriate referral for angiography.

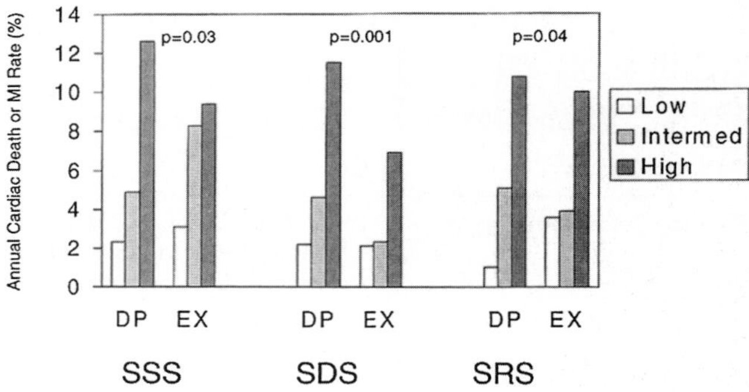


**Figure 22–1** Annual rates of mortality/recurrent MI in patients with initial uncomplicated MI, according to the results of either dipyridamole (DP) or submaximal exercise (EX) myocardial perfusion scintigraphy. SSS, summed stress perfusion defect score; SDS, summed difference between stress and rest segmental scores; SRS, summed rest perfusion defect score. Low SSS and SRS values were defined by scores of 0–4; intermediate (Intermed) values by scores of 5–8; high values by scores >8. Low SDS values were defined by scores of 0–2; intermediate values by 3–7, and high values by scores >7. Higher perfusion defect scores were associated with higher event rates, and dipyridamole stress imaging provided better risk stratification than submaximal exercise perfusion scintigraphy. (Reproduced by permission from Brown KA et al. Early dipyridamole $^{99m}$Tc-sestamibi single photon emission computed tomographic imaging 2 to 4 days after acute myocardial infarction predicts in-hospital and postdischarge cardiac events. Comparison with submaximal exercise imaging. *Circulation*. 1999;100:2060–2066.)

### *Risk Assessment after Non–ST-Elevation Myocardial Infarction*

Updated ACC/AHA guidelines for the management of patients with unstable angina and non–ST-elevation myocardial infarction (NSTEMI) recommend an early invasive approach for those with a high-risk profile who have no significant co-morbidities (12). However, the guidelines also suggest that stable patients without high-risk indicators might be managed using either a conservative or an early invasive strategy. Several studies have demonstrated the utility of myocardial perfusion imaging for the risk stratification of patients following NSTEMI. The presence of perfusion defects (fixed or reversible) on stress testing in stabilized NSTEMI patients is predictive of future events. In one study of 126 men who underwent a Tc-99m sestamibi stress SPECT myocardial perfusion study prior to hospital discharge, the event-free survival in patients with a normal scan was about 90% in the 18-month follow-up period, as compared to 55% in those with abnormal scans. Patients with reversible defects fared less favorably, with an event-free survival of only 30%. The rate of death and recurrent MI in this group was 40%, as compared to 20% for all patients with abnormal scans.

In those with unstable angina or NSTEMI, current AHA/ACC/ASNC imaging guidelines indicate that stress SPECT myocardial perfusion imaging is appropriate for the identification of inducible ischemia in (a) patients at intermediate or low risk for major adverse cardiac events, (b) patients whose angina is stabilized with medical therapy or in those in whom the diagnosis is uncertain, and (c) patients who have coronary stenoses of uncertain hemodynamic consequence on coronary angiography. Use of rest gated myocardial perfusion imaging can also be considered for determination of the left ventricular function.

### *Patients with Suspected or Established Chronic Coronary Artery Disease*

#### Detection of Coronary Stenoses

Myocardial perfusion imaging has the highest clinical utility for the detection of flow-limiting coronary arterial stenoses in patients with an intermediate pretest probability of disease (7). The pretest probability of disease can be estimated using a Bayesian statistical model incorporating variables such as age, sex, symptoms, presence of cardiac risk factors, findings on the resting electrocardiogram, and the results of prior stress testing (13). For the patient with an intermediate pretest probability of disease, a positive imaging study effectively stratifies the individual to a high risk of having obstructive coronary artery disease. On the other hand, a negative imaging study indicates that the patient has a low likelihood of having obstructive coronary disease. Thus, regardless of whether the imaging study is negative or positive, the patient's posttest probability of disease has been substantially influenced by the results of the test.

In contrast, consider those patients who have either a low or a high pretest probability of disease. In those with a low pretest likelihood of disease, correlative angiographic studies indicate that the posttest probability of obstructive disease remains low, regardless of whether the study is negative or positive (odds favor a false positive imaging study). On the other hand, the patient with a high pretest probability of disease is stratified to an even higher likelihood of disease if the study is positive, and he or she is still is left with a high probability of disease even if the study is negative (odds favor a false negative imaging study). For either type of patient, a positive or negative imaging study does not appreciably alter the posttest likelihood of disease and little clinical diagnostic benefit isaachieved by performing the test.

The reported sensitivity of exercise myocardial perfusion SPECT imaging for detecting coronary stenoses of ≥50% ranges from 71% to 97% (average 87%), whereas specificity ranges from 36% to 100% [average 73% (20)]. For vasodilator (adenosine or dipyridamole) stress SPECT, reported sensitivity ranges from 72% to 93% (average 89%), whereas specificity ranges from 28% to 100% (average 75%). For myocardial perfusion imaging with positron emission tomography, reported sensitivities range from 83% to 100% (average 97%), whereas specificities range from 73% to 100% (average 87%). In general, reported sensitivities and specificities of PET perfusion studies tend to be slightly higher than for SPECT studies, resulting in greater diagnostic accuracy (14). The higher diagnostic accuracy likely reflects several factors, including the use of transmission images to correct the myocardial images for attenuation and the superior spatial resolution afforded by the PET imaging technique. Although it is not widely used in current clinical practice, recent studies suggest that the use of attenuation correction in conjunction with SPECT myocardial perfusion might enhance its diagnostic accuracy. At the present time, studies directly comparing attenuation corrected SPECT versus PET for the detection of coronary artery disease are lacking.

Myocardial perfusion imaging is especially useful for the detection of disease in individuals in whom the electocardiographic changes with stress are nondiagnostic. These include patients taking digoxin, and those with left ventricular hypertrophy, ventricular pacemakers, left bundle branch block, or Wolff–Parkinson–White syndrome. In those with left bundle branch block, both reversible and fixed perfusion defects have been reported in the absence of obstructive disease on coronary angiography (15). False positive perfusion defects are more common when exercise is used for stress, and for this reason pharmacologic vasodilator stress imaging is preferred in those with left bundle branch block (7). The perfusion defects are usually localized in the interventricular septum and may reflect actual abnormalities in regional blood flow. The cause of the septal perfusion defects is not clear, but it may reflect compression of perforating septal branch arteries due to the delayed onset of septal contraction resulting in a relative reduction in septal perfusion.

#### Identifying Disease Severity, Risk and Prognosis

Increasingly, myocardial perfusion imaging is being used to gauge the risk of cardiac events in patients with known or suspected coronary artery disease. Some have argued that the use of prognostic endpoints is a better measure of the clinical utility of a test than a direct comparison with the disease severity on angiography. Still others have proposed that myocardial perfusion imaging should serve a "gatekeeper" function, identifying the individuals most likely to benefit from referral to cardiac catheterization, and thereby reducing medical costs. In a multicenter trial involving 11,372 patients with stable angina, an aggressive strategy with direct assignment to cardiac catheterization was compared to a conservative strategy using SPECT myocardial perfusion imaging to selectively refer patients to coronary angiography (16). In both patient cohorts, rates of myocardial infarction and cardiac death were similar for those at low, intermediate, and high risk prior to study entry. Rates of coronary revascularization were reduced by almost one half in the patients managed using the conservative strategy employing nuclear imaging, and there was a significant reduction in per-patient cost, with the savings averaging $1,320, $1,275, and $1,229, respectively, in the low-, intermediate-, and high-risk groups. A review of the cost-effectiveness of SPECT myocardial perfusion imaging is now available online from the American Society of Nuclear Cardiology (17).

The factors associated with adverse outcomes on myocardial perfusion imaging studies include a large perfusion defect on the stress images (a summed stress score greater than 8), a large fixed perfusion defect due to prior myocardial infarction, a large area of reversible ischemia (especially if identified in multiple vascular territories), a left ventricular ejection fraction <40%, stress-induced ventricular dyssynergy, transient ischemic dilatation of the left ventricle, and increased pulmonary uptake of the perfusion tracer (18). An additional report indicates that there is an incremental prognostic value in assessing poststress left ventricular volumes on the gated SPECT perfusion images, with end systolic volumes >70 mL denoting a poorer prognosis.

Markers reflecting left ventricular function, such as the extent of myocardial scar, ventricular ejection fraction, and transient ischemic dilatation of the ventricle appear to be more predictive of cardiac death (18). In contrast, markers of inducible ischemia, such as exertional symptoms, electrocardiogram (ECG) changes, the extent and severity of a reversible perfusion defect, and associated inducible ventricular dysfunction, appear to be more predictive of an acute ischemic event, that is, the need for urgent coronary revascularization, progression from stable to unstable angina, and acute myocardial infarction.

The patients most likely to benefit from myocardial perfusion imaging for risk stratification are those with an intermediate pretest risk of a cardiac event over the ensuing year. Low-risk, intermediate-risk, and high-risk categories have typically been defined as <1%, 1% to 2%, and >2% risk of a cardiac event per year, respectively. However, these values also need to be considered in light of the population being considered. In the very elderly, for example, a 2% risk might more appropriately be considered a low risk, given the higher mortality risk of coronary revascularization in these individuals. Patients at low or high risk are already adequately risk stratified for clinical decision making, and nuclear imaging in this population is not cost-effective. There is no survival benefit of revascularization in patients with minimal symptoms who are at low risk (<1%), because the mortality risk from coronary artery bypass grafting (CABG) or percutaneous coronary intervention (PCI) is at least 1%. On the other hand, patients with minimal symptoms and a >3% annual mortality rate can potentially derive a survival benefit from coronary revascularization.

In general, patients with an intermediate pretest risk who have a normal cardiac SPECT scan have a low annual risk of cardiac events, of the order of 0.6% per year. Several more recent studies have suggested an even lower rate of cardiac death and nonfatal myocardial infarction in those with a normal cardiac SPECT scan, about 0.2% year. In these latter studies, individuals with an established history of coronary artery disease and a normal SPECT perfusion scan had an event rate about 0.9% per annum. *In general, the absolute risk associated with a normal SPECT myocardial perfusion scan reflects the specific patient population under consideration.* That is, stratification of patient risk depends on the anticipated pretest cardiac event rate in that specific population (Fig. 22–2). A patient with a higher pretest risk, such as a patient with established coronary artery disease, diabetes, or peripheral vascular disease, would have a greater absolute posttest risk, as a result of greater disease and co-morbidity burden. In individuals with a somewhat higher pretest risk, the adverse cardiac event rate associated with a normal perfusion scan is of the order of 1% to 2% per year. By contrast, a low-risk SPECT study in a patient from a population with a very high cardiac event profile (e.g., about 10% per year) would stratify that individual to a posttest risk of about 2% to 3% per year (Fig. 22–2).

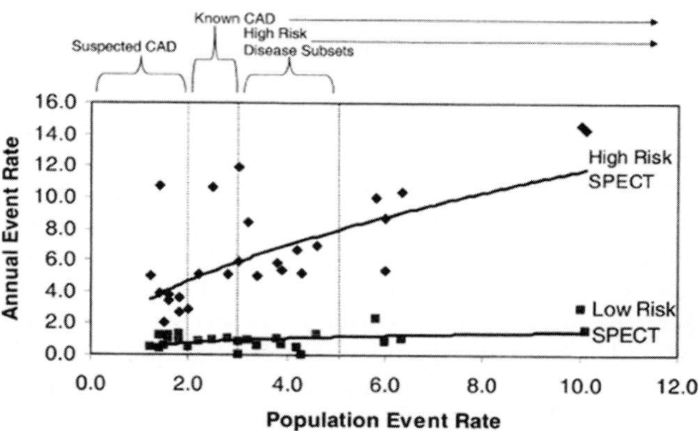


**Figure 22–2** Meta-analysis of the posttest likelihood of a cardiac event, according to the findings on SPECT myocardial perfusion scintigraphy. The data points associated with a high-risk scan are shown by diamonds; those indicating a low-risk scan are shown by squares. The posttest event rate associated with a high- or low-risk myocardial SPECT perfusion scan reflects the pretest event rate in the population that best reflects the patient's clinical characteristics. A low-risk SPECT study in a patient from a population in which there is a larger naturally occurring pretest event rate (e.g., a diabetic patient) results in a posttest likelihood of a cardiac event that is somewhat higher than that in a patient from a pretest population with a low event rate. Conversely, a high-risk scan in a patient from a population with a low event rate is associated with a smaller absolute risk than that in a patient from a population with a higher frequency of cardiac events. (Reproduced by permission from Shaw LJ, Iskandrian AE. Prognostic value of gated myocardial perfusion SPECT. *J Nucl Cardiol.* 2004;11:171–185.)

For patients with abnormal scans, the risk of a cardiac event increases as the degree of the scan abnormality increases. This was demonstrated in a prospective study of 5,183 consecutive patients who underwent rest and stress myocardial perfusion imaging. In this investigation, patients with normal scans had a <0.5% annual rate of cardiac death and myocardial infarction over the ensuing 642 ± 226 days. Those with mildly abnormal scans had a low risk of cardiac death but an intermediate risk of myocardial infarction (0.8% versus 2.7% per year), whereas those with moderately abnormal scans had an intermediate risk of cardiac death and myocardial infarction (2.3% versus

2.9% per year). The risk of cardiac death and myocardial infarction was intermediate to high (2.9% versus 4.2% per year) in the patients with severely abnormal scans.

Although individual authors may vary slightly in their definition of a high-risk myocardial perfusion scan, the annual rate of death or nonfatal myocardial infarction is about 5.9% in those with high-risk scans. In an individual belonging to a population with a very high pretest cardiac event rate (e.g., about 10% per year), a high-risk scan would stratify the patient to an even higher posttest risk of about 14% to 15% per year (Fig. 22–2).

Other factors also modulate cardiac risk. For both low-risk and high-risk perfusion scans, the risk of cardiac death or nonfatal MI is higher for pharmacologic stress studies than for exercise studies. With exercise, a low-risk SPECT study has about a 0.7% annual event rate, whereas that for pharmacologic stress is about 1.2% per year. The annual event rate associated with a high-risk SPECT scan with exercise is about 5.6% per year, and is about 8.3% per year for a pharmacologic stress study (18). Some authors therefore consider the necessity to use pharmacologic stress for myocardial perfusion imaging (a reflection of a poor functional class) an independent prognostic risk factor.

Gender also influences risk stratification. Although there is little difference between the sexes in the event rates associated with a low-risk SPECT scan, women with a high-risk SPECT scan have an annual cardiac event rate of approximately 6.2%, whereas that for men is about 5.3%. Diabetic patients also have higher event rates, for both low-risk (about 2% per year) and high-risk scans (about 9.5% per year). Therefore, diabetic women constitute the highest-risk patient cohort.

## Specific Populations and Situations

The use of myocardial perfusion imaging in selected patient populations and situations merits consideration.

### *Before and after Coronary Revascularization*

*Myocardial Perfusion Imaging before Percutaneous Coronary Intervention.* In a patient with atypical symptoms and an equivocal coronary lesion, the stenosis identified on angiography might not be the proximate cause of the individual's symptoms. Stress myocardial perfusion imaging is useful to characterize the physiologic effects of equivocal coronary lesions and thereby establish a link between the patient's symptoms and the angiographic findings (7). Myocardial perfusion imaging can also be used to identify the "culprit" vessel(s) in those with mild to moderate lesions in multiple arteries who have clinical evidence for stress-induced ischemia. In order to adequately characterize the flow reserve characteristics of a coronary lesion, it is important to insure that adequate hyperemia has been achieved during stress (above). In patients who are unable to achieve at least 85% of their maximum predicted heart rate, pharmacologic stress testing is a practical alternative.

*Myocardial Perfusion Imaging after Percutaneous Coronary Interventions.* Symptoms are not reliable indicators of restenosis, as up to 25% of asymptomatic patients with recent percutaneous coronary intervention (PCI) have signs of ischemia on exercise testing. In the first few months after PCI, routine myocardial perfusion imaging is usually not indicated because only about a third of patients with recurrent chest pain will have angiographically significant restenosis. Some have advocated myocardial perfusion imaging 3 to 12 months after PCI, because the presence of stress-induced myocardial ischemia, with or without symptoms, is associated with a poorer prognosis. The ACC/AHA 2002 Guideline Update for Exercise Testing suggests that stress testing be performed in the first 12 months after PCI only in high-risk patients (19). High-risk patients include those with left ventricular dysfunction, multivessel coronary disease, proximal disease of the left anterior descending coronary artery, previous sudden death, diabetes mellitus, hazardous occupations, and those with suboptimal PCI results. Late following successful PCI, the main indication for myocardial perfusion imaging is recurrence of symptoms. The appropriate utilization of myocardial perfusion imaging in this population, however, merits additional study.

*Myocardial Perfusion Imaging after CABG.* Myocardial perfusion imaging can readily demonstrate the location, extent, and severity of rest and stress-induced perfusion defects in individuals with prior coronary artery bypass surgery. However, interpretation of the perfusion images should be performed considering the alterations in coronary anatomy resulting from the bypass procedure. Inducible ischemia might reflect obstructive disease in a bypass graft, a local problem with a graft anastamosis, or progression of a lesion in a native vessel distal to the insertion of a bypass graft (7). Ischemia can sometimes be identified in myocardial regions proximal to the insertion of a bypass graft. On gated perfusion images, abnormal septal motion is commonly noted in the post–CABG patient. This may reflect the loss of pericardial constraint as a result of the prior surgical procedure, rather than an intrinsic abnormality in contractile function, as systolic thickening is usually well preserved in those without prior injury.

The prognostic value of myocardial perfusion imaging has been demonstrated in clinical studies of patients early and late following CABG. In a study of 873 asymptomatic post–CABG patients, Lauer and colleagues found that exercise capacity and thallium perfusion defects were strong and independent predictors of death and nonfatal MI (20). They reported that 12% of those with reversible thallium perfusion defects died, and 13% had a major cardiovascular event during the 3-year follow-up period. In contrast, 5% of those without ischemia died, and 7% had a major event in that time interval. After adjusting for baseline clinical variables, surgical variables, the time interval from CABG, and standard cardiovascular risk factors, thallium perfusion defects were independently predictive of death (relative risk 2.78) and major cardiovascular events (relative risk 2.63). In studies of patients >5 years after CABG, several variables have been linked to an adverse outcome: the extent and severity of inducible ischemia (as measured by the summed reversibility score), perfusion defects in multiple vascular territories, the extent of fixed perfusion defects, and increased pulmonary uptake of thallium (7).

***Preoperative Testing prior to Noncardiac Surgery.*** Myocardial perfusion imaging is used prior to noncardiac surgery to identify individuals at risk for perioperative ischemia, infarction, and death (21). Despite advances in medical care, reported mortality rates for perioperative myocardial infarction are as high as 26%. Moreover, the costs of perioperative morbidity and mortality are of the order of $12 billion per year in the United States. Appropriate treatment can reduce perioperative morbidity and mortality, and improve the long-term prognosis of the patient. These facts underscore the need for identification of high-risk surgical patients, in order to weigh the potential benefits of an operation against the risk of a cardiac event.

Several clinical scoring systems have been utilized to assess cardiac risk in patients prior to noncardiac surgery. Most of these scoring systems, however, were derived from and applied to general surgical populations with a relatively low prevalence (<10%) of coronary artery disease. Use of these scoring systems in populations with a higher prevalence of coronary disease (as, for example, in those with peripheral vascular disease, in whom the prevalence of coronary artery disease may be as much as 60%), underestimates the risk of cardiac events.

Noninvasive preoperative stress testing has its highest utility in patients with intermediate clinical predictors of cardiac risk. These include mild angina, a history of prior myocardial infarction, compensated congestive heart failure, and diabetes mellitus. Current practice guidelines suggest that the patients most likely to benefit from preoperative risk stratification are those with poor functional capacity (able to achieve less than 4 METS with exercise) who are scheduled to undergo intermediate- (abdominal, carotid endarterectomy) or high-risk (abdominal aortic aneurysm repair) surgical procedures (21).

The positive predictive value of myocardial perfusion imaging for perioperative cardiac ischemia is low (4% to 20%), but the negative predictive value is very high (96% to 100%). Patients with reversible defects have a greater risk of perioperative ischemia than those with fixed defects, and the relative risk increases in proportion to the extent of inducible ischemia on the perfusion imaging study. The evaluation of left ventricular function on gated SPECT perfusion images is important in patients with signs and/or symptoms of heart failure, because reduced ventricular systolic function is correlated with the risk of perioperative heart failure.

***Nuclear Stress Testing in Women.*** More women die of cardiovascular disease each year in the United States than from any other cause (22). Although the prevalence of coronary artery disease in nondiabetic women <45 years of age is low, it increases significantly following menopause, and is similar to that in men by the seventh decade. Although deaths from coronary artery disease are declining in men, the same is not true for women. Coronary artery disease claims the lives of more than 240,000 women each year in the United States and is a significant cause of morbidity and disability. Women are more likely to die from an acute myocardial infarction than their male counterparts and are more likely to sustain recurrent infarction. Therefore, early identification of women with coronary heart disease affords the best opportunity for intervention and, ultimately, a reduction in cardiovascular mortality.

Current guidelines rely on a Bayesian approach to gauge the relative value of stress testing for the detection of coronary artery disease in women. In asymptomatic premenopausal women, there is a low prevalence of coronary disease, cardiovascular risk is low, and the clinical utility of stress testing is generally of limited benefit. However, women with diabetes or peripheral vascular disease are the exception, because there is an intermediate or higher risk of coronary artery disease. Stress testing in these women is appropriate, even in the absence of symptoms, because of the greater pretest probability of disease. In symptomatic women, those with an intermediate or high pretest likelihood of disease (<50 years of age with typical angina, 50 years or older with typical or atypical chest pain, two or more cardiac risk factors) can be expected to benefit from stress testing.

The diagnostic accuracy of exercise stress electrocardiography for the detection of coronary artery disease in women is somewhat limited. ST-segment changes with stress have been reported to be less accurate for the detection of coronary artery disease than in men, as a consequence of a higher prevalence of ST–T-wave changes on the resting electrocardiogram, lower electrocardiographic voltages, and poorly understood hormonal effects on vascular tone (22). Women are generally older when they present for evaluation, and may be limited in their ability to achieve an adequate level of stress because of lower exercise capacity. Reported average sensitivities and specificities of stress electrocardiography for coronary artery disease detection in women are about 61% and 70%, respectively as compared to 72% and 77% for men. Current ACC/AHA guidelines suggest that stress electrocardiography be used as a first-line test for coronary artery disease detection in women with an intermediate pretest likelihood of disease who have a normal resting electrocardiogram and who are capable of achieving an adequate level of stress. In those with baseline ST–T changes on the electrocardiogram, or in those in whom an adequate level of stress is unlikely to be achieved, myocardial perfusion imaging provides an incremental benefit over the stress electrocardiogram, for both the diagnosis of coronary artery disease and risk stratification. Cardiac imaging is also suggested for women in whom the stress electrocardiogram is indeterminate or suggests an intermediate level of risk, as well as in those with an intermediate-risk Duke treadmill score.

In early clinical studies employing SPECT thallium-201 scintigraphy, reported sensitivities for the detection of single vessel disease in women were lower than in men. This was attributed to smaller left ventricular chamber sizes in women and to the physical characteristics of the isotope itself. In addition, breast attenuation often resulted in anterior wall defects and false positive tests. With the advent of technetium-99m–labeled tracers and gated imaging, the diagnostic accuracy of myocardial perfusion imaging has improved significantly in female populations. For example, adenosine sestamibi imaging has been reported to be 91% sensitive and 86% specific for the detection of coronary stenoses. Although the diagnostic accuracy of SPECT myocardial perfusion imaging in women may be slightly less than that in men, there is a substantial incremental benefit of myocardial perfusion imaging over the routine clinical variables and stress electrocardiography for risk stratification in female patients.

***The Patient with Coronary Calcification on CT.*** The presence of coronary calcification on electron beam CT (EBCT) or multidetector CT (MDCT) is related to the amount and extent of atherosclerotic plaque on coronary angiography. In general, the higher the CT coronary calcium score in a given patient, the poorer the prognosis. In a study of 4,151 asymptomatic men and 1,484 asymptomatic women followed for a mean of 3 years, the risk of cardiac events was eightfold greater in the men with the highest quartile of calcium scores, relative to those with the lowest quartile of scores. In women, the risk of cardiac events in those with the highest quartile of calcium scores was 10-fold greater than in those in the lowest quartile group. In other studies, coronary artery calcification has been shown to be an independent predictor of death relative to other clinical variables, with the mortality risk increasing linearly as the coronary artery calcium score increases.

Despite its proposed clinical utility, the coronary calcium score may be an incomplete descriptor of the disease state in patients with coronary atherosclerosis. As a result of outward remodeling of coronary arterial plaques, the presence of calcium in a lesion is not always indicative of a stenosis that encroaches on luminal blood flow. Conversely, immature plaques that encroach on the coronary lumen and are flow limiting may contain little or no calcification. Therefore, the information provided by CT and myocardial perfusion imaging is considered by some to be complementary. In general, the higher the coronary calcium score, the greater is the probability that a perfusion defect will be identified on SPECT myocardial perfusion imaging. For patients with coronary calcium scores $<100$, the prevalence of perfusion defects on myocardial perfusion imaging has been reported to be $<1.8\%$ (23). For patients with scores between 100 and 400, the reported prevalence of SPECT perfusion defects is 5.2%, whereas that for patients with calcium scores $>400$ is 15% to −40%. Thus, some authors have proposed that stress myocardial perfusion imaging should be considered for patients with coronary scores $>400$, especially if the patient is symptomatic, as this score places the patient at an intermediate risk for a cardiac event. Conversely, the reported prevalence of coronary calcification in those with a normal SPECT myocardial perfusion study is relatively high (24). Normal SPECT myocardial perfusion studies have been reported in about half of patients with calcium scores $>100$, 20% of those with scores between 400 and 999, and in about 10% of those with scores $>1{,}000$. Further clinical studies are needed to determine if the extent of coronary artery calcification contributes to the risk stratification of those with normal myocardial perfusion studies.

## NUCLEAR CARDIAC IMAGING IN HEART FAILURE

### Role of Nuclear Imaging in Congestive Heart Failure

In individuals with congestive heart failure, nuclear imaging can assist in clinical management of the patient by (a) helping to define the etiology of the ventricular dysfunction, (b) characterizing right and left ventricular function and volumes, (c) determining the relative contributions of myocardial stunning and scar to left ventricular dysfunction, and (d) distinguishing myocardial hibernation from scar in those with chronic ischemic heart disease. Although echocardiography has largely supplanted nuclear imaging for assessing diastolic ventricular function, and for characterizing cardiac performance in hypertrophic and valvular heart disease, nuclear imaging techniques remain extremely useful for the evaluation of patients with systolic heart failure. By the use of nuclear imaging, the clinician is afforded insights into the etiology and prognosis of heart failure in the patient, and perhaps more important, whether coronary revascularization in a high-risk individual is likely to improve symptoms and survival.

### Etiology of Heart Failure: Ischemic versus Nonischemic Cardiomyopathy

In patients with impaired systolic function, it is crucial to distinguish myocardial dysfunction due to coronary artery disease (ischemic cardiomyopathy) from other causes of dilated heart failure (nonischemic dilated cardiomyopathy). In selected individuals with ischemic cardiomyopathy, coronary revascularization can provide both symptomatic and prognostic benefit, and noninvasive identification of these patients is key for optimal clinical management (25). Myocardial perfusion imaging is helpful for distinguishing between those with and without ischemic cardiomyopathy, and for the identification of those with ischemic cardiomyopathy who might benefit from coronary revascularization.

Generally, patients with left ventricular dysfunction due to coronary artery disease have either extensive fixed perfusion defects, or a modest number of fixed defects with large reversible stress-induced perfusion defects [suggesting dysfunction on the basis of myocardial stunning (20)]. Six studies have shown that the sensitivity of myocardial perfusion imaging for the detection of coronary artery disease in heart failure patients is 100%, with a homogeneous pattern of perfusion having a predictive value of 100% for a nonischemic cardiomyopathic process. However, a fixed perfusion defect does not preclude the possibility of a nonischemic cardiomyopathic process, for patchy myocardial fibrosis can sometimes be manifest as a fixed defect. In addition, coronary flow reserve can be abnormal in nonischemic cardiomyopathy and reversible perfusion defects have also been reported in these individuals. The specificity of myocardial perfusion imaging for the identification of ischemic cardiomyopathy in dilated heart failure patients is therefore only about 40% to 50%.

## Assessment of Ventricular Function

In addition to gated myocardial perfusion imaging, assessment of right and left ventricular function and volumes can also be achieved using radionuclide ventriculography. Right ventricular function can be evaluated using a first-pass imaging study, in which a series of images is obtained rapidly as a radioactive tracer is administered intravenously. It is useful for visualizing right ventricular function without the confounding influence of activity in other nearby vascular structures. Alternatively, tomographic equilibrium-gated blood pool imaging can also be used to assess right ventricular function.

Left ventricular function can be evaluated using equilibrium-gated blood pool radionuclide ventriculography. In this technique, an intravenously administered radioactive tracer such as technetium-99m pertechnetate is used to label the patient's red blood cells. Once the label is uniformly distributed throughout the vascular space, a set of images synchronized to the patient's electrocardiogram is obtained over multiple cardiac cycles. These images depict different times in the cardiac cycle (see Chapter 9). Because background corrected left ventricular counts are proportional to ventricular volume, the ejection fraction can be calculated by subtracting end-systolic counts from end-diastolic counts and dividing by the end-diastolic counts. Unlike echocardiography or contrast ventriculography, computation of the left ventricular ejection fraction is independent of any assumptions about the shape of the ventricle.

Radionuclide ventriculography can be performed in nearly anyone with a stable cardiac rhythm, including those with obstructive pulmonary disease and marked obesity.

**TABLE 22–3**
**INDICATIONS FOR RADIONUCLIDE VENTRICULOGRAPHY**

| |
|---|
| Determination of left ventricular function in STEMI and non-STEMI/unstable angina patients |
| Initial evaluation of RV and LV function in patients with congestive heart failure |
| Baseline measurement and serial monitoring of left ventricular function during therapy with cardiotoxic drugs (e.g., adriamycin) |
| Quantitation of rest RV and LV function in valvular heart disease |
| Initial and serial assessment of RV and LV function in adults with congenital heart disease |

Most of the available computer programs for the analysis of the gated images use automated edge-detection algorithms to define the border of the ventricular cavity in a consistent manner, resulting in left ventricular ejection fraction measurements that are very reproducible. In patients with congestive heart failure, the severity of global and regional systolic dysfunction can easily be defined with this imaging technique. Because of the high reproducibility of the left ventricular ejection fraction measurements made with this imaging technique, it is also used to monitor the effects of cardiotoxic drugs such as doxorubicin. Serial left ventricular ejection fraction determinations allow the clinician to maximize the dose of the chemotherapeutic agent given to the patient while minimizing the risk of congestive heart failure due to drug toxicity. The indications for radionuclide ventriculography are listed in Table 22–3.

## Perfusion and Metabolic Imaging for Reversible Left Ventricular Dysfunction

In patients with ischemic cardiomyopathy, regional dysfunction associated with normal resting myocardial perfusion generally represents viable myocardium that is likely to benefit from coronary revascularization. These areas frequently demonstrate a perfusion defect with stress, suggesting that the regional dysfunction results from recent or repetitive myocardial stunning. Individuals with the largest amounts of ischemia may be expected to derive the greatest functional benefit from coronary revascularization.

For patients with regional left ventricular dysfunction and fixed perfusion defects, additional imaging is warranted to identify the presence or absence of viability (myocardial hibernation) in that region. Coronary revascularization can improve regional and global left ventricular function in those with viable but dysfunctional myocardial tissue, and thereby benefit heart failure symptoms and quality of life. Usually, an improvement in the global left ventricular ejection can be anticipated if the extent of hibernating myocardium exceeds 20% to 25% of the ventricle. Even more important, coronary revascularization in patients with myocardial viability benefits survival (25). The survival benefit could conceivably reflect factors besides an improvement in ventricular function, including

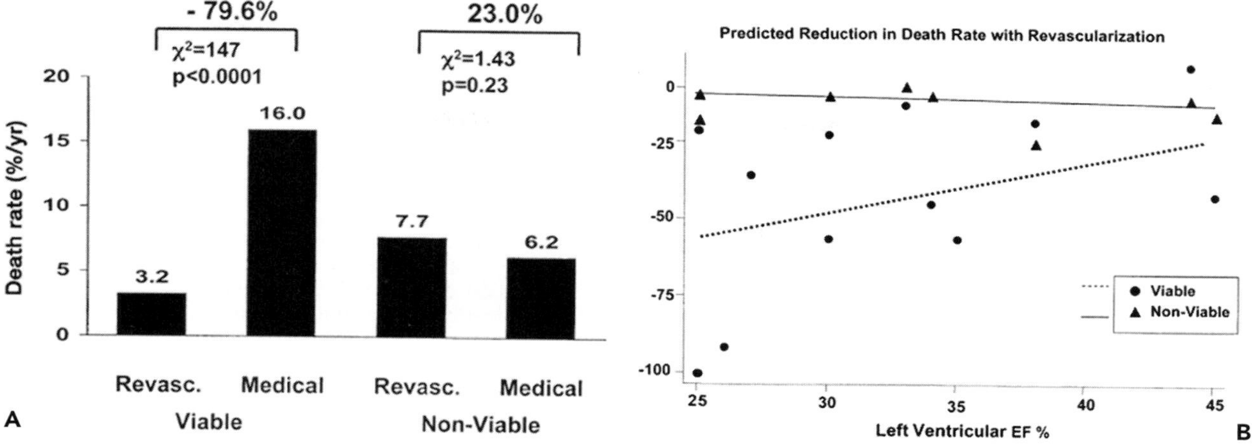


**Figure 22–3** Results of a meta-analysis examining the influence of coronary revascularization on survival in patients with and without viability in dysfunctional myocardial regions. **A:** In patients with myocardial viability and left ventricular dysfunction, coronary revascularization (Revasc) provided nearly an 80% reduction in mortality as compared to medical therapy. In contrast, no survival benefit was noted if revascularization was performed in patients with completed infarction. **B:** The expected improvement in survival due to coronary revascularization, according to the preoperative left ventricular ejection fraction. Those with myocardial viability on noninvasive imaging are depicted by circles, whereas those with completed scar are shown by triangles. In the patients with scar, there is little survival benefit conferred by coronary revascularization. In the individuals with ventricular dysfunction and myocardial viability, the greater the reduction in the preoperative left ventricular ejection fraction, the greater the survival benefit accruing from coronary revascularization. (Reproduced with permission from Allman KC, Shaw LJ, Hachamovitch R, Udelson JE. Myocardial viability testing and impact of revascularization on prognosis in patients with coronary artery disease and left ventricular dysfunction: a meta-analysis. *J Am Coll Cardiol.* 2002;39:1151–1158.)

prevention of myocardial infarction and ventricular remodeling, and a reduction in ventricular arrhythmogenesis. In a meta-analysis of 3,088 patients with coronary artery disease and left ventricular dysfunction (mean LVEF = 32 ± 8%) followed for 25 ± 10 months, patients with myocardial viability who had coronary revascularization experienced an 80% reduction in annual mortality compared to those who were treated medically (16% versus 3.2%, $p < 0.0001$) (Fig. 22–3A) (25). By contrast, annual mortality rates were comparable in those without viability who were treated either surgically (7.7%) or medically (6.2%, $p = \text{NS}$). Moreover, in the patients with viability, those who had the most severe reduction in left ventricular function prior to surgery derived the greatest survival benefit from coronary revascularization (Fig. 22–3B).

Several nuclear imaging options can be used to identify myocardial viability. Markers of viability that have been proposed include the fill-in of a perfusion defect on late (24-hour) thallium-201 redistribution or reinjection images, reversibility of a rest perfusion defect on 3- to 4-hour redistribution images, and demonstration of residual tissue glucose metabolic activity in hypoperfusion myocardial regions (a perfusion–metabolism mismatch) on PET images obtained using the glucose analog F-18 2-fluoro-2-deoxyglucose (FDG). Some have proposed that a relative perfusion tracer concentration >55% to 60% of maximal myocardial activity on rest perfusion images can be used to identify myocardial viability. In a meta-analysis, radionuclide techniques and dobutamine echocardiography had similar positive and negative predictive values for identifying segments with improvement in wall motion following revascularization (26). The nuclear imaging techniques appeared to be slightly more sensitive in identifying viability, as defined by an improvement in function following revascularization, whereas dobutamine echocardiography appeared to be slightly more specific.

## SUMMARY

Nuclear cardiac imaging techniques have become an integral component of the practice of clinical cardiology. As with any diagnostic tool, the physician must have a working knowledge of the strengths and limitations of the imaging technology in order to utilize this technology for optimum clinical benefit. In appropriately selected patients, myocardial perfusion imaging is very useful for identifying obstructive coronary artery disease, for characterizing the functional significance of equivocal coronary stenoses, and for risk stratification. In those with coronary artery disease and systolic ventricular dysfunction, nuclear imaging techniques can be used to quantitate the severity of the ventricular dysfunction and to monitor the myocardial response to treatment noninvasively. Perhaps even more important, nuclear imaging techniques can reliability identify those individuals with ischemic cardiomyopathy who are likely to benefit functionally and prognostically from coronary revascularization.

## ACKNOWLEDGMENTS

The authors would like to thank Dr.Wael Jaber and Dr. Manuel Cerqueira for their thoughtful review of this chapter.

## REFERENCES

1. Di Carli M, Czernin J, Hoh CK, et al. Relation among stenosis severity, myocardial blood flow, and flow reserve in patients with coronary artery disease. *Circulation.* 1995;91:1944–1951.
2. Medrano R, Lowry RW, Young JB, et al. Assessment of myocardial viability with $^{99m}$Tc sestamibi in patients undergoing cardiac transplantation. A scintigraphic/pathological study. *Circulation.* 1996;94:1010–1017.
3. Canty JM, Fallavollita JA. Hibernating myocardium. *J Nucl Cardiol.* 2005;12:104–119.
4. Travin MI, Bergmann SR. Assessment of myocardial viability. *Semin Nucl Med.* 2005;35:2–16.
5. Hendel RC, Jamil T, Glover DK. Pharmacologic stress testing: new methods and new agents. *J Nucl Cardiol.* 2003;10:197–204.
6. Lapeyre AC, Goraya TY, Johnston DL, Gibbons RJ. The impact of caffeine on vasodilator stress perfusion studies. *J Nucl Cardiol.* 2004;11:506–511.
7. Klocke FJ, Baird MG, Lorell BH, et al. ACC/AHA/ASNC guidelines for the clinical use of cardiac radionuclide imaging—executive summary: a report of the American College of Cardiology/American Heart Association Task Force on Practice Guidelines (ACC/AHA/ASNC Committee to Revise the 1995 Guidelines for the Clinical Use of Cardiac Radionuclide Imaging). *J Am Coll Cardiol.* 2003;42:1318–1333.
8. Wackers FJT, Brown KA, Heller GV, et al. American Society of Nuclear Cardiology position statement on radionuclide imaging in patients with acute ischemic syndromes in the emergency department or chest pain center. *J Nucl Cardiol.* 2002;9:246–250.
9. Antman EM, Anbe DT, Armstrong PW, et al. ACC/AHA guidelines for the management of patients with ST-elevation myocardial infarction: a report of the American College of Cardiology/American Heart Association Task Force on Practice Guidelines (Committee to Revise the 1999 Guidelines for the Management of Patients with Acute Myocardial Infarction). 2004. Available at www.acc.org/clinical/guidelines/stemi/index.pdf.
10. Mahmarian JJ, Dwivedi G, Lahiri T. Role of nuclear cardiac imaging in myocardial infarction: postinfarction risk stratification. *J Nucl Cardiol.* 2004;11:186–209.
11. Brown KA, Heller GV, Landin RS, et al. Early dipyridamole $^{99m}$Tc-sestamibi single photon emission computed tomographic imaging 2 to 4 days after acute myocardial infarction predicts in-hospital and postdischarge cardiac events. Comparison with submaximal exercise imaging. *Circulation.* 1999;100:2060–2066.
12. Braunwald E, Antman EM, Beasly JW, et al. ACC/AHA 2002 guideline update for the management of patients with unstable angina and non-ST-segment elevation myocardial infarction: a report of the American College of Cardiology/American Heart Association Task Force on Practice Guidelines (Committee on the Management of Patients with Unstable Angina). 2002. Available at www.acc.org/clinical/guidelines/unstable/unstable.pdf.
13. Gibbons RJ, Chatterjee K, Daley, J, et al. ACC/AHA 2002 guideline update for the management of patients with chronic stable angina: a report of the American College of Cardiology/American Heart Association Task Force on Practice Guidelines (Committee to Update the 1999 Chronic Stable Angina Guidelines). 2002. Available at www.acc.org/clinical/guidelines/stable/stable_clean.pdf.
14. Machac J. Cardiac positron emission tomography imaging. *Semin Nucl Med.* 2005;35:17–36.
15. Hansen HL. The conundrum of left bundle branch block [editorial]. *J Nucl Cardiol.* 2004;11:90–92.
16. Shaw LJ, Hachamovitch R, Berman DS, et al., for the Economics of Noninvasive Diagnosis (END) Multicenter Study Group. The economic consequences of available diagnostic and prognostic strategies for the evaluation of stable angina patients: an observational assessment of the value of precatheterization ischemia. *J Am Coll Cardiol.* 1999;33:661–669.
17. Des Pres RD, Gillespie RL, Jaber WA, et al. Cost-effectiveness of myocardial perfusion imaging: a summary of the currently available literature. Informational statement posted by the American Society of Nuclear Cardiology, September 2005. Available at www.asnc.org.
18. Shaw LJ, Iskandrian AE. Prognostic value of gated myocardial perfusion SPECT. *J Nucl Cardiol.* 2004;11:171–185.
19. Gibbons RJ, Balady GJ, Bricker JT, et al. ACC/AHA 2002 guideline update for exercise testing: a report of the American College of Cardiology/American Heart Association Task Force on Practice Guidelines (Committee on Exercise Testing). 2002. Available at www.acc.org/clinical/guidelines/exercise/dirindex.htm.
20. Lauer MS, Lytle B, Pashkow F, et al. Prediction of death and myocardial infarction by screening with exercise—thallium testing after coronary-artery bypass grafting. *Lancet.* 1998;351:615–622.
21. Brown KA. Advances in nuclear cardiology. Preoperative risk stratification. *J Nucl Cardiol.* 2004;11:335–348.
22. Mieres JH, Shaw LJ, Arai A, et al. Role of noninvasive testing in the clinical evaluation of women with suspected coronary artery disease. Consensus statement from the Cardiac Imaging Committee, Council on Clinical Cardiology, and the Cardiovascular Imaging and Intervention Committee, Council on Cardiovascular Radiology and Intervention, American Heart Association. *Circulation.* 2005;111:682–696.
23. Berman DS, Wong ND, Gransar H, et al. Relationship between stress-induced ischemia and atherosclerosis measured by coronary calcium tomography. *J Am Coll Cardiol.* 2004;44:923–930.
24. Thompson RC, McGhie AI, Moser KW, et al. Clinical utility of coronary calcium scoring after nonischemic myocardial perfusion imaging. *J Nucl Cardiol.* 2005;12:392–400.
25. Allman KC, Shaw LJ, Hachamovitch R, Udelson JE. Myocardial viability testing and impact of revascularization on prognosis in patients with coronary artery disease and left ventricular dysfunction: a meta-analysis. *J Am Coll Cardiol.* 2002;39:1151–1158.
26. Bax JJ, Poldermans D, Elhendy A, et al. Sensitivity, specificity, and predictive accuracy of various noninvasive techniques for detecting hibernating myocardium. *Curr Probl Cardiol.* 2001;26:141–188.

## QUESTIONS

**1.** A 65-year-old man with a 45-pack-year smoking history, hyperlipidemia, intermittent claudication, and hypertension has been experiencing shortness of breath with exertion for 3 months. He is referred for an adenosine cardiac SPECT study for symptom evaluation. His medications include metoprolol, lisinopril, aspirin, theophylline, and simvastatin. During the adenosine infusion, the patient does not report any chest pain, nor are there any ST-segment changes on the electrocardiogram. High-degree atrioventricular block develops 30 seconds following the start of the adenosine infusion, prompting the cardiology fellow attending the stress test to stop the infusion. The SPECT perfusion images are interpreted as normal, with no regional ischemia. Despite continuation of medical therapy the patient's symptoms persist, and 6 weeks later he is referred for cardiac catheterization. At catheterization there is a proximal 75% right coronary artery stenosis, a 75% to 80% proximal left anterior descending artery stenosis, and a 70% to 75% stenosis of the proximal circumflex artery. Possible reasons for the absence of a reversible perfusion defect on the cardiac SPECT study include all of the following *except*:

a. Ingestion of a chocolate bar 3 hours before the test was performed
b. Right bundle branch block on the resting electrocardiogram
c. Provocation of "balanced ischemia" by the adenosine stress
d. Failure to withhold the patient's medications prior to the test
e. Termination of the adenosine infusion at 30 seconds

Answer is b: Appropriate patient preparation is crucial for successful nuclear stress imaging. Recent ingestion of chocolate and/or theophylline could have blunted the hyperemic effects of adenosine, resulting in a falsely negative study. A 30-second infusion of adenosine might not have delivered a sufficient amount of the drug to produce adequate myocardial hyperemia. Alternatively, in a patient with proximal stenoses of nearly equal severity in each of the major coronary vessels, "balanced ischemia" is also a consideration; in this situation, a regional disparity in myocardial perfusion on the stress images is not identified because the impairment in flow reserve is similar in each of the three vascular territories. Right bundle branch block itself would not be expected to cause a false negative perfusion study.

**2.** Which of the following individuals is likely to benefit most from nuclear stress imaging?

a. A 25-year-old man with midline chest pain, which is tender to the touch and intermittently responsive to ibuprofen.
b. A 30-year-old woman who gets chest discomfort after eating highly seasoned food, but who has no trouble when she plays tennis three times a week.
c. A 39-year-old male smoker with shortness of breath on exertion and a mildly elevated LDL cholesterol level. His father died suddenly at age 45, and his 42-year-old brother recently had two stents placed in one of his coronary arteries. The resting electrocardiogram shows nonspecific ST–T-wave changes.
d. A 76-year-old man, former smoker, with hypertension and recent inferior wall myocardial infarction treated by placing two stents in the right coronary artery. He was awakened by an episode of chest pain that lasted almost 20 minutes and that has not responded to sublingual nitroglycerin.
e. A 55-year-old female with hypercholesterolemia, hypertension, frequent heartburn, and increasing shortness of breath on exertion. On echocardiography, there is moderate left ventricular hypertrophy, and aortic valvular calcification with an estimated aortic valve area of 0.69 $cm^2$.

Answer is c: The 39-year-old smoker has several cardiac risk factors and is in an intermediate-risk category for an adverse cardiac event. This patient is the one most likely to benefit from diagnostic testing, for a positive stress perfusion study will put him into a high-risk category, whereas a negative stress perfusion study will stratify him into a low-risk patient population. The young man and woman in a and b have noncardiac chest pain; they are in a low-risk population and are unlikely to derive a benefit from stress myocardial perfusion imaging. The patient in d has known coronary artery disease and an unstable clinical picture following recent coronary stenting, and would more appropriately be referred directly for repeat coronary angiography. The patient in e has moderately severe aortic stenosis, and would more appropriately be referred for cardiac catheterization and coronary angiography.

**3.** A 58-year-old male executive is seen for left-sided chest pain. He has a history of bilateral thumb pain for which he took a cox-II inhibitor for 2 years before switching to naproxen. He works long hours and admits to fatigue and loss of libido. He has an elevated lipoprotein a (Lpa) level but an otherwise normal lipid profile. The hs-CRP level is normal and a cardiac SPECT study 3 years earlier was normal. He undergoes an exercise cardiac SPECT and exercises to 10 METs on the Bruce protocol, achieving 106% of his MPHR. With exercise he experiences fatigue but no angina. No ST-segment changes are noted with stress. The myocardial perfusion images from the exercise study are shown below.

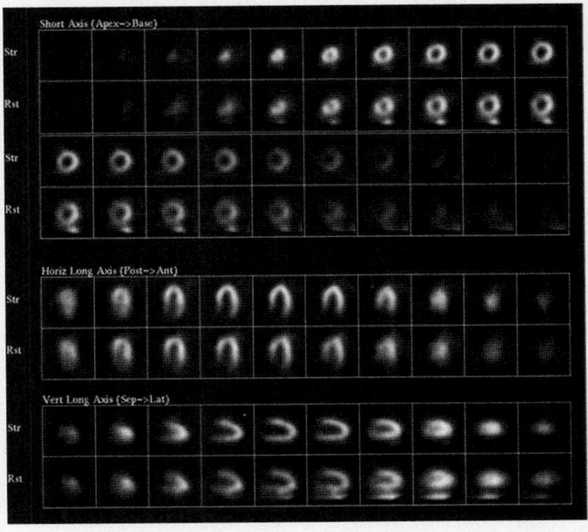

Based on the results of this scan, his cardiac mortality over the next 3 years can be estimated as

a. ≤1.5%
b. 3%
c. 5%
d. 6%
e. >9%

Answer is a: The myocardial perfusion images in this middle-aged man with atypical chest pain and two cardiac risk factors (male sex, elevated lipoprotein a level) are normal. The risk of a cardiac event over the next 3 years in this patient is ≤1.5% (≤0.5%/year), according to one study.

**4.** A 71-year-old man with a history of hyperthyroidism, hypertension, and remote pulmonary embolism is referred for treatment of new-onset atrial fibrillation. He underwent a rest rubidium/dipyridamole stress rubidium-82 perfusion study.

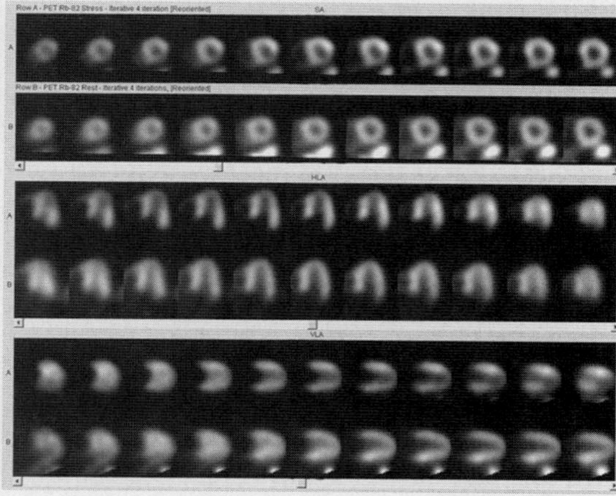

The myocardial perfusion images are most consistent with

a. Inferior ischemia
b. Apical and inferior ischemia
c. Anterior wall ischemia
d. Diaphragmatic attenuation
e. Normal perfusion scan

Answer is b: Reversible perfusion defects are identified involving the apical and inferior myocardial regions. In PET imaging, transmission images are used to correct the emisson images for attenuation, thus attenuation by the diaphragm should not influence the tracer concentration in the inferior wall.

**5.** A 36-year-old woman presents to the Emergency Room with atypical chest pain. She smokes and there is a family history of coronary artery disease. The electrocardiogram shows a normal sinus rhythm with early repolarization. Cardiac enzymes are negative and the patient is referred for stress myocardial perfusion imaging. The patient undergoes treadmill exercise using the Bruce protocol. She is able to complete Stage 2 of the exercise protocol (7 METS), being limited by leg fatigure. She does not experience chest pain with exercise. She achieves 92% of her maximal age-predicted heart rate. During stress, the electrocardiogram shows a new left bundle branch block. Rest thallium-201 and stress Tc-99m tetrofosmin images were obtained:

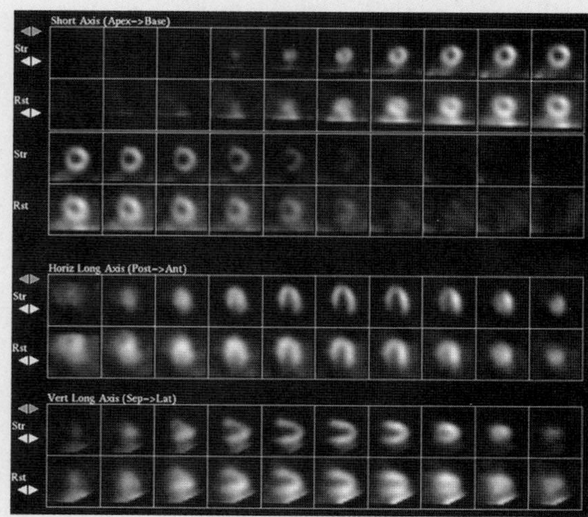


The myocardial perfusion images demonstrate

a. Normal study with breast attenuation
b. A fixed septal perfusion defect
c. A reversible septal perfusion defect, indicating disease in the left anterior descending coronary artery
d. A reversible septal perfusion defect, reflecting the development of left bundle branch block with exercise
e. A reversible septal perfusion defect of uncertain etiology

Answer is e: A reversible septal perfusion defect is identified on the myocardial perfusion images. The reversible defect could reflect either the onset of left bundle branch block with stress *or* obstructive coronary disease in the left anterior descending artery *or* both. Therefore, the findings are equivocal for coronary artery disease. The patient had CT coronary angiography following the nuclear imaging study, and this did not reveal any coronary lesions.

**6.** An 80-year-old man is referred for a second opinion regarding the need for cardiac surgery. He sustained an inferior myocardial infarction 12 years ago. Over the last 4 years he has had increasing shortness of breath, but no angina. Nine months ago he had an echocardiogram that showed mild calcific aortic stenosis, with a left ventricular ejection fraction of 60%. Three months prior to presentation he was hospitalized for congestive heart failure. Echocardiogram again showed mild aortic stenosis, with a LVEF of 25%. Cardiac catheterization confirmed mild aortic stenosis and on coronary angiography there was multivessel coronary artery disease. Rest and stress rubidium-82 perfusion images, and $^{18}$FDG metabolic PET images, were obtained:

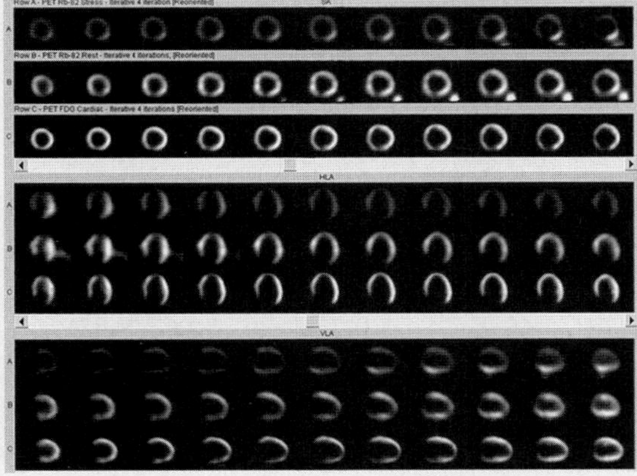

The PET scan demonstrates

a. A small inferior scar
b. Extensive septal, anterior, apical, and lateral ischemia
c. A small inferior scar, with extensive septal, anterior, apical, and lateral ischemia
d. Extensive myocardial hibernation involving the septal, anterior, apical, and lateral regions, with a small inferior scar
e. Normal regional perfusion and metabolism findings suggest nonischemic dilated cardiomyopathy

Answer is c: Extensive reversible perfusion defects are noted in the septal, anterior, apical, and lateral regions, and there is a small scar in the inferior region that is best identified on the short-axis images. Because of the extensive ischemia, the patient was referred for coronary revascularization.

**7.** In a patient with ischemic cardiomyopathy, which of the following scintigraphic findings suggests that abnormal regional function is unlikely to improve if coronary revascularization is performed?

a. A defect on rubidium-82 PET images with preserved uptake on $^{18}$F-fluorodeoxyglucose PET images in the same area.
b. A reversible stress-induced perfusion defect in the same region on rest thallium-201/stress Tc-99m sestamibi SPECT images.
c. The region exhibits a Tc-99m sestamibi SPECT perfusion defect with a relative tracer concentration of 55% of maximal myocardial activity. Relative tracer activity on PET images with $^{18}$F-fluorodeoxyglucose is 95% of peak maximal myocardial activity.
d. A resting thallium-201 perfusion defect in which the relative tracer concentration is 40% of peak myocardial uptake, and which then increases to 90% of peak myocardial uptake on images obtained following thallium-201 reinjection.
e. A matching defect on $^{13}$N-ammonia and $^{18}$F-fluorodeoxyglucose PET images.

Answer is e: A matching defect on $^{13}$N-ammonia and $^{18}$F-fluorodeoxyglucose PET images is indicative of myocardial scar, and there is little chance that the region will exhibit improved function if revascularization is performed. Regions with perfusion–metabolism mismatches, or hibernating myocardium, as exemplified by the findings in a and c, are likely to improve functionally if revascularization is performed. Dysfunctional regions with reversible perfusion defects, whether in response to stress (b) or on rest/reinjection thallium-201 images (d), are also likely to benefit functionally from coronary revascularization.

**8.** A 57-year-old man with a history of coronary artery disease, prior myocardial infarction, and remote coronary artery bypass surgery was referred for evaluation for coronary revascularization because of recurrent angina and heart failure symptoms. There was a history of hyperlipidemia, hypertension, and deep venous thrombosis. An AICD had been placed 2 years before because of ventricular arrhythmias. On echocardiography, there is global left ventricular systolic dysfunction, with an LVEF of 20%. Rest and stress rubidium-82 perfusion and $^{18}$F-fluorodeoxyglucose PET images were obtained:

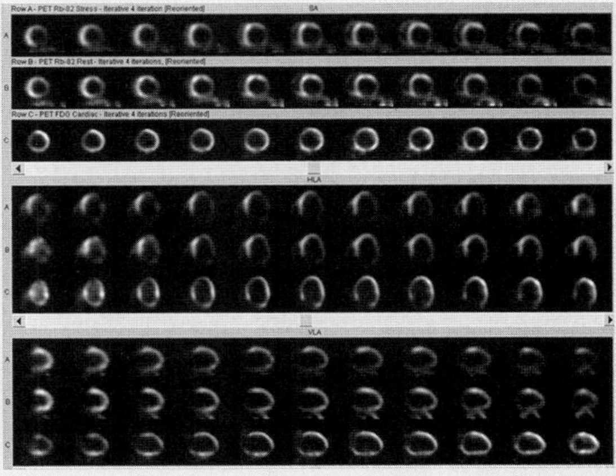

Which of the following statements is true regarding the scintigraphic findings?

a. Left ventricular dysfunction is probably due to a nonischemic cardiomyopathy.
b. On contrast magnetic resonance imaging, pronounced late enhancement will probably be observed in the lateral wall.
c. A reversible perfusion defect is identified in the anterior wall.
d. Coronary revascularization would be unlikely to improve the patient's heart failure symptoms.
e. On histopathologic examination, extensive myocardial fibrosis would be expected if a biopsy of the lateral wall of the left ventricle were obtained.

Answer is c: A reversible perfusion defect is identified in the anterior wall. On the rest rubidium-82 perfusion and $^{18}$F-fluorodeoxyglucose images, there is an extensive perfusion–metabolism "mismatch" consistent with myocardial hibernation involving the anterolateral and inferolateral walls, as well as a portion of the inferior wall. There is a small inferior scar. The findings indicate that the patient would benefit from coronary revascularization. Prior histopathologic studies indicate that there is minimal fibrosis in areas with hibernating tissue, and therefore extensive late enhancement on contrast magnetic resonance imaging would not be anticipated.

# Stress Echocardiography 23

**L. Leonardo Rodriguez** **Daniel Sauri**

Stress echocardiography (SE) is one the main diagnostic modalities used in the evaluation of patients with known or suspected coronary artery disease (CAD). Stress echo permits an integral evaluation of global and regional ventricular function, valvular integrity, and, most important, myocardial response to stress. The class I indications for stress echocardiography in chronic ischemic heart disease are diagnosis of ischemia in symptomatic individuals and the assessment of myocardial viability (hibernating myocardium) for planned revascularization (dobutamine echo).

The accuracy of SE is superior to stress electrocardiography (ECG) and comparable to that of nuclear stress testing. In general, SE is less sensitive for single vessel CAD, but more specific than perfusion imaging.

Numerous studies have validated the prognostic significance of SE, with a negative test carrying a very low risk (<1%) of major cardiac events over the subsequent 4 to 5 years. SE can also distinguish viable from scarred myocardium. The accuracy of dobutamine stress echocardiography (DSE) to detect viability is comparable to the more contemporary modalities of positron emission tomography (PET) imaging and magnetic resonance imaging (MRI). More important, it is able to predict which patients with left ventricular dysfunction will benefit from modern revascularization techniques. Within the realm of valvular heart disease, SE has an increasing role in predicting the functional significance of a variety of valvular lesions. Compared to other noninvasive modalities, SE is safe, widely available, relatively inexpensive, and avoids radiation exposure. However, its interpretation remains subjective and requires a considerable learning curve with substantial interobserver variability.

SE detects ischemia earlier in the ischemic cascade than ECG and before symptoms appear, by identifying new regional wall motion abnormalities (RWMA) (Fig. 23–1). SE adds to exercise ECG particularly when the baseline ECG limits ST-segment assessment such as in LBBB, intraventricular conduction delay, paced rhythms, left ventricular hypertrophy (LVH), and digitalis effect.

## FORMS OF STRESS

### Exercise Echocardiography

The most physiologic form of stress testing remains exercise. In addition to the echocardiographic data, exercise provides important physiologic information for prognosis and risk stratification. Exercise echo can be done using a treadmill or bicycle. The advantage of bicycle exercise is that imaging can be performed during stress. For treadmill exercise, patients must be taken off the treadmill and the echo images acquired within 1 minute of peak exercise. However, bicycle exercise is more effort dependent and therefore less reliable in reaching a target heart rate. Exercise is also preferred for noncoronary indications such as valvular heart disease or hypertrophic cardiomyopathy.

### Dobutamine Echocardiography

Approximately 30% of patients are unable to exercise for reasons such as peripheral vascular disease, obstructive lung disease, or musculoskeletal problems. For these patients, pharmacologic stress echocardiography can be performed. There are three options for pharmacologic stress echocardiography: (a) sympathomimetic agents such as dobutamine, (b) vasodilator agents such as adenosine, and (c) atrial pacing.

Of the sympathomimetic agents, dobutamine has the largest clinical experience. It produces stress through an increase in myocardial oxygen demand via its positive inotropic and chronotropic effects. At low doses, it has positive inotropic effects mediated through cardiac $\alpha$ and $\beta_1$ receptors. At high doses it possesses chronotropic effects through the $\beta_2$ receptor. Dobutamine can be combined

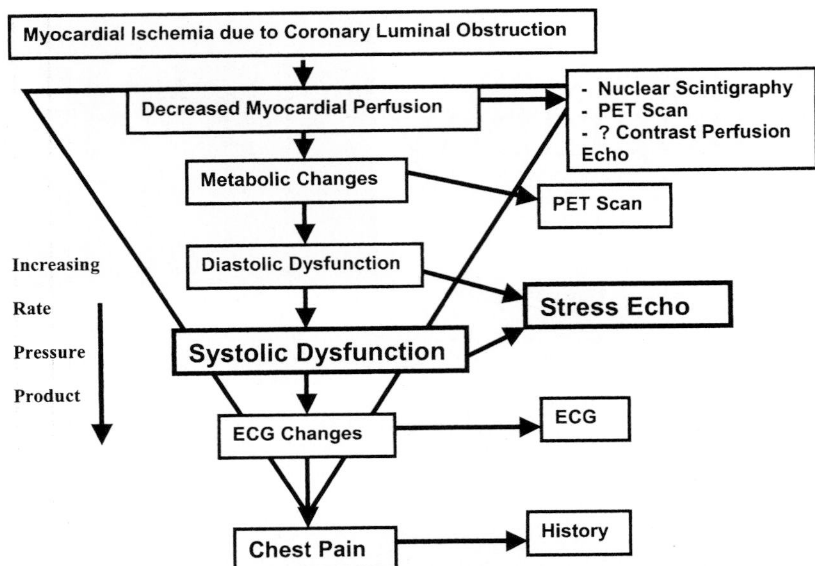


**Figure 23–1** Ischemic cascade. (From The Cleveland Clinic Foundation. *Manual of Cardiovascular Medicine.* 2nd ed. Philadelphia: Lippincott Williams & Wilkins; 2004, Figure 46.1.)

with atropine to achieve a target heart rate of 85% of age-predicted maximum heart rate. Contraindications to atropine use include glaucoma, severe benign prostatic hypertrophy, or severe reactive airway disease. In patients who are morbidly obese without other viable noninvasive options for risk stratification, dobutamine has been combined with transesophageal echo to avoid the potential morbidity of cardiac catheterization. When assessing viability, dobutamine is preferred, for assessment of contractile reserve at low doses.

Vasodilators, such as adenosine or dipyridamole, induce ischemia via a coronary steal effect that preferentially shunts blood away from myocardial segments supplied by stenotic coronary arteries. These agents have a shorter half-life with fewer side effects than dobutamine. Given their shorter duration of action, the echo findings are also less pronounced, resulting in a decreased sensitivity of approximately 50% to 60%, and a decreased ability to detect small amounts of ischemia in patients with single-vessel disease.

Atrial pacing, either by transvenous or transesophageal routes, has been used to achieve stress. The small increases in rate/pressure product and general poor tolerability of pacing have prevented this method from having general acceptance.

## IMAGING TECHNIQUE

The typical treadmill protocol involves acquiring a series of resting images: parasternal long-axis, parasternal short-axis, apical four-chamber and apical two-chamber views. These images are stored digitally and then compared side by side with similar views acquired immediately poststress. During bike stress echo testing, images are recorded at rest and after each increment under load.

The dobutamine echo protocol starts with resting images in the same parasternal and apical views already mentioned. The infusion is started at 10 $\mu$g/kg/min, and this dose is increased every 3 minutes to 20, 30, and 40 $\mu$g/kg/min. Atropine is administered if the patient does not achieve >85% of predicted maximal heart rate (PMHR) and handgrip can also be added.

Harmonic imaging is now used routinely for better endocardial definition. Furthermore, imaging contrast should be used liberally for patients with suboptimal images to improve visualization of endocardial thickening, as this is the most specific marker for ischemia.

## INTERPRETATION OF STRESS ECHO

Responses to stress echo and their interpretations are summarized in Table 23–1. Results are reported graphically in bull's-eye form (Fig. 23–2), with segments assumed to correspond to a particular coronary distribution (Fig. 23–3). Each wall segment is graded subjectively as normal, mildly hypokinetic, severely hypokinetic, akinetic, or dyskinetic in both the rest and stress images. A normal response to stress echo involves a global increase in contractility and hyperdynamic wall motion, and a gradual increase in heart rate. This is manifested by increased wall thickness, increased endocardial excursion, and a reduction in cavity size with stress.

At rest, akinetic or dyskinetic segments generally represent a transmural infarct, particularly if the wall is also thin (<6 mm). Hypokinetic segments demonstrate a partial infarct or viable myocardium. A decrease in overall ejection fraction with left ventricular dilation post stress is an abnormal response that usually represents global ischemia. There are, however, other causes of global hypokinesis, such as a hypertensive response and severe valvular regurgitant lesions.

Dobutamine stress echo typically displays each view at rest and at 10, 30, and 40 $\mu$g. The normal response to

**TABLE 23–1**
**STRESS ECHOCARDIOGRAPHIC RESPONSES AND INTERPRETATION**

| Interpretation | Resting or Baseline Function | Response to Low-Dose Pharmacologic Stress | Peak and Poststress Function |
|---|---|---|---|
| Normal | Normal | Normal | Hyperdynamic |
| Ischemic | Normal | Normal; decreased in severe ischemia (new wall motion abnormality) | Decreased (new wall motion abnormality); left ventricular dilatation (severe ischemia) |
| Scar | Decreased | Decreased | Decreased |
| Viable and ischemic (hibernating) | Decreased | Improved | Decreased (bibhasic response) |
| Viable and not ischemic (stunned) | Decreased | Improved | Improved |
| Nonspecific | Decreased | Decreased | Improved |

*Source:* From The Cleveland Clinic Foundation. *Manual of Cardiovascular Medicine.* 2nd ed. Philadelphia: Lippincott Williams & Wilkins; 2004, Table 46.3.

dobutamine is a marked reduction in cavity size and an increase in endocardial thickening. Systolic cavity obliteration is not uncommon, and it decreases the sensitivity of the test. Another finding with little clinical significance is the development of systolic anterior motion of the mitral valve with a dynamic LVOT gradient.

Reproducibility of SE within centers is generally very good, yet concordance may be less than 80% between different centers, especially for technically difficult studies or mild CAD. Importantly, the prognostic implications of stress echo hold up across these differences.

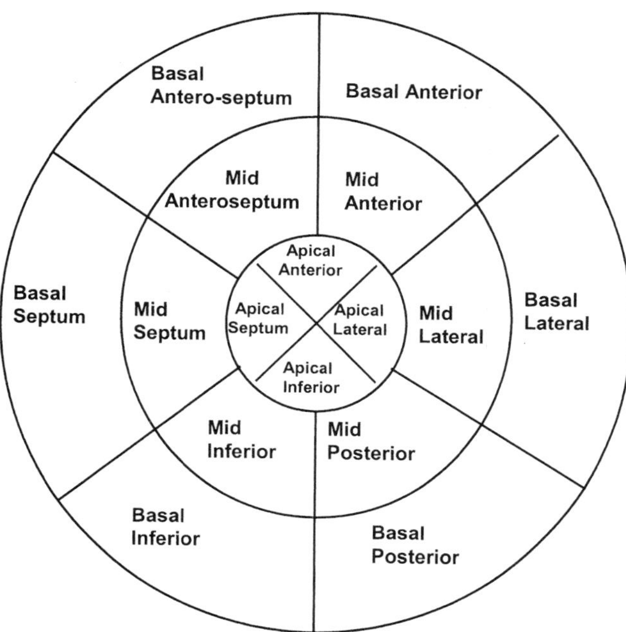


**Figure 23–2** Typical bull's-eye representation used for reporting the 16 myocardial segments model. (From The Cleveland Clinic Foundation. *Manual of Cardiovascular Medicine.* 2nd ed. Philadelphia: Lippincott Williams & Wilkins; 2004, Figure 46.3.)

## USES FOR STRESS ECHO

Traditionally, SE has been used for the diagnosis of CAD, but other uses include the assessment of myocardial viability with DSE, determining functional significance of valvular heart lesions, and prognosis of patients with known or suspected CAD.

### Diagnosis of CAD

The diagnosis of CAD is made when regional wall motion abnormalities are present. Ischemia is diagnosed when *new* areas of wall motion abnormalities develop with stress. The accuracy of stress echo for the detection of CAD is greater than that of ECG exercise stress testing alone and equivalent to that obtained with myocardial perfusion. The sensitivity ranges from 75% to 87%, and the specificity ranges from 74% to 80%, depending on disease prevalence. As with all noninvasive modalities, SE is less sensitive for single-vessel disease than for multivessel disease. Table 23–2 lists causes of false-positive and false-negative SE.

Compared to exercise ECG, SE is more sensitive and specific, as would be predicted based on the ischemic cascade in which regional wall motion abnormalities (WMA) occur prior to ECG changes (see Fig. 23–1). Compared to nuclear stress testing, SE is less sensitive, because perfusion precedes the development of WMA, but is more specific.

DSE has a sensitivity of 68% to 76% and a specificity of 80% to 85%, which is comparable to that of exercise echocardiography. Vasodilator SE with adenosine demonstrates a significant decrease in sensitivity of 50% to 75%, but with slightly increased specificity of 80% to 100%.

### Role of DSE to Assess Viability

In patients with CAD and left ventricular dysfunction, it is important to assess for myocardial viability. This is a Class I indication for the use of dobutamine echocardiography.

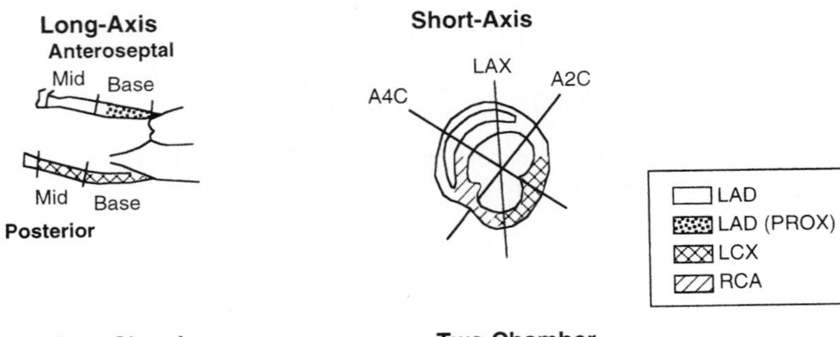


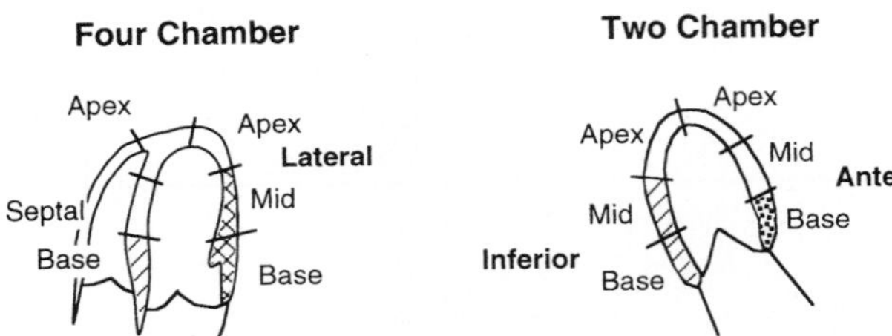


**Figure 23–3** Relationships among the 16 myocardial segments in the American Society of Echocardiography (ASE) classification system and their coronary artery supplies. The four standard views are used to delineate the associations between coronary artery distribution and the segments. (From The Cleveland Clinic Foundation. *Manual of Cardiovascular Medicine.* 2nd ed. Philadelphia: Lippincott Williams & Wilkins; 2004, Figure 46.2.)

For viability evaluation, the dobutamine protocol is modified and an additional set of images is acquired at 5 $\mu$g/kg/min. The diagnosis of viability using this technique is based on the presence of contractile reserve, defined as an increase in wall thickening at low-dose dobutamine (5 or 10 $\mu$g/kg/min). An abnormal myocardial segment at rest can respond to dobutamine in a different way (see Table 23–1). The segment can improve at low dose and then become abnormal at peak. This is called biphasic response. The segment can improve at low dose and continue improving at peak, so-called uniphasic improvement. If the segment does not improve at all with low dose or peak dose it is considered irreversibly damaged, or a scar. The biphasic and uniphasic responses to dobutamine suggest the presence of viable myocardium. Of the two, a biphasic response is the most predictive of recovery after revascularization. The number of segments with contractile reserve is important in predicting an increase in ejection fraction after revascularization. DSE has 80% sensitivity and 80% specificity to detect functional recovery after revascularization. The accuracy of DSE to predict recovery after revascularization is similar to that of PET, with less sensitivity but greater specificity. DSE is substantially more specific than thallium redistribution imaging for viability. The accuracy of DSE compared to MRI is also similar. If there are >25% viable segments or an increase in ejection fraction with low-dose dobutamine, then DSE demonstrates >80% accuracy to predict significant improvement of EF postrevascularization.

## Prognostic Role

Stress echo provides information about the two most important aspects of cardiovascular prognosis, left ventricular function and the severity and extent of ischemia.

Exercise echo offers incremental prognostic information particularly in patients with intermediate risk probability. The total number of abnormal segments both at rest and exercise induced is important in predicting mortality. In patients with known or suspected disease, a negative test pertains to a low risk of subsequent events (<1% per year), whereas a positive study has a 10% to 30% 1-year event rate of MI, PCI, CABG, or death.

Marwick et al. (2001) demonstrated that exercise echo is an independent predictor of death and provides incremental evidence to the traditional Duke treadmill score. It is particularly useful in further stratifying yearly mortality in those with intermediate Duke treadmill scores. Patients with an intermediate Duke treadmill score but normal SE had a 5-year mortality of 1.7%. For those with single-vessel ischemia the mortality was 3.6%, and for those with multivessel disease, 6.7%.

For DSE, ECG changes and hypotension are relatively insensitive markers of ischemia, but regional WMA with stress are analogous to ischemia development with exercise. A risk score based on clinical and echocardiographic data may be used to quantify the risk of events in patients undergoing DSE given a lack of exercise data:

$$\begin{aligned}\text{DSE risk} = {} & (\text{age} \times 0.02) + (\text{heart failure} + \text{rate} \\ & - \text{pressure product} < 15{,}000) \times 0.4 \\ & + (\text{ischemia} + \text{scar}) \times 0.6\end{aligned}$$

Using cutoff values of 1.2 and 2.6, patients are classified into groups with 5-year event-free survivals of >95%, 75% to 95%, and <75%. This prognostic information may help facilitate rational decision making about medical management based on the likelihood of an adverse outcome, rather than a binary approach of whether the test is positive or negative.

Scar pertains to an intermediate prognosis between ischemia (high risk) and a normal study (low risk). In post-MI patients, the extent of LV dysfunction is more important

**TABLE 23–2**
**CAUSES OF FALSE-POSITIVE AND FALSE-NEGATIVE STRESS ECHOCARDIOGRAPHIC TEST RESULTS**

| Causes of False Stress Echocardiographic Results | Factors Reducing Specificity or Sensitivity |
|---|---|
| **False-Positive Results** | |
| Abnormal septal motion (LBBB, after cardiac surgery) | Reduced or abnormal septal excursion with normal septal thickness |
| Nonischemic cardiomyopathy | May develop regional WMAs (exact cause unknown) |
| Hypertensive response to exercise (SBP > 230 mm Hg, DBP > 120 mm Hg) | Nonischemic WMAs or LV dilatation |
| Poor image quality | |
| Overinterpretation | Observer bias may result in a lower threshold for calling a positive study; important to be blinded |
| Basal inferior or septal wall segments | Areas most likely to be overcalled; reduced excursion due to annular tethering effects |
| **False-Negative Results** | |
| Single-vessel disease | More likely to have subtle, rapidly resolving WMA than multivessel disease |
| Inadequate level of stress (more likely with b-blockers) | Important to stress maximally; reach at least 85% of age-predicted maximum heart rate |
| LV cavity obliteration (more likely to occur with dobutamine) | Makes segmental wall motion analysis difficult |
| Poor image quality | |
| Left circumflex disease | Lateral wall drop-out; more likely to miss ischemia |

DBP, diastolic blood pressure; LBBB, left bundle branch block; LV, left ventricular; SBP, systolic blood pressure; WMAs, wall motion abnormalities.
*Source:* From The Cleveland Clinic Foundation. *Manual of Cardiovascular Medicine.* 2nd ed. Philadelphia: Lippincott Williams & Wilkins; 2004, Table 46.4.

than the extent of ischemic/viable myocardium, suggesting that with modern revascularization techniques, the long-term risk is more related to the inability to recover LV function.

For patients undergoing major noncardiac surgery, a positive DSE is associated with a risk of 7% to 25% for hard events (i.e., death and MI). The negative predictive value of DSE for this patient group is 93% to 100%. Questions remain as to whether preoperative revascularization can alter these event rates. A meta-analysis concluded that nuclear stress testing and SE had comparable levels of accuracy for preoperative risk assessment, but that SE was significantly cheaper.

## Stress Echo in Valvular Heart Disease

SE helps determine the hemodynamic and functional significance of valvular lesions such as aortic stenosis, mitral regurgitation, mitral stenosis, and hypertrophic cardiomyopathy.

DSE is useful in assessing the presence of contractile reserve in patients with aortic stenosis and severe LV dysfunction. Lack of LV function improvement with dobutamine suggests a poor prognosis even after aortic valve replacement. An increase in valve gradients with dobutamine infusion with no change in aortic valve area suggests that the aortic stenosis is the main contributor to low output, and that valve replacement may alter the patient's long-term prognosis. In some patients this technique may help to differentiate pseudostenosis from true aortic stenosis when severe LV dysfunction is present.

SE helps predict latent LV dysfunction in patients with normal LV function at baseline, severe MR, and little or no symptoms. Patients with increased LV size with stress present an increased risk of LV dysfunction post-valve repair. In patients with symptomatic moderate mitral stenosis or in those who are asymptomatic with apparent severe mitral stenosis, stress echo can evaluate the patient's functional response to exercise. SE can determine functional capacity as well as peak arterial pressures at peak stress, which can assist with surgical timing. SE can help explain exertional symptoms in a patient with hypertrophic cardiomyopathy with mild or no resting gradients. Furthermore, important prognostic and hemodynamic information, such as hypotension with peak stress, can be gained from SE in this patient population.

## BIBLIOGRAPHY


**Bax JJ, Cornel JH, Visser FC, et al.** Prediction of myocardial dysfunction after revascularization. Comparison of fluorine-18 fluorodeoxyglucose/thallium-201 SPECT, thallium-201 stressreinjection SPECT and dobutamine echocardiography. *J Am Coll Cardiol.* 1996;28:558–564.

**Bonow RO.** Identification of viable myocardium. *Circulation.* 1996;94:2674–2680.

**Cornel JH, Bax JJ, Ehendy A, et al.** Biphasic response to dobutamine predicts improvement of global left ventricular dysfunction after surgical revascularization in patients with stable coronary artery disease: implications of time course of recovery on diagnostic accuracy. *J Am Coll Cardiol.* 1998;31:1002–1010.

**Decena BF 3rd, Tischler MD.** Stress echocardiography in valvular heart disease. *Cardiol Clin.* 1999;17:555–572.

**Fleischmann KE, Hunink MG, Kuntz KM, et al.** Exercise echocardiography or exercise SPECT imaging? A meta-analysis of diagnostic performance. *JAMA.* 1998;280:913–920.

**Marwick TH, Case C, Sawada S, et al.** Prediction of mortality by exercise echocardiography: a strategy for combination with Duke treadmill score. *Circulation.* 2001;103:2566–2571.

**Marwick TH, Case C, Poldermans D, et al.** A clinical and echocardiographic score for assigning risk of major events after dobutamine echocardiograms. *J Am Coll Cardiol* 2004;43:2102–2107.

**Picano E, Lattanzi F, Orlandini A, et al.** Stress echocardiography and the human factor: the importance of being expert. *J Am Coll Cardiol.* 1991;17:666–669.

**Secknus MA, Marwick TH.** Evolution of dobutamine echocardiography protocols and indications: safety and side effects in 3,011 studies over 5 years. *J Am Coll Cardiol.* 1997;29:1234–1240.

# Valvular Heart Disease

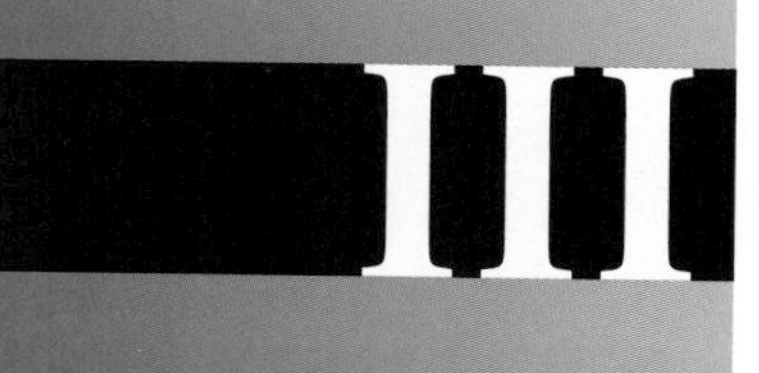

# Aortic and Pulmonary Valve Disease

24

***Christian Gring    Brian Griffin***

## NORMAL AORTIC VALVE ANATOMY

Normal aortic valves are tricuspid—with right, left, and noncoronary cusps—and have a valve area of 2 to 3 cm$^2$. However, congenital variations in this anatomy are relatively common, particularly bicuspid valves. Most commonly, bicuspid valves result from fusion of the right and left coronary cusps, although any two cusps may be fused. More rare are unicuspid and quadricuspid valves, with one and four cusps, respectively (Fig. 24–1). Although some congenitally abnormal valves function normally and are clinically silent, they more frequently result in symptomatic aortic stenosis or aortic insufficiency by middle age.

## AORTIC STENOSIS

Aortic stenosis (AS) is one of the most frequent valve pathologies encountered in clinical cardiology. The etiology can be varied, and may include subvalvular, valvular, or supravalvular lesions, but the pathophysiologic and hemodynamic responses to fixed outflow obstruction are usually predictable.

### Pathophysiology of Aortic Stenosis

Aortic stenosis, regardless of degree, creates a pressure overload on the left ventricle. Over time, the ventricle develops a compensatory concentric hypertrophy, which allows left ventricular (LV) wall stress, or afterload, to remain normal, despite increased systolic pressures. This relationship is expressed by the law of Laplace, which states that wall stress is proportional to the chamber radius divided by its thickness. Thus, in compensated aortic stenosis, LV hypertrophy functions to normalize afterload and helps to maintain normal LV contractile function. The hypertrophy does, however, lead to increased LV mass and end-diastolic pressures, which in turn may precipitate diastolic heart dysfunction and myocardial ischemia. The degree of hypertrophy may vary dramatically among individuals, and gender differences have also been noted. Classically, women develop more hypertrophy with a small-to-normal LV cavity size, whereas men develop a lesser degree of hypertrophy, a dilated LV cavity, and earlier systolic dysfunction (1). Ultimately, compensatory mechanisms fail and patients develop symptoms due to progressive diastolic dysfunction, systolic dysfunction, compromised cardiac output, or myocardial ischemia.

### Etiologies of Aortic Stenosis

There are multiple etiologies of aortic stenosis, the most common of which are discussed below.

*Degenerative aortic stenosis* is the most common etiology of AS in the United States. Once believed to be a passive process of calcification due to years of "wear and tear," degenerative AS is now understood to be a dynamic process involving a robust inflammatory response of macrophages, T cells, and fibroblasts. The exact precipitants for AS are not clear, but observational evidence suggests the process may share some risk factors with atherosclerosis. In retrospective studies, statins have attenuated progression of aortic stenosis (2,3); however, no prospective studies have shown that medical therapy is effective in delaying progression of AS.

*Rheumatic heart disease* is a common cause of AS is less developed countries, but its incidence in developing countries has declined over the past 30 years.

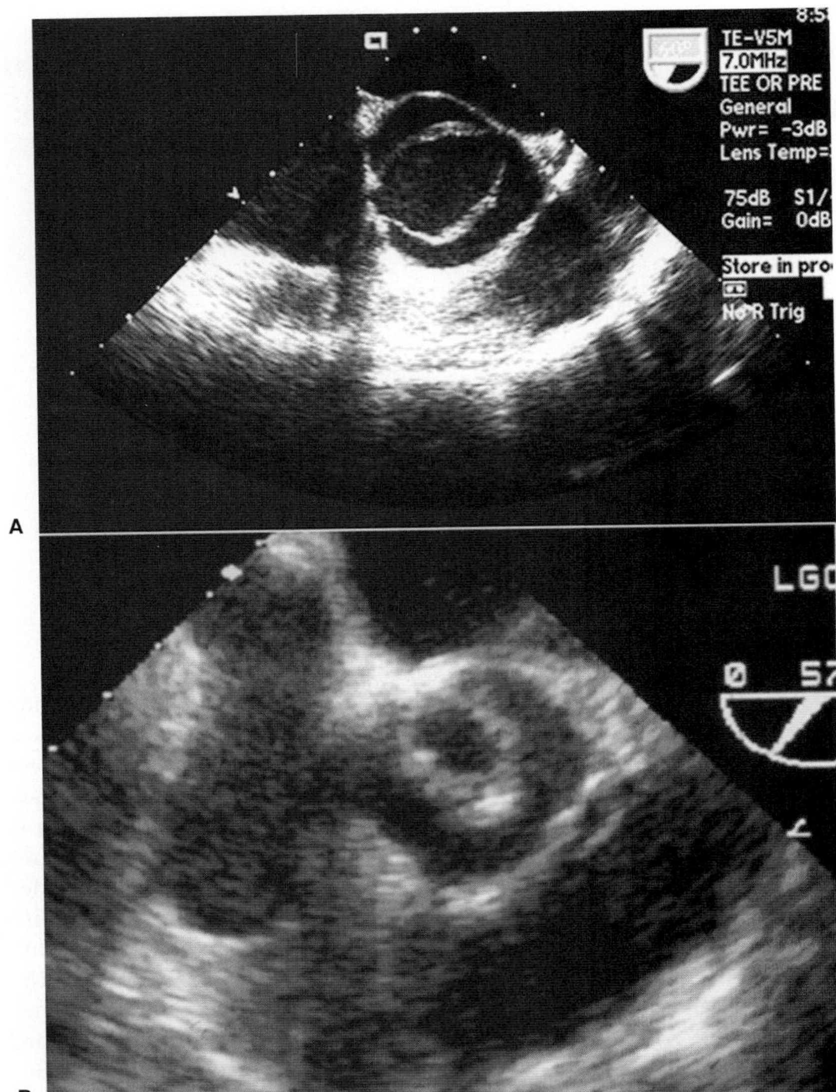


**Figure 24–1** Transesophageal echocardiography short-axis images of bicuspid aortic valve **(A)** and unicuspid valve **(B)**.

*Congenital valve disease* may result in bicuspid or unicuspid valves, which are a frequent cause of symptomatic AS in younger patients (Fig. 24–1) Bicuspid valves (BAV) have a prevalence of 1% to 2% in the population, and are associated with other congenital abnormalities (especially coarctation) in 20% of cases. Up to 80% of patients with coarctation have BAV. Bicuspid valves are also associated with aortic root dilatation and an aortopathy that resembles cystic medial necrosis. Unicuspid valves are inherently stenotic, and usually cause symptoms by the third decade of life. Like bicuspid valves, unicuspid valves also are associated with an aortopathy.

*Radiation heart disease* may occur in patients who have a history of mediastinal radiation as treatment for lymphoma, breast, or esophageal cancers. Such patients have an increased tendency to aortic and mitral valve disease. Usually, radiation-associated aortic disease is mixed stenosis and regurgitation.

*Subvalvular aortic stenosis* is a rare form of AS, and may be due to a tunnel of muscular tissue or a discrete band or membrane. Subvalvular stenosis should be suspected in any patient who has symptoms of AS or high left ventricular outflow velocities on echo cardiography, but whose aortic valve is structurally normal. Subvalvular stenosis also presents as a component of the Shone complex: multiple left-sided heart obstructions, including supravalvular mitral stenosis, parachute mitral valve, subvalvular AS, BAV, and aortic coarctation. Additionally, subaortic stenosis may be associated with a patent ductus and ventricular septal defects. Over time, the jet from subvalvular stenosis will damage the native aortic valve and will lead to aortic insufficiency. For this reason, early surgical repair of asymptomatic subvalvular stenosis is often recommended.

*Supravalvular aortic stenosis* is a rare variant of AS that is classically associated with Williams syndrome (childlike facies, peripheral pulmonary stenosis, hypercalcemia) and familial dyslipidemias. A mutation in the gene for elastin has been linked to Williams syndrome. Other cardiovascular associations of supravalvular stenosis include coarctation of the thoracic or abdominal aorta and renal artery stenosis.

## Clinical Findings in Aortic Stenosis

The history of patients with AS varies with the etiology of the stenosis. Patients with rheumatic heart disease or bicuspid aortic valves frequently have a long history of a heart murmur. They also are more likely to present with symptomatic disease at a younger age. In contrast, patients with degenerative AS usually are older, in their seventh or eighth decade, and may present with symptoms without prior knowledge of aortic valve pathology.

The symptoms of AS are most frequently the direct result of the heart's compensatory changes. Initially, patients develop diastolic heart dysfunction, which often manifests as exertional dyspnea. With stress, patients with AS may become significantly symptomatic because their cardiac output cannot augment adequately and left ventricular end-diastolic pressure (LVEDP) markedly increases. Dyspnea and early fatigability result. As the AS progresses, the classic symptoms of angina, syncope, and heart failure develop. This triad of symptoms has been well studied and allows a rough estimate of disease severity and prognosis: if untreated, survival in patients with angina approximates 5 years, with syncope is 3 years, and with heart failure is <2 years.

Angina is very common in severe AS and may be due to concomitant coronary disease, demand ischemia, or both. Interestingly, up to 50% of patients with angina and severe AS have no obstructive coronary disease. The angina is usually typical substernal pain, worsened with exertion or stress, and relieved with rest. Anginal equivalents, such as dyspnea on exertion, are also common. Syncope or presyncope most often results from exertional cerebral hypoperfusion; with exercise, the systemic arterial tree vasodilates but the cardiac output remains relatively fixed. Arrhythmias may also precipitate syncope, especially atrial fibrillation or ventricular tachycardia. Congestive heart failure symptoms such as pulmonary edema, paroxysmal nocturnal dyspnea, and orthopnea are late findings in AS and signify advanced disease with very poor prognosis if untreated.

Less common manifestations of aortic stenosis include cardiac cachexia in very advanced cases and gastrointestinal bleeds from atriovenous (AV) malformations. Cardiac cachexia and debilitation result from a profound, long-standing low-output state. The mechanism for gastrointestinal bleeding from arteriovenous malformations is presumed to be destruction of large multimers of von Willebrand factor as they are sheered through the aortic valve. These larger multimers are apparently critical to the initial phases of hemostasis.

### *The Physical Exam*

#### Vascular Findings

The carotid pulsations in patients with severe AS are characterized by a delayed and weakened upstroke, the *pulsus parvus et tardus*. In long-standing critical AS, the peripheral pulses also may be weak, and signs of poor perfusion may be present.

#### Cardiac Findings

On palpation, one may feel a systolic thrill in cases of severe AS. The Apex may be laterally displaced if the heart has begun to dilate. The cardiac exam in AS is notable for a crescendo–decrescendo murmur, heard best in the right upper sternal border and radiating to the carotids. Occasionally, the murmur may instead radiate to the apex and mimic mitral regurgitation; this is known as the Gallavardin phenomenon. As AS progresses, the murmur peaks increasingly later in systole until S2 is obliterated, suggesting severe disease. The grade of the murmur correlates with severity of the stenosis, and the presence of a thrill (Grade IV/VI), suggests critical stenosis. An S4 is also frequently appreciated. An ejection click suggests the presence of a bicuspid aortic valve.

The physical exam may be useful in differentiating valvular AS from hypertrophic cardiomyopathy (HCM) and subaortic stenosis. In HCM, the carotid pulsation is on time and is bifid, with a two-component, "spike and dome" contour. This is caused by the presystolic closure of the aortic valve. The PMI pulsation in HCM patients classically has three components, which correspond to atrial filling and the two components of systolic ejection. The murmur in HCM can be differentiated from AS by several maneuvers. Decreasing either preload or afterload will accentuate the murmur of HCM, but will soften the murmur of valvular AS. Thus, a Valsalva maneuver or arising from squatting to standing will accentuate a HCM murmur, but will decrease the murmur of AS. Amyl nitrate will similarly decrease afterload and preload, resulting in marked increase in the HCM murmur.

The murmur of subvalvular stenosis resembles valvular AS. Clues that the murmur might be due to subvalvular stenosis include a younger patient age, the presence of aortic insufficiency, and the absence of an ejection click. In supravalvular AS, blood flow preferentially is directed into the innominate artery, so the murmur of supravalvular stenosis classically radiates to the right neck and subclavian, and may be associated with a thrill over the right carotid. The blood pressure in the right arm may be slightly higher than in the left. Careful auscultation of the lung fields may reveal murmurs associated with peripheral pulmonary stenosis.

### *Key Diagnostic Studies*

#### Electrocardiogram

The electrocardiogram (ECG) in patients with severe AS may show left ventricular hypertrophy (LVH) with concomitant strain pattern, left atrial abnormality, or interventricular conduction delay. Transient third-degree heart block has been described, and has been ascribed to aortic annular calcification impinging on the AV nodal conduction system.

### Chest x-Ray

The chest x-ray (CXR) is often normal in patients with AS, especially because LVH frequently is unaccompanied by dilation early in the disease. With advanced disease, left ventricular hypertrophy and enlargement, aortic dilation, and aortic valvular calcification may be appreciated.

### Transthoracic Echocardiogram

Echocardiography has become the gold standard for diagnosis and quantification of aortic valve disease. Key data that are attained from a transthoracic echocardiogram (TTE) assessment include the following.

***LV Size and Systolic Function.*** Systolic function is usually normal until late in the disease. The left ventricle will show variable hypertrophy, with overall normal size.

***Diastolic Function.*** Early in the disease process, LV compliance decreases and the atrial component of diastolic filling becomes increasingly prominent. Over time, left atrial (LA) pressure rises, and ultimately, patients with long-standing AS may develop restrictive diastolic filling patterns.

***Assessing Aortic Valve Morphology.*** Echocardiography is paramount in identifying the etiology of AS. Standard transthoracic images usually can identify bicuspid or unicuspid valves, can suggest a rheumatic etiology, or can quantify the degree of valvular calcification.

***Assessing the Severity of Aortic Stenosis.*** There are several methods to estimate the severity of AS. Multiple methods should be used in each patient to ensure accurate data.

*Jet velocity:* Peak aortic valve jet velocity provides a rough measure of valve severity and also provides a measure of prognosis. A normal outflow velocity is approximately 1 m/s. Studies have suggested that asymptomatic patients with outflow gradients in excess of 4 m/s will most likely develop symptoms within 2 years (4).

*Valve gradients:* Peak transaortic valve gradients can be estimated using the jet velocity and the modified Bernoulli equation: peak gradient $= 4v^2$, where $v$ is the peak velocity across the valve. Mean gradients are calculated using the velocity time integral (VTI).

*Aortic valve area (AVA):* Aortic valve area most frequently is estimated using planimetry on a parasternal short-axis image of the aortic valve or by using the continuity equation (Fig. 24–2).

*The dimensionless index:* The dimensionless index refers to the ratio of the left ventricular outflow VTI to

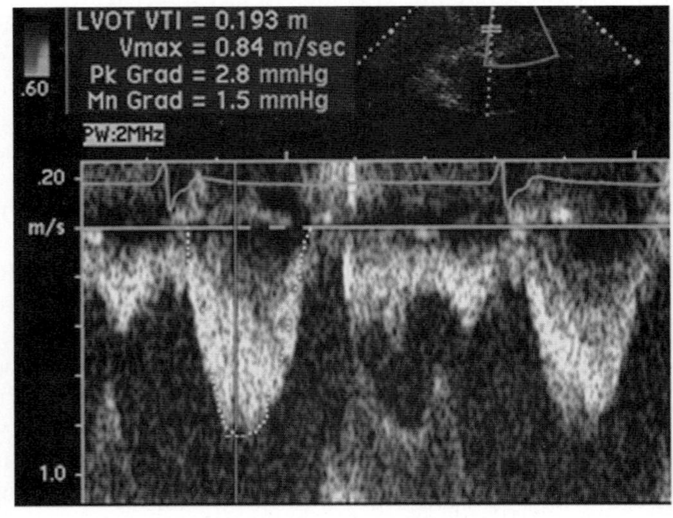


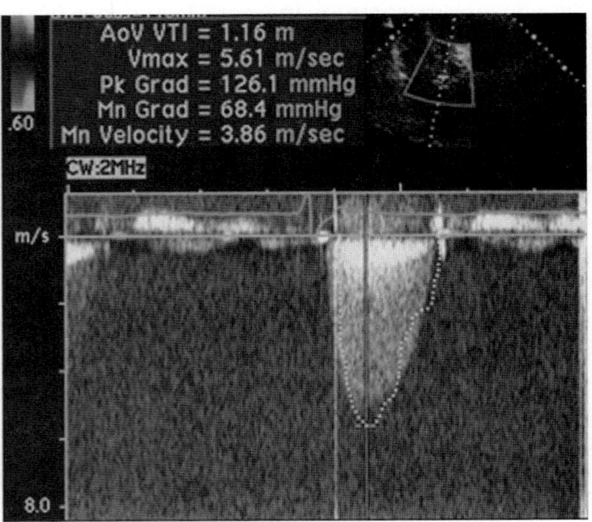


**Figure 24–2** Pulse-wave Doppler flow through the left ventricular outflow tract (LVOT) **(A)** and continuous–wave Doppler flow through the aortic valve **(B)**. The continuous-wave flow allows simple calculation of the peak transaortic gradient: peak $= 4v^2$, where $v$ is equal to the maximum flow across the aortic valve. In this case, $v = 5.6$ m/s, and the peak gradient is given as 126 mm Hg. The aortic valve area can be calculated from the continuity equation, $A_{LVOT}(VTI)_{LVOT} = A_{AV}(VTI)_{AV}$, where $A$ is area and $VTI$ is the velocity time integral, or the flow velocity integrated over the systolic ejection period. In this example, assuming the LVOT diameter is 2 cm,

$$\begin{aligned} A_{AV} &= A_{LVOT}(VTI)_{LVOT}/(VTI)_{AV} \\ &= 3.14\ \text{cm}^2(0.193\ \text{m})/(1.16\ \text{m}) \\ &= 0.55\ \text{cm}^2 \end{aligned}$$

the aortic valve VTI. This ratio allows for a quick, semiquantitative assessment of valve stenosis. An index <25% is consistent with severe stenosis.

Several caveats must be kept in mind when using echo cardiography to assess the severity of AS. First, Doppler echocardiography can underestimate the peak AS gradient if the echo beam is not accurately aligned with the aortic outflow. Therefore, multiple echo windows must be assessed to find the highest transvalvular velocities. Additionally, the modified Bernoulli equation assumes an LVOT velocity of 1 m/s, which may not always be true. If the true LVOT velocity is >1 m/s, then the modified Bernoulli equation will overestimate stenosis severity. Finally, continuous-wave Doppler cannot assess stenoses in series, such as dynamic LVOT obstruction and valvular AS, or subvalvular and valvular AS. In such instances, the use of the continuity equation can be erroneous.

### Invasive Assessment of the Aortic Stenosis

Echocardiography usually is sufficient to determine the severity of AS; however, invasive assessment of AS is sometimes necessary, particularly in cases in which clinical symptoms are not congruent with echo data. (see ACC/AHA Guidelines [6]). During right heart catheterization, Fick cardiac outputs are preferable to thermodilution because they are more reliable in low-output states. During left heart catheterization, simultaneously measured LV and ascending aortic pressures are ideal, although a pullback gradient may be used if the patient is in sinus rhythm. The femoral artery waveform should not be used to estimate aortic pressures. The AVA can be estimated with the Hakki equation: $AVA = CO/\sqrt{(\text{peak or mean transvalvular gradient})}$. A formal calculation can be done with the Gorlin equation (Fig. 24–3).

Invasive hemodynamic assessment measures a peak LV-to-peak aortic gradient across the aortic valve, which is invariably lower than the peak gradient on echocardiography. This is due to the fact that Doppler echocardiography measures the peak instantaneous velocity. The mean transvalvular gradients by echo and catheterization correlate well, however. Occasionally, Doppler gradients greatly exceed gradients on catheterization, which may be due to the phenomenon of pressure recovery. In effect, substantial turbulent flow of blood through the valve may cause the pressure in the aorta to be artificially low immediately distal to the valve. Several centimeters into the proximal aorta, however, laminar flow is restored, and pressure "recovers." Doppler echocardiography detects the maximum pressure gradient between the left ventricle and the proximal aorta. Pressure recovery usually is not an issue with native aortic valves, but can be problematic especially with smaller prosthetic valves.

## Classifications of Severity of Aortic Stenosis

Normal aortic valve area: 2 to 3 $cm^2$
Mild AS: >1.5 $cm^2$
Moderate AS: 1.0 to 1.5 $cm^2$
Severe AS: <1.0 $cm^2$
Mean transvalvular gradient: >50 mm Hg

## Treatment of Patients with Aortic Stenosis

### *Asymptomatic Patients*

Patients with aortic stenosis who have no symptoms may be managed expectantly, as the risk of adverse events—for example, sudden death, cardiac death, or all-cause mortality—is very low in asymptomatic patients (5). Medical therapy includes appropriate endocarditis prophylaxis. Vasodilators should be avoided. According to ACC guidelines (6), serial echocardiography is recommended only every 5 years for patients with mild AS, and every 2 to 3 years for patients with moderate AS, as long as they are clinically stable. For patients with severe AS, surveillance echocardiography may be appropriate on an annual basis or even more frequently.

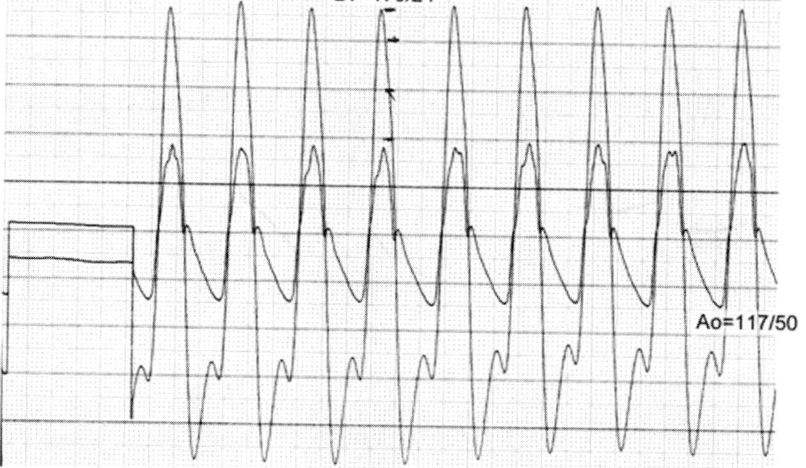


**Figure 24–3** Simultaneous pressure recordings of the left ventricle and aorta. Peak-to-peak gradient is approximately 53 mm Hg. If one knows the cardiac output (*CO*), the Aortic Valve Area (*AVA*) can be estimated with the Hakki equation: $AVA = CO/(\text{peak gradient})^{1/2}$. Assume that the $CO = 4$ L/m. Then

$$AVA = 4/(53)^{1/2} = 4/7.2 = 0.55 \text{ cm}^2$$

(Courtesy of D. Vivek.)

Patients with mild AS are encouraged to keep physically active and may participate in competitive sports. For patients with moderate AS, aerobic activity is permissible; however, competitive contact sports or heavy lifting is not advised. The ACC guidelines suggest evaluating moderate AS patients with a stress test prior to engaging in strenuous activities. Patients with severe AS should not engage in strenuous activity or competitive sports.

Progression of aortic stenosis is highly variable, but on average, valve area decreases approximately 0.1 $cm^2$/year. Progression of AS has been associated with risk factors for coronary artery disease (CAD) (diabetes, hypercholesterolemia, hypertension) in observational studies, and thus treatments of these conditions may be important is AS therapy as well. A more rapid rate of change (>0.3 m/s per year increase in velocity) (7) or a peak jet velocity >4 m/s suggest that patients have <2 years before symptoms will develop (4,7). Heavily calcified valves are also associated with a higher likelihood of symptomatic disease.

Any patient with severe AS should be aware that dyspnea, angina, or presyncope merits prompt evaluation. Symptoms of AS may be insidious, however, and patients may be unaware of a decline in functional capacity. In such cases, stress echocardiography can be useful to assess functional capacity, ventricular function, transvalvular gradients with stress, and the pulmonary artery pressure responses to stress. Such variables may alter the threshold to pursue AVR.

### *Patients with Rheumatic Fever*

Rheumatic fever is an important cause of both aortic and mitral valve disease. Its prevalence has decreased over the past 30 years, largely because of better diagnosis and treatment of group A streptococcal pharyngitis. Acute rheumatic fever is recognized as a serious complication of pharyngeal streptococcal infections, and is due to an autoimmune phenomenon triggered by group A streptococcal M proteins, which mimic cardiac myosin.

Primary prevention of rheumatic fever includes prompt diagnosis of group A streptococcal infections and treatment with appropriate antibiotics, usually a penicillin derivative or macrolide. Patients who develop acute rheumatic fever require long-term secondary prophylaxis, usually with monthly intramuscular injections of benzathine penicillin (Table 24–1).

**TABLE 24–1**
**RECOMMENDATIONS FOR SECONDARY PROPHYLAXIS OF RHEUMATIC FEVER**

| Indication | Recommendation |
|---|---|
| 1. Rheumatic fever with carditis and persistent valvular disease | >10 y or at least until age 40, whichever is longer. Consider life-long prophylaxis if high risk (e.g., health care worker, teacher) |
| 2. Rheumatic fever with carditis but without valve disease | 10 y, or "well into adulthood," whichever is longer. |
| 3. Rheumatic fever without carditis or valve disease | 5 y, or until age 21, whichever is longer. |

*Source:* From The AHA/ACC Task Force Report. *J Am Coll Cardiol.* 1998; 32:1486–1588.

### *Symptomatic Patients*

For patients with severe AS who develop symptoms or experience a decline in LV systolic function, aortic valve replacement is the therapy of choice. The risk of AVR increases with patient age; however, because the prognosis for untreated, severe symptomatic AS is abysmal, age should not be used to exclude patients from valve surgery. Low ejection fraction, heart failure, renal failure, female gender, and atrial fibrillation also are adverse predictors in patients undergoing aortic valve surgery.

Additional ACC/AHA Class I indications (6) for AVR in AS include patients undergoing open-heart surgery for another reason (e.g., valve surgery, coronary artery bypass grafting (CABG), aortic surgery). Class IIa indications for aortic valve replacement (AVR) include patients with moderate AS who are undergoing open-heart surgery for another reason, or patients who have severe asymptomatic AS and abnormal response to exercise or LV dysfunction (Table 24–2). Aortic valve surgery in patients with asymptomatic critical AS is currently a Class IIb recommendation. Nevertheless, in patients with severely calcified valves or with rapidly progressing AS, elective AVR in patients with critical AS seems reasonable, especially as mortality from AVR continues to decline. Recent series report perioperative mortality rates of 3% to 5% in patients <75 year of age who undergo AVR ± CABG (1).

**TABLE 24–2**
**INDICATIONS FOR AORTIC VALVE SURGERY IN PATIENTS WITH SEVERE AS**

| Indication | AHA/ACC Class |
|---|---|
| 1. Patients with symptomatic, severe AS | I |
| 2. Patients with severe AS undergoing open-heart or aortic surgery for another reason | I |
| 3. Patients with moderate AS undergoing open-heart or aortic surgery for another reason | IIa |
| 4. Asymptomatic patients with severe AS and | |
| LV dysfunction | IIa |
| Hypotension with exercise | IIa |
| Ventricular tachycardia | IIb |
| Moderate–severe LVH (>1.5 cm) | IIb |
| Critical AS with AVA <0.6 $cm^2$ | IIb |
| 5. Asymptomatic patients with severe AS and none of the above modifiers | III |

*Source:* From The AHA/ACC Task Force Report. *J Am Coll Cardiol.* 1998; 32:1486–1588.

### *Valve Replacement Options*

#### Mechanical Valves

Mechanical prostheses have excellent longevity but require systemic anticoagulation. For patients with normal ejection fractions, bileaflet or single-leaflet Medtronic Hall valves require an INR of 2 to 3. Older-generation valves should be anticoagulated to an INR of 2.5 to 3.5. Additionally, any patient with atrial fibrillation, depressed LV function, prior thromboembolism, or a hypercoagulable state should have a target INR of 2.5 to 3.5. Mechanical valves should especially be considered in younger patients (<65 years of age), patients with renal disease, and those with calcium-handling metabolic disorders. Younger women who wish to have children are better served with a biologic valve until after their child-bearing years.

#### Biologic Valves

Porcine valve or bovine pericardial tissue valves do not require anticoagulation, but have shorter life spans than mechanical valves. In older patients, tissue valves may be expected to last 10 to 15 years, but have an expected lifespan of <10 years in younger patients. Therefore, tissue valves should be considered for patients >age 65 years, and in patients for whom anticoagulation is problematic. All patients with tissue valves should be treated with aspirin (81 mg daily).

#### Homografts

Cadaveric homografts are the valve of choice for patients with active infective endocarditis because they may resist infection more than tissue or mechanical valves. Additionally, they do not require long-term anticoagulation. However, the durability of homografts is no better than that of tissue valves, and reoperation is much more challenging with homografts than with mechanical or other tissue valves.

#### Ross Procedure

The Ross procedure transplants the pulmonic valve into the aortic position and places a homograft in the pulmonic position. This operation may be appropriate at experienced centers for younger patients who have not completed their growth cycle, as studies suggest that the native pulmonic valve (autograft) may grow with the patient when implanted at the aortic position. However, in the long term it creates double-valve pathology from a single-valve problem, and therefore has a limited role in aortic valve disease.

#### Balloon Valvuloplasty

Balloon valvuloplasty may be a very effective therapy for children or very young adults with congenital, noncalcific AS (Table 24–3). However, because of a high rate of major complications and poor intermediate- to long-term results, this intervention has a very limited role in the treatment of adults with aortic stenosis. Patients may experience short-term (<6 months) symptomatic and hemodynamic benefit from balloon valvuloplasty; however, most redevelop significant symptoms by 6 to 12 months postprocedure. Balloon valvuloplasty may be beneficial in temporizing symptoms until a definitive valve surgery can be performed—for example, in patients with cardiogenic shock who are too ill to undergo immediate surgery, or in patients with severe symptomatic AS who need an urgent noncardiac surgery. Nevertheless, balloon valvuloplasty can never be considered a replacement therapy for valve surgery. Current indications for valvuloplasty in adult, calcific AS are limited and are listed in Table 24–4.

**TABLE 24–3**
**RECOMMENDATIONS FOR BALLOON VALVULOPLASTY IN YOUNG PATIENTS WITH NONCALCIFIC AS**

| Indication | ACC/AHA Class |
|---|---|
| 1. Symptomatic patients with peak gradient >50 mm Hg | I |
| 2. Peak gradient >60 mm Hg, regardless of symptoms | I |
| 3. ECG abnormalities suggestive of ischemia and peak gradient >50 mm Hg | I |
| 4. Peak gradient >50 mm Hg in a patient wishing to play competitive sports or desiring pregnancy | IIa |
| 5. Asymptomatic gradient <50 mm Hg | III |

*Source:* From The AHA/ACC Task Force Report. *J Am Coll Cardiol.* 1998; 32:1486–1588.

## LOW-GRADIENT AORTIC STENOSIS VERSUS PSEUDO-STENOSIS

Patients with LV dysfunction and aortic stenosis present a challenging diagnostic dilemma. Because gradients across

**TABLE 24–4**
**INDICATIONS FOR BALLOON VALVULOPLASTY IN ADULT PATIENTS WITH SEVERE, CALCIFIC AS**

| Indication | ACC/AHA Class |
|---|---|
| 1. Temporizing hemodynamically unstable patients who are at high risk for AVR until definitive valve surgery can be performed | IIa |
| 2. Palliation therapy for patients who are not operative candidates | IIb |
| 3. Temporizing patients who require urgent noncardiac surgery | IIb |
| 4. Alternative to AVR in patients who are operative candidates for valve surgery | III |

*Source:* From The AHA/ACC Task Force Report. *J Am Coll Cardiol.* 1998; 32:1486–1588.

the valve are proportional to flow and inversely proportional to valve area, an abnormally low flow state can cause low gradients regardless of valve stenosis. In patients who have LV dysfunction, low transvalvular gradients, and suspected severe AS, it is critically important to determine if the poor cardiac output is due in part to severe AS, because these patients will benefit from AVR. However, if there is intrinsic myocardial dysfunction, the LV may not generate sufficient flow to maximally open a mildly stenotic valve. In such patients, the measured gradients may overestimate stenotic severity, leading to "pseudo-stenosis." These patients have a poor prognosis and should not undergo AVR. Dobutamine echocardiography has been used to differentiate low-gradient AS from pseudo-stenosis and to assess LV contractile reserve. In the presence of true stenosis, dobutamine will increase or normalize cardiac output, improve LV contractile function and ejection fraction, and lead to increased transvalvular gradients. In true AS, the dimensionless index and valve area will not change significantly with increased cardiac output. Conversely, in patients with pseudo-stenosis, an increase in cardiac output will augment LVOT velocities more so than transvalvular velocities, leading to an increase in both the dimensionless index and the calculated valve area. Therefore, after administration of dobutamine, indications to proceed to AVR include a significant increase in transvalvular gradients, an increase in LV ejection fraction >5%, and no significant change in the dimensionless index or calculated AVA.

## AORTIC INSUFFICIENCY

### Pathophysiology of Aortic Insufficiency

Whereas AS is purely an LV pressure overload, aortic insufficiency (AI) provokes both pressure and volume overload, creating the largest increase in afterload of any valvular condition. The volume overload is a direct result of the aortic insufficiency. In turn, the regurgitation leads to an increased stroke volume through a relatively fixed outflow orifice and into the relatively high-pressure aorta, resulting in chronic pressure overload. Initially, LV compliance rises and the cavity dilates to maintain adequate forward stroke volume. Concomitantly, the LV hypertrophies eccentrically to minimize wall stress. LVEDP thus remains normal early in the disease. As the AI progresses, the ventricle progressively dilates and outpaces hypertrophy, leading to increased EDP and afterload. Ultimately, the LV ejection fraction declines, and irreversible myocardial dysfunction results.

### Etiology of Aortic Insufficiency

It is useful to divide causes of AI into primary (valvular) and secondary (aortic) causes.

#### Valvular Causes of Aortic Insufficiency

*Bicuspid aortic valves* are a common cause of AI, and especially are associated with aortic root dilatation.

*Infective endocarditis* can cause acute AI, particularly in patients with pre-existing valve pathology, such as a bicuspid valve.

*Rheumatic heart disease* AS, AI or a combination of both.

*Radiation heart disease.*

*Subaortic stenosis* is a rare cause of severe AI. The turbulent jet flow caused by the subvalvular stenosis frequently leads to progressive destruction of the aortic valve.

*Drugs:* Anorectic drugs such as fenfluramine and phentermine have been shown to cause thickening of aortic and mitral valve leaflets, leading to regurgitation. Likewise, ergots have been shown to cause a similar pathology.

#### Secondary Causes of Aortic Insufficiency

*Aortic root dilatation:* There are multiple causes of aortic root dilatation that may lead to severe AI. Some of the most clinically relevant include bicuspid aortic valve and Marfan disease, both of which cause root dilatation via cystic medial necrosis. Aortitis due to syphilis and collagen-vascular disease (e.g., Takayasu disease, ankylosing spondylitis, giant-cell arteritis) also may precipitate AI.

*Aortic dissection:* Type A aortic dissections are a major cause of severe acute AI.

*VSD:* Supracristal VSDs can lead to aortic insufficiency by causing aortic leaflet prolapse. Even if they are small, these VSDs should be closed early on to prevent aortic valve pathology.

### Clinical Findings

#### Acute Aortic Insufficiency

Acute aortic insufficiency most often results from infective endocarditis, trauma, or aortic dissection. On history, patients may have conditions that predispose them to these complications, such as a biscuspid valve, Marfan disease, or a known aortic aneurysm. The physical exam frequently shows profound hemodynamic compromise, with hypotension, tachycardia, and heart failure. It may be difficult to appreciate a diastolic murmur, because aortic diastolic pressure and LVEDP equilibrate very rapidly. Thus, unlike chronic AI, the murmur is only early diastolic. Because the LV does not have time to dilate and increase stroke volume, physical findings of a displaced PMI and wide pulse pressure are absent.

#### Chronic Aortic Insufficiency

Chronic AI, even when severe, is usually well tolerated for many years. Thus, many patients have AI diagnosed before the onset of symptoms. Early symptoms most often include dyspnea on exertion and a decline in exercise capacity. More progressive disease may lead to frank symptoms of heart failure, particularly as the LV function begins to decline. As with AS, patients with chronic AI may develop angina, regardless of obstructive coronary lesions.

## Physical Exam

### *Vascular Findings*

The peripheral vascular hallmark of severe AI is a widened pulse pressure characterized by a brisk systolic upstroke followed by a rapid diastolic collapse, which corresponds to reversal of flow in the aorta. Multiple eponyms have been ascribed to this phenomenon, and include Corrigan pulses ("waterhammer" carotid pulsation) and Quincke pulses (systolic blushing of the nail beds). A bisferiens carotid pulsation, with two systolic peaks, may also be appreciated in severe AI. (Chapter 5)

### *Cardiac Findings*

On palpation, one may appreciate a laterally displaced PMI or a thrill. The classic AI auscultatory signs include a diminished mitral closing sound, and a decrescendo, blowing, holodiastolic murmur, appreciated best at end-expiration with the patient leaning forward. Classically, a diastolic murmur at the right sternal border indicates aortic dilation with secondary AI, and a left sternal border location indicates primary valvular AI. A soft systolic murmur may also be heard at the aortic position as a result of increased flow across the valve. Occasionally, severe AI creates a low-pitched, mitral stenosis–like murmur, the Austin–Flint murmur. The exact mechanism of this murmur is not clear, but it occurs when the AI jet hits the anterior leaflet of the mitral valve. An ejection click suggests a bicuspid valve.

## Key Studies

### *Electrocardiogram*

The ECG classically shows LVH.

### *Chest X-ray*

Chronic severe AI leads to an increase in LV size and mass. Thus, the CXR frequently shows cardiomegaly with an enlarged LV. The aorta may be aneurysmal in patients with secondary AI.

### *Echocardiography*

As with most valvular disease, the most useful noninvasive assessment is with Doppler echocardiography. When assessing a patient with substantial aortic insufficiency, there are several key considerations.

1. *LV size and ejection fraction:* In patients with severe, asymptomatic AI, both LV size and function must be carefully monitored, because both parameters may guide decisions for valve surgery.
2. *Aortic pathology:* Particularly in patients with secondary AI, a careful assessment for aortic pathology is mandatory. In many patients, progressive dilation of the aorta dictates AVR and aortic surgery before the aortic insufficiency becomes severe.
3. *Aortic valve morphology:* Careful assessment of the valve itself may give clues to the etiology of regurgitation. Bicuspid valves, leaflet prolapse, presence of vegetations, and rheumatic changes all can be diagnosed or suggested by transthoracic images.
4. *Assessing the severity of AI:* There are multiple methods for assessing AI severity. No single measurement is definitive, so several methods should be used to evaluate the AI severity.
   a. Regurgitant jet width (vena contracta) in the parasternal long-axis view: A vena contracta width >50% of the LVOT width suggests severe AI.
   b. Presence of a proximal isovelocity surface area (PISA): a PISA suggests at least moderate AI, and allows calculation of a regurgitant orifice area. An ROA >0.3 cm$^2$ suggests severe AI.
   c. Pressure half-time: Pressure half-time (PHT) refers to how fast the pressure gradient across the aortic valve in diastole is reduced by half. Rapid reduction in the pressure gradient (PHT <250 milliseconds) suggests severe AI, whereas slow degradation of the gradient (PHT >400 milliseconds) suggests milder disease. PHT is dependent on multiple variables, including systemic vascular resistance and LV and aortic compliance, and thus changes in these variables reduce the utility of PHT.
   d. Diastolic flow reversal in the descending aorta: If the reversed flow is pan-diastolic and exceeds 25 cm/s, severe AI is likely (Fig. 24–4).
   e. M-mode echocardiography: On classic M-mode imaging, fluttering of the mitral valve is seen with moderate to severe AI. Fluttering may be seen in both acute and chronic AI. In severe acute AI, premature closure of the mitral valve is also seen. Diastolic mitral regurgitation may be noted on color M-mode or color Doppler (Fig. 24–5).

## Treatment of Aortic Insufficiency

### *Acute Aortic Insufficiency*

Because acute severe AI is poorly tolerated, emergency or urgent surgery is advised. If a delay is necessary before surgery, IV vasodilators become the treatment of choice. Increasing the heart rate will decrease the diastolic period, anmay temporize the hemodynamic effects of acute severe AI. Intra-aortic balloon pumps are absolutely contraindicated in severe AI.

### *Chronic Aortic Insufficiency*

#### Asymptomatic Patients

Chronic AI is usually well tolerated for years before symptoms develop. In asymptomatic patients with normal LV function and severe compensated AI, the progression rate

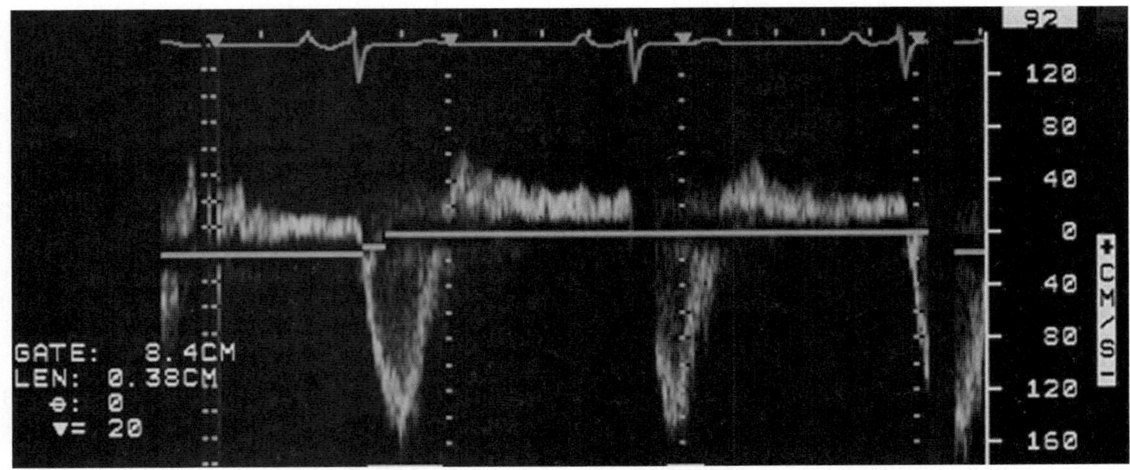


**Figure 24–4** Continuous-wave Doppler flow profile in the descending aorta, showing flow reversal at approximately 30 cm/s. This profile suggests severe aortic insufficiency.

to symptoms is 4% per year, and the progression to LV dysfunction is 1.3% per year. The risk of sudden death is very low in asymptomatic patients (<0.2% per year). Once LV dysfunction develops, symptoms will likely follow within 3 years. Once symptoms develop, the rate of mortality increases to 10% per year.

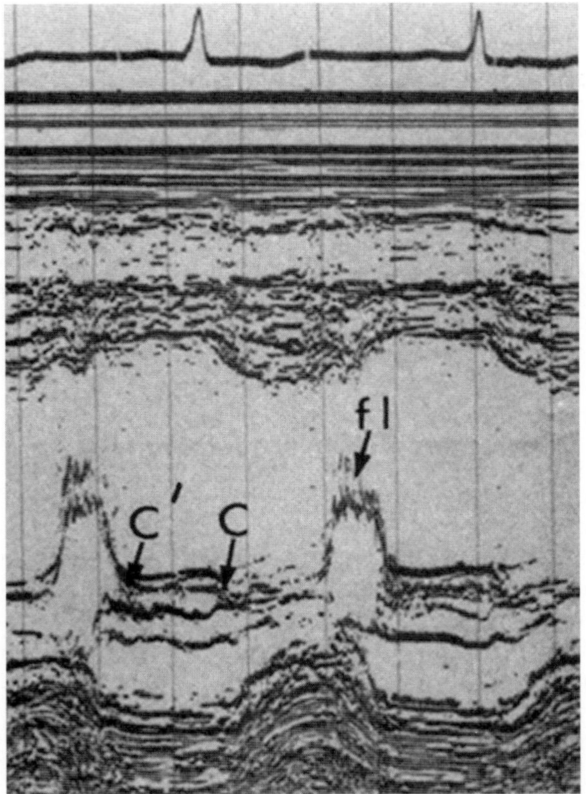


**Figure 24–5** M-mode image through the mitral valve in a patient with severe acute AI. Classic findings shown include fluttering of the anterior leaflet (fl) and early closure of the mitral valve (c′).

### Medical Treatment

Medical therapy for patients with severe AI includes endocarditis prophylaxis and afterload reduction with vasodilators. Vasodilators carry an ACC/AHA Class I recommendation for patients with severe AI, normal LV function, and mild–moderate LV dilatation. They also should be used in patients with AI who have hypertension (Table 24–5). Dihydropyridine calcium channel blockers are first-line agents, although ACE inhibitors are frequently used as well. For patients with mild–moderate AI, yearly exams and biannual echocardiograms are sufficient follow-up if clinical symptoms are stable. For patients with severe AI, follow-up with echocardiography should be done every 6 months.

**TABLE 24–5**
**INDICATIONS FOR VASODILATOR THERAPY IN PATIENTS WITH SEVERE AORTIC INSUFFICIENCY**

| Indication | ACC/AHA Class |
|---|---|
| 1. Severe AI with LV dysfunction when surgery is not possible | I |
| 2. Severe asymptomatic AI with normal systolic function, but mild–moderate LV dilatation | I |
| 3. Treatment of hypertension in patients with any AI | I |
| 4. Long-term ACE inhibitor therapy in patients post-AVR with persistent LV dysfunction | I |
| 5. Long-term therapy in asymptomatic patients with normal systolic function and mild–moderate AI | III |
| 6. Long-term therapy in patients who have indication for AVR instead of valve surgery | III |

*Source:* From The AHA/ACC Task Force Report. *J Am Coll Cardiol.* 1998;32:1486–1588.

For patients with mild–moderate secondary AI due to aortic root dilatation (>4.5 cm), beta-blockers can be used carefully to decrease aortic wall stress. Relative bradycardia, however, may worsen the AI. On follow-up exams, care must be taken to ensure that aortic process is stable.

## Indications for Surgery

Patients with severe AI who have symptoms, LV dilatation or dysfunction, or (in the case of secondary AI) who have enlarging aortas should undergo valve surgery. ACC/AHA indications for aortic valve surgery for aortic insufficiency are listed in Table 24–6. Class I indications for AVR include New York Heart Association (NYHA) Class III–IV patients with normal LV and NYHA Class II patients who have normal LV but evidence of progressive LV dilatation. In addition, patients who have angina, or who are undergoing open-heart surgery for another reason, should have valve surgery performed. Patients with mild symptoms (Class II) but without evidence of LV dilation have a Class IIa indication for AVR. If patients develop a declining LVEF (<50%) or severe LV dilatation with end-systolic diameter >55 mm and end-diastolic diameter >75 mm, valve surgery should be initiated.

**TABLE 24–6**
**INDICATIONS FOR AORTIC VALVE SURGERY IN PATIENTS WITH AORTIC INSUFFICIENCY**

| Indication | AHA/ACC Class |
|---|---|
| 1. Patients with NYHA Class III–IV and normal systolic function | I |
| 2. Patients with NYHA Class II and normal systolic function but progressive dilatation of LV, declining functional capacity, or declining left ventricular function on serial testing | I |
| 3. Patients with angina | I |
| 4. Patients with mild–moderate LV dysfunction, regardless of symptoms | I |
| 5. Patient undergoing open-heart surgery for another reason | I |
| 6. Patients with NYHA Class II symptoms, normal systolic function and stable LV dimensions, functional capacity, and ventricular function on serial testing | IIa |
| 7. Patient who are asymptomatic but who have severe LV dilatation (LV end-diastolic diameter >75 mm, end-systolic diameter >55 mm) | IIa |
| 8. Patients with severe LV dysfunction (EF <25%) | IIb |
| 9. Asymptomatic patients with normal EF and moderate LV cavity dilatation (LVEDd 70–75 mm, ESd 50–55 mm) | IIb |
| 10. Asymptomatic patients with normal LV at rest, but with: | |
| Decrease in EF on stress nuclear study | IIb |
| Decrease in EF on stress echo | III |
| 11. Asymptomatic patients with normal EF and no or mild LV cavity dilatation (LVEDd <70 mm, LVESd <50 mm) | III |

*Source:* From The AHA/ACC Task Force Report. *J Am Coll Cardiol*. 1998; 32:1486–1588.

For patients with aortic root dilatation and significant AI, progression of the aortic diameter >50 mm is generally accepted as an indication for aortic root and aortic valve surgery (6). Lower thresholds (>45 mm) should be considered for patients with Marfan syndrome or bicuspid aortic valves, particularly if the rate of aortic dilatation is accelerating.

Surgical options for AI include valve repair or replacement. Valve repair may be considered for noncalcified bicuspid valves with substantial AI. Repair results for regurgitant trileaflet valves have been disappointing. For valve replacement, the decision to use mechanical versus bioprosthetic valves is based on a number of considerations (see discussion above, for AS). By guidelines, patients younger than age 65 years, and patients with end-stage renal disease or other disorders that affect calcium metabolism, should receive mechanical valves.

# PULMONIC VALVE DISEASE

## Pulmonic Stenosis

Pulmonic stenosis (PS) is nearly always a congenital defect, although very rare cases of acquired disease have been reported with rheumatic heart disease and carcinoid heart disease. PS may be a component of more complex congenital diseases, where it is often associated with a VSD; most frequently, however, PS is an isolated congenital defect (8). Noonan syndrome is classically associated with isolated PS.

### *History and Physical Exam*

Symptoms with PS are rare unless the transvalvular gradient exceeds 50 mm Hg, so mild–moderate stenosis is often subclinical. When symptoms are present, they relate to decreased cardiac output and usually include fatigue, dyspnea on exertion, and decreased functional capacity. With more severe disease, presyncope and syncope may develop.

The hallmark of PS on jugular venous examination is a prominent A wave, which reflects increased right ventricular end-diastolic pressure.

The classic auscultatory findings include a widely split S2, and a crescendo–decrescendo systolic murmur at the pulmonic position. When murmurs are associated with peripheral pulmonary stenoses, they may be heard over the lateral chest wall, the axillae, or in the back. An ejection click may also be appreciated, which moves earlier in systole as the severity of stenosis increases. Signs of severe stenosis include a late-peaking systolic murmur, decreasing intensity of P2, and the complete disappearance of the ejection click. Unlike other right-sided valvular lesions, respiration tends to decrease the intensity of the murmur. Clinical signs of RVH or RV failure do not present until late in the disease.

**TABLE 24–7**
**RECOMMENDATIONS FOR VALVE INTERVENTION IN PATIENTS WITH PULMONIC STENOSIS**

| Indication | AHA/ACC Class |
|---|---|
| 1. Symptomatic PS | I |
| 2. Asymptomatic PS with: | |
| Peak gradient >50 mm Hg | I |
| Peak gradient 40–49 mm Hg | IIa |
| Peak gradient 30–39 mm Hg | IIb |
| Peak gradient <30 mm Hg | III |

*Source:* From The AHA/ACC Task Force Report. *J Am Coll Cardiol.* 1998; 32:1486–1588.

### *Diagnostic Studies*

The *chest x-ray* classically shows asymmetric pulmonary artery enlargement, with a prominent left pulmonary artery. The heart size is usually normal.

The key finding on *echocardiography* is the transpulmonic gradient, which is calculated from the peak jet velocity across the pulmonic valve.

### *Treatment of Pulmonic Stenosis*

Patients with asymptomatic pulmonic stenosis and gradients <50 mm Hg can be followed expectantly. They should receive infective endocarditis (IE) prophylaxis. For patients with elevated gradients or with symptoms, balloon valvotomy is the treatment of choice. Indications for balloon valvotomy are listed in Table 24–7. Class I indications for intervention include symptoms or a resting gradient >50 mm Hg. PS with transvalvular gradients <30 mm Hg should be managed medically.

## Pulmonary Insufficiency

The main etiologies of significant pulmonary insufficiency (PI) are annular dilation due to pulmonary hypertension, dilation of the PA (which may be idiopathic or secondary to Marfan syndrome), a late complication of tetralogy of Fallot repair, or a primary valve disorder, caused by carcinoid, rheumatic disease, or endocarditis.

Mild PI is quite common in normal hearts, and even moderately severe PI is hemodynamically well tolerated. Over long periods of time, however, severe PI may create a volume and pressure overload on the RV, which leads eventually to RV dilation and failure.

### *Physical Findings*

Pulmonic insufficiency is frequently very difficult to appreciate on physical exam, particularly if the pulmonary pressures are normal. On chest palpation, one may appreciate a hyperdynamic RV. On auscultation, PI may be heard as a low-pitched diastolic murmur along the left sternal border, which accentuates with respiration.

In the setting of pulmonary hypertension, PI results in a Graham–Steel murmur, a high-pitched, decrescendo murmur heard best along the left sternal border. It immediately follows an accentuated P2. With respiration, this murmur also increases in intensity.

### *Diagnostic Studies*

The *chest x-ray* may variably show RV enlargement.

Key data to be obtained from *transthoracic echocardiography* include RV size and function, PA size and pressures, and the degree of PI. Stress echocardiography may be used to assess right ventricular function and reserve.

### *Treatment for Pulmonary Insufficiency*

Pulmonary insufficiency usually requires valve surgery only if there is progressive evidence of RV dilatation and failure. Biologic prostheses or homografts are favored because of lower associated thrombotic risk as compared to mechanical prostheses at this position.

## REFERENCES


1. Otto C. Aortic stenosis. In: Otto C. *Valvular Heart Disease*. 2nd ed. Philadelphia: Elsevier; 2004:197–246.
2. Bellamy MF, Pellikka PA, Klarich KW, et al. Association of cholesterol levels, hydroxymethylglutaryl coenzyme-A reductase inhibitor treatment, and progression of aortic stenosis in the community. *J Am Coll Cardiol*. 2002;40:1723–1730.
3. Novaro GM, Tiong IY, Pearce GL, et al. Effect of hydroxymethylglutaryl coenzyme a reductase inhibitors on the progression of calcific aortic stenosis. *Circulation*. 2001;104:2205–2209.
4. Otto CM, Burwash IG, Legget ME, et al. Prospective study of asymptomatic valvular aortic stenosis. Clinical, echocardiographic, and exercise predictors of outcome. *Circulation*. 1997;95(9):2262–2270.
5. Kelly TA, Rothbart RM, Cooper CM, et al. Comparison of outcome of asymptomatic to symptomatic patients older than 20 years of age with valvular aortic stenosis. *Am J Cardiol*. 1988;61(1):123–130.
6. The ACC/AHA guidelines for the management of patients with valvular heart disease. *J Am Coll Cardiol*. 1998;32:1486–588.
7. Rosenhek R, Binder T, Porenta G, et al. Predictors of outcome in severe, asymptomatic aortic stenosis. *N Engl J Med*. 2000;343(9):611–617.
8. Otto C. Right-sided valve disease. In: Otto C. *Valvular Heart Disease*. 2nd ed. Philadelphia: Elsevier; 2004:415–436.


## QUESTIONS

1. A 42-year-old man with hypertension, but no prior cardiac history, presents with increasing dyspnea on exertion. Physical exam reveals a heart rate of 75 beats/min and blood pressure of 175/67. The jugular venous pattern (JVP) is unremarkable. S1 is soft, S2 is normal, and there

is an early systolic sound. There is a soft II/VI SEM at RUSB radiating to the neck, and a III/VI decrescendo, holodiastolic murmur near LLSB. There is also a low-pitched diastolic rumble heard at the apex. The PMI is laterally displaced. Carotid pulsations are brisk and have a rapid upstroke, immediately followed by a second systolic pulsation. Femoral pulses are normal, and are slightly delayed compared to the radial pulse.

Which of the following findings would you *not* expect to see on transthoracic echocardiography?

a. Fluttering of the anterior mitral leaflet on M-mode echocardiography
b. Mitral stenosis
c. Bicuspid aortic valve
d. Dilated LV cavity
e. Coarctation of the aorta

Answer is b: This patient is fairly young and has hypertension with a wide pulse pressure. The cardiac exam suggests a diagnosis of bicuspid aortic valve (younger patient with aortic insufficiency and an ejection click) with significant AI. The holodiastolic murmur is characteristic of chronic AI, and the displaced PMI suggests long-standing disease that has dilated the left ventricle. Likewise, bounding carotids and a bisferiens pulse are classic findings of AI. BAV usually results from fusion of the right and left coronary cusp leaflets, which then causes a posteriorly directed AI jet. This jet frequently hits the anterior leaflet of the mitral valve, which is manifested on M-mode echocardiography as fluttering of the anterior mitral leaflet and on exam as an Austin–Flint murmur. A history of hypertension in a young patient with AI should prompt an evaluation for aortic coarctation, because up to 20% of patients with BAV also have coarctation. On physical exam, the slightly weaker and delayed femoral pulsations suggest that coarctation might be present.

2. You see a 17-year-old male adolescent in clinic, who is referred to you for evaluation of a murmur. He is well developed and physically active. His heart rate is 62 beats/min, and his blood pressure is 110/70. His JVP is normal. The cardiac exam shows normal S1 and S2. There is no third heart sound. There is a III/VI systolic ejection murmur (SEM) at the right upper sternal border (RUSB), which radiates to the carotids, and a soft diastolic murmur along the left sternal border. With Valsalva, the murmur softens. The carotid pulses are slightly delayed. Which of the following diagnoses is most likely?

a. Bicuspid aortic valve
b. Supravalvular AS
c. Subvalvular AS
d. Hypertrophic cardiomyopathy

Answer is c: This patient has typical exam findings of subvalvular stenosis. In practice, subvalvular stenosis can easily be mistaken for native-valve AS. In younger patients, bicuspid or unicuspid valves are the main differential diagnoses—both of which can have findings of AS and AI. However, the absence of any ejection sound argues against aortic valvular pathology. Hypertrophic cardiomyopathy should also be considered in a patient this age; the slight delay in the carotids and the failure of the murmur to augment with Valsalva make HCM less likely.

3. You see a 25-year-old woman in clinic for a murmur. She is mildly mentally retarded but is sociable and conversational. Her eyes are widely spaced and her ears are low set. Her neck is webbed, and you note that she is rather short. Her jugular venous pattern has a prominent A wave. She has a pectus excavatum deformity of her chest. Cardiac exam reveals a sternal lift and a III/VI SEM at the LUSB, radiating to the left neck, which decreases with inspiration. You cannot appreciate any clicks. Which of the following statements is *not* true regarding this woman's condition?

a. The mode of transmission is autosomal dominant.
b. The genetic defect is linked to elastin.
c. This valvular abnormality is not easily treated with valvuloplasty.
d. ASD is a commonly associated cardiac abnormality.

Answer is b: This patient has Noonan syndrome, an autosomal dominant disease characterized by mild mental retardation, characteristic facial features, and a variety of cardiac abnormalities—the most common of which are pulmonary stenosis, peripheral pulmonary stenosis, ASDs, and hypertrophic cardiomyopathy. The physical exam findings are typical of PS with increased a wave, RV left, and a systolic ejection murmur. Unlike other cases of congenital PS, patients with Noonan syndrome tend to have dysplastic pulmonary leaflets that do not cause an ejection click. They also are frequently not amenable to balloon valvuloplasty. Mutations in the gene for elastin are associated with supravalvular AS.

4. A 75-year-old man with prior bypass surgery is referred to you for shortness of breath and heart failure symptoms. He has a past history of hypertension and chronic obstructive pulmonary disease (COPD). His $FEV_1$ is 1.6 L. He also complains of occasional exertional angina. A recent adenosine nuclear scan revealed a fixed defect in the inferior wall, but no reversible defects. On gated images, the ejection fraction was 25%.

On physical exam, his heart rate is 80 beats/min and his blood pressure is 110/80. He appears fatigued and somewhat frail. His JVP is elevated to 10 cm. He has bibasilar rales on pulmonary exam. Cardiac exam shows a normal S1 and a paradoxically split S2. There is a harsh III/VI SEM at the LSB, which peaks very late in systole and radiates to the carotids. A II/VI HSM is appreciated at the apex that radiates to the axilla. Carotid pulsations are delayed.

You order an echocardiogram that confirms the severe LV systolic dysfunction. His LV is mildly dilated. The entire inferior and basal posterior walls are akinetic and thinned. The LAD and LCx territory is hypokinetic and hypertrophied. The aortic valve is heavily calcified and has poor leaflet excursion. Peak and mean gradients across the aortic valve are 27 and 17 mm Hg, respectively. By continuity, the AVA is 0.8 $cm^2$. There is 2+ mitral regurgitation due to posterior leaflet restriction. What is your next step in this patient's management?

a. Suggest left heart catheterization to pursue percutaneous balloon valvuloplasty.
b. Refer for cardiac surgery for AVR and MV repair.
c. Institute diuretic therapy and afterload reduction to treat his congestive heart failure (CHF).
d. Order dobutamine stress echocardiography.

Answer is d: This patient has low-gradient AS with moderately severe LV dysfunction. His chief complaint is consistent with AS, but could be secondary to CHF or COPD. His physical exam, with narrow pulse pressure, paradoxically split S2, and SEM radiating to the carotids, all suggest AS. Loss of A2 is also consistent with severe AS. The nuclear stress test argues against ischemia. A relatively small fixed defect on nuclear study and preserved wall thickness in the left coronary territory both suggest that the LV dysfunction may be out of proportion to CAD, and may be secondary to valvular disease. For patients with low-gradient AS, dobutamine echo can be very helpful in assessing true stenosis versus pseudo-stenosis. In this patient, we would expect dobutamine to result in an increased EF (contractile reserve), increased gradients across the valve, and a valve area that remained severe. If he has pseudo-stenosis and a cardiomyopathy unrelated to the valve disease, dobutamine will increase cardiac output, but will not result in significant increases in the transaortic gradient or AVA. Patients with LV dysfunction who have contractile reserve and severe AS should undergo AVR. This patient has no contraindications to surgery, and thus valvuloplasty should not be considered definitive treatment.

**5.** A 37-year-old woman with an active history of IV drug abuse presents to the Emergency Department with abrupt-onset shortness of breath. She is tachycardic to 110 beats/min and has a systolic blood pressure of 95 mm Hg. Her boyfriend reports that over the past 7 days she has been febrile and anorectic. He also adds that the patient was "born with an abnormal" aortic valve. Which of the following findings is inconsistent with acute AI?

a. Diminished S1 on auscultation
b. Diastolic MR on echocardiography
c. A holodiastolic murmur heard at the left sternal border.
d. Premature closure of the mitral valve on 2-D echocardiography

Answer is c: Acute AI typically has a brief, early diastolic murmur. Rapid equilibration of aortic and LVED pressures causes termination of the murmur by mid-diastole. All of the remaining answers are typical of acute AI. A diminished S1 may be seen in acute or chronic AI.

# Mitral and Tricuspid Valve Disease

25

*Mehdi H. Shishehbor* *William J. Stewart*

Mitral valve disease is a common valvular abnormality, resulting from various etiologies and having well-understood, varied, and interesting clinical manifestations. Tricuspid valve disease is less common, occurring most often as a functional result of left-sided heart disease and/or pulmonary hypertension.

## MITRAL VALVE ANATOMY

The mitral valve apparatus consists of anterior and posterior leaflets, chordae tendineae, anterolateral and posteromedial papillary muscles, and mitral annulus. To be inclusive, it also includes the atrial and ventricular myocardium. Mitral valve dysfunction may result from aberrations of any portion of the mitral valve apparatus, as a result of mechanical, traumatic, infectious, degenerative, congenital, or metabolic causes.

## MITRAL VALVE PROLAPSE

Mitral valve prolapse (MVP) is found in approximately 2% of the population and occurs equally commonly in men and women. It is the most common cause of mitral regurgitation in the United States. Most such patients have a minor amount of mitral regurgitation and therefore a benign prognosis, with no significant cardiovascular symptoms or manifestations such as congestive heart failure. The diagnosis of MVP is made usually by bedside physical examination, finding a mid-to-late systolic click or multiple clicks, sometimes associated with a late systolic or pansystolic murmur. The murmur becomes earlier and louder with standing and the Valsalva maneuver, resulting from reduction in preload, which brings the mitral leaflets closer together before left ventricular contraction. The murmur of mitral prolapse becomes softer and later with squatting due to an increase in preload.

The diagnosis of MVP is best confirmed echocardiographically. The best two-dimensional echocardiogram criterion is leaflet displacement beyond the line of the mitral annulus in the long-axis view. Because of the saddle-shaped configuration of the mitral valve, caution must be taken when MVP is diagnosed only from apical four- and two-chamber views. Hence, a parasternal or apical long-axis view is required for diagnosis of MVP. M-mode criteria require 2 or 3 mm of displacement, either as late systolic or holosystolic hammocking (Fig. 25–1). The presence of an eccentric jet direction of mitral regurgitation makes the diagnosis of MVP more likely. In general, prolapse with leaflet thickness greater than 5 mm is considered "classic" MVP, whereas prolapse with thinner valve leaflets, less than 5 mm in thickness, is considered "nonclassic prolapse."

Accepted indications (1) for performing echocardiographic study in mitral prolapse include establishing the diagnosis, determining the severity of mitral regurgitation, evaluating leaflet morphology, and defining left ventricular (LV) size and function. The list implies that echo cardiography should be used when it can add information to findings available from history and the physical examination. Indications for echo cardiography may also include exclusion of mitral valve prolapse in patients diagnosed with mitral valve prolapse when there is no clinical evidence to support the diagnosis (Table 25–1). Subsequent or serial echocardiograms are not usually necessary if the patient is asymptomatic, unless there are clinical indications of

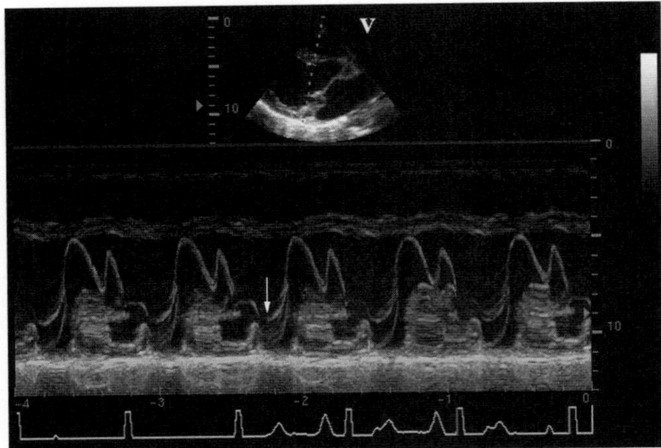

**Figure 25–1** M-mode echocardiography showing late-systolic prolapse of the mitral valve.

severe or worsening mitral regurgitation. Most patients with mitral prolapse should have antibiotic prophylaxis for endocarditis if there is a murmur, or if the echocardiogram shows significant mitral regurgitation (Table 25–2).

The natural history of MVP is frequently benign. Follow-up studies in large population samples show that most patients with MVP do quite well, without developing significant congestive heart failure, atrial fibrillation, stroke, or syncope (2). After a prolonged asymptomatic interval, a small percentage of patients develop more severe mitral regurgitation (MR), ruptured mitral valve chordae (flail), left atrial and ventricular enlargement, or atrial fibrillation. In addition, with gradual progression of mitral regurgitation, LV dilatation and dysfunction may occur, leading to congestive heart failure. In addition, patients with MVP have a significantly increased risk of developing infective endocarditis. Predictors of infective endocarditis in patients MVP include male gender, age >45 years, the presence of mitral regurgitation, and leaflet thickening and redundancy. Patients with MVP also have an increased risk of sudden death, most likely secondary to ventricular tachyarrhythmias, when they also have systolic dysfunction, moderate to severe mitral regurgitation, and redundant chordae.

Mitral valve prolapse has been associated with multiple nonspecific symptoms such as palpitations, atypical chest pain, syncope, and anxiety, and the constellation of these findings has been frequently termed "MVP syndrome." No such associations have been found in multiple studies, but a small group of patients may have a complex set of symptoms associated with MVP. For example, a few studies have shown a pattern of autonomic dysfunction, with increased catecholamines and decreased vagal tone, in patients with MVP.

A substantial negative effect on survival has been seen in patients who develop left ventricular dysfunction, atrial fibrillation, left atrial enlargement, age >50 years, and flail mitral leaflet (3). Recently, quantitatively severe regurgitation has also been associated with adverse prognosis (4).

The mainstay of medical management of patients with MVP is reassurance. Beta-Blockers are the treatment of choice for patients with increased adrenergic symptoms such as palpitations, chest pain, or anxiety. In patients with MVP and transient ischemic attacks (TIA) or stroke, the treatment is usually just aspirin (81 to 325 mg/day).

**TABLE 25–1**

**RECOMMENDATIONS FOR ECHOCARDIOGRAPHY IN MITRAL VALVE PROLAPSE (MVP)**

| Indication | Class |
|---|---|
| 1. Diagnosis, assessment of hemodynamic severity of mitral regurgitation, leaflet morphology, and ventricular compensation in patients with physical signs of MVP | I |
| 2. To exclude MVP in patients who have been given the diagnosis when there is no clinical evidence to support the diagnosis | I |
| 3. To exclude MVP in patients with first-degree relatives with known myxomatous valve disease | IIa |
| 4. Risk stratification in patients with physical signs of MVP or known MVP | IIa |
| 5. To exclude MVP in patients in the absence of physical findings suggestive of MVP or a positive family history | III |
| 6. Routine repetition of echocardiography in patients with MVP with mild or no regurgitation and no change in clinical signs or symptoms | III |

*Source:* From the ACC/AHA Guidelines for the Clinical Application of Echocardiography, (reference 1).

**TABLE 25–2**

**RECOMMENDATIONS FOR ANTIBIOTIC ENDOCARDITIS PROPHYLAXIS FOR PATIENTS WITH MITRAL VALVE PROLAPSE (MVP) UNDERGOING PROCEDURES ASSOCIATED WITH BACTEREMIA[a]**

| Indication | Class |
|---|---|
| 1. Patients with characteristic systolic click-murmur complex | I |
| 2. Patients with isolated systolic click and echocardiographic evidence of MVP and mitral regurgitation | I |
| 3. Patients with isolated systolic click, echocardiographic evidence of high-risk MVP | IIa |
| 4. Patients with isolated systolic click and equivocal or no evidence of MVP | III |

[a]These procedures are defined in the American Heart Association Guidelines for prevention of endocarditis and in the full-text version of these guidelines, (reference 1).

Warfarin may be indicated in some patients with MVP and recurrent TIA or stroke. In addition, in patients with atrial fibrillation from mitral valve disease or any other etiology, there should be a low threshold for instituting anticoagulation, individualized for the patient's risks of stroke versus bleeding. In general, patients <65 of age with no cardiovascular risk factors can be treated with aspirin only; however, warfarin should be added for those with multiple cardiac risk factors or those >65 years old.

Surgical consideration for MVP with regurgitation is similar to that for other forms of nonischemic severe mitral regurgitation and is discussed later. The timing of surgery depends on heart failure symptoms, severity of MR, LV function, presence or absence of arrhythmias such as atrial fibrillation, and the dimensions of LV at end-systole. When it is feasible, mitral valve repair is the operation of choice for individuals with severe MR due to prolapse that requires surgery.

## ACUTE MITRAL REGURGITATION

Acute mitral regurgitation is an uncommon medical condition of grave importance, requiring urgent medical and surgical intervention. Acute disruption of mitral valve leaflets, chordae tendineae, or papillary muscles can result from infective endocarditis, acute myocardial infarction, trauma, or rheumatic fever. The most common cause is probably myocardial ischemia leading to severe mitral regurgitation and acute pulmonary edema, as part of an acute coronary syndrome.

High left atrial pressure and reduced left atrial compliance secondary to severe mitral regurgitation are the mechanisms of pulmonary edema. A less common complication of severe acute MR is reduced forward flow and cardiogenic shock. Acute MR usually presents as sudden and marked increased in congestive heart failure symptoms, with weakness, fatigue, dyspnea, and sometimes respiratory failure and shock. Peripheral vasoconstriction, pallor, and diaphoresis are usually associated presenting signs. In some patients, a loud systolic murmur and a diastolic rumble or third heart sound are heard. In others, no murmur is heard, because the lack of atrial compliance leads to equalization of pressures between the left atrium and ventricle midway through systole. In addition, the acute nature of the condition obscures the mitral murmur by other aspects of the patient's distress, including orthopnea, precluding a good exam in the left lateral decubitus position.

Echocardiography is the diagnostic procedure of choice. In acute coronary syndromes, emergency catheterization and cardiac surgery are life saving. There is little use for contrast left ventricular angiography, except in cases where there is discrepancy in clinical and noninvasive findings. In some cases, hemodynamic measurements and monitoring may also be helpful in management.

Acute mitral regurgitation after myocardial infarction is discussed in detail in another chapter of this book. It is the cause of about 7% of cases of cardiogenic shock after myocardial infarction. The onset of the MR is most commonly between days 2 and 7 after myocardial infarction. It most often involves the posteromedial papillary muscle, which derives its blood supply solely from the right coronary artery, as opposed to the anterolateral papillary muscle, which has a dual blood supply from the circumflex and left anterior descending arteries. Despite the devastating effects of acute MR, the infarct size is sometimes limited (<25% of LV) with a mild to moderate enzyme leak.

Hemodynamic stabilization with prompt surgical intervention is the most effective therapy for most cases of acute mitral regurgitation. Vasodilator therapy with intravenous nitroprusside and nitroglycerine may lead to decreased MR, increased forward flow, and reduced pulmonary congestion. If there is no appreciable aortic regurgitation, intra-aortic balloon counterpulsation reduces regurgitant volume and LV filling pressure, while increasing forward output and mean arterial pressure, and is frequently used for initial stabilization, as a bridge to prompt surgical intervention.

## CHRONIC MITRAL REGURGITATION

The physiology of mitral regurgitation includes a number of classical features (Fig. 25–2). The patient with mitral regurgitation of any cause usually has a pansystolic murmur, best audible at the apex, often radiating to the axilla. In severe MR, this murmur also may be heard in the left paravertebral area of the back. The pulmonic component of the second heart sound may be louder than normal if there is pulmonary hypertension. An inflow sound (a third heart sound or an early diastolic rumble) at the apex may be heard in some patients if the mitral regurgitation is severe. The apical impulse is enlarged, displaced laterally, and exaggerated, reflecting the hyperdynamic left ventricular motion. Left atrial pressure (and pulmonary capillary wedge pressure) is elevated by the regurgitant flow, with an associated systolic V wave, though its height is not a reliable measure of the severity of MR. The left atrium and the diastolic size of the left ventricle are enlarged. As pulmonary venous pressure becomes elevated, dyspnea or even pulmonary congestion may occur. In the later phase, pulmonary hypertension may develop, causing pulmonary artery dilation, right-sided heart failure, and systemic venous congestion.

Untreated chronic mitral valve abnormalities often lead to a common endpoint, with left atrial enlargement, pulmonary hypertension, atrial fibrillation, myocardial dysfunction, and left-sided congestive heart failure (5). If the situation is not corrected, it may progress to include left atrial thrombosis, hemoptysis, and right-sided heart failure. Cardiac output is usually normal in the early phases,

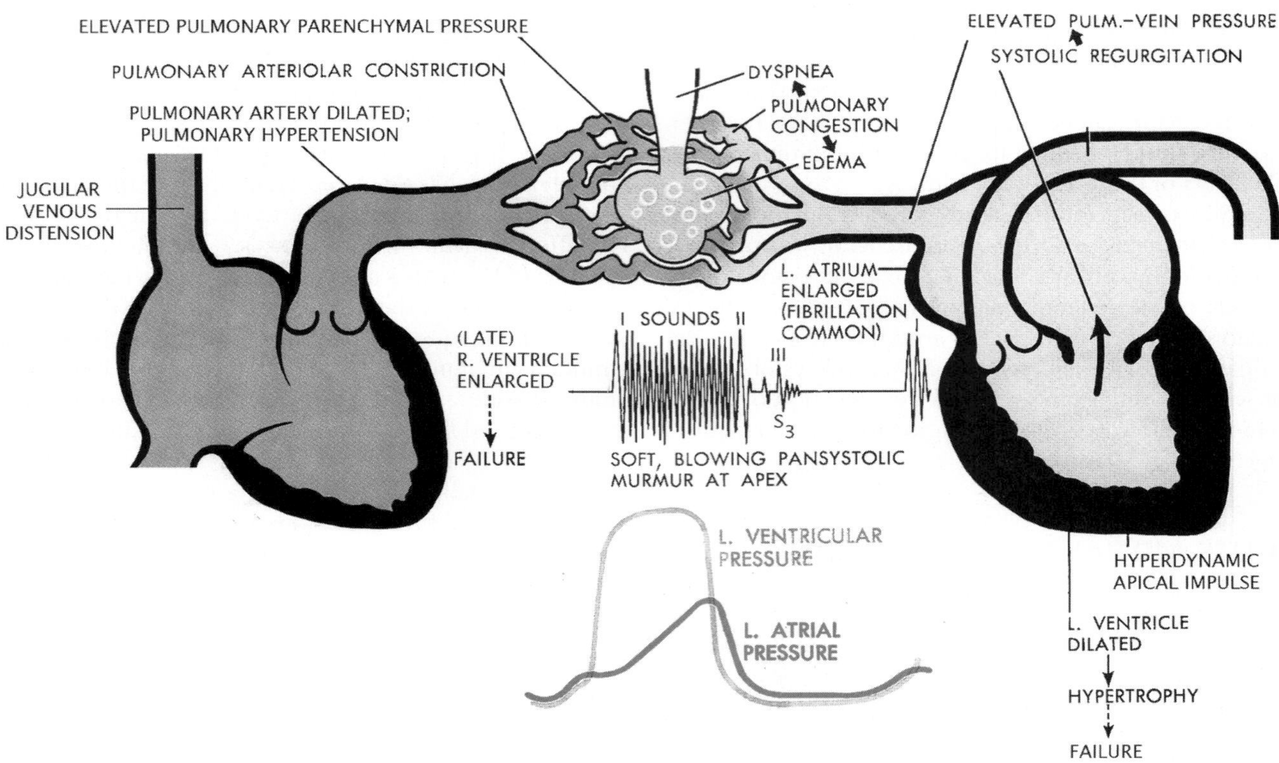


**Figure 25–2** Schematic diagram representing pathologic complications of chronic mitral regurgitation. (Adapted from Netter's volume 5, section II, plate 49, and page 88.)

but is reduced in the later phases of the disease if the MR goes untreated.

The natural history of chronic mitral regurgitation may involve many years of being asymptomatic, the so-called compensated phase of MR. In early years, chronic mitral regurgitation leads to increased LV size and mass and increased LV end-diastolic volume associated with a normal or elevated ejection fraction. At this stage there are few or no symptoms, because the dilated and compliant left atrium and LV allow accommodation of the regurgitant volume at normal filling pressures. However, as these mechanical changes progress, LV contractile dysfunction and hemodynamic derangements occur, including pulmonary congestion, heart failure symptoms, and increases in LV end-systolic and end-diastolic diameter. Reduced forward flow is a very late occurrence.

The chest x-ray often shows left atrial enlargement with a double-density and widened carina, with no other findings early in the course of chronic MR. Later, the left ventricle dilates and there may be signs of pulmonary venous congestion. The lateral chest x-ray may show posterior protrusion of the left atrial cavity, a prominent pulmonary trunk, or small pleural effusions.

After clinical evaluation, a transthoracic echocardiogram is useful for determining the MR severity, mechanism, etiology, presence of flail, left ventricular size and function, left atrial size, abnormalities of other valves, and right ventricular systolic pressure (Table 25–3). It is also useful for assessing serial changes in left ventricular size

**TABLE 25–3**
**RECOMMENDATIONS FOR TRANSTHORACIC ECHOCARDIOGRAPHY IN MITRAL REGURGITATION**

| Indication | Class |
|---|---|
| 1. For baseline evaluation to quantify severity of MR and LV function in any patient suspected of having MR | I |
| 2. For delineation of mechanism of MR | I |
| 3. For annual or semiannual surveillance of LV function (estimated by ejection fraction and end-systolic dimension) in asymptomatic severe MR | I |
| 4. To establish cardiac status after a change in symptoms | I |
| 5. For evaluation after MVR or mitral valve repair to establish baseline status | I |
| 6. Routine follow-up evaluation of mild MR with normal LV size and systolic function | III |

MR, mitral regurgitation; LV, left ventricular; MVR, mitral valve repair. (reference 1)

**TABLE 25–4**
**RECOMMENDATION FOR TRANSESOPHAGEAL ECHOCARDIOGRAPHY IN MITRAL REGURGITATION**

| Indication | Class |
|---|---|
| 1. Intraoperative transesophageal echocardiography to establish the anatomic basis for MR and to guide repair | I |
| 2. For evaluation of MR patients in whom transthoracic echocardiography provides nondiagnostic images regarding severity of MR, mechanism of MR, and/or status of LV function | I |
| 3. In routine follow-up or surveillance of patients with native-valve MR | III |

MR, mitral regurgitation; LV, left ventricular. (reference 1)

and function, and evaluating the patient after a change in symptoms. Occasionally a transesophageal echocardiogram may be needed to better assess the severity and etiology of MR (Table 25–4). A stress echocardiogram is often useful for determining the severity and effect of the disease on the patient's exercise hemodynamics. Left ventriculography and hemodynamic measurements including magnetic resonance imaging are helpful in rare specific conditions; however, the routine use in management of patients with chronic mitral regurgitation in unproven (Fig. 25–3).

## MECHANISM OF MITRAL REGURGIATION

The mechanism of mitral regurgitation can be determined by looking at leaflet motion and color Doppler jet direction (6). First, the patient's leaflets are categorized by two-dimensional echocardiography into those with normal, excessive, or restricted motion. Then additional information is gained by looking at the size, location, and direction of the regurgitant jet by color Doppler.

Mitral valve disease may have numerous causes, including myxomatous degeneration, ischemic, rheumatic, congenital, endocarditis, autoimmune disorders, and seroto nin-mediated valve lesions. In the last half-century, there has been a remarkable increase of the frequency of myxomatous degeneration in surgical populations, with a decline in postinflammatory (rheumatic) cases, while ischemic– and infective endocarditis–associated mitral regurgitation have continued at a relatively low frequency.

In myxomatous degeneration, the most significant abnormality is abnormal elasticity with redundancy and enlargement of various portions of the mitral valvular apparatus, including the mitral annulus, chordae tendinae, and leaflets. In long-axis views, it is easy to see which leaflet is moving into the atrial side of the coaptation line in systole, showing prolapse or flail. Thereafter, the direction of the regurgitant jet provides supplemental diagnostic information. In excessive leaflet motion, the jet is directed to the opposite side of the most affected leaflet. Short-axis and intercommissural views (apical two-chamber and mid-esophageal transesophageal views aligned parallel to the intercommissural line) are useful for determining which portion of a leaflet is abnormal.

Rheumatic heart disease is characterized by leaflet thickening, diastolic mitral doming, valvular and subvalvular fibrosis, and various degrees of systolic and diastolic restriction of leaflet motion. In most cases of restriction involving both leaflets, the jet of mitral regurgitation is central. In some patients, the posterior leaflet is more restricted and the jet direction is posterior.

Ischemic mitral regurgitation is the result of remodeling, enlargement, and "sphericalization" of the left ventricle. Functional mitral regurgitation from nonischemic cardiomyopathy is very similar. Both are caused by apical tethering of normal leaflets (Fig. 25–4). The length of mitral tissue, including the leaflets, chordae, and papillary muscle, is fixed. As the left ventricle dilates, often after myocardial infarction, the LV wall and papillary muscles are displaced outward, which tethers the coapting surfaces of the

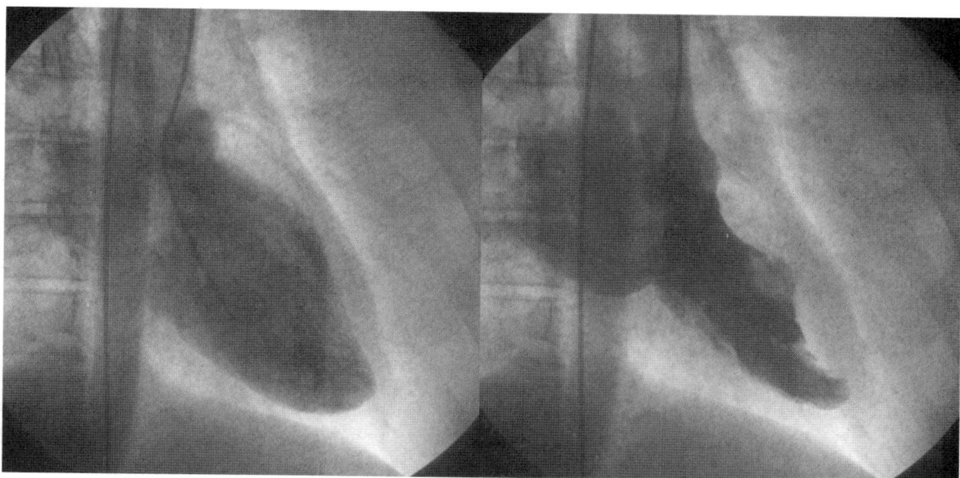

**Figure 25–3** Left ventriculogram in the RAO projection in diastole **(left)** and systole **(right)**, showing severe mitral regurgitation that completely fills the left atrium.

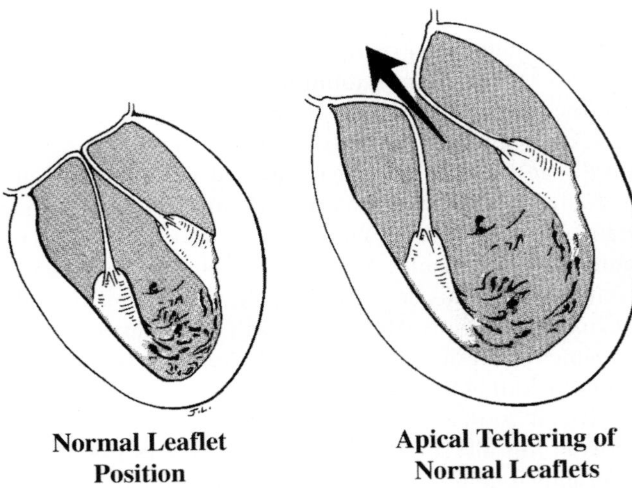


**Figure 25–4** Mechanism of functional mitral regurgitation, often due to ischemic heart disease, contrasting systolic leaflet coaptation in a normal mitral valve **(left)** with the pattern of apical tethering of normal leaflets due-to-left ventricular enlargement **(right)**, as occurs in patients with ischemic left ventricular enlargement and dysfunction.

mitral valve downward, reducing the amount of leaflet tissue available for coaptation. In many cases, the result is a central, or in some cases a posterior direction of the mitral regurgitation jet. In rare cases, a focal infarction may cause elongation or disruption of the papillary muscle, leading to excessive leaflet motion (often involving both leaflets) most commonly the medial side of both leaflets from medial papillary muscle abnormalities.

Mitral valve endocarditis can cause leaflet or chordal disruption, flail, and perforations. These often cause mitral regurgitation with associated nodular hypermobile densities (vegetations) that are the echocardiographic hallmarks of the disease. Care should be taken to look at adjacent valves and the perivalvular tissue looking for abscess formation or paravalvular leakage. Mitral regurgitation secondary to the phospholipid antibody syndrome is associated with symmetric thickening of leaflets, with noninfected vegetations, causing mitral regurgitation.

## QUANTITATION OF MITRAL REGURGITATION

Mitral regurgitation may be quantitated using a variety of echo and Doppler methods, including spatial mapping, flow convergence, pulmonary vein velocity patterns, vena contracta width, continuous-wave Doppler density and shape, and quantitation of antegrade valvular flow volumes. We often use a "weighted average" of multiple methods, emphasizing more the methods that have good-quality data in that patient (7).

The flow convergence method, also called the proximal isovelocity surface area (PISA) method, involves assessing the color images on the left ventricular side of the mitral regurgitation (Fig. 25–5) (8). This flow convergence zone is the location where the blood is accelerating as the flow

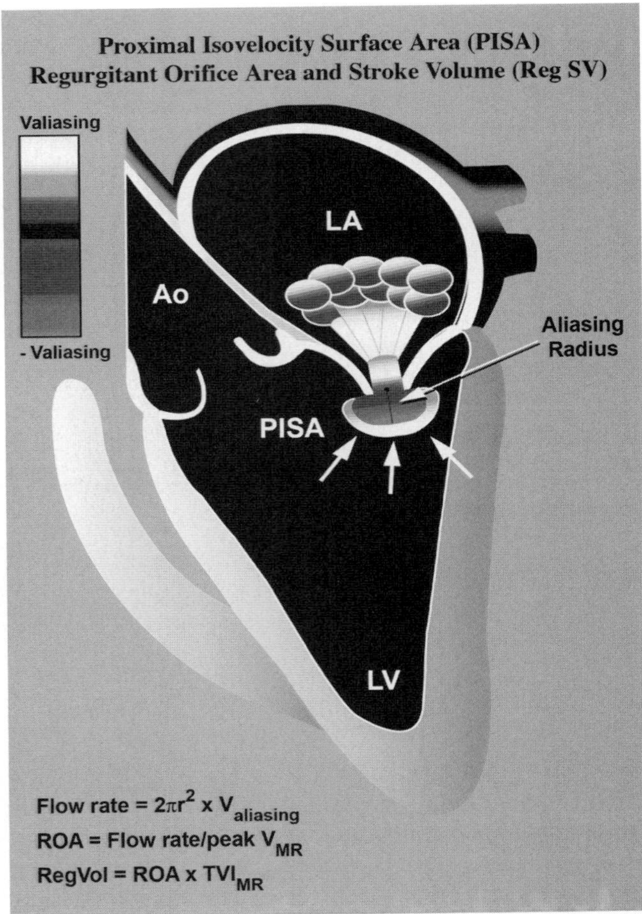


**Figure 25–5** Method of quantifying the severity of mitral regurgitation using the proximal isovelocity surface area (PISA) method (see text for details). (Adapted from Savage R et al. Chapter 28, page 512, 2005.)

stream narrows progressively to the regurgitant orifice, as it undergoes a pressure drop from left ventricular pressure to left atrial pressure. With this area of flow acceleration, color Doppler tracks the location of increases in velocity and shows this as a proximal zone of color aliasing. Analysis of this convergence zone when its shape is hemispheric allows estimation of the surface area of the hemisphere, which is derived from a measurement of the radius ($R$) and the aliasing velocity ($V$), extracted from the "color bar," reflecting machine settings. When this is combined with the maximum velocity, the size of the regurgitant orifice can be calculated according to the formula $2\pi R^2 V$ divided by maximum systolic velocity through the valve obtained by continuous-wave Doppler. The advantage of this formula is that it calculates the actual size of the regurgitant lesion, a fundamental parameter of valve integrity, which may be less load dependent than other methods. A regurgitant orifice area $>0.4$ cm$^2$ is indicative of severe regurgitation, whereas $<0.2$ cm$^2$ is considered mild.

Pulmonary vein flow profiles (Fig. 25–6) are also useful for determination of severity of mitral regurgitation (9). The normal pulmonary vein pattern is for velocity during

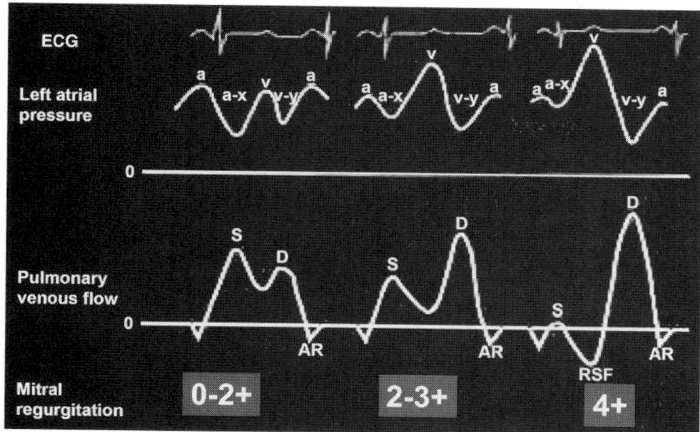


**Figure 25–6** Stylistic ECGs, left atrial pressure waveforms, and pulmonary vein pulsed Doppler recordings, in three patients: normal; moderate, 2–3+ MR; and severe, 4+ MR. Note the reversal of systolic flow (RSV) associated with severe mitral regurgitation, which results from the systolic V wave in the left atrial pressure. (Adapted from Klein et al, *J Am Coll Cardiol* 1991;18:518–26.)

ventricular systole to be higher than antegrade velocity during diastole, a pattern that persists in mild and sometimes moderate mitral regurgitation. When the regurgitation is moderate or moderately severe, pulmonary vein systolic velocity is blunted, with systolic velocity less than diastolic velocity. With even more MR, there is cessation of systolic flow. In patients with severe mitral regurgitation, there is often reversal of systolic flow, with flow away from the left atrium during ventricular systole (Fig. 25–7). This occurs because of the large V wave in the left atrial pressure, which transiently becomes higher than pulmonary parenchymal pressure.

Medical management of patients with MR includes diuresis to correct any volume overload. Rate and rhythm control, often with beta-blockers, is appropriate because many patients have atrial fibrillation. Aggressive blood-pressure control and risk-factor modification should be a routine part of management of these patients.

There are no randomized studies of surgical management of mitral regurgitation. Patients who have symptoms due to the MR should undergo surgery before LV

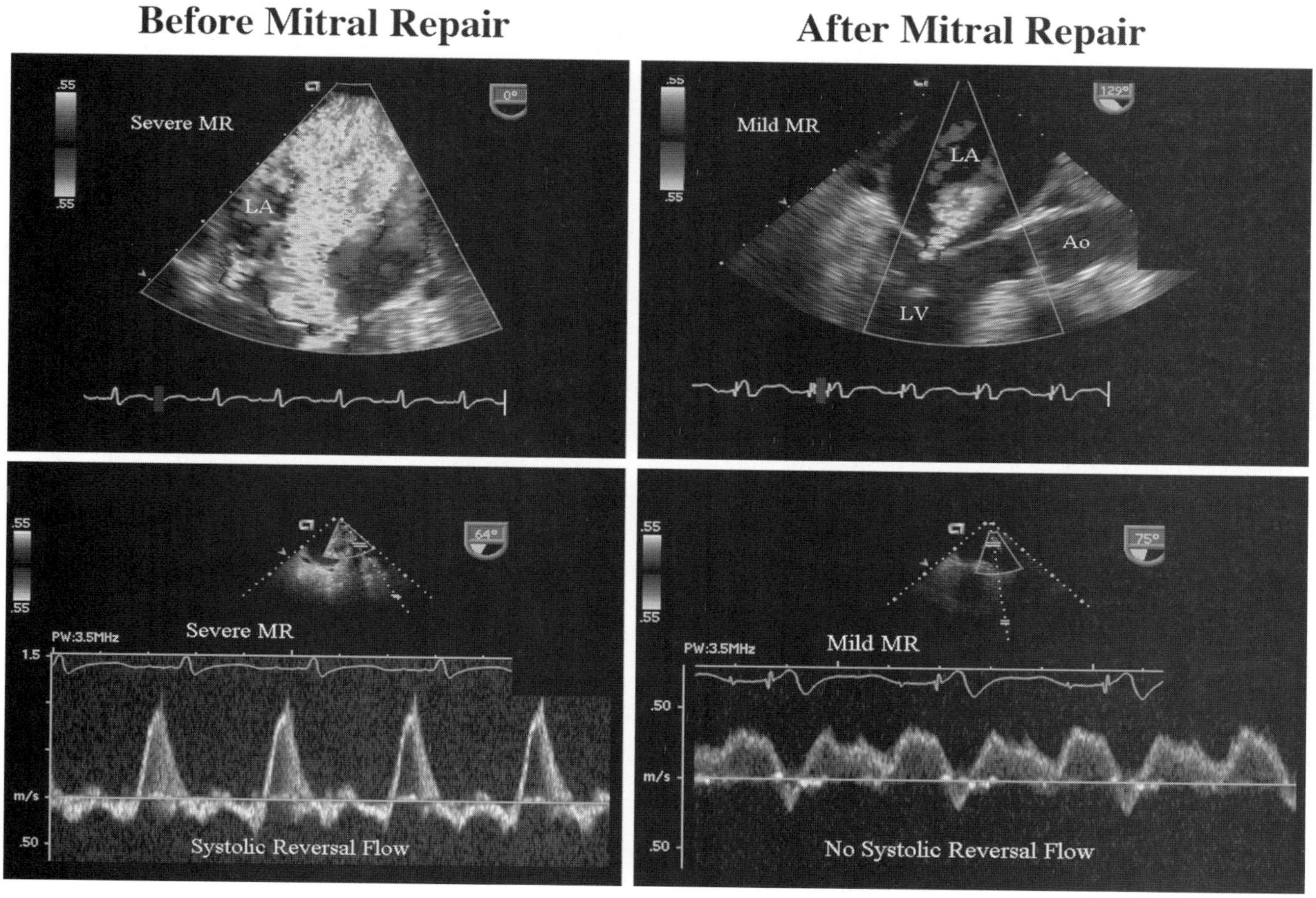

**Figure 25–7** **Upper left:** Still frame of posterior mitral valve prolapse with an anteriorly directed jet of severe mitral regurgitation by color Doppler before repair. **Lower left:** Left upper pulmonary vein pulsed Doppler showing systolic flow reversal, a sign of severe mitral regurgitation. **Upper right:** still frame of mild mitral regurgitation by color Doppler after mitral valve repair. **Lower right:** pulmonary vein pulsed Doppler showing resolution of pulmonary vein pattern to normal after repair. Ao, aorta; LA, left atrium; LV, left ventricle; MR, mitral regurgitation.

**TABLE 25–5a**
**RECOMMENDATIONS FOR MITRAL VALVE SURGERY IN NONISCHEMIC SEVERE MITRAL REGURGITATION**

| Indication | Class |
|---|---|
| 1. Acute symptomatic MR in which repair is likely | I |
| 2. Patients with NYHA functional Class II, III, or IV symptoms with normal LV function defined as ejection fraction >0.60 and end-systolic dimension <45 mm | I |
| 3. Symptomatic or asymptomatic patients with mild LV dysfunction, ejection fraction 0.50–0.60, and end-systolic dimension 45–50 mm | I |
| 4. Symptomatic or asymptomatic patients with moderate LV dysfunction, ejection fraction 0.30–0.50, and/or end-systolic dimension to 55 mm | I |
| 5. Asymptomatic patients with preserved LV function and atrial fibrillation | IIa |
| 6. Asymptomatic patients with preserved LV function and pulmonary hypertension (pulmonary artery systolic pressure >50 mm Hg at rest or >60 mm Hg with exercise | IIa |
| 7. Asymptomatic patients with ejection fraction 0.50–0.60 and end-systolic dimension <45 mm and asymptomatic patients with ejection fraction >0.60 and end-systolic dimension of 45–55 mm | IIa |
| 8. Patients with severe LV dysfunction (ejection fraction <0.30 and/or end-systolic dimension >55 mm) in whom chordal preservation is highly likely | IIa |
| 9. Asymptomatic patients with chronic MR with preserved LV function in whom mitral valve repair is highly likely | IIb |
| 10. Patients with MVP and preserved LV function who have recurrent ventricular arrhythmias despite medical therapy | IIb |
| 11. Asymptomatic patients with preserved LV function in whom significant doubt about the feasibility of repair exists | III |

Adapted from reference 1.

dysfunction occurs (1). There are no randomized surgical studies in asymptomatic patients with severe mitral regurgitation. If the patient has repairable MR that is truly severe quantitatively, most experts agree that mitral valve surgery should be recommended if the patient has developed any decrease in LV ejection fraction, significant dilation of end-systolic LV size (>4.5 cm systolic diameter), atrial fibrillation, or significant pulmonary hypertension. In addition, many centers recommend mitral valve surgery for selected patients with severe mitral regurgitation when they also have a flail mitral leaflet (10), or when there is exercise echo evidence of "latent LV dysfunction," defined by a declining EF or increasing ESV with exercise (11).

American College of Cardiology/American Heart Association (ACC/AHA) guidelines do not advocate mitral valve surgery for patients with ejection fraction <30% (Table 25–5). However, selected symptomatic patients with severe

**TABLE 25–5b**
**INDICATIONS FOR SURGERY FOR SEVERE MITRAL REGURGITATION**

Symptoms of heart failure

*or*

Asymptomatic with a repairable valve and

- Concomitant coronary artery disease
- LV-enlargement LVIDs >4.5 cm
- Systolic dysfunction EF <55%
- Pulmonary HTN RVSP >55
- Recurrent atrial fibrillation
- Exercise echo with "latent LV dysfunction" (declining EF or increasing ESV)
- Flail mitral leaflet
- ROA >0.6 $cm^2$ (exact threshold is not yet determined)

LVIDs, left ventricular internal diameter systolic; EF, ejection fraction; HTN, hypertension; RVSP, right ventricular systolic pressure; ESV, end systolic volume; ROA, regurgitant orifice area.
Adapted from reference 1.

LV dysfunction may benefit from mitral valve operation, particularly if they have ventricular dilation and very severe regurgitation (Fig. 25–8).

Mitral valve repair is now the surgical management of choice (5) for most cases of mitral regurgitation, which spares the patient from chronic anticoagulation. In addition, preservation of the mitral apparatus leads to improved LV function and survival compared to mitral valve replacement with loss of chordal integrity. However, for many conditions, such as rheumatic mitral valve disease or in those with significant subvalvular thickening and major loss of leaflet substance, mitral valve replacement is necessary. If so, it should be done with preservation of as much as possible of the mitral valve chordal apparatus.

Based on the ACC/AHA guidelines (1), cardiac catheterization is indicated in patients with angina or previous myocardial infarction, individuals with one or more cardiac risk factors, and when ischemia is the cause of mitral regurgitation. Patients <35 years of age with no clinical suspicion of coronary artery disease do not need to undergo coronary angiography (Table 25–6).

## MITRAL VALVE STENOSIS

The primary cause of mitral stenosis (MS) is rheumatic heart disease, a chronic, postinfectious, inflammatory condition that leads to fusion and fibrosis of commissural, cuspal, and chordal portions of the mitral valve apparatus. Less commonly, MS is a complication of malignant carcinoid, radiation, systemic lupus erythematosus, rheumatoid arthritis, Whipple disease, and rare connective tissue diseases. The normal mitral valve area is 4.0 to 5.0 $cm^2$. Symptomatic mitral valve stenosis occurs when the valve area is <1.5 to 2.0 $cm^2$. Symptoms often begin with mild exercise intolerance and accelerate when the patient develops atrial fibrillation, particularly when the ventricular rate

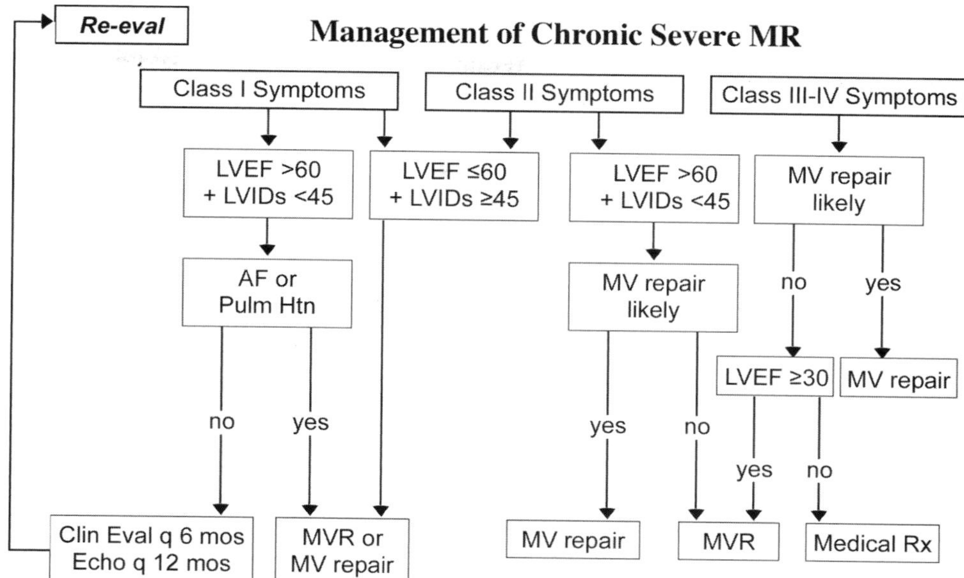


**Figure 25–8** Flow chart summarizing management of chronic mitral regurgitation. (Adapted from reference 1.)

is rapid. The natural history of MS is a life-long, continuous, and slow process (Fig. 25–9). It usually takes 20 to 40 years after occurrence of a streptococcus infection and rheumatic fever for the patient to develop symptoms of rheumatic valve disease. Dyspnea with exertion may occur several years before the patient experiences decompensated heart failure. Patients with MS and atrial fibrillation can occasionally present with neurologic sequela, which results from embolization of clot, occurring due to blood stasis in the left atrium. With progression of disease and increased left atrial pressure, orthopnea, paroxysmal nocturnal dyspnea, and occasionally hemoptysis may occur.

A loud first heart sound, an opening snap, and a diastolic rumble are the classic auscultatory features of mitral stenosis. The intensity of the pulmonic component of second heart sound is important in the bedside estimate of the severity of secondary pulmonary hypertension. The opening snap (OS) is caused by sudden tensing of the valve leaflet and occurs about 50 to 120 milliseconds after the A2 component of the second heart sound. The time between A2 and OS is inversely associated with severity of mitral stenosis; therefore, a short A2–OS interval is a bedside indication of severe mitral stenosis. However, patients with severe immobility of the mitral valve often have no opening snap despite significant MS.

**TABLE 25–6**
**RECOMMENDATIONS FOR CORONARY ANGIOGRAPHY IN MITRAL REGURGITATION**

| Indication | Class |
|---|---|
| 1. When mitral valve surgery is contemplated in patients with angina or previous myocardial infarction | I |
| 2. When mitral valve surgery is contemplated in patients with ≥1 risk factor for CAD | I |
| 3. When ischemia is suspected as an etiologic factor in MR | I |
| 4. To confirm noninvasive tests in patients no suspected of having CAD | IIb |
| 5. When mitral valve surgery is contemplated in patients aged <35 y and there is no clinical suspicion of CAD | III |

CAD, coronary artery disease; MR, mitral regurgitation. Adapted from reference 1.

The electrocardiographic (ECG) features of MS include left atrial enlargement, and occasionally right ventricular enlargement. Atrial fibrillation is a frequent arrhythmia in these patients. Radiographic features of mitral stenosis included enlarge left atrium, enlarged pulmonary arteries, mitral valve calcium, and congestive heart failure, and occasional Kerley B lines.

Although the history, physical exam, chest x-ray (Fig. 25–10), and ECG may help to suggest mitral stenosis, two-dimensional (2-D) echo and Doppler echocardiography are the tools of choice for its diagnosis. The characteristic findings of mitral stenosis on the 2-D echo are restriction of diastolic motion, with doming in diastole of the anterior and posterior leaflets (Fig. 25–11). There is often contraction and fibrosis of the various components of the mitral apparatus, often with thickening of the submitral chordae and papillary muscles. In the parasternal short-axis view, the mitral valve can be planimetered to determine the effective mitral valve area. To do so, one must scan up and down the mitral valve short axis, searching for the smallest flow-limiting orifice, at the time during early diastole when the diastolic opening is at its maximum (Fig. 25–12). In order to provide accurate measurements, the gain settings must not be too high or too low. In addition, echo imaging assesses the degree of valve thickening, decreased mobility, calcification, and subvalvular disease (the "splittability index"), which helps to predict the success and durability of percutaneous balloon valvotomy versus surgical options (12). Echo is also essential for exclusion of other valvular

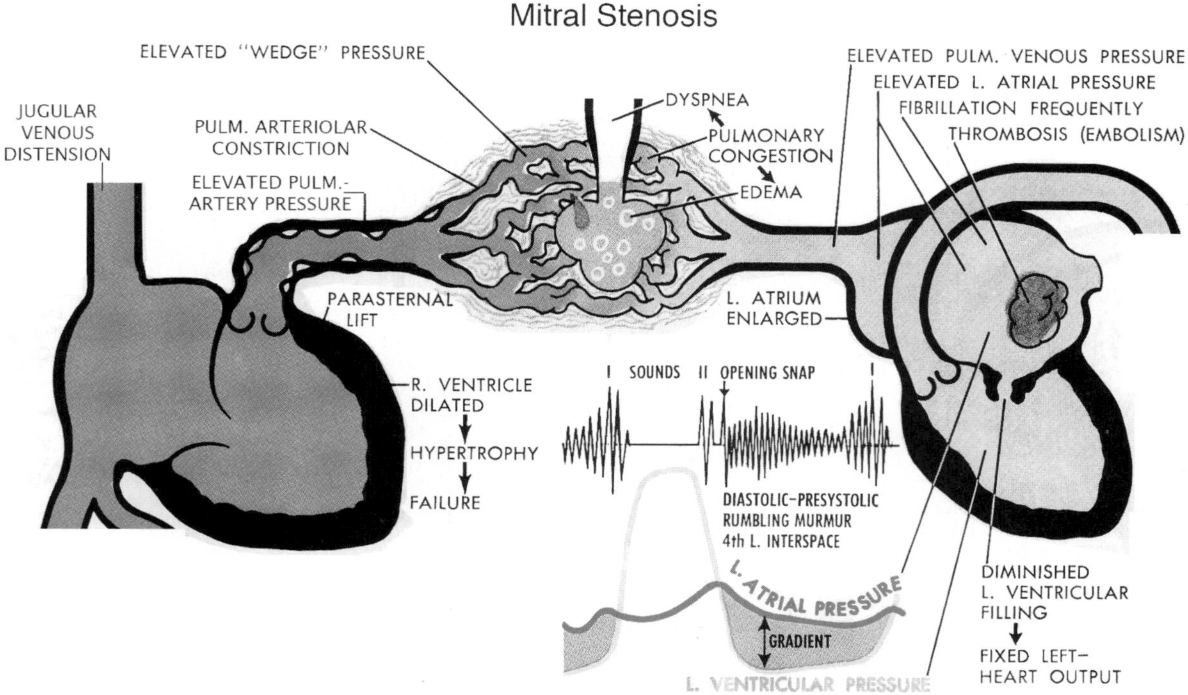


**Figure 25–9** Schematic diagram representing pathologic complications of mitral stenosis. (Adapted from Netter's volume 5, section II, plate 48, and page 87.)

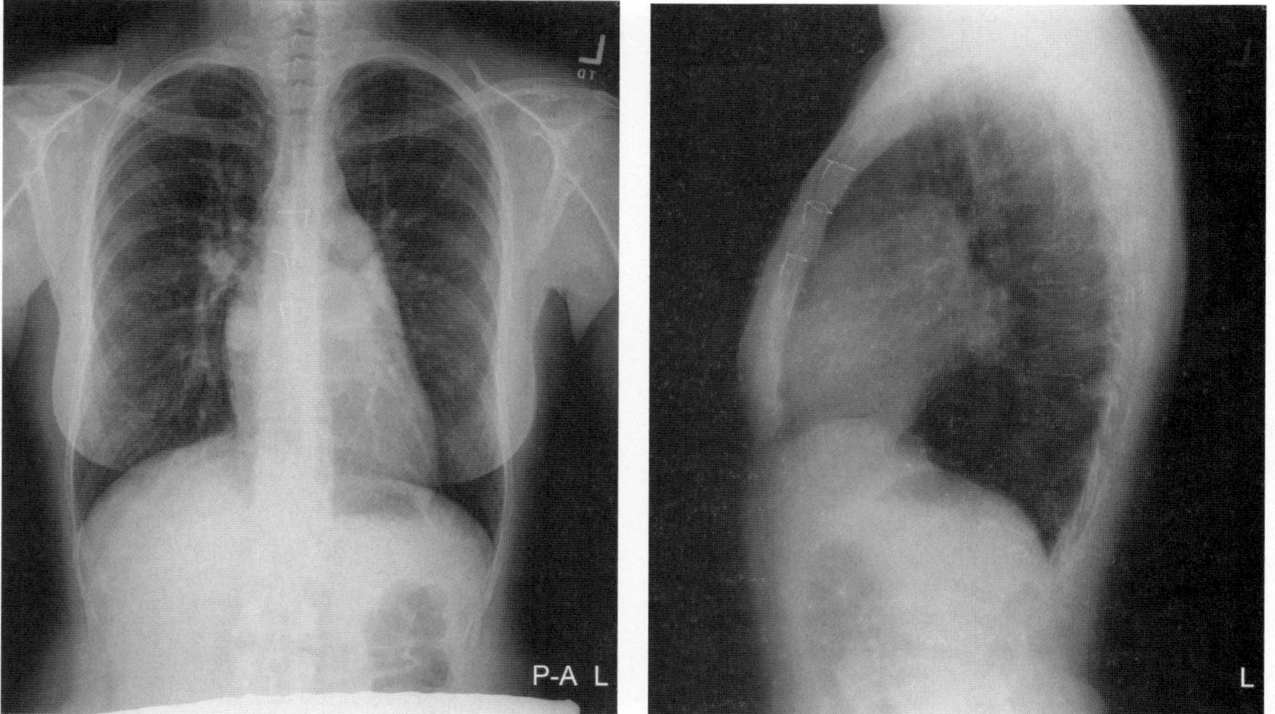


**Figure 25–10** Posteroanterior chest x-ray showing typical features of rheumatic mitral stenosis, with and enlarged left atrium (note the widened carina), and prominent bilateral pulmonary artery shadows, with normal left ventricular size. This patient was not in heart failure at the time of the study, but had mid-sternal wires from a previous thoracotomy **(A).** Lateral chest x-ray showing prominent pulmonary arteries and left atrial enlargement protruding from the cardiac silhouette posteriorly **(B).**

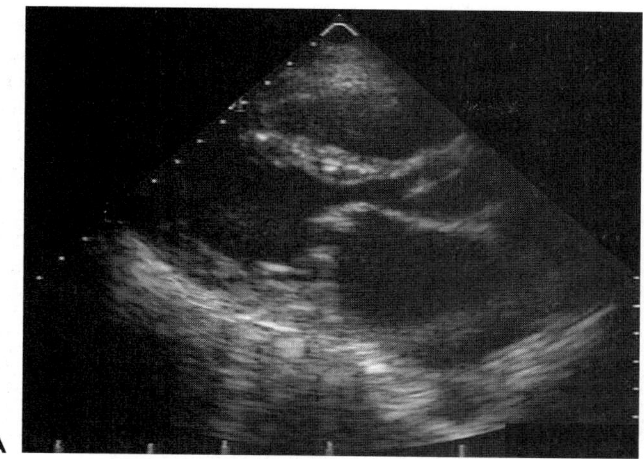

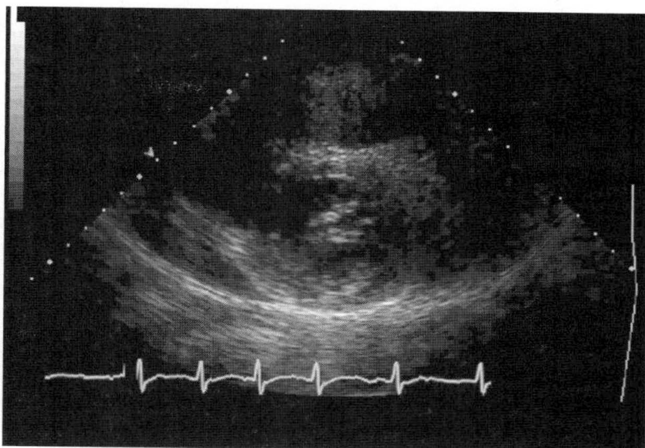

**Figure 25–11** Parasternal long-axis **(A)** and short-axis **(B)** views of a patient with rheumatic mitral valve stenosis. Note the diastolic doming, the leaflet thickening, the left atrial enlargement, and the normal LV size.

lesions, because it is common for patients with rheumatic mitral disease to have concomitant aortic and/or tricuspid valve disease.

Apical or midesophageal (transesophageal echo) recording of diastolic antegrade mitral flow are also characteristic and useful for quantitation of severity. Doppler accurately estimates mean mitral gradient, mitral valve area, and estimation of right ventricular systolic pressure. The mean mitral gradient is the temporal average of instantaneous gradients throughout diastole, using the modified Bernoulli equation ($4V^2$). However, this particular measurement is very subject to changes with increased heart rate, which reduces the diastolic interval and increases the mean mitral gradient. It is also subject to concomitant mitral regurgitation (which increases antegrade flow) and other changes in cardiac output (with low cardiac output causing a lower mitral gradient). Severity of MS can also be judged using the mitral pressure half-time (the time in milliseconds that it takes the maximum transmitral velocity to fall to its initial velocity, divided by the square root of 2). Mitral valve area is calculated from the formula: 220/pressure half-time (Fig. 25–13). In general, a valve area of 4 to 6 $cm^2$ is normal, 1.6 to 2.0 $cm^2$ is mild, 1.1 to 1.5 $cm^2$ is moderate, and $\leq 1.0$ $cm^2$ is severe mitral stenosis (Fig. 25–14). Estimation of right ventricular systolic pressure is made from the maximum tricuspid regurgitation velocity.

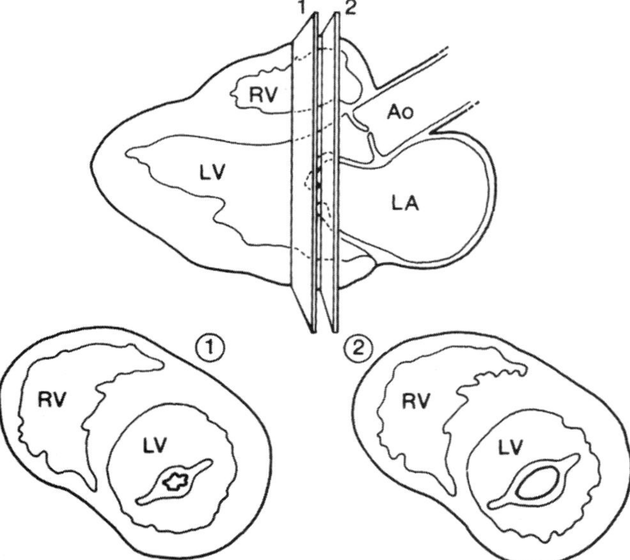


**Figure 25–12** Artistic diagram illustrating the technique of obtaining the optimum parasternal short axis images. Planimetry to measure the severity of mitral stenosis would obtain a larger orifice area in image plane (2) than in image plane (1), because of the funnel-shaped mitral valve. RV, right venticle. (Adapted from Salcedo; Atlas of Echocardiography 1985, page 73.)

Although often supplanted by a complete Doppler study, an invasive right and left heart catheterization should be reserved for patients with discrepancy between Doppler-derived hemodynamics and clinical symptoms or when there is elevation of pulmonary artery pressures out of proportion to mitral valve area or diastolic gradients (Table 25–7). Simultaneous Doppler and catheterization studies, using a transseptal measurement of left atrial pressure, has revealed that Doppler-derived mean mitral gradients and pressure half-times are accurate in most circumstances. Use of the pulmonary capillary wedge technique may overestimate the mitral gradient because of incomplete wedging and hence overestimation of the left atrial pressure.

Medical management of patients with mitral stenosis involves antibiotic prophylaxis for infective endocarditis and aggressive anticoagulation in patients at high risk. Patients who have atrial fibrillation or previous systemic embolic events should definitely be anticoagulated with warfarin. The ACC/AHA guidelines recommend anticoagulation in all patients with mitral stenosis with paroxysmal

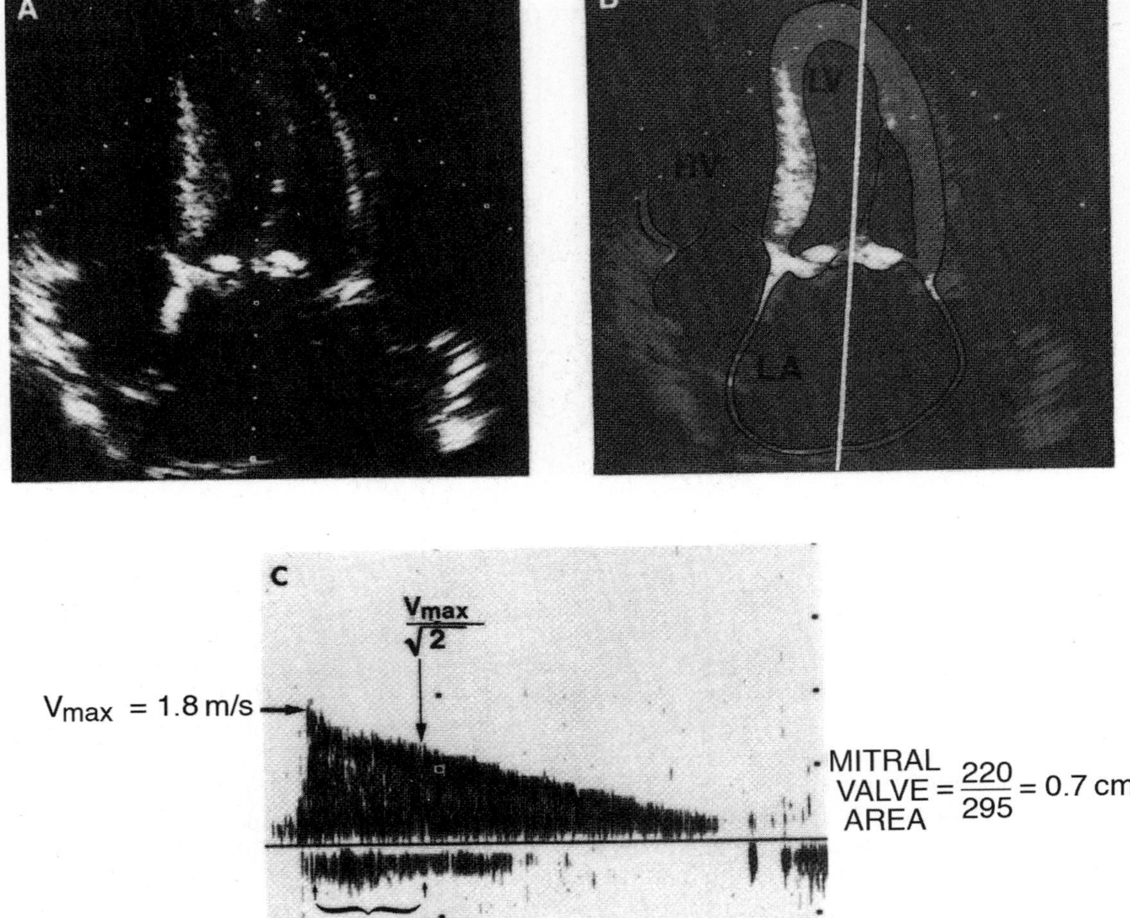


**Figure 25–13** Apical four-chamber echo image **(A)** and artistic drawing **(B)** for recording continuous-wave Doppler of mitral antegrade velocity profiles **(C)** in mitral stenosis. Pressure half-time ($t_{1/2}$) in milliseconds is divided into 220 milliseconds, to derive mitral valve area, in square centimeters. (Adapted from Stewart et al in *Pohost GM Cardiac Imaging*, Yearbook Inc, Chicago, 1986, page 76.)

and chronic atrial fibrillation, and in those with prior embolic events (Table 25–8).

Patients with moderate or greater degree of mitral stenosis should avoid strenuous physical activity sufficient to cause severe symptoms. In those with exertional symptoms, beta-blockers or calcium channel blockers may be beneficial to increase the duration of diastole, especially if symptoms occur with rapid heart rate. Salt restriction and diuretic use are necessary components for management of pulmonary congestion in these patients. The incidence of atrial fibrillation is around 30% to 40% in patients with mitral stenosis, and, as mentioned, anticoagulation is an important part of medical management.

Atrial fibrillation (AF) causes loss of the atrial component of ventricular filling. When AF is rapid, there is a decrease in diastolic filling period per minute, increasing the average gradient across the stenotic mitral valve. Therefore, anything that accelerates ventricular rate has deleterious hemodynamic consequences in mitral stenosis, because diastole takes up a smaller portion of the heart cycle at more rapid rates. In patients with rapid AF and hemodynamic instability or evidence of shock with ongoing end-organ underperfusion, direct-current cardioversion should be performed without delay.

At the onset of AF in any patient with MS, rapid assessment and management with agents such as beta-blockers, calcium channel blockers, or intravenous digoxin may be necessary. In general, stable patients should undergo transesophageal echocardiography to look for thrombus, or be anticoagulated for 3 weeks prior to cardioversion. In addition, all patients should be anticoagulated continuously during and after the cardioversion.

The decision to intervene with surgery or catheter-based therapy in patients with mitral stenosis depends largely on

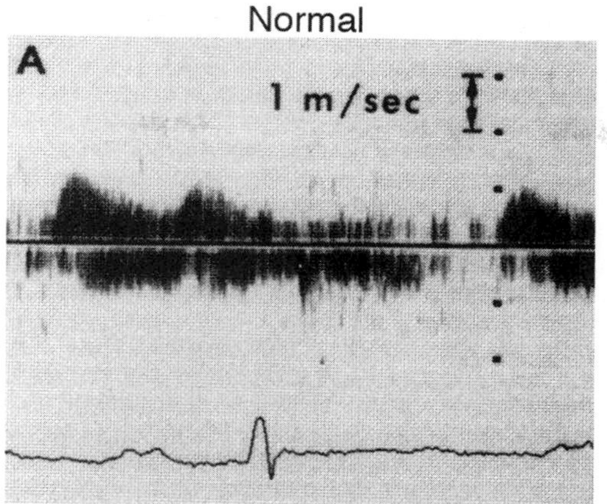


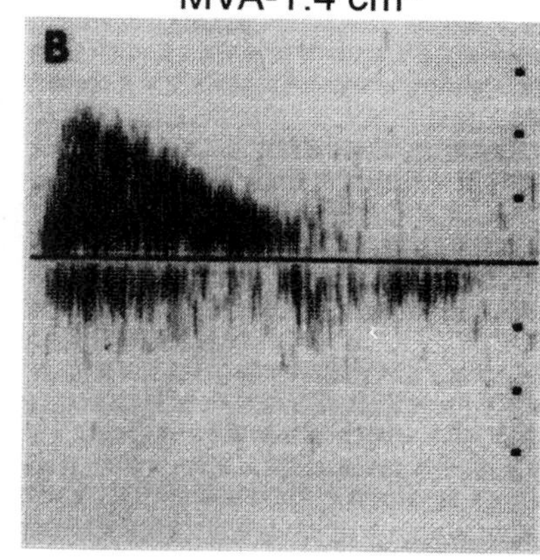


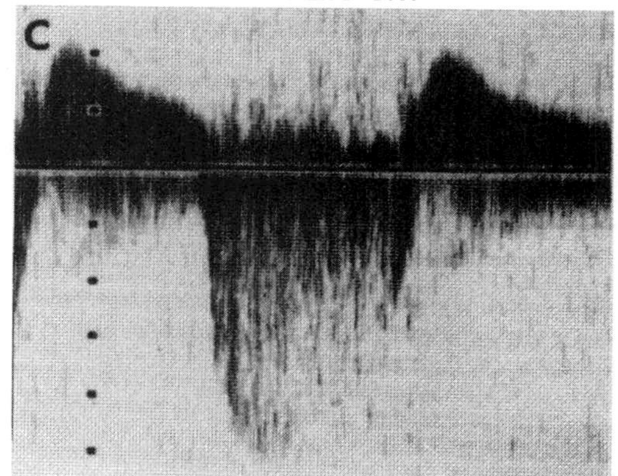


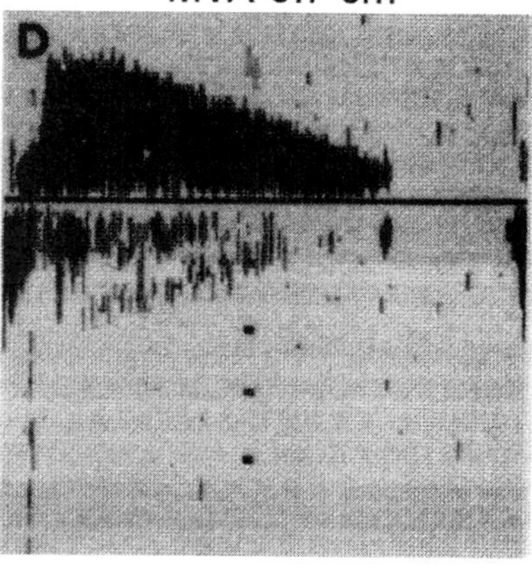


**Figure 25–14** Continuous-wave Doppler recordings from apical four-chamber view showing a normal patient **(A)** and three different degrees of severity of mitral valve stenosis **(B).** (Adapted from Stewart et al. in *Pohost GM Cardiac Imaging*, Yearbook Inc, Chicago, 1986, page 77.)

the severity of symptoms, but also depends on the quantitative severity of MS, the level of pulmonary hypertension, the history of atrial arrhythmias, and thromboembolic complications. Congestive heart failure that is New York Heart Association (NYHA) Class II or above, with severe mitral stenosis, $<1.0$ cm$^2$ valve area, is a clear indication for intervention. The presence of pulmonary hypertension, with systolic pressures above 55 at rest or above 60 mm Hg with exercise, is considered an indication for intervention even without symptoms.

## TABLE 25–7
## RECOMMENDATIONS FOR ECHOCARDIOGRAPHY IN MITRAL STENOSIS

| Indication | Class |
|---|---|
| 1. Diagnosis of MS, assessment of hemodynamic severity (mean gradient, mitral valve area, pulmonary artery pressure), and assessment of right ventricular size and function | I |
| 2. Assessment of valve morphology to determine suitability for percutaneous mitral balloon valvotomy | I |
| 3. Diagnosis and assessment of concomitant valvular lesions | I |
| 4. Re-evaluation of patients with known MS with changing symptoms or signs | I |
| 5. Assessment of hemodynamic response of mean gradient and pulmonary artery pressures by exercise Doppler echocardiography in patients when there is a discrepancy between resting hemodynamics and clinical findings | IIa |
| 6. Re-evaluation of asymptomatic patients with moderate to severe MS to assess pulmonary artery pressure | IIb |
| 7. Routine re-evaluation of the asymptomatic patient with mild MS and stable clinical findings | III |

Adapted from reference 1.

## TABLE 25–8
## RECOMMENDATIONS FOR ANTICOAGULATION IN MITRAL STENOSIS

| Indication | Class |
|---|---|
| 1. Patients with atrial fibrillation, paroxysmal or chronic | I |
| 2. Patients with a prior embolic event | I |
| 3. Patients with severe MS and left atrial dimension $\geq$55 mm by echocardiography | IIb |
| 4. All other patients with MS | III |

Adapted from reference 1.

**TABLE 25–9**
**RECOMMENDATIONS FOR PERCUTANEOUS MITRAL BALLOON VALVOTOMY**

| Indication | Class |
|---|---|
| 1. Symptomatic patients (NYHA functional Class II, III, or IV), moderate or severe MS (mitral valve area ≤1.5 cm$^2$), and valve morphology favorable for percutaneous balloon valvotomy in the absence of left atrial thrombus or moderate to severe MR | I |
| 2. Asymptomatic patients with moderate or severe MS (mitral valve area ≤1.5 cm$^2$) and valve morphology favorable for percutaneous balloon valvotomy who have pulmonary hypertension (pulmonary artery systolic pressure >50 mm Hg at rest or 60 mm Hg with exercise), in the absence of left atrial thrombus or moderate to severe MR | IIa |
| 3. Patients with NYHA functional Class III-IV symptoms, moderate or severe MS (mitral valve area ≤1.5 cm) and a nonpliable calcified valve who are at high risk for surgery in the absence of left atrial thrombus or moderate to severe MR | IIa |
| 4. Asymptomatic patients, moderate or severe MS (mitral valve area 1.5 cm), and valve morphology favorable for percutaneous balloon valvotomy who have new onset of atrial fibrillation in the absence of left a trial thrombus or moderate to severe MR. | IIb |
| 5. Patients in NYHA functional Class III-IV, moderate or severe MS (mitral valve area ≤1.5 cm$^2$) and a nonpliable calcified valve who are low-risk candidates for surgery | IIb |
| 6. Patients with mild AS | III |

Adapted from reference 1.

Based on these criteria, intervention may take the form of balloon valvotomy, open commissurotomy, or mitral valve replacement (Table 25–9). Balloon valvotomy is a therapeutic technique done through a transseptal catheterization that can accomplish enlargement of the mitral orifice in patients with mitral stenosis who have suitable anatomy. Balloon valvotomy is more likely to be feasible if the echo "splittability index" is below about 9, based on moderate or less criteria for the severity of mitral calcification, valve thickening, restricted mobility, and subvalvular disease. Balloon valvotomy is reasonably safe and has results similar to that of open mitral commissurotomy based on published studies. Prior to a transcatheter therapeutic procedure, transesophageal echo is warranted to exclude left atrial thrombus and moderately severe (3+ on a scale of 4+) or more mitral regurgitation, both of which are contraindications to the balloon valvotomy technique. In general, mitral valve area typically doubles with a successful balloon valvotomy procedure in which both commissures are split.

Patients with a left atrial thrombus, significant mitral regurgitation, or a high echo splittability index should be considered for valve repair or valve replacement rather than balloon procedures. Mitral valve repair can be accomplished in selected patients with mitral stenosis, particularly when the valve has a moderate or lower splittability index, and is the procedure of choice when there is concomitant substantial mitral regurgitation, especially if there is a contraindication to anticoagulation.

**TABLE 25–10**
**RECOMMENDATIONS FOR MITRAL VALVE REPLACEMENT FOR MITRAL STENOSIS**

| Indication | Class |
|---|---|
| 1. Patients with moderate or severe MS (mitral valve area ≤1.5 cm$^2$), and NYHA functional Class III–IV symptoms who are not considered candidates for percutaneous balloon valvotomy or mitral valve repair | I |
| 2. Patients with severe MS (mitral valve area ≤1 cm$^2$), and severe pulmonary hypertension (pulmonary artery systolic pressure >60–80 mm Hg) with NYHA functional Class I–II symptoms who are not considered candidates for percutaneous balloon valvotomy or mitral valve repair | IIa |

Adapted from reference 1.

Mitral valve replacement (MVR) is an alternative procedure for patients who are not candidates for percutaneous mitral valvotomy or surgical commissurotomy (Table 25–10). In heavily calcified, immobile, fibrotic valves that have a high splittability index, percutaneous mitral valvotomy or surgical commissurotomy may not be feasible and MVR is the best option. Traditionally a mechanical valve is used for most patients having mitral replacement who are <65 years of age, whereas older patients undergo bioprosthetic valve replacement.

## TRICUSPID VALVE REGURGITATION

Tricuspid regurgitation (TR) is a very common valvular abnormality, but it is often mild or moderate in severity, and in those cases, usually asymptomatic. In severe tricuspid regurgitation, right-sided heart failure often occurs, and the patients develop ascites, hepatic congestion, and peripheral edema (Fig. 25–15). In addition, patients may complain of fatigue, shortness of breath, and exercise intolerance as a result of an inability to augment cardiac output because of the severe tricuspid regurgitation.

On physical exam, patients often have distended jugular veins, leg and pedal edema, and an enlarged liver. The jugular vein profile and the right atrial pressure waveform shows a positive systolic V wave from the effects of the TR. On cardiac auscultation, there may or may not be a holosystolic murmur, which may be high pitched, much lower pitched, or absent. The murmur is often heard best at the right or left sternal border, and classically increases with inhalation, though this is not a reliable finding. Maneuvers that increase venous return, such as leg raising, augment the intensity of the tricuspid regurgitation murmur. In severe TR, an S3 or an early diastolic rumble may be heard. When there is associated pulmonary hypertension, the second heart sound may be loud. Palpation of the heart

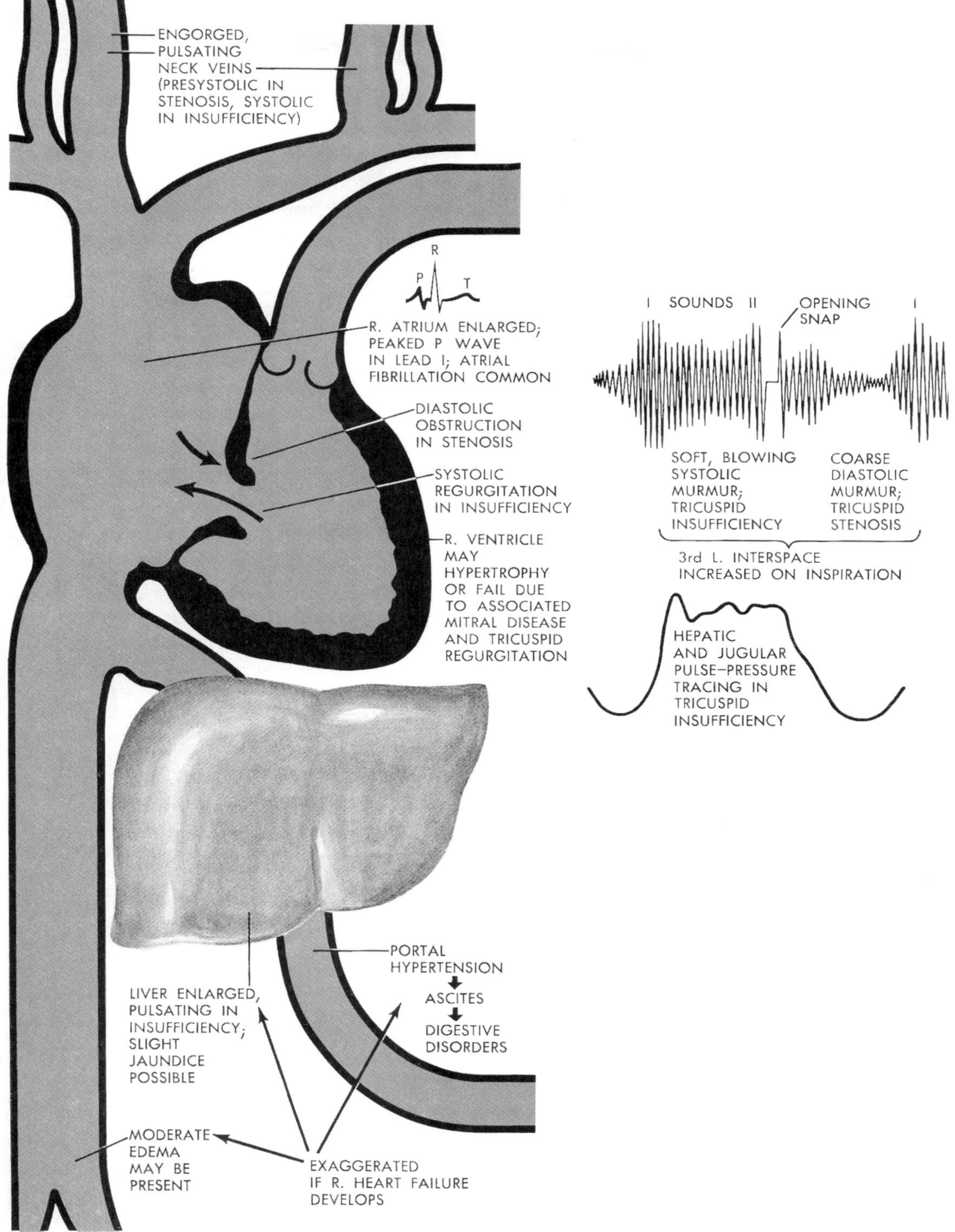


**Figure 25–15** Schematic diagram representing pathologic complications of stenosis and regurgitation. (Adapted from Netter's volume 5, section II, plate 52, and page 91.)

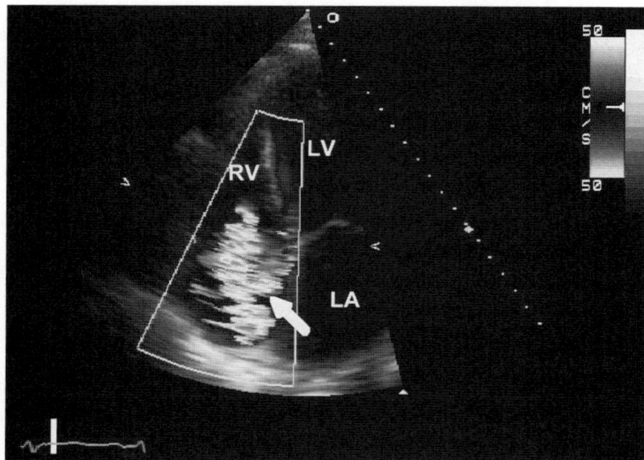


**Figure 25–16** Apical four-chamber color flow Doppler image of a patient with severe tricuspid regurgitation (arrow). RV, right ventricle; LV, left ventricle; RA, right atrium.

often reveals a right ventricular lift or heave. Palpation of the liver reveals pulsatile hepatomegaly, which may achieve vast proportions. In severe, long-standing TR, chronic passive congestion of the liver occurs, and the patient may develop numerous secondary phenomena. These include abdominal bloating and tenderness, early satiety, jaundice, and other "digestive symptoms." Variable diffuse elevations of blood tests of liver function, cardiac cirrhosis, and progressive cachexia may also occur. Many patients with severe tricuspid regurgitation have been misdiagnosed as having various gastrointestinal disorders.

The most useful diagnostic modality is echocardiography. Color Doppler can define the severity and presence of the regurgitant flow (Fig. 25–16). Care should be give to the Nyquist setting in color imaging, as severe intrinsic TR may be low velocity and not show color aliasing at the usual Nyquist settings. Two-dimensional echocardiography may identify other structural abnormalities that may have caused the tricuspid regurgitation, such as leaflet prolapse, flail, fibrosis, or annular dilation. The cardiac chambers usually show enlargement of the right atrium and right ventricle. Other findings include paradoxical septal motion as a result of right ventricular diastolic overload, and reversal of flow during ventricular systole in the inferior vena cava or hepatic veins by pulsed Doppler. Continuous-wave Doppler is used to define the severity of pulmonary hypertension.

There are no specific electrocardiographic changes associated with tricuspid regurgitation; however, with severe pulmonary hypertension, the ECG pattern of right ventricular hypertrophy may be seen. When right atrial enlargement is present, the ECG may show large P waves in the pattern "P pulmonale," but in the chronic phase, most patients have atrial fibrillation. Chest x-ray often reveals cardiomegaly due to right ventricular and right atrial enlargement, coupled with the findings that reflect their left-sided heart disease, if present.

**TABLE 25–11**

**RECOMMENDATIONS FOR SURGERY FOR TRICUSPID REGURGITATION**

| Indication | Class |
|---|---|
| 1. Annuloplasty for severe TR and pulmonary hypertension in patients with mitral valve disease requiring mitral valve surgery | I |
| 2. Valve replacement for severe TR secondary to diseased/abnormal tricuspid valve leaflets not amenable to annuloplasty or repair | IIa |
| 3. Valve replacement or annuloplasty for severe TR with mean pulmonary artery pressure <60 mm Hg when symptomatic | IIa |
| 4. Annuloplasty for mild TR in patients with pulmonary hypertension secondary to mitral valve disease requiring mitral valve surgery | IIb |
| 5. Valve replacement or annuloplasty for TR with pulmonary artery systolic pressure N60 mm Hg in the presence of a normal mitral valve, in asymptomatic patients, or in symptomatic patients who have not received a trial of diuretic therapy | III |

Adapted from reference 1.

Regarding etiology, the most common type of tricuspid regurgitation is called "functional," because it results from right ventricular and tricuspid annular dilatation. Any cause of pulmonary hypertension may cause this type of TR, including left-sided heart failure due to left ventricular dysfunction, mitral stenosis or regurgitation, or, less commonly, aortic valve disease. Functional tricuspid regurgitation also results from right ventricular hypertension or enlargement caused by intrinsic pulmonary disease, primary pulmonary hypertension, pulmonic valve abnormalities, or left-to-right shunts. Right heart dilation also occurs directly as a result of various disorders of the right ventricular (RV) myocardium, including RV infarction or dilated cardiomyopathy.

Regurgitation from intrinsic tricuspid valvular dysfunction is less common than functional TR. These etiologies include infective endocarditis, myxomatous degeneration (prolapse), rheumatic fever, Ebstein anomaly, carcinoid syndrome, papillary muscle dysfunction or rupture, connective tissue disorders, trauma, rupture of chordae tendineae, marantic endocarditis, and endomyocardial fibrosis.

Treatment of tricuspid regurgitation involves correcting the primary cause. For example, if a correctable cause of acute or chronic pulmonary hypertension can be found, TR may resolve. For example, diuresis of a patient in left heart failure may also diminish the severity of tricuspid regurgitation. Rhythm and rate control also are beneficial to patient well-being in appropriate patients. In some patients, vasodilator therapy may help by dilation of venous capacitance beds, or by reducing pulmonary arteriolar resistance.

Annuloplasty is the most frequent surgical treatment used for tricuspid regurgitation. However, when valve leaflets themselves are destroyed or diseased, and a prosthesis is needed, a biologic valve is usually used as there is a high prevalence of valve thrombosis with mechanical valves in the tricuspid position. The indications for tricuspid valve surgery are listed in Table 25–11. Surgical correction of mitral valve dysfunction may relieve the right ventricular dilation sufficient to correct the TR, but there should be low threshold for annuloplasty for any patient who has 2 to 3+ TR or more on a scale of 4+, at any time prior to surgery.

## TRICUSPID VALVE STENOSIS

The primary cause of tricuspid valve stenosis (TS) is rheumatic heart disease. Stenosis is a complication of the chronic rheumatic fibrosis, as discussed above for MS, occurring many years after the episode of acute rheumatic fever. It is almost never seen as an isolated valvular lesion and frequently presents later in the phase of rheumatic mitral and aortic valve disease. By the time TS is apparent, most patients have a long history of heart failure and most have already had mitral valve disease long enough to have had one or more cardiac surgical procedures. TS almost always is accompanied by severe tricuspid regurgitation.

The symptoms and hemodynamic effects of TS are typically those of prolonged right-sided congestive failure, and cannot be distinguished easily from those resulting from TR, and the frequent concomitant mitral and aortic valve dysfunction. Patients often complain of chronic progressive dyspnea, weakness, fatigue, edema, and anorexia. On physical exam, peripheral cyanosis, elevated jugular venous pressure, a right ventricular lift, ascites, peripheral edema, and diastolic rumble on auscultation are common findings. There is seldom a tricuspid opening snap. Electrocardiogram shows atrial fibrillation in most patients. The rare patient in sinus rhythm has abnormal P waves from left and right atrial enlargement. Chest x-ray often shows massive cardiomegaly, where the dilated right atrium is eclipsed by severe left atrial enlargement.

The findings by echocardiography include diastolic doming, thickening, and restricted motion of tricuspid leaflets. Valve area and pressure gradients can be obtained by Doppler echocardiography, similar to mitral stenosis, although the accuracy of these measurements is not as well validated.

Surgical correction is the mainstay of therapy, and this is clinically successful primarily when combined with mitral and/or aortic valve surgery. Correcting the tricuspid valve without fixing the left-sided problems may lead to pulmonary congestion and edema. Open or balloon valvotomy, especially to relieve the fusion at the commissure between the anterior and septal leaflets and between the posterior and septal leaflets, can relieve the stenosis, but the clinical results are often poor because of persistence of tricuspid regurgitation. Often tricuspid valve replacement is necessary to treat the patient with significant TS-TR adequately.

## REFERENCES

1. Bonow RO, Carabello B, de Leon AC Jr, et al. Guidelines for the management of patients with valvular heart disease: executive summary. A report of the American College of Cardiology/American Heart Association Task Force on Practice Guidelines (Committee on Management of Patients with Valvular Heart Disease). *Circulation*. 1998;98:1949–1484.
2. Freed LA, Levy D, Levine RA, et al. Prevalence and clinical outcome of mitral-valve prolapse. *N Engl J Med*. 1999;341:1–7.
3. Avierinos JF, Gersh BJ, Melton LJ 3rd, et al. Natural history of asymptomatic mitral valve prolapse in the community. *Circulation*. 2002;106:1355–1361.
4. Enriquez-Sarano M, Avierinos JF, Messika-Zeitoun D, et al. Quantitative determinants of the outcome of asymptomatic mitral regurgitation. *N Engl J Med*. 2005;352:875–883.
5. Cosgrove DM, Stewart WJ. Mitral valvuloplasty. *Curr Probl Cardiol*. 1989;14:359–415.
6. Stewart WJ, Currie PJ, Salcedo EE, et al. Evaluation of mitral leaflet motion by echocardiography and jet direction by Doppler color flow mapping to determine the mechanisms of mitral regurgitation. *J Am Coll Cardiol*. 1992;20:1353–1361.
7. Zoghbi WA, Enriquez-Sarano M, Foster E, et al. Recommendations for evaluation of the severity of native valvular regurgitation with two-dimensional and Doppler echocardiography. *J Am Soc Echocardiogr*. 2003;16:777–802.
8. Pu M, Vandervoort PM, Griffin BP, et al. Quantification of mitral regurgitation by the proximal convergence method using transesophageal echocardiography. Clinical validation of a geometric correction for proximal flow constraint. *Circulation*. 1995;92: 2169–2177.
9. Pu M, Griffin BP, Vandervoort PM, et al. The value of assessing pulmonary venous flow velocity for predicting severity of mitral regurgitation: a quantitative assessment integrating left ventricular function. *J Am Soc Echocardiogr*. 1999;12:736–743.
10. Grigioni F, Enriquez-Sarano M, Ling LH, et al. Sudden death in mitral regurgitation due to flail leaflet. *J Am Coll Cardiol*. 1999;34: 2078–2085.
11. Stewart WJ. Myocardial factor for timing of surgery in asymptomatic patients with mitral regurgitation. *Am Heart J*. 2003; 146:5–8.
12. Abascal VM, Wilkins GT, O'Shea JP, et al. Prediction of successful outcome in 130 patients undergoing percutaneous balloon mitral valvotomy. *Circulation*. 1990;82:448–456.
13. Leung DY, Griffin BP, Stewart WJ, et al. Left ventricular function after valve repair for chronic mitral regurgitation: predictive value of preoperative assessment of contractile reserve by exercise echocardiography. *J Am Coll Cardiol*. 1996 Nov 1;28(5):1198–1205.

## QUESTIONS

1. Mitral valve prolapse is associated with which of the following?
   a. Heart failure
   b. Atrial fibrillation
   c. Stroke
   d. Pulmonary hypertension
   e. None of the above

Answer is e: In a study by Freed et al. (2) of 84 subjects with mitral valve prolapse and 3,407 patients with no mitral valve prolapse, there was no significant association between presence of mitral valve prolapse and congestive heart failure, atrial fibrillation, cerebrovascular disease, or syncope.

**2.** What is the effect of successful mitral regurgitation repair on left ventricular ejection fraction?

a. Stays the same
b. Goes up
c. Goes down

Answer is c: In a study by Leung et al. (13) of 139 patients with isolated mitral regurgitation and no evidence of coronary artery disease, of whom 74 underwent uncomplicated valve repair, mitral regurgitation repair was associated with decreased left ventricular ejection fraction and end-diastolic volume. However, end-systolic volume was preserved.

**3.** What level of regurgitant orifice area (ROA) is the criterion for severe (4+) mitral regurgitation?

a. >60 cc
b. $>0.4$ cm$^2$
c. >200 cc/s
d. $>400$ mm$^2$
e. $>0.6$ cm$^2$

Answer is b: The following cut points have been established for severe mitral regurgitation when using proximal isovelocity surface area (PISA) to calculate regurgitant surface area (ROA) (7):

$<0.19$ cm$^2$ is mild
0.2–0.29 cm$^2$ is moderate
0.3–0.39 cm$^2$ is moderately severe
$>0.4$ cm$^2$ is severe

**4.** What is the most common etiology of tricuspid regurgitation?

a. Rheumatic disease
b. Prolapse or flail
c. Trauma
d. Carcinoid
e. Left-sided heart failure

Answer is e: The most common etiology of tricuspid regurgitation is left sided heart disease.

# Infective Endocarditis

# 26

***Ravindran A. Padmanabhan*** ***Steven M. Gordon***

The clinical spectrum of infective endocarditis (IE) has undergone dramatic changes (1). These include:

- A shift in the at-risk population
- The underlying cardiac defects predisposing a patient to IE
- The clinical presentation itself
- The etiologic agents of IE

There has been an upward shift in the age of the population at risk for IE. This has been linked to the advances in the field of cardiothoracic surgery, which have enabled patients to undergo valve replacement at older ages. The underlying cardiac defect has also shifted from rheumatic valvulitis to mitral valve prolapse. In the older population, lesions such as calcific aortic stenosis, calcified mitral annulus, degenerative aortic valve disease on either a previously normal or on a bicuspid valve, or a mural thrombus following myocardial infarction predispose to IE. In most urban areas, patients who are intravenous drug users (IDUs) account for a majority of IE, most commonly caused by *Staphylococcus aureus.* Such patients tend to present more acutely with fever and sepsis syndromes rather than as the classic Oslerian presentation of fever of unknown origin, Roth spots, Janeway lesions, Osler nodes, or regurgitant valvulitis. In an etiologic sense, too, there has been a shift of agents. For instance, the majority of cases in the 1960s and 1970s were caused by viridans Streptococci, whereas 15% of cases were due to Staphylococci. In more recent studies, Staphylococci have surpassed Streptococci as the most common cause of IE.

## EPIDEMIOLOGY

Infective endocarditis is still a rare phenomenon. The epidemiology of IE of native valves in the developed world is as follows.

The incidence of community-acquired native valve endocarditis is 1.7 to 6.2 per 100,000 person-years (2). The incidence of IE associated with injected drug use is 150 to 2,000 per 100,000 person-years (2). The incidence of IE associated with mitral valve prolapse is 100 per 100,000 person-years (2). The incidence of prosthetic valve endocarditis (PVE) was 0.94 per 100,000 patient-years in metropolitan Philadelphia. The risk for PVE increases with duration, and studies have revealed this to be approximately 1% at 1 year and 2% to 3% at 5 years.

## DEFINITIONS

Infective endocarditis is defined as a microbial infection of the endocardial surface of the heart. Acute and subacute endocarditis are further subdivisions based on the tempo and severity of the infection (2). Onset of PVE within 2 months after surgery is defined as early, and infections that are acquired after this period are defined as late. Mechanical heart valves are at higher risk for infection than are bioprosthetic valves during the first 3 months following surgery. After this period, both types of prosthetic valves are at equal risk for infection.

## HEALTH CARE–ASSOCIATED INFECTIVE ENDOCARDITIS

Hospital-acquired infective endocarditis constitutes 9% to 29% of all cases of IE and has increased in frequency in recent years owing to greater use of invasive procedures. Hospital-acquired IE has been defined as either IE with onset of symptoms >72 hours after hospitalization or IE occurring from 4 to 8 weeks after discharge from the hospital if an invasive procedure was performed during hospitalization. Methicillin Resistant Staphylococcus Aureus (MRSA), coagulase-negative Staphylococci and gram-negative bacilli tend to predominate as causative agents in

**TABLE 26–1**
**RISK FACTORS FOR INFECTIVE ENDOCARDITIS**

| High Risk | Moderate Risk |
|---|---|
| Prosthetic cardiac valves, including bioprosthetic and homograft valves | Most other congenital cardiac malformations (other than to the left) |
| Previous bacterial endocarditis | Acquired valvular dysfunction (e.g., rheumatic heart disease) |
| Complex cyanotic congenital heart disease (e.g., single ventricle states, transposition of the great arteries, tetralogy of Fallot) | Hypertrophic cardiomyopathy |
| Surgically constructed systemic pulmonary shunts or conduits | Mitral valve prolapse with valvular regurgitation and/or thickened leaflets |

nosocomial IE. Mortality rates are as high as 40% to 60% for IE acquired in the hospital.

## RISK FACTORS

Important cardiac risk factors (3) for IE are shown in Table 26–1.

## PATHOGENESIS

Four main mechanisms (4,5) are responsible for the initiation and localization of infection of the endocardium:

1. A previously damaged cardiac valve or a situation in which a jet effect is produced by blood flowing from a region of high pressure to one of low pressure (e.g., ventricular septal defect (VSD))
2. A sterile platelet fibrin thrombus
3. Bacteremia, even transient
4. High titer of agglutinating antibody for the infecting organism

## MICROBIOLOGY AND THE ROLE OF BLOOD CULTURES

In recent times, Staphylococci, particularly *Staph. aureus*, have overtaken viridans Streptococci as the most common cause of infective endocarditis (2).Fowler et al. (6) recruited 324 patients with *Staph. aureus* bacteremia (SAB) caused by an infected intravascular device to define patient and bacterial characteristics associated with the development of hematogenous complications (including endocarditis). On multivariable analysis, symptom duration, hemodialysis dependence, presence of a long-term intravascular catheter or a non–catheter device, and infection with Methicillin Resistant Staphylococcus Aureus (MRSA) placed the patients at a higher risk of developing hematogenous complications. In the future, we foresee a further shift in IE being caused by *Staph. aureus*.

Coagulase-negative Staphylococci are the most common pathogens in early prosthetic-valve endocarditis (2). *Staphylococcus lugdunensis*, a coagulase-negative organism, tends to cause a particularly virulent form of IE with high rates of perivalvular extension and metastatic seeding (2). The most common Streptococci isolated from patients with endocarditis are *Streptococcus sanguis, Strep. bovis, Strep. mutans,* and *Strep. mitis* (2). *Strep. bovis* infective endocarditis is prevalent among the elderly and is associated with preexisting colonic lesions (2) Polymicrobial infective endocarditis is encountered most often in the setting of injected drug use and is uncommon (2).

Blood cultures are excellent traditional tools, not only for diagnosis but also for the determination of antibiotic susceptibility to guide therapy. According to Towns et al. (7), best practice guidelines for blood cultures include:

- Obtaining blood cultures before starting antimicrobials whenever possible
- Exercising strict aseptic technique and optimal skin preparation when collecting blood cultures
- In acute presentations, obtaining at least two or preferably three sets of blood cultures rapidly within 5 to 10 minutes of each other prior to starting antibiotic therapy
- In subacute presentations, obtaining three separate blood cultures spaced 30 minutes apart
- Obtaining 20 mL of blood for each sample drawn

The most common cause of "culture-negative endocarditis" is prior administration of antibiotics. To overcome this problem, special blood culture media have been devised to inhibit the effects of antibiotics (7). When blood cultures from patients with IE remain negative at 48 to 72 hours, the lab should be alerted for prolonged incubation or for plating of subcultures on enriched media. A list of organisms that cause culture-negative endocarditis is provided in Table 26–2.

**TABLE 26–2**
**ORGANISMS CAUSING CULTURE-NEGATIVE ENDOCARDITIS**

| Organism | Approach |
|---|---|
| Abiotrophia species (previously classified as nutritionally variant streptocooci) | Grow in thioglycolate medium of blood culture and as satellite colonies around *Staphylococcus aureus* on blood agar or on medium supplemented with pyridoxal hydrochloride or L-cysteine |
| Bartonella species (usually *Bartonella hensla* or *B. quintane*) | Serologic tests<br>Lysis-centrifugation system for blood cultures<br>PCR of valve or embolized vegetations; special culture techniques available, but organisms are slow-growing and may require a month or more for isolation |
| *Coxiella a burnetii (Q fever)* | Serologic tests<br>PCR, Giemsa stain, or immunohistologic techniques on operative specimens |
| HACEK organisms | Blood cultures positive by day 7; occasionally require prolonged incubation and subculturing |
| Chlamydia species (usually *Chlamydia psittaci*) | Culture from blood has been described<br>Serologic tests<br>Direct staining of tissue with use of fluorescent monoclonal antibody |
| *Tropheryma whipplei* | Histologic examination (silver and PAS stains) of excised heart valve; PCR or culture of vegetation |
| Legionella species | Subculture from blood cultures, lysis-centrifugation pellet from blood cultures or operative specimens on BCYE agar; direct detection on heart valves with fluorescent antibody<br>Serologic tests |
| Brucella species (usually *Brucella melitensis* or *B. abortus*) | Serologic tests<br>Prolonged incubation of standard or lysis-centrifugation blood cultures |
| Fungi | Regular blood cultures often positive for candida species; lysis-centrifugation system with specific fungal medium can increase yield; testing urine for *Histoplasma capsulatum* antigen or serum for *Cryptococcus neoformans* polysaccharide capsular antigen can be helpful<br>Accessible lesions (such as emboli) should be cultured and examined histologically for fungi |

PCR, polymerase chain reaction; HACEK organisms *Haemophilus* species (*H. parainfluenzae, H. aphrophilus,* and *H. paraphrophilus*), *Actinobacillus actinomycctcomitans, Cardiobacterium hominis, Eikenella corrodens,* and *Kingella kingae*; PAS, periodic acid–Schiff; BCYE, buffered charcoal yeast extract.
*Source:* Reproduced from Mylonakis E, Calderwood SB. Infective endocarditis in adults. *N Engl J Med.* 2001;345(18):1318–1330, with permission.

*Coxiella burnetii* is the cause of Q fever and is a common cause of IE in parts of the world where sheep, cattle, and goat farming are common. *Coxiella* tends to infect prosthetic valves or previously damaged aortic and mitral valves and causes small subendothelial vegetations that are often missed by echocardiography. The organism resides in the acidic phagolysosome, where antibiotic activity may be inhibited.

*Brucellae* infect humans through the ingestion of contaminated meat or unpasteurized milk, the inhalation of infectious aerosols, or direct contact with infected tissues. This is mainly a disease of farmers, abattoir workers, veterinarians, and shepherds. Because vegetations are large and valve destruction commonly occurs, most patients require a combination of antimicrobial therapy and valve replacement.

*Legionella* IE presents as a febrile illness that has been present over many months. Most patients have prosthetic valves. Embolic events are unusual with this organism, and it requires special media to grow. *Pseudomonas aeruginosa* is a rare cause of IE and occurs in the setting of intravenous drug use.

Fungal IE is usually caused by *Aspergillus* or *Candida* species. Fungal IE usually is manifested by large and bulky vegetations, perivalvular extension of infection, metastatic seeding, and embolization to large blood vessels. Predisposing factors for fungal IE are injected drug use, prolonged antibiotic therapy, immunosuppression, intravenous catheters, pacemaker implantation, prior or concomitant bacterial endocarditis, and disseminated fungal infection. The rate of recovery of filamentous fungi such as *Aspergillus* is <30% even with the lysis centrifugation system.

## Role of PCR Amplification in Clinical Specimens

The diagnosis of IE is straightforward in a patient with typical signs and symptoms and a positive blood culture with a characteristic microorganism. It can be more difficult when blood cultures are sterile, either because of prior antimicrobial therapy or because of the fastidious nature of the pathogen.

More recently, a range of microorganisms including *T. whipplei, C. burnetii, B. henselae,* and *B. Quintana* have been identified using a broad-range polymerase chain reaction (PCR) in valvular specimens. Using universal primers, species-specific genetic sequences can be identified directly from tissue samples. This technique is culture independent, and almost all bacteria can be detected in a single reaction. Species-specific PCR primers are also available for many bacterial genera, including *T. whipplei, Chlamydia spp, Brucella spp, Legionella,* mycobacteria, and *Mycoplasma spp.*

In a recent study by Greub et al., (12) culture, histologic examination, and broad-range PCR were performed on valve samples taken from 127 patients with definite and possible IE (determined prior to valve surgery according to modified Duke criteria) and from 118 patients without IE. The sensitivity of PCR was 61%, whereas that of histology was 63% and that of valve culture was 13%. The specificity of both PCR and histology were 100%.

### The Important Role of *Staph. aureus* Bacteremia

The issue of IE in patients with prosthetic valves and SAB has been recently addressed in a study by Fadi El-Ahdab et al. (8). In this prospective study, approximately 50% of patients with prosthetic valves who developed *Staph. aureus* bacteremia had definite endocarditis. The authors recommend that all such patients undergo transesophageal echocardiography whenever possible. The authors also found a high rate of mortality (60%) in those patients who were managed medically. We have already alluded to the study by Fowler et al. (6), in which the authors found that 42 of 324 patients with SAB caused by intravascular device infection developed a hematogenous complication. Of these 42 patients, 31 had IE.

## CLINICAL FEATURES

In patients manifesting with classic features such as bacteremia or fungemia, active valvulitis, peripheral emboli, and immunologic vascular phenomena, the diagnosis of IE is straightforward. Fever is the most common symptom and sign; however, it may be absent or minimal in patients with congestive heart failure, severe debility, chronic renal or liver failure, previous use of antimicrobial drugs, or infective endocarditis caused by less virulent organisms. Other common symptoms of subacute infective endocarditis include anorexia, weight loss, malaise, and night sweats. Joint complaints are an early symptom in subacute IE, ranging from low-back pain and myalgias to frank septic arthritis. A chronic wasting disease similar to that seen in HIV or cancer may develop in a proportion of patients with subacute IE. Pulmonary findings such as pneumonia may be the dominant feature in isolated right-sided infective endocarditis. The onset of nosocomial infective endocarditis is usually acute, and signs of endocarditis are infrequent.

The presentation of infective endocarditis often includes extracardiac manifestations or findings that are associated with intracardiac extension of infection. Most patients with infective endocarditis have a heart murmur (most commonly pre-existing), and patients may have petechiae on the skin, conjunctivae, or oral mucosa, as well as splenomegaly and other peripheral manifestations. A murmur or other evidence of valvular disease, especially aortic or mitral regurgitation, may be a common sign in subacute IE.

Splinter hemorrhages (Fig. 26–1) are 1- to 2-mm brown streaks under the nails and are of greater significance when seen in the proximal nail bed. Osler nodes (Fig. 26–2) are red, painful, indurated lesions between 2 and 15 mm, found on the palms and soles. Janeway lesions (Fig. 26–3) are red, painless macules that appear on the palms and soles. Roth's spots are retinal hemorrhages with a pale center. Embolization of small vegetations to the distal extremities may result in "blue toe syndrome," which resolves in most cases without sequelae. Acute IE presents as severe sepsis with high fevers, lethargy, shock, and rapid cardiac deterioration. In acute aortic regurgitation, signs such as a widened pulse pressure are not usually present. In acute

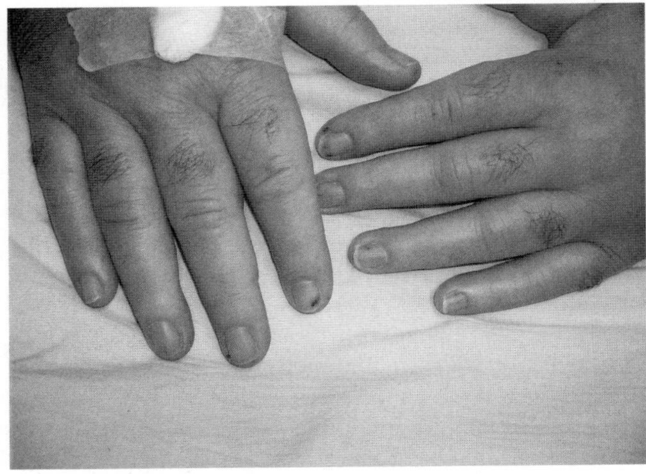

**Figure 26–1** Splinter hemorrhages.

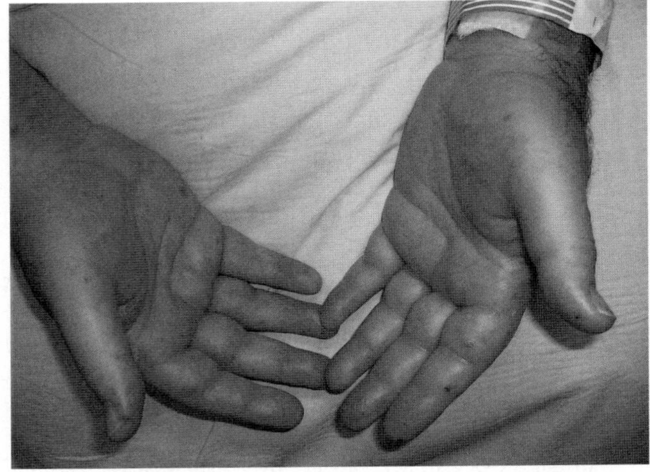

**Figure 26–2** Osler nodes.

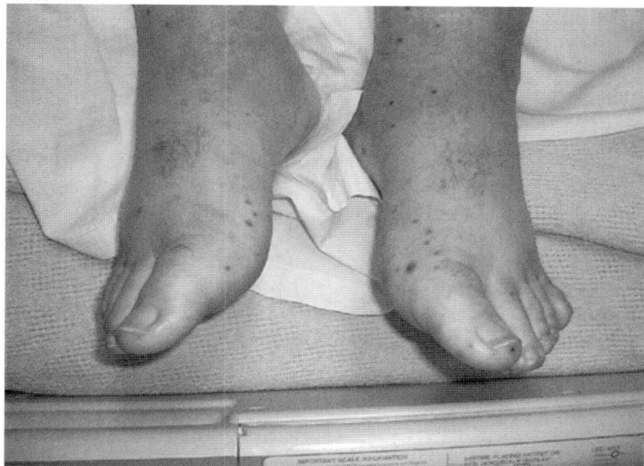
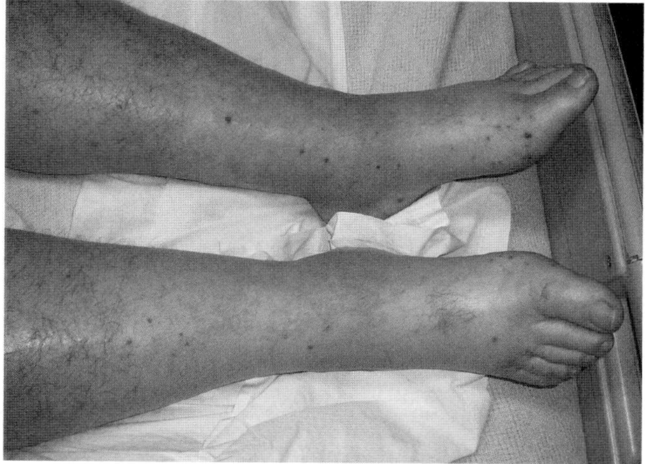

**Figure 26–3** Janeway lesions.

mitral regurgitation, a fourth heart sound may develop rather than the typical third heart sound seen in chronic mitral regurgitation. A rapid destruction of left-sided valves occurs, leading to heart failure and circulatory collapse. Metastatic infection can also occur in any organ of the body.

Prosthetic valve endocarditis may be manifested as an indolent illness with low-grade fever or it can be an acute febrile and toxic illness. The high frequency of invasive infection in prosthetic valve endocarditis results in higher rates of new or changing murmurs and of congestive heart failure. Unexplained fever in a patient with a prosthetic valve should prompt careful evaluation for prosthetic valve endocarditis.

Other signs and symptoms related to the complications of IE include cerebral vascular accident (CVA), lethargy, confusion, frank psychosis, and ruptured mycotic aneurysm causing hemorrhage in an intracranial location, renal failure from severe sepsis, embolization, or immune complex deposition. Embolization to peripheral arteries may present as an acutely ischemic limb, a splenic infarct causing abdominal pain, a kidney embolus causing flank pain, or a coronary embolus causing myocardial infarction.

## DIAGNOSIS

A substantial proportion of patients with IE do not present with the classic Oslerian manifestations because of the acute nature of their illness. The diagnosis of infective endocarditis requires the assimilation of clinical, laboratory, and echocardiographic data.

Nonspecific laboratory abnormalities may be present, including anemia, leukocytosis, abnormal urinalysis results (hematuria, proteinuria, or red cell casts), and an elevated erythrocyte sedimentation rate and C-reactive protein level. New atrioventricular, fascicular, or bundle branch block, particularly in the setting of aortic valve endocarditis, suggests perivalvular invasion, and such patients may need cardiac monitoring until they are stable.

### The Duke Criteria

The variability of illness in IE mandates a diagnostic strategy that is both sensitive and specific. In 1981, von Reyn et al. proposed very stringent criteria called the Beth Israel criteria to aid in the diagnosis of IE. More recently, in 1994, a group at Duke University proposed standardized criteria for assessing patients with suspected infective endocarditis (9). These criteria integrated factors predisposing patients to the development of infective endocarditis, the blood-culture isolate and persistence of bacteremia, and echocardiographic findings with other clinical and laboratory information. In a review of the individual value of each component of the Duke criteria, the major microbiologic criteria had the highest relative importance. This further stresses the importance of obtaining adequate blood cultures in a patient suspected of having IE, preferably prior to the administration of antibiotics.

The Duke criteria classify patients into three categories: definite cases identified either clinically or pathologically, possible cases, and rejected cases. Numerous studies have validated the usefulness of the Duke criteria. Misclassification of culture-negative cases, the increasing role of transesophageal echocardiography, the relative risk of endocarditis in *Staph. aureus* bacteremia, and the overly broad categorization of casesas "possible" were problems with the original criteria. A modified version of the Duke criteria has recently been proposed (10) (Table 26–3).

### Echocardiography

Transthoracic echocardiography (TTE) is rapid, noninvasive, and has excellent specificity for vegetations (98%) (1). However, TTE may be inadequate in up to 20% of adult

**TABLE 26–3**
**MODIFIED DUKE CRITERIA**

| Criteria | Comments |
|---|---|
| Major criteria | |
| Microbiologic | |
| Typical microorganism isolated from two separate blood cultures: viridans streptococci, *Streptococcus bovis,* HACEK group, *Staphylococcus aureus,* or community acquired enterococcal bacteremia without a primary focus<br>or | In patients with possible infective endocarditis, at least two sets of cultures of blood collected by separate venipunctures should be obtained within the first 1 to 2 hours of presentation. Patients with cardiovascular collapse should have three cultures of blood obtained at 5 to 10 minute intervals and thereafter receive empirical antibiotic therapy |
| Microorganism consistent with infective endocarditis isolated from persistently positive blood cultures<br>or | |
| Single positive blood culture for *Coxiells burnetii* or phase 1 IgG antibody titer to *C. burnetii* >1:800 | *C. burnetii* is not readily cultivated in most clinical microbiology laboratories |
| Evidence of endocardial involvement | |
| New valvular regurgitation (increase or change in preexisting murmur not sufficient)<br>or | |
| Positive echocardiogram (transesophageal echocardiogram recommended in patients who have a prosthetic valve, who are rated as having at least possible infective endocarditis by clinical criteria, or who have complicated infective endocarditis) | Three echocardiographic findings quality as major criteria: a discrete, echogenic, oscillating intracardiac mass located at a site of endocardial injury; a periannular abscess; and a new dehiscence of a prosthetic valve |
| Minor criteria | |
| Predisposition to infective endocarditis that includes certain cardiac conditions and injection drug use | Cardiac abnormalities that are associated with infective endocarditis are classified into three groups:<br>High risk conditions: previous infective endocarditis,[46] aortic valve disease, rheumatic heart disease, prosthetic heart valve, coarctation of the aorta, and complex cyanotic congenital heart diseases<br>Moderate risk conditions: mitral valve prolapse with valvular regurgitation or leaflet thickening, isolated mitral stenosis, tricuspid valve disease, pulmonary stenosis, and hypertrophic cardiomyopathy<br>Low or no risk conditions: secundum atrial septal defect, ischemic heart disease, previous coronary artery bypass graft surgery, and mitral valve prolapse with thin leaflets in the absence of regurgitation |
| Fever | Temperature >38°C (100.4°F) |
| Vascular phenomena | Petechiae and splinter hemorrhages are excluded<br>None of the peripheral lesions are pathognomonic for infective endocarditis |
| Immunologic phenomena | Presence of rheumatoid factor, glomerulonephritis, Osler's nodes, or Roth spots |
| Microbiologic findings | Positive blood cultures that do not meet the major criteria<br>Serologic evidence of active infection; single isolates of coagulase negative staphylococci and organisms that very rarely cause infective endocarditis are excluded from this category. |

Cases are defined clinically as definite if they fulfill two major criteria, one major criterion plus three minor criteria, or five minor criteria; they are defined as possible if they fulfill one major and one minor criterion, or three minor criteria. HACEK, *Haemophilus* species (*H. parainfluenzae, H. aphriphilus,* and *H. paraphrophilus*), *Actinobacillus actinomyoctomcomitants, Cardiobacterium hominis, Eikenella corrodens, and Kingella kingae.*
*Source:* Reproduced from Mylonakis E, Calderwood SB. Infective endocarditis in adults. *N Engl J Med.* 2001;345(18):1318–1330, with permission.

patients because of obesity, chronic obstructive pulmonary disease, or chest-wall deformities; the overall sensitivity for vegetations may be less than 60% to 70% (1). Additionally, TTE cannot exclude several important aspects of IE, including infection on prosthetic valves, periannular abscess, leaflet perforation, and fistulae (1).

Transesophageal echocardiography images utilize higher ultrasonic frequencies and hence possess higher spatial resolution with decreased interference from interposed tissues. Transesophageal echocardiography is more costly and invasive but increases the sensitivity for detecting vegetations to 75% to 95% while maintaining a specificity of 85% to 98%. Transesophageal echocardiography is particularly useful in patients with prosthetic valves and for the evaluation of myocardial invasion. A negative transesophageal echocardiogram has a negative predictive value for infective endocarditis of >92%.

Transesophageal echocardiography (TEE) is more sensitive (76% to 100%) and more specific (94%) than transthoracic echocardiography for defining perivalvular extension of infective endocarditis and the presence of a myocardial abscess. Transesophageal echocardiography with spectral and color-flow Doppler techniques can also demonstrate the distinctive flow patterns of fistulas, pseudoaneurysms, or unruptured abscess cavities and is more sensitive than transthoracic echocardiography for identifying valve perforations.

Recent guidelines suggest that, among patients with suspected infective endocarditis, transthoracic echocardiography should be used in the evaluation of those with native valves who are optimal imaging candidates (11). In fact, the appropriate use of echocardiography depends on the prior probability of infective endocarditis. If this probability is less than 4%, a negative transthoracic echocardiogram is cost effective and clinically satisfactory in ruling out infective endocarditis. For patients whose prior probability of infective endocarditis is 4% to 60%, the initial use of transesophageal echocardiography is more cost effective and diagnostically efficient than initial use of transthoracic echocardiography, which, if negative, is followed by transesophageal echocardiography. This category of intermediate prior probability includes patients with unexplained bacteremia with a gram-positive coccus, those with catheter-associated *Staph. aureus* bacteremia, and those admitted with fever or bacteremia in the setting of recent injection-drug use. The category of low prior probability (<2%) includes patients with gram-negative bacteremia with a clear non-cardiac source and patients with firm alternative diagnoses or those in whom the "endocarditis" syndrome resolves within 4 days.

There has been considerable controversy as to whether vegetation size as measured by echocardiography is a prognostic indicator for embolism or even an indication for surgery. Table 26–4 summarizes the echocardiographic features that suggest the potential need for surgical intervention.

Figure 26–4 is a suggested algorithm for the use of TEE or TTE in the diagnosis of IE.

**TABLE 26–4**
**ECHOCARDIOGRAPHIC FEATURES THAT SUGGEST POTENTIAL NEED FOR SURGICAL INTERVENTION**

| |
|---|
| Vegetation |
| Persistent vegetation after systemic embolization |
| Anterior mitral leaflet vegetation, particularly with size >10 mm[a] |
| 1 embolic events during first 2 wk of antimicrobial therapy[a] |
| Increase in vegetation size despite appropriate antimicrobial therapy[a,b] |
| Valvular dysfunction |
| Acute aortic or mitral insufficiency with signs of ventricular failure[b] |
| Heart failure unresponsive to medical therapy[b] |
| Valve perforation or rupture[b] |
| Perivalvular extension |
| Valvular dehiscence, rupture, or fistula[b] |
| New heart block[b,c] |
| Large abscess or extension of abscess despite appropriate antimicrobial therapy[b] |

See text for more complete discussion of indications for surgery based on vegetation characterizations.
[a]Surgery may be required because of risk of embolization.
[b]Surgery may be required because of heart failure or failure of medical therapy.
[c]Echocardiography should not be the primary modality used to detect or monitor heart block.
*Source:* From Baddour LM, Wilson WR, Bayer AS, et al. Infective endocarditis: diagnosis, antimicrobial therapy, and management of complications. *Circulation.* 2005;111:e394.

## COMPLICATIONS

Certain conditions place patients at increased risk for complications from IE. These are summarized in Table 26–5. Complications of IE may be classified as follows:

- Cardiac, including congestive heart failure (CHF), paravalvular extension
- Neurologic, including stroke
- Systemic emboli, including splenic abscess
- Mycotic aneurysms, intracranial and extracranial

CHF may develop acutely as a result of valve perforation, rupture of mitral chordae, mechanical blockage of valve orifice by bulky vegetation, advanced heart block, or fistulization of cardiac chambers (2). CHF may occur in a more gradual fashion as a result of worsening valvular insufficiency. CHF as a result of IE is associated with a grave prognosis, and delaying surgery to the point of total ventricular decompensation increases operative mortality. In addition, poor surgical outcomes are portended by New York Heart Association (NYHA) Class III or IV, renal insufficiency, and advanced age. Aortic valve infection is more commonly associated with CHF than is mitral valve infection. The left ventricle alone bears the brunt of the overload in the case of moderate to severe acute aortic valve infection as opposed to acute mitral valve regurgitation, in which the left atrium and the pulmonary vascular bed accommodate the regurgitant volume. Hence, new-onset, moderate to severe aortic incompetence due to IE usually requires surgery. The indications for surgery in right-sided IE are less clear cut. Tricuspid incompetence and pulmonary incompetence are well tolerated as long as there is no pre-existing increased pulmonary vascular resistance.

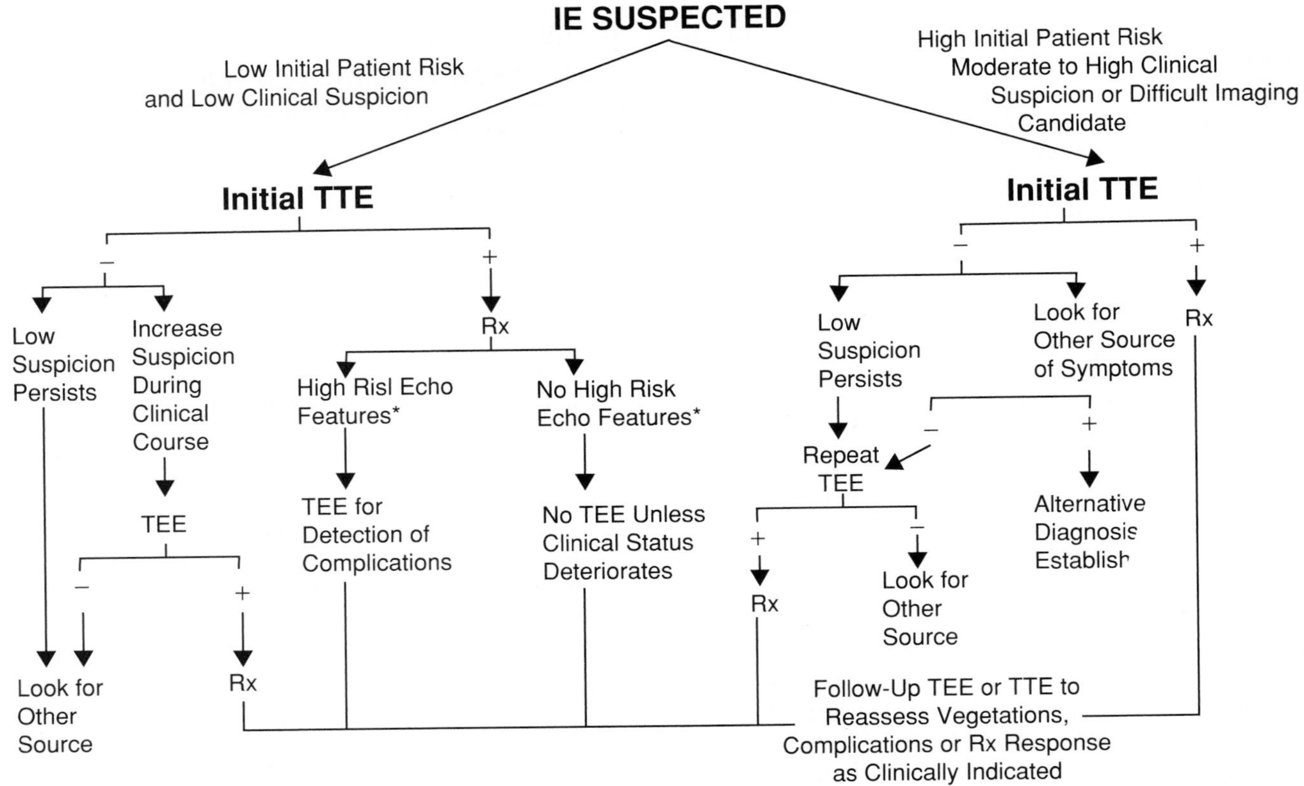


**Figure 26–4** Algorithm for the use of TEE or TTE in the diagnosis of IE. (From Baddour LM, Wilson WR, Bayer AS, et al: Infective endocarditis: diagnosis, antimicrobial therapy, and management of complications. A statement for healthcare professionals from the Committee on Rheumatic Fever, Endocarditis and Kawasaki Disease, Council on Cardiovascular Disease in the Young, and the Councils on Clinical Cardiology, Stroke, and Cardiovascular Surgery and Anesthesia, American Heart Association, and endorsed by the Infectious Diseases Society of America. *Circulation*. 2005;111:e394.

Extension of infection beyond the valve annulus is associated with higher mortality, more frequent CHF, and the need for cardiac surgery. This complication occurs in 10% to 40% of all native valve IE, and in 56% to 100% of all PVE IE. In native aortic valve IE, the extension tends to happen at the weakest portion of the annulus, which resides near the membranous septum and atrioventricular node. This is the reason why abscesses and heart blocks are more frequent in this location (1). Clinical parameters or the size of the vegetation do not predict the possibility of perianular extension. Development of new atrial valve block has a 77% positive predictive value for abscess formation, but the sensitivity is only 42%. TEE is the modality of choice when perivalvular extension is suspected. Urgent surgery is usually indicated for this condition and involves drainage of abscess cavities, excision of necrotic tissue, and closure of fistulous tracts in addition to valve replacement.

Neurologic complications develop in up to 40% of all patients with IE (2). These may include embolic stroke with or without hemorrhage, transient ischemic attacks, ruptured intracranial mycotic aneurysm, meningitis, and encephalopathy. The majority of emboli lodge in the middle cerebral artery distribution (1). The management of a patient with neurologic complications in the acute phase of IE is a controversial area. Any patient with IE and neurologic symptoms should have a preoperative CT of the head. A ruptured mycotic aneurysm should be clipped, resected, or embolized prior to cardiac surgery for IE. In patients

**TABLE 26–5**
**CLINICAL SITUATIONS CONSTITUTING HIGH RISK FOR COMPLICATIONS FOR IE**

Prosthetic cardiac valves
Left-sided IE
*Staphylococcus aureus* IE
Fungal IE
Previous IE
Prolonged clinical symptoms (≥3 mo)
Cyanotic congenital heart disease
Patients with systemic to pulmonary shunts
Poor clinical response to antimicrobial therapy

*Source:* Reproduced from Bayer AS, Bolger AF, Taubert KA, et al. Diagnosis and management of infective endocarditis and its complications. *Circulation*. 1998;98(25):2936–2948, with permission.

with a hemorrhagic infarct, the current recommendation is to wait for 2 to 3 weeks between the neurologic event and cardiac surgery because of two concerns: the risk of intracranial bleeding during cardiopulmonary bypass, and the risk related to anticoagulation post–cardiac surgery.

Systemic embolization most commonly involves the spleen, kidney, liver, and the iliac or mesenteric arteries (2). Splenic abscess is a rare complication of IE and develops as a result of bacteremic seeding of a bland infarct caused by a splenic artery embolus, or by direct seeding of the splenic tissue by an infected vegetation (1). It occurs in 5% of all splenic infarctions, with viridans Streptococci and *Staph. aureus* being the major causes. The diagnosis must be suspected in any patient with IE and flank, back, or abdominal tenderness in the left upper quadrant (1). Abdominal CT or MRI are the most sensitive modalities to diagnose this complication, and definitive treatment is splenectomy with antibiotics before valve surgery, unless valve replacement is more urgent (1).

Mycotic aneurysms (MAs) may be intra or extracranial. They are uncommon complications of IE and result from septic embolization of vegetations first to the vasa vasorum, then into the intima, and finally through the outer layer of the vessel wall. The most common sites are the branching points of arteries and occur, in decreasing order, in intracranial arteries, visceral arteries, and arteries of the lower and upper extremities.

Intracranial MAs occur in 1.2% to 5% of patients with IE and carry a high mortality rate of 60%. The bifurcations of the distal MCA are the most commonly involved arteries. Symptoms may include severe headache, altered mental status, hemianopia, or cranial neuropathies. Sudden hemorrhage may occur in the absence of other premonitory symptoms (1,2). Routine screening for intracranial MAs is not recommended in the absence of neurologic symptoms or signs. Contrast-enhanced CT, MRI, and MRA are all useful techniques to diagnose intracranial MAs, but the current "gold standard" is four-vessel cerebral angiography. Decisions concerning the medical versus surgical treatment of intracranial MAs need to be tailored according to the individual patient. A single MA distal to the first bifurcation of a major intracranial artery should be monitored closely with serial angiograms and must be excised if it enlarges or bleeds. In the case of multiple aneurysms, close monitoring is required with angiograms or CT scans, and if more than one aneurysm enlarges, prompt surgical excision is required (1). A less invasive alternative to surgery, especially in a distally or peripherally located aneurysm, is coil embolization (1).

Extracranial (1) MAs, intrathoracic or intra-abdominal, are often asymptomatic. However, the appearance of a new, painful, pulsatile mass with IE should prompt the diagnosis of extracranial MA. Hematuria and hypertension should suggest the rupture of a renal artery MA. Massive bloody diarrhea should suggest the rupture of an intra-abdominal MA into the bowel. Hematemesis, hematobilia, and jaundice should suggest rupture of a hepatic artery MA. Mortality in patients with IE is high, and revascularization should be established through extra-anatomic routes via uninfected tissue planes. Long-term suppressive antibiotic therapy will probably be required, as patients are at high risk of recurrence of infection, especially in the interposed vascular grafts in previously infected areas.

## TREATMENT

Certain principles are important when considering treatment of infective endocarditis (1). The regimen must be bactericidal. Prolonged therapy is often necessary. Vancomycin is less rapidly bactericidal than semisynthetic penicillins and first-generation cephalosporins. IE is one of the conditions for which skin testing should be performed on patients with a questionable history of immediate hypersensitivity reactions to penicillin.

The American Heart Association's recommendations for the treatment of IE due to Streptococci, Enterococci, Staphylococci, and HACEK have recently been updated (1). These are summarized in Table 26–6.

### Caveats for the Common Causes of IE

Minimum inhibitory concentrations (MIC) should be determined for Streptococci against penicillin, as treatment is dependent on the values obtained (2). A 2-week regimen may be appropriate in certain situations, such as those cases of uncomplicated IE caused by highly penicillin-susceptible viridans Streptococci and *Strep. bovis* in those patients at low risk for complications from gentamicin therapy. For patients who are allergic to $\beta$-lactams, vancomycin is an effective alternative.

*Enterococcus faecium* and *E. faecalis* (1) are the two major enterococcal causes of IE. These organisms are relatively resistant to penicillin, expanded-spectrum penicillins, and vancomycin. They are also uniformly resistant to cephalosporins and relatively resistant to aminoglycosides. The combination of penicillin, vancomycin, or ampicillin with aminoglycosides is necessary to exhibit a synergistic bactericidal effect on these isolates, and standard therapy should continue for 4 weeks. All enterococcal isolates that cause IE must be screened for antimicrobial susceptibility against penicillin, ampicillin, vancomycin, gentamicin-and streptomycin. Optimal therapy has not been determined for isolates with high level resistance to both gentamicin and streptomycin.

For organisms with intrinsic high-level resistance to penicillin (MIC $>16$ $\mu$g/mL), vancomycin is the preferred agent for combination. Vancomycin may enhance the nephrotoxic potential of aminoglycosides. Serum levels of aminoglycosides should be carefully monitored during therapy of enterococcal endocarditis. Peak levels of gentamicin should not exceed 3 and trough levels should not

**TABLE 26–6**
**THERAPY OF NATIVE VALVE ENDOCARDITIS CAUSED BY HIGHLY PENICILLIN-SUSCEPTIBLE VIRIDANS GROUP STREPTOCOCCI AND *Streptococcus bovis***

| Regimen | Dosage[a] and Route | Duration (wk) | Strength of Recommendation | Comments |
|---|---|---|---|---|
| Aqueous crystalline penicillin G sodium | 12 to 18 million U/24 h IV, either continuously or in 4 or 6 equally divided doses | 4 | IA | Preferred in most patients >65 y or patients with impairment of eighth cranial nerve function or renal function |
| *or* | | | | |
| Ceftriaxone sodium | 2 g/24 h IV/IM in 1 dose<br>*Pediatric dose*[b]: penicillin 200 000 U/kg per 24 h IV in 4 to 6 equally divided doses; ceftriaxone 100 mg/kg per 24 h IV/IM in 1 dose | 4 | IA | |
| Aqueous crystalline penicillin G sodium | 12 to 18 million U/24 h IV either continuously or in 6 equally divided doses | 2 | IB | 2-wk regimen not intended for patients with known cardiac or extracardiac abscess or for those with creatinine clearance of <20 mL/min, impaired eighth cranial nerve function, or *Abiotrophia, Granulicatella*, or *Gemella* spp infection; gentamicin dosage should be adjusted to achieve peak serum concentration of 3 to 4 μg/mL and trough serum concentration of <1 μg/mL when 3 divided doses are used; nomogram used for single daily dosing[d] |
| *or* | | | | |
| Ceftriaxone sodium | 2 g/24 h IV/IM in 1 dose | 2 | IB | |
| *plus* | | | | |
| Gentamicin sulfate[c] | 3 mg/kg per 24 h IV/IM in 1 dose<br>*Pediatric dose*: penicillin 200 000 U/kg per 24 h IV in 4 to 6 equally divided doses; ceftriaxone 100 mg/kg per 24 h IV/IM in 1 dose; gentamicin 3 mg/kg per 24 h IV/IM in 1 dose or 3 equally divided doses[e] | 2 | | |
| Vancomycin hydrochloride[f] | 30 mg/kg per 24 h IV in 2 equally divided doses not to exceed 2 g/24 h unless concentrations in serum are inappropriately low<br>*Pediatric dose*: 40 mg/kg per 24 h IV in 2 to 3 equally divided doses | 4 | IB | Vancomycin therapy recommended only for patients unable to tolerate penicillin or ceftriaxone; vancomycin dosage should be adjusted to obtain peak (1 h after infusion completed) serum concentration of 30 to 45 μg/mL and a trough concentration range of 10 to 15 μg/mL |

Minimum inhibitory concentration 0.12 μg/mL.
[a]Dosages recommended are for patients with normal renal function.
[b]Pediatric dose should not exceed that of a normal adult.
[c]Other potentially nephrotoxic drugs (e.g., nonsteroidal anti-inflammatory drugs) should be used with caution in patients receiving gentamicin therapy.
[d]See reference 280 in full statement.
[e]Data for once-daily dosing of aminoglycosides for children exist, but no data for treatment of IE exist.
[f]Vancomycin dosages should be infused during course of at least 1 h to reduce risk of histamine-release "red man" syndrome.
*Source:* From Baddour LM, Wilson WR, Bayer AS, et al. Infective endocarditis: diagnosis, antimicrobial therapy, and management of complications. *Circulation.* 2005;111:e394.

exceed 1. Note that these levels are not as high as those when aminoglycosides are used in the synergistic treatment of gram-negative systemic infections. Daptomycin has proven in vitro activity against MRSA, MRSE, glycopeptide intermediate SA and VRE faecium in an in vitro pharmacodynamic model with simulated endocardial vegetations.

For methicillin-susceptible staphylococci native valve IE, nafcillin or oxacillin must be used with a brief 3- to 5-day course of gentamicin. Though the aminoglycoside offered no significant mortality or morbidity benefit, it shortened the duration of positive blood cultures in a multicenter collaborative study while harmful side effects were reduced. For methicillin-susceptible staphylococcal IE in prosthetic valves, nafcillin or oxacillin with rifampin for 6 weeks plus gentamicin for the first 2 weeks is recommended. For methicillin-resistant staphylococcal native valve IE, Vancomycin, usually with gentamicin added for the first 3 to

**TABLE 26–7**
**INDICATIONS FOR SURGERY IN PATIENTS WITH INFECTIVE ENDOCARDITIS**

| Indication | Evidence Based |
|---|---|
| Emergency indication for cardiac surgery (same day) | |
| 1. Acute AR with early closure of mitral valve | A |
| 2. Rupture of a sinus Valsalva aneurysm into the right heart chamber | A |
| 3. Rupture into the pericardium | A |
| Urgent indication for cardiac surgery (within 1 to 2 d) | |
| 4. Valvular obstruction | A |
| 5. Unstable prosthesis | A |
| 6. Acute AR or MR with heart failure, NYHA III-IV | A |
| 7. Septal perforation | A |
| 8. Evidence of annular or aortic abscess, sinus or aortic true or false aneurysm, fistula formation, or new onset conduction disturbances | A |
| 9. Major embolism + mobile vegetation >10 mm + appropriate antibiotic therapy <7 to 10 d | B |
| 10. Mobile vegetation >15 mm + appropriate antibiotic therapy <7 to 10 d | C |
| 11. No effective antimicrobial therapy available | A |
| Elective indication for cardiac surgery (earlier is usually better) | |
| 12. Staphylococcal prosthetic valve endocarditis | B |
| 13. Early prosthetic valve endocarditis (≤2 mo after surgery) | B |
| 14. Evidence of progressive paravalvular prosthetic leak | A |
| 15. Evidence of valve dysfunction and persistent infection after 7 to 10 d of appropriate antibiotic therapy, as indicated by presence of fever or bacteremia, provided there are no noncardiac causes for infection | A |
| 16. Fungal endocarditis caused by a mold | A |
| 17. Fungal endocarditis caused by a yeast | B |
| 18. Infection with difficult-to-treat organisms | B |
| 19. Vegetation growing larger during antibiotic therapy >7 d | C |

A strong evidence or general agreement that cardiac surgery is useful and effective; AR, aortic regurgitation; B, Inconclusive or conflicting evidence or a divergence of opinion about the usefulness/efficacy of cardiac surgery, but weight of evidence/opinion of the majority is in favor; C, Inconclusive or conflicting evidence or a divergence of opinion; lack of clear consensus on the basis of evidence/opinion of the majority. MR, mitral regurgitation; NYHA, New York Heart Association classification.
*Source:* Reprinted from Olaison L, Pettersson G. Current best practices and guidelines. Indications for surgical intervention in infective endocarditis. *Cardiol. Clin.* 2003;21(2):235–251, Copyright 2003, with permission from Elsevier.

5 days of therapy, is the standard. For methicillin-resistant staphylococcal IE on prosthetic valves, combination therapy is advocated, with vancomycin and rifampin for 6 weeks plus gentamicin for the first 2 weeks.

The benefit of rifampin in MRSA endocarditis has been derived from the ability of this drug to sterilize "foreign body infection" in an experimental animal model. Coagulase-negative staphylococci are now the most common cause of prosthetic valve IE, particularly in the first 12 months following surgery. The organisms are usually methicillin resistant, and treatment should be the combination described. If the organism is resistant to gentamicin, an aminoglycoside to which susceptibility is demonstrated should be chosen. If the isolate is resistant to all aminoglycosides, this component should be omitted from the regimen.

In the situation of right-sided native valve IE caused by methicillin-susceptible *Staph. aureus* in intravenous drug users, limited data suggest that a 2-week course of nafcillin or oxacillin with gentamicin may be sufficient. This regimen may not be suitable in IDUs with left-sided IE, metastatic IE such as lung abscess, underlying HIV, or vegetations >1 to 2 cm.

HACEK organisms should be considered ampicillin resistant, and monotherapy with this drug is no longer recommended. Limited data suggest that a third-generation cephalosporin such as ceftriaxone or cefotaxime sodium should be used for 4 weeks in native valve and for 6 weeks in prosthetic valve IE. Aztreonam, trimethoprim–sulfamethoxazole (TMP-SMX), or the fluoroquinolones are the recommended alternative agents for patients with HACEK IE who are unable to tolerate cephalosporins.

## Caveats for Some Uncommon Causes of IE

*Coxiella burnetii* IE is usually treated with a combination of doxycycline and rifampin, TMP-SMX, or fluoroquinolones. The optimal duration of therapy is unknown. Valve replacement is indicated only for CHF, PVE, or uncontrolled infection. Many experts recommend long-term and possibly indefinite therapy in this setting. Yet others have suggested a minimum of 3 years of therapy once phase I IgG antibody titers drop to <1:4,000 and phase I IgA antibody is undetectable.

Few patients with *Brucella* IE have been cured with antimicrobial therapy alone. Most require valve replacement in addition to the following: doxycycline plus either streptomycin or gentamicin *or* doxycycline plus either TMP-SMX or rifampin. Again, the optimal duration of therapy is unknown, but authorities recommend this regimen for 8 weeks to 10 months following valve replacement.

In *Legionella* IE, cure has been obtained by prolonged parenteral therapy with either doxycycline or erythromycin followed by an oral course for a prolonged period. The total duration of therapy is usually 6 to 17 months.

*Pseudomonas aeruginosa* IE of the right side usually requires the combination of high doses of an antipseudomonal penicillin (piperacillin) and an aminoglycoside (tobramycin). Left-sided pseudomonal IE rarely responds to medical therapy alone, and surgery is considered mandatory.

In fungal IE caused by *Aspergillus* or *Candida* species, amphotericin B has poor penetration into vegetations. Most vegetations are bulky and metastatic complications, including periannular extension and embolization to large blood vessels, are frequent. Virtually all complicated cases of *Candida* IE need surgery, and mortality is 90% to 100% in *Aspergillus* IE without surgery.

## INDICATIONS FOR SURGERY IN IE

The decision regarding surgery in the treatment of infective endocarditis is multidisciplinary (input from surgeon, cardiologist, and infectious disease clinicians) and should be individualized (1).

Table 26–7 summarizes the indications for surgical intervention in IE. Surgical therapy in IE has contributed to the overall decrease in mortality, especially in patients with CHF, complicated perivalvular extension, and in PVE. The general preoperative condition of the patient, chronic hemodialysis, ongoing antibiotic treatment, timing of surgery, surgical techniques, postoperative care, and follow-up are important influences of outcome. Preoperative NYHA class, age, and preoperative renal failure are the variables that foretell operative mortality in logistic regression analysis.

## CONCLUSIONS

The incidence of IE continues to rise. It is now the fourth most common cause of death among life-threatening infectious diseases. Clinical manifestations of IE are so varied that the patient may present to any of the medical subspecialties. The successful management of these infections requires close cooperation between medical and surgical teams. Even with advanced diagnostic and management strategies in the 21st century, it still is a life-threatening disease.

## REFERENCES


1. Baddour LM, Wilson WR, Bayer AS, et al: Infective endocarditis: diagnosis, antimicrobial therapy, and management of complications. A statement for healthcare professionals from the Committee on Rheumatic Fever, Endocarditis and Kawasaki Disease, Council on Cardiovascular Disease in the Young, and the Councils on Clinical Cardiology, Stroke, and Cardiovascular Surgery and Anesthesia, American Heart Association, and endorsed by the Infectious Diseases Society of America. *Circulation.* 2005;111:e394. Available at http://circ.ahajournals.org/cgi/content/full/111/23/e394. Accessed November 18, 2005.
2. Mylonakis E, Calderwood SB. Infective endocarditis in adults. *N Engl J Med.* 2001;345(18):1318–1330.
3. Dajani AS, Taubert KA, Wilson W, et al. Prevention of bacterial endocarditis. Recommendations by the American Heart Association. *Circulation.* 1997;96(1):358–366.
4. Weinstein L, Schlesinger JJ. Pathoanatomic, pathophysiologic and clinical correlations in endocarditis (first of two parts). *N Engl J Med.* 1974;291(16):832–837.
5. Weinstein L, Schlesinger JJ. Pathoanatomic, pathophysiologic and clinical correlations in endocarditis (second of two parts). *N Engl J Med.* 1974;291(21):1122–1126.
6. Fowler VG Jr, Justice A, Moore C, et al. Risk factors for hematogenous complications of intravascular catheter-associated *Staphylococcus aureus* bacteremia. *Clin Infect Dis.* 2005;40(5):695–703.
7. Towns ML, Reller LB. Diagnostic methods. Current best practices and guidelines for isolation of bacteria and fungi in infective endocarditis. *Cardiol. Clin.* 2003;21(2):197–205.
8. El-Ahdab F, Benjamin DK Jr, Wang A, et al. Risk of endocarditis among patients with prosthetic valves and *Staphylococcus aureus* bacteremia. *Am J Med.* 2005;118:225–229.
9. Durack DT, Lukes AS, Bright DK. New criteria for diagnosis of infective endocarditis: utilization of specific echocardiographic findings. *Am J Med.* 1994;96:200–209.
10. Li JS, Sexton DJ, Mick N et al. Proposed modifications to the Duke criteria for the diagnosis of infective endocarditis. *Clin Infect Dis.* 2000;30(4):633–638.
11. Cheitlin MD, Alpert JS, Armstrong WF, et al. ACC/AHA guidelines for the clinical application of echocardiography: executive summary: a report of the American College of Cardiology/American Heart Association Task Force on Practice Guidelines (Committee on Clinical Application of Echocardiography): developed in collaboration with the American Society of Echocardiography. *J Am Coll Cardiol.* 1997;29:862–879.


## QUESTIONS

1. All the following are true statements *except*:
   a. By definition, "early" prosthetic valve endocarditis refers to the development of infection within 90 days of surgery.
   b. Aztreonam is an acceptable alternative for the treatment of HACEK endocarditis.
   c. Gram-negative bacilli are important causative agents in hospital-acquired endocarditis.

d. Endocarditis with *Streptococcus bovis* should prompt a search for a colonic neoplasm.
e. Surgery is rarely necessary in IE with *Brucella* organisms.

Answer is a: Early-onset prosthetic valve endocarditis is usually attributed to pathogens from perioperative contamination (health care–associated), and therefore the cutoff is 90 days from implant of the valve. Aztreonam (gram-negative organism only) will not be active against HACEK organisms. *Staphylococcus aureus* is the most common health care–associated cause of infective endocarditis (not gram-negative organisms). *Brucella* IE almost always requires surgery for cure.

**2.** All the following are false statements *except*:

a. Mitral valve prolapse is a risk factor for the development of IE.
b. Mechanical valves are as equally at risk as are native valves for IE during the first 90 days following surgery.
c. MSSA is a common causative agent of hospital-acquired endocarditis.
d. In persons with *Staphylococcus aureus* bacteremia, hemodialysis dependence has been shown to be a risk factor for the development of IE.
e. Rheumatic valvulitis is still the most common predisposing factor for IE in the elderly in developed nations.

Answer is d: *Staphylococcus aureus* is recognized as the most common health care–associated pathogen causing infective endocarditis. Patients receiving hemodialysis with indwelling vascular catheters are at particular risk for *S. aureus* bacteremia and subsequent endocarditis (Fowler VG et al., *JAMA*. 2005;293:3012). Mitral valve prolapse without regurgitation is not a high-risk condition for IE. Methicillin-resistant *S. aureus* is more common than methicillin-susceptible *S. aureus* as a cause of nosocomial IE in the United States. Rheumatic valvulitis is not the most common predisposing factor for IE in the developed world.

**3.** All the following are correctly matched associations *except*:

a. *Brucella*—abattoir workers
b. *Coxiella*—sheep farmers
c. *Pseudomonas* IE—intravenous drug users
d. Fungal IE—prolonged antibiotic exposure
e. HACEK IE—veterinarians

Answer is e: HACEKorganisms are not particularly associated with veterinarians. *Brucella* is a zoonosis and associated with abattoir workers. Similarly, *Coxiella burnetii* (agent of Q fever) is associated with parturient sheep. *Pseudomonas* has been associated with injected drug users (contamination with processing), and nosocomial fungal IE can follow prolonged antibiotic use (risk factor for fungemia).

**4.** The cutoff MIC for a penicillin-susceptible *Streptococcus viridans* is

a. $\leq 0.5\ \mu g/mL$
b. $\leq 0.05\ \mu g/mL$
c. $\leq 0.01\ \mu g/mL$
d. $\geq 0.1\ \mu g/mL$
e. $\leq 0.1\ \mu g/mL$

Answer is e: The NCCLS cutoff for *S. viridans* penicillin susceptibility is $0.1\ \mu g/mL$.

**5.** Regarding the complications of IE, all of the following are true *except*:

a. Four-vessel cerebral angiography is the current gold standard for diagnosing intracranial mycotic aneurysms.
b. Mitral valve infection is a more common cause of congestive heart failure in IE than aortic valve infection.
c. The definitive treatment of a splenic abscess resulting from embolization in IE is splenectomy.
d. Transthoracic echocardiogram is inferior to transesophageal echocardiogram in detecting paravalvular extension of IE.
e. Extracranial mycotic aneurysms are more common in the visceral arteries than in the upper-extremity arteries.

Answer is b: Mitral valve IE is not more often associated with complications of CHF than aortic valve IE. MRA is not as sensitive as four-vessel angiogram for detection of mycotic aneurysms.

# Prosthetic Valvular Disease

27

*Daniel Sauri*    *Mario J. Garcia*

About 50 years ago, the development of valve prostheses dramatically improved the prognosis of patients with valvular heart disease. There are two major classes of prosthetic valves: (a) mechanical and (b) bioprostheses (Fig. 27–1). Each specific valve within these groups has unique features that provide differences in hemodynamics, durability, and thromboembolic risk.

## MECHANICAL VALVES

The advantages of mechanical prosthesis are high durability and better hemodynamic performance. There main disadvantage is higher thrombogenicity, requiring the use of long-term anticoagulation. Two subgroups of mechanical valves are available: (a) ball/disc-and-cage, and (b) tilting disc valves.

Ball/disc-and-cage valves, such as the Starr Edwards, consist of a moving silicone/metal ball or disc within a cage, attached to a metallic alloy ring. Flow is diverted around the ball/disc, as a result of which the hemodynamic profile is unfavorable and worse than with a tilting disc prosthesis. Ball/disc-and-cage valves also demonstrate a higher incidence of thromboembolic complications, requiring higher levels of anticoagulation. Although they have the longest proven durability among all prosthetic valves, the aforementioned problems limit their clinical use today.

Tilting disc valves have either one or two discs mounted in a ring. Single tilting disc valves such as the Bjork–Shiley, Medtronic Hall, and Omniscience valves, consist of a metallic sewing ring attached to a tilting disc that rotates about an off-centered pivot axis with a range of about 60 to 85 degrees from occluded to open position. At the open position there are two orifices—a major orifice downstream and a minor orifice that opens proximally. Early models of the Bjork-Shiley valve, >29 mm in size and with opening angles >70 degrees, demonstrated a high degree of strut fracture (~2% per year) and embolization of the disc, resulting in withdrawal of these valves from the market, and prophylactic valve replacement in those whose risk of embolization exceeded the risk of reoperation. Older Bjork-Shiley and Omniscience valves have greater thrombosis risk (3% per year) than newer Medtronic-Hall valves, in which a small orifice in the center permits regurgitant flow to "wash" potentially thrombogenic material from the disc. The St. Jude's Medical and the Carbomedics valves are bileaflet tilting disc valves. Their semicircular leaflets open to an 85% angle, leaving two larger lateral orifices and a narrow rectangular slit between them. The symmetric flow across the bileaflet system provides excellent hemodynamics, and the rates of mechanical failure and thromboembolism with these valves are very low. These characteristics have resulted in bileaflet valves being the most commonly used mechanical prostheses in the United States during the past 15 years.

## BIOPROSTHETIC VALVES

Bioprosthetic valves fall into one of two categories: heterografts, or non–human tissue valves, such as Carpentier–Edwards and Hancock bioprostheses; and aortic homografts, which are cadaveric human aortic valves implanted within a small portion of the donor's aortic root for support. As a class, bioprosthetic valves require less anticoagulation than mechanical valves, but they are less durable than mechanical valves. Stented heterografts resemble native valves but have less optimal hemodynamic

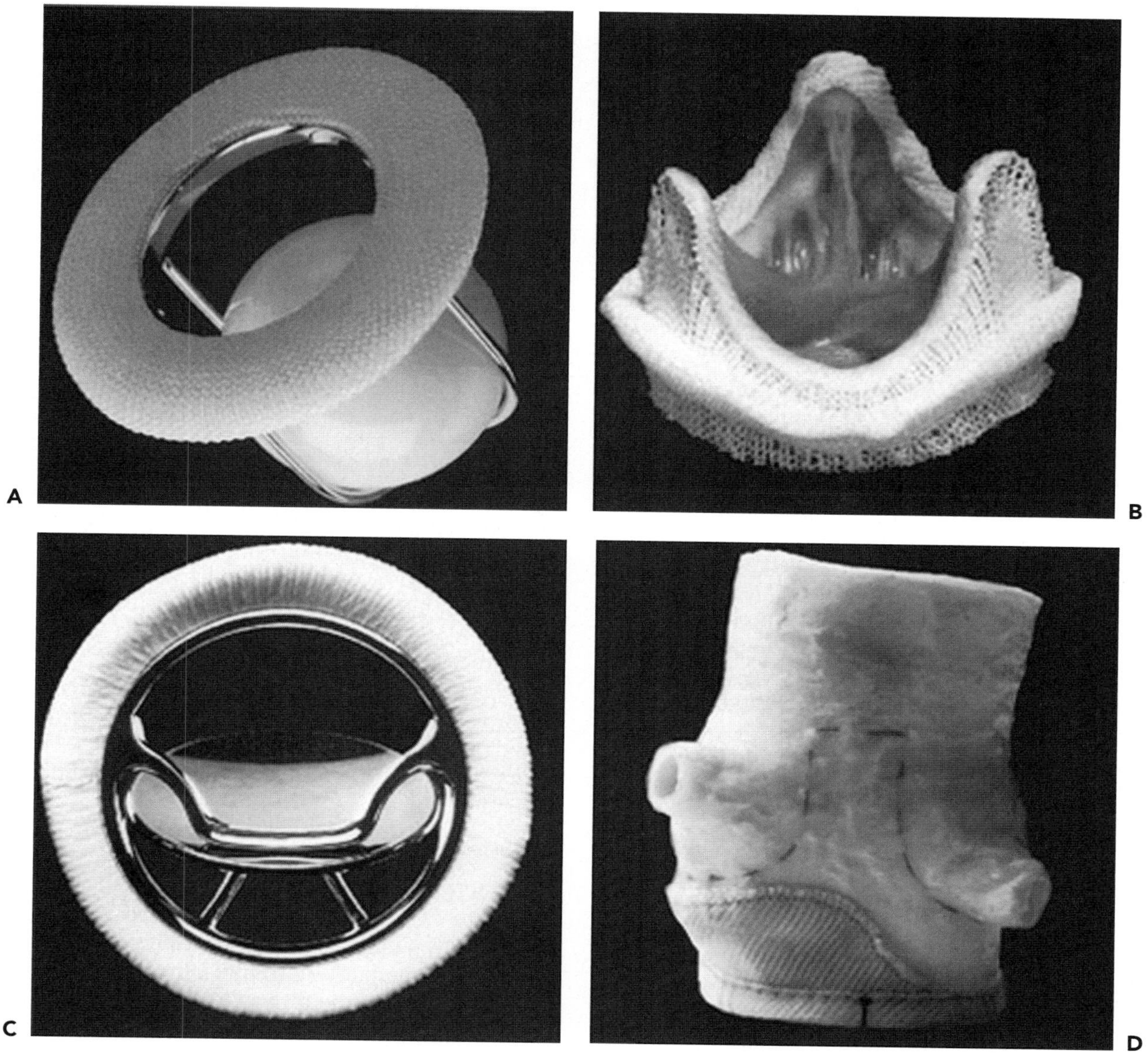

A B C D

**Figure 27–1** **A:** Ball-and-cage Starr–Edwards valve. **B:** Stented porcine valve. **C:** Single tilting disc Bjork-Shiley valve. **D:** Stentless aortic heterograft.

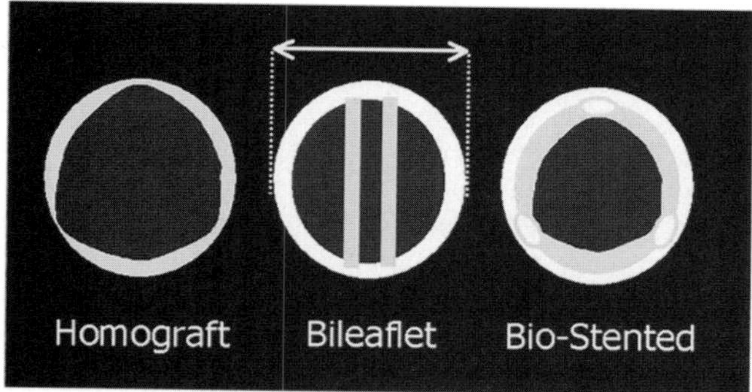


**Figure 27–2** Although mechanical and bioprosthetic valves have similar external diameters, the figure demonstrates that the stented bioprosthetic valves have a smaller internal diameter and thus a more unfavorable hemodynamic profile.

performance because of decreased flow profile as a result of interposed stents and the sewing ring (Fig. 27–2). These valves are manufactured from porcine valvular tissue or bovine pericardium. The durability of porcine valves has been improved with changes in design and preservation techniques. In older patients, bovine pericardial valves have demonstrated 85% freedom from structural dysfunction at 15 years and generally demonstrate greater longevity than porcine valves. Stentless porcine bioprostheses consist of a tubular segment of a porcine ascending aorta containing the aortic valve *in situ*, which is sutured proximally to the aortic annulus and distally to the mid ascending aorta. Surgical implantation of these valves is more demanding, but these valves have the potential advantage of improved hemodynamic performance compared to stented valves. However, it remains to be proven whether their superior hemodynamics will translate into improved clinical outcome. Aortic homografts are harvested from cadaveric hearts and cryopreserved. Similar to stentless heterografts, they are supported by a short segment of the donor's aortic root, in which the recipient's coronary arteries are reimplanted. Antigenicity is reduced by antibacterial sterilization and cryopreservation, resulting in less leaflet degeneration. Reported freedom from structural valve degeneration at 10, 15, and 20 years is 81%, 62%, and 31%, respectively. Younger donor homografts have greater durability than older donors' homografts. Although the durability of homograft prostheses may be slightly higher than that of heterografts in younger adults, the complexity of reoperation (need for reimplantation of the coronary arteries) has led to a decrease from the initial excitement for their use. Homografts do have a reduced rate of reinfection and are the valve of choice in aortic valve endocarditis.

## SELECTION OF VALVE TYPE

Multiple factors need to be considered in selecting a prosthetic valve, including the age of the patient, the probability of future pregnancy, life expectancy, occupation, and lifestyle. The risk of future reoperation should also be considered, possibly being greater after more extensive surgery such as a stentless valve or allograft replacement.

When it is feasible, valve repair should always be considered prior to surgery. Mitral valve repair offers several potential advantages over replacement, including preservation of left ventricular (LVa) function via conservation of the subvalvular apparatus, lower operative mortality, higher long-term survival rate, and freedom from anticoagulation. An aortic valve with predominant regurgitation due to prolapse or redundancy, but without severe stenosis or calcification, can also be repaired. If repair is not feasible, with the exception of very few circumstances such as the patient already receiving chronic anticoagulation and anticipated short life expectancy, there is no absolute advantage for a specific valve type.

Mechanical valves are more durable than bioprothetic valves, but they require a commitment to chronic anticoagulation. They are generally recommended for patients younger than age 60 years who have no contraindications to anticoagulation and are expected to be medically compliant. The relative benefit-to-risk ratio shifts later for mitral than for aortic mechanical valves, given the more rapid deterioration of bioprostheses in the mitral position. Bioprostheses are indicated for patients with a contraindication to chronic anticoagulation and are preferred for patients older than 70 years of age because of their reasonable durability, favorable hemodynamic profile, and freedom from anticoagulation. The incidence of bioprosthetic failure rates is age dependent, further advocating their use in older patients (Table 27–1). With the increased durability of bovine bioprosthesis, the recommended earlier age limit for placement of these valves continues to decrease. Two large studies have both demonstrated that the risk of death and combined major complications including systemic embolization, bleeding, endocarditis, valve thrombosis, and valve deterioration are comparable at long-term follow-up. In the Edinburg Heart valve trial, 541 patients were randomized to Bjork–Shiley 60-degree tilting disc valves versus Carpentier–Edwards porcine valves. In the VA cooperative study, 575 were randomized to Bjork–Shiley or Hancock bioprostheses. Although the mechanical valves led to more bleeding complications, the bioprosthetic valves required more reoperations. Rates of embolism and endocarditis were similar.

**TABLE 27–1**
**HETEROGRAFT VALVE FAILURE RATE 10 YEARS AFTER VALVE REPLACEMENT RELATIVE TO THE PATIENT'S AGE**

| Patient's Age (y) | Failure Rate at 10 y (%) |
|---|---|
| <40 | 40 |
| 40–49 | 30 |
| 50–59 | 20 |
| 60–69 | 15 |
| ≥70 | 10 |

*Source:* Modified from Vongpatanasin W, Hillis D, et al . Prosthetic heart valves. *N Engl J Med.* 1996;335:412, by permission of The Massachusetts Medical Society.

## ANTICOAGULATION

Thromboembolism represents one of the most important causes of morbidity and mortality for patients with prosthetic valves. The embolic event rates are greater for mitral than for aortic prostheses. The incidence of thromboembolic events is significantly higher with mechanical prosthesis in nonanticoagulated patients, ranging from 7% to 34% per year. Patient-related contributing factors include older age, atrial fibrillation, and LV dysfunction. Table 27–2 summarizes the recommended targets for anticoagulation therapy in patients with mechanical prosthetic valves. With respect to mechanical valves, Starr–Edwards valves have the highest rate of embolism, followed by single tilting disc valves. Bileaflet tilting disc valves have the lowest reported rates of thromboembolism, because of the built-in regurgitation, which acts to "clean" debris off the valve. Regardless of the type of valve, at appropriate levels of anticoagulation the incidence of thromboembolism is less than 1% in those maintained on therapeutic anticoagulation. The majority of patients who experience thromboembolic complications have subtherapeutic international normalizing ratio (INR) at the time of the event. Chronic anticoagulation therapy increases the long-term hemorrhagic complications, with an incidence of major bleeding occurring at a

**TABLE 27–2**
**RECOMMENDED ANTICOAGULATION THERAPY FOR PATIENTS WITH MECHANICAL PROSTHETIC VALVES**

| Level of Risk | Prosthesis Type | Recommended INR |
|---|---|---|
| Low | Single-tilting disc | 3.0–4.0 |
| | Double-tilting disc | 2.5–3.0 |
| High[a] | Caged disc | 3.0–4.5 |
| | Caged ball | 3.0–4.5 |
| | Multiple prostheses | 3.0–4.5 |

INR, International Normalizing Ratio.
[a]Patients with atrial fibrillation, left atrial thrombus, severe left ventricular dysfunction, or previous embolic events.
*Source:* From Cleveland Clinic Foundation. *Manual of Cardiovascular Medicine.* 2nd ed. Philadelphia: Lippincott Wilkins; Table 18.4.

rate of 1.4 per 100 patient-years and 2% to 4% per year for minor bleeding. Both hemorrhagic and thromboembolic complications are more frequent in older patients (~5% to 6%).

Antiplatelet therapy may be combined with warfarin in patients with mechanical heart valves. It has been demonstrated that low-dose aspirin in combination with warfarin can reduce the annualized risk of death and major systemic thromboembolic events from 11.7% to 4.2%. This is at a cost of increased minor bleeding, from 22% to 35%, but with a similar incidence of major bleeding. The additive benefit of aspirin appeared to be greater in patients with previous embolic events and who were at higher risk for thromboembolism per year after the age of 70 years.

In the early postoperative period, the approach to anticoagulation for mechanical prostheses varies widely. Early anticoagulation increases the risk of bleeding and tamponade. One approach is warfarin, but not heparin, starting 3 to 4 days following surgery, when epicardial wires are removed. Others advocate low-dose heparin after surgery until chest tubes are removed, followed by full-dose heparin and initiation of warfarin. The need for anticoagulation with bioprosthetic valves is controversial. The risk for embolism is greatest early postoperatively and declines after 3 months. It is greater for mitral prostheses (7%) than for aortic prostheses (3%). A reasonable approach is to anticoagulate patients with mitral prosthesis for 3 months and then change to aspirin, 325 mg daily. Patients with aortic prostheses should receive 325 mg of aspirin daily for 3 months unless there is another reason for anticoagulation. Patients with prior embolic events, atrial fibrillation, or LV dysfunction should be anticoagulated long term.

For patients with mechanical valves who require major noncardiac surgery with anticipated substantial blood loss, warfarin should be stopped 3 days prior to the procedure, to achieve an INR level of 1.6 or less. Hospital admission with initiation of heparin is recommended for patients with ball/disc-and-cage valves, atrial fibrillation, documented left atrial thrombus, severe LV dysfunction, previous embolization, or mitral prostheses. Postoperatively, intravenous heparin should be restarted when it is considered safe and continued until therapeutic anticoagulation is achieved with warfarin. For minor procedures, in which blood loss is minimal, anticoagulation can be continued.

Pregnant women have an increased incidence of thromboembolic complications, given the hypercoagulable state associated with pregnancy. Given its teratogenic effects, warfarin should be discontinued when pregnancy is considered or detected during the first trimester, when the risk of embryopathy is as high as 30% and the risk of spontaneous abortion is 25% to 30%. Subcutaneous heparin with 17,500 to 20,000 U twice a day, with a target activated partial thromboplastin time of 1.5 to 2.0 times the control 6 hours after injection, should be administered until at least the second trimester of pregnancy. At that time warfarin may be restarted and continued until the middle of the third trimester. Subcutaneous heparin is then administered twice a day until 24 hours prior to delivery, when heparin should be stopped. Low-dose aspirin can be used in conjunction with anticoagulation therapy for women at higher risk of thromboembolism. The role of low-molecular-weight heparin is not supported in this setting, and recent reports suggest that it may not provide optimal anticoagulation in the hypercoaguable pregnancy state. Nursing mothers can use both heparin and warfarin safely, because they do not appear to secrete it into breast milk.

## COMPLICATIONS OF VALVE PROSTHESES

It is important to define normal Doppler findings with prosthetic valves to be able to identify pathology. Table 27–3 provides average transvalvular gradients across different types of prostheses. Conditions with increased cardiac output such as anemia, tachycardia, pregnancy, hyperthyroidism, or severe prosthetic leak can lead to higher-than-normal gradients and give the false impression of prosthetic stenosis. Ball-and-cage valves and bileaflet tilting disc valves can exhibit the phenomenon of pressure recovery (Fig. 27–3). With this, the highest pressure gradient recorded through the prosthesis by Doppler overestimates the true pressure gradient by approximately one third, as a result of flow acceleration through a narrowed orifice. This phenomenon occurs especially with small mechanical bileaflet prostheses in the aortic position. Given the need to follow transvalvular gradients to exclude pannus, thrombus, or stenosis secondary to increasing calcification, it is critical to obtain a baseline echocardiogram early postoperatively for future reference. Many mechanical valves have physiologic regurgitation to help clean off debris, but it should be no more than mild and should

**TABLE 27–3**

**NORMAL DOPPLER VELOCITY AND GRADIENTS FOR PROSTHETIC VALVES**

| Prosthetic Valve | Peak Velocity (m/s) | Mean Gradient (mm Hg) |
|---|---|---|
| Aortic Position | | |
| Starr–Edwards | 3.1 ± 0.5 | 24 ± 4 |
| Björk–Shiley | 2.5 ± 0.6 | 14 ± 5 |
| St. Jude | 3.0 ± 0.8 | 11 ± 6 |
| Medtronic–Hall | 2.6 ± 0.3 | 12 ± 3 |
| Aortic homograft | 0.8 ± 0.4 | 7 ± 3 |
| Hancock | 2.4 ± 0.4 | 11 ± 2 |
| Carpentier–Edwards | 2.4 ± 0.5 | 14 ± 6 |
| Mitral position | | |
| Starr–Edwards | 1.8 ± 0.4 | 5 ± 2 |
| Björk–Shiley | 1.6 ± 0.3 | 5 ± 2 |
| St. Jude | 1.6 ± 0.3 | 5 ± 2 |
| Medtronic–Hall | 1.7 ± 0.3 | 3 ± 1 |
| Hancock | 1.5 ± 0.3 | 4 ± 2 |
| Carpentier–Edwards | 1.8 ± 0.2 | 7 ± 2 |

*Source:* Modified from Nottestad SY, Zabalgoitia M. In: Otto CM, ed. *The Practice of Clinical Echocardiography*. Philadelphia: WB Saunders; 1997:803, by permission of W.B. Saunders Company.

not be paravalvular in origin. Regurgitation from mechanical valves in the mitral position is often underestimated by transthoracic echocardiography because of acoustic shielding. Indirect evidence of increased flow across the valve can be obtained in the presence of severe regurgitation if peak gradients are elevated. Transesophageal echocardiography remains the best way to detect and quantify prosthetic mitral regurgitation.

The diagnosis of structural valve degeneration relies primarily on echocardiographic findings, but physical exam findings can sometimes provide clues to complications (Fig. 27–4). By echo, interrogation of a prosthetic valve requires appreciation of the prosthetic apparatus, peak and mean gradients, and regurgitant flow. Transesophageal echo (TEE) generally supplements transthoracic images in patients with symptoms or those suspected of having endocarditis. Accoustic shadowing and reverberation can limit the assessment of prosthetic valves, particularly mitral prosthesis shadowing the aortic valve by transthoracic echo. Prosthetic valve degeneration occurs more commonly with bioprosthetic valves. The leaflets gradually become thickened and calcified, resulting in both stenosis and regurgitation. Elevated gradients across the valve support the diagnosis and define the severity. Prosthetic valve degeneration occurs gradually with bioprosthetic valves. Replacement in this setting is usually done once symptoms appear. Prosthetic degeneration can be gradual for mechanical prostheses, resulting from thrombosis, encroachment by pannus, or abrasion of a silastic ball occluder (Fig. 27–5). Abrupt failure can be fatal, although rare, occurring as a result of strut fracture or disc dislodgement.

The annual incidence of prosthetic valve thrombosis is ~0.5% to 1.5%. The highest incidence is at the tricuspid position, followed by the mitral and then the aortic position. Thrombus is suspected in patients with acute onset of symptoms, embolic event, or inadequate anticoagulation. TEE is the most widely used diagnostic technique, although cinefluoroscopy can be used to document restriction in occluder mobility. No imaging modality can clearly differentiate thrombus from pannus, and frequently they coexist. Echocardiographic features suggestive of thrombus include

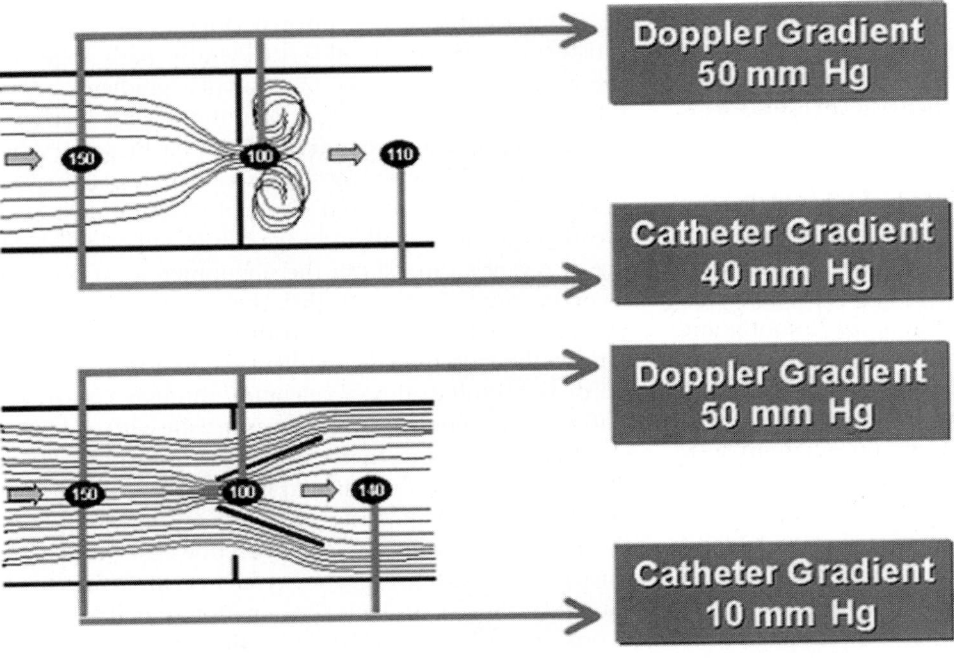


**Figure 27–3** Demonstration of pressure recovery. The higher pressure gradient recorded through a prosthesis by Doppler overestimates the true pressure gradient as a result of flow acceleration through a narrowed orifice. Pressure recovers distally, at the position of the catheter recording. This occurs primarily with small mechanical bileaflet prostheses in the aortic position.

| Type of Valve | Aortic Prosthesis | | Mitral Prosthesis | |
|---|---|---|---|---|
| | Normal Findings | Abnormal Findings | Normal Findings | Abnormal Findings |
| Caged-Ball (Starr-Edwards) | OC $S_1$ CC $P_2$ SEM | Aortic diastolic murmur Decreased intensity of opening or closing click | CC OC $S_2$ SEM | Low-frequency apical diastolic murmur High-frequency holosystolic murmur |
| Single-Tilting-Disk (Bjork–Shiley or Medtronic-Hall | OC $S_1$ CC $P_2$ SEM DM | Decreased intensity of closing click | CC $S_2$ OC DM | High-frequency holosystolic murmur Decreased intensity of closing click |
| Bileaflet-Tilting-Disk (St. Jude Medical) | OC $S_1$ CC $P_2$ SEM | Aortic diastolic murmur Decreased intensity of closing click | CC $S_2$ OC DM | High-frequency holosystolic murmur Decreased intensity of closing click |
| Heterograft Bioprosthesis (Hancock or Carpentier–Edwards | $S_1$ AC $P_2$ SEM | Aortic diastolic murmer | MC $S_2$ MO SEM DM | High-frequency holosystolic murmur |

**Figure 27–4** Accoustic characteristics of various mechanical and bioprosthetic valves. (From Cleveland Clinic Foundation. *Manual of Cardiovascular Medicine*. 2nd ed. Philadelphia: Lippincott Williams & Wilkins; Fig. 18.2.)

a soft, irregular, or mobile mass. The valve type or suspected duration of valve thrombosis does not affect the indication for treatment, although the location of the prosthetic valve does. Heparin is usually initiated early in the course. Fibrinolytic therapy is considered the treatment of choice for right-sided prosthetic valve thrombosis, because the consequences of distal embolization are less severe than for left-sided prostheses. Streptokinase and urokinase are the most commonly used agents. Fibrinolytic therapy has an initial success rate of 82%, an overall thromboembolism rate of 12%, and a 5% incidence of major bleeding episodes. Similar rates of success and complications (stroke ~10%) have been described for left-sided prosthetic valve thrombosis.

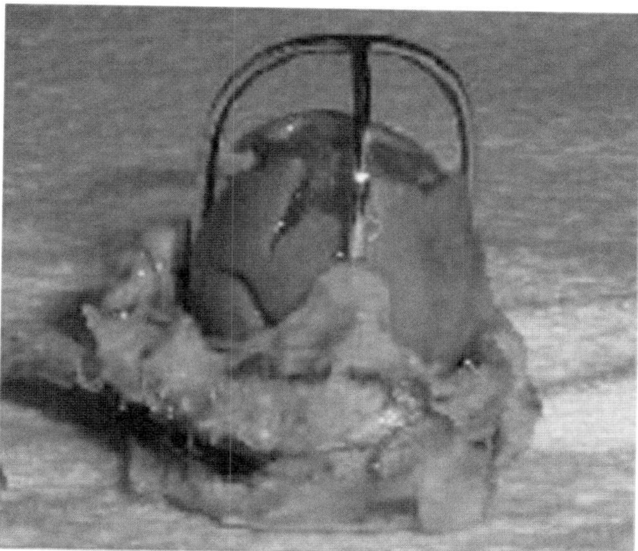

**Figure 27–5** Starr–Edwards valve showing degeneration of silicone ball and pannus invasion of the suture ring.

The recommended dosage of streptokinase is a 250,000-U bolus given over 30 minutes, followed by an infusion of 100,000 U/h. Urokinase is given as an infusion of 4,400 U/kg per hour. Duration of therapy varies and can be given up to 5 days; however, thrombolysis should be stopped if there is no hemodynamic improvement after 1 to 3 days. TEE can be used to follow progression of the thrombus burden. Anticoagulation alone with heparin is generally recommended for small thrombi (<5 mm) with no hemodynamic consequence with higher doses of heparin and a PT/INR of 2.5 to 3.5 on coumadin. Surgery is generally preferred for left-sided prosthetic valve thrombosis unless the thrombus is small or the patient has a prohibitive surgical risk. Surgery is also indicated in the case of unsuccessful thrombolysis 24 hours following discontinuation of the infusion.

Approximately 3% to 6% of patients with prosthetic heart valves will experience endocarditis (PVE). PVE is typically associated with large vegetations, because microorganisms are sheltered from the host defense mechanisms. Early PVE (<2 months following implantation) is typically caused by *Staphylococcus epidermidis*. The clinical course is often fulminating, with mortality as high as 50% to 70%. Surgery is almost universally required for effective treatment. Late PVE occurs most commonly in patients with multiple prostheses and bioprosthetic valves, especially in the aortic position. Its clinical course resembles that of native-valve endocarditis, and the most common infectious agents are Streptococci, followed by gram-negative bacteria, Enterococci, and *S. epidermidis*. The general therapy for patients with PVE is surgery. The mortality of patients with antibiotic therapy alone is 61%, versus 38% for those having repeat surgery. Medical cure of PVE caused by Staphylococci, gram-negative organisms, or fungi is very rare. Streptococcal PVE responds to medical therapy alone in 50%

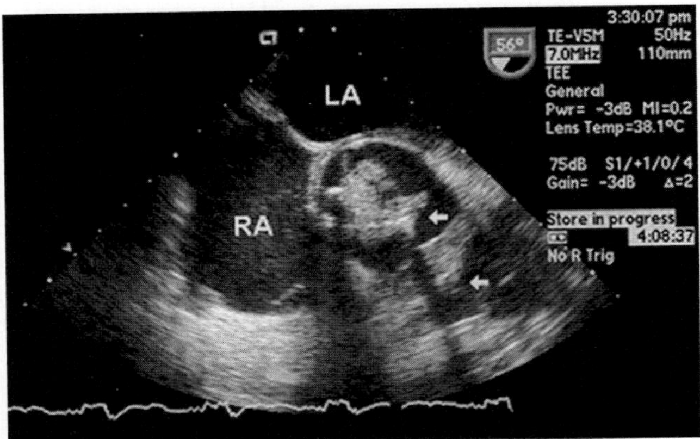


**Figure 27–6** Prosthetic aortic valve demonstrating large vegetation and surrounding abscess. RA, right atrium; LA, left atrium.

of cases. Patients with PVE should also continue to receive anticoagulation. PVE is associated with a 50% incidence of stroke in the absence of anticoagulation, as opposed to a 10% incidence with anticoagulation, and there is no compelling evidence of increased hemorrhage with warfarin in patients with PVE. Surgery is clearly indicated in patients with persistent bacteremia despite IV antibiotics, tissue invasion or fistula formation, recurrent embolization, fungal infection, prosthetic valve dehiscence or obstruction, new or worsening heart block, or medically refractory congestive heart failure (Fig. 27–6). Of course, as discussed above, the cure rates with medical therapy in PVE are considerably lower, and repeat surgery should be a consideration for all appropriate candidates.

Subclinical hemolysis is present in many patients with mechanical valves but rarely results in significant anemia. Clinical hemolysis occurs in ~10% of patients with ball/disc-and-cage valves but is uncommon with normal bioprostheses or tilting disc valves. Clinical hemolysis is associated with multiple prosthetic valves, small prostheses, periprosthetic leaks, and prosthetic valve endocarditis. Mechanisms involved in the generation of hemolysis include high shear stress or turbulance across the prosthesis. Diagnosis is made various laboratory tests and echo imaging. Hemolysis is likely in the presence of an elevated LDH, reticulocyte count, unconjugated bilirubin, urinary haptoglobin, and schistocytes on blood smear. Echocardiography can demonstrate abnormal rocking of the prosthesis or regurgitant jets of high shear stress such as periprosthetic regurgitant jets or those impacting on a solid surface such as the left atrial appendage. Mild anemia from hemolysis can be managed with iron, folic acid, and occasional blood transfusions. Beta-blockade and blood-pressure control may reduce the severity of hemolysis. Surgical therapy is recommended for those with periprosthetic leaks in patients with severe anemia requiring repeated transfusions or those with congestive heart failure.

Dehiscence of the sewing ring from the annulus may occur in the early postoperative period because of poor surgical techniques, excessive annular calcification, chronic steriod use, fragility of the valvular tissue (particularly following prior valve operations), or infections. Late dehiscence occurs mainly by infectious endocarditis. Abnormal rocking of the prosthesis on echo or cinefluoroscopy is an indication for urgent surgery, but some rocking may occur with preservation of the mitral valve apparatus.

The use of antibiotic prophylaxis is recommended for all patients with prosthetic valves, although its effectiveness remains to be proven. Guidelines established by the American Medical Association cover the administration of oral or intravenous antibiotics for dental and for invasive medical procedures, and the use of alternative drugs for patients with established allergies.

## BIBLIOGRAPHY

**Acar J, Iung B, et al.** Multicenter randomized comparison of low-dose versus standard-dose anticoagulation in patients with mechanical prosthetic heart valves. *Circulation.* 1996;94:2107–2112.

**Bloomfield P, Wheatley DJ.** Twelve-year comparison of a Bjork-Shiley mechanical heart valve with porcine bioprostheses. *N Engl J Med.* 1991;324(9):573–579.

**Cannegieter SC, Rosendaal FR, et al.** Optimal oral anticoagulation therapy in patients with mechanical heart valves. *N Engl J Med.* 1995;333(1):11–17.

**Davis EA, Greene PS, et al.** Bioprosthetic versus mechanical prosthesis for aortic valve replacement in the elderly. *Circulation.* 1996;94:II-121–II-125.

**Garcia MJ.** Prosthetic heart valves. In: Topol EJ, ed. *Textbook of Cardiovascular Medicine.* 2nd ed. Philadelphia: Lippincott Williams & Wilkins; 2002:463–482.

**Ginsberg JS, Hirsh J.** Use of antithrombotic agents during pregnancy. *Chest.* 1995;108(4 suppl):305S–311S.

**Hammermeister KE, Seithi GK, et al.** A comparison of outcomes in men 11 years after heart-valve replacement with a mechanical valve or bioprosthesis. Veterans Affairs Cooperative Study on Valvular Heart Disease. *N Engl J Med.* 1993;328(18):1289–1296.

**Rahimtoola SH.** Prosthetic heart valve performance: long term follow-up. *Curr Probl Cardiol.* 1992;334–406.

**Saour JN, Sieck JO, et al.** Trial of different intensities of anticoagulation in patients with prosthetic heart valves. *N Engl J Med.* 1990; 322(7):428–432.

**Turpie AG, Gent M, et al.** A comparison of aspirin with placebo in patients treated with warfarin after heart-valve replacement. *N Engl J Med.* 329(8):524–529.

**Vongpatanasin W, Hillis LD, et al.** Prosthetic heart valves. *N Engl J Med.* 1996;335:407–416.

**Zabalgoitia M.** Echocardiographic assessment of prosthetic heart valves. *Curr Probl Cardiol.* 1992;270–325.

## QUESTIONS

1. What is the recommended anticoagulation therapy for each of the following valves?
   a. Carbomedics aortic valve
   b. St. Jude mitral valve

c. Mitral bioprosthetic valve
d. Starr-Edwards aortic valve
e. Aortic bioprosthetic valve
f. Single tilting Bjork Shiley mitral valve

Answer: Embolic event rates are higher for mitral valves than for aortic valves and therefore generally require higher anticoagulation therapy. Caged ball and single tilting valves also carry greater embolic risk than double tilting mechanical valves. Bioprosthetic valves generally carry the lowest risk of embolization, yet according to AMA guidelines, anticoagulation is still recommend in the first 3 months after placement, although this varies according to institution. Thus,

a. INR of 2 to 3 for life of valve
b. INR of 2.5 to 3.5 for life of valve
c. Anticoagulation therapy with INR of 2.5 to 3.5 for first 3 months, then aspirin therapy thereafter
d. INR of 3.5 to 4.5 for life of valve
e. Anticoagulation therapy with INR of 2 to 3 for first 3 months, then aspirin therapy thereafter
f. INR of 3 to 4 for life of valve

**2.** What is the preferred valve choice in each of the following clinical situations?

a. A 45-year-old man with aortic valve endocarditis and aortic root abscess in the presence of a bicuspid aortic valve
b. A 30-year-old man with a nonrepairable aortic bicuspid valve in the setting of severe symptomatic aortic insufficiency
c. A 68-year-old woman with chronic lymphocytic leukemia, who has rheumatic mitral stenosis that is not amenable to valvuloplasty
d. A 30-year-old woman with a nonrepairable aortic bicuspid valve in the setting of severe symptomatic aortic insufficiency

Answers:

a. In the setting of infection and, in particular, aortic root abscess, an aortic homograft is generally considered the best choice to prevent subsequent immediate reinfection. The durability of homografts was once thought to be superior to that of bioprosthetics, but recent experience has demonstrated this not to be the case. Furthermore, the difficulty of reoperation in such a patient (coronary reimplantation and subsequent extensive calcification) should be taken into account.
b. A mechanical aortic valve with the lowest thromboembolic risk, such as a St. Jude or Carbomedics, is preferred, given its durability and potential to prevent future reoperation. The risk of anticoagulation for the patient must also be taken into consideration.
c. Given the co-morbidity of chronic lymphocytic leukemia, which carries a decreased life expectancy yet not imminent death, a bioprosthetic valve is probably a good option. Of course, there are surgical considerations to the placement of a bioprosthetic, such as the larger profile of the valve secondary to its struts. If possible, however, the risk of anticoagulation should be avoided, given the low potential for reoperation in this patient. Recent data with bovine pericardial bioprosthetic valves demonstrate a higher-than-expected durability of ~85% at 15 years, which may ultimately shift the threshold for bioprosthetic valves to patients in their 50s and 60s.
d. It is critical in such a situation to discuss valve selection with the patient. A young woman who would still like to have children should be informed of the risk of anticoagulation during pregnancy. Of course, a bioprosthetic valve in a young patient also carries a high risk of reoperation within the next 5 to 10 years. Some women may prefer to have a bioprosthetic valve, bear children in a timely fashion, and then later undergo a more definitive mechanical valve reoperation, to avoid the risks of anticoagulation during pregnancy. A homograft is not a good choice in this case, given that its durability is not much greater than that of a bioprosthetic, but the reoperation is significantly more difficult.

**3.** Which of the following statements regarding prosthetic valve thrombosis (PVT) is false?

a. The annual incidence of PVT is ~0.5% to 1%.
b. Incidence is highest for the tricuspid position, followed by the mitral position, then the aortic position.
c. Valve replacement and débridement is generally performed for left-sided prosthetic valve thrombosis unless the thrombus is small or the patient has prohibitive surgical risk.
d. Surgery is generally considered the treatment of choice for right-sided PVT.
e. Cinefluoroscopy is a good option to determine restriction in occluder mobility.

Answer is d: Fibrinolytic therapy is considered the treatment of choice for right-sided PVT because the consequences of distal embolization are less severe than in a left-sided prosthesis. Streptokinase and urokinase are the most common agents, and the success rate is ~82%, with a 12% rate of thromboembolism and 5% incidence of major bleeding for right-sided PVT.

**4.** When assessing transvalvular gradients across a prosthetic valve, all of the following can lead to a false assessment of prosthetic valve stenosis *except:*

a. Patient–prosthesis mismatch
b. Anemia
c. Sepsis
d. Regurgitation
e. Pressure-recovery phenomenon

Answer is a: Patient–prosthesis mismatch implies a true physiologic stenosis that is a result of the placement of a relatively small prosthesis, typically in the aortic position, that leads to a reduction in cardiac output. All prosthetic valves have an inherent relative stenosis, but when an inappropriately small prosthesis is placed, a patient can be left with a true gradient that is similar to that prior to the operation. Anything that increases cardiac output, such as anemia, as in the postoperative period, or sepsis, will increase flow through the prosthesis and produce higher-than-normal transvalvular gradients. Similarly, increased regurgitation, such as mitral regurgitation, which is often shielded on surface echo by prosthetic valves, will increase flow across the valve and produce a picture of pseudo-stenosis. Pressure-recovery phenomenon describes a false elevation in gradients that is obtained by echocardiography, typically as a result of turbulent flow just above a mechanical valve, which dissipates in the ascending aorta.

**5.** A 30-year-old woman with a history of an aortic mechanical aortic valve is found to be pregnant. She is thought to be 3 weeks pregnant. The best course of action for managing her anticoagulation during the pregnancy is

a. Terminate the pregnancy, given the risk of warfarin embryopathy.
b. Stop coumadin, admit her to the hospital, place her on IV heparin to a PTT two times normal, and once the PTT goal is achieved at steady state, send her home with IV heparin for the duration of her pregnancy until shortly prior to delivery, when the heparin will be stopped.
c. Stop coumadin and place her on lovenox for the duration of the pregnancy.
d. Stop coumadin, place her lovenox for the first trimester, then restart coumadin for the second trimester, and continue coumadin until the middle of the third trimester. Restart lovenox at that point and stop 12 hours prior to delivery.
e. Stop coumadin, admit her to the hospital for IV heparin, and then convert to SQ heparin to get a consistent PTT of two times the control. Restart coumadin in the second trimester and continue until the middle of the third trimester. Restart SQ heparin again at that point until just prior to delivery

Answer is e: Warfarin therapy during pregnancy carries a risk to both the fetus and the mother. The risk of warfarin embryopathy is ~30% in the first trimester. In addition, the risk of miscarriage or stillbirth is ~40%; thus, warfarin is an absolute contraindication in the first trimester of pregnancy. During the second and third trimesters, the risk of coumadin is less related to the embryopathy than fetal hemorrhage or placental compromise. Therefore, the risks of coumadin during this time period, although still somewhat high, are much more expectable. Lovenox therapy has limited data, but recent data suggest that low-molecular-weight heparin may not provide optimal anticoagulation in a hypercoagulable pregnancy. Continuous IV heparin therapy is not a practical option.

# Congestive Heart Failure and Cardiomyopathy

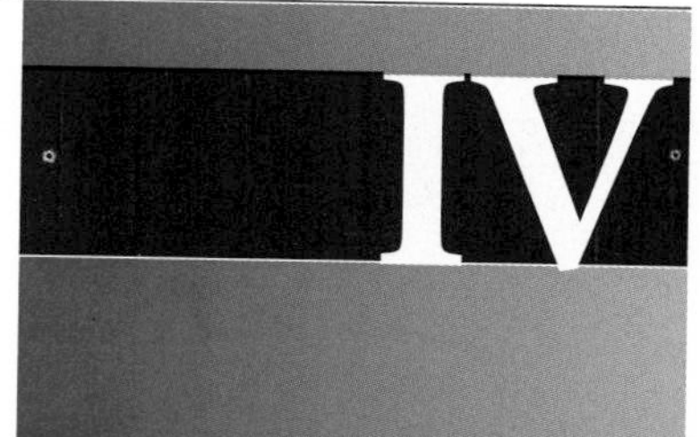

# Pathophysiology of Congestive Heart Failure

28

***Anne Kanderian*** ***Gary S. Francis***

## HOW TO PREPARE FOR THE BOARDS PERTAINING TO CONGESTIVE HEART FAILURE

Heart failure is the single most common reason for patients over the age of 65 years to be admitted to the hospital, so one can expect to be asked questions about it. Some questions will undoubtedly relate to the many large clinical trials, but there will be some attempt to probe your knowledge regarding fundamental pathophysiologic principles. One should have an understanding of the definition, how the syndrome begins, the various hemodynamic profiles that emerge, the underpinnings of myocardial remodeling, how the periphery is affected, the clinical manifestations of the syndrome, and the important prognostic features.

How does one study and learn such material? There are thousands of manuscripts, book chapters, books, and CDs about heart failure. This review chapter will be limited to the pathophysiology of systolic heart failure, thus reducing the material to a single type of heart failure (so-called diastolic heart failure is discussed in another chapter). It would be prudent to read the description of pathophysiology of heart failure in the latest editions of the major cardiovascular textbooks. Standard internal medicine textbooks and review articles (see bibliography) should also be consulted. It will be more meaningful if one can integrate the pathophysiology with the treatment and the results of large clinical trials, as they are historically linked. That is, when it became apparent that the sympathetic nervous system and the renin–angiotensin–aldosterone system played integral roles in heart failure, drugs designed specifically to block these systems began to undergo testing in large clinical trials and later proved to be the cornerstone of treatment.

There are a few "must review" topics: demographics, mechanisms of left ventricular (LV) remodeling, hemodynamic profiles in dilated versus restrictive versus constrictive physiology, hemodynamic differences between systolic and diastolic heart failure, the clinical manifestations of heart failure, and prognostic features.

## DEFINITION OF HEART FAILURE

There are multiple definitions of heart failure, but it is fundamentally a clinical syndrome. Similar to anemia or acute renal failure, heart failure is not a "stand-alone" diagnosis, but rather, always possesses an etiology. In some cases, however, the etiology cannot be determined. Virtually any form of heart disease can lead to heart failure. The definition of heart failure is as follows: a clinical syndrome characterized by shortness of breath and fatigue at rest or with exertion in the presence of underlying structural and/or functional heart disease. In advanced cases, salt and water retention are manifested by edema and organ dysfunction.

## DEMOGRAPHICS OF HEART FAILURE

Some demographics of heart failure include:

- 995,000 annual hospitalizations as a primary diagnosis

- 20% of all hospital admissions in patients over 65 years of age
- 164% increase in hospitalization rate over the past 15 years
- 2.5 million annual hospitalizations as a secondary diagnosis
- 12 to 15 million physician visits annually
- 6.5 million annual hospital days
- In-hospital mortality 5% to 8%

In addition:

- One-year mortality can be as high as 40% to 60%.
- The average patient takes six medications.
- 78% of patients have at least two hospitalizations per year.
- 20% of patients are readmitted within 6 months.
- Heart failure constitutes the single highest volume diagnosis-related group for patients over age 65 years.
- Estimated direct costs in 2004 were $23.7 billion.
- Prevalence increases with age.
- African Americans have 25% higher prevalence of heart failure.

## THE INDEX EVENT

Heart failure always begins with an "index event" (Fig. 28–1). The event may be obvious, such as a sudden loss of a large mass of contractile tissue (i.e., an acute myocardial infarction), or it may be completely silent, such as the early expression of a mutant gene. In many cases, such as familial cardiomyopathy and the onset of valvular heart disease or hypertension, heart failure occurs after a lengthy latency period; or it may come on acutely, such as from acute aortic insufficiency due to bacterial endocarditis. The index event could take the form of acute lymphocytic myocarditis, and manifest as heart failure only many months or years later. There are infinite genetic and environmental influences, which is why the natural history of heart failure and the pace at which it unfolds is so variable among individual patients. Uncertainty about the index event or etiology also makes the prognosis for any individual patient unclear. Even when the etiology and index event are clear, the prognosis for individual patients is ambiguous because of variations in natural history, such as

- Hypertension
- Ischemia
- Idiopathic, familial, hereditary
- Diabetes mellitus
- Myocarditis
- Infiltrative
- Substance use
- Peripartum
- Connective tissue disease
- Doxorubicin and other chemotherapy toxicity
- HIV
- Other miscellaneous pathologies

## ADAPTIVE RESPONSES TO THE HEART FAILURE SYNDROME

The circulation adapts to a perceived disruption in homeostasis with both short-term and long-term adaptations. Short-term adaptations include activation of the Frank–Starling mechanism and activation of the sympathetic nervous system (SNS). Long-term adaptations include heightened activity of the renin–angiotensin–aldosterone system (RAAS) and alterations in the size and the shape of the heart (LV remodeling). Although these adaptations may be somewhat protective in the short- term, over time they become counterproductive and contribute importantly to the pathogenesis of heart failure.

The Frank–Starling mechanism acts to increase the force of heart muscle contraction in response to an increase in end-diastolic volume (Fig. 28–2). In heart failure, however,

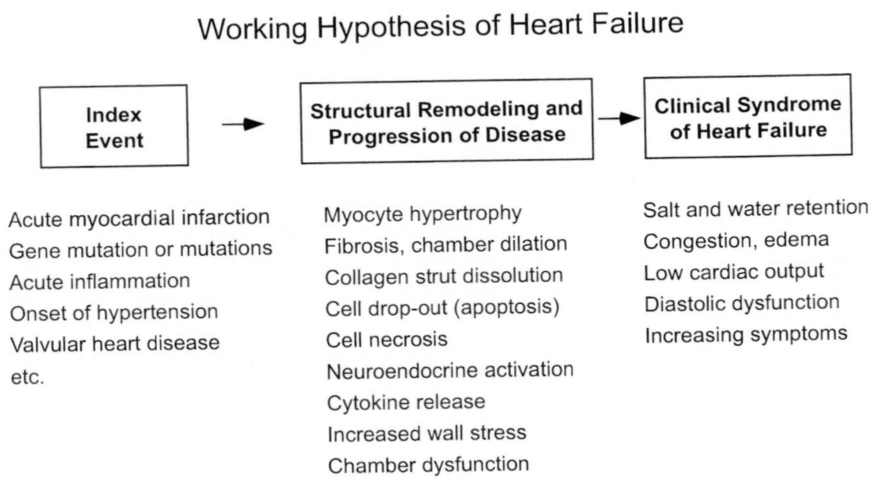

**Figure 28–1** Heart failure begins with an "index event" and progresses through stages of remodeling. Ultimately, the clinical syndrome of chronic heart failure is expressed.

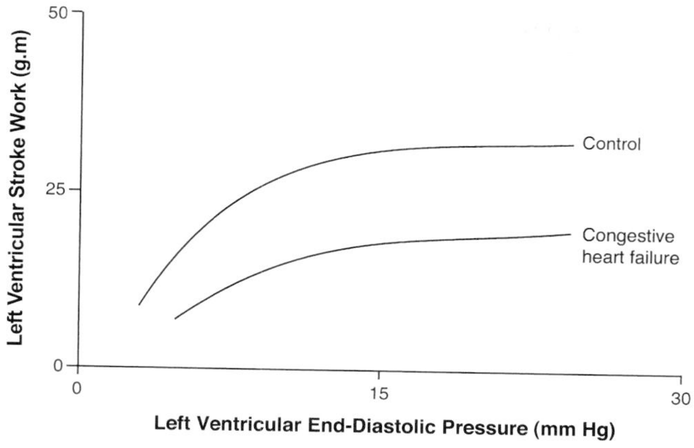


**Figure 28–2** Heart failure is characterized by a diminished ability to increase the cardiac output or cardiac work in response to an increase in preload—Starling's law of the heart.

this response is blunted, both at rest and during exercise. The force–frequency response is also attenuated in the failing heart, secondary to decreased norepinephrine stores and $\beta$-receptor density, which produces a decreased inotropic response to exercise so that less contractile force is generated in response to an increase in heart rate. Patients with heart failure can still call on the Frank–Starling mechanism, albeit at a reduced operational level. The inability to raise the stroke volume during exercise may be one reason why patients have reduced exercise capacity.

## THE SYMPATHETIC NERVOUS SYSTEM

The SNS is activated early in the syndrome of heart failure, before overt signs and symptoms occur. Elevated plasma norepinephrine levels are observed and are an important marker of a poor prognosis. The mechanism that activates the SNS in heart failure is unknown. Increased local levels of synaptic norepinephrine in the heart increase the force of contraction and heart rate, offering early support for the failing heart. But this may also be the source of dysrhythmias, and likely is responsible for the down-regulation of $\beta$-adrenergic receptors. The failing heart tissue is itself also relatively depleted of norepinephrine, thus rendering the heart less responsive to sympathetic stimulation. There is less myocardial reserve in response to inotropic stimulation. The SNS also drives some of the increase in myocyte size, thus contributing to the LV remodeling process. Finally, the SNS activates the RAAS via $\beta$-receptors in the kidney, adding further to heightened peripheral resistance, salt and water retention, and LV remodeling. In summary, early activation of the SNS in heart failure is "protective" by increasing heart rate, force of contraction, myocardial mass, and by protecting blood pressure, but there is a price to pay in the long run. Ultimately, excessive SNS activity is directly toxic to the heart and contributes importantly to the pathogenesis of heart failure.

## RENIN–ANGIOTENSIN–ALDOSTERONE SYSTEM

The RAAS is active in the circulation and in the tissue in heart failure. Probably 90% of the activity of the RAAS is embedded in the various tissues, including the heart, brain, and vasculature. This system, in conjunction with the SNS, plays a key role in the pathogenesis of the syndrome.

The RAAS is known to be activated by numerous mechanisms:

- Volume contraction
- Low cardiac output
- Decreased renal blood flow
- Hyponatremic perfusate to the macula densa
- $\beta$-Adrenergic stimulation to the kidney
- Diuretics
- Salt and water restriction

Angiotensin-II (Ang II) is a small, potent peptide produced by the cleavage of angiotensin-I by angiotensin-converting enzyme (ACE). Ang-II has a vast array of biologic activities, most of which contribute importantly to the pathogenesis of heart failure:

- Vasoconstriction
- Vascular and cardiac myocyte growth, hypertrophy
- Activation of fibroblasts with increased collagen production
- Facilitation of norepinephrine release
- Stimulation of aldosterone release
- Volume expansion
- Thirst stimulation
- Arginine vasopressin release
- Proinflammatory activity
- Direct toxicity to the myocardium when present in excessive quantities
- Mesangial hypertrophy in the kidney
- Increased intraglomerular hydraulic pressure via post–glomerular efferent arteriole vasoconstriction

## COUNTERREGULATORY SYSTEMS (B-TYPE NATRIURETIC PEPTIDE)

B-type natriuretic peptide is released from the myocardium during heart failure in response to increased myocardial wall tension. It circulates in quantities relative to the severity of heart failure, and is widely used as a marker for the diagnosis and severity of heart failure. The biologically active moiety, BNP, is a modest vasodilator with some diuretic and natriuretic properties. It also has antigrowth activity and reduces collagen synthesis in vitro. BNP also tends to offset activity of the SNS and the RAAS. This unique profile of BNP has prompted the development of nesiritide, human BNP produced by recombinant DNA techniques, for the intravenous treatment of patients with severe heart failure. This endogenous counterregulatory peptide is not able to stem the tide of forces that drive the progression of severe heart failure, and very high levels of plasma BNP and NT-pro-BNP are observed in patients with acute decompensation. It is possible, however, that the release of BNP in the early stages of heart failure may forestall the onset of more severe signs and symptoms, and may be more counterregulatory toward the SNS and RAAS.

## OTHER NEUROHORMONES ACTIVE IN HEART FAILURE

There are numerous additional neurohormones, peptides, and cytokines that are active in the heart failure syndrome, many of them participating in the pathophysiology of heart failure:

- Renin
- Angiotensin-II
- Aldosterone
- Tumor necrosis factor-$\alpha$
- Interleukin-6
- Epinephrine
- Arginine vasopressin
- Endothelin
- Adrenomedullin
- Dopamine
- Growth hormone
- Urodilantin
- Insulin
- Vasoactive intestinal peptide
- Neuropeptide Y

Many of these "neurohormones" are important in the progression of heart failure, including LV remodeling. They are more slow-acting systems, like the RAAS. Over many months, neurohormones may contribute to increased interstitial matrix of the heart and vasculature, and to hypertrophy of smooth muscle cells and cardiac myocytes. The SNS and use of the Frank–Starling mechanism are more quick-acting systems, but over time the SNS also contributes to LV remodeling, including increased LV mass and cardiac myocyte elongation leading to chamber dilation. The RAAS and the SNS clearly represent the dominant neurohormones that are most important in the pathogenesis of heart failure, and their pharmacologic blockade has led to substantial improvement in patient survival. This has not been true of other neurohormones and cytokines. It is likely that all of these systems evolved over millions of years, and in some cases led to a survival advantage via conservation of salt and water, volume repletion, and protection of blood pressure and perfusion to vital organs. In heart failure, these systems become maladaptive, become part of the problem, and contribute importantly to progression of disease. This is the so-called *neurohumoral hypothesis* of heart failure.

## RENAL RETENTION OF SALT AND WATER

A hallmark of advanced heart failure is retention of salt and water. This leads to the well-recognized signs and symptoms of tissue congestion, such as pulmonary edema, ascites, and leg edema. The mechanism of salt and water retention early in the natural history of heart failure is still not well understood. In the later stages, reduction in renal blood flow undoubtedly contributes to the problem. The kidney somehow perceives a reduction in effective circulating volume, and unleashes a host of mechanisms, including activation of the RAAS, to conserve and expand circulating volume. Glomerular filtration rate (GFR) is protected early in heart failure by vasoconstriction of the efferent glomerular arterioles. This is due to Ang-II, which also stimulates the release of aldosterone from the adrenal cortex and contributes to sodium reabsorption and water retention. Eventually, this adaptation wanes, intraglomerular hydraulic pressure falls, and GFR is reduced. The development of renal insufficiency heralds the onset of a dwindling prognosis. Salt and water retention are further aggravated by intense activation of the SNS, causing edema and congestion. Increased release of arginine vasopressin diminishes free water clearance, leading to hyponatremia and more vasoconstriction. Eventually the "goal" of volume expansion is met, but at the expense of circulatory and tissue congestion. Circulatory homeostasis is not achieved.

## AUTONOMIC NERVOUS SYSTEM DYSFUNCTION

Reflex control mechanisms are abnormal in heart failure (Fig. 28–3). Peripheral vascular resistance is increased, there is defective parasympathetic control, an abnormal response to orthostasis, a blunted heart rate response to exercise and to pharmacologic vasodilation, impaired heart rate recovery from exercise, reduced heart-rate variability, and altered baroreceptor function. These abnormalities may improve following heart transplantation, suggesting that these are functional and not structural changes. They are rarely normalized. The precise cause of these abnormal reflex control mechanisms is not clear, but they may be the result of evolutionary forces that are acting to redistribute blood flow to more vital organs.

## LEFT VENTRICULAR REMODELING

Another hallmark of heart failure is that the heart gradually changes size and shape as the syndrome progresses. LV mass increases, cells drop out, myocytes slip away from each other, collagen increases, the heart becomes more stiff, the myocytes become larger and elongate, the chamber dimension increases, wall tension increases adding to reduced performance (the law of Laplace), and the heart

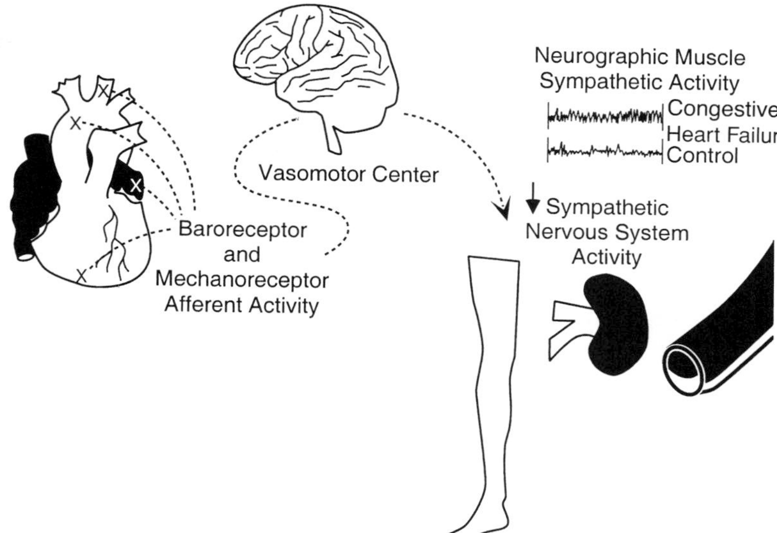


**Figure 28–3** Baroreceptor and mechanoreceptor activation occurs when the heart is distended due to volume overload. This signal is processed by the brain, and in the setting of heart failure, fails to reduce sympathetic activity (the normal response). The result is enhanced sympathetic traffic to the periphery, vasoconstriction, and reduced renal blood flow. These are hallmarks of advanced heart failure.

simply becomes less efficient over time. The failing heart is exquisitely sensitive to higher afterload (Fig. 28–4), consistent with the notion that the dilated heart performs more poorly. In a sense, these changes define heart failure at the organ level. The remodeling process is due to a confluence of forces, including perverse loading conditions and unrelenting activity of various neurohormones. As the heart hypertrophies, capillary density is reduced, leading to a form of "energy starvation" from oxygen deprivation. High-energy phosphate use is altered. Eventually, myocardial contractility is reduced. The following processes, currently under intense study, contribute to the remodeling of the heart:

- Increased myocardial mass (hypertrophy)
- Increased myocyte size (elongation and increased width)
- Cellular necrosis and apoptosis (cell drop-out)

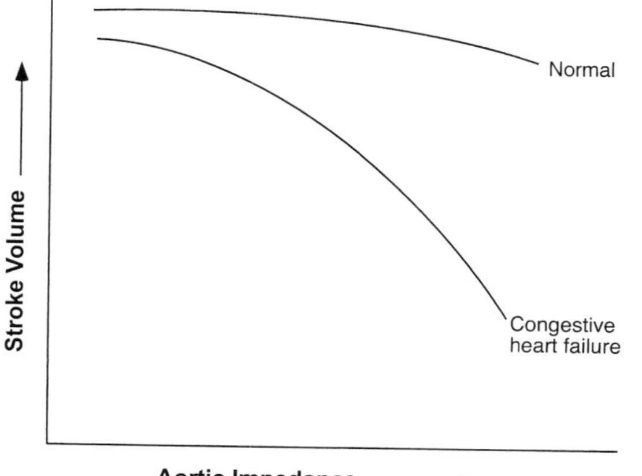


**Figure 28–4** The failing heart is exquisitely sensitive to afterload. As impedance to ejection increases (increased vascular resistance, increased wall tension, etc.), the performance of the left ventricle diminishes proportionately. On the contrary, acute vasodilation with nitroprusside leads to a marked increase in cardiac output.

- Collagen deposition (reactive and replacement)
- Myocyte slippage (increased matrix metalloproteinases [MMPs], decreased tissue inhibitors of MMPs or TIMPs)
- Chamber enlargement
- Increased wall tension
- Decreased myocardial performance
- Impaired filling due to increased muscle and chamber stiffness
- Reversion to the fetal genetic program (enhanced BNP synthesis, pro-growth)
- Activation of neurohormones
- Increased synthesis and release of counterregulatory hormones (i.e., BNP)
- Perverse loading conditions

## ABNORMAL CELLULAR MECHANISMS

Important changes occur at the cellular level in the setting of heart failure. These abnormalities undoubtedly contribute to reduced contractility, as they are imbedded in the contractile units, i.e., the sarcomere and the myocyte itself. Many of these abnormalities have been observed in vitro, in the laboratory setting only, but some have been derived from failing human hearts extirpated at the time of heart transplantation. It is not entirely clear whether these molecular abnormalities are primary features that contribute quantitatively to the failing heart, or whether they are secondary or so-called epiphenomena that occur as a consequence or a result of the heart failure syndrome. Nevertheless, it is important to consider them:

- Decreased $\beta$-receptor density in the heart
- Increased Gi coupling protein in the heart
- $\alpha$- to $\beta$-myosin heavy-chain transition (decreased myosin ATPase enzyme velocity) in the myocytes
- Defect in sarcolemma calcium uptake

- Defect in calcium-ATPase (SERCA) and phospholamban ($Ca^{2+}$ exchange)
- Abnormal contractile proteins

These changes, observed at the molecular level, likely contribute to reduced inotropy and may serve as a substrate for rhythm disturbances. They may be a vestige of evolutionary forces that initially allow the heart to operate in a more economical manner in the face of excessive inotropic stimulation. Over time, these "adaptations" contribute to impaired organ function.

## PERIPHERAL VASCULAR AND SKELETAL MUSCLE ADAPTATIONS IN HEART FAILURE

Profound changes occur in the periphery in the setting of heart failure, and these likely are responsible for the impaired exercise tolerance and fatigue that commonly plagues patients. In addition to exercise intolerance, sleep disturbances occur, often in the form of obstructive and central sleep apnea. Blood flow is redistributed to the brain and skeletal muscles, away from the kidneys and the splanchnic beds. Abnormalities in reflex control underlie these changes. Skeletal muscles begin to atrophy, which contributes to fatigue. The causes of exercise intolerance are multiple and complex:

- Endothelial dysfunction (decreased nitric oxide [NO] in the periphery)
- Reduced nutritive flow to skeletal muscles
- Skeletal muscle atrophy
- Inability to increase stroke volume in response to exercise
- Chronotropic incompetence
- Reduced myocardial force–frequency response
- Deconditioning
- Decreased $\beta$-adrenergic myocardial receptor density
- Skeletal muscle shift from slow- to fast-twitch fibers, atrophy of fast-twitch fibers
- Reduced skeletal muscle mitochondrial size
- Reduced skeletal muscle mitochondrial enzymes
- Excessive ventilatory drive in response to exercise
- Reduced lung compliance

## PROGNOSIS

It is important to identify where an individual patient is situated in the natural history of heart failure, providing needed optimism for those in the early stages while allowing for advanced directives for patients in the end stages. However, data regarding prognosis are nearly always derived retrospectively from large data bases, and represent group data that may not apply to an individual patient. For example, a low ejection fraction is not a powerful risk factor in a group of patients with advanced disease, as all of the ejection fractions cluster at a low end in this group. Physicians need to keep this in mind when interacting with patients and their families, who frequently ask about prognosis. Clearly, the overall prognosis has improved for heart failure over the past 10 to 15 years with many new and effective treatments. Nonetheless, heart failure is usually not "cured", but it can be managed. Many prognostic factors associate with a poor prognosis, including:

- Reduced ejection fraction
- Reduced exercise capacity (peak $VO_2 \leq 14$ mL/kg/min)
- New York Heart Association (NYHA) functional class IV
- Renal insufficiency or chronic kidney disease
- Markedly dilated LV chamber size
- Markedly increased plasma BNP and plasma norepinephrine levels
- Depression
- Severe ascites and tissue congestion
- Cheyne–Stokes breathing pattern
- Syncope
- Symptomatic ventricular arrhythmias
- Anemia
- Cardiac cachexia
- Hyponatremia
- Widening QRS complex
- Associated comorbid conditions

## SUMMARY

Heart failure is a complex syndrome, and its pathophysiology is inherently complex. Nevertheless, there are some unifying features. There are signs and symptoms of dyspnea, fatigue, and sometimes tissue congestion. There are underlying structural and/or functional abnormalities of the heart. The heart "adapts" to an index event to maintain circulatory homeostasis in the short term, but over the long term there is further progression of heart failure, in part driven by these "adaptive" mechanisms. The heart enlarges, becomes more globular, and more inefficient. Excitation contraction becomes abnormal. Rhythm disturbances occur. LV performance diminishes, and often mitral and tricuspid insufficiency occur. Exercise tolerance is diminished, salt and free water are retained, renal function deteriorates, and signs and symptoms worsen. We now have a much better understanding of how these events unfold, and treatment has improved markedly. However the natural history of heart failure is highly variable in individual patients, making prognosis difficult to determine.

## BIBLIOGRAPHY

**Anand IS, Chandrashekhar Y, Ferrari R, et al.** Pathogenesis of congestive state in chronic obstructive pulmonary disease. *Circulation*. 1992;86:1992:12–21.

**Anand IS, Chandrashekhar Y, Ferrari R, et al.** Pathogenesis of edema in chronic severe anemia: studies of hemodynamic variables, and plasma hormones. *Br Heart J*. 1993;70:357–362.

**Cohn JN.** From hypertension to heart failure. *Eur Heart J Suppl*. 2000; 2(suppl A):A2–A5.

Harris P. Evolution and the cardiac patient. *Cardiovasc Res*. 1983;17: 1–22.
Harris P. Congestive cardiac failure: central role of the arterial blood pressure. *Br Heart J*. 1987;58:190–203.
Mann DL. Mechanisms and models in heart failure. *Circulation*. 1999; 100:999–1008.
Packer M. The neurohormonal hypothesis: a theory to explain the mechanism of disease progression in heart failure. *J Am Coll Cardiol*. 1992;20:20:248–254.
Tang WHW, Francis GS. Natural history of heart failure. In: Kukin ML, Fuster V, eds. *Oxidative Stress and Cardiac Failure*. Armonk, NY: Futura; 2003:3–47.

## QUESTIONS

**1.** Which of the following statements about heart failure is true?

a. It is a clinical syndrome.
b. It can be caused by any form of heart disease.
c. It is diagnosed primarily by history and physical exam.
d. All of the above

Answer is d: Heart failure, like renal failure or anemia, is a clinical syndrome with a constellation of signs and symptoms. It has many possible etiologies, since virtually any form of heart disease can lead to heart failure. Patients must have signs and symptoms (i.e., a low ejection fraction does not equal heart failure) that usually consist of dyspnea and fatigue at rest or with exertion. There must be underlying cardiac structural and/or functional abnormalities. There is no laboratory test for heart failure (i.e., a history and physical exam are necessary), though a plasma BNP level may help facilitate the diagnosis in certain settings.

**2.** The principal features of heart failure include all of the following *except*:

a. Activation of the RAAS and SNS
b. Left ventricular remodeling
c. The ability to mount a reflex tachycardia
d. Downregulation of $\beta$-adrenergic receptors

Answer is c: Patients with heart failure have well-documented disturbances of the autonomic nervous system, and are unable to mount a reflex tachycardia in response to upright tilt, orthostasis, intense vasodilation, or other volume-depleting stimuli. In fact, the extent of this blunted sympathetic response is coupled to the severity of heart failure and is predictive of a poor prognosis. Similarly, patients with heart failure do not fully activate the parasympathetic arm of the autonomic nervous system in response to systemic pressor activity with phenylephrine (there is less vagal-induced slowing of the heart rate). Heart-rate variability is also blunted in patients with heart failure, and is also associated with a poor prognosis.

**3.** The inability to exercise properly in heart failure is due to all of the following *except*:

a. Reduced ejection fraction
b. Skeletal muscle atrophy
c. Endothelial dysfunction in peripheral vessels
d. Inability to increase stroke volume and heart rate

Answer is a: There has been a very reproducible and consistently poor relationship noted between resting ejection fraction (EF) and exercise capacity ($r = 0.20$–25) in patients with chronic heart failure. This is likely because exercise capacity is limited in patients with chronic heart failure, not by abnormal central hemodynamics, but by peripheral factors such as deconditioning and atrophy of skeletal muscles, changes in skeletal muscle oxidative enzymes, redistribution of blood flow away from skeletal muscles to more vital organs, and endothelial dysfunction in the peripheral vasculature due to a relative deficiency of local nitric oxide synthesis in blood vessels.

**4.** Which of the following statements about the prognosis for heart failure is true? (Select the best answer.)

a. It is fairly easy to predict in individual patients.
b. It is commonly assessed by measuring peak $VO_2$ during exercise.
c. It is closely coupled to ejection fraction in individual patients.
d. It is commonly estimated by measuring neurohormones.

Answer is b: There are almost as many "prognostic factors" in heart failure as there are stars in the clear night sky. Many of them are related to each other, and their independent contributions to prognosis are difficult to measure. Determining how much exercise the patient can do is perhaps the closest "factor" we have to a true "gold standard" for estimating prognosis. For example, the $VO_2$ max should be less than 14 Ml/kg/min for a patient to be considered for heart transplantation. Preserved exercise tolerance is a very powerful predictor of a better prognosis in patients with chronic heart failure.

**5.** Which of the following characterizes heart failure?

a. Downregulation of $\beta_1$- and $\beta_2$-receptors
b. Downregulation primarily of $\beta_1$-receptors, with little change in $\beta_2$-receptors
c. Downregulation of G proteins and $\beta_1$- and $\beta_2$-receptors
d. Increase in myocardial norepinephrine stores
e. Intact baroreceptor function

Answer is b: In chronic heart failure it is primarily the $\beta_1$-receptor that is downregulated. The density of cardiac $\beta_2$-receptors is much less than that of the $\beta_1$-receptors, and the $\beta_2$-receptors may be less important in modulating positive inotropy. In addition to relatively selective

$\beta_1$-receptor downregulation that occurs in chronic heart failure, there is important uncoupling of the G-stimulating protein from the $\beta$-receptors, leading to a reduction in positive inotropic state.

6. All of the following neurohormones are associated with vasoconstriction, cell growth, hypertrophy, and sodium retention *except*:
   a. Angiotensin-II
   b. Norepinephrine
   c. Brain natriuretic peptide
   d. Endothelin
   e. Arginine vasopressin

Answer is c: Natriuretic peptides modulate sodium and water (volume) regulation, vasodilation, natriuresis, antifibroblast proliferation, and anticollagen deposition, and have antiremodeling activity. Their biologic activities are nearly opposite those of angiotensin-II, norepinephrine, endothelin, and arginine vasopressin.

# 29 Medical Treatment of Heart Failure

*Hsuan-Hung Chuang* *Randall C. Starling*

Treatment plans for patients with heart failure (HF) should take into account the complexity of the syndrome, including comorbid conditions, presence or absence of systolic dysfunction and its severity, symptomatology, and etiology.

All patients with symptomatic or asymptomatic left ventricular (LV) systolic dysfunction, regardless of etiology, should be started on an angiotensin-converting enzyme (ACE) inhibitor unless contraindicated or not tolerated, and in most patients a beta-blocker.

## DISEASE AND DEFINITIONS

Traditionally, heart failure management was directed toward symptom control and improving survival. The American College of Cardiology (ACC) and the American Heart Association (AHA) published guidelines in 2001, introducing a classification system, with four stages, which emphasizes both the evolution and progression of HF (1). It is hoped that early detection of LV dysfunction and determination of the underlying etiology will lead to early intervention and prevention of progressive dysfunction, thereby reducing the incidence and mortality of HF. The four stages are as follows:

*Stage A* identifies the patient who is at high risk for developing HF (e.g., one with essential hypertension).

*Stage B* refers to a patient with a structural disorder of the heart but who has never developed symptoms of HF (e.g., one with asymptomatic mitral regurgitation).

*Stage C* refers to a patient with past or current symptoms of HF associated with underlying structural heart disease.

*Stage D* denotes a patient with end-stage disease who requires specialized treatment strategies, such as continuous inotropic infusion, mechanical circulatory support (MCS), cardiac transplantation, or even hospice care.

Evaluation of the newly diagnosed HF patient is performed to elucidate the underlying etiology of the syndrome, to identify precipitating causes of decompensation, and to search for potentially reversible factors. ACE inhibitors and beta-blockers form the cornerstone of standard medical therapy. Antiarrhythmic drugs, warfarin, aspirin, and nutritional supplements are controversial. Treatment of myocardial ischemia, valvular dysfunction, cardiac arrhythmias, anemia, thyroid disease, and sleep apnea is important. An implantable defibrillator will improve survival in certain patients. Biventricular pacing may be considered for symptomatic patients with LV dyssynchrony to improve symptoms and survival (CARE Heart Failure Trial). Multidisciplinary HF management programs are useful in preventing cardiac decompensation leading to hospital admissions. Education is provided about compliance with medications, diet, exercise, fluid restriction, self-care, weight reduction, smoking cessation, avoidance of alcohol, and cardiac rehabilitation (2–7).

## MANAGEMENT OF CHRONIC HEART FAILURE

### Pharmacological Therapy for Heart Failure Caused by Systolic Dysfunction

#### *Angiotensin-Converting Enzyme Inhibitors (ACE Inhibitors)*

The renin–angiotensin system plays a key role in the development of HF. ACE inhibitors inhibit the conversion of angiotensin-I to angiotensin-II in the vasculature by blocking the angiotensin-converting enzyme. They enhance the vasodilatory actions of kinins, inhibit aldosterone and inflammatory cytokines, and augment kinin-mediated prostaglandin synthesis. Cardiovascular (CV) effects include reductions in right and left heart filling pressures, increased cardiac output (CO) without reflex tachycardia, and attenuation of myocardial hypertrophy and fibrosis. These benefits appear to be a class effect, and have made ACE inhibitors the cornerstone of medical therapy from asymptomatic LV dysfunction to end-stage HF.

Multiple large randomized trials using several different ACE inhibitors have demonstrated an 18% to 40% reduction in overall mortality, decreased mortality secondary to HF and sudden cardiac death (SCD), and lower HF hospitalization rates. The Cooperative North Scandinavian Enalapril Survival Study (CONSENSUS) demonstrated that enalapril reduced 6-month mortality by 40% and 1-year mortality by 31% in patients with New York Heart Association (NYHA) Class III–IV HF, with an average risk reduction of 30% over the 10-year duration. The larger Studies of Left Ventricular Dysfunction (SOLVD) Treatment trial showed that enalapril reduced mortality by 16% over an average follow-up of 41 months in symptomatic NYHA Class II–III HF. When compared with another vasodilator combination (hydralazine and isosorbide dinitrate) in the first Vasodilator Heart Failure Trial (V-HeFT I) trial, the mortality rate was lower with enalapril (18% versus 25%).

ACE inhibitors improve the outcome in patients with asymptomatic LV dysfunction or overt HF occurring after an acute myocardial infarction (MI). In the Survival and Ventricular Enlargement (SAVE) trial, captopril therapy in asymptomatic patients with post-MI LV dysfunction was associated with a 19% decrease in mortality, a 37% reduction in the incidence of severe HF, a 22% reduction in hospitalization for HF, and a 25% reduction in the incidence of recurrent MI, at a mean follow-up of 42 months. In the Acute Infarction Ramipril Efficacy (AIRE) study, ramipril likewise was associated with a 27% decrease in mortality, a 23% reduction in incidence of severe HF, and a 30% reduction in sudden death among recruited patients with post-infarct HF. In an analysis from the Trandolapril Cardiac Evaluation (TRACE) study of patients with LV dysfunction and sinus rhythm after an acute MI, trandolapril significantly reduced the incidence of subsequent atrial fibrillation (AF). The chronic use of ACE inhibitors in patients with stable coronary artery disease and normal or slightly reduced LV systolic function did not demonstrate additional benefit in the Prevention of Events with Angiotensin Converting Enzyme Inhibition (PEACE) trial when background modern conventional medical therapy was utilized.

The use of ACE inhibition in diastolic HF is being evaluated. ACE inhibitors may be beneficial in such patients, especially those with hypertensive heart disease or concomitant systolic dysfunction. The Heart Outcomes Prevention Evaluation (HOPE) study indicates that ACE inhibitors reduce the risk of coronary events in patients with preserved LV function and such risk factors as diabetes, peripheral vascular disease, and coronary artery disease.

In general, it is believed that administering target doses of ACE inhibitors is beneficial. In the Assessment of Treatment with Lisinopril and Survival (ATLAS) trial, compared to the low-dose regimens, high-dose lisinopril reduced mortality by an insignificant 8%, although it significantly lowered the combined endpoint of mortality and hospitalization for any cause by 12%, and HF hospitalizations by 24%. The minimal incremental benefits were offset by more adverse side effects.

It is known that increased kinin levels may contribute to the observed benefit seen with ACE inhibitors, possibly through enhanced release of vasodilator prostaglandins. Some studies have shown that aspirin, a prostaglandin synthesis inhibitor, attenuates the beneficial effect of enalapril mediated on systemic vascular resistance (SVR) and CO in patients with severe HF. Systematic reviews suggest that aspirin does not significantly attenuate the beneficial effects of ACE inhibitors and the combination should be used in appropriate patients with coronary artery disease.

Six ACE inhibitors are currently approved for heart failure treatment: captopril, enalapril, lisinopril, quinapril, trandolapril, and fosinopril. Ramipril is approved for heart failure following MI. Dose titration to target levels is desirable to achieve maximal clinical benefit (150 mg of captopril daily, 20 to 40 mg of enalapril daily, 40 mg of lisinopril daily, 20 mg of ramipril daily, 40 mg of quinapril daily, and 4 mg of trandolapril daily).

ACE inhibitors, often given in combination with diuretics, should ideally be initiated before aggressively performing diuresis. ACE inhibitors should not be prescribed to patients with acute renal failure, bilateral renal artery stenosis, a history of angioedema, or during pregnancy. ACE intolerance (10% to 20%) is manifested by hypotension, azotemia, hyperkalemia, cough, angioedema, or agranulocytosis. Generally, electrolytes and renal function should be checked approximately a week after initiation or change in dosage. Although cough is poorly tolerated, ensure that the cough is not related to fluid overload or underlying pulmonary disease before drug discontinuation.

- All patients with symptomatic or asymptomatic LV dysfunction (LV ejection fraction $\leq$40%), regardless of etiology, should be started on an ACE inhibitor, unless contraindicated or not tolerated.
- ACE inhibitors should be prescribed as soon as safely possible following acute myocardial infarction.

### *Angiotensin-II Receptor Blockers*

Angiotensin-II receptor blockers (ARBs) prevent the effects of angiotensin II (including those generated through non-ACE pathways) at the angiotensin-II type 1 receptor. Clinical trials have shown that ARBS are better tolerated, improve exercise performance, have similar hemodynamic and neurohormonal effects, but probably are not equivalent or superior to ACE inhibitors in managing heart failure. Angiotensin-converting enzyme inhibitors remain the therapy of choice for all levels of HF. The most common reason for changing from an ACE inhibitor to an ARB is cough; rarely, angioedema may necessitate substitution.

In the Evaluation of Losartan in the Elderly (ELITE I) trial, losartan was reported to have a lower mortality rate compared with captopril in patients with CHF. This finding was not confirmed in the larger ELITE II study, which showed that losartan was not superior to captopril in reducing mortality, but was better tolerated. In the Valsartan Heart Failure Trial (Val-HeFT), the added benefit of valsartan to standard therapy for heart failure was evaluated. There was no difference in mortality between valsartan and placebo, but there was an improved quality of life and fewer hospitalizations. The addition of valsartan resulted in a 28% reduction in HF hospitalization. An adverse effect on mortality and morbidity observed in the group receiving ACE inhibitor and beta-blocker plus valsartan raised concern regarding the safety of this specific combination. The Candesartan in Heart Failure Assessment of Reduction in Mortality and Morbidity (CHARM) program is a set of three parallel studies comparing candesartan to placebo in three different HF populations: those with preserved ejection fraction (EF) (CHARM-Preserved), those unable to tolerate ACE inhibitors (CHARM-Alternative), and those already on a stable HF regimen that included an ACE inhibitor (CHARM-Added). In the CHARM-Alternative, after a mean follow-up of 33.7 months, the candesartan group experienced a lower rate of CV death or HF hospitalization than the placebo group, which was attributed largely to a reduction in HF hospitalizations. In the CHARM-Preserved, the use of candesartan did not result in significant difference in CV death; however, a moderately positive effect on hospital admissions was shown. In the CHARM-Added trial, 37.9% of those taking candesartan died due to CV causes or were admitted to the hospital for HF, compared with 42.3% of those in the placebo group. Although subgroup analysis of Val-HeFT suggested that there was a trend toward increased mortality in patients receiving valsartan, ACE inhibition, and beta-blockers, the CHARM-Added trial did not confirm this adverse interaction. Candesartan significantly reduces all-cause mortality, cardiovascular death, and heart failure hospitalizations in patients with CHF and left ventricular ejection fraction (LVEF) ≤40% when added to standard therapies including ACE inhibitors, beta-blockers, and an aldosterone antagonist. Routine monitoring of blood pressure, renal function, and electrolytes is advised. The U.S. Food and Drug Administration has approved the use of candesartan for use with an ACE inhibitor in the treatment of NYHA Class II–IV HF on the basis of the CHARM-Added trial, which showed that the addition of candesartan produced a 15% relative risk reduction in cardiovascular death or HF hospitalizations. On the basis of the CHARM-Alternative study, candesartan is also approved for use in patients with systolic heart failure who cannot tolerate an ACE inhibitor. In summary, the use of an ARB should be considered in patients with (a) progressive systolic heart failure despite maximally titrated ACE inhibitor and beta-blocker medications; and (b) patients with systolic heart failure with intolerance to ACE inhibitors or for whom ACE inhibitors are contraindicated.

The Optimal Trial in Myocardial Infarction with the Angiotensin II Antagonist Losartan (OPTIMAAL) randomized >5,000 patients with clinical HF or LVEF <35% following acute MI within 10 days of their qualifying event to receive 50 mg of captopril three times a day or 50 mg of losartan daily. There was a nonsignificant mortality trend favoring captopril. In the Valsartan in Acute Myocardial Infarction Trial (VALIANT), after a median follow-up of 24.7 months, the all-cause mortality was 19.9% in the valsartan group, 19.5% in the captopril group, and 19.3% in the combination group. Secondary endpoints of CV death, MI, and HF hospitalization were also similar in the three treatment groups. Thus, the VALIANT trial showed that valsartan is as effective as captopril in reducing fatal or nonfatal CV events in these high-risk postinfarct patients. However, combining valsartan with captopril increased adverse events without improving survival. Therefore, current evidence does not recommend ARBs as routine therapy for patients following acute MI, and ACE inhibitors remain the drugs of choice early after a myocardial infarction.

ARB selection and utilization should be based on evidence from clinical trials. Both candesartan and valsartan are dose-dependent inhibitors of the AT1 receptor, with respective affinities that are approximately 80 to 100 times that of losartan. The bioavailability of valsartan drops by 40% if it is taken with food. Losartan is a relatively weaker receptor blocker, but its active metabolite is capable of insurmountable receptor blockade. ARB dose is likely very important, and the ongoing Heart Failure End-Point Evaluation with the Angiotensin II Antagonist Losartan (HEAAL) study will address this issue.

- ACE inhibitors rather than ARBs continue to be the agents of choice in HF. Patients who are truly intolerant to ACE inhibitors should be considered for treatment with an ARB and/or the combination of hydralazine and isosorbide dinitrate.
- Currently the most compelling indication for combination therapy is in patients who remain symptomatic despite standard therapy, including target doses of ACE inhibitors and beta-blockers. Combined therapy with ACE inhibitor and ARB is without merit in acute postinfarct LV dysfunction (evidence on basis of VALIANT trial).

### *Beta-Adrenergic Blockers*

The first observation suggesting that beta blockade might be beneficial in HF was made in 1975, when the administration of metoprolol to seven patients with congestive cardiomyopathy resulted in improvements in LVEF and overall clinical status. Currently, beta-blockers are of paramount importance in treating HF of all etiologies. Multiple benefits include improved survival (30% to 35% across trials), decreased hospitalizations, increased LVEF, improvement in quality of life, decreased hospitalizations, enhanced exercise performance, lowered blood pressure (BP), decreased ischemia, and reduced sudden cardiac death incidence. Simply reducing the heart rate allows longer diastolic filling time, lowers myocardial energy expenditure, and lengthens coronary perfusion. More important, beta-blockers inhibit the deleterious effects of sustained $\beta_1$-adrenergic stimulation, such as myocyte cell death (e.g., necrosis and apoptosis), alterations in "fetal" gene expression, as well as further activation of the renin–angiotensin cascade.

The first beta-blocker trial in HF patients was the Metoprolol Dilated Cardiomyopathy (MDC) trial, which examined only younger patients with nonischemic cardiomyopathy. Although it did not demonstrate statistical significance as being associated with reduced mortality, use of metoprolol was associated with significant improvements in exercise capacity, functional capacity, and the ability to remove patients from a heart transplant list. The U.S. Carvedilol Trial randomized >1,000 patients with Class II–IV HF and LVEF <35% who were receiving ACE inhibitors, digitalis, and diuretics to carvedilol or placebo. The study was terminated early when interim analysis revealed a 65% overall mortality reduction. There was also a 26% reduction in hospitalization for CV causes and a 38% reduction in combined risk of death or CV hospitalization. The Metoprolol Cr/XL Randomized Intervention Trial in Congestive Heart Failure (MERIT-HF) trial demonstrated a 34% relative reduction in all-cause mortality, a 38% reduction in CV mortality, a 40% reduction in SCD, and a 49% reduction in the risk of progressive HF with long-acting metoprolol. A similar benefit of beta-blockers was demonstrated in the two Cardiac Insufficiency Bisoprolol Study (CIBIS-I and CIBIS-II) trials. In the CIBIS-II trial, there was a 34% reduction in all-cause mortality, a 42% reduction in sudden death, and a 32% reduction in HF hospitalizations. More recently, the use of carvedilol in patients with severe HF was further explored in the Carvedilol Prospective Randomized Cumulative Survival (COPERNICUS) trial, which showed a significant 35% reduction in mortality at 1 year, 41% reduction in death and HF hospitalizations, and 24% reduction in death and total hospitalizations. With a carvedilol withdrawal rate less than placebo, COPERNICUS demonstrated the safety and efficacy of treating patients with severe HF with carvedilol. The Carvedilol Post Infarction Survival Control in Left Ventricular Dysfunction (CAPRICORN) trial showed a 15% to 20% absolute reduction in all-cause mortality with the use of carvedilol versus placebo in patients with post–MI LV dysfunction, even in the modern era when thrombolytics, ACE inhibitors, statin therapy, and aspirin are prescribed. Thus a beta-blocker and an ACE inhibitor should be given to patients with impaired LV function following MI, regardless of their functional class. The U.S. Food and Drug Administration has approved the post-MI indication based on the evidence cited.

The first trial that failed to demonstrate a benefit of beta-blockers in HF was the Beta-Blocker Evaluation of Survival Trial (BEST). Failure of bucindolol to demonstrate a benefit may be related to higher representation in this trial by African American patients, who have a much higher incidence of hypertension as the cause of HF (which is often a low renin state and not particularly responsive to beta-blockade). Conversely, the Caucasian population in this trial had a relatively favorable outcome. These data caution against the extrapolation of trial data to all patients with HF and suggest racial heterogeneity, likely related to genetic polymorphism and differing pharmacokinetics.

Can the effects of beta-blockers in HF be attributed to the entire class of agents? In general, three agents (carvedilol, metoprolol, and bisoprolol), both selective and nonselective beta-receptor antagonists, are currently advocated for use in HF. The Carvedilol or Metoprolol European Trial (COMET) trial compared generic metoprolol tartrate (50 mg twice a day) with carvedilol (25 mg twice a day). Carvedilol was found to be superior to metoprolol tartrate, with a 17% relative reduction in all-cause mortality after approximately 5 years of follow-up. The trial has been criticized for use of metoprolol tartrate rather than metoprolol succinate, at inadequate doses and incorrect dosing intervals. The degree of beta-blockade may not have been equivalent, as the carvedilol arm had significantly greater reductions in heart rate and systolic BP.

At present, it remains difficult to declare which beta-blocker is superior. Does the dose matter? The Multicenter Oral Carvedilol Heart Failure Assessment (MOCHA) trial demonstrated that even at a dose of 6.25 mg of carvedilol twice daily, there was a reduction in mortality compared to placebo when added to standard therapy. There were dose-dependent improvements in LV function and mortality, although there was no difference in submaximal exercise performance.

Beta-blockers are prescribed to euvolemic patients with LV dysfunction, starting with low doses and slowly uptitrating to target levels over weeks to months. Occasionally, beta-blockade may be associated with decreased LVEF and increased LV volume, causing fatigue, fluid retention, or overt cardiac decompensation. However, within weeks to months, EF increases and reverse LV remodeling often occurs, resulting in functional improvement. Side effects may include hypotension, lightheadedness, fluid retention, cardiac decompensation, and bradycardia. Titration to target doses is desirable but may not be achieved in some patients due to side effects. Beta-blockers can potentially cause bronchoconstriction and vasoconstriction, and may mask hypoglycemic symptoms. However, a retrospective review of the use of carvedilol in community practice demonstrated tolerance rates in patients with diabetes, chronic obstructive pulmonary disease (COPD) or asthma, and peripheral vascular disease that were similar to the overall population. The choice of beta-blocker must be individualized, with consideration for the potential risks and benefits. Temporary reduction and gradual cessation of beta-blocker therapy is required if HF exacerbation is characterized by hypoperfusion, bradycardia, or the requirement for inotropic drugs. Inotropes that act independent of the beta-adrenergic receptor, such as the phosphodiesterase inhibitor milrinone, may be preferable in this setting. Dobutamine is an alternative, but higher than expected doses are required to achieve equivalent hemodynamic effects. Gradual reintroduction of the beta-blocker should occur if the patient stabilizes.

- Beta-blocker therapy should be routinely administered to patients with stable NYHA Class II–III HF and LVEF ≤40% who are on standard therapy, and for asymptomatic LV dysfunction post–MI.
- Beta-blockers should be considered for patients with stable Class IV HF.
- Beta-blocker therapy should be initiated at low doses and titrated up slowly.

### *Aldosterone Antagonists*

Aldosterone, released from the adrenal cortex following stimulation by angiotensin-II, promotes sodium and water retention with potassium and magnesium loss. Plasma aldosterone levels may be elevated by 20-fold in patients with HF as a result of the combination of increased adrenal production and decreased hepatic clearance. Aldosterone antagonists, such as spironolactone and eplerenone, act by binding to and antagonizing the mineralocorticoid receptors. They are known to increase diuresis and natriuresis and to lower blood pressure in patients with essential hypertension, while sparing potassium. The nonrenal effects of aldosterone blockade, including effects on vascular inflammation, vascular remodeling and compliance, ventricular hypertrophy and fibrosis, endothelial dysfunction, myocardial norepinephrine uptake, heart-rate variability, baroreceptor function, fibrinolysis, and platelet activation have been demonstrated in recent years and may in large part be responsible for its beneficial effects.

The Randomized Aldactone Evaluation Study (RALES) studied the role of spironolactone in patients with NYHA Class III–IV HF and LVEF ≤35%. Over a mean follow-up of 2 years, spironolactone was associated with a significant 30% reduction in all-cause mortality, a 35% reduction in hospitalization for HF, a 36% reduction in death from progressive HF, and a 29% reduction in SCD. The side effects of spironolactone are attributed to its binding to glucocorticoid, progesterone, and androgen receptors and include gynecomastia (10%), breast tenderness or pain, impotence, and oligomenorrhea. Aldosterone-blocking agents have the potential to worsen creatinine and cause hyperkalemia, so diligent monitoring of serum potassium levels is necessary during the first week of therapy and regularly thereafter. The physician may need to decrease or discontinue potassium supplementation when spironolactone is administered. The benefits of aldosterone blockade in mild HF are uncertain because of the lack of data.

Eplerenone, a selective aldosterone blocker, was studied in the Eplerenone Post-Acute Myocardial Infarction Heart Failure Efficacy and Survival Study (EPHESUS). Compared to placebo, there was a 13% relative reduction in mortality, a 15% relative decrease in HF hospitalization, and a 21% relative reduction in SCD. The less robust results for the EPHESUS trial compared with the RALES trial may be explained by the inclusion of less sick patients and a greater percentage being treated with beta-blockade. There was no excess of gynecomastia, breast pain, or impotence in males, attesting to the selectivity of eplerenone for the mineralocorticoid receptor in comparison to spironolactone, which also binds to androgen and progesterone receptors. Eplerenone is currently approved for use in post-MI patients with either diabetes or signs of HF and LVEF ≤40%. At present, it would not be reasonable to extrapolate the findings in RALES and EPHESUS to those patients with HF caused by preserved systolic function and those with asymptomatic LV dysfunction.

- Aldosterone antagonism is indicated for all patients with LV systolic dysfunction and Class III–IV symptoms. Its use in patients with milder degrees of HF may be considered on an individual basis. Eplerenone is indicated in two categories of postinfarction patients with reduced ejection fraction: diabetics and nondiabetics with symptomatic heart failure.

### *Diuretics*

Diuretics relieve congestion and provide rapid symptomatic improvement. Despite this, diuretics possess no proven mortality benefit. They are useful in both systolic and diastolic dysfunction in conjunction with an ACE inhibitor and are important for the efficacy of other drugs, especially beta-blockers. They act by inhibition of sodium reabsorption at various sites in the renal tubules, thereby promoting fluid and sodium excretion, leading to the lowering of intracardiac pressure and improvement of exercise tolerance. Loop diuretics (e.g., furosemide, bumetanide, and torsemide) inhibit sodium reabsorption in the thick ascending segment in the loop of Henle. Thiazides, including metolazone, prevent sodium reabsorption in the distal convoluted tubule. Spironolactone has its primary site of action in the collecting duct. Most HF patients require a loop diuretic combined with a reduced-sodium diet.

Diuretics have numerous metabolic sequelae, including electrolyte imbalance with low sodium, potassium, and magnesium levels, hypotension, azotemia, and neurohormonal activation. Loop diuretics may be given with a thiazide (e.g., metolazone) to patients with severe fluid retention. Torsemide, which has better absorption but is more costly than furosemide, may be useful for refractory fluid retention. The aldosterone antagonists, spironolactone and eplerenone, are weak diuretics when used independently.

- Use the minimal dose of diuretics needed to control congestion. Overdiuresis leads to further neurohormonal activation and may result in hypotension, prerenal azotemia, hyponatremia, hypokalemia, and hypomagnesemia.

### *Digitalis*

Digitalis is a centrally acting neurohormonal modulating agent that exerts its effect primarily by binding and inhibiting membrane-bound $\alpha$ subunits of sodium–potassium ATPase (sodium pump), mainly but not exclusively located in the human myocardium. This inhibition promotes sodium–calcium exchange, which increases the intracellular calcium concentration that is available to the contractile proteins, resulting in an increase in the force of myocardial contraction. Digitalis improves LVEF and reduces pulmonary capillary wedge pressure (PCWP) in patients with impaired systolic function. It increases cardiac output both at rest and during exercise. Exercise tolerance and maximal exercise capacity (as measured by peak oxygen consumption) improve with digitalis. Digitalis exerts an antiadrenergic effect by augmenting parasympathetic tone and reducing sympathetic outflow with improvement in the pathologic baroreceptor response in patients with HF. Digitalis may also be beneficial in patients with rapid AF by inducing partial atrioventricular (AV) block to slow the ventricular rate. In the kidney, inhibition of sodium–potassium ATPase leads to decreased renin release.

The Prospective Randomized Study of Ventricular Failure and the Efficacy of Digoxin (PROVED) and Randomized Assessment of Digoxin on Inhibitors of the Angiotensin-Converting Enzyme (RADIANCE) trials demonstrated that withdrawal of digitalis in patients with reduced LVEF and symptomatic HF led to a significant increased risk of recurrent HF, deterioration in quality of life, increased body weight, and higher heart rate. The subsequent National Institutes of Health (NIH)–sponsored DIG trial showed that there was absolutely no difference in survival between patients with NYHA Class II–III HF, although there was a 28% reduction in HF hospitalization. In the DIG ancillary study, which enrolled nearly 1,000 patients with diastolic HF, digitalis therapy was associated with a reduction in worsening HF but not mortality.

Digitalis has a low therapeutic-to-toxic range, and the dose should be decreased with advanced age, renal dysfunction, amiodarone, calcium channel blockers, and propafenone. Toxic effects include the induction of arrhythmias, conduction disturbances, and constitutional symptoms such as nausea and visual disturbances. Post-hoc data analysis from the DIG trial indicated that digitalis may be associated with increased mortality in women and that mortality was increased in men at higher serum digitalis concentrations. Doses that achieve a serum concentration of $<0.9$ ng/mL are recommended. Digitalis should be avoided or used with extreme caution in Wolff–Parkinson–White syndrome, severe conduction abnormalities, restrictive or hypertrophic cardiomyopathy, amyloid heart disease, renal failure, and acute coronary syndromes. Experimentally, digitalis can cause coronary artery constriction, mediated directly via coronary arterial smooth muscle.

- Digitalis should be considered for patients who have NYHA Class III–IV symptoms caused by LV systolic dysfunction despite optimal therapy. Therapeutic drug monitoring and appropriate serum levels are required.
- No benefit has been shown for digitalis use in asymptomatic patients with left ventricular systolic dysfunction and normal sinus rhythm.

### *Calcium Channel Blockers*

There is no survival advantage in using calcium channel blockers (CCBs) in HF. Short-acting CCBs are contraindicated. They depress LV function, worsen symptoms, increase neurohormones, and increase mortality. The Vasodilator Heart Failure Trial III (V-HeFT III), which examined felodipine, and the Prospective Randomized Amlodipine Survival Evaluation (PRAISE) trial, which examined amlodipine, a dihydropyridine vasodilating CCB, similarly showed no beneficial effect on survival. Subgroup analysis of the PRAISE trial demonstrated a significant mortality benefit in response to amlodipine in patients with a nonischemic congestive heart failure etiology, which was not, however, borne out in the subsequent PRAISE-2 trial. In view of their neutral effect on survival, felodipine and amlodipine may be considered for treatment of angina pectoris or hypertension associated with HF. The Antihypertensive and Lipid-Lowering Treatment to Prevent Heart Attack Trial (ALLHAT) suggested that hypertensive patients treated with CCBs are at increased risk for HF. Therefore, one should try to maximize the other standard HF regimens before using CCBs.

### *Hydralazine and Isosorbide Dinitrate*

Hydralazine and nitrates are respectively arterial and venous vasodilators, together reducing afterload and preload. Hydralazine has antioxidant properties and nitrates inhibit remodeling. The Veterans Administration Cooperative Vasodilator Heart Failure Trial (V-HeFT I) showed that this combination improved survival and LV function compared to placebo. This combination was associated with a higher mortality rate than enalapril in the Second Veterans Administration Cooperative Heart Failure Trial (V-HeFT II) (25% versus 18% at 2 years). Most of the benefit from ACE inhibitors was due to reduced incidence of SCD, but hydralazine and nitrates improved ejection fraction and exercise tolerance more than ACE inhibitors. Hydralazine and nitrates may be added to ACE inhibitors for improved vasodilation and when using hemodynamic monitoring to "tailor" medical therapy. The combination is also useful in patients who cannot tolerate ACE inhibitors or ARBs because of renal impairment.

The African American Heart Failure Trial (A-HeFT) reported that the combination when added to standard heart failure therapies resulted in a significant survival benefit in those with Class III–IV symptoms (6.2% versus 10.2%, $p = 0.02$). There was a 43% improvement in survival with a hazard ratio of 0.57 ($p = 0.01$) with a mean duration of follow-up of 10 months. Patients were treated with ACE inhibitors or ARBs (>85%), beta-blockers (>70%), and other therapies for 3 months and then randomized to receive isosorbide dinitrate/hydralazine given three times daily or placebo.

- The combination of hydralazine and isosorbide dinitrate should not be used for HF treatment in patients who have no prior use of an ACE inhibitor and should not substitute for ACE inhibitors in patients who are ACE-inhibitor tolerant.

## Pharmacologic Therapy for Heart Failure Caused by Diastolic Dysfunction

Thirty to fifty percent of patients with symptomatic HF demonstrate diastolic rather than systolic dysfunction. It is more common in patients with diabetes and hypertension, women, and the elderly. No medical treatment that conclusively reduces mortality in the presence of diastolic dysfunction is currently available. The cornerstone of treatment is regulation of ventricular filling pressure by diuretics, allowing for adequate cardiac output in the absence of congestion. ACE inhibitors and/or spironolactone make diuretic management easier by preventing excessive activation of the renin–angiotensin–aldosterone system (8,9). In patients with tachycardia, beta-blockers may be used to slow heart rate and prolong filling time, and also prevent supraventricular arrhythmias. The CHARM-Preserved trial demonstrated a modest 18% reduction in HF hospitalizations in the candesartan group, without a beneficial effect on the primary endpoint of cardiovascular mortality or HF hospitalization or all-cause mortality. Because myocardial ischemia can cause diastolic dysfunction, the guidelines offer support for consideration of use of coronary revascularization in patients with coronary disease, although the syndrome may not be completely ameliorated even after effective revascularization. The treatment of hypertensive heart disease is likewise a cornerstone of therapy for diastolic dysfunction with an associated etiology.

- The current recommendations for management of patient in this class reflect the lack of conclusive data on effective therapies. The major strategies are control of hypertension, treatment of ischemia, control of ventricular rate in patients with AF, and use of diuretics to control pulmonary congestion. Candesartan should also be considered.

## Adjunctive Therapies in Heart Failure Management

### *Antiarrhythmic Agents*

Patients with HF are at high risk for SCD, presumably from arrhythmias. Most antiarrhythmic agents possess negative inotropic effects and are proarrhythmic, especially in the setting of ventricular dysfunction. In general, Class IA, IC, and some Class III agents (such as sotalol) are contraindicated in HF. In general, antiarrhythmics are reserved for symptomatic arrhythmias or for control of the ventricular response to atrial fibrillation (AF). Amiodarone, a type III antiarrhythmic with antiadrenergic properties, is the preferred drug for treating AF or ventricular tachycardia (VT), but its use is limited by the high incidence of pulmonary, thyroid, liver, and other toxicities. Amiodarone has negative inotropic effects and may be poorly tolerated in patients with advanced HF. In the GESICA study, there were fewer deaths and HF hospitalizations in the amiodarone group. In the recent Sudden Cardiac Death in Heart Failure Trial (SCD-HeFT), amiodarone was associated with a nonsignificant 6% increase in mortality compared with placebo. Its use should be accompanied by careful adverse effect surveillance.

Dofetilide, a Class III antiarrhythmic agent, is effective for maintaining sinus rhythm but does not improve survival in patients with heart failure. In the Danish Investigations of Arrhythmia and Mortality on Dofetilide Study in Congestive Heart Failure, dofetilide did not affect all-cause mortality but significantly reduced the risk of HF hospitalization and recurrence of AF. Dofetilide has restricted use because of a narrow therapeutic index, a complex dosing regimen, and potential toxicity (including torsade de pointes in 3% of cases), especially when renal dysfunction is present.

Catheter-based ablation and implantable defibrillators are increasingly being used in the management of arrhythmias in HF patients. Current indications for device therapy in heart failure and sudden cardiac death are covered in another chapter.

- Amiodarone is the preferred drug when antiarrhythmic therapy is indicated in patients with heart failure for supraventricular tachycardia not controlled by digoxin or beta-blocker or for patients with life-threatening ventricular arrhythmia who are not candidates for ICD placement.
- Amiodarone is not recommended for the primary prevention of death in patients with chronic heart failure.

### *Anticoagulation*

Because the risk of thromboembolic events in patients with HF in sinus rhythm is low (1% to 3% per year), prophylactic use of warfarin is controversial. Warfarin may be indicated in HF patients with AF, LV thrombi (especially mobile), LV aneurysms, hypercoagulable states, history of thromboembolism, and patent foramen ovale. Aspirin is indicated in patients with ischemic left ventricular dysfunction. There is no evidence supporting the routine use of aspirin in patients devoid of coronary obstructive disease. The Warfarin and Antiplatelet Therapy in Heart Failure Trial (WATCH) was stopped early because of low enrollment and found no difference in mortality, MI, stroke, HF, unstable angina pectoris, or emboli in patients treated with aspirin, warfarin, or clopidogrel. Compared to aspirin, there were more bleeding episodes but fewer HF hospitalizations in the warfarin group. It was suggested that inhibition of prostaglandin by aspirin may worsen heart failure. At present, the risk/benefit ratio does not justify the routine administration of aspirin or warfarin in the heart failure patient group.

### *Treatment of Sleep Apnea*

Sleep apnea is an underrecognized comorbidity in patients with heart failure. Forty percent of HF patients have central sleep apnea (CSA) and 10% have obstructive sleep apnea (OSA). Sleep apnea causes nocturnal catecholamine surges, hypertension, and cardiac arrhythmias and may represent an independent risk factor for increased mortality and sudden cardiac death in HF patients. Patients suspected of having sleep apnea should undergo polysomnography. CSA improves with intensification of HF therapy, and nocturnal oxygen may be helpful in some cases. Sleep apnea should be treated with continuous positive airway pressure (CPAP) when efficacy is documented in the sleep lab. OSA may improve with weight loss and avoidance of alcohol and sedatives.

### *Treatment of Anemia*

Anemia occurs in 10% to 20% of HF patients, is associated with symptomatic impairment, decreased exercise capacity, increased risk for hospitalizations, and a worse prognosis. The cause of anemia is often multifactorial. Low cardiac output impairs bone marrow function, and chronic renal insufficiency and ACE inhibitors may decrease erythropoietin production. Cytokines suppress bone marrow function and inhibit erythropoietin effects. Poor nutrition, GI blood loss, and iron deficiency may contribute to low hemoglobin. Treatment of anemia with erythropoietin alone or in combination with iron therapy may improve the natural history of heart failure, quality of life, functional class, and exercise capacity. Single-center studies suggest that erythropoietin therapy can improve outcomes in chronic heart failure. Adequately powered randomized clinical trials have not been completed. Unresolved issues are the threshold level for initiating therapy and the target level of hemoglobin as a therapeutic endpoint (10).

### *Ultrafiltration*

Severe HF may require treatment with high-dose IV diuretics, combination loop and thiazide diuretics, or continuous diuretic infusion. When ascites and edema persist in the setting of rising creatinine and hyponatremia, ultrafiltration may be utilized. Ultrafiltration removes fluid from the blood at a rate proportional to fluid refill from the extravascular tissue space. This balanced diuresis maintains plasma volume and avoids hypotension. Clinical trials are in progress to fully delineate the role of ultrafiltration in heart failure management.

### *Enhanced External Counterpulsation*

Enhanced external counterpulsation (EECP) involves the sequential compression of the lower extremities by inflatable pneumatic cuffs synchronized with the patient's electrocardiogram (ECG). EECP functions as a noninvasive circulatory assist device, similar to an intra-aortic balloon pump. Hemodynamic effects consist of diastolic augmentation and systolic unloading, which increase blood flow to the heart and coronary arteries while reducing afterload. The Prospective Evaluation of Enhanced External Counterpulsation in Congestive Heart failure (PEECH) study was designed to evaluate improvements in exercise capacity and quality of life in HF patients refractory to medical therapies. Preliminary results were reported at the American College of Cardiology annual meeting in 2005. The patients treated with a 7-week course of EECP improved their duration of treadmill exercise time but did not increase peak oxygen consumption, yielding a somewhat equivocal benefit. The conclusion was that in optimally treated NYHA Class II–III patients, EECP improves exercise duration, quality of life, and NYHA functional class.

## Novel Therapies for Heart Failure Management

### *Immunosuppressive Therapy*

Patients with dilated cardiomyopathy who had evidence of myocarditis on biopsy and increased expression of HLA were randomly assigned to therapy with prednisone and azathioprine or placebo. There was no difference in the primary endpoint of death, transplantation, or rehospitalization at two years. However, immunosuppressive therapy was associated with a significant reduction in LV chamber dimensions, increase in LVEF, and clinical improvement. The Myocarditis Treatment trial randomized 111 patients with histologically proven myocarditis to placebo versus immunosuppressive therapy with the primary endpoint of LVEF. There was no significant difference in improvement in ejection fraction or survival in the two groups. Currently, neither endomyocardial biopsy nor immunosuppressive therapy is routinely indicated for acute cardiomyopathy.

### *Intravenous Immune Globulin*

Small clinical studies have shown that immunomodulation with intravenous immune globulin increased the plasma levels of anti-inflammatory mediators and produced a significant elevation in LVEF. However, this positive result has not been duplicated in other studies.

### Immunoadsorption

Antibodies against cardiac cell proteins have been identified in dilated cardiomyopathy, including antibodies against mitochondrial proteins, contractile proteins, and $\beta$-receptors. They are thought to be detrimental, and their removal with immunoadsorption might improve cardiac hemodynamics. The subclass of immunoglobulin removed may be important in antibody-mediated DCM. In one study, immunoadsorption completely eliminated the anti-$\beta_1$-adrenoceptor autoantibodies with improvement in LVEF and LV end-diastolic volume after 1 year of therapy. There were no changes in antibody levels or LV function in patients undergoing only standard medical therapy. The improvement in LV function with immunoadsorption has been associated with reduced myocardial inflammation and reduced oxidative stress.

### Antiproinflammatory Cytokines

Experimental and human studies suggest that drugs that inhibit tumor necrosis factor-alpha (TNF-$\alpha$) might be beneficial. However, large clinical trials with Etanercept in the Randomized Etanercept North American Strategy to Study Antagonism of Cytokines (RENAISSANCE), Research into Etanercept Cytokine Antagonism in Ventricular Dysfunction (RECOVER), and the Randomized Etanercept Worldwide Evaluation (RENEWAL—long term follow-up of the RECOVER and RENAISSANCE), and a pilot trial with Infliximab (ATTACH), failed to show any benefit in clinical HF, morbidity, or mortality.

### Neutral Endopeptidase Inhibitors

Neutral endopeptidase inhibitors simultaneously inhibit both neutral endopeptidase, which slows down the metabolism of endogenous atrial natriuretic peptide (ANP), and angiotensin-converting enzyme. They reduce systolic and mean BP and renal vascular resistance, reduce LV wall stress and increase LVEF, and increase renal blood flow and sodium excretion in mild HF. The Omapatrilat Versus Enalapril Randomized Trial of Utility in Reducing Events (OVERTURE) trial compared omapatrilat to enalapril in patients with Class II–IV HF and LVEF $\leq$30%, and showed no mortality or morbidity benefit.

### Vasopressin Antagonists

Vasopressin levels are increased in HF, and the levels correlate with both disease severity and the presence of hyponatremia. Release of vasopressin could be precipitated by hypotension, a low cardiac output state, angiotensin-II, and catecholamines. There are two main receptors for vasopressin: the $V_{1a}$ and $V_2$ receptors. $V_1$ receptors are found primarily in vascular smooth muscle, and $V_2$ receptors in kidneys. Activation of the $V_{1a}$ receptor appears to modulate myocardial fibrosis, hypertrophy, and vasoconstriction, whereas water retention and hyponatremia result from activation of the $V_2$ receptor. Tolvaptan was shown to be an effective aquaretic for hospitalized patients with HF and is now being studied to determine its impact on survival.

### Endothelin Receptor Antagonists

Endothelin, a more potent vasoconstrictor than angiotensin-II or norepinephrine, is frequently elevated in patients with severe HF. Randomized trials using oral and intravenous endothelin receptor antagonists have shown no benefit in patients with either acute or chronic HF.

### Antimetabolites

Abnormalities of energy metabolism are often cited as key elements in the progression of worsening LV dysfunction, and myocardial metabolic manipulation using drugs such as trimetazidine, ranolazine, carnitine, and others may offer a new therapeutic approach to the treatment of heart failure. It is suggested that the protective effects of trimetazidine and ranolazine are obtained at the cellular level by shifting the energy substrate reference from fatty acid oxidation to glucose oxidation. Carnitine plays a key role in the oxidation of long-chain fatty acids, and facilitates the aerobic metabolism of carbohydrates. Neither coenzyme-$Q_{10}$ nor antioxidants have demonstrated any clinical effectiveness in patients with HF. Allopurinol, an antioxidant, is currently being studied in a randomized controlled clinical trial.

## MANAGEMENT OF ACUTE HEART FAILURE

Acute heart failure (AHF) is a clinical syndrome with reduced cardiac output, tissue hypoperfusion, increase in the pulmonary capillary wedge pressure (PCWP), and tissue congestion. Although the current ACC/AHA Guidelines have not addressed the management of acute heart failure, this has been discussed in a recently published statement by the European Society of Cardiology (11–13). The initial goals of managing AHF are to correct hypoxia and increase cardiac output, renal perfusion, sodium excretion, and urine output. Specific therapies should be administered based on the clinical and hemodynamic characteristics of the patient. This may include the use of vasodilators, inotropes, or calcium sensitizers. Once the patient is stabilized, the goal shifts to maintaining compensation and improving long-term outcomes, including the prevention of rehospitalization and mortality. Therapies that slow the progression of heart failure, including patient education and disease management, are essential before hospital discharge.

### Pharmacologic Therapy for Acute Heart Failure

#### Diuretics

Diuretics are the first agents administered to patients with acute pulmonary edema. They decrease pulmonary vascular congestion, jugular venous distension, ascites, and edema, thus providing rapid symptomatic benefit. Intravenous diuretics are usually reserved for hospitalized patients. Continuous infusion may be needed for patients with diuretic resistance and provide improved diuresis and natriuresis.

### Milrinone

Milrinone is a phosphodiesterase III inhibitor. This enzyme, located in the myocyte sarcoplasmic reticulum, degrades cyclic adenosine monophosphate (cAMP), the second messenger for inducing contractility. Milrinone prevents the breakdown of cAMP, thus increasing cAMP concentration and its duration of action. Milrinone, an inotropic and vasodilating agent, is a more potent vasodilator than dobutamine. Milrinone is typically administered intravenously at a dose of 0.25 to 0.75 $\mu$g/kg/min and possesses a half-life of 2.4 hours. It has minimal chronotropic properties, mildly increases myocardial oxygen consumption, and has arrhythmogenic potential. The drug has been used to treat patients with hypotensive HF and cardiogenic shock.

In the Outcomes of a Prospective Trial of Intravenous Milrinone for Exacerbations of Chronic Heart Failure (OPTIME CHF) study, patients hospitalized with decompensated HF who received 48 hours of IV milrinone had no improvement in length of stay, readmission rates, mortality, HF scores, or treatment failures, but had increased morbidity due to arrhythmias and hypotension. Continuous rather than intermittent infusion milrinone is occasionally used as palliative therapy for end-stage HF.

### Dobutamine

Dobutamine is a positive inotropic agent that directly stimulates $\beta_1$-receptors in the myocardium. It increases cardiac output and has minimal vasodilating effects. At standard doses, dobutamine increases adenylate cyclase, which converts ATP to cAMP. Cyclic AMP acts as a second messenger that releases calcium from the sarcoplasmic reticulum, leading to enhanced contractility. Dobutamine has positive inotropic and chronotropic properties that increase myocardial oxygen consumption, and may provoke ischemia and arrhythmias. The drug is administered by continuous infusion, with doses ranging from 2 to 15 $\mu$g/kg/min. The onset of action is within 1 to 2 minutes, and the half-life is 2 minutes.

Dobutamine is used to treat patients in cardiogenic shock, hypotensive patients with HF, and may serve as a bridge to cardiac transplant or LV-assist devices. Mortality is high in patients who are inotrope dependent and require continuous infusions. There are no placebo-controlled data documenting improved survival from either intermittent or continuous dobutamine. Eosinophilic myocarditis, often accompanied by peripheral eosinophilia, has been occasionally reported in patients with prolonged dobutamine use, and may be related to an allergic reaction to the sodium bisulfite stabilizer in the solution. The inotropic response to dobutamine is markedly blunted in patients treated with beta-blockers.

### Dopamine

Dopamine is a sympathomimetic amine and the immediate precursor of norepinephrine. It has dose-dependent physiologic effects when administered intravenously. At low doses, dopamine acts via dopaminergic receptors in the mesenteric arteries to produce renal vasodilation. At medium doses, increased concentrations of norepinephrine are released from sympathetic neurons that stimulate cardiac $\beta$-receptors, producing an inotropic response. At high doses, peripheral $\alpha$-receptors are activated, causing vasoconstriction.

### Nitroprusside

Sodium nitroprusside is an IV vasodilator that lowers systemic arterial BP, PCWP, pulmonary artery pressure (PAP), and RA pressure. It is used to treat acute pulmonary edema or hypertensive crises in an ICU setting with invasive hemodynamic monitoring. Nitroprusside is rapidly metabolized by the liver into nitric oxide and cyanide. Nitric oxide activates guanylate cyclase in smooth muscle and epithelial cells, which increases the intracellular concentration of cyclic guanosine monophosphate (cGMP), resulting in smooth muscle relaxation and vasodilation. The drug is administered intravenously by a continuous infusion at a dose of 0.3 of 10 $\mu$g/kg/min. Its onset of action is 2 to 5 minutes, and its half-life is 3 minutes.

Nitroprusside must be protected from light. Hypotension is a common side effect, mandating frequent BP measurements. It may cause coronary steal syndrome and should be avoided in active ischemia. Nitroprusside has been associated with rebound worsening of hemodynamics when the infusion is discontinued. Prolonged infusions, particularly in patients with hepatic or renal dysfunction, have been associated with cyanide or thiocyanate toxicity manifested by lethargy, confusion, psychosis, seizures, hyperreflexia, acidosis, and renal compromise. Nitroprusside can also cause intrapulmonary shunting and hypoxemia.

### Nitroglycerin

Nitroglycerin is a commonly used IV vasoactive drug for the treatment of acute heart failure. It is a venodilator at low doses and an arterial vasodilator at high doses. It is biotransformed into nitric oxide that activates guanylate cyclase and increases cGMP, causing smooth muscle relaxation and vasodilation. Intravenous nitroglycerin improves pulmonary congestion by lowering PCWP, PAP, and RAP. It relieves myocardial ischemia by coronary artery dilation and improved collateral flow.

Nitroglycerin is infused at 5 to 10 $\mu$g/min and titrated upward to achieve hemodynamic parameters. Its half-life is 3 minutes. Long-term use is limited by tachyphylaxis occurring within 24 hours as a result of sulfhydryl depletion.

**TABLE 29–1**
**HEART FAILURE MANAGEMENT RECOMMENDATION FOR PATIENTS IN VARIOUS STAGES OF DISEASE**

| Stage of HF | ACC/AHA Guidelines Recommendations for Management of HF |
|---|---|
| Stage A | Class I<br>■ Control of systolic and diastolic hypertension in accordance with recommended guidelines (A)<br>■ Treatment of lipid disorders, in accordance with recommended guidelines (B)<br>■ Avoidance of patient behaviors that may increase the risk of HF (e.g., smoking, alcohol consumption, and illicit drug use) (C)<br>■ ACE inhibition in patients with a history of atherosclerotic vascular disease, diabetes mellitus, or hypertension and associated cardiovascular risk factors (B)<br>■ Control of ventricular rate in patients with supraventricular arrhythmias (B)<br>■ Treatment of thyroid disorders (C)<br>■ Periodic evaluation for signs and symptoms of HF (C)<br>Class IIa<br>■ Noninvasive evaluation of left ventricular function in patients with a strong family history of cardiomyopathy or in those receiving cardiotoxic interventions (C) |
| Stage B | Class I<br>■ ACE inhibition in patients with a recent or remote history of myocardial infarction regardless of ejection fraction (A)<br>■ ACE inhibition in patients with a reduced ejection fraction, whether or not they have experienced a myocardial infarction (B)<br>■ Beta-blockade in patients with a recent myocardial infarction regardless of ejection fraction (A)<br>■ Beta-blockade in patients with a reduced ejection fraction, whether or not they have experienced a myocardial infarction (B)<br>■ Regular evaluation for signs and symptoms of HF (C)<br>■ Measures listed as Class I recommendations for patients in Stage A<br>Class IIb<br>■ Long-term treatment with systemic vasodilators in patients with severe aortic regurgitation (B) |
| Stage C | Class I<br>■ Diuretics in patients who have evidence of fluid retention (A)<br>■ ACE inhibition in all patients, unless contraindicated (A)<br>■ Beta-adrenergic blockade in all stable patients, unless contraindicated. Patients should have no or minimal evidence of fluid retention and should not have required treatment recently with an intravenous positive inotropic agent (A)<br>■ Digitalis for the treatment of symptoms of HF, unless contraindicated (A)<br>■ Withdrawal of drugs known to adversely affect the clinical status of patients (e.g., nonsteroidal anti-inflammatory drugs, most antiarrhythmic drugs, and most calcium channel blocking drugs) (B)<br>■ Measured listed as Class I recommendations for patients in stages A and B<br>Class IIa<br>■ Spironolactone in patients with recent or current Class IV symptoms, preserved renal function, and a normal potassium concentration (B)<br>■ Exercise training as an adjunctive approach to improve clinical status in ambulatory patients (A)<br>■ Angiotensin receptor blockade in patients who are being treated with digitalis, diuretics, and a beta-blocker and who cannot be given an ACE inhibitor because of cough or angioedema (A)<br>■ A combination of hydralazine and a nitrate in patients who are being treated with digitalis, diuretics, and a beta-blocker and who cannot be given an ACE inhibitor because of hypotension or renal insufficiency (B)<br>Class IIb<br>■ Addition of an angiotensin-receptor blocker to an ACE inhibitor (B)<br>■ Addition of a nitrate (alone or in combination with hydralazine) to an ACE inhibitor in patients who are also being given digitalis, diuretics, and a beta-blocker (B) |
| Stage D | Class I<br>■ Meticulous identification and control of fluid retention (B)<br>■ Referral for cardiac transplantation in eligible patients (B)<br>■ Referral to an HF program with expertise in the management of refractory HF (A)<br>■ Measures listed as Class I recommendations for patients in Stages A, B, and C.<br>Class IIb<br>■ Pulmonary artery catheter placement to guide therapy in patients with persistently severe symptoms (C)<br>■ Mitral valve repair or replacement for severe secondary mitral regurgitation (strength of evidence C)<br>■ Continuous intravenous infusion of a positive inotropic agent for palliation of symptoms (C) |

*Source:* Adapted from Hunt SA et al. ACC/AHA guidelines for the evaluation and management of chronic heart failure in the adult: a report of the American College of Cardiology/American Heart Association Task Force on Practice Guidelines (Committee to Revise the 1995 Guidelines for the Evaluation and Management of Heart Failure), 2001.

**TABLE 29–2**
**ACC/AHA GUIDELINES FOR MANAGEMENT OF CONCOMITANT DISEASES IN PATIENTS WITH HEART FAILURE**

| Class | Indication | Strength of Evidence |
|---|---|---|
| I | 1. Control of systolic and diastolic hypertension in patients with HF in accordance with guidelines | A |
| | 2. Nitrates and beta-blockers (in conjunction with diuretics) for the treatment of angina in patients with HF | B |
| | 3. Coronary revascularization in patients who have both HF and angina | A |
| | 4. Anticoagulants in patients with HF who have paroxysmal or chronic atrial fibrillation or a previous thromboembolic event | A |
| | 5. Control of the ventricular response in patients with HF and atrial fibrillation with a beta-blocker (or amiodarone, if the beta-blocker is contraindicated or not tolerated) | A |
| | 6. Beta-adrenergic blockade (unless contraindicated) in patients with HF to reduce the risk of sudden death. Patients should have no or minimal fluid retention and should not have recently required treatment with an intravenous positive inotropic agent | A |
| | 7. Implantable cardioverter-defibrillator (alone or in combination with amiodarone) in patients with HF who have a history of sudden death, ventricular fibrillation, or hemodynamically destabilizing ventricular tachycardia | A |
| IIa | 1. Antiplatelet agents for prevention of myocardial infarction and death in patients with HF who have underlying coronary artery disease | B |
| | 2. Digitalis to control the ventricular response in patients with HF and atrial fibrillation | A |
| IIb | 1. Coronary revascularization in patients who have HF and coronary artery disease but no angina | B |
| | 2. Restoration of sinus rhythm by electrical cardioversion in patients with HF and atrial fibrillation | C |
| | 3. Amiodarone to prevent sudden death in patients with HF and asymptomatic ventricular arrhythmias | B |
| | 4. Anticoagulation in patients with HF who do not have atrial fibrillation or a previous thromboembolic events | B or C |
| III | 1. Routine use of an implantable cardioverter-defibrillator in patients with HF | C |
| | 2. Class I or III antiarrhythmic drugs (except amiodarone) in patients with HF for the prevention or treatment of asymptomatic ventricular arrhythmias | A |
| | 3. Ambulatory electrocardiographic monitoring for detection of asymptomatic ventricular arrhythmias | A |

*Source:* Adapted from Hunt SA et al. ACC/AHA guidelines for the evaluation and management of chronic heart failure in the adult: a report of the American College of Cardiology/American Heart Association Task Force on Practice Guidelines (Committee to Revise the 1995 Guidelines for the Evaluation and Management of Heart Failure), 2001.

Possible adverse reactions include headache, hypotension, and methemoglobinemia.

### *Nesiritide*

Nesiritide is the generic name for synthetic brain natriuretic peptide (BNP). It is a balanced vasodilator potentially with modest concomitant diuretic properties. Diuretic effects have not been clearly established at the current, clinically utilized doses. Nesiritide is approved for patients with acute heart failure without cardiogenic shock or systemic hypoperfusion. It acts via natriuretic peptide receptors on the cell surface of smooth muscle and endothelial cells, increasing concentrations of cGMP, a second messenger that causes smooth muscle relaxation and vasodilation. The onset of action is within 15 minutes, and the half-life is 18 minutes. Nesiritide may offer benefits in the management of AHF when compared to other available vasodilators. Vasodilators such as nitroglycerin often require dosing adjustments because of tolerance with prolonged use. Nitroprusside may cause problems due to precipitous drops in blood pressure and requires invasive hemodynamic monitoring.

The Vasodilation in the Management of Acute Congestive Heart Failure (VMAC) study showed that, when added to standard therapy, the reduction in PCWP with nesiritide was significantly better than with placebo or nitroglycerin. Recent contentious meta-analyses have indicated that nesiritide, when given at doses higher than recommended, is associated with an increased incidence of worsening renal function and mortality when compared with other standard therapies. Additional studies examining the efficacy and safety of nesiritide in acute heart failure with mortality and rehospitalization endpoints are needed.

## Nonpharmacologic Therapy for Acute HF

Patients with refractory AHF should be considered for further support, where indicated, including intra-aortic balloon pump, mechanical ventilation, or ventricular assist devices as bridge to recovery or transplantation. In a setting of HF secondary to infarction, the goal is to establish and maintain patency of the infarct artery in the most expeditious manner. Intervention, such as angioplasty or urgent cardiac surgery, may be needed (14).

## CURRENT ACC/AHA GUIDELINES

It is important to note that the strength of evidence may not reflect the strength of a recommendation in the current ACC/AHA Guidelines (Table 29–1). For those patients at high risk of developing HF (Stage A), control of CV risk factors, including hypertension, hyperlipidemia, diabetes, alcohol use, and cigarette smoking. is essential.

The main goal of management in Stage B HF is to minimize the progression of LV dysfunction. Aggressive risk-factor modification coupled with ACE inhibitor and beta-blocker administration is warranted. Surgical correction of valvular disease and control of tachyarrhythmias should be considered when indicated.

In patients with symptomatic LV dysfunction (Stage C), Class I measures recommended for Stages A and B patients are still applicable. Physical activity should be individualized. ACE inhibitors and beta-blockers are essential, and spironolactone can be added for Class III–IV HF symptoms. ARBs or hydralazine/nitrate combinations may be used in patients who are intolerant of ACE inhibitors. Withdrawal of calcium channel blockers, nonsteroidal anti-inflammatory agents, and most antiarrhythmic drugs is advised.

In Stage D HF, patients may need specialized treatments, such as mechanical circulatory support, referral for cardiac transplantation, and even hospice care. The use of ACE inhibitors and beta-blockers for this group of patients should be done with caution, especially in patients with significant hypotension or peripheral hypoperfusion. Spironolactone is beneficial, but electrolyte levels should be closely monitored, especially in those with impaired renal function. Continuous IV inotropic support rather than an intermittent infusion may be useful for some as a bridge to transplantation.

Differences in responses to medical treatment may exist among the different patient subsets, such as women, minorities, and the elderly. Coexisting medical conditions, including hypertension, ischemic heart disease, diabetes, renal insufficiency, thromboembolism, and arrhythmias, must be taken into consideration in disease management (Table 29–2). The potential beneficial impact of ICDs for primary prevention of sudden cardiac death in HF patients has been substantiated by recently released clinical trials with utilization of biventricular pacing strategies meriting consideration in symptomatic patients with LV dyssynchrony. In Stage C, ARBs (specifically, candesartan and valsartan) could be considered for patients with reduced LV systolic function and ACE inhibitor intolerance. Candesartan can also be considered beneficial when added to an ACE inhibitor for patients with depressed LVEF as well as for individuals with HF and preserved LVEF. Multidisciplinary HF management programs are useful in preventing cardiac decompensation leading to hospital admissions. Successful heart failure management mandates education of patients and caregivers, and patients must accept the responsibility to manage their disease holistically, similar to the approach taken by diabetics. Medication compliance, dietary restrictions, symptom awareness, diuretic titration, exercise, and avoidance of alcohol and tobacco are all essential to successful outcomes.

## REFERENCES


1. Hunt SA, Baker DW, Chin MH, et al. ACC/AHA Guidelines for the evaluation and management of chronic heart failure in the adult: executive summary. A report of the American College of Cardiology/American Heart Association Task Force on Practice Guidelines (Committee to Revise the 1995 Guidelines for the Evaluation and Management of Heart Failure): developed in collaboration with the International Society for Heart and Lung Transplantation; endorsed by the Heart Failure Society of America. *Circulation*. 2001;104:2996–3007.
2. Jessup M, Brozena S. Heart failure. *N Engl J Med*. 2003;348:2007–2018.
3. Swedberg K, Cleland J, Dargie H, et al. Guidelines for the diagnosis and treatment of chronic heart failure: executive summary (update 2005): The Task Force for the Diagnosis and Treatment of Chronic Heart Failure of the European Society of Cardiology. *Eur Heart J*. 2005;26:1115–1140.
4. Yan AT, Yan RT, Liu PP. Narrative review: pharmacotherapy for chronic heart failure: evidence from recent clinical trials. *Ann Intern Med*. 2005;142:132–145.
5. DiBianco R. Update on therapy for heart failure. *Am J Med*. 2003;115:480–488.
6. McMurray J, Pfeffer MA. New therapeutic options in congestive heart failure: Part I. *Circulation*. 2002;105:2099–2106.
7. McMurray J, Pfeffer MA. New therapeutic options in congestive heart failure: Part II. *Circulation*. 2002;105:2223–2228.
8. Angeja BG, Grossman W. Evaluation and management of diastolic heart failure. *Circulation*. 2003;107:659–663.
9. Aurigemma GP, Gaasch WH. Clinical practice. Diastolic heart failure. *N Engl J Med*. 2004;351:1097–1105.
10. Colonna P, Sorino M, D'Agostino C, et al. Nonpharmacologic care of heart failure: counseling, dietary restriction, rehabilitation, treatment of sleep apnea, and ultrafiltration. *Am J Cardiol*. 2003;91:41F–50F.
11. Jain P, Massie BM, Gattis WA, et al. Current medical treatment for the exacerbation of chronic heart failure resulting in hospitalization. *Am Heart J*. 2003;145:S3–S17.
12. Nohria A, Lewis E, Stevenson LW. Medical management of advanced heart failure. *JAMA*. 2002;287:628–640.
13. Nieminen MS, Bohm M, Cowie MR, et al. Executive summary of the guidelines on the diagnosis and treatment of acute heart failure: the Task Force on Acute Heart Failure of the European Society of Cardiology. *Eur Heart J*. 2005;26:384–416.
14. Vitali E, Colombo T, Fratto P, et al. Surgical therapy in advanced heart failure. *Am J Cardiol*. 2003;91:88F–94F.


## QUESTIONS

**1.** A 49-year-old man with dilated cardiomyopathy is admitted to the coronary care unit (CCU) for heart failure exacerbation. On examination, his respiratory rate is 30, with distended neck veins and a prominent S3. In addition to aggressive diuresis, a decision was made to start nesiritide.

After the infusion, you notice hemodynamic changes. Which of the following changes is not related to the effects of nesiritide?

a. Decrease in heart rate
b. Decrease in BP
c. Reduction in pulmonary capillary wedge pressure (PCWP)
d. No change in stroke volume index
e. All of the above
f. None of the above

Answer is a: BNP increases HR. All of the others are hemodynamic effects of BNP.

2. You have a 40-year-old man with a LVEF of 20%, ready to be discharged after treatment for HF exacerbation. At discharge, you explain to him the benefits of lisinopril, simvastatin, aspirin, digitalis, and furosemide. Finally, you want to explain the benefit of spironolactone to him. What will you tell the patient?

   a. Spironolactone in addition to standard therapy (ACE inhibitor, diuretic) does not decrease mortality or morbidity
   b. Spironolactone in addition to standard therapy (ACE inhibitor, diuretic) only decreases rehospitalization; it does not improve NYHA functional class
   c. Spironolactone in addition to standard therapy (ACE inhibitor, diuretic) decreases mortality and rehospitalization
   d. Spironolactone only benefits patients who are not on standard therapy.

Answer is c: Spironolactone in addition to standard therapy decreases mortality and rehospitalization.

3. An 80-year-old woman with hyperlipidemia, hypertension, and diabetes mellitus has been well on enalapril, aspirin, simvastatin, glipizide, and metformin. Her friend tells her that losartan is better than enalapril. She wants your opinion. How would you advise her?

   a. Because the patient has no history of CHF, there is no reason to change her medication
   b. Losartan showed no significant reduction in the composite of mortality and morbidity from cardiovascular causes in diabetic, hypertensive patients, so there is no need to switch medications.
   c. Losartan did not show any mortality benefit but decreased the risk of MI; so she should have her prescription changed.
   d. Losartan did show mortality benefit—but only in patients younger than 60 years.

Answer is b: Losartan showed a reduction in first hospitalization for heart failure in the RENAAL study. Losartan showed no effect on the rate of death. The composite of morbidity and mortality from cardiovascular causes was similar in the two groups, although the rate of first hospitalization for heart failure was significantly lower with losartan (risk reduction, 32%; $p = 0.005$). The reduction in MI was not statistically significant.

4. According to the ACC/AHA Practice Guidelines for Chronic Heart Failure, which of the following statements is false?

   a. A patient with a history of hypertension who does not have structural heart disease is classified as Stage A.
   b. A critically important aspect of the new "Staging Classification" is the increased focus on patients at high risk for the development of heart failure (Stage A).
   c. An asymptomatic patient with a prior MI and an ejection fraction of 25% is considered Stage B.
   d. A patient with severe mitral regurgitation and an ejection fraction of 45%, who complains of dyspnea upon exertion, is considered Stage C.
   e. None of the above

Answer is e: None of the statements is false. Stage A is underlying predisposing disease without clinical or structural evidence of heart failure. The new criteria focus on disease treatment to prevent the development of heart failure. The patient with prior MI and no symptoms fits Stage B. The patient with mitral regurgitation and abnormal ejection fraction with symptoms fits the description of Stage C.

# Heart Transplantation

# 30

*Celeste T. Grant* *David O. Taylor*

## ORGAN ALLOCATION

In the United States, the United Network for Organ Sharing (UNOS) has the government contract for the procurement and distribution of cadaveric organs. UNOS operates by dividing the United States into 11 geographic regions. Each region is further divided into multiple procurement organizations whose main responsibility is to communicate with local hospitals, identify potential donors, and coordinate the transplant process.

## THE DONOR

The organ procurement organization, also known as the OPO, is responsible for the initial identification and screening of the potential donor. Once consent for donation is obtained, the primary screening consists of confirming brain death, age, body size, and ABO blood type of the potential donor. The initial evaluation also includes obtaining routine laboratory tests, serologic tests (hepatitis B and C, HIV), identifying the presence of active malignancies, clinical course, and the etiology of death. Cardiac screening includes an electrocardiogram, chest x-ray, transthoracic echocardiogram (if inadequate, transesophageal echocardiogram), and determination of prolonged hypotension or cardiopulmonary resuscitation. A cardiac catheterization may be performed, depending on the age and the presence of coronary artery disease risk factors. Generally, if the potential donor is male and >45 years of age or female and >50 years of age, a cardiac catheterization is recommended.

Once the screening is completed, the donor is entered into the UNOS database and a "rank list" is obtained for each organ. The OPO contacts the recipient transplant centers in order of rank on the list. Candidates are ranked by a variety of factors, including ABO blood group compatibility, geographic proximity between donor and transplanting hospitals, status of the potential recipient, and length of time spent on the waiting list. Currently, the highest priority is given to Status 1A patients, who are considered to be urgent. Status 1A is defined as patients limited to the intensive care units who are dependent on mechanical circulatory support devices (mechanical assist device, intra-aortic balloon pump, extracorporeal membrane oxygenator) or high-dose intravenous inotropes plus Swan-Ganz catheter. Patients who are mechanically ventilated or have ventricular-assist device-related complications such as a thromboembolism, or a device infection, are also listed as Status 1A. Status 1B includes patients on continuous intravenous inotropes or patients with ventricular-assist devices for more than 30 days. A patient who does not meet criteria for Status 1A or 1B is listed as Status 2. Patients listed as Status 7 are considered temporarily unsuitable to receive a transplant (Table 30–1). If the OPO is unable to find a local Status 1A recipient, the organ is offered next to the Status 1B candidates, followed by the Status 2 candidates. With few exceptions, the allocation of hearts is first within the local OPO, then outside the OPO in 500-mile concentric rings with the donor hospital in the center of the rings.

The final screen is completed by the harvesting surgeon and involves a review of the locally obtained data as well as a visual inspection of the donor heart. The surgeon looks for contusions, palpates for any obvious atherosclerotic lesions in the epicardial vessels, and reassesses cardiac function.

After brain death has been established and up to the time the organ is procured, the goal of medical management is to maintain hemodynamic stability of the potential donor. Brain death is associated with a high adrenergic state causing fluctuation in blood pressure, peripheral vasoconstriction, and end-organ underperfusion. Therefore, continuous monitoring of arterial pressure, central venous pressure, and urinary output is essential. The targeted systolic blood pressure is >100 mm Hg, central venous pressure between 8 and 12 mm Hg, urinary output >100 mL/h but <300 mL/h, and hematocrit >30%. Close attention

**TABLE 30–1**
**UNOS STATUS DEFINITIONS**

*Status 1A:* A patient listed Status 1A has at least one of the following devices or therapies in place.
- Mechanical circulatory support that includes one of the following:
  - LVAD and/or RVAD (max 30 d)
  - Total artificial heart
  - Intra-aortic balloon pump
  - ECMO
- Mechanical circulatory support with objective medical evidence of significant device-related complications such as
  - Thromboembolism, device infection, mechanical failure, and/or life-threatening ventricular arrhythmias
  - Mechanical ventilation
  - High-dose single intravenous inotrope, or multiple intravenous inotropes, in addition to Swan-Ganz catheter

*Status 1B:* A patient listed as Status 1B has at least one of the following devices or therapies in place.
- LVAD and/or RVAD
  - Continuous infusion of intravenous inotropes

*Status 2:* A patient listed as Status 2 is one who does not meet criteria of Status 1A or 1B.

*Status 7:* A patient listed as Status 7 is considered temporarily unsuitable to receive a transplant.

must be made to maintaining normal electrolytes, acid–base balance, and oxygenation. The goal is to optimize cardiac output of the donor heart to achieve blood flow that promotes organ function with the least amount of vasoactive drug support. However, inotropic or vasopressor agents (dopamine, dobutamine, and epinephrine) may be needed. Some centers recommend the use of hormone replacement therapy (i.e., corticosteroids and thyroid hormone); however this remains controversial.

## THE RECIPIENT

The incidence of heart failure continues to increase worldwide. It has been estimated that there are close to 5 million people in the United States with heart failure. Despite optimal medical therapy, the 1-year survival of patients with New York Heart Association (NYHA) functional Class IV heart failure averages 50% to 80%. In contrast, the 1-year survival after transplantation averages 85% to 90% at most U.S. centers. Clearly, the benefit of cardiac transplantation is substantial; however, the availability of donor organs is limited by donor supply. The number of suitable cardiac donors has plateaued at 2,100 to 2,200 per year. In 2002, approximately 4,000 cardiac transplantations were performed worldwide, of which 2,155 were performed in the United States (1). The potential need has been estimated at 10,000 to 40,000 per year. With this great disparity, the process of patient selection and allocation must be examined closely. It is crucial that transplant centers allocate organs to patients with the greatest need and the greatest chance to derive maximal benefit.

The current indication for cardiac transplantation is end-stage, Class III–IV heart failure (or the rare patient with refractory angina and high-risk anatomy or ventricular arrhythmias) who has failed medical and/or surgical therapies. Potential recipients must undergo a thorough evaluation in an attempt to identify any condition that could potentially adversely affect the recipient's survival or quality of life after transplantation. Listed in Table 30–2 is the recommended evaluation prior to cardiac transplantation. The initial screening should include a complete history and physical, routine laboratory tests, infectious disease

**TABLE 30–2**
**RECOMMENDED EVALUATION PRIOR TO TRANSPLANTATION**

Complete history and physical examination

Laboratory data:
- Complete blood count (CBC) with differential, complete metabolic panel,
- Thyroid function studies
- Liver function panel, creatinine clearance
- Lipid profile, hemoglobin A1c, urinalysis

Cardiovascular data:
- Electrocardiogram, chest x-ray, echocardiogram
- Exercise test with oxygen consumption
- Right and left heart catheterization, myocardial biopsy[a]

Immunologic data:
- Blood type and antibody screen
- Human leukocyte antigen (HLA) typing
- Panel of reactive antibodies (PRA) screen

Serology for infectious diseases:
- Hepatitis HBsAg HBsAb, HBcAb, HepCAb
- Herpes group virus
- Human immunodeficiency virus
- Cytomegalovirus (CMV) IgG antibody
- Toxoplasmosis
- Varicella and rubella titers
- Ebstein–Barr virus IgG and IgM antibodies
- Venereal Disease Research Laboratory (VDRL) or Rapid Plasma Reagin (RPR)

Vascular assessment:
- Carotid Dopplers
- Peripheral vascular assessment
- Abdominal ultrasound
- Ophthalmology exam[a]

Cancer screening:
- Prostate-specific antigen[a]
- Papanicolaou smear, mammography[a]
- Colonoscopy[a]

Psychosocial evaluation:
- Support system
- Substance abuse history
- Psychiatric history

Baseline:
- Dental examination
- Bone density scan
- Pulmonary function tests

[a]If appropriate.

**TABLE 30–3**
**EXCLUSION CRITERIA FOR CARDIAC TRANSPLANTATION**

| |
|---|
| Irreversible pulmonary parenchymal disease |
| Renal dysfunction with Cr >2.0–2.5 or CrCl <30–50 mL/min (unless combined heart–kidney transplant) |
| Irreversible hepatic dysfunction |
| Severe peripheral and cerebrovascular obstructive disease |
| Insulin-dependent diabetes with end-organ damage |
| Acute pulmonary embolism |
| Irreversible pulmonary hypertension (PVR >3.0–4.0 after vasodilators) |
| Psychosocial instability or substance abuse |
| Severe obesity |
| Severe osteoporosis |
| Active infection |
| Coexisting neoplasm |

background data, cancer screening, and basic cardiovascular data including a right heart catheterization with a detailed hemodynamic evaluation. The patient also needs immunologic testing including ABO blood typing, tissue typing for determination of human leukocyte antigens (HLA), and screening for preformed anti-HLA antibodies (PRA). It is imperative that a careful psychosocial evaluation be performed to identify patients with substance abuse, noncompliance, or any behavioral trait that would lead to adverse posttransplant outcomes.

Historically, many programs had a list of "absolute" contraindications to cardiac transplantation (Table 30–3). However, most "absolute" contraindications have been overcome by some program at some time. Most cardiac surgeons and transplant cardiologists now agree that there are very few "absolute" contraindications to transplantation and that there are primarily "relative" contraindications. Each co-morbid condition must be looked at closely and in context to the potential recipient in question. The "relative" contraindications to transplantation are simply risk factors for high early or late mortality found after analyzing data from the International Society for Heart and Lung Transplantation (ISHLT), the Cardiac Transplant Research Database (CTRD), and several single-center studies. Risk factors include age, short-term ventricular-assist device use (<30 days), irreversible high pulmonary vascular resistance (PVR >4 Wood units), mechanical ventilation at the time of transplantation, active infection, diabetes mellitus, particularly if end-organ damage is present, peripheral vascular disease, cerebrovascular disease, renal or hepatic insufficiency, and active smoking. In the final analysis, it is the pooled risk from the variety of risk factors (both positive and negative) that determines eligibility of the potential recipient.

Determining the timing of listing for transplantation is based on several factors. The NHYA classification is a subjective way to classify the functional capacity of heart failure patients. Cardiopulmonary exercise testing, which measures the peak oxygen uptake (VO2) during maximal exercise is a more objective test to determine functional status. The peak VO2 value is very helpful in determining the timing of listing for transplantation by predicting survival in ambulatory heart failure patients. In 1991, Mancini and colleagues found that cardiac transplantation can be safely deferred in patients with a peak VO2 >14 mL/kg/min (2). Several studies have suggested that a peak VO2 less than 50% predicted is a significant predictor of cardiac death within 1 to 3 years regardless of absolute peak VO2. This test not only provides an objective assessment of functional capacity but also provides valuable prognostic information to heart failure patients. The goal is to list a patient for transplantation after all medical and surgical options have been exhausted, but before the patient becomes debilitated with end-organ damage that may compromise posttransplant survival.

## REJECTION

Rejection involves both cellular and humoral (antibody-mediated) immune injury to the allograft once it is recognized as non-self. Rejection is often classified into four major types: hyperacute, acute cellular, antibody-mediated (humoral), and chronic (cardiac allograft vasculopathy).

Hyperacute rejection is an antibody-mediated event, which occurs minutes to hours after transplantation and is caused by pre-existing recipient antibodies against the donor's human leukocyte antigens (HLA) present on the vascular endothelial cells. The histological hallmark of hyperacute rejection is leaky capillaries, endothelial swelling, microthrombosis, polymononuclear infiltrate, and, subsequently, tissue necrosis. Immunohistochemical studies show deposition of immunoglobulin and complement within the vessel walls. Clinically there is profound hemodynamic compromise and graft failure. Even with aggressive treatment, hyperacute rejection almost always leads to rapid graft loss. The catastrophic effects of hyperacute rejection can generally be prevented by PRA screening and by donor–recipient HLA and ABO blood-group cross-matching prior to transplantation.

Unlike hyperacute rejection, acute cellular rejection is primarily a T-lymphocyte–mediated process, which can occur from the first week after transplantation up to many years out. Monitoring for acute cellular rejection primarily involves surveillance endomyocardial biopsies. The vast majority are performed via the right internal jugular vein, and four to five samples are taken from the right ventricular septum with a cardiac bioptome. Functional studies such as echocardiography with detailed diastolic function evaluation have been found to be useful but not accurate enough to eliminate the need for biopsies entirely. The ISHLT has adopted a histologic grading system that classifies the severity of cellular rejection based on the amount of inflammatory infiltrate and presence or absence of myocyte

**TABLE 30–4**
**WORKING FORMULATION OF THE INTERNATIONAL SOCIETY OF HEART AND LUNG TRANSPLANTATION**

Grade 0 (no acute rejection):
- No evidence of lymphocyte infiltrates
- No myocyte damage on biopsy specimen

Grade 1A (focal, mild acute rejection):
- Focal perivascular or interstitial infiltrates of lymphocytes
- No myocyte damage on biopsy specimen

Grade 1B (diffuse, mild acute rejection):
- Diffuse perivascular or interstial infiltrates of lymphocytes
- No myocyte damage on biopsy specimen

Grade 2 (focal, moderate acute rejection):
- One focus of lymphocytes that is sharply circumscribed
- Myocyte damage and architectural distortion within the focus

Grade 3A (multifocal, moderate rejection):
- Multiple foci of large aggressive lymphocytes
- Myocyte damage and architectural distortion present

Grade 3B (diffuse, borderline severe rejection):
- Diffuse aggressive inflammatory infiltrates within several biopsy specimens
- Myocyte damage
- Eosinophils and occasional neutrophils

Grade 4 (severe acute rejection):
- Diffuse, aggressive polymorphous infiltrate (lymphocytes, eosinophils, neutrophils)
- Myocyte necrosis
- Edema, hemorrhage, vasculitis usually present

necrosis (Table 30–4). This classification system helps guide immunosuppressive therapy. The consensus of most transplant centers is that rejection is considered significant when the biopsy is graded 3A or higher or if there is any evidence of hemodynamic compromise regardless of grade. Many advanced grades of rejection (such as ISHLT grade 3A and 3B) may be present for prolonged periods (weeks) prior to the development of allograft dysfunction, thus the rationale for "surveillance" biopsies to detect rejection prior to the progression to significant allograft compromise. Because most rejection episodes occur within the first 3 to 6 months after transplantation, the frequency of biopsies is greater early on. A typical schedule might be weekly for 1 month, every other week for 1 month, every 3 to 4 weeks for next 1 to 2 months, every 4 to 6 weeks for 1 to 2 months, every 6 to 8 weeks until 1 year after transplant, and then every 3 to 6 months for the next 1 to 3 years while immunosuppression is being altered. Many programs stop routine surveillance biopsies after 3 to 5 years if the patient is stable on maintenance immunosuppression. Obviously, endomyocardial biopsy is indicated for unexplained acute graft dysfunction regardless of time posttransplant or if major changes in the immunosuppressive regimen are required.

Antibody-mediated rejection, also known as humoral rejection, is initiated by alloantibodies directed against donor human leukocyte antigens or endothelial cell antigens (3). Antibody-mediated rejection is much less common than acute cellular rejection, occurring in less than 10% of transplanted patients. The biopsy reveals prominent capillaries and endothelial swelling by light microscopy and deposition of immunoglobulin and complement within the vessel walls by immunoflourescence. Episodes of antibody-mediated rejection are more severe than acute cellular rejection and are usually associated with greater hemodynamic compromise, increased incidence of accelerated coronary artery vasculopathy, and graft failure, with an overall poorer prognosis. Patients at the highest risk for developing humoral rejection include women, patients with high panel reactive antibodies and/or a positive donor–recipient cross-match, CMV seropositivity, and patients with sensitization to OKT3 (4).

Cardiac allograft vasculopathy (CAV), often called chronic rejection, remains a major limiting factor to long-term survival following cardiac transplantation. It is an aggressive form of coronary artery disease that occurs months to years after transplantation. It has been reported that as many as 50% of the transplant recipients have angiographically confirmed CAV by 5 years after transplantation (1). The histologic changes seen in CAV are not uniform and show a broad spectrum of abnormalities, which often differ from traditional atherosclerosis. CAV is elicited by endothelial injury, which causes release of pro-fibrotic cytokines, leading to recruitment of circulating leukocytes, proliferation of smooth muscle cells, and deposition of extracellular matrix protein within the walls of intramural and epicardial coronary arteries, causing luminal occlusion (5). CAV is more diffuse than native CAD, even occurring in the coronary veins. Often the small intramyocardial vessels are severely involved.

Both immune and nonimmune factors contribute to the pathogenesis of CAV. The ISHLT Registry looked at >5,700 transplants performed from 1996 through June 2000 to determine risk factors for developing early CAV (within 3 years) and late CAV (within 7 years). Early CAV risk factors include pretransplant coronary artery disease, increase in donor age, donor body mass index (BMI), and a history of donor hypertension, while lesser risks for developing early CAV were seen in female donors and recipients. Late CAV risk factors include donor hypertension, hospitalization during the first year posttransplant for rejection, pretransplant coronary artery disease, HLA-DR mismatch, decreasing recipient age, and increasing donor age.

Unfortunately, the clinical diagnosis of CAV is usually made after the disease is advanced. Many times, the first clinical manifestation of CAV is ventricular arrhythmias, congestive heart failure, or sudden death. The surgical denervation of the heart prevents the pain associated with myocardial ischemia or infarction, particularly in the first 5 to 10 years after transplant. Because of the absence of symptoms, annual angiograms are often performed to detect CAV. Angiograms are somewhat insensitive because of the poor visualization of the concentric lesions that affect distal and small vessels before they become apparent in the main epicardial vessels. Coronary angiograms have been shown to underestimate the presence of disease as demonstrated by histopathologic studies and intracoronary ultrasound (IVUS). Studies have shown IVUS to be a more sensitive tool in detecting and following the progression of CAV; however, its increased cost and invasiveness limits its use.

Angioplasty of CAV lesions, if discrete, may provide short-term palliation; however, restenosis rates are high. Coronary artery bypass has limited use because CAV usually involves distal vessels and thus provide poor targets for bypassing. Retransplantation is an option, but the risk is higher than at the first transplant.

The mainstay of therapy for CAV is prevention and modification of coronary artery disease risk factors, including weight loss, lipid reduction, and controlling hypertension and diabetes. All these may contribute to endothelial injury and the proliferation of smooth muscle cells and thus progression of CAV. Along with risk-factor modification, some therapeutic modalities have been shown to be of some benefit in the prevention and progression of CAV. Statins not only lower cholesterol, they also downregulate cytokine expression, lower plasma levels of C-reactive protein, and improve endothelial function. Calcium channel blockers have been found to stabilize the endothelium and decrease platelet aggregation with a decrease in release of platelet-derived growth factor. Single-center studies have suggested that supplementation with vitamin C and E may retard early progression of transplant-associated arteriosclerosis. Two newer immunosuppressive agents, sirolimus and everolimus, have potent antiproliferative and antimigratory actions on vascular smooth muscle cells and may reduce the incidence of CAV.

## IMMUNOSUPPRESSIVE AGENTS

### Polyclonal Antibodies

Antilymphocyte antibodies are used immediately posttransplantation and to treat rejection episodes refractory to high-dose steroids or in patients with rejection associated with hemodynamic compromise. Polyclonal antithymocyte antibodies are antibodies derived from horse (*ATGAM*) or rabbit (*Thymoglobulin*). These antibodies are directed against multiple T-cell surface antigens (CD2, CD3, CD4, and CD8) and B-cell surface antigens (CD19, CD20, and CD21). The polyclonal antibodies bind to the surface antigens, leading to cell depletion, and are considered efficacious when the CD3/CD2 counts are reduced to less than 10% of the pretreatment values. Complications can include febrile reactions, which usually occur during the initial infusion, and, rarely, serum sickness. The development of leukopenia or thrombocytopenia may require a reduction in dose or termination of therapy. Studies have shown an increased incidence in viral infections (CMV), and perhaps posttransplant lymphoproliferative disease associated with polyclonal antibody use.

### Monoclonal Antibodies

Muromonab-CD3 (*OKT3*) is used for induction therapy in recipients with greater risk of rejection and for episodes of steroid-resistant rejection. OKT3 is an antiCD3 monoclonal antibody that prevents the activation of the CD3-TCR receptor, which is required to generate the intracellular signals to activate T cells. However, OKT3 itself binds to the CD3-TCR complex on the surface of the T cell, activates the T cell, and cytokines are released. As the antibody remains bound to the receptor, further activation and proliferation of T cells are inhibited. Fever, chills, wheezing, chest pain, and hypotension characterize the cytokine release syndrome, which can be potentially life threatening. Symptoms are minimized by premedication with acetominephen, IV steroids, and antihistamines. CD3+ T cells are generally undetectable during OKT3 therapy; however, within 12–24 hours after cessation of OKT3, CD3+ T cells reappear in circulation, unlike after treatment with ATG preparations, with which the lymphocyte depletion is present for weeks. There is an increased risk of developing HSV and CMV infections, especially in patients who are CMV donor positive and recipient negative. Also, latent Epstein–Barr virus (EBV) may reactivate, leading to lymphoproliferative disorders including malignant monoclonal B-cell lymphomas. OKT3 is occasionally associated with aseptic meningitis or encephalopathy.

The interleukin-2 (IL-2) receptor antibodies *basiliximab* (Simulec) and *daclizumab* (Zenapax) selectively inhibit T-cell proliferation by binding to the IL-2 receptor of activated T cells, preventing clonal expansion and activation of T cells. In heart transplant recipients, IL-2 receptor antagonists reduce the risk of rejection without increasing the incidence of infections during the early postoperative period. These monoclonal antibodies are used during induction to delay the introduction of calcineurin inhibitors. This approach creates a window to improve renal dysfunction exacerbated by ischemic-reperfusion injury. Basiliximab and daclizumab are considered to be nondepleting induction agents because they do not affect resting lymphocytes. Basiliximab is a chimeric antibody, whereas dacliximab is a humanized antibody, both designed to be less immunogenic than a fully murine monoclonal antibody. The IL-2 receptor antibodies appear to offer some advantage in heart transplant recipients, including the lack of the cytokine release syndrome and no reported increased risk of infections or malignancies. Additional research is needed to clarify their role in this population.

### Calcineurin Inhibitors

In the early 1980s, cyclosporine (CsA), a lipophilic endacapeptide calcineurin inhibitor derived from a plant fungus, was first introduced as an immunosuppressant. Its use resulted in a dramatic reduction in the incidence of acute rejection in heart transplant recipients. Today, the calcineurin inhibitors are the cornerstone of therapy after heart transplantation, in conjunction with an antiproliferative agent and corticosteroids (so-called, triple-drug therapy).

Calcineurin, a calcium-dependent serine-threonine-phosphatase, is a vital enzyme in the transcription of interleukin-2 and other cytokine genes. The interaction of IL-2 with its receptor on activated T cells induces T-cell proliferation, which triggers the emergence of effector cells responsible for tissue destruction, resulting in clinical acute rejection. The T-cell receptor (TCR) is activated in response to alloantigens, causing an increase in intracellular calcium, which in turn activates the cytosolic protein, calmodulin. $Ca^{2+}$-calmodulin interacts with calcineurin, activating its phosphatase moiety. Calcineurin is then able to dephosphorylate the nuclear factor of activated T cells (NFAT). NFAT translocate into the cells nucleus and cause transcription of T-cell–dependent lymphokines, such as interleukin-2 and its receptor, interferon-$\gamma$, and tumor necrosis factor-$\alpha$.

The calcineurin inhibitors (*cyclosporine* and *tacrolimus*) exert their effects by binding to cytosolic proteins called immunophilins upon entry into the T cell. Cyclosporin binds to cyclophilin and tacrolimus binds to FK-binding protein-12 (FKBP-12). Binding of cyclosporine and tacrolimus to its respective immunophilin enhances the immunophilins affinity to calcineurin. The immunophilin-drug complex inhibits the phosphatase activity of calcineurin, thereby preventing translocation of NFAT into the nucleus and therefore preventing the transcription of IL-2 and other cytokine genes.

The early preparation of cyclosporine (Sandimmune) was oil based and its bioavailability was unpredictable, ranging from 1% to 67% but averaging around 30%. This variability has been attributed to suboptimal gastrointestinal absorption and a significant first-pass effect through the enterohepatic circulation with extensive hepatic metabolism via the enzyme cytochrome 3A-4 system, a member of the cytochrome p450 enzyme system. Therefore the intravenous dose is generally one third of the oral dose. Neoral, the new microemulsion formulation of cyclosporine, has demonstrated greater bioavailability and more predictable pharmacokinetics than Sandimmune.

The side effects and toxicities of cyclosporine include nephrotoxicity, hypertension, gingival hyperplasia, hirsutism, neuropathy, hyperlipidemia, and hyperkalemia. Drug-level monitoring is helpful in lessening the risk of toxicity while maintaining anti-rejection efficacy. Target CsA levels are measured trough levels. Because rejection is more prevalent early posttransplantation, higher levels of CsA are generally targeted (Table 30–5).

*Tacrolimus* (Tac), formerly called FK506, is a highly immunosuppressive calcineurin inhibitor. Tac is about 100

**TABLE 30–5**
**DRUG THERAPY IN CARDIAC TRANSPLANTATION**

| Drug | Target Level (ng/dL) [mo] | Interactions | Toxicities |
|---|---|---|---|
| Cyclosporine | 300–400 [0–3]<br>250–300 [3–6]<br>200–250 [6–12]<br>100–200 [>12] | ↑ cyclo levels via cyt P450: erythromycin, ketoconazole, diltiazem, cimetidine<br>↓ cyclo levels: isoniazid, rifampin, phenytoin | Nephrotoxcity<br>Hypertension<br>Hypomagnesemia<br>Hypertrichosis<br>Gout<br>Gingival hyperplasia<br>Hyperlipidemia |
| Tacrolimus | 12–17 [0–1]<br>10–15 [1–3]<br>8–12 [3–12]<br>8–10 [>12] | Same as cyclosporine | Nephrotoxicity<br>Neurotoxicity<br>HTN < cyclosporine<br>↑ lipids < cyclosporine<br>Glucose intolerance<br>Alopecia<br>Diarrhea |
| Mycophenolate-mofetil | 2.0–4.0 | ↓ absorption in the presence of antacids containing magnesium or aluminum hydroxide | Anemia<br>Diarrhea<br>Nausea |
| Rapamycin | 5–15 | Same as cyclosporine | Hyperlipidemia<br>Thrombocytopenia<br>Anemia<br>Neutropenia<br>Diarrhea |
| Azathioprine | Levels not monitored | Allopurinol—↑ levels | Myelosuppression, leukopenia<br>Keep WBC >3,000/mL |

times more potent than CsA. Like CsA, it is metabolized via the cytochrome p450 3A-4 system, and its intravenous dose is one fourth to one fifth of its oral dose. Toxicities include nephrotoxicity, neurotoxicity, hyperuricemia, hypomagnesemia, gastrointestinal symptoms, diabetes, hyperkalemia, hyperlipidemia, and alopecia. Drug monitoring is very important to lessen the toxic effects while maintaining efficacy (see Table 30–5).

Clinical trials have compared the performance of Tac and conventional CsA among heart transplant patients while receiving azathioprine and steroids. No significant differences in the two calcineurin inhibitors were found with regard to rejection, nephrotoxicity, or incidence of diabetes. However, several studies have shown the effectiveness of replacing CsA with Tac in cases of refractory rejection, gingival hyperplasia, or hirsutism. The calcineurin inhibitor chosen is often dependent on the patient, the side-effect profile, and the institutional experience.

## Antiproliferative Agents

*Azathioprine* (Imuran) is a purine analog that impairs DNA synthesis and acts as an antiproliferative agent. It suppresses both T- and B-cell synthesis. It is well absorbed in the upper gastrointestinal (GI) tract and metabolized in the liver. Some of its metabolites are broken down via xanthine oxidase. A xanthine oxidase inhibitor such as allopurinol can increase the azathioprine levels to four times. The usual dose is 1 to 3 mg/kg per day, with the aim of keeping the white blood cell count >3,000 and the platelet count >100,000. Myelosuppression is the major toxicity, and it is generally dose dependent. Withdrawal of azathioprine usually reverses myelosuppression within 7 to 10 days. Other side effects include hepatotoxicity and pancreatitis. Malignancies, especially cutaneous malignancies, may be more common when compared to other, newer agents.

*Mycophenolate mofetil* (MMF, Cellcept), also an antiproliferative agent, blocks the *de novo* pathway of purine synthesis in T and B lymphocytes that lack a robust salvage pathway. Mycophenolic acid (MPA), a product of a *Penicillin* fungus, is the active metabolite of MMF. It is readily absorbed across the GI tract; however, the absorption of MPA is decreased in the presence of antacids containing magnesium and aluminum hydroxides. Toxicities of MMF include gastrointestinal symptoms (nausea, vomiting, and diarrhea) and myelosuppression. The incidence of these adverse events is higher in patients receiving >3 g/day. Most symptoms will resolve with reduction of dose. It is important to monitor serum level of mycophenolic acid, the active metabolite of MMF (see Table 30–5). The serum levels of MPA are higher when this drug is administered with Tac compared to CsA, thus is advisable to empirically reduce the dosage of MMF when switching from CsA to Tac. Comparing MMF to azathioprine on background of CsA and prednisone, there appears to be a 3-year survival advantage and a reduction of grafts loss to rejection with MMF, thus it has become has become the dominant antiproliferative agent (6).

## TOR Inhibitors

*Rapamycin* (Sirolimus) is a macrolide antibiotic with a similar structure to tacrolimus. It is in the class of immunosuppressants called TOR (target of rapamycin) inhibitors. The TOR enzyme is a cytoplasmic protein responsible for connecting signals from the surface of the T cell to the nucleus for stimulation of growth and proliferation of the T lymphocytes. Rapamycin binds to TOR and inhibits cell proliferation stimulated by growth factors. It is known to inhibit platelet-derived growth factor and basic fibroblast growth factors, which inhibit arterial smooth muscle cells and endothelial cell proliferation, respectively. Studies have shown a decrease in the incidence of coronary allograft vasculopathy in heart transplant recipients receiving this immunosuppressant. Common side effects include hyperlipidemia and thrombocytopenia. When rapamycin is used alone there appears to be no adverse effects on kidney function; however, when it is used in combination with calcineurin inhibitors there is a potentiation of the calcineurin inhibitor–induced nephrotoxicity. Therefore, the dose and target levels of the calcineurin inhibitor must be reduced substantially.

*Everolimus* (RAD: Certican) is a derivative of sirolimus with an identical mechanism of action. RAD, like rapamycin, inhibits clonal expansion of T cells but does not inhibit T-cell activation. It exerts its affects by forming a complex with FKBP-12 to inhibit the cyclin-dependent kinases termed the target of rapamycin (TOR), causing G1 S-phase cell cycle arrest. Everolimus has a shorter half-life (30 hours compared to rapamycin at 60 hours) as well as a relative higher bioavailability. Like the calcineurin inhibitors, RAD and rapamycin are biotransformed through the cytochrome P450, 3A-4 system. Also similar to rapamycin, the relevant side effects include hyperlipidemia and an exacerbation of CsA-induced nephrotoxicity. As with sirolimus, everolimus has been associated with a significant reduction in allograft vasculopathy measured by IVUS at 1 year (7).

Corticosteroids are important to induction, maintenance, and treatment of rejection in heart transplant recipients. Corticosteroids have immunosuppressive and anti-inflammatory effects. Corticosteroids affect the number, distribution, and function of T cells, B cells, macrophages, as well as endothelial cells. The usual treatment for moderate rejection (grade 3A or 3B) without hemodynamic compromise is pulse-dose steroids (250 to 1,000 mg solumedrol intravenously daily for 3 days). Most rejection episodes respond to initial therapy. Steroids are associated with many side effects, including cataracts, diabetes, myopathy, osteopenia, growth retardation in children, aseptic necrosis, hirsutism, cushingnoid appearance, and dermatologic problems. Steroids may also exacerbate hypertension and hyperlipidemia, and cause adrenal insufficiency. Thus, it is important to give stress doses of hydrocortisone when indicated (illness, surgical procedures) to patients on chronic corticosteroids.

## POSTTRANSPLANT COMPLICATIONS

### Infection

Preventing allograft rejection with immunosuppressive agents increases the risk of infection posttransplantation. Infections continue to be one of the leading causes of death after cardiac transplantation. Knowing the timetable of common infections following solid-organ transplant will aid in formulating a differential diagnosis and determining the timing of the various preventative strategies.

The pretransplant infectious disease evaluation is used to identify any condition that would disqualify a potential recipient for transplantation, update immunizations, identify and treat active infections, and define the risk of infection in order to determine the strategy for preventing posttransplant infections.

During the first 30 days after transplantation there are generally three types of infections that occur: (a) active infection transmitted with the allograft, (b) untreated pretransplant infection in the recipient, and (c) nosocomial infections, which are commonly related to surgical wounds or indwelling catheters. More than 95% of the nosocomial infections during this period are bacterial or fungal (*Candida* species). In contrast, late infections that occur 1 to 6 months following transplantation are generally caused by opportunistic organisms such as *Pneumocystis carinii* (PCP), *Aspergillosis* species, *Nocardia asteroids*, and *Listeria monocytogenes* and viral infections such as cytomegalovirus (CMV) or Epstein–Barr virus (EBV), which are by far the most common. After 6 months posttransplantation, most patients require decreasing levels of immunosuppression and thus their infectious disease risks become similar to those of the general population. The majority of patients require antiviral, antibacterial, and antifungal prophylaxis for 6 to 12 months posttransplantation. Approximately 5% to 10% of transplant recipients experience recurrent rejection episodes and thus are still at risk of developing opportunistic infections secondary to increased immunosuppressive therapy.

### Viral Infections

Cytomegalovirus (CMV) remains the most important infection affecting the morbidity and mortality of heart transplant recipients. The serologic (presence of antibody to CMV) status of the donor and the recipient is the most significant predictor of posttransplant events. Donor seropositive (D+), recipient seronegative (R−) bears the greatest risk of developing CMV clinical disease, which can present as leukocytopenia, pneumonia, colitis, gastritis, esophagitis, hepatitis, or myocarditis. With D+/R− status there is an increased incidence of tissue invasive CMV, recurrent CMV, ganciclovir-resistant CMV, and CAV. Table 30–6 shows the risks of clinical CMV disease based on donor and recipient status. Patients at highest risk receive prophylaxis with oral valgancyclovir with or without CMV hyperimmune globulin (CMV-IVIG, Cytogam). Active CMV disease must be treated with intravenous gancyclovir with or without CMV-IVIG, depending on whether or not invasive CMV is present.

**TABLE 30–6**
**RISK OF CYTOMEGALOVIRUS CLINICAL DISEASE**

| Donor | Recipient | Immunosuppression | Risk (%) |
|---|---|---|---|
| + | − | Standard[a] | >50 |
| +/− | + | Standard | 15–20 |
| +/− | + | Induction ALA[b] + standard | 25–35 |
| +/− | + | Antirejection ALA + standard | 65 |
| − | − | Any | 0 |

[a]Cyclosporine or FK 506, aziathioprine or mycophenolate-mofetil, and prednisone.
[b]Antilymphocyte antibodies.

### Fungal Infections

*Candida* species and aspergillosis are the most common fungal infections after transplantation. Oral clotrimazole or nystatin is used during the first 3 to 6 months or during periods of enhanced immunosuppression, when there is an increased risk of opportunistic infections.

### Protozoa Infections

Trimethoprim-sulfamethoxazole (TMP-SMX) is highly effective against *Pneumocystis carinii* (PCP) as well as *Nocardia* infections. Prior to the institution of PCP prophylaxis, approximately 10% of cardiac transplant recipients developed PCP, with a mortality rate up to 40%. Nowadays, with TMP-SMX prophylaxis, PCP is exceedingly rare. Toxoplasmosis is also a concern in heart transplant recipients. A *Toxoplasma*-seronegative recipient of a *Toxoplasma*-seropositive donor is at highest risk of developing toxoplasmosis posttransplant. Prophylaxis with trimethoprim-sulfamethoxazole is also effective posttransplantation and during episodes of increased immunosuppression therapy (steroid-resistant rejection). Active toxoplasmosis can present as myocarditis and is treated with pyrimethamine and sulfonamide.

### Malignancies

Posttransplant lymphoproliferative disease (PTLD) is a unique type of lymphoma that occurs in approximately

3.4% of all heart transplant recipients (8). Approximately 90% of all PTLDs are associated with EBV. These tumors are B cell in origin and range from a benign polyclonal process to a highly malignant monoclonal lymphoma. Typically the tumor arises 12 to 18 months following transplant and is most commonly located intra-abdominally. The patient may have a mononucleosis-like presentation. Risk factors for developing PTLD include EBV-seropositive donor to EBV-seronegative recipient, type of organ transplanted (lung and heart have the highest incidence), preceding CMV infection, and the level and type of immunosuppression used posttransplantation. PTLDs have variable prognoses, with treatment strategies geared toward drastically decreasing background immunosuppressant drug therapy. This tactic may lead to a regression of PTLD in 23% to 50% of the patients (8). Malignant lymphomas (even if EBV initiated) usually require cytotoxic chemotherapy as well, and despite aggressive therapy, have poor response rates (<50%).

Cutaneous premalignant and malignant lesions are the most commonly seen tumors after cardiac transplantation and account for nearly 40% of *de novo* cancers (1). Posttransplantation, the incidence of squammous cell carcinoma and basal cell carcinoma is increased, with basal cell carcinoma being the most common type—unlike the general population, in which squamous cell carcinoma is the most common type of skin cancer.

## Chronic Renal Dysfunction

Renal dysfunction remains an important complication. Data from the ISHLT Registry indicate that about 20% of patients have some degree of renal dysfunction 1 year following cardiac transplantation. By year 7, approximately 10% of survivors have a creatinine >2.5 mg/dL while 4% are on chronic dialysis (1).

Risk factors for late renal dysfunction include chronic administration of calcineurin inhibitors (cyclosporine and tacrolimus), pre-existing renal dysfunction, diabetes, hypertension, and generalized atherosclerosis. The renal toxicity associated with calcineurin inhibitors includes early functional nephrotoxicity and late structural nephrotoxicity. The early form of nephrotoxicity occurs when calcineurin inhibitors are administered for the first time. The calcineurin inhibitors cause vasoconstriction of the afferent arterioles, resulting in a decrease in renal blood flow and a decrease in glomerular filtration rate; both are dose related and reversible. The late form of renal dysfunction is thought to be caused by a combination of the acute renovascular effects plus direct toxic effects on renal tubular epithelial cells. Cyclosporine has been shown experimentally to cause apoptosis in tubular and interstitial cells, potentially inducing tubular atrophy and subsequent fibrosis. The management of chronic renal insufficiency is to minimize the dosage of calcineurin inhibitors, which may or may not halt the progression of the renal dysfunction. Another alternative is to switch to a sirolimus-based regimen, which may have renal-sparing effects if initiated before renal dysfunction is progressive.

## Hypertension

The use of cyclosporine is linked directly to the development of posttransplant hypertension. Three proposed mechanisms are direct sympathetic activation, increased responsiveness to circulating neurohormones, and direct vascular effects. A common endpoint of these proposed mechanisms is vasoconstriction of the renal vasculature, leading to sodium retention and an elevated plasma volume. Hypertension has been found to be less common in patients receiving tacrolimus than in those receiving cyclosporine. Steroids also play a role in the development of hypertension posttransplant. The mineralocorticoid activity causes sodium retention and also contributes to the increase in plasma volume. The denervated transplanted heart may not respond well to the increased afterload, and persistent hypertension may lead to left ventricular hypertrophy and subsequent left ventricular systolic and diastolic dysfunction. Initial nonpharmacologic therapy should be sodium restriction. First-line pharmacologic agents include calcium channel blockers and ACE inhibitors. Diltiazem has the advantage of increasing the cyclosporine level by competing with cytochrome P450, thereby decreasing the cyclosporine dose and thus the drug cost. Unfortunately, monotherapy is effective in <50% of patients posttransplantation, and multiple agents are often needed to achieve adequate blood pressure control. Diuretics are often used. Historically, beta-blockers have been avoided, secondary to concerns about excessive bradycardia or exercise intolerance due to the denervated heart; however, if they are needed, they are effective antihypertensive agents.

## Hyperlipidemia

Approximately 3 months after heart transplantation, recipients frequently demonstrate an increase in total cholesterol, low-density lipoprotein (LDL) cholesterol, apolipoprotein B, and triglyceride levels. The etiology of dyslipidemia in heart transplant recipients is multifactorial, including genetic predisposition, high-fat diets, and immunosuppressive agents. In particular, corticosteroids and cyclosporine have been found to be important immunomodulating drugs that contribute to the development of hyperlipidemia posttransplant. Cyclosporine decreases bile acid synthesis from cholesterol and thus increases serum cholesterol levels. Corticosteroids increases acetyl coenzyme A (CoA) carboxylase activity and free fatty acid synthesis, which is a precursor to cholesterol synthesis. The statins have been found to reduce the LDL cholesterol levels in heart transplant recipients. In particular, pravastatin has been shown to cause not only a significant reduction in cholesterol levels at 3, 6, 9, and 12 months posttransplantation but also a reduction in rejection episodes associated with hemodynamic compromise, a decrease in the incidence of cardiac allograft vasculopathy, and an increased overall 1-year survival (9). Current recommendations are to prescribe a low-dose statins to all transplant recipients early after transplantation, regardless of their lipid levels, as long as liver function tests are normal. A critical interaction between the statins and cyclosporine or tacrolimus (via cytochrome P450-3A inhibition) increases the risk of myositis and rhabdomyolysis. Thus statins are started at lower doses in transplant patients and titrated up carefully.

### Tricuspid Regurgitation

Tricuspid regurgitation (TR) is not uncommon in the transplanted heart. Mild TR is present in virtually all transplanted hearts, and moderate–severe TR is present in up to 50% of transplant patients who live >5 years. Mechanical torsion on the tricuspid annulus due to the biatrial anastamosis accounts for at least mild–moderate regurgitation. The more anatomically correct, bicaval anastamotic technique has decreased the incidence but not prevented it. Recipients with pre-existing pulmonary artery hypertension often experience acute right ventricular dysfunction and subsequent chronic dilation, which contributes to the regurgitation. More important, repeated endomyocardial biopsies with damage to the valve, chordal apparatus, and papillary muscles account for the majority of severe cases of tricuspid regurgitation. Generally, even severe TR is well tolerated, but in a small minority of patients with progressive right heart failure due to TR, tricuspid replacement is needed (<3% of all heart transplants).

### Osteoporosis

Osteoporosis remains a common problem in heart transplant recipients, contributing to fracture-associated immobility that may compromise quality of life posttransplantation. The risk factors for osteoporosis may begin well before transplantation. Patients awaiting heart transplantation have a mean average reduction in bone mineral density (BMD) up to 10% compared to age-matched healthy individuals. Contributing factors to bone loss in severe heart failure patients include reduced exercise or immobilization, cardiac cachexia, smoking, alcohol, low calcium intake, heparin administration, and loop diuretics.

Bone loss is most rapid during the first 6 months following transplant, which coincides with the period of aggressive immunosuppression. Glucocorticoids are known to cause accelerated bone loss and are associated with a higher-than-normal incidence of vertebral fractures. Glucocorticoids reduce bone density by direct inhibition of osteoblast function and impairment of collagen and new bone formation. Shane et al. showed that at 2 years after cardiac transplant, severe osteoporosis was detected in the lumbar spine in 28% of patients and within the femoral neck in 20% of patients (10). It is common to perform routine screening of transplant candidates with baseline bone mineral density study prior to transplantation to identify and correct any secondary causes of bone loss. A regimen of elemental calcium, vitamin D supplementation, with or without bisphosphonates, and proper exercise training is indicated pretransplantation, and most programs routinely add bisphosphonates for all posttransplant patients receiving corticosteroids.

## SURVIVAL

In the current era, the 1-year survival after cardiac transplantation exceeds 85% and approaches 90% at most institutions. The greatest mortality occurs in the first year posttransplantation. After year 1, the annual mortality rate is approximately 3.6%, such that the 5- and 10-year survival rates are approximately 70% to 75% and 50% to 60% respectively (1). The survival for retransplantation has improved drastically if the patient is undergoing retransplantation at least 12 months after the initial transplant. Currently, the 1-year survival in this group of patients is approximately 82%.

The ISHLT registries have looked at the breakdown of causes of death from transplant recipients from January 1992 through June 2003 and divided them into time intervals. Graft failure was found to be the primary cause of death during the first 30 days posttransplantation, accounting for 41% of the deaths, followed by non-CMV infections (14%) and multiorgan failure (13%). After the first month and up until day 365, non-CMV infections account for almost 35% of deaths, followed by graft failure (19%) and acute rejection (12%). After 5 years posttransplantation, cardiac allograft vasculopathy and graft failure combined account for 30% of deaths, while malignancies account for 24% and non-CMV infections for 10% (1).

## REFERENCES


1. Taylor DO, Edwards LB, Boucek MM, et al. The Registry of the International Society for Heart and Lung Transplantation: Twenty-first Official Adult Heart Transplant Report—2004. *J Heart Lung Transplant.* 2004;23:796–803.
2. Mancini DM, Eisen H, Kussmahl W, et al. Value of peak exercise oxygen consumption for optimal timing of cardiac transplantation in ambulatory patients with heart failure. *Circulation.* 1991;83:778–786.
3. Hammond EH, Yowell RL, Nunoda S, et al. Vascular (humoral) rejection in heart transplantation: pathologic observations and clinical implications. *J Heart Lung Transplant.* 1989;8:430–443.
4. Micheals PJ, Espejo ML, Kobashigawa J, et al. Humoral rejection in cardiac transplantation: risk factors, hemodynamic consequences and relationship to transplant coronary artery disease. *J Heart Lung Transplant.* 2003;22(1):58–69.
5. Waller J, Brook NR, Nicholson ML. Cardiac allograft vasculopathy: current concepts and treatment. *Transplant Int.* 2003;16:367–375.
6. Kobashigawa AJ, Miller L, Renlund D, et al. A randomized active-controlled trial of mycophenolate mofetil in heart transplant recipients. *Transplantation.* 1998;66:507–515.
7. Eisen HJ, Tuzcu EM, Dorent R, et al. Everolimus for the prevention of allograft rejection and vasculopathy in cardiac transplant recipients. *N Engl J Med.* 2003;349:847.

8. Cockfield SM. Identifying the patient at risk for post-transplant lymphoprolierative disorder. *Transplant Infect Dis.* 2001;3:70–80.
9. Kobashigawa J, Katznelson S, Laks H, et al. Effect of pravastatin on outcomes after transplantation. *N Engl J Med.* 1995;333:621.
10. Shane E, Rivas M, Silverberg SJ, et al. Osteoporosis and bone morbidity in cardiac transplant recipients. *Am J Med.* 1993;94: 257–264.

## SUGGESTED READING

**Cimato TR, Jessup M.** Recipient selection in cardiac transplantation: contraindications and risk factors for mortality. *J Heart Lung Transplant.* 2002;21:1161–1173.

**Kirklin JK, Young JB, McGiffin DC, eds.** *Heart Transplantation.* Philadelphia: Churchill Livingstone; 2002.

## QUESTIONS

**1.** A 28-year-old man underwent heart transplantation 5 years ago for a presumed postviral dilated cardiomyopathy. He is seen at an urgent care clinic with complaints of a nonproductive cough, sore throat, and low-grade fever. He is diagnosed with an upper respiratory tract infection and prescribed clarithromycin, 500 mg twice daily for 10 days. Two weeks later, after completing antibiotics, he returns to the Transplant Clinic with complaints of generalized fatigue, shortness of breath, and a persistent nonproductive cough. His current immunosuppressive regimen includes prednisone, 10 mg daily; mycophenolate mofetil, 750 mg twice daily; and tacrolimus, 2 mg twice daily.

*Physical exam:* Sick-appearing man. Blood pressure is 142/92 mm Hg, heart rate is 98 beats/min and regular. Oropharynx is clear. Chest with bibasilar crackles. His abdomen shows no organomegaly or ascites. There is 3+ peripheral edema.
*ECG:* normal sinus rhythm, biatrial enlargement, incomplete right bundle branch block.
*Laboratory studies:* Hematocrit 36%; white cell count 4,100/μL; BUN 60 mg/dL; creatinine 5.3 mg/dL (baseline 1.3); tacrolimus level 29 ng/mL; MMF 4.5 ng/mL.

Which of the following is the most likely explanation of the patient's current condition?

a. Humoral rejection with hemodynamic compromise
b. Interaction of tacrolimus with mycophenolate mofetil, causing cellular rejection and thus acute renal failure
c. Immunocompromised patient with a viral syndrome
d. Interaction of tacrolimus with clarithromycin, resulting in acute renal failure
e. Noncompliance

Answer is d: The patient's clinical picture is most likely secondary to tacrolimus (Tac) toxicity resulting in acute renal failure. Clarithromycin inhibits the cytochrome P450 system, causing increased levels of calcineurin inhibitors (tacrolimus and cyclosporine). The target trough level of tacrolimus >12 months posttransplant is 8 to 10 ng/mL. The patient should discontinue tacrolimus until target trough levels are obtained. This clinical scenario could represent a rejection episode; however with the given history, tacrolimus toxicity is most likely the culprit. Tacrolimus taken with mycophenolate mofetil (MMF) is a common immunosuppression regimen. There is no increased incidence of renal failure or episodes of cellular rejection with this particular regimen. When taking Tac with MMF, the MMF dose should be decreased to lessen the likelihood of developing MMF toxicity (myelosuppression). The patient is definitely compliant, secondary to elevated trough levels of immunosuppressants.

**2.** A 23-year-old woman is seen for routine monthly posttransplant follow-up. She underwent an orthotopic cardiac transplantation 9 months ago for familial dilated cardiomyopathy. She has returned to college and reports that she saw an internist 3 weeks ago and was taken off of diltiazem, 60 mg twice daily, secondary to severe ankle swelling. She reports that her ankle swelling has improved and she is able to walk an hour a day without becoming fatigued or dyspneic. Current medications include prednisone, 10 mg daily; mycophenolate mofetil, 500 mg twice daily; cyclosporine, 75 mg twice daily; and bactrim, 1 tablet daily.

*Physical examination:* Blood pressure 110/78 mm Hg; heart rate 95 beats/min; RR 18/min. Chest is clear, PMI nondisplaced, normal S1 and S2. Extremities: no edema.
*ECG:* Normal sinus rhythm at 95, with nonspecific ST–T abnormalities.
*Laboratory:* Hematocrit 37%; white blood cell count 8,400/μL, platelets 220,000/μL; BUN 30 mg/dL; creatinine 1.1 mg/dL; cyclosporine 45 ng/mL; MMF level 2.2 ng/mL. Right ventricular biopsy shows prominent lymphocytic infiltrate with associated areas of myocyte necrosis with ISHLT Grade 3A rejection.

Which of the following statements is false?

a. Cyclosporine dose should be increased to achieve adequate trough levels.

b. This rejection episode is most likely secondary to the discontinuation of diltiazem.
c. There is no need to treat this rejection episode; the patient feels great and is hemodynamically stable.
d. Patients should report all changes in medications to the Transplant Clinic.

Answer is c: The patient's episode of rejection is most likely secondary to discontinuing diltiazem 3 weeks earlier. Diltiazem inhibits the cytochrome P450 system, causing increased levels of cyclosporine and therefore requiring lesser dosages to achieve trough levels. Once diltiazem was discontinued, the dose of cyclosporine should have been increased. Almost all rejection episodes Grade 3A and higher and all rejection episodes that show hemodynamically instability (regardless of grade) are treated with augmented immunosuppression. It is important for transplant recipients to communicate any changes in medications to the Transplant Clinic, so these complications can be avoided.

**3.** All of the following are risk factors for posttransplant mortality *except*:

a. Diabetes with end-organ damage
b. Reversible pulmonary hypertension
c. Active smoking
d. Left ventricular assist device <30 days
e. Active infection

Answer is b: Risk factors for posttransplant mortality include but are not limited to short-term ventricular assist device use (<30 days), irreversible pulmonary vascular resistance (PVR >4 Wood units), mechanical ventilation at the time of transplant, active infection, active smoking, diabetes particularly with end-organ damage, and hepatic or renal insufficiency.

**4.** What is the most sensitive tool in detecting cardiac allograft vasculopathy posttransplantation?

a. Serial echocardiography
b. Intracoronary vascular ultrasound
c. Positron emission scanning
d. RV endomyocardial biopsy
e. Coronary angiogram

Answer is b: Serial echocardiograms are important for following graft function posttransplant; however, they are not very sensitive for detecting early CAV. Periodic right ventricular biopsy is the standard method of surveillance for cellular rejection, but adds little to the diagnosis of CAV. Positron emission scans are used to detect ischemia, and scarred and hibernating myocardium; however, they suffer from poor sensitivity in detecting CAV. Studies have shown intracoronary ultrasound (IVUS) to be the most sensitive tool in detecting and following the progression of CAV, compared to coronary angiograms.

**5.** Which of the following is true regarding posttransplant lymphoproliferative disease (PTLD)?

a. Treatment includes reduction in immunosuppression therapy.
b. It occurs in approximately 90% of all cardiac transplant patients.
c. The highest-risk group for developing PTLD is recipients who are Epstein–Barr virus (EBV) seronegative who receive an EBV-seronegative heart.
d. The lymphomas that arise in PTLD are usually T cell in origin.
e. The tumor usually arises 1 month after transplantation, with the cervical lymph nodes being the most common site.

Answer is a: Posttransplant lymphoproliferative disease (PTLD) is a unique polyclonal B-cell lymphoma that occurs in approximately 3.4% of all heart transplant recipients. Ninety percent of PTLDs are associated with EBV; with EBV D+/R– being a high-risk group for developing PTLD. These tumors usually arise 12 to 18 months following transplant, after a mononucleosis-like illness (fever, sore throat, myalgias, and lymphadenopathy) and commonly are located intra-abdominally. Treatment includes decreasing the level of immunosupression, surgical debulking, cytotoxic chemotherapy, and radiation therapy if indicated; however, the response rate of advanced disease to treatment is poor (<50%).

# Devices for Heart Failure

31

*Drew Allen James B. Young*

Over the past two decades, mechanical circulatory support devices have improved such that some are now standard for care for patients with advanced, life-threatening heart failure that is unresponsive to standard medical therapies, serving as a bridge to cardiac transplantation (1–7). In some cases, use of these devices has been approved for "destination" therapy (as an alternative to heart transplantation). The evolution has been dramatic and must continue because of substantial remaining limitations. Nonetheless, "device therapy" for select patients with devastating heart failure generally means one form or another of mechanical circulatory support. It is important to understand the role and the limitations of these devices possess in heart failure patients. It is also wise to have some insight into the clinical settings in which devices can be deployed successfully, the variety of devices currently available, the indications for insertion of a device, and the expected outcomes, including morbidity associated with mechanical circulatory support. This overview addresses these critical issues and provides a framework for preparing answers to expected Board certification questions.

## IMPORTANT CONSIDERATIONS REGARDING MECHANICAL CIRCULATORY SUPPORT DEVICES

Mechanical circulatory support devices were initially developed to bridge patients to "recovery," then as a bridge, or alternative, to transplantation. Dr. Michael E. DeBakey, in the early 1960s, was the first to report successes with insertion of rudimentary left ventricular assist prototypes. This was a time when open heart surgery was evolving rapidly, but substantial limitations to cardiopulmonary bypass were present. In an effort to transiently support patients who were unable to be weaned from cardiopulmonary bypass after cardiotomy and open heart surgery, pneumatically displaced pulsatile devices were used haltingly. Slowly, devices evolved with improvements that allowed successful bridging to recovery from cardiogenic shock postcardiotomy and cardiopulmonary bypass, and in patients with acute myocarditis or in the peri-infarction period, when stunning of potentially viable myocardial tissue had occurred. Use of these devices initially for patients with more chronic and advanced "end-stage" heart failure subsequently became more frequent as an option to stabilize a patient before cardiac transplantation. In some patients, though infrequently, recovery of ventricular function occurred and device removal was possible.

Table 31–1 summarizes issues to consider when mechanical circulatory support devices may be possible treatment options. Clinical settings that should prompt consideration of device use commonly include cardiopulmonary bypass wean failure, acute cardiogenic shock (usually in the setting of an acute coronary syndrome with massive myocardial infarction or fulminant myocarditis), and in the chronic, severely decompensated heart failure patient (American College of Cardiology (ACC)/American Heart Association (AHA), Heart Failure Stage D) as a bridge to transplantation or as an alternative to transplantation. Rarely, mechanical circulatory support devices are inserted during resuscitative efforts in individuals with the sudden cardiac death syndrome.

When clinicians are making decisions regarding the type of mechanical circulatory support, consideration of the support system role becomes important. This is generally related to whether total heart function replacement is necessary or individual ventricular assistance (or replacement)

**TABLE 31–1**
**MECHANICAL CIRCULATORY SUPPORT DEVICES: CONSIDERATIONS**

Clinical setting
- Cardiopulmonary bypass wean failure
- Acute cardiogenic shock (usually acute coronary syndrome or fulminant myocarditis setting)
- Chronic severely decompensated heart failure (ACC/AHA Stage D)
- Sudden cardiac death syndrome

Circulatory support system role
- Total heart function replacement
- Left and/or right ventricular function replacement
  - Reduced preload and/or afterload
  - Augmentation of systemic blood flow

Anatomic focus
- Peripheral circulation
- Total heart
- Left ventricle (and/or)
- Right ventricle

Clinical goal
- Bridge to more sophisticated bridge
- Bridge to clinical improvement
- Bridge to recovery
- Bridge to improvement to transplant
- Bridge to transplant
- Permanent insertion ("destination" or home therapy as an alternative to transplant)

is the goal. Total artificial heart systems focus on the biatrial and biventricular anatomy. Left and/or right ventricular function assistance produces reduced preload and/or afterload with augmentation of systemic blood flow, but really contributes "assistance" to the ventricle rather than functional replacement. Left and/or right ventricular function replacement requires more powerful units capable of sustaining the entire cardiac circulatory load.

The anatomic focus of mechanical circulatory support varies from the peripheral circulation, to the total heart, or the left and/or right ventricle. The intra-aortic balloon counterpulsation pump, for example, focuses on the peripheral circulation, as do temporary centrifugal-flow cardiopulmonary bypass systems, which support blood flow from large venous structures into large arterial structures to augment cardiac output.

As alluded to, clinical goals with mechanical circulatory support devices vary. For example, an individual who cannot be weaned from cardiopulmonary bypass may have a temporary support device implanted as a bridge to a more sophisticated and perhaps more permanent device. This subsequent device can also become a bridge to clinical improvement and cardiac recovery, allowing device removal, or bridge to improvement so that transplant can subsequently be done safely. Finally, the option of permanent insertion of a mechanical circulatory support device is now available. Sometimes this is referred to as "destination" or "homebound" therapy or as an "alternative" to cardiac transplantation.

## PATIENT SELECTION

When referring patients for mechanical circulatory support, one must weigh the risk of a major operation in a patient who has tenuous circulatory stability and often high mortality risk. Knowing the relative contraindications to device insertion as well as which patients are likely to gain the most benefit is critical. The U.S. Food and Drug Administration (FDA) has approved several ventricular assist devices for implantation only as a "bridge-to-cardiac transplant," but in reality that is not how the devices are actually used. A much broader utilization of devices, as alluded to in Table 31–1, is accepted by clinicians. Though no complete consensus exists regarding patient selection, generally these individuals have systolic blood pressures <80 to 90 mm Hg (mean arterial blood pressure <65 mm Hg), pulmonary capillary wedge pressure >20 mm Hg, systemic vascular resistance >2,000 dynes, falling urine outputs despite diuretics (<20 cc/h in an adult), and a cardiac index of $<2/L/min/m^2$ despite aggressive use of inotropic agents, vasopressers, and sometimes an intra-aortic balloon pump (IABP). Many factors must be weighed, and certain ones will affect device selection, as we will review. There is an art to matching patient characteristics to individual devices, and it is important to realize that "one size does not fit all." Devices come in an array of physiologic types, anatomic configurations, and sizes.

## AVAILABLE MECHANICAL CIRCULATORY SUPPORT DEVICES

The most commonly used mechanical circulatory support device is the intra-aortic counterpulsation displacement balloon device (Table 31–2). This is a relatively simple device that can be inserted percutaneously through the femoral or axillary artery (on occasion it is inserted intraoperatively and in other configurations) and that produces short-term diastolic blood flow augmentation that is particularly beneficial in acute coronary syndromes. The device unloads the heart during systole and augments diastolic retrograde perfusion of the coronary arteries by inflating at precisely timed moments within the diastolic cardiac cycle. Often, placement of the IABP is a bridge to a more sophisticated mechanical circulatory support device. IABPs can be used only for several days before risk of arterial trauma, infection, device failure, or thrombotic complications force their removal. Flow augmentation is not substantial with these devices, but afterload reduction and increased coronary perfusion frequently is of enough benefit to see patients recover significant ventricular function and survive cardiogenic shock. Advantages of IABPs

**TABLE 31–2**
**MECHANICAL CIRCULATORY SUPPORT: DEVICES AVAILABLE**

- Aortic counterpulsation displacement
  - Intra-aortic balloon counter pulsation (IABP)
  - Extra-aortic (balloon/mechanical) counter pulsation (experimental)
- Extracorporeal devices
  - Continuous flow
    - Axial flow (impellar driven)
    - Centrifugal flow
  - Pulsatile flow
    - Pneumatic displacement (diaphragmatic)
    - Electric motor displacement (pusher plate)
- Intracorporeal devices
  - Complete component implantation
  - Partial component implantation
  - Intrathoracic
    - Continuous flow
    - Pulsatile flow
  - Subdiaphragmatic
    - Continuous flow
    - Pulsatile flow

include their ready availability, ease of insertion, simplistic design, and relatively low cost.

Extracorporeal support devices (Table 31–2) include continuous-flow axial or centrifugal pumps that can be inserted percutaneously or during an operative procedure to expose, most commonly, the femoral arteries and veins. The most frequently used continuous-flow extracorporeal device in an acute emergency situation is the Biomedicus continuous-flow device, which is sometimes coupled with an oxygenator to provide cardiopulmonary bypass. Indeed, at the bedside, placing an oxygenator between the device and the arterial input cannula is the configuration referred to as extracorporeal membrane oxygenator support. More sophisticated extracorporeal devices are placed at the time of thoracotomy and cardiotomy and generally are pneumatic or electric motor displacement devices with pumping chambers connected paracorporeally to exteriorized cannula. The cannula can be set up in a variety of configurations so that left ventricular, right ventricular, or biventricular bypass can be achieved. Interestingly, the first successful use of a ventricular assist device was by Dr. Michael E. DeBakey in 1966, when an extracorporeal pneumatically displaced pulsatile device was used in a patient who could not be weaned from cardiopulmonary bypass after valvular heart surgery for rheumatic heart disease and severe heart failure (8). A cannula was placed in the left atrium for inflow into the device, with the arterial outflow cannula anastomosed to the right axillary artery. The patient survived the operative procedure, was extubated without complications, and native heart recovery occurred. The device was removed in the intensive care unit under local anesthesia, with the cannula being occluded subcutaneously and then allowed to thrombose. The patient survived hospital discharge and led an active life until being mortally injured in an automobile accident.

Intracorporeal devices have been a desirable goal because of the potential for complete component implantation (Table 31–2). With a completely implantable system, violation of the infection barrier with percutaneous connections is eliminated and the risk of sepsis is markedly reduced. This remains problematic, however, as multiple controlling elements must be buried within the patient, including the pump itself, cardiac and arterial conduits, a compliance chamber (for pulsatile devices), a pump controller, and a power system with transcutaneous capabilities for energy transfer. Because of the complexity surrounding development of such a device, present intracorporeal devices are, for the most part, only partially component-implanted devices. These devices can be implanted intrathoracically or subdiaphragmatically and are either continuous-flow or pulsatile units. Continuous-flow systems include impeller-driven devices and centrifugal devices that are currently in clinical trials.

## COMPONENTS AND CONFIGURATIONS OF MECHANICAL CIRCULATORY ASSIST DEVICES

The IABP, the least sophisticated mechanical circulatory support device, requires an obturator that allows gas displacement into and out of a balloon that surrounds the ridged internal device central frame. This device is usually inserted percutaneously through the femoral artery and connected to an external controlling device that monitors arterial pressure and electrocardiographic recordings. Mechanical features of the device integrate these measurements and trigger inflation and deflation of the device at the onset of electromechanical diastole, effecting subsequent hemodynamic benefits as summarized previously.

Table 31–3 summarizes more sophisticated pump system components. The pump itself must be affixed to inflow and outflow conduits and valves to control blood direction, with the pump chamber itself located between the valves and conduits. The interior of the pump represents the blood component–device interface, where many problems such as thrombosis and hemolysis begin. The pump controller is linked to circulatory pressure and an electrocardiographic monitor. Sophisticated electronics regulate a pressure–rhythm pump interface system that usually controls the amount of flow and pressure a device generates. The pump driver or activator is the actual flow-generating system and is either a pneumatically displaced diaphragm or an electric motor moving pusher plates back and forth. The pump requires a power source, and this must come from wall-socket alternating current or some form of a battery pack. Interestingly, from an historic standpoint, some

**TABLE 31–3**
**MECHANICAL CIRCULATORY SUPPORT DEVICES COMPONENTS AND CONFIGURATIONS: SYSTEM REQUIREMENTS AND OPTIONS**

Pump (pulsatile or continuous flow)
- Inflow/outflow conduits
- Inflow/outflow valves
- Pump chamber
- Blood component–device interface

Controller
- Circulatory pressure/electrocardiographic monitors
- Pressures–rhythm–pump interface system

Pump driver (activator) for pulsatile systems
- Pneumatic displacement
- Electric motor pusher plate
- Impellar motor
- Centrifugal motor

Driver power source
- Wall-socket alternating current
- Battery pack

Air-displacement system for pulsatile systems
- External venting line
- Implanted compliance chamber

of the earliest mechanical circulatory support devices intended to be completely implantable were developed with nuclear energy identified as the power source. These devices are no longer being pursued. Because pneumatic pulsatile devices require displacement of gas-driven volume, one form or another of air-displacement management system is necessary, and this can be accomplished with either an external venting line or an implanted compliance chamber. External venting lines are yet another blow to the skin barrier, as they represent a second externalized access for infection. Implanted compliance chambers have problems with obstruction and breakage of the constantly moving membrane. Because continuous-flow devices do not require air-displacement systems and possess smaller drive lines, they may have some advantage.

## MECHANICAL CIRCULATORY SUPPORT DEVICES CURRENTLY AVAILABLE OR UNDER EVALUATION

Many devices have entered clinical trials (Table 31–4). Nonetheless, only a few devices are currently available for use. Of note is the Jarvik device, a total artificial heart system, which was first implanted at the University of Utah in Dr. Barney Clark. It is a large device with large external components and renders the patient relatively immobile, though portable component systems have improved this greatly in later iterations. This device is associated with significant infection and embolism risk. It has been used successfully as a bridge to transplantation in patients who require complete left and right ventricular replacement rather than simply left ventricular assistance. Another experimental total artificial heart, the Abiomed device, is also totally implantable and very recently entered clinical trials, with the main difficulty seeming to be thrombosis and emboli. The Penn State total artificial heart entered clinical trials but appears to have been abandoned recently.

The Biomedicus centrifugal-flow pump mentioned earlier is a short-term device that can be used for biventricular support and linked to an oxygenator for extracorporeal membrane oxygenation. It is relatively easy to insert, but its utilization time is limited because of risks of thrombosis, blood trauma, and infection. A smaller, perhaps more suitable centrifugal-flow device is the Arrow-CCF unit, which has recently entered clinical trials. This is a small, surgically implantable device suitable for longer-term support as a bridge to recovery or transplantation.

The Abiomed external pneumatic device is a short-term device that can be put into a left and/or right ventricular assist configuration. It is easy to insert and is probably the most commonly used device today for cardiopulmonary bypass pump wean failure. Unfortunately, the device requires the patient to be hospital bound, and generally bed bound, with complications including bleeding and thrombosis.

The Thoratec device is an example of an external pneumatic-powered system that can be used for much longer periods and also has biventricular assist device capabilities. It has proved to be an excellent bridge to cardiac transplantation, though for the most part, patients who have these external pumps are generally hospital bound. Complications of bleeding, infection, and emboli are seen with some frequency. Because of its external-component nature, the device is relatively easy to insert at the time of thoracotomy, but the external chest pumps can produce disconcerting problems.

Three electric pusher plate devices are available: the Berlin heart in Europe, and the HeartMate vented electric and Novacor systems in North America. These devices are characterized by an electric pusher plate system, with the HeartMate and Novacor being devices that can be implanted in the abdomen and are suitable for long-term use. It is difficult to use these devices in a biventricular mode, with only the Berlin heart having biventricular capabilities. The Berlin heart in particular can be used for patients who are of smaller body mass. These pusher plate devices are for the most part quite reliable but are still plagued with problems of infection and peripheral emboli.

The Jarvik and Heart Mate II are completely implantable axial-flow devices designed for long-term support. The DeBakey/MicroMed axial-flow device is also implantable, long term, and clinically available in Europe. These devices all have characteristics of small device size, small drive lines, and are nonpulsatile. Whether pulsatility matters in the end with respect to cardiovascular physiology in patients with advanced heart failure is a contentious subject. These

**TABLE 31–4**
**MECHANICAL CIRCULATORY SUPPORT DEVICES: TYPES**

| Class | Device | Implantable | Long Term? | BiVAD Capable | Comments |
|---|---|---|---|---|---|
| TAH | CardioWest | + | + | + | Clinically available<br>Immobility of patient<br>Infection<br>Emboli |
| TAH | Abiomed (Exp) | + | + | + | Totally implantable<br>Emboli |
| TAH | Penn State (Exp) | + | + | + | Totally implantable<br>Large |
| Centrifugal flow | Biomedicus | | | + | Simple, easy, inexpensive<br>Bleeding<br>Emboli<br>Device failure<br>Bed bound<br>Perfusionist required |
| Centrifugal flow | Arrow-CCF | + | + | + | Small<br>Easier to insert<br>Small drive lines<br>Hemolysis |
| External pneumatic | Abiomed | | | + | Easier to insert<br>Most common<br>Flow limit 6 L<br>Thrombosis<br>Bleeding<br>Hospital bound |
| External pneumatic | Thoratec | | + | + | Only approved long-term BiVAD<br>Hospital bound<br>BSA limitation<br>Bleeding<br>Infection<br>Embolus |
| Pusher plate | Berlin heart | | + | + | Low-BSA compatible<br>Pump cleaning required |
| Pusher plate | HeartMate VE | + | + | | Low CVA rate<br>Infection<br>BSA >1.5 |
| Pusher plate | Novacor | + | + | | Reliable<br>Infection<br>BSA limit<br>CVA |
| Axial flow | Jarvik (Exp) | + | + | | Small size<br>Small drive line<br>Nonpulsatile |
| Axial flow | Heart Mate II (Exp) | + | + | | Small size<br>Small drive line<br>Nonpulsatile |
| Axial flow | DeBakey/Micromed | + | + | | Small size<br>Small drive line<br>Nonpulsatile |

BiVAD, ; TAH, ; Exp, experimental; BSA, ; CVA, .

axial-flow devices as well as the previously discussed centrifugal-flow devices are ventricular "assist" devices rather than ventricular "replacement" devices because of the lesser degree of support provided and inherent characteristics of continuous flow.

## IDEAL LONGER-TERM MECHANICAL CIRCULATORY SUPPORT SYSTEM PARAMETERS

In general, effective pressure and blood flow sustenance is required for circulatory support systems (Table 31–5). Ultimately, this is the issue with severe advanced heart failure and the most important parameter that will correlate with resuscitation of compromised organs. Time and again, during effective flow support, reversal of substantive hepatic insufficiency, renal insufficiency, and even cardiac failure is observed. The major challenge is trying to determine when seemingly irreversible failure in fact is not present. Another important parameter is the potential for removing the device if ventricular recovery occurs. This is not possible with total artificial heart implantation, as there has been extirpation of most essential cardiac structures.

Small devices are more attractive because they can be completely implanted with less surgical intervention and render more efficient power-source utilization. Small devices do suffer from limitations of producing inadequate circulatory support and, particularly with impeller-driven devices or centrifugal-flow devices, can precipitate substantive blood component trauma.

Other important parameters include reliability and durability. Having a high risk of device failure increases the complexity of support and creates extraordinary anxiety in patients and their families. Also, if devices fail completely or there is component failure, frequent reinsertion is not practical nor often possible.

Because of the external conduits, infection is a tremendous risk with both implantable and extracorporeal circulatory assist systems. Inadequate understanding of the blood–device interface has resulted in inability to control adequately for thrombus development. A low thromboembolic risk is extremely important, as is minimal blood component trauma. Finally, the device should be nonimmunogenic, as activation of the immune system can lead to a procoagulable state and other general medical complications.

**TABLE 31–5**
**IDEAL LONGER-TERM MECHANICAL CIRCULATORY SUPPORT SYSTEMS: IMPORTANT PARAMETERS**

- Effective pressure and flow support
- Potential for removal if ventricle recovers
- Small
  - Efficient power source
  - Completely implantable
- Reliable
- Durable
- Low infection risk
- Low thromboembolic risk
- Minimal blood component trauma
- Nonimmunogenic

## PROBLEMATIC SITUATIONS: CHALLENGES THAT CAN COMPROMISE OUTCOMES

Many clinical situations can create challenges that may ultimately compromise beneficial outcomes after device implantation (Table 31–6). Most implantable pulsatile left ventricular assist systems require a reasonable-sized body habitus to make the device fit without compromising internal organ function. Patients with a body surface area $<1.5$ m$^2$ have a limited choice of devices, usually restricted to extracorporeal or small continuous-flow systems. Larger individuals, those with a body surface area $>2.5$ m$^2$ or an ideal body weight of $>150\%$, also are problematic because of technical challenges posed during the operation and, in some situations, limited length of available driveline tubing. Hemodynamically significant aortic insufficiency limits effectiveness of left ventricular bypass and support. Mechanical aortic valve prostheses are at risk for thrombosis if the valve remains closed during complete ventricular bypass and support. Sometimes pulsatile left ventricular assist devices are implanted in these patients with the mechanical prostheses replaced by biologic prostheses. Because of the risk of thrombosis and emboli, most devices require

**TABLE 31–6**
**PROBLEMATIC SITUATIONS: CHALLENGES THAT MAY COMPROMISE OUTCOMES**

- Body surface area $<1.5$ m$^2$ or $>2.5$ m$^2$
- Weight $>150\%$ ideal
- Highly calcified aorta (particularly at proposed site of outflow cannula anastomosis)
- Hemodynamically significant aortic insufficiency
- Mechanical aortic valve prosthesis
- Inability to anticoagulate patient
- Significant "fixed" pulmonary hypertension
- Recent pulmonary embolus
- Chronic ventilator dependence
- Impaired pulmonary function ($FEV_1$ $<50\%$ predicated or $<1.5$ L)
- Aortic aneurysm
- Peripheral vascular disease
- Cerebrovascular disease
- Active infection (particularly systemic)
- Psychosocial issues that might impair compliance
- Irreversible and significant end-organ dysfunction (see Table 31–7)

aggressive anticoagulation. If patients cannot be anticoagulated effectively, mechanical circulatory assist becomes compromised. Because of the sensitivity of the right ventricle to significant pulmonary hypertension, fixed pulmonary pressures in a setting of a dilated and failing right ventricle with associated tricuspid insufficiency makes left ventricular assist device insertion alone problematic and prone to failure. Recent pulmonary emboli cause the same challenges and can be linked to the presence of pulmonary hypertension. Though some patients on a ventilator do well after mechanical circulatory device insertion, most patients who have demonstrated chronic ventilator dependence have become colonized with unhealthy micro-organisms and have substantial risk of systemic infection and sepsis. Also, patients who are ventilator dependent usually have profound cachexia and problems such that they cannot be weaned from the ventilator. In aggregate, these situations predispose patients to less than optimal outcomes. Peripheral vascular disease, including cerebral vascular disease and aortic aneurysms, set the stage for failure. An aortic aneurysm, when confronted with the sheer stress generated by a pulsatile ventricular assist device, is much more likely to expand and rupture postinsertion. An active infection, particularly a systemic infection, may set the stage for device infection, which can be devastating and impossible to cure. "Endopumpitis" is one of the most feared complications of mechanical circulatory support. Many psychosocial issues appear during chronic diseases, and because of the extraordinary challenges these devices present, any psychosocial instability will lead to a compromised outcome. Finally, irreversible significant end-organ dysfunction will clearly cause problems post–device insertion.

Table 31–7 summarizes end-organ compromise that should prompt avoidance of device insertion. They include any evidence of hepatic cirrhosis or persistent hepatic enzymes elevation >3 times the upper limit of normal or bilirubin >3.0 mL/dL (despite aggressive hemodynamic resuscitation efforts). Likewise, a platelet count <50,000 or primary coagulopathy indicate serious difficulties that should prompt avoidance of device implantation. Further indicating coagulopathy or hepatic dysfunction is a prothrombin time or activated partial thromboplastin time greater than twice control values or international normalizing ratio (INR) >1.8 in patients who are not anticoagulated. Also problematic is a serum creatinine >3.0 mg/dL or creatine clearance <30 mL/h.

**TABLE 31–7**

**PROBLEMATIC END-ORGAN DYSFUNCTION: CHALLENGES THAT MAY COMPROMISE OUTCOMES**

Any hepatic cirrhosis
Liver enzymes >3 times upper limit of normal or bilirubin >3.0 mL/dL
Prothrombim time or activated partial thromboplastin time > twice control values or INR > 1.8 in patients not anticoagulated
Platelet count <50,000
Primary coagulopathy
Prothrombim time or activated partial thromboplastin time >2 times control values or INR >1.8 in patients not anticoagulated
Serum creatinine >3.0 mg/dL or creatine clearance <30 mL/h

INR, international normalizing ratio.

**TABLE 31–8**

**ISHLT MCSD 2005 REGISTRY ANALYSIS (*N* = 655): RISK FACTORS FOR DEATH POSTIMPLANT[a]**

| Risk Factor | RR | *p* Value |
|---|---|---|
| Early hazard phase | | |
| Concurrent RVAD | 4.89 | <0.0001 |
| Age (older) | 3.13 | <0.0001 |
| Female | 2.53 | 0.0003 |
| Platelet count (lower) | 2.13 | 0.02 |
| WBC count (higher) | 2.01 | 0.01 |
| Longer-term hazard phase | | |
| Diabetes | 2.01 | 0.01 |
| Preimplant ventilator | 1.84 | 0.03 |
| Creatine (higher) | 1.64 | 0.03 |

ISHLT, International Heart Lung Transplant Society; MCSD, mechanical circulatory support device; RR, relative risk (by multivariable hazard analysis); WBC, white blood cell count; RVAD, right ventricular assist device.
[a]Patients censored at time of transplant.

The International Society for Heart and Lung Transplantation Mechanical Circulatory Database Report for 2005 includes an elegant analysis of risk factors for death post–device implantation (excluding IABP). As Table 31–8 summarizes, the highest risk for early postoperative death occurs in individuals who are receiving concurrent right ventricular assist, who are older, female, and have a lower platelet count and a higher white blood cell count. Significant longer-term hazard is noted in diabetics, individuals on a ventilator, and those with higher creatinine levels.

Table 31–9 summarizes the postimplantation patient-related events seen in the International Society for Heart and Lung Transplantation Mechanical Circulatory Support Device 2005 Registry. Infection and bleeding were two of the most often occurring adverse events. Infection was seen in approximately one third of patients, with almost 30% having significant bleeding episodes. Neurologic dysfunction was observed in 14% of the registry patients. This points to the challenges and the frailty of patients receiving mechanical circulatory support.

## OUTCOMES AFTER CIRCULATORY SUPPORT IMPLANTATION

In 655 patients analyzed in the ISHLT-MCSD Registry (entered between January 2002 and December 2004),

**TABLE 31–9**
**ISHLT MCSD 2005 REGISTRY ANALYSIS ($N = 655$): POSTIMPLANTATION PATIENT-RELATED EVENTS**

| Event | No. of Patients | Percentage of All Patients |
|---|---|---|
| Infection | 134 | 32.5 |
| Bleeding | 115 | 27.8 |
| Arrhythmia | 100 | 24.2 |
| Renal dysfunction | 85 | 20.6 |
| Respiratory dysfunction | 66 | 16.0 |
| Neurologic dysfunction | 58 | 14.0 |
| Right ventricular dysfunction | 44 | 10.7 |
| Hepatic dysfunction | 30 | 7.2 |
| Cardiac tamponade | 22 | 5.3 |
| Thrombotic vascular complication | 10 | 2.4 |
| Hematoma | 10 | 2.2 |
| Pleural effusion | 9 | 2.2 |
| Internal organ compromise | 5 | 1.2 |
| Pacemaker implanted | 2 | 0.5 |

1-month survival was 83% and 12-month survival was 50%, sensoring patients at the time of transplantation. Age played a significant factor in outcomes, with an individual 40 years of age having a predicted 6-month mortality of about 5%, versus a 70-year-old patient with a predicted mortality of almost 20% after a left ventricular assist device alone was implanted. With the combination of a left and right ventricular assist device during the same operation, for a 50-year-old individual the mortality approaches 20%, compared to a little over 5% for a left ventricular assist device alone. In individuals under the age of 30 years receiving mechanical circulatory support as a bridge to transplant, 51% were transplanted at the 6-month mark, with 33% alive and still waiting transplantation and 10% dying before transplant. This should be compared to those individuals >50 years of age who, at the 6-month mark, saw only 39% transplanted, with a 33% pretransplant mortality and 27% of patients still waiting for transplant. Interestingly, though recovery sometimes occurs and mechanical circulatory support devices can be explanted, this is a rare event in patients >50 years of age, with only a 0.4% recovery–explantation rate noted over a 12-month period of time, compared to a 6-month explanted–recovery rate observed in patients <30 years of age of 3%. Complications such as bleeding episodes and thromboembolism were most frequent in the first 30 days after transplantation, leveling off after this point. This is in contrast to infection episodes, which saw a constant rise throughout the observation period.

Though only 78 patients received a device as "destination" therapy and were entered into the ISHLT-MCSD analysis, 65% of these patients were alive at the 6-month mark and 34% at 12 months, with a 12-month mortality rate of 55%.

## CLINICAL TRIALS OF DEVICE THERAPY

Because mechanical circulatory support systems are generally utilized only in desperate situations, particularly in situations where a patient is being bridged from cardiogenic shock and near certain death to either recovery or transplantation, randomized clinical trials of devices have not been performed. For destination therapy, on the other hand, a seminal trial demonstrated that longe-term survival as well as improved quality of life did occur with a left ventricular assist device implantation in select patients. The Randomized Evaluation of Mechanical Assistance for the Treatment of Congestive Heart Failure (the REMATCH Trial) randomized 129 patients who were not considered transplant candidates to either "best medical therapy" or a HeartMate left ventricular assist device. All patients had New York Heart Association (NYHA) Class IV symptoms, with very advanced heart failure characterized by a mean ejection fraction of 17%, a mean systolic blood pressure of 102 mm Hg, an elevated mean creatinine of 1.8 mg/dL, and dependency on intravenous inotropic support in 70% of patients. The 1- and 2-year survival rates were 52% versus 25% ($p = 0.002$) and 23% versus 8% ($p = 0.09$) for the left ventricular assist device versus medical therapy groups, respectively. This translates into a 48% reduction in the risk of death from any cause in the left ventricular assist device group compared to the medical therapy group. Indeed, of the 54 deaths in the medical therapy group, 50 were due to heart failure, compared to only one death due to heart failure in 41 deaths noted in the HeartMate group. Minnesota Living with Heart Failure quality-of-life scores were better in the left ventricular assist device group.

Despite these observations, destination therapy in advanced heart failure patients with this left ventricular assist device has not been enthusiastically embraced. This probably relates to relatively short-term improvement in outcomes and the fact that morbidity was high, with stroke, infection, and device failures, all noted with some frequency and paralleling what was seen in the ISHLT MCSD Registry (Table 31–9).

## CONCLUSION

Mechanical circulatory support devices have matured in robust fashion over four decades but still remain problematic. Nonetheless, they possess great potential for rehabilitating patients with end-stage terminal heart failure. They are most effective when used in the proper clinical setting (severe heart failure without co-morbidities likely to compromise postoperative outcomes) and most frequently allow a successful bridge to cardiac transplantation.

## HOW TO PREPARE FOR THE BOARDS

Certification and recertification Cardiovascular Disease Board questions on the topic of cardiac circulatory support will likely not require a detailed knowledge of ventricular assist device nuances. The questions are more apt to focus on appropriate selection of patients who might benefit from short-term or long-term device support. In particular, diagnoses that predispose to adverse outcomes or are associated with substantive clinical problems postoperatively need to be known. Also important is knowledge regarding device complications, including infection, bleeding, right ventricular failure, thromboembolism, and renal insufficiency. The knowledge base regarding mechanical circulatory support devices should be linked to that focused on managing NYHA Class IV, ACC/AHA Stage D patients.

## REFERENCES


1. Hunt SA, Abraham WT, Chin MH, et al. ACC/AHA 2005 guidelines for the diagnosis and management of chronic heart failure in the adult. *Circulation*. 2005; DOI 10.116/Circulation AHA. 105.167587.
2. Stevenson LW, Kormos RL, Bourge RC, et al. Mechanical cardiac support 2000: current applications in future trial design. *J Am Coll Cardiol*. 2001;37:340–370.
3. Williams MR, Oz MC. Indications and patient selection for mechanical ventricular assistance. *Ann Thorac Surg*. 2001;71:S86–S91.
4. Dang MC, Edwards LD, Hertz MI, et al. Mechanical circulatory support device database of the Internal Society for Heart and Lung Transplantation: 3rd annual report—2005. *J Heart Lung Transplant*. 2005;24:1182–1187.
5. Rose EA, Moskowitz AJ, Pecker M, et al. The REMATCH trial: rationale, design, and endpoints. Randomized evaluation of mechanical assistance for treatment of congestive heart failure. *Ann Thorac Surg*. 1999;67:723–730.
6. Rose EA, Gelijns AC, Moskowitz AJ, et al. Long term use of left ventricular assist device for end stage heart failure. *N Engl J Med*. 2001;345:1435–1443.
7. Young JB. Healing the heart the heart with ventricular assist device therapy: mechanisms of cardiac recovery. *Ann Thorac Surg*. 2001; 71:S210–S219.
8. The Committee on Trauma, Division of Medical Sciences, National Academy of Sciences, National Research Council. *Mechanical Devices to Assist the Failing Heart*. National Academy of Sciences Publication 1283. Washington DC: National Academy of Sciences; 1966.


## QUESTIONS

**1.** The patient most likely to benefit from an implantable pulsatile ventricular assist device as a bridge to cardiac transplantation is

a. A patient found to be in full cardiac arrest in the coronary care unit after being admitted with an acute coronary syndrome.

b. A New York Heart Association Class II outpatient with ischemic congestive cardiomyopathy and atrial fibrillation, a QRS-complex duration of 130 milliseconds, moderate symptoms, physical findings of congestion, and a blood pressure of 140/80 mm Hg despite treatment with an angiotensin-converting enzyme inhibitor, aldosterone antagonist, and an angiotensin-receptor antagonist.

c. A middle-aged-man with idiopathic dilated cardiomyopathy status post–biventricular pacemaker/ICD insertion who is hypotensive in response to oral medication therapies and requires continuous dobutamine infusion to maintain reasonable renal function but who is having intermittent and still problematic episodes of ventricular tachycardia.

d. A postoperative coronary artery bypass patient who suffers a sudden ischemic event and, though resuscitated, has steadily increasing inotropic requirements, with blood pressure falling to 50 mm Hg despite polypharmacy with inotropic agents and vasopressers. He has not awakened postsurgery, and his mental status is questionable.

e. A 30-year-old woman who develops pulmonary edema 1 week after a normal delivery and is admitted to the coronary care unit with a blood pressure of 90/50, a heart rate of 110 beats/min, atrial fibrillation, and profound respiratory distress. Hepatic and renal function are normal.

Answer is c: Appropriate selection of patients for ventricular assist device insertion as a bridge to transplantation is best described for this patient. This gentleman appears to have had aggressive therapies, including insertion of a biventricular pacemaker/ICD unit, but he remains compromised with hypotension and is inotropic dependent. Ventricular arrhythmias are compromising his current status. Insertion of a ventricular assist device will likely allow withdrawal of the inotrope, restore adequate systemic perfusion, and often in these cases, improve the ventricular arrhythmias as well as other organ function. This would then allow for successful cardiac transplantation. The patient described in (a) is in a very difficult situation, and because of the uncertainties regarding central nervous system integrity after a full cardiac arrest, is not the best candidate for aggressive mechanical circulatory support intervention. Sometimes, in newly presenting patients who are young and otherwise healthy, a temporary percutaneous Biomedicus pump or Biomedicus pump with extracorporeal oxygenation is used to see if the patient will in fact awaken and improve. The patient in (b) appears to be a bit "too well" for heart transplantation, and many things can be done, including insertion of a cardiac resynchronization device and intensification of medical therapies, to lower his blood pressure and treat the heart failure syndrome more optimally. The patient described in (d) resembles, in some ways, the patient described in (a). Using a smaller, less sophisticated temporizing device may be more prudent than implantation of a more permanent, and large, complex pulsatile system. The patient described in (e) is likely a peripartum cardiomyopathy patient who, in all likelihood, will have a reasonable response to medication therapies and correction of her atrial fibrillation. She may require transient intubation, but it is unlikely a device will be required.

**2.** Clinical goals that should be considered when mechanical circulatory support devices are inserted include:

a. Bridge to a more sophisticated bridge
b. Bridge to clinical improvement
c. Permanent implantation without the goal of heart transplant
d. None of the above, as the only consideration is bridge to transplant
e. All of the above

Answer is e: No longer should mechanical circulatory support be considered simply as a bridge to heart transplant. Many options now exist. Mechanical circulatory support devices can be used as a bridge to more sophisticated device implantation. They can also be used as a bridge to clinical improvement that perhaps will allow bridging to transplantation, even bridging the patient to recovery, with device removal or use of the device as a permanent alternative to transplantation.

**3.** A contraindication to mechanical circulatory support device implantation is

a. Systolic blood pressure of 80 mm Hg on dobutamine at 10 $\mu$g/kg/min
b. A serum creatinine of 2.8 mL/dL
c. A platelet count consistently of 75,000
d. Hepatic cirrhosis on liver biopsy, with normal liver enzymes and bilirubin
e. Presence of insulin-requiring diabetes

Answer is d: One of the more feared difficulties after circulatory support device implantation is hepatic failure, which can quickly lead to coagulopathy and systemic organ failure. Even when liver enzymes and bilirubin levels are normal, the finding of hepatic cirrhosis on liver biopsy generally renders a patient at excessive risk for device implantation. This is the sole absolute contraindication included in this question.

**4.** Risk factors for death post–circulatory support device implantation include:

a. Lower platelet count
b. Higher white blood cell count
c. Female sex
d. All of the above
e. None of the above

Answeris d: According to the International Society for Heart and Lung Transplantation Mechanical Circulatory Support Database, female sex contributes to significant risk post–circulatory support device implantation. Reasons for this are not entirely clear, but it is more likely for an advanced female heart failure patient to be allosensetized, which will often prevent bridging to successful transplantation. Women are generally of smaller build, rendering implantation of some of the larger devices more technically challenging, with more frequent pulmonary hypertension.

**5.** The most common complication after mechanical circulatory support device implantation is

a. Neurologic dysfunction
b. Atrial fibrillation
c. Bleeding requiring transfusion
d. Right ventricular dysfunction
e. Systemic infection requiring antibiotics

Answer is e: According to the International Society for Heart and Lung Transplantation Mechanical Circulatory Support Device Registry, systemic infection requiring parenteral antibiotic therapy is the most common complication after device insertion and rises in continuous risk fashion over time (Table 31–9).

# Hypertrophic Cardiomyopathy

32

*Michael S. Chen* *Harry M. Lever*

## PREVALENCE AND DEFINITION

Hypertrophic cardiomyopathy (HCM) is the most common genetic cardiovascular disease (1). The prevalence in the general adult population for people with phenotypic evidence of HCM is estimated at 1 per 500 (2). In young adults, including competitive athletes, HCM is the most common etiology for sudden cardiac death (3,4).

Hypertrophic cardiomyopathy (HCM) has traditionally been defined as myocardial hypertrophy of ≥1.5 cm without an identifiable cause (Figs. 32–1 and 32–2). Other etiologies of increased left ventricular thickness, such as long-standing hypertension and aortic stenosis, as well as rarer causes such as subvalvular stenosis, supravalvular stenosis, amyloidosis, Fabry disease (5), and Friedrich ataxia, must be excluded before diagnosing HCM. HCM is also known as muscular subaortic stenosis (MSS), hypertrophic obstructive cardiomyopathy (HOCM), and idiopathic hypertrophic subaortic stenosis (IHSS). The World Health Organization (WHO) recommends that HCM be used as the term for the disease. As our understanding of the genetics of HCM progresses, HCM will be diagnosed in the future by genetic testing, with echocardiography used to assess the phenotypic manifestations and clinical severity of the disease.

## CLASSIFICATION

HCM can be classified as obstructive or nonobstructive, depending on whether a significant left ventricular outflow tract (LVOT) gradient is present, either at rest or with provocative maneuvers. Most HCM patients do not have LVOT gradients under resting conditions. However, approximately 70% of subjects with HCM have LVOT gradients ≥30 mm Hg at rest or with exercise (6). Obstruction may be either subaortic, caused by systolic anterior motion of the mitral valve leaflet, or mid-cavity, caused by cavity obliteration of the myocardial walls.

Anatomic variants of HCM exist, and these can be categorized based on the location of the hypertrophy (e.g., proximal septal, apical, or diffuse). Apical hypertrophy is also known as Yamaguchi's disease (Fig. 32–3). Additionally, distinct forms of HCM appear to exist, depending on age. Younger patients tend to have reversal of septal curvature and more diffuse hypertrophy (see Fig. 32–1), whereas older patients generally have focal proximal septal hypertrophy (see Fig. 32–2) (7). It is believed that these are two different disease processes. The majority of elderly HCM (diagnosed at >50 years of age) were negative for mutations for HCM, especially when a sigmoid septum was present, whereas younger subjects with HCM were more likely to have mutations for HCM (8).

## PATHOPHYSIOLOGY AND HISTOLOGY

Ventricular hypertrophy usually involves the proximal portion of the interventricular septum. As the septum thickens, it may narrow the outflow tract. In addition, systolic anterior motion of the mitral valve may occur (Fig. 32–4) and result in left ventricular outflow tract obstruction and mitral regurgitation (Fig. 32–5). When systolic anterior motion occurs, the mitral valve leaflets are pulled or dragged anteriorly toward the ventricular septum (9), producing LVOT obstruction. The left ventricle thus must generate higher pressures to overcome the obstruction and to pump blood systemically. Premature closure of the aortic valve

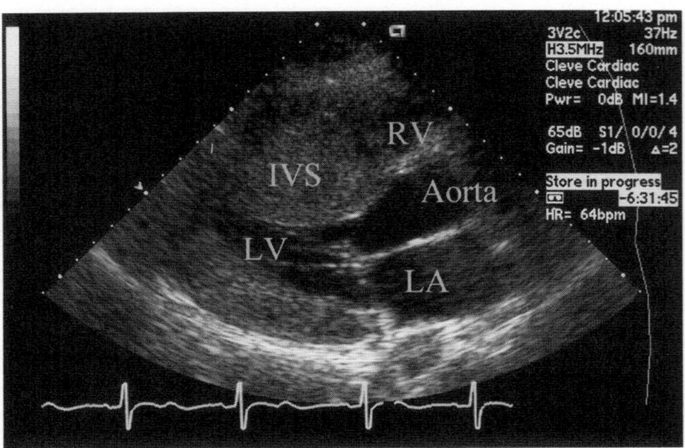


Figure 32–1 Transthoracic echocardiogram of hypertrophic cardiomyopathy in the young—diffuse hypertrophy. Parasternal long-axis view depicts a markedly thickened interventricular septum. The thickening is diffuse, extending from base to beyond the mid-ventricle. LV, left ventricle; RV, right ventricle; LA, left atrium; IVS, interventricular septum.

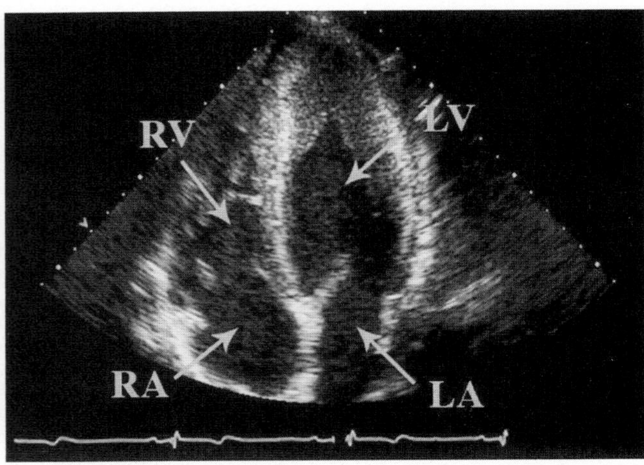


Figure 32–3 Transthoracic echocardiogram of apical variant of hypertrophic cardiomyopathy (Yamaguchi). Apical four-chamber view depicts ventricular thickening of the apex. LV, left ventricle; LA, left atrium; RV, right ventricle; RA, right atrium.

frequently occurs, caused by the decline in pressure distal to the LVOT obstruction.

Dynamic obstruction occurs with HCM, whereas, in contrast, fixed obstruction occurs with aortic stenosis and subvalvular aortic membranes. In dynamic obstruction, the degree of obstruction depends to a larger extent on cardiac contractility and loading conditions, whereas in fixed obstructions, cardiac contractility and preload have little effect on the degree of obstruction. An underfilled left ventricle results in greater obstruction because there is less separation between the interventricular septum and the mitral valve. Augmenting cardiac contractility also increases LVOT obstruction, because a more vigorous contraction is more likely to cause the obstructing components to come into contact. Recently, a systole–diastole mismatch in HCM has been described during dobutamine infusion, in which the systolic period lengthens abnormally and the diastolic period shortens abnormally (10). Consequently, less time exists for coronary filling to occur. This mismatch may contribute to symptoms described with LVOT obstruction.

Histologically, HCM manifests as hypertrophied, disorganized cardiac myocytes present throughout the myocardium. The abnormal cells may take on bizarre shapes, and the connections among cells are often in disarray. Myocardial scarring and growth of the collagen matrix also occur (1). Scarring and disarray may then form the substrate for arrhythmias. These pathologic abnormalities are not necessarily confined to the septum, for areas of the

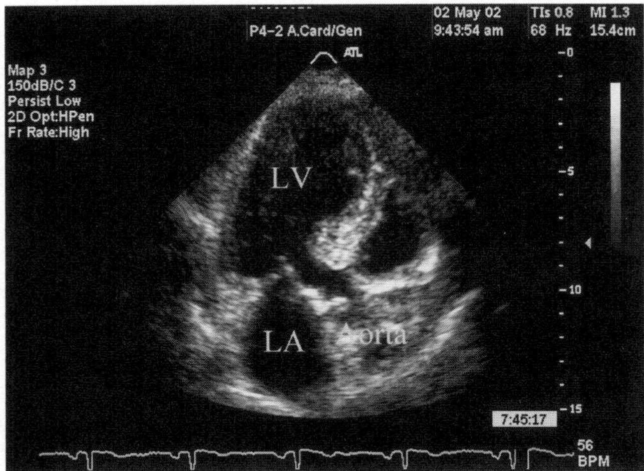


Figure 32–2 Transthoracic echocardiogram of hypertrophic cardiomyopathy in the elderly—proximal septal hypertrophy. Apical three-chamber view depicts focal thickening of the interventricular septum at its base. The mid-ventricle appears to be uninvolved. LV, left ventricle; LA, left atrium.

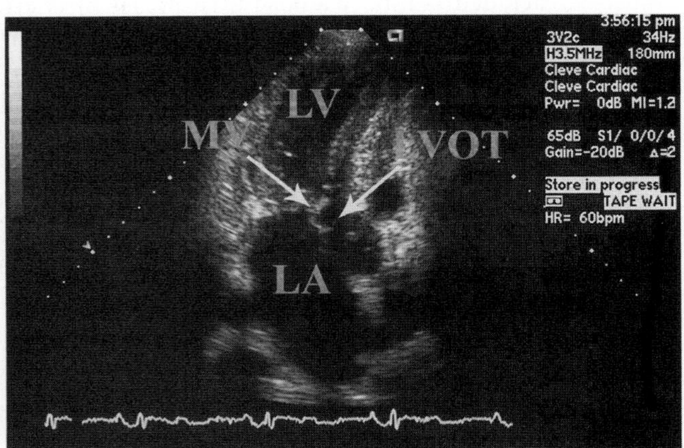


Figure 32–4 Transthoracic echocardiogram of systolic anterior motion of mitral valve. Apical three-chamber view illustrates systolic anterior motion of the mitral valve, resulting in obstruction of the left ventricular outflow tract. LV, left ventricle; LA, left atrium; MV, mitral valve; LVOT, left ventricular outflow tract.

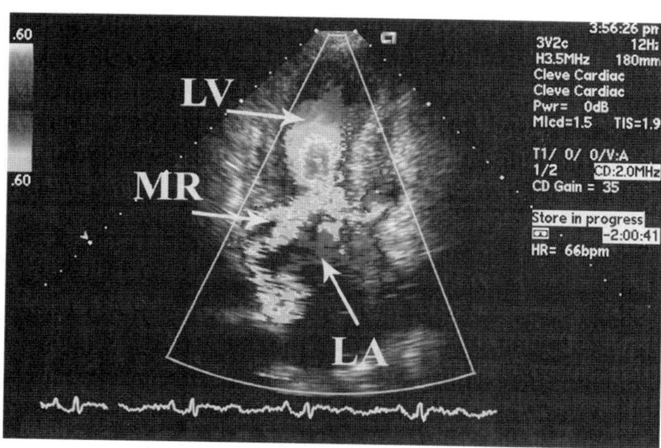


**Figure 32–5** Transthoracic echocardiogram of mitral regurgitation in HCM. Apical three-chamber view illustrates the classic posterolaterally directed mitral regurgitation jet in HCM. The jet direction occurs secondary to systolic anterior motion of the mitral valve. LV, left ventricle; LA, left atrium; MR, mitral regurgitation jet.

heart that appear grossly normal may have these pathologic findings.

## SYMPTOMS AND CLINICAL COURSE

Most patients with HCM are asymptomatic (11). For those HCM patients who develop symptoms, the symptoms do not necessarily correlate with the magnitude of LVOT gradient. For instance, some patients may remain asymptomatic for years with a gradient of 70 mm Hg, whereas others may have severe symptoms with only a 30-mm Hg gradient.

The most common symptom of HCM is dyspnea on exertion. Patients may also complain of chest pain with exertion, syncope or near-syncope, or palpitations. Eating may make symptoms worse because of splanchnic vasodilation and the resulting decrease in systemic vascular resistance (12). Symptoms may be more closely related to diastolic dysfunction (4). With diastolic dysfunction, the increased chamber thickness in HCM results in increased left ventricular stiffness and impaired filling and relaxation. These diastolic abnormalities result in elevated left atrial, left ventricular end-diastolic, and pulmonary pressures. Symptoms may also be caused by mitral regurgitation from systolic anterior motion of the mitral valve, left ventricular outflow tract obstruction, arrhythmias such as atrial fibrillation, and myocardial ischemia.

The clinical course of HCM is variable. In one community cohort, 23% of subjects with HCM had normal life expectancy (13). Other patients may have premature death. Annual mortality rate from HCM is approximately 1% (1). Congestive heart failure and atrial fibrillation may be part of the natural history of HCM. Unfortunately, HCM can also present as sudden cardiac death (SCD). SCD tends to occur in younger patients and may occur during heavy exertion, light exertion, or even at rest. In an unselected, community-based population with HCM, the estimated incidence of SCD is approximately 0.1% to 0.7% per year (14,15).

Subjects with LVOT obstruction (gradient >30 mm Hg) are at increased risk for progression to New York Heart Association (NYHA) Class III–IV symptoms as well as death, when compared to those with no or mild LVOT obstruction (16). However, the magnitude of LVOT obstruction >30 mm Hg does not correlate with increased risk (16).

## PHYSICAL EXAMINATION

The physical examination may provide several clues that suggest HCM. With LVOT obstruction, a harsh systolic murmur exists at the upper sternal border. It is important that this murmur be differentiated from that of mitral regurgitation, which can also be present in HCM secondary to systolic anterior motion of the mitral valve. In contrast, in nonobstructive HCM, there generally is no systolic murmur. Palpation of the carotid pulse aids in distinguishing HCM from aortic stenosis or the presence of a subvalvular aortic membrane. With HCM, little difficulty exists during early systole in ejecting the blood through the LVOT into the aorta; therefore, the carotid upstroke is brisk. As systole progresses, LVOT obstruction occurs, resulting in a collapse in the pulse and then a secondary rise as left ventricular pressure increases to overcome the obstruction. This sign is known as a *bisferiens,* or spike-and-dome, pulse. In contrast, because the fixed obstruction of aortic stenosis or a subvalvular aortic membrane is present during the entire cardiac cycle, the carotid upstroke in these entities is the classic *parvus et tardus* pulse, a carotid pulse with delayed amplitude and upstroke. Therefore, if any patient carrying a diagnosis of HCM has decreased carotid pulses, this should prompt thoughts of a mistaken diagnosis and further investigation into a fixed obstruction of the LVOT.

Unless congestive heart failure has developed, the lungs are clear and the jugular venous pressure is normal. The point of maximal impulse is often forceful and sustained, and a palpable S4 gallop may be present. Occasionally, a bifid apical impulse may be palpated; the first impulse represents forceful atrial contraction and the second impulse represents sustained ventricular contraction.

The classic auscultatory finding for HCM is a crescendo–decrescendo systolic murmur along the left sternal border that increases with the Valsalva maneuver. Almost all cardiac murmurs decrease in intensity during Valsalva, with the exception of HCM, so this maneuver is a crucial part of the cardiac examination if HCM is suspected. The Valsalva maneuver decreases preload, which results in decreased filling of the left ventricle. An underfilled left ventricle results in increased obstruction. Similarly, a change in position from squatting to standing decreases left ventricular

**TABLE 32–1**
**THE RESPONSE IN HCM TO VARIOUS PHYSIOLOGIC AND PHARMACOLOGIC MANEUVERS**

| | Ventricular Volume | LVOT Gradient | Murmur Intensity |
|---|---|---|---|
| Valsalva | Decrease | Increase | Increase |
| Amyl nitrite | Decrease | Increase | Increase |
| Isoproterenol | Decrease | Increase | Increase |
| Hand grip | Increase | Decrease | Decrease |
| Phenylephrine | Increase | Decrease | Decrease |
| Beta-blocker | Increase | Decrease | Decrease |

LVOT, left ventricular outflow tract.

preload and increases the murmur intensity. Finally, amyl nitrite results in vasodilation, decreased preload, and a reflex tachycardia, all of which result in a louder murmur because of greater obstruction. The effect of various physiologic and pharmacologic maneuvers on the intensity of the HCM murmur is illustrated in Table 32–1.

During the cardiac examination, it is also imperative to listen carefully for a mitral regurgitation murmur; such a finding may indicate systolic anterior motion of the mitral valve with accompanying mitral regurgitation. The remainder of the physical examination is generally unremarkable in HCM.

## DIAGNOSTIC TESTING

### Labs, Chest x-Ray and Electrocardiogram

Blood work generally is unremarkable, with the exception of plasma B-type natriuretic peptide (BNP); BNP levels may be elevated, and BNP levels are associated with NYHA functional class (17). The chest x-ray is often normal, because the hypertrophy in HCM involves the ventricular septum. The electrocardiogram (ECG) should show left ventricular hypertrophy. Occasionally, a pseudo-infarct pattern (with Q waves in the anterolateral leads) may be present on ECG. Figure 32–6 illustrates this pseudo-infarct pattern in a patient with HCM, normal left ventricular (LV) systolic function, and no known coronary artery disease. In the apical variant of hypertrophic cardiomyopathy, the ECG may have deep T-wave inversions in the anteroapical leads (Fig. 32–7). Left atrial abnormality may be present if the patient has had long-standing mitral regurgitation from systolic anterior motion of the mitral valve. Atrial fibrillation may also be present.

### Echocardiography

Transthoracic echocardiography (TTE) is currently the primary clinical modality for diagnosing HCM. The septum should be visualized and measured in the parasternal long-axis, apical long-axis, apical four-chamber, and

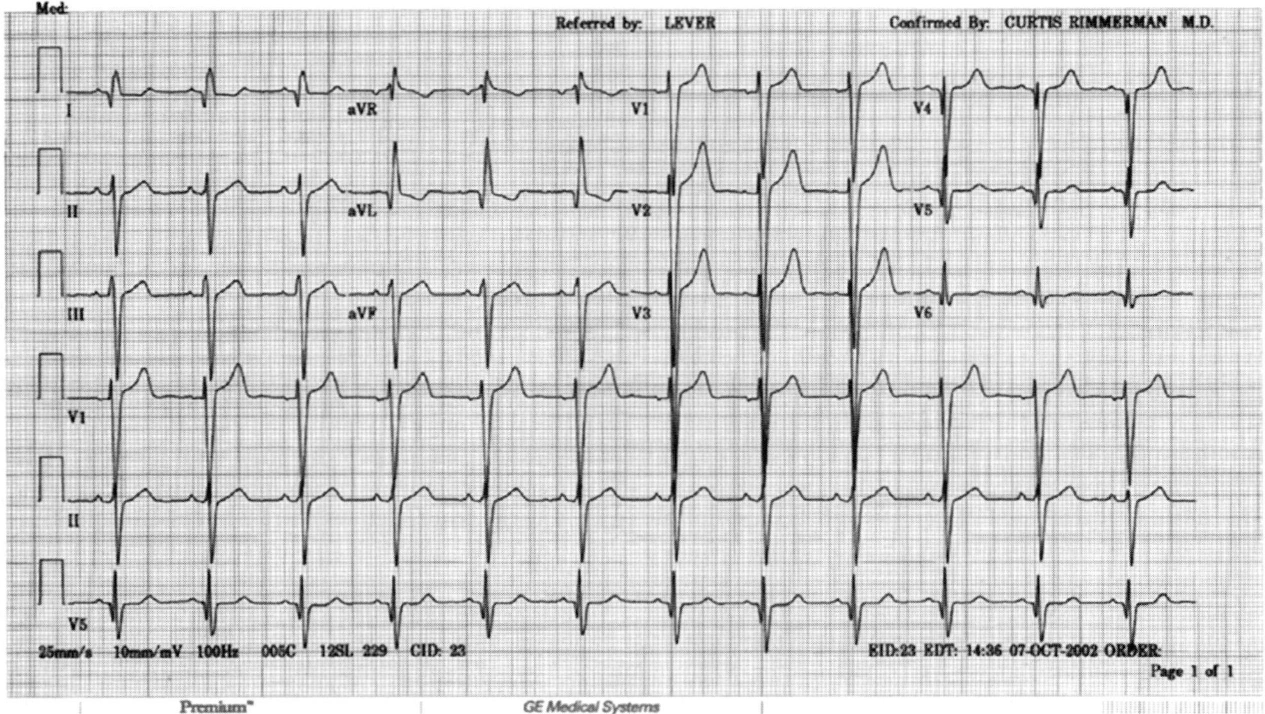


**Figure 32–6** Pseudo-infarct pattern on ECG in HCM. In HCM, a pseudo-infarct pattern (Q waves in lateral leads) may sometimes be noted. This patient had normal left ventricular systolic function and normal coronary arteries.

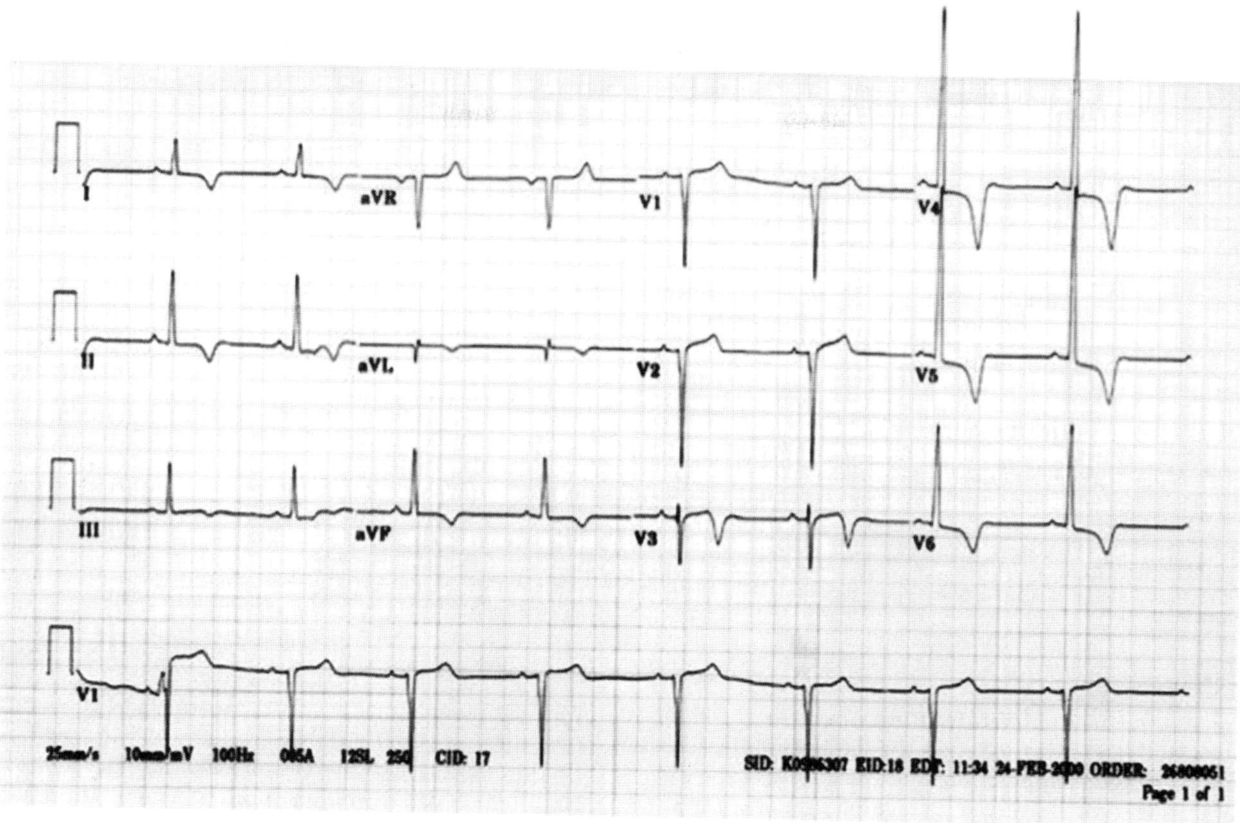


**Figure 32–7** ECG in apical HCM (Yamaguchi). The classic ECG for apical HCM has deep anteroapical T-wave inversions.

parasternal short-axis views. The major diagnostic criterion for HCM is left ventricular wall thickness of ≥15 mm in the absence of other causes for increased ventricular thickness (4). The left ventricle is no-dilated and hyperdynamic. Figures 32–1 and 32–2 are TTE images from HCM patients with marked hypertrophy of the interventricular septum. Figure 32–4 illustrates systolic anterior motion of the mitral valve and resulting LVOT obstruction. During TTE, particular attention should be paid to the septal thickness; location and pattern of hypertrophy; site and magnitude of left ventricular outflow tract obstruction; presence of systolic anterior motion of the mitral valve; and presence of premature closure of the aortic valve.

Some patients have no or minimal resting gradients but develop substantial gradients with exercise. In patients with HCM or suspected HCM, if no resting obstruction is present, subjects should undergo provocative testing during TTE with amyl nitrite, Valsalva, or exercise (treadmill or bicycle) to determine whether latent obstruction exists. Amyl nitrite is a vasodilator that decreases preload to the left ventricle, followed by a compensatory increase in heart rate. Exercise results in an increase in contractility and an increase in heart rate. The physiologic effects of amyl nitrite and exercise thus result in an increase in LVOT gradient. In our experience, supervised exercise stress tests in patients with HCM are safe, with a major complication rate of 0.04% (18). Dobutamine is generally not recommended for the purposes of provoking LVOT gradients, for gradients provoked by dobutamine are of questionable clinical significance (4).

Pulse-wave Doppler should be performed to record left ventricular and left atrial inflows to assess diastolic function. Diastolic abnormalities, which are common in HCM secondary to the thickness and stiffness of the left ventricle, are unfortunately not specific for the diagnosis of HCM. One promising modality is tissue Doppler, which is sensitive for identifying reduced shortening velocities and may help differentiate between HCM and athlete's heart (19), as well as between nonobstructive HCM and hypertensive heart disease with left ventricular hypertrophy (20).

The mitral valve should be interrogated in multiple views to assess for the presence of mitral regurgitation, which is commonly present when systolic anterior motion of the mitral valve leaflet is present (see Fig. 32–4). Systolic anterior motion (SAM) of the mitral valve has a classic appearance in M mode, where the mitral valve leaflets can be seen to approach and often contact the interventricular septum (Fig. 32–8). In HCM, the mitral valve leaflets may be elongated and anterior displacement of the papillary muscles of the mitral valve may occur. With SAM, the mitral

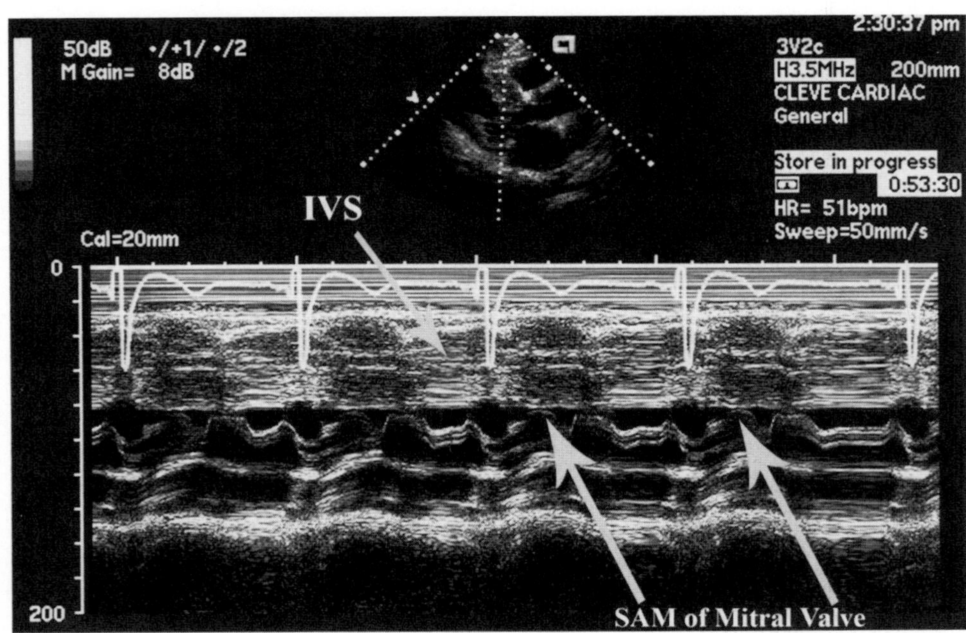


**Figure 32–8** M mode of systolic anterior motion (SAM) of mitral valve in HCM. With SAM of the mitral valve, the mitral leaflet contacts the interventricular septum during systole in a patient with HCM, as illustrated in this transthoracic M-mode echocardiograph. Normally, the mitral leaflets should be well away from the septum during ventricular systole. IVS, interventricular septum; SAM, systolic anterior motion.

regurgitation may range from mild to severe and is posteriorly and laterally directed in the left atrium because of incomplete leaflet apposition (see Fig. 32–5). If the direction of the color jet of mitral regurgitation is central or anterior, then suspicion should be raised for intrinsic abnormalities of the mitral valve.

Fixed obstructions such as aortic stenosis, subvalvular aortic membrane, and supravalvular aortic membrane can result in secondary hypertrophy of the interventricular septum, as distinct from HCM, which is primary hypertrophy of the septum. In aortic stenosis, the aortic valve is calcified and has restricted mobility, whereas in HCM, the obstruction occurs below the aortic valve, and the aortic valve structure and function are preserved. Subvalvular aortic membranes (Fig. 32–9) and supravalvular aortic membranes may be difficult to visualize on TTE, in which case transesophageal echocardiography may need to be performed to assess for the presence of these structures.

Continuous-wave Doppler imaging aids in the differentiation of HCM from fixed obstructions. The modified Bernoulli equation [pressure $= 4 \times (\text{velocity})^2$] is used with the continuous-wave Doppler tracing through the LVOT to calculate the LVOT gradient. Figure 32–10 illustrates the difference between continuous-wave Doppler signals from HCM and from fixed obstructions. During early systole, blood still flows through the LVOT in HCM; however, with continued contraction of the left ventricle, exacerbated by systolic anterior motion of the mitral valve, an outflow tract gradient develops. Thus, with HCM, the continuous Doppler signal classically is described as having a late systolic dagger shape, because the obstruction is late peaking as a result of its dynamic nature. In contrast, a fixed obstruction is present during all of systole. Thus, the continuous-wave Doppler signal for fixed obstructions is a smoother contour that peaks earlier.

The continuous-wave Doppler profile of HCM also must be differentiated from that of mitral regurgitation. The mitral regurgitation jet is generally higher velocity (approximately 6 m/s), whereas the LVOT obstruction jet is often in the 4- to 5-m/s range. The mitral regurgitation velocity tracing also has a smoother, symmetric contour, unlike the dagger-shaped profile of HCM. The mitral regurgitation jet

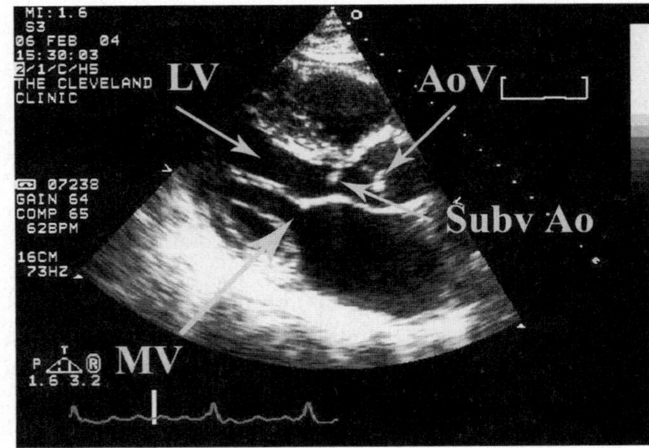


**Figure 32–9** Subvalvular aortic membrane. Subvalvular aortic membranes must be distinguished from HCM, for both can result in a thickened septum and a left ventricular outflow tract gradient. Although subvalvular aortic membranes may sometimes be difficult to visualize by transthoracic echocardiography, in this example a membrane below the aortic valve is clearly seen. LV, left ventricle; MV, mitral valve; AoV, aortic valve; Subv Ao, subvalvular aortic membrane.

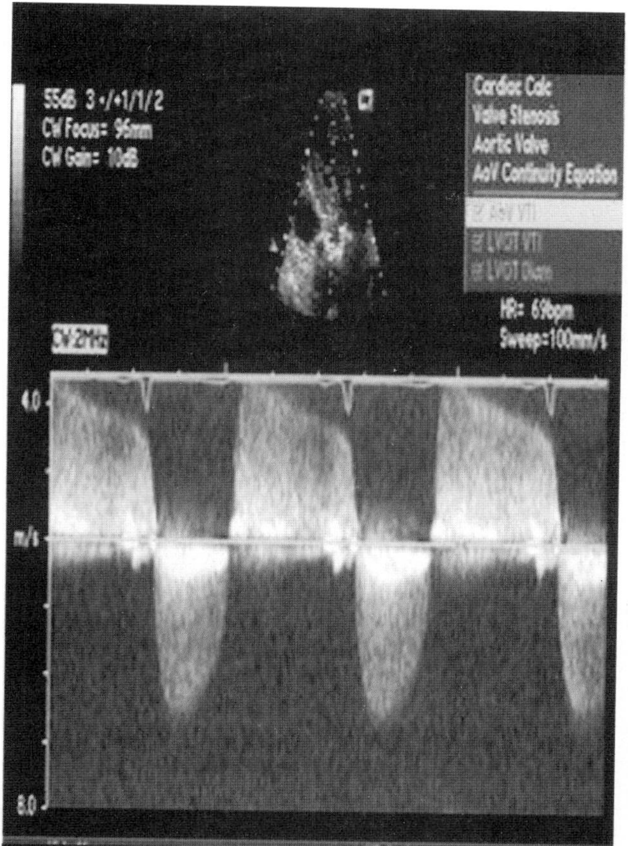


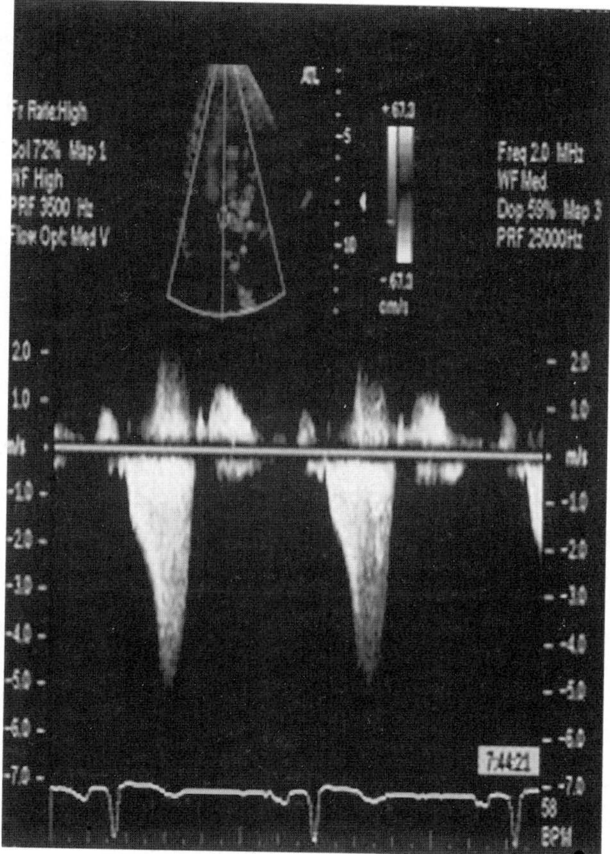


**Figure 32–10** Continuous-wave Doppler profile comparison of aortic stenosis and HCM. Continuous-wave Doppler profiles from transthoracic echocardiography for aortic stenosis **(left)** and HCM **(right)** are illustrated. The Doppler profile in aortic stenosis has a smooth, symmetric contour because the obstruction is fixed, whereas the Doppler profile in HCM has a late-peaking, dagger-shaped appearance as a result of the dynamic nature of the obstruction, with its peak in mid-late systole.

may be late peaking because mitral regurgitation may not occur until systolic anterior motion has occurred, which occurs partway through systole. However, the mitral regurgitation tracing should extend beyond aortic valve closure, up to the point at which mitral forward flow occurs with diastole. In contrast, the LVOT obstruction signal ends at aortic valve closure.

### *Transthoracic Echocardiogram—Distinguishing HCM from Athlete's Heart*

Because preathletic screening is one means by which the diagnosis of HCM is raised, it is imperative to distinguish HCM from athlete's heart. Several findings on echocardiography help distinguish HCM from athlete's heart. In HCM, the septal thickness is usually >15 mm, whereas in an athlete's heart, septal thickness is <15 mm. Left atrial enlargement often occurs with HCM secondary to long-standing mitral regurgitation from systolic anterior motion of the mitral valve and/or diastolic dysfunction, whereas in an athlete's heart, the left atrial size should be normal. The left ventricle should not be dilated in end diastole in HCM, whereas in athletes, it is common for left ventricular end diastolic diameter to be >45 mm. Finally, diastolic dysfunction often exists in HCM as a result of the increased ventricular thickness and stiffness, whereas diastolic function should be normal in athletes. If it is still not certain whether a patient has HCM or athlete's heart, the athlete should stop training; after 3 to 6 months, ventricular hypertrophy will persist with HCM, whereas with athlete's heart, hypertrophy should regress.

## Cardiac Catheterization

Cardiac catheterization has limited utility in diagnosing HCM, for advances in echocardiography have made the latter method the predominant means by which HCM is diagnosed. Right heart catheterization may be performed to measure pulmonary artery pressures, which can then provide information concerning the severity and chronicity of mitral regurgitation. Coronary angiography is indicated prior to septal myectomy if the patient is >40 years old or if coronary artery disease is otherwise suspected, to determine whether concomitant coronary artery bypass graft surgery should be performed. Coronary angiography also needs to be performed prior to alcohol ablation, to delineate the size and course of the septal perforators and ensure that an adequate target exists for alcohol ablation.

Patients with HCM often have no obstructive coronary artery disease. However, they may have thickened vessels and small-vessel disease from increased collagen deposition in the intima and media (1). The mismatch between myocardial oxygen supply and demand, driven primarily by the increased myocardial mass, may then cause myocardial ischemia. Microvascular dysfunction is present in HCM patients and is associated with worse clinical outcomes (21).

The left ventriculogram demonstrates cavity obliteration and a hyperdynamic left ventricle. LVOT gradients can be assessed by positioning a JR4 or multipurpose diagnostic catheter near the left ventricular apex and recording ventricular pressures during slow catheter pullback. A pigtail catheter may not give accurate gradient measurements because there are multiple side holes extending along the distal portion of the catheter, in contrast to the JR4 and multipurpose catheters, which provide true end-hole measurements.

The Brockenbrough response to a premature ventricular contraction (PVC), which suggests HCM, is illustrated in Fig. 32–11. In the beat after a PVC, there is increased filling of the left ventricle from the compensatory pause. The augmented preload results in augmented contractility. In patients with HCM, the increased contractility results in subsequent worsening of the LVOT obstruction. Thus, during the beat after the PVC, there is an increase in left ventricle systolic pressure, a decrease in aortic systolic pressure, and thus an increase in the gradient between left ventricle and aorta. In contrast, in normal subjects, the increased contractility associated with the post-PVC beat results in an increase in *both* left ventricle systolic and aortic systolic pressure, and there is no gradient between the left ventricle and aorta.

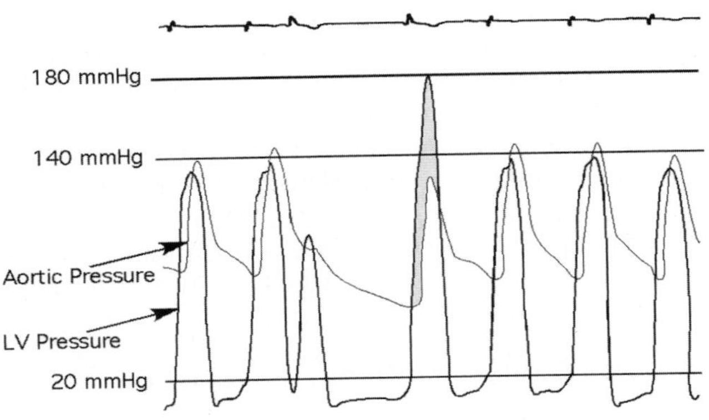


**Figure 32–11** The Brockenbrough response to a premature ventricular contraction (PVC). In normal subjects, a PVC results in a compensatory pause, increased ventricular filling, and subsequent increased cardiac contractility. There is no left ventricle–aortic gradient, either at rest or in the beat post-PVC. The aortic pulse pressure in the beat post-PVC usually increases because of the increased contractility. In contrast, as illustrated in the figure, the Brockenbrough response in the post-PVC beat (fourth beat) suggests HCM. In HCM, the increased contractility occurring with the post-PVC beat results in increased LVOT obstruction and a subsequent increase in the left ventricle–aorta gradient (shaded) as well as decreased aortic pulse pressure during the post-PVC beat.

## GENETICS OF HCM

More than 200 mutations in 10 genes have been identified as causes of HCM (22,23). The mutations associated with HCM are inherited in an autosomal dominant pattern. These mutations primarily involve the myosin, actin, or troponin components of the cardiac sarcomere. The most common mutations that cause HCM involve the $\beta$-myosin heavy chain (chromosome 14), myosin-binding protein C (chromosome 11), and cardiac troponin-T (chromosome 1), which together comprise over half of all of the genotyped HCM patients to date (4). However, having the HCM genotype does not necessarily imply that subjects will have the phenotypic traits of HCM. Variable penetrance exists, and environmental factors as well as modifier genes affect whether a particular subject will manifest HCM phenotypically.

DNA analysis is the most definitive method for diagnosing HCM (4). However, genetic testing remains expensive, time consuming, and not widely available. Results of genetic testing often do not alter management. Although genetic counseling may be considered for HCM patients and their families, we presently do not recommend widespread genetic testing for HCM. Thus, TTE will continue to play a major role in diagnosis of HCM.

One area of promise for genetic testing is in risk stratification for sudden cardiac death in subjects with HCM. Five of the >200 mutations are considered especially malignant in light of their propensity for sudden cardiac death. However, a recent study of 293 HCM patients at the Mayo Clinic assessed the prevalence of these malignant mutations and found that only three patients, or approximately 1%, had one of the malignant mutations for HCM (24).

## SCREENING OF FAMILY MEMBERS

Traditionally, it has been recommended that first-degree relatives of HCM patients be screened on a 12- to 18-month basis, beginning at age 12 years, with a 12-lead electrocardiogram and TTE. The recommended screening interval reflects the fact that latent HCM may be unmasked by growth spurts and subsequent worsening hypertrophy during adolescence. After approximately age 21 years, when growth has ceased, it has been believed that the serial echocardiograms can be discontinued. However, recent evidence of late-onset ventricular hypertrophy occurring well into adulthood has spurred a push toward continuing serial echocardiograms past adolescence and into middle age for HCM relatives (23). It is now recommended that adult relatives of HCM patients undergo screening transthoracic echocardiograms at a minimum of every 5 years.

## THERAPY

Treatment options for HCM include pharmacologic therapy, septal myectomy, percutaneous alcohol septal ablation, and heart transplantation. Additionally, pacemaker implantation has been performed, but randomized trials have indicated a substantial placebo effect.

### Medical Therapy

Treatment with beta-blockers is considered first-line therapy (4). By decreasing contractile force, beta-blockers decrease the outflow gradient during exercise and decrease oxygen demand. Beta-blockers also lengthen diastolic filling by slowing the heart rate, thus improving any component of myocardial ischemia. We generally start patients on metoprolol, 50 mg twice a day, or Toprol XL, 50 mg daily. If the patient continues to be symptomatic, the dose of metoprolol or Toprol XL can be increased further by 25-mg increments every few weeks. Alternative beta-blocker choices include propranolol, 200 to 400 mg/day, nadolol, or atenolol. Beta-blockers improve symptoms (25) and exercise intolerance.

Second-line therapy includes the calcium channel blocker verapamil and the Class IA antiarrhythmic agent disopyramide. Both calcium channel blockers and disopyramide exert a negative inotropic effect and improve ventricular relaxation. The extended-release formulation of verapamil can be started at 240 mg daily and increased by 60 mg every few weeks up to 480 mg daily. Calcium channel blockers have been shown to decrease symptoms in comparison to placebo (25). Verapamil should not be used in patients with severe pulmonary hypertension, because this subgroup may develop excessive vasodilation that worsens LVOT obstruction and cardiac output, resulting in pulmonary edema or even death (26). Diltiazem has been used in HCM patients, but there are few data on its effectiveness.

The extended-release formulation of disopyramide may be started at 150 mg twice a day. Disopyramide improves diastolic function and lowers the LVOT gradient (27). Anticholinergic side effects may occur with disopyramide. Concomitant therapy with beta-blockers is recommended because disopyramide may cause accelerated A–V nodal conduction, which may be deleterious, especially during episodes of atrial fibrillation.

Certain pharmacologic agents should be avoided or used with caution in HCM. Nifedipine, amlodipine, and felodipine should be avoided because they cause peripheral vasodilation, which may result in decreased left ventricular filling and worsening of outflow tract obstruction. Angiotensin-converting enzyme inhibitors and angiotensin-receptor blockers, which also cause peripheral vasodilation, should be avoided. Diuretics, if deemed necessary, should be used cautiously, because subjects with HCM often have stiff ventricles that require high filling pressures. Digoxin is not favored in HCM because its positive inotropic effect may worsen LVOT obstruction.

### Septal Myectomy

Septal myectomy is considered the most definitive treatment for patients with medically refractory, symptomatic, obstructive (resting or latent gradient of 50 mm Hg or more) HCM (4). In contrast, subjects with gradients >50 mm Hg but no or only mild symptoms are generally treated medically until more severe symptoms manifest (4). A subgroup of HCM patients who may be considered for septal myectomy despite the lack of significant symptoms is young patients with marked LVOT obstruction (gradient ≥75 mm Hg) (4). In assessing risk and benefit of septal myectomy, the young age of this subgroup decreases the operative risk. Septal myectomy is not indicated in mid-cavity obstruction.

Septal myectomy involves resecting part of the proximal septum through an aortotomy so that the outflow tract obstruction is lessened (Fig. 32–12). Sometimes myectomy

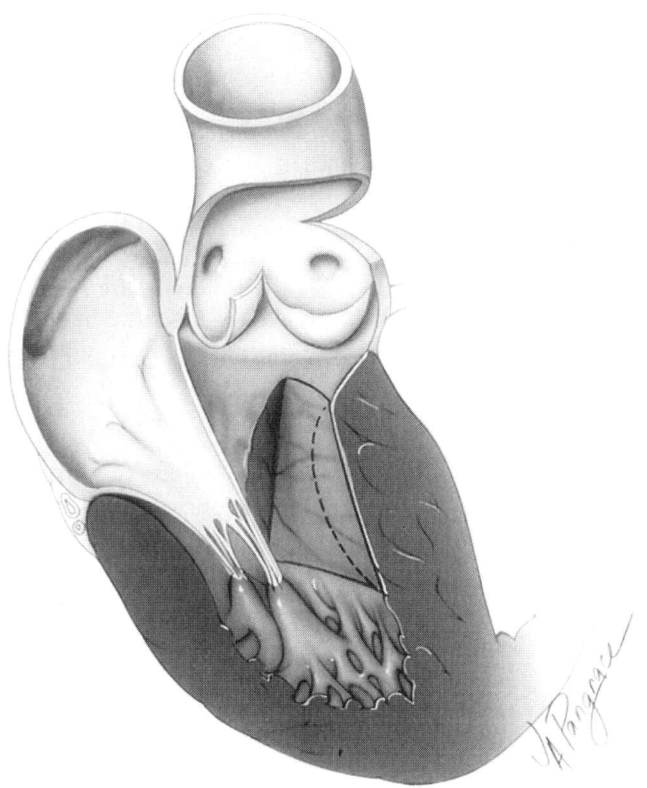

**Figure 32–12** Septal myectomy. Septal myectomy involves resecting a portion of the proximal septum.

may be combined with other cardiac surgery such as coronary artery bypass surgery, mitral valve repair, or mitral valve replacement.

Operative mortality for isolated myectomy is low, at approximately 0 to 4% (28–33). Increasing age and concomitant cardiac procedures may increase the surgical risk. Septal myectomy is associated with high success rates in decreasing LVOT gradients (32,34,35) and in improving symptoms (31–33,35) and exercise capacity (34). Symptom improvement occurs from decreasing the LVOT gradient as well as decreasing the severity of any associated mitral regurgitation. Results postmyectomy are durable. Rarely is reoperation needed secondary to recurrence of LVOT obstruction (4).

Long-term survival in HCM patients undergoing isolated myectomy is 93% to 96% at 5 years and 83% to 87% at 10 years (36,37). Multivariate predictors of overall mortality include age ≥50 years at time of surgery, concomitant coronary artery bypass graft surgery, female gender, history of preoperative atrial fibrillation, and left atrial diameter of ≥46 mm (38). For patients undergoing a myectomy combined with other cardiac surgery, primarily coronary artery bypass graft surgery or valve surgery, 5-year survival was 80% and 10-year survival was also 80% (37).

Retrospective, nonrandomized data suggest that long-term survival for HCM subjects undergoing myectomy does not differ significantly when compared to the age- and sex-matched general population (36). Furthermore, myectomy patients had higher survival rates than obstructive HCM patients who did not undergo surgery (36). Thus, myectomy patients appear to fare no worse than the general population. Although randomized comparisons are needed, nonrandomized data suggest that survival may actually be improved in HCM patients who undergo myectomy (36).

Pre-existing conduction abnormalities influence the likelihood of needing permanent pacemakers postmyectomy. Left bundle branch block is common after surgical myectomy, occurring in 93% of subjects (39). Thus, subjects with pre-existing right bundle branch block are at high risk for requiring a permanent pacemaker postmyectomy. In subjects with normal conduction systems on ECG, there was a 2% rate of permanent pacemaker implantation postmyectomy, whereas for patients with pre-existing conduction abnormalities, there was a 10% incidence of permanent pacemaker implantation (39).

## Percutaneous Alcohol Septal Ablation

For patients with medically refractory HCM and resting or provocative gradients ≥50 mm Hg who are poor surgical candidates or for those who choose not to undergo open heart surgery, alcohol septal ablation is another option. In the late 1990s, unbridled enthusiasm for alcohol ablation resulted in the fact that by 2000, >3,000 alcohol ablations had been performed for HCM, more than the number of myectomies performed since the introduction of myectomies approximately 40 years ago (40). This optimism has been tempered recently, and presently, alcohol ablation is considered second-line therapy behind myectomy for medically refractory, obstructive HCM (41).

Review of the patient's cardiac anatomy is critical in selecting subjects for alcohol ablation. In order for alcohol ablation to succeed, LVOT obstruction needs to be secondary to contact of the mitral valve with the proximal septum. If the LVOT obstruction actually occurs in the mid-distal LV cavity, then alcohol ablation will not be of benefit.

Alcohol septal ablation is performed in the cardiac catheterization laboratory. First, a temporary pacing wire is placed in the right ventricle in case heart block occurs during alcohol ablation. Next a coronary guidewire is advanced into the first major septal perforator (or the perforator that supplies the proximal septum) of the left anterior descending artery and a balloon is inflated in the septal perforator (Fig. 32–13). Prior to alcohol injection, myocardial contrast echocardiography is performed, with injection of contrast through the distal lumen of the coronary balloon and subsequent imaging by transthoracic echocardiography to visualize the amount and location of myocardium supplied by the particular septal perforator. This contrast

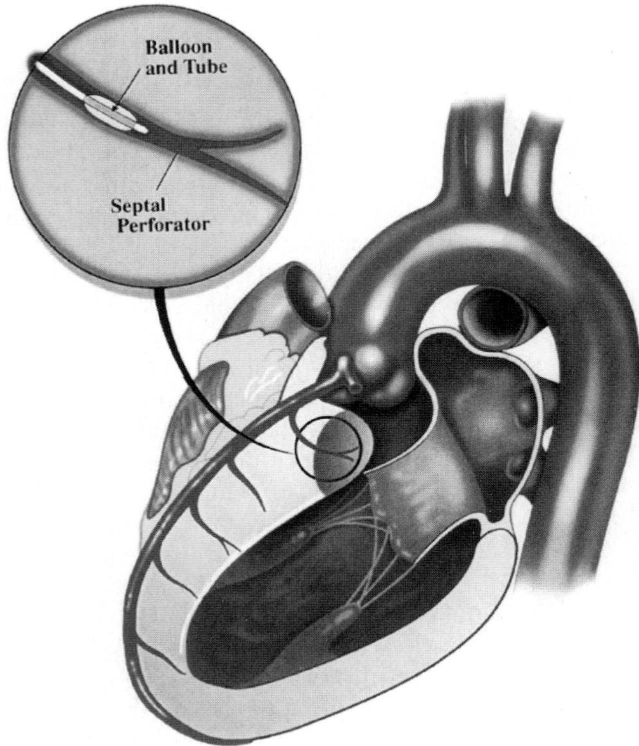


**Figure 32–13** Alcohol septal ablation. In alcohol septal ablation, a balloon is inflated in the proximal septal perforator and alcohol is injected into the septal artery through the distal port of the balloon. The goal is to create a controlled myocardial infarction of the proximal septum, resulting in shrinkage of the septum and lessening of the LVOT obstruction.

injection also helps verify that no leakage is occurring proximal to the inflated balloon in the septal perforator. Any leakage could potentially be disastrous, for it would result in alcohol flowing antegrade in the left anterior descending artery and cause an anterior myocardial infarction.

After verification of the territory supplied by the septal perforator and ruling out any leaks retrograde in the septal perforator, 1 to 3 cc of desiccated ethanol is instilled into the septal perforator through the distal lumen of the balloon. Alcohol acts as a toxic agent to the coronary artery and surrounding myocardium, resulting in a controlled myocardial infarction of the cardiac muscle supplied by the septal perforator. Consequently, the proximal septum shrinks, LVOT obstruction lessens, and any associated systolic anterior motion is also decreased. In comparison with the effects of septal myectomy on LVOT obstruction, which are instantaneous, the effects of alcohol ablation on LVOT obstruction take longer to occur, because necrosis of the proximal septum needs to occur. After alcohol ablation, the patient is observed in the cardiac intensive care unit for 2 days. Creatine kinase (CK) and CK-MB are measured, and CK elevations generally range from 400 to 2,500 units (3% to 10% of the LV or 20% of the septum) (4). Despite the myocardial infarction, global LV function is usually not impaired.

Because of the lack of randomized controlled trials and a suitable control population, alcohol ablation has not been shown to improve survival. Alcohol ablation does result in decreased LVOT gradients (42–45) and an improvement in symptoms (42–45), with persistence of benefit at 2 to 3 years (46). Effectiveness of alcohol ablation extends to include the elderly population (47). There is also a decrease in LV filling pressures (51) and a decrease in septal thickness (44,48). In 3-month follow-up data, we reported a decrease in LVOT gradient from 64 to 28 mm Hg and an improvement in NYHA class from 3.5 to 1.9 after alcohol ablation (44). Predictors of unsatisfactory outcomes after alcohol septal ablation include a residual LVOT gradient after ablation of >25 mm Hg in the cardiac catheterization lab as well as a peak creatinine kinase (CK) of <1,300 U/L (49).

At the Cleveland Clinic, most alcohol ablations have been performed on elderly, suboptimal surgical candidates. We generally prefer that the septum be between 1.8 and 2.5 cm, to provide a safety margin; if the septum is too thick, favorable ablation results may be difficult to attain, whereas if it is too thin, the patient is at higher risk for development of a ventricular septal defect. A septum <1.8 cm thick in a patient with the clinical picture of HCM often indicates that mitral valve abnormalities, such as long leaflets, abnormal insertion of the papillary muscles, or anterior displacement of the mitral valve apparatus may be the primary etiology for the left ventricular outflow tract obstruction. Such mitral valve abnormalities contraindicate alcohol septal ablation.

Complications of alcohol ablation include right bundle branch block (39,45,50), complete heart block (requiring a permanent pacemaker), a large anterior wall myocardial infarction, ventricular tachycardia or fibrillation, and pericarditis. The risks of alcohol ablation include a 2% to 4% procedural mortality rate and a 9% to 27% incidence of patients requiring permanent pacemakers (39,46,48,50–52).

Alcohol ablation, unlike septal myectomy, results in myocardial scar. Thus, a theoretical risk exists that alcohol ablation may increase the risk of sudden cardiac death, especially in light of the fact that an arrhythmogenic substrate is already present with HCM. One study of 71 HCM patients who already had implantable cardioverter-defibrillators for primary prevention of sudden cardiac death and were undergoing alcohol ablation found that alcohol ablation was not proarrhythmic, although they did report an 8% appropriate ICD firing rate at nearly 2 years (53). However, sudden cardiac death has been reported several months after successful alcohol ablation (54).

## Comparison of Septal Myectomy and Alcohol Ablation

Overall, comparisons between myectomy and alcohol ablation indicate that both are effective in reducing LVOT gradient and improving symptoms, but there appears to be a slight advantage to septal myectomy (Table 32–2). A comparison of the two modalities at the Cleveland clinic suggested slight superiority of myectomy on the basis of larger and more consistent reductions in LVOT gradient (44). This nonrandomized study of 51 HCM patients who underwent either myectomy or alcohol ablation found that of the 26 patients who underwent septal myectomy, LVOT gradient was significantly reduced, from 62 mm Hg premyectomy to 7 mm Hg postmyectomy. In the 25 alcohol ablation subjects, LVOT gradient was significantly reduced from 64 mm Hg preablation to 28 mm Hg. New York Heart Association class improved significantly, from 3.3 to 1.5 in the myectomy group and from 3.5 to 1.9 in the alcohol ablation group (44). In our study, five patients underwent myectomy secondary to persistent provocable gradients from alcohol ablation.

Another nonrandomized cohort study of 44 patients found similar improvements in LVOT gradients and NYHA classification after either myectomy or ablation (55). However, in this study, myectomy was noted to have superior results with respect to exercise parameters, including peak oxygen consumption and peak work rate achieved (55).

A third nonrandomized study compared 41 alcohol ablation patients from Baylor to an age- and gradient-matched cohort of myectomy patients performed at the Mayo Clinic (52). The functional and hemodynamic changes after 1 year were similar in the two groups, although the alcohol ablation group did have a significantly higher incidence of permanent pacing (52).

Associated severe coronary artery disease or valvular abnormalities that warrant surgical intervention are factors that further tip the balance toward myectomy over alcohol

**TABLE 32–2**
**COMPARISON OF SEPTAL MYECTOMY AND PERCUTANEOUS ALCOHOL SEPTAL ABLATION**

| | Surgical Myectomy | Percutaneous Alcohol Septal Ablation |
|---|---|---|
| Invasiveness | Invasive | Noninvasive |
| Onset of reduction in LVOT gradient | Instantaneous | Some effect instantly, but more often 6–12 mo for full effect |
| Procedural mortality (4,40) | 1–2% | 1–2% |
| Effect on LVOT gradient (4,40) | Decreases to <10 mm Hg | Decreases to <25 mm Hg |
| Conduction abnormality postprocedure (41,53) | Left bundle branch block | Right bundle branch block |
| Recovery time | 1 wk | A few days |
| Need for permanent pacemaker—all patients (41,48,53) | 3–10% | 12–27% |
| Need for permanent pacemaker if no pre-existing conduction abnormalities (41) | 2% | 13% |
| Length of follow-up | 30–40 y | 6–8 y |
| Success rate | >95% | >85% |

LVOT, left ventricular outflow tract.

ablation, for concomitant cardiac surgery can be performed at the time of myectomy. It is crucial to completely assess the degree and etiology of any mitral regurgitation that exists. A subject with HCM and severe mitral regurgitation secondary to SAM could potentially be a candidate for either septal myectomy or alcohol ablation if the primary abnormality is the septal thickness, and it is believed that reducing the septal thickness will alleviate the SAM. In contrast, a subject with HCM and severe mitral regurgitation secondary to intrinsic valvular abnormalities would not be a good candidate for alcohol ablation because in this instance, decreasing the septal thickness would not affect the intrinsic etiology for the mitral regurgitation and the mitral regurgitation would remain even after alcohol ablation.

### Permanent Pacemaker Implantation

Pacemaker implantation has been used historically to alleviate the symptoms of HCM, but this procedure has fallen out of favor. It was hypothesized that initiating ventricular contraction at the right ventricular apex and distal septum would alter the sequence of ventricular contraction such that the outflow gradient would be decreased and symptoms improved.

Although initial nonrandomized, unblinded studies reported symptomatic improvement, subsequent double-blind, randomized crossover trials with dual-chamber pacing demonstrated no significant change in exercise capacity but a small decrease in LVOT gradient (56,57). In addition, patients both with and without active pacing noted subjective improvement in exercise capacity. Thus, placebo effect accounts for the improvement in symptoms attributed to pacemakers (57). Furthermore, in a nonrandomized, concurrent cohort study, 39 patients either underwent surgical myectomy or received permanent pacemakers (58). Surgical myectomy was unquestionably superior in this study, with larger decreases in LVOT gradient (76 to 9 mm Hg versus 77 to 55 mm Hg) and larger improvements in symptoms and exercise duration than permanent pacing (58).

American College of Cardiology/American Heart Association (ACC/AHA) guidelines consider pacemaker implantation for medically refractory, symptomatic HCM with a significant LVOT gradient to be a Class IIb indication (59). Class IIb means there is conflicting evidence for the particular intervention, and its usefulness and efficacy is less well established by the available evidence and expert opinion. We do not recommend a permanent pacemaker specifically for treatment of HCM.

## INFECTIVE ENDOCARDITIS PROPHYLAXIS

According to ACC/AHA guidelines, patients with HCM should receive prophylactic antibiotics for endocarditis prior to dental or invasive procedures (60). Turbulent flow through the LVOT striking the aortic valve as well as mitral regurgitation from systolic anterior motion of the mitral valve predispose to infective endocarditis. The site of infection most commonly is the thickened anterior mitral valve leaflet (4). One study found that in 810 patients evaluated for HCM, infective endocarditis occurred in eight patients (61). Infective endocarditis occurred only in HCM subjects with LVOT obstruction, and the presence of mitral valve abnormalities, manifest as atrial dilation, also predisposed to endocarditis (61).

## SUDDEN CARDIAC DEATH

The most serious complication of HCM is sudden cardiac death (SCD), with an incidence of 0.1% to 0.7% per year (14,15). The first presentation of HCM may be SCD, generally from ventricular arrhythmias. Among subjects with HCM, SCD is more common in adolescents and young adults (62), but it can occur at any age.

Holter monitors have been recommended as a means of risk stratification for primary prevention of SCD. Ventricular arrhythmias are very common, with 88% of HCM patients having premature ventricular contractions and 31% of HCM patients having nonsustained ventricular tachycardia on 24-hour Holter monitoring (63). Nonsustained ventricular tachycardia had a 95% negative predictive value and 9% positive predictive value for sudden cardiac death (63). Thus, the absence of nonsustained ventricular tachycardia on 24-hour Holter is reassuring, but if it is present, such a finding is nonspecific. Electrophysiologic testing has not been shown to be predictive of SCD in HCM, and presently has little role in risk stratification in HCM (4).

A survivor of SCD warrants an implantable cardioverter-defibrillator (ICD). Primary prevention of SCD in HCM patients is not as well defined. An ICD firing rate of 11% per year has been reported in ICDs implanted for secondary prevention and 5% per year when implanted for primary prevention of SCD (64). ACC/AHA/North American Society of Pacing and Electrophysiology 2002 guidelines designate ICD implantation for secondary prevention to be a Class I indication, whereas ICD implantation for primary prevention in HCM is a Class IIb indication (59). Antiarrhythmic therapy for primary prevention generally is not recommended in asymptomatic patients.

Major risk factors for SCD in HCM include a left ventricular wall thickness >30 mm (65); prolonged or repetitive episodes of nonsustained ventricular tachycardia on Holter monitor (66); family history of SCD; no change or a decrease in blood pressure with exercise (67); and syncope or nearsyncope (68,69). A LVOT gradient of ≥30 mm Hg is considered a minor risk factor for SCD (16). It has been suggested that HCM patients with two or more major risk factors should receive an ICD for primary prevention, and those with one major risk factor should be considered on an individualized basis.

Genotype testing holds great promise in risk stratification for primary prevention of SCD. For example, some $\beta$-myosin heavy-chain mutations are associated with a higher incidence, whereas certain mutations in myosin-binding protein C and $\alpha$-tropomyosin are associated with a more favorable prognosis (22). However, presently, genetic testing will generally not alter management in the prevention of SCD.

## HCM AND ATHLETICS

Patients with HCM should be restricted from competitive athletics or strenuous athletic activity because of the risk for SCD (70,71). Low-level exercise is acceptable.

## ATRIAL FIBRILLATION AND HCM

Atrial fibrillation, which occurs in 28% of HCM subjects, is the most prevalent sustained arrhythmia in HCM (14). HCM subjects with atrial fibrillation have lower long-term survival rates compared to those in sinus rhythm (14,72). One study attributed the lower survival to an excess of heart failure-related deaths as opposed to sudden cardiac death (72). A specific $\beta$-myosin heavy-chain mutation, Arg663 His mutation, has been associated with an increased incidence of atrial fibrillation (73).

Atrial fibrillation is a significant cause of morbidity in HCM. Strokes occur in 6% of subjects with HCM, nearly all of whom have atrial fibrillation (74). Medical treatment of persistent atrial fibrillation in HCM includes anticoagulation with warfarin and rate control, preferably with beta-blockers.

HCM patients who develop atrial fibrillation may present with acute clinical deterioration. The hypertrophied ventricle is stiff and may require atrial contraction for optimal filling. Losing the atrial contribution to ventricular filling may result in decreased cardiac output and potentially pulmonary edema. The substantial morbidity and increased mortality associated with atrial fibrillation in the setting of HCM justifies an aggressive approach to attempting to maintain sinus rhythm.

One should attempt to restore normal sinus rhythm with direct-current cardioversion and/or antiarrhythmic agents. If atrial fibrillation has been present for >48 hours or the duration of atrial fibrillation is uncertain, then one of two approaches may be undertaken. Transesophageal echocardiogram (TEE) may be performed to ensure that there is no left atrial or left atrial appendage clot, and if clot is absent, then, in the presence of therapeutic anticoagulation, electrical or chemical attempts at restoring sinus rhythm may be performed. Alternatively, anticoagulation with warfarin for at least 4 weeks may be performed prior to any electrical or chemical attempts at restoration of sinus rhythm. The second alternative does not warrant TEE prior to cardioversion. However, HCM patients often tolerate atrial fibrillation poorly, and expeditious TEE followed by electrical cardioversion is generally the preferred approach. Amiodarone or sotalol is the preferred therapy for pharmacologic conversion to sinus rhythm or maintenance of sinus rhythm in HCM patients. Digoxin should be avoided in HCM patients, particularly in those with resting or latent obstruction, because of its positive inotropic effect. Atrial fibrillation ablation or a maze procedure may be considered for those with refractory, highly symptomatic atrial fibrillation. In a small number of patients with severe HCM and atrial fibrillation, we have performed combined maze-myectomy procedures (75).

## HCM AND PREGNANCY

Although pregnant women with HCM are at slightly higher risk for maternal or fetal complications than the average pregnant woman, the absolute morbidity and mortality rate for pregnant women with HCM is low (76,77). Generally, such women do not need to undergo Caesarean section and can deliver vaginally. Adequate fluid intake during pregnancy should be emphasized in pregnant women with HCM, to ensure that the left ventricle does not become underfilled.

## NONOBSTRUCTIVE HCM

Nonobstructive HCM is diagnosed when there is ventricular thickness of >15 mm in the absence of other etiologies, and when no significant LVOT obstruction exists (i.e., LVOT gradient <30 mm Hg with provocation). Approximately 30% of HCM patients do not have LVOT obstruction. Provocative maneuvers used to exclude latent obstruction include Valsalva, amyl nitrite, and exercise. Because some patients have difficulty performing a Valsalva, we generally challenge patients with amyl nitrite when we are trying to exclude latent obstruction.

The treatment of patients with nonobstructive hypertrophic cardiomyopathy is difficult and less effective than in those with obstructive disease. Pharmacologic therapy is the primary modality of treatment. Beta-blockers may be used to control heart rate and decrease contractility, and calcium channel blockers may improve diastolic function. Alcohol ablation and septal myectomy are not performed in subjects who do not have LVOT obstruction. Over time, hypertrophic cardiomyopathy may become "burned out" and evolve into a picture similar to a dilated cardiomyopathy, with decreased left ventricular systolic function and a dilated left ventricle. Such a subset comprises approximately 5% of all HCM subjects (4). In patients with symptoms and signs of congestive heart failure, standard heart failure therapy such as beta-blockers, diuretics, ACE inhibitors, and digoxin may be necessary. Heart transplantation is an option for end-stage nonobstructive HCM.

## CONCLUSIONS

HCM is the most common genetic cardiovascular disorder and the most common cause of SCD in young adults. A harsh systolic murmur along the left sternal border that increases with Valsalva in conjunction with brisk carotid upstrokes strongly suggests HCM. Transthoracic echocardiography is presently the preferred modality for diagnosing HCM, although in the near future, HCM may be diagnosed by genetic testing. Beta-blockers are first-line medical therapy for HCM, with verapamil and disopyramide as alternatives. Septal myectomy is first-line therapy for obstructive HCM (generally, LVOT gradient >50 mm Hg) that is refractory to medical therapy, whereas alcohol septal ablation should be reserved for subjects with obstructive HCM that is refractory to medical therapy who are deemed poor operative candidates. Our armamentarium of therapeutic options for HCM is associated with high success rates in improving symptoms and decreasing LVOT gradients in combination with low mortality rates.

## REFERENCES


1. Maron BJ. Hypertrophic cardiomyopathy: a systematic review. *JAMA*. 2002;287:1308–1320.
2. Maron BJ, Gardin JM, Flack JM, et al. Prevalence of hypertrophic cardiomyopathy in a general population of young adults. Echocardiographic analysis of 4111 subjects in the CARDIA Study. Coronary Artery Risk Development in (Young) Adults. *Circulation*. 1995;92:785–789.
3. Maron BJ, Shirani J, Poliac LC, et al. Sudden death in young competitive athletes. Clinical, demographic, and pathological profiles. *JAMA*. 1996;276:199–204.
4. Maron BJ, McKenna WJ, Danielson GK, et al. American College of Cardiology/European Society of Cardiology clinical expert consensus document on hypertrophic cardiomyopathy. A report of the American College of Cardiology Foundation Task Force on Clinical Expert Consensus Documents and the European Society of Cardiology Committee for Practice Guidelines. *J Am Coll Cardiol*. 2003;42:1687–1713.
5. Chimenti C, Pieroni M, Morgante E, et al. Prevalence of Fabry disease in female patients with late-onset hypertrophic cardiomyopathy. *Circulation*. 2004;110:1047–1053.
6. Maron MS, Olivotto I, Zenovich AG, et al. Evidence that hypertrophic cardiomyopathy is a disease characterized by predominantly left ventricular outflow tract obstruction. *J Am Coll Cardiol*. 2005;45(suppl A).
7. Lever HM, Karam RF, Currie PJ, et al. Hypertrophic cardiomyopathy in the elderly. Distinctions from the young based on cardiac shape. *Circulation*. 1989;79:580–589.
8. Binder JA, Ommen SR, Gersh BJ, et al. Echocardiography-Guided Genetic Testing in Hypertrophic Cardiomyopathy: Septal Morphological Features Predict the Presence of Myofilament Mutations. *Mayo Clin Proc*. 2006;81(4):459–467.
9. Sherrid MV, Chu CK, Delia E, et al. An echocardiographic study of the fluid mechanics of obstruction in hypertrophic cardiomyopathy. *J Am Coll Cardiol*. 1993;22:816–825.
10. Arshad W, Duncan AM, Francis DP, et al. Systole-diastole mismatch in hypertrophic cardiomyopathy is caused by stress induced left ventricular outflow tract obstruction. *Am Heart J*. 2004; 148:903–909.
11. Spirito P, Seidman CE, McKenna WJ, et al. The management of hypertrophic cardiomyopathy. *N Engl J Med*. 1997;336:775–785.
12. Gilligan DM, Chan WL, Ang EL, et al. Effects of a meal on hemodynamic function at rest and during exercise in patients with hypertrophic cardiomyopathy. *J Am Coll Cardiol*. 1991;18: 429–436.
13. Maron BJ, Casey SA, Hauser RG, et al. Clinical course of hypertrophic cardiomyopathy with survival to advanced age. *J Am Coll Cardiol*. 2003;42:882–888.
14. Cecchi F, Olivotto I, Montereggi A, et al. Hypertrophic cardiomyopathy in Tuscany: clinical course and outcome in an unselected regional population. *J Am Coll Cardiol*. 1995;26:1529–1536.
15. Maron BJ, Casey SA, Poliac LC, et al. Clinical course of hypertrophic cardiomyopathy in a regional United States cohort. *JAMA*. 1999;281:650–655.

16. Maron MS, Olivotto I, Betocchi S, et al. Effect of left ventricular outflow tract obstruction on clinical outcome in hypertrophic cardiomyopathy. *N Engl J Med*. 2003;348:295–303.
17. Maron BJ, Tholakanahalli VN, Zenovich AG, et al. Usefulness of B-type natriuretic peptide assay in the assessment of symptomatic state in hypertrophic cardiomyopathy. *Circulation*. 2004; 109:984–989.
18. Drinko JK, Nash PJ, Lever HM, et al. Safety of stress testing in patients with hypertrophic cardiomyopathy. *Am J Cardiol*. 2004; 93:1443–1444, A12.
19. Rajiv C, Vinereanu D, Fraser AG. Tissue Doppler imaging for the evaluation of patients with hypertrophic cardiomyopathy. *Curr Opin Cardiol*. 2004;19:430–436.
20. Kato TS, Noda A, Izawa H, et al. Discrimination of nonobstructive hypertrophic cardiomyopathy from hypertensive left ventricular hypertrophy on the basis of strain rate imaging by tissue Doppler ultrasonography. *Circulation*. 2004;110:3808–3814.
21. Cecchi F, Olivotto I, Gistri R, et al. Coronary microvascular dysfunction and prognosis in hypertrophic cardiomyopathy. *N Engl J Med*. 2003;349:1027–1035.
22. Seidman JG, Seidman C. The genetic basis for cardiomyopathy: from mutation identification to mechanistic paradigms. *Cell*. 2001;104:557–567.
23. Maron BJ, Seidman JG, Seidman CE. Proposal for contemporary screening strategies in families with hypertrophic cardiomyopathy. *J Am Coll Cardiol*. 2004;44:2125–2132.
24. Ackerman MJ, VanDriest SL, Ommen SR, et al. Prevalence and age-dependence of malignant mutations in the beta-myosin heavy chain and troponin T genes in hypertrophic cardiomyopathy: a comprehensive outpatient perspective. *J Am Coll Cardiol*. 2002;39:2042–2048.
25. Gilligan DM, Chan WL, Joshi J, et al. A double-blind, placebo-controlled crossover trial of nadolol and verapamil in mild and moderately symptomatic hypertrophic cardiomyopathy. *J Am Coll Cardiol*. 1993;21:1672–1679.
26. Wigle ED, Rakowski H, Kimball BP, et al. Hypertrophic cardiomyopathy. Clinical spectrum and treatment. *Circulation*. 1995; 92:1680–1692.
27. Matsubara H, Nakatani S, Nagata S, et al. Salutary effect of disopyramide on left ventricular diastolic function in hypertrophic obstructive cardiomyopathy. *J Am Coll Cardiol*. 1995;26:768–775.
28. Heric B, Lytle BW, Miller DP, et al. Surgical management of hypertrophic obstructive cardiomyopathy. Early and late results. *J Thorac Cardiovasc Surg*. 1995;110:195–206; discussion 206–208.
29. Merrill WH, Friesinger GC, Graham TP Jr, et al. Long-lasting improvement after septal myectomy for hypertrophic obstructive cardiomyopathy. *Ann Thorac Surg*. 2000;69:1732–1735; discussion 1735–1736.
30. Robbins RC, Stinson EB. Long-term results of left ventricular myotomy and myectomy for obstructive hypertrophic cardiomyopathy. *J Thorac Cardiovasc Surg*. 1996;111:586–594.
31. McCully RB, Nishimura RA, Tajik AJ, et al. Extent of clinical improvement after surgical treatment of hypertrophic obstructive cardiomyopathy. *Circulation*. 1996;94:467–471.
32. ten Berg JM, Suttorp MJ, Knaepen PJ, et al. Hypertrophic obstructive cardiomyopathy. Initial results and long-term follow-up after Morrow septal myectomy. *Circulation*. 1994;90:1781–1785.
33. Schulte HD, Borisov K, Gams E, et al. Management of symptomatic hypertrophic obstructive cardiomyopathy—long-term results after surgical therapy. *Thorac Cardiovasc Surg*. 1999;47:213–218.
34. Redwood DR, Goldstein RE, Hirshfeld J, et al. Exercise performance after septal myotomy and myectomy in patients with obstructive hypertrophic cardiomyopathy. *Am J Cardiol*. 1979;44: 215–220.
35. Mohr R, Schaff HV, Danielson GK, et al. The outcome of surgical treatment of hypertrophic obstructive cardiomyopathy. Experience over 15 years. *J Thorac Cardiovasc Surg*. 1989;97:666–674.
36. Ommen SR, Olivotto I, Maron MS, et al. Long-term effects of surgical myectomy on survival in patients with obstructive hypertrophic cardiomyopathy. *J Am Coll Cardiol*. 2005;46:470–476.
37. Minami K, Boethig D, Woltersdorf H, et al. Long term follow-up of surgical treatment of hypertrophic obstructive cardiomyopathy (HOCM): the role of concomitant cardiac procedures. *Eur J Cardiothorac Surg*. 2002;22:206–210.
38. Woo A, Williams WG, Choi R, et al. Clinical and echocardiographic determinants of long-term survival after surgical myectomy in obstructive hypertrophic cardiomyopathy. *Circulation*. 2005;111:2033–2041.
39. Qin JX, Shiota T, Lever HM, et al. Conduction system abnormalities in patients with obstructive hypertrophic cardiomyopathy following septal reduction interventions. *Am J Cardiol*. 2004;93: 171–175.
40. Maron BJ. Role of alcohol septal ablation in treatment of obstructive hypertrophic cardiomyopathy. *Lancet*. 2000;355:425–426.
41. Maron BJ, Dearani JA, Ommen SR, et al. The case for surgery in obstructive hypertrophic cardiomyopathy. *J Am Coll Cardiol*. 2004; 44:2044–2053.
42. Knight C, Kurbaan AS, Seggewiss H, et al. Nonsurgical septal reduction for hypertrophic obstructive cardiomyopathy: outcome in the first series of patients. *Circulation*. 1997;95:2075–2081.
43. Lakkis NM, Nagueh SF, Dunn JK, et al. Nonsurgical septal reduction therapy for hypertrophic obstructive cardiomyopathy: one-year follow-up. *J Am Coll Cardiol*. 2000;36:852–855.
44. Qin JX, Shiota T, Lever HM, et al. Outcome of patients with hypertrophic obstructive cardiomyopathy after percutaneous transluminal septal myocardial ablation and septal myectomy surgery. *J Am Coll Cardiol*. 2001;38:1994–2000.
45. Shamim W, Yousufuddin M, Wang D, et al. Nonsurgical reduction of the interventricular septum in patients with hypertrophic cardiomyopathy. *N Engl J Med*. 2002;347:1326–1333.
46. Faber L, Meissner A, Ziemssen P, et al. Percutaneous transluminal septal myocardial ablation for hypertrophic obstructive cardiomyopathy: long term follow up of the first series of 25 patients. *Heart*. 2000;83:326–331.
47. Gietzen FH, Leuner CJ, Obergassel L, et al. Transcoronary ablation of septal hypertrophy for hypertrophic obstructive cardiomyopathy: feasibility, clinical benefit, and short term results in elderly patients. *Heart*. 2004;90:638–644.
48. Gietzen FH, Leuner CJ, Raute-Kreinsen U, et al. Acute and long-term results after transcoronary ablation of septal hypertrophy (TASH). Catheter interventional treatment for hypertrophic obstructive cardiomyopathy. *Eur Heart J*. 1999;20:1342–1354.
49. Chang SM, Lakkis NM, Franklin J, et al. Predictors of outcome after alcohol septal ablation therapy in patients with hypertrophic obstructive cardiomyopathy. *Circulation*. 2004;109:824–82.
50. Talreja DR, Nishimura RA, Edwards WD, et al. Alcohol septal ablation versus surgical septal myectomy: comparison of effects on atrioventricular conduction tissue. *J Am Coll Cardiol*. 2004;44: 2329–232.
51. Seggewiss H, Faber L, Gleichmann U. Percutaneous transluminal septal ablation in hypertrophic obstructive cardiomyopathy. *Thorac Cardiovasc Surg*. 1999;47:94–100.
52. Nagueh SF, Ommen SR, Lakkis NM, et al. Comparison of ethanol septal reduction therapy with surgical myectomy for the treatment of hypertrophic obstructive cardiomyopathy. *J Am Coll Cardiol*. 2001;38:1701–1706.
53. Crawford FA, Killip D, Franklin J, et al. Implantable cardioverter-defibrillators for primary prevention of sudden cardiac death in patients with hypertrophic obstructive cardiomyopathy after alcohol ablation. *Circulation*. 2003;108:386–387.
54. Hirata K, Wake M, Asato H, et al. Sudden death of a case of hypertrophic obstructive cardiomyopathy 19 months after successful percutaneous transluminal septal myocardial ablation. *Circ J*. 2003;67:559–561.
55. Firoozi S, Elliott PM, Sharma S, et al. Septal myotomy-myectomy and transcoronary septal alcohol ablation in hypertrophic obstructive cardiomyopathy. A comparison of clinical, haemodynamic and exercise outcomes. *Eur Heart J*. 2002;23:1617–1624.
56. Nishimura RA, Trusty JM, Hayes DL, et al. Dual-chamber pacing for hypertrophic cardiomyopathy: a randomized, double-blind, crossover trial. *J Am Coll Cardiol*. 1997;29:435–441.
57. Maron BJ, Nishimura RA, McKenna WJ, et al. Assessment of permanent dual-chamber pacing as a treatment for drug-refractory symptomatic patients with obstructive hypertrophic cardiomyopathy. A randomized, double-blind, crossover study (M-PATHY). *Circulation*. 1999;99:2927–2933.
58. Ommen SR, Nishimura RA, Squires RW, et al. Comparison of dual-chamber pacing versus septal myectomy for the treatment of

patients with hypertropic obstructive cardiomyopathy: a comparison of objective hemodynamic and exercise end points. *J Am Coll Cardiol.* 1999;34:191–196.
59. Gregoratos G, Abrams J, Epstein AE, et al. ACC/AHA/NASPE 2002 guideline update for implantation of cardiac pacemakers and antiarrhythmia devices—summary article: a report of the American College of Cardiology/American Heart Association Task Force on Practice Guidelines (ACC/AHA/NASPE Committee to Update the 1998 Pacemaker Guidelines). *J Am Coll Cardiol.* 2002;40:1703–1719.
60. Bonow RO, Carabello B, de Leon AC, et al. ACC/AHA guidelines for the management of patients with valvular heart disease. executive summary. a report of the American College of Cardiology/American Heart Association Task Force on Practice Guidelines (Committee on Management of Patients with Valvular Heart Disease). *J Heart Valve Dis.* 1998;7:672–707.
61. Spirito P, Rapezzi C, Bellone P, et al. Infective endocarditis in hypertrophic cardiomyopathy: prevalence, incidence, and indications for antibiotic prophylaxis. *Circulation.* 1999;99:2132–2137.
62. Maron BJ, Olivotto I, Spirito P, et al. Epidemiology of hypertrophic cardiomyopathy-related death: revisited in a large non-referral-based patient population. *Circulation.* 2000;102:858–864.
63. Adabag AS, Casey SA, Kuskowski MA, et al. Spectrum and prognostic significance of arrhythmias on ambulatory Holter electrocardiogram in hypertrophic cardiomyopathy. *J Am Coll Cardiol.* 2005;45:697–704.
64. Maron BJ, Shen WK, Link MS, et al. Efficacy of implantable cardioverter-defibrillators for the prevention of sudden death in patients with hypertrophic cardiomyopathy. *N Engl J Med.* 2000; 342:365–373.
65. Spirito P, Bellone P, Harris KM, et al. Magnitude of left ventricular hypertrophy and risk of sudden death in hypertrophic cardiomyopathy. *N Engl J Med.* 2000;342:1778–1785.
66. Monserrat L, Elliott PM, Gimeno JR, et al. Non-sustained ventricular tachycardia in hypertrophic cardiomyopathy: an independent marker of sudden death risk in young patients. *J Am Coll Cardiol.* 2003;42:873–879.
67. Lim PO, Morris-Thurgood JA, Frenneaux MP. Vascular mechanisms of sudden death in hypertrophic cardiomyopathy, including blood pressure responses to exercise. *Cardiol Rev.* 2002;10: 15–23.
68. Elliott PM, Poloniecki J, Dickie S, et al. Sudden death in hypertrophic cardiomyopathy: identification of high risk patients. *J Am Coll Cardiol.* 2000;36:2212–2218.
69. McKenna WJ, Behr ER. Hypertrophic cardiomyopathy: management, risk stratification, and prevention of sudden death. *Heart.* 2002;87:169–176.
70. Maron BJ. Sudden death in young athletes. *N Engl J Med.* 2003; 349:1064–1075.
71. Maron BJ, Isner JM, McKenna WJ. 26th Bethesda conference: recommendations for determining eligibility for competition in athletes with cardiovascular abnormalities. Task Force 3: hypertrophic cardiomyopathy, myocarditis and other myopericardial diseases and mitral valve prolapse. *J Am Coll Cardiol.* 1994;24: 880–885.
72. Olivotto I, Cecchi F, Casey SA, et al. Impact of atrial fibrillation on the clinical course of hypertrophic cardiomyopathy. *Circulation.* 2001;104:2517–2524.
73. Gruver EJ, Fatkin D, Dodds GA, et al. Familial hypertrophic cardiomyopathy and atrial fibrillation caused by Arg663His beta-cardiac myosin heavy chain mutation. *Am J Cardiol.* 1999;83: 13H–18H.
74. Maron BJ, Olivotto I, Bellone P, et al. Clinical profile of stroke in 900 patients with hypertrophic cardiomyopathy. *J Am Coll Cardiol.* 2002;39:301–307.
75. Chen MS, McCarthy PM, Lever HM, et al. Effectiveness of atrial fibrillation surgery in patients with hypertrophic cardiomyopathy. *Am J Cardiol.* 2004;93:373–375.
76. Thaman R, Varnava A, Hamid MS, et al. Pregnancy related complications in women with hypertrophic cardiomyopathy. *Heart.* 2003;89:752–756.
77. Autore C, Conte MR, Piccininno M, et al. Risk associated with pregnancy in hypertrophic cardiomyopathy. *J Am Coll Cardiol.* 2002; 40:1864–1869.

## QUESTIONS

**1.** All of the following increase the gradient in hypertrophic cardiomyopathy *except:*

a. Valsalva maneuver
b. Squatting
c. Amyl nitrite
d. Isoproterenol
e. Standing

Answer is b: The Valsalva maneuver decreases venous return and thus decreases ventricular volume, thus accentuating the SAM and thus increasing the gradient. Amyl nitrite causes peripheral vasodilation and tachycardia. Both of these factors cause the left ventricle to decrease in size and thus increase the gradient. Isoproterenol increases the contractility and thus decreases ventricular volume, which increases the gradient. Standing decreases venous return and decreases ventricular volume. Squatting increases the vascular resistance and venous return, thus increasing ventricular volume and reducing the SAM, which reduces the gradient.

**2.** Which of the following are symptoms of left ventricular outflow tract obstruction?

a. Dyspnea on exertion
b. Syncope
c. Chest pain
d. Sudden death
e. All of the above

Answer is e: All of the above are classic symptoms of left ventricular outflow tract obstruction.

**3.** All of the following are true of the Brockenbrough response *except:*

a. There is increased filling of the left ventricle with the compensatory pause.
b. The premature beat causes a decrease in contractility in HCM but not in normal individuals.
c. There is an increase in ventricular pressure in both normal individuals and in patients with hypertrophic cardiomyopathy.
d. The is a decrease in aortic pressure in HCM.
e. There is an increase in aortic pressure in normal individuals.

Answer is b: The Brockenbrough maneuver causes the contractility to increase in both normal individuals and in patients with HCM. All of the other statements are true.

**4.** Echocardiography is the primary clinical modality for diagnosing hypertrophic cardiomyopathy. Which of the following findings is (are) commonly seen in HCM?

a. A septum >15mm
b. Preclosure of the aortic valve
c. Anterior displacement of the papillary muscles
d. Elongated mitral leaflets
e. All of the above

Answer is e: The definition for the diagnosis of HCM is that the septum must be 15 mm or greater in the absence of any disease know to cause hypertrophy. Preclosure of the aortic valve is commonly seen on a M-mode echo of the aortic valve in the presence of left ventricular outflow tract obstruction. Anterior displacement of the papillary muscles is frequently seen in HCM and contributes to the development of outflow tract obstruction. Elongated mitral leaflets have been recognized for some time in HCM but are now more easily seen with better instrumentation.

**5.** All of the following drugs are useful in the treatment of HCM *except:*

a. Metoprolol
b. Disopyramide
c. Enalapril
d. Diltiazem
e. Phenylephrine

Answer is c: Enalapril is an angiotensin-converting enzyme inhibitor, and it can worsen obstruction by causing peripheral vasodilation. Metoprolol is a beta-blocker and thus, by slowing the heart rate, may allow for prolonging diastolic filling and lessen the provocable outflow tract gradient. It is also a negative inotrope. It is somewhat less helpful if there is resting obstruction. Disopyramide has a negative inotropic effect on the left ventricle and thus frequently diminishes left ventricular outflow tract obstruction. Diltiazem is a calcium channel blocker that has some negative inotropic and may lessen left ventricular outflow tract obstruction. In addition, it improves diastolic filling. Phenylephrine may be life saving in the treatment of hypotension-associated severe left ventricular outflow tract obstruction. It is a pure vascular constrictor and does not increase the contractility of the heart.

**6.** Which of the following is a risk factor for sudden death in HCM?

a. Septal thickness >30mm
b. Prolonged or repetitive episodes of nonsustained ventricular tachycardia
c. Family history of sudden death
d. Syncope or near- syncope
e. No change or a decrease in blood pressure with exercise
f. All of the above

Answer is f: Although all these factors have been shown to have a high negative predictive accuracy, the positive predictive accuracy is low.

# Myocarditis and Dilated Cardiomyopathy

33

**W. H. Wilson Tang**

## MYOCARDITIS

Myocarditis is broadly defined as an inflammatory infiltration of the myocardium with associated necrosis and/or degeneration (1). The disease is also known as "inflammatory cardiomyopathy" or "myocarditis with cardiac dysfunction" when left ventricular systolic dysfunction is evident. Although it is often associated with the acute onset of profound cardiac dysfunction leading to rapidly progressive heart failure and arrhythmia in an otherwise healthy young person, there is a tremendously wide spectrum of clinical presentation.

### Epidemiology and Classification

The exact incidence and prevalence of myocarditis is unclear because the majority of cases of myocarditis may be subclinical in presentation. Nevertheless, myocarditis usually affects younger individuals (median age of 42 years). The estimated incidence of myocarditis is 1 to 10 per 100,000 persons from military recruits and autopsy studies, and about 1% to 5% of patients with acute viral infections may have some involvement in the myocardium (2). The incidence of biopsy-proven myocarditis ranges from 9% to 11% in adults (3) and up to 38% in children with acute-onset heart failure.

The terminology of myocarditis is confusing, but myocarditis is often described according to the description of the disease course as "fulminant," "acute," or "chronic" (4) (Table 33–1). With the availability of endomyocardial biopsy techniques in the 1970s, a technical (histologic) definition has been standardized by pathologists:

1. *The Dallas criteria* (1987) (5) describe the quantity and distribution patterns of lymphocyte infiltrates, and classify myocarditis into three main types: (a) myocarditis (with or without fibrosis); (b) borderline myocarditis; or (c) no myocarditis. A second, follow-up biopsy may allow further stratification into "ongoing myocarditis," "resolving/healing myocarditis," or "resolved myocarditis."
2. *The World Heart Foundation Marburg Criteria* (1996) (6) stratify according to a quantitative assessment of lymphocyte density (with the cutoff at 14 cells/mm$^2$). Recent modifications have been proposed using immunohistologic quantification and characterization of immunocompetent infiltrates and cell adhesion molecule expression found in 50% of patients with dilated cardiomyopathy (7).

### Etiologies and Pathophysiology

Many infectious and noninfectious agents can cause myocarditis (Table 33–2) (2), although enteroviruses can cause >50% of myocarditis episodes in developed countries. The precise pathogenic mechanisms of the disease are generally not well understood, and may vary according to the causative agent and host factors. The majority of the cases are presumed to be due to a common pathway of host-mediated autoimmune-mediated injury, although direct cytotoxic effects of the causative agent and damages due to cytokine expression in the myocardium may play some role. Clinically, myocardial damage follows the expected course of inflammatory response (2):

- *Acute phase* (0 to 3 days) is characterized by myocyte destruction as a direct consequence of the offending agent from cytokine expression and macrophage activation, leading to cell-mediated cytotoxicity and cytokine

**TABLE 33–1**
**CLINICOPATHOLOGIC CLASSIFICATION OF MYOCARDITIS**

| | Fulminant | Acute | Chronic Active | Chronic Persistent |
|---|---|---|---|---|
| Prevalence | 17% | 65% | 11% | 7% |
| Symptom onset | Distinct | Indistinct | Indistinct | Indistinct |
| Presentation | Shock | CHF | CHF | Non-CHF |
| LV function | Severe LVD | LVD | LVD | Normal |
| Biopsy findings | Multiple foci of active myocarditis | Active or borderline myocarditis | Active or borderline myocarditis | Active or borderline myocarditis |
| Natural history | Complete recovery or death | Partial recovery or DCM | DCM | Non-CHF, normal LV function |
| Histologic evaluation | Complete resolution | Complete resolution | Ongoing or resolving myocarditis | Ongoing or resolving myocarditis |
| Immunosuppression | No benefit | Sometimes beneficial | No benefit | No benefit |
| Long-term survival[a] | | | | Unknown |
| 1 y | 93% | 85% | | |
| 11 y | 93% | 45% | | |

CHF, congestive heart failure; LV, left ventricular; LVD, LV dysfunction; DCM, dilated cardiomyopathy.
[a]Long-term survival data from 147 biopsy-proven myocarditis cases followed at the Johns Hopkins Hospital from 1984 to 1997 (16).
*Source:* Adapted from Lieberman EB, Hutchins GM, Herskowitz A, et al. Clinicopathologic description of myocarditis. *J Am Coll Cardiol.* 1991;18:1617–1626.

release and contributing to myocardial damage and dysfunction. In viral myocarditis, viremia is often present, although detection may sometimes be difficult.

- *Subacute phase* (4 to 14 days) involves continuing cytokine production plus myocyte destruction by nonspecific autoimmune-mediated injury by cytotoxic T- and B-lymphocytes and natural killer cells. Active viral clearing occurs in this stage.
- *Chronic phase* (>14 days) involves a repair process characterized by fibrosis, persistence of autoantibodies, and sometimes with persistence of the viral genome in the myocardium but without significant inflammation (unless chronic active or persistent subtypes). Cardiac dilatation and heart failure may ensue.

In viral myocarditis, viral isolates differ in tissue tropism and virulence. For example, coxsackie A9 is a self-limiting myocarditis, whereas coxsackie B3 causes severe myocarditis with a high mortality. In addition, the induction of the coxsackie-adenovirus receptor (CAR) and the complement-deflecting protein decay-accelerating factor (DAF, CD55) may allow efficient internalization of the viral genome (8). These key molecular determinants for cardiotropic viral infections can be found in up to two thirds of patients with dilated cardiomyopathy (DCM). Viral replication may lead to further disruption of metabolism and perturbation of inflammation and its response. Vasospasm induced by endothelial cell viral infection may also contribute to further damage. New evidence of dystrophin disruption by expression of enteroviral protease 2A points to yet another unique pathogenic mechanism (9).

## Clinical Presentation

Myocarditis can be totally asymptomatic or can present with chest pain syndromes ranging from mild persistent chest pain of acute myopericarditis (35%) to severe symptoms that mimic acute myocardial infarction (2). About 60% of patients may have antecedent arthralgias, malaise, fevers, sweats, or chills consistent with viral infections (pharyngitis, tonsillitis, upper respiratory tract infection) usually about 1 to 2 weeks prior to onset. The hallmark symptoms of acute or fulminant myocarditis are those of acute-onset heart failure in a person without known cardiac dysfunction or with low cardiac risks. The diagnosis is usually presumptive, based on patient demographics and the clinical course (spontaneous recovery following supportive care). In some instances, patients may present with arrhythmia in the form of syncope, palpitations caused by heart block (Stokes–Adams attack), ventricular tachyarrhythmia, or even sudden cardiac death. Patients often present with signs of acute decompensated heart failure including an $S_3$ gallop, central and peripheral edema, jugular venous distension, and tachycardia. An audible pericardial friction rub may accompany concomitant myopericarditis.

Additional findings may accompany specific forms of myocarditis. In patients with acute rheumatic fever, associated signs include erythema marginatum, polyarthralgia, chorea, and subcutaneous nodules (Jones criteria for rheumatic fever). In cases of sarcoid myocarditis, lymphadenopathy and arrhythmias are common (up to 70% of affected individuals). Chagas cardiomyopathy also presents with arrhythmias and heart blocks. Hypersensitive or eosinophilic myocarditis often comes with a pruritic

**TABLE 33–2**
**CAUSES OF MYOCARDITIS**

**Infective Causes of Myocarditis**

Viral:

- Enteroviruses—coxsackievirus A and B, echovirus, influenza virus, poliovirus
- Herpesviruses—human herpes virus 6
- Adenovirus, mumps, rubella, rubeola
- Hepatitis B or C viruses
- Human immunodeficiency virus (HIV)

Rickettsial

Fungal: cryptococcosis, aspergillosis, coccidioidomycosis, histoplasmosis

Protozoan: *Trypanosomiasis cruzi* (Chagas disease), *Toxoplasmosis gondii*

Helminthic: trichinosis, schistosomiasis

Bacterial: legionella, clostridium, streptococci, staphylococci, salmonella/shigella

Spirochetal: *Borrelia burgdorferi* (Lyme disease)

**Noninfective Causes of Myocarditis**

Hypersensitive reaction ("eosinophilic myocarditis"):

- Antibiotics (ampicillin, chloramphenicol, tetracycline, sulfisoxazole)
- Diuretics (hydrochlorothiazide, spironolactone)
- Anticonvulsives (phenytoin, carbamazepine)
- Others (lithium, clozapine, indomethacin)
- Tetanus toxoid or smallpox vaccines

Cardiotoxic drugs:

- Catecholamines (especially dobutamine, amphetamines, cocaine)
- Chemotherapeutic drugs (anthracyclines, fluorouracil, streptomycin, cyclophosphamide, interleukin-2, trastuzumab)

Collagen vascular diseases:

- Systemic lupus erythematosus ("lupus carditis")
- Wegener granulomatosis
- Churg–Strauss syndrome (eosinophilic myocarditis)
- Dermatomyositis/polymyositis
- Scleroderma

Systemic illnesses:

- Sarcoidosis
- Giant-cell myocarditis
- Kawasaki disease
- Large-vessel vasculitis (polyarteritis nodosa, takayasu arteritis)
- Inflammatory bowel diseases (ulcerative colitis, Crohn disease)

Acute rheumatic fever

Bites/stings: scorpion venom, snake venom, wasp venom, black widow spider venom

Chemicals: hydrocarbons, carbon monoxide, thallium, lead, arsenic, cobalt

Physical injury: radiation, heatstroke, hypothermia

Peripartum cardiomyopathy

maculopapular rash (and history of offending drug use) and eosinophilia in the blood work. The typical presentation of a patient with giant-cell myocarditis involves sustained ventricular tachycardia in rapidly progressive heart failure leading to cardiogenic shock. These features have low specificities, but are often useful and may raise the suspicion of underlying myocarditis.

## Evaluation

Inflammation is the hallmark feature of myocarditis. Clinically, an early onset, fever, tachycardia, hypotension, reduced right ventricular function, increased cardiac enzymes (CK-MB/cardiac troponins), elevated acute-phase reactants (erythrocyte sedimentation rate or high-sensitivity C-reactive protein), and leukocytosis are predictive of myocarditis. The presence of eosinophilia may suggest hypersensitive (eosinophilic) myocarditis. Novel inflammatory markers that are still under investigation include tumor necrosis factor (TNF)-$\alpha$, interleukins, serum-soluble Fas and soluble Fas-ligand levels (10). Elevation of these markers portends a worse prognosis, although they are rarely used in the clinical setting. Serum viral antibody titers are usually increased fourfold or more acutely and gradually fall during convalescence. However, measurement of viral antibody titers is rarely indicated. Because of their low specificity, measurement of anticardiac antibody titers is not indicated (only 62% of myocarditis cases have titers $\geq$1:40). Screening antinuclear antibodies and rheumatoid factor are often indicated to rule out common rheumatologic problems. Disease-specific testing is indicated if specific conditions such as systematic lupus erythematosus, polymyositis, Wegner granulomatosis, or scleroderma are suspected.

The electrocardiogram often reveals sinus tachycardia, although sometimes the presence of ST-segment deviation may represent focal or global ischemia. In some cases, fascicular block or atrioventricular conduction disturbances as well as ventricular tachyarrhythmias may be hemodynamically significant. A complete echocardiogram is standard procedure for patients with suspected myocarditis in order to (a) exclude alternative causes of heart failure, (b) detect the presence of intracardiac thrombi and associated valvular disease, and (c) quantify the degree of left ventricular dysfunction to monitor response to therapy. Occasionally, focal wall motion abnormalities and presence of pericardial fluid may prompt further work-up or intervention. Fulminant myocarditis is often characterized by near-normal diastolic dimensions and increased septal wall thickness, whereas acute myocarditis often has increased diastolic dimensions but normal septal wall thickness (11). Coronary angiography is often performed to rule out coronary disease as a cause of new-onset heart failure, as the clinical presentation of myocarditis may mimic myocardial infarction ("pseudo-infarct pattern"), especially with the presence of focal wall motion abnormalities and localizing electrocardiographic changes. Several specialized imaging procedures are available to detect the presence of myocarditis, although they are rarely used clinically. Antimyosin scintigraphy using indium-III monoclonal antimyosin antibody provides identification of myocardial inflammation, with a high sensitivity (91% to 100%) and negative predictive value (93% to 100%) but relatively low specificity (28% to 33%) in detecting myocarditis. Gallium scanning has been utilized to identify severe myocardial cellular infiltration with high specificity (98%) but low sensitivity (36%) (2). Gadolinium-enhanced magnetic resonance imaging is another reliable method to detect the presence of myocarditis, although it is rarely indicated.

Histology remains the "gold standard" for the diagnosis of myocarditis. Endomyocardial biopsy, however, is insensitive and not without risks. False-positive rates are high (even with multiple biopsy samples) because of the small number of lymphocytes reviewed, the difficulties in distinguishing cell types, and the wide interobserver variability. In cases with suspected myocarditis, endomyocardial biopsy is reserved for patients who may have giant-cell myocarditis, such as those presenting with rapidly progressive heart failure symptoms despite conventional therapy, or new-onset frequent ventricular tachyarrhythmia or conduction disturbances. In patients with "idiopathic" dilated cardiomyopathy, up to 25% may have either ongoing (chronic active) inflammation or evidence of viral genome materials on their biopsy samples, indicating antecedent myocarditis as their probable cause (12). Therefore, in the clinical setting, other than in a small number of instances (such as the identification of giant cells), the histologic criteria provide only confirmation of the diagnosis, and perhaps some prognostic information. It is also important to recognize that the farther away from illness onset to biopsy, the lower the yield of the biopsy specimens.

## Treatment and Prognosis

There are no hard-and-fast rules for managing myocarditis once the acute events have occurred. In general, patients are treated in the same manner as if they had chronic heart failure. Clinical follow-up should be close, as persistent chronic inflammation may lead to dilated cardiomyopathy (initially, 1- to 3-month intervals for drug and physical activity titration). Serial echocardiographic assessment of ventricular structure and function is often performed, although there is no agreement regarding the frequency of echocardiographic assessment following myocarditis. There is a theoretical increased risk of myocardial inflammation and necrosis, cardiac remodeling, and death with exercise in animal models. Therefore, patients suffering from myocarditis are usually advised to abstain from vigorous exercise for several months in order to limit myocardial demands. Depending on the clinical presentation, standard heart failure therapy with diuretics, angiotensin-converting enzyme (ACE) inhibitors, beta-blockers, and/or aldosterone antagonists should be use to delay or reverse disease progression of cardiac dysfunction. Although not proven in human studies, proarrhythmic properties of digoxin have been observed in animal models of myocarditis, and therefore should be avoided. Anticoagulation is often indicated to prevent thromboembolic events, and is usually recommended in patients with apical aneurysm with thrombus (such as in Chagas cardiomyopathy), atrial fibrillation, and prior embolic episodes. Permanent pacemakers should be implanted for persistent heart block or bradyarrhythmia. Implantable cardioverter-defibrillators (ICDs) are indicated only after medical stabilization in the chronic phase with persistent cardiac dysfunction or ventricular tachyarrhythmia refractory to medical therapy. Inotropic therapy often is reserved for those experiencing severe hemodynamic compromise (particularly in fulminant myocarditis). Sometimes, intra-aortic balloon counterpulsation can be used for hemodynamic support and afterload reduction to prevent further deterioration. Mechanical assist devices (LVADs) and even extracorporeal membrane oxygenation (ECMO) have been used in cases of fulminant myocarditis with the hope for recovery and/or bridge to transplantation. Early consideration for cardiac transplantation should be given especially in severe, progressive, biopsy-proven giant-cell myocarditis or peripartum cardiomyopathy. Data from the ISHLT registry suggest that patients with myocarditis may have increased rejection and reduced survival after heart transplantation as compared to those without, and myocarditis may recur in allograft in less severe forms.

Table 33–3 summarizes the major clinical trials on immunosuppression therapy for myocarditis and inflammatory cardiomyopathy. Routine immunosuppression therapy (including steroids), antiviral regimens, and nonsteroid anti-arrhythmic agents are not warranted. The findings from the Myocarditis Treatment Trial (with oral prednisone and cyclosporine) (13) and the IMAC study (with intravenous immunoglobulin) (3) indicated that routine immunosuppression therapy may not be effective. Therefore, at present there is no regimen that is U.S. Food and Drug Administration (FDA) approved for the treatment for acute or chronic myocarditis. Immunosuppression or immunomodulation therapy is reserved for refractory patients with chronic myocarditis, or biopsy-proven giant-cell myocarditis. Patients with fulminant myocarditis should not be routinely immunosuppressed, but rather supported. Some reports have suggested that eosinophilic or sarcoid myocarditis may respond to high-dose steroid therapy. Specific therapy for underlying collagen vascular diseases may be used.

The role of viral persistence and tailored therapy for myocarditis has recently been debated. Recent studies have suggested potential benefits of targeted therapy with azathioprine and prednisone in patients with recent-onset DCM. An ongoing multicenter European Study on the Epidemiology and Treatment of Cardiac Inflammatory Disease (ESETCID) may provide further insight (14). There is likely a category of patients who have an active immune process for whom immunosuppression, immune absorption, or immune regulation will ultimately provide benefit.

Many patients may have full spontaneous clinical recovery, even after weeks of medical and mechanical support (including intra-aortic balloon counterpulsation and

**TABLE 33–3**
**MAJOR CLINICAL TRIALS OF MYOCARDITIS AND INFLAMMATORY CARDIOMYOPATHY**

| | NHLBI Study | Myocarditis Treatment Trial | Multicenter IMAC Trial | Polish Study | Italian Cohort |
|---|---|---|---|---|---|
| Authors | Parillo et al. (26) | Mason et al. (13) | McNamara et al. (3) | Wojnicz et al. (27) | Frustaci et al. (28) |
| Year | 1989 | 1995 | 2001 | 2001 | 2003 |
| Drug | Prednisone | Prednisone & cyclosporine | IVIG | Prednisone & azathioprine | Prednisone & azathioprine |
| Sample size | 102 | 111 | 62 | 84 | 41 |
| Study population | Idiopathic DCM | EMB-proven myocarditis, EF <40% | Recent-onset DCM, EF <40% | DCM with upregulated HLA | EMB-proven myocarditis with CHF |
| Primary endpoint | Change in LV function at 3 mo | Change in LV function at 7 mo | Change in LV function at 6 mo | Change in LV function at 24 mo | Change in LV function at 12 mo |
| Outcomes (treatment vs. placebo) | No benefit (4.3% vs. 2.1%) | No benefit (10% vs. 7%) | No benefit (14% vs. 14%) | Benefit (20% vs. 6%) | Benefit (21% vs. 0%) |

NHLBI, National Heart, Lung & Blood Institute; IVIG, intravenous immunoglobulin; DCM, dilated cardiomyopathy; EMB, endomyocardial biopsy; EF, ejection fraction; HLA, human leukocyte antigen; CHF, congestive heart failure; LV, left ventricular.

mechanical assist devices). In the Myocarditis Treatment Trial, 1-year mortality was 20% and 4-year mortality was 56% (13). Interestingly, long-term outcomes do not differ significantly between active and borderline myocarditis by the Dallas criteria. Severe heart block requiring permanent pacemaker placement occurs in 1% patients. Unfavorable factors for survival include extremes of age (very old or very young), electrocardiographic abnormalities (QRS alterations, atrial fibrillation, low voltages), syncope, and specific etiologies (peripartum cardiomyopathy, giant-cell myocarditis). On the other hand, favorable factors for survival include preserved cardiac function, shorter clinical history, or survivors of fulminant presentation at onset. In fact, the prognosis for patients with secondary myocarditis, when compared with patients with idiopathic myocarditis, seems to be most affected by the primary disease processes (15). Nevertheless, for unclear reasons, survivors of fulminant myocarditis experienced better long-term outcomes than those presenting with acute myocarditis (16). Adults may present with heart failure years after the initial index event of myocarditis (up to 12.8% of patients with idiopathic DCM had presumed prior myocarditis in one case series). Up to half of patients with myocarditis develop subsequent DCM over a range of 3 months to 13 years.

## SPECIFIC FORMS OF CARDIOMYOPATHY RELATED TO MYOCARDITIS

### Chagas Heart Disease

It is estimated that 16 to 18 million persons in South and Central America are infected with *Trypanosoma cruzi*. Although most patients recover from the acute inflammatory phases of the infection, cardiac involvement usually appears decades after initial treatment, and is the leading cause of death in persons aged 30 to 50 years in endemic areas. The hallmark of Chagas cardiomyopathy is arrhythmia, often presenting with symptoms of palpitations, syncope, chest pain, and, subsequently, heart failure (17). Frequent complex ectopic beats and ventricular tachyarrhythmia occur in 40% to 90% affected, with sudden cardiac death occurring in 55% to 65% affected. Bundle branch block is also frequently seen, sometimes with bradyarrhythmia and high-grade atrioventricular block requiring pacemaker placement. Heart failure is predominantly right sided, can be found in 25% to 30% of those affected, sometimes with cerebral or pulmonary thromboembolism. Apical left ventricular aneurysm, ventricular dilatation, and cardiac fibrosis are commonly found in autopsies.

There are several types of serological tests to confirm the presence of exposure to *T. cruzi*. Cardiac lesions can be confirmed by *in situ* polymerase chain reaction in biopsy specimens. Echocardiographic findings may include left ventricular aneurysm with or without thrombi, posterior basal akinesis or hypokinesis with preserved septal contraction, and diastolic dysfunction. Antibiotic therapy with benznidazole or nifurtimox may help to reduce parasitemia and prevent complications.

### Giant-Cell Myocarditis

Giant-cell myocarditis (also known as pernicious myocarditis, Fiedler myocarditis, granulomatous myocarditis, or idiopathic interstitial myocarditis) is a rare disorder with unclear etiology. The hallmark feature is the presence of fused, multinucleated (>20 nuclei) epithelioid "giant cells" of histocytic origin within a diffuse, intramyocardial inflammatory infiltrate with lymphocytes. Giant-cell myocarditis often presents with an aggressive clinical course, with progression over days to weeks. Rapidly progressive heart failure occurs in 75% of those affected and sustained ventricular tachyarrhythmia in >50% of those affected. Giant-cell myocarditis is often refractory to standard medical therapy, although small observational series have suggested potential benefits of immunosuppressive therapy (18). Consideration for early cardiac transplantation is appropriate (5-year survival is 71% following successful transplantation). Often, mechanical support may be required as a temporary bridge to recovery or transplantation. The prognosis is often dismal without intervention such as cardiac transplant (1-year mortality up to 80%, with median survival 5.5 months from symptom onset). Therefore, early identification of giant-cell myocarditis by means of endomyocardial biopsy may permit prompt referral for cardiac transplantation. A 20% to 25% rate of histologic recurrence in surveillance endomyocardial biopsies has been observed following transplantation, but without substantial impact on the clinical course.

### Hypersensitive/Eosinophilic Myocarditis

Eosinophilic endomyocardial disease (also known as Löffler endomyocardial fibrosis) occurs as a major complication of idiopathic hypereosinophilic syndrome as a result of direct toxic damage caused by eosinophil granule proteins within the heart (19). Drug-induced eosinophilic myocarditis is independent of cumulative dose and duration of therapy. Common drugs include catecholamines, chemotherapeutic agents, ampicillin, and tetanus toxoid (see Table 33–1). The absence of peripheral eosinophilia does not rule out eosinophilic myocarditis. Although observational series suggest potential clinical benefits of corticosteroid therapy, the best strategy is to remove the causative agent when it can be identified.

### Peripartum Cardiomyopathy (See also Chapter 55)

Peripartum cardiomyopathy will be discussed in Chapter 55.

## DILATED CARDIOMYOPATHY

The World Health Organization (WHO) has defined dilated cardiomyopathy as myocardial disease characterized by dilatation and impaired contraction of the left ventricle or both the left and right ventricles (Table 33–4) (1). Intracardiac filling pressures are invariably high in symptomatic patients. Dilated cardiomyopathy is a heterogeneous disease and shares the same common pathophysiologic processes of myocyte apoptosis and necrosis, fibrosis, and neurohormonal upregulation with other specific cardiomyopathies. The clinical presentation of dilated cardiomyopathy ranges from asymptomatic to heart failure, stroke from thromboembolism, arrhythmias, and sudden cardiac death—almost parallel to that of myocarditis. Although classification schemes are largely academic and the general diagnostic and therapeutic strategy follows that of all heart failure etiologies, several specific forms of cardiomyopathy are worth mentioning, because they possess unique clinical features and specific treatment options.

### Idiopathic Dilated Cardiomyopathy

Strict diagnostic criteria and epidemiology for idiopathic dilated cardiomyopathy (IDCM) are lacking because many cases go undiagnosed, and many patients who experience heart failure do not undergo an extensive evaluation. It has been estimated that the prevalence of IDCM is 0.4 per 1,000 in the general population. However, as more diagnostic techniques become available, specific causes of dilated cardiomyopathy can be identified and fewer cases will

**TABLE 33–4**
**MAJOR FORMS OF CARDIOMYOPATHY AND THEIR CLASSIFICATION**

| Clinicopathologic Pattern | Primary Cardiomyopathy | Specific Heart Muscle Disease (Secondary Cardiomyopathy) | Other Cardiovascular Disorders |
|---|---|---|---|
| Dilated cardiomyopathy (systolic dysfunction) | Idiopathic<br>Familial | Inflammatory myocarditis<br>Alcohol/toxic<br>Peripartum<br>Metabolic | Ischemic<br>Valvular<br>Hypertensive<br>Congenital |
| Hypertrophic cardiomyopathy (diastolic dysfunction) | Familial (50%)<br>Idiopathic | Amyloidosis | Hypertensive<br>Aortic stenosis |
| Restrictive cardiomyopathy (diastolic dysfunction) | Idiopathic<br>Familial | Amyloidosis<br>Radiation/endomyocardial fibrosis | Pericardial constriction |
| Arrhythmogenic right ventricular cardiomyopathy | Idiopathic<br>Familial | | |

*Source:* Adapted from Richardson P, McKenna W, Bristow M, et al. Report of the 1995 World Health Organization/International Society and Federation of Cardiology Task Force on the definition and classification of cardiomyopathies. *Circulation*. 1996;93:841–842.

be deemed "idiopathic." For example, histologic evidence of myocarditis is seen in 4% to 10% of endomyocardial biopsies of IDCM patients. Indeed, it has been estimated that >50% of patients with acute myocarditis may develop dilated cardiomyopathy (20). Recent reports of molecular diagnosis of viral involvement even suggested a viral etiology in up to two thirds of IDCM cases (21).

Metabolic cardiomyopathies include amino acid, lipid, and mitochondrial disorders, as well as storage diseases. Certain metabolic deficiencies, such as selenium, carnitine, phosphate, calcium, and vitamin B deficiencies (especially in chronic diuresis) can all result in dilated cardiomyopathy, as often seen in patients with anorexia nervosa. Many endocrine disorders (adrenocortical insufficiency, thyroid abnormalities, acromegaly, and pheochromocytoma) also cause secondary cardiomyopathies. However, in cases of metabolic cardiomyopathies such as hemochromatosis, amyloidosis, glycogen storage diseases, and Fabry–Anderson disease, restrictive physiology is the hallmark presentation. Identification of the underlying etiology may aid the appropriate treatment (e.g., phlebotomy and chelation therapy for hemochromatosis, $\alpha$-galactosidase replacement therapy for Fabry cardiomyopathy).

Several forms of dilated cardiomyopathy may develop in early childhood. Noncompacted myocardium occurs as a result of an arrested endomyocardial morphogenesis, and usually presents in childhood with persisting myocardial sinusoids, prominent trabeculations, and evidence of patchy "spongy" morphology of the embryonic heart. Endocardial fibroelastosis can lead to thickening of left ventricle and left-sided cardiac valves, leading to dilated or restrictive cardiomyopathy.

## Inherited Forms of Dilated Cardiomyopathy

Although familial dilated cardiomyopathy accounts for at least 20% to 30% of dilated cardiomyopathy cases, genetic screening is rarely performed. Mutations in genes encoding for cytoskeletal proteins (lamin A/C, phospholamban, dystrophin) as well as sarcomeric proteins (myosin heavy chain, cardiac troponin-T, actin) have been described (22–24). Interestingly, the latter mutations are similar to those found in hypertrophic cardiomyopathy (see Chapter 32). Furthermore, patients with ion channelopathy (such as long and short QT syndromes, Brugada syndrome, catecholaminergic polymorphic ventricular tachyarrhythmia) often develop dilated cardiomyopathy. The autosomal form of familial dilated cardiomyopathy is the most prevalent. The clinical expression and penetrance of these inherited gene defects is variable and may encompass skeletal myopathies (including Duchenne, Becker-type, and myotonic dystrophies), neuromuscular disorders (include Friedreich ataxia, Noonan syndrome, and lentiginosis), cardiac conduction system abnormalities, and progression to end-stage heart failure. The risk of sudden cardiac death is less clearly defined as compared with hypertrophic cardiomyopathy, but appears to be increased, particularly in patients with sarcomere protein mutations. Family members may be asymptomatic early in the course of disease, but identification of affected individuals with serial echocardiography is important, as early treatment may improve prognosis. Patients with familial dilated cardiomyopathy, particularly those with inherited forms of systolic dysfunction with minimal dilatation (without restrictive physiology), may carry a poor prognosis.

Arrhythmogenic right ventricular cardiomyopathy (ARVC) emerged as a unique entity in the 1995 WHO classification scheme. It is an autosomal dominant disease predominantly affecting the right ventricle by massive or partial replacement of myocardium by fatty or fibro-fatty tissue, and can be detected by magnetic resonance imaging or by endomyocardial biopsy (often sparing the trabeculae and the septum) (25). More than 50% of cases are inherited with an autosomal dominant pattern, and mutations in the plakoglobin and desmoplakin genes (recessive form of ARVC known as Naxos disease) have been associated with familial ARVC. Residual islands or strands of myocytes are often electrically unstable, leading to widespread ventricular tachyarrhythmias and sudden death of young individuals. Clinically, they may present in early adulthood with tachyarrhythmias or with right-sided heart failure (sometimes extending to the left ventricle). Echocardiography may demonstrate localized right ventricle (RV) aneurysm or isolated RV failure, and the electrocardiogram may show slurred ST segments and inverted T-waves in the anterior leads (epsilon waves) without right bundle branch block. Aggressive treatment with antiarrhythmic drugs, radiofrequency ablation, and ICDs is indicated. Heart failure is difficult to manage, and cardiac transplantation can be considered in selective cases.

Mitochondrial cardiomyopathy represents a special form of maternally inherited cardiomyopathy due to mutations in mitochondrial DNA with resultant abnormalities in oxidative phosphorylation. Indeed, the MELAS syndrome (mitochondrial encephalopathy, lactic acidosis, and strokelike syndrome) can manifest as a cardiomyopathy. Electron microscopy of muscle biopsy specimens may reveal giant mitochondria, concentric cristae, and intramitochondrial inclusions. There have also been reports of the association of mutations of the hereditary hemochromatosis (HFE) gene with IDCM.

## REFERENCES

1. Richardson P, McKenna W, Bristow M, et al. Report of the 1995 World Health Organization/International Society and Federation of Cardiology Task Force on the definition and classification of cardiomyopathies. *Circulation.* 1996;93:841–842.
2. Feldman AM, McNamara D. Myocarditis. *N Engl J Med.* 2000;343: 1388–1398.
3. McNamara DM, Holubkov R, Starling RC, et al. Controlled trial of intravenous immune globulin in recent-onset dilated cardiomyopathy. *Circulation.* 2001;103:2254–2259.

4. Lieberman EB, Hutchins GM, Herskowitz A, et al. Clinicopathologic description of myocarditis. *J Am Coll Cardiol*. 1991;18:1617–1626.
5. Aretz HT, Billingham ME, Edwards WD, et al. Myocarditis. A histopathologic definition and classification. *Am J Cardiovasc Pathol*. 1987;1:3–14.
6. Maisch B, Portig I, Ristic A, et al. Definition of inflammatory cardiomyopathy (myocarditis): on the way to consensus. A status report. *Herz*. 2000;25:200–209.
7. Noutsias M, Pauschinger M, Poller WC, et al. Current insights into the pathogenesis, diagnosis and therapy of inflammatory cardiomyopathy. *Heart Fail Monit*. 2003;3:127–135.
8. Liu PP, Mason JW. Advances in the understanding of myocarditis. *Circulation*. 2001;104:1076–1082.
9. Badorff C, Knowlton KU. Dystrophin disruption in enterovirus-induced myocarditis and dilated cardiomyopathy: from bench to bedside. *Med Microbiol Immunol (Berl)*. 2004;193:121–126.
10. Fuse K, Kodama M, Okura Y, et al. Predictors of disease course in patients with acute myocarditis. *Circulation*. 2000;102:2829–2835.
11. Felker GM, Boehmer JP, Hruban RH, et al. Echocardiographic findings in fulminant and acute myocarditis. *J Am Coll Cardiol*. 2000;36:227–232.
12. Felker GM, Hu W, Hare JM, et al. The spectrum of dilated cardiomyopathy. The Johns Hopkins experience with 1,278 patients. *Medicine (Balt)*. 1999;78:270–283.
13. Mason JW, O'Connell JB, Herskowitz A, et al. A clinical trial of immunosuppressive therapy for myocarditis. The Myocarditis Treatment Trial Investigators. *N Engl J Med*. 1995;333:269–275.
14. Hufnagel G, Pankuweit S, Richter A, et al. The European Study of Epidemiology and Treatment of Cardiac Inflammatory Diseases (ESETCID). First epidemiological results. *Herz*. 2000;25:279–285.
15. Pulerwitz TC, Cappola TP, Felker GM, et al. Mortality in primary and secondary myocarditis. *Am Heart J*. 2004;147:746–750.
16. McCarthy RE 3rd, Boehmer JP, Hruban RH, et al. Long-term outcome of fulminant myocarditis as compared with acute (nonfulminant) myocarditis. *N Engl J Med*. 2000;342:690–695.
17. Rassi A Jr, Rassi A, Little WC. Chagas' heart disease. *Clin Cardiol*. 2000;23:883–889.
18. Cooper LT Jr, Berry GJ, Shabetai R. Idiopathic giant-cell myocarditis—natural history and treatment. Multicenter Giant Cell Myocarditis Study Group Investigators. *N Engl J Med*. 1997; 336:1860–1866.
19. Spodick DH. Eosinophilic myocarditis. *Mayo Clin Proc*. 1997; 72: 996.
20. D'Ambrosio A, Patti G, Manzoli A, et al. The fate of acute myocarditis between spontaneous improvement and evolution to dilated cardiomyopathy: a review. *Heart*. 2001;85:499–504.
21. Kuhl U, Pauschinger M, Noutsias M, et al. High prevalence of viral genomes and multiple viral infections in the myocardium of adults with "idiopathic" left ventricular dysfunction. *Circulation*. 2005;111:887–893.
22. Hughes SE, McKenna WJ. New insights into the pathology of inherited cardiomyopathy. *Heart*. 2005;91:257–264.
23. Arbustini E, Morbini P, Pilotto A, et al. Familial dilated cardiomyopathy: from clinical presentation to molecular genetics. *Eur Heart J*. 2000;21:1825–1832.
24. Pasotti M, Repetto A, Tavazzi L, Arbustini E. Genetic predisposition to heart failure. *Med Clin North Am*. 2004;88:1173–1192.
25. Gemayel C, Pelliccia A, Thompson PD. Arrhythmogenic right ventricular cardiomyopathy. *J Am Coll Cardiol*. 2001;38:1773–1781.
26. Parrillo JE, Cunnion RE, Epstein SE, et al. A prospective, randomized, controlled trial of prednisone for dilated cardiomyopathy. *N Engl J Med*. 1989;321:1061–1068.
27. Wojnicz R, Nowalany-Kozielska E, Wojciechowska C, et al. Randomized, placebo-controlled study for immunosuppressive treatment of inflammatory dilated cardiomyopathy: two-year follow-up results. *Circulation*. 2001;104:39–45.
28. Frustaci A, Chimenti C, Calabrese F, et al. Immunosuppressive therapy for active lymphocytic myocarditis: virological and immunologic profile of responders versus nonresponders. *Circulation*. 2003;107:857–863.

## QUESTIONS

A 45-year-old woman came to see you because of intermittent chest pain and progressive shortness of breath for the last 3 days. She was seen last week by her primary physician because of sinusitis and was placed on azithromycin for 5 days without relief.

Exam: Blood pressure 110/80 mm Hg, pulse 110 beats/min regular, jugular venous pressure 10 cm $H_2O$, bibasilar rales, $S_3$ gallop, 1–2+ pedal edema
Electrocardiogram: Sinus tachycardia, nonspecific T-wave changes
Echocardiography: Left ventricular ejection = 25%, 1–2+ mitral regurgitation

**1.** Which of the following is *not* an appropriate next course of action?

a. Cardiac catheterization
b. Endomyocardial biopsy to rule out acute lymphocytic myocarditis
c. Start diuretics and ACE inhibitors
d. Blood testing for thyroid function tests

Answer is b: New-onset heart failure in a relatively young woman who had a recent bout of upper respiratory tract infection can be a potential clinical presentation of acute myocarditis. That being said, the usual course of action should involve cardiac catheterization to rule out coronary ischemia, blood testing to rule out reversible causes of heart failure such as hypo- or hyperthyroidism, and commencing therapy with diuretics, ACE inhibitors, and beta-adrenergic blockers. Routine endomyocardial biopsy, even though it may provide the definitive diagnosis, does not change the patient management, and should be reserved for when patients require further evaluation because of decompensation.

The patient's blood work and autoimmune work-up were negative. Cardiac catheterization revealed normal coronary arteries. Her clinical course deteriorated rapidly over the course of the next few days, requiring hospital admission for decompensated heart failure. She was found to be in cardiogenic shock, requiring inotropic support for stabilization. An endomyocardial biopsy was performed, and the preliminary results suggested acute lymphocytic myocarditis according to the Dallas criteria. Her cardiac index and hemodynamics were stable other than frequent nonsustained ventricular tachyarrhythmia.

**2.** Based on this information, what is the appropriate therapeutic intervention?

a. Intravenous Solu-Medrol
b. Implantable cardioverter-defibrillator (ICD)
c. Plasmapheresis
d. No additional therapy at this point

Answer is d: The patient now presents with fulminant myocarditis, requiring inotropic support. She should remain on supportive therapy, and there is no supporting evidence to recommend immunosuppression therapy at this stage. It would also be inappropriate for her to receive an ICD in this acute setting.

**3.** What is her 5-year prognosis if she survives this acute event?

a. 93%
b. 80%
c. 65%
d. 45%

Answer is a: McCarthy and colleagues (16) compared the long-term prognosis between fulminant and acute myocarditis, and found a 93% survival for those suffering from fulminant myocarditis at 1-year follow-up, which was maintained for the next 10 years. This is significantly better from those presenting with acute myocarditis (45% at 11 years).

**4.** Which of the following patients would have a worse prognosis?

a. A 29-year-old man with giant-cell myocarditis
b. A 27-year-old woman with fulminant myocarditis
c. A 3-year-old man with idiopathic restrictive cardiomyopathy
d. A 25-year-old woman with postpartum cardiomyopathy

Answer is a: All the choices have poor prognosis except for fulminant myocarditis if supported, but giant-cell myocarditis has the worst prognosis, and cardiac transplantation should be considered.

# Pulmonary Hypertension

34

***W. H. Wilson Tang***

Pulmonary hypertension (PH) is defined as mean pulmonary artery pressure >25 mm Hg at rest, or >30 mm Hg with exercise (1). The pulmonary vascular bed is a high-capacitance, low-resistance system. Therefore, in the setting of persistent raised pulmonary vascular resistance (>3 Woods units), pulmonary hypertension can lead to biologic changes in the pulmonary vasculature, right ventricular hypertrophy, and ultimately failure (cor pulmonale). In general, PH (in particular, pulmonary arterial hypertension) is a devastating disease, not only because it affects relatively young individuals, but because the therapeutic options are somewhat limited. According to the National Institute of Health Pulmonary Hypertension Registry (2), untreated mean survival in patients with Class III symptoms is 2.5 years, and mean survival in patients with Class IV symptoms is 6 months.

## CLASSIFICATION

Pulmonary hypertension encompasses a heterogeneous group of diseases with a common clinical manifestation. The true scope of the problem is not known, since many people have unrecognized PH. The terms "primary" (idiopathic or familial) and "secondary" pulmonary hypertension have been abandoned. The latest classification scheme (2003 Venice Third World Symposium on Pulmonary Arterial Hypertension)(3) outlined five major categories of PH (4):

1. Pulmonary arterial hypertension (PAH)
2. Pulmonary hypertension related to left heart disease
3. Pulmonary hypertension related to lung disease or hypoxemia
4. Chronic thrombotic or embolic pulmonary hypertension
5. Miscellaneous

### Idiopathic or Familial Pulmonary Arterial Hypertension

Fortunately, idiopathic or familial PAH (previously known as "primary pulmonary hypertension") is rare (about 1 to 2 cases per million). It is estimated that there are 100,000 PAH patients with Class III–IV symptoms in the United States, with about 300 new cases diagnosed each year (3). Familial cases account for 5% to 10% of all PH cases. Mutations in the bone morphogenetic protein receptor II (BMPR2) gene have been identified in about 50% of patients with familial PAH, and in 25% of patients with sporadic, idiopathic PAH (5). Other families with PAH have demonstrated linkage to the same chromosome region where BMPR2 resides (2q32). Lack of a functional BMPR2 gene appears to affect antiproliferative pathways of vascular cells. Other genetic mutations have also been identified, including the activin-receptor-like kinase 1 (ALK-1), changes in cellular $K_v$ channel expression and function, and polymorphisms involving the serotonin transporter (5-HTT), plasminogen activator inhibitor-1 (PAI-1), and endothelial nitric oxide synthase (ecNOS) genes (1,5). Relatives of patients with familial idiopathic PAH should be advised about the availability of genetic testing and counseling in addition to echocardiographic screening (1,6).

### Pulmonary Hypertension in Pregnancy

Several patient populations with higher risks of developing PH are worth mentioning—those with pregnancy, systemic sclerosis, and liver cirrhosis. The blunted pulmonary vascular reactivity cannot adequately compensate for the increase in blood volume during pregnancy in patients with pre-existing PH (i.e., without any pulmonary vasoreactivity reserve) (see Chapter 55). Maternal mortality rates may be as high as 35% to 50% in patients with PH, and therefore pregnancy should be avoided. However, there is no consensus regarding the safety of hormonal contraceptive agents in patients with PH.

### Pulmonary Hypertension in Connective Tissue Disorders

Up to 50% of patients with limited systemic sclerosis (or CREST syndrome) may develop PH (7). In contrast, in patients with diffuse systemic sclerosis (scleroderma), PH develops in association with pulmonary fibrosis and a decrease in lung diffusion capacity. Therefore patients with these disorders should be screened regularly with pulmonary function tests.

### Portopulmonary Hypertension

Approximately 2% to 10% of cirrhotic patients develop proliferative pulmonary arteriopathy and plexiform lesions, often referred to as "portopulmonary hypertension." The development of PH in this population is poorly understood and may portend poor survival (median 6 months) and high transplant mortality (8,9). Medical interventions and liver transplantation may sometimes reverse mild to moderate portopulmonary hypertension.

## PATHOPHYSIOLOGY

The pulmonary circulation capacity is approximately one tenth of the circulating blood volume, and can be increased by both recruitment and distention to increase pulmonary blood flow up to fourfold without an appreciable change in pulmonary artery pressures. This low-pressure, low-resistance, and high-compliance vascular bed is regulated by a balance of vasodilators (including prostacyclin, nitric oxide, natriuretic peptides, and adrenomedullin) and vasoconstrictors (thromboxane A2, endothelin-1, angiotensin-II, and serotonin). Various external and host genetic factors may influence this intricate balance.

Pulmonary vasoconstriction is believed to be an early component of the pulmonary hypertensive process. Excessive vasoconstriction has been related to abnormal function or expression of potassium channels in the smooth muscle cells. In many forms of PH, vascular remodeling is mediated by (a) distal extension of smooth muscle cells in to the small, peripheral, nonmuscular branches of the pulmonary arterial tree and (b) formation of neointima by myofibroblasts and extracellular matrix (10). Angiopoietin-1, an angiogenic factor essential for vascular lung development, seems to be upregulated in cases of PH, correlating directly with the severity of the disease. In addition, inflammatory cells are ubiquitous in PAH and can further cause pulmonary vascular damage and endothelial dysfunction by cytokine release and cytotoxic effects. A reduction of prostacyclin synthase expression as well as prothrombotic abnormalities in the pulmonary arteries has also been demonstrated in PH patients (Fig. 34–1). The

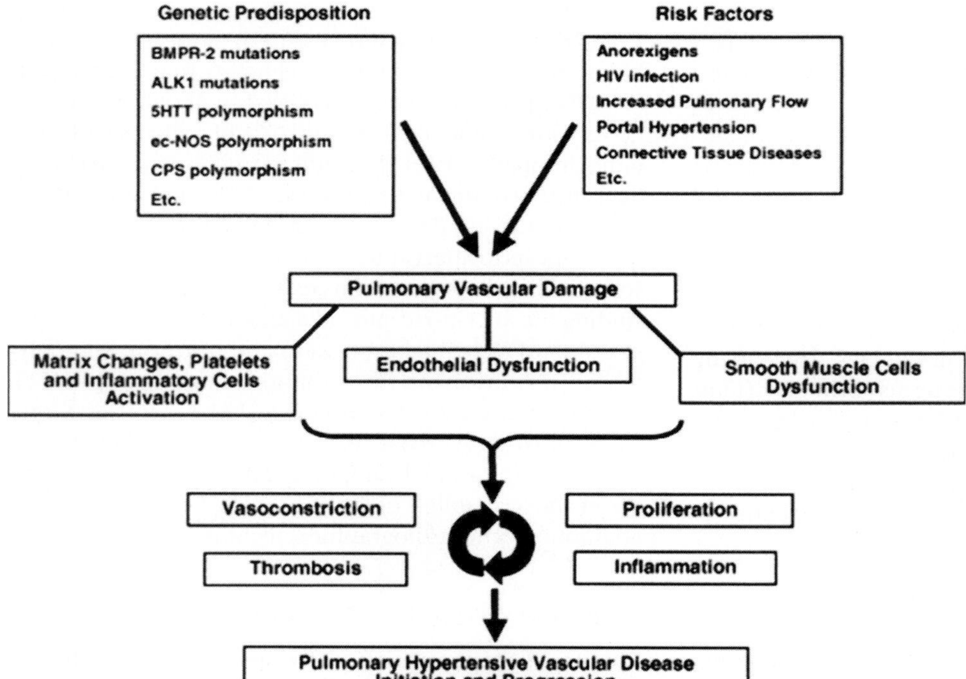


**Figure 34–1** Pathophysiology of pulmonary hypertension. Abbreviations: BMPR-2, bone morphogenetic protein receptor II; ALK-1, activin-receptor-like kinase 1; 5HTT, serotonin transporter; ec-NOS, endothelial cell nitric oxide synthase; CPS, carbamyl-phosphate synthase; HIV, human immunodeficiency virus. (Reproduced from Galie N, Torbicki A, Barst R, et al. Guidelines on diagnosis and treatment of pulmonary arterial hypertension. The Task Force on Diagnosis and Treatment of Pulmonary Arterial Hypertension of the European Society of Cardiology. *Eur Heart J.* 2004; 25:2243–2278.)

precise cellular and molecular process is not well understood, but endothelin-1 (ET-1) and nitric oxide (NO) have been well established as major players in the pathophysiology (as well as the therapeutic targets) in pulmonary arterial hypertension.

### Endothelin

Endothelin-1 belongs to a family of vasoconstrictor peptides that plays an important role in vascular control. It is produced and released from endothelial cells as Big ET-1, and converted to vasoactive ET-1 by endothelin-converting enzymes, ECE-1A (in endothelial cells) and ECE-1B (in smooth muscle cells). In patients with PH, ET-1 levels are often increased, and ET-A receptors are abundant (11). ET-1 causes vasoconstriction and has a mitogenic effect on vascular smooth muscles via their ET-A receptors.

### Nitric Oxide

Nitric oxide is also produced in endothelial cells from L-arginine by nitric oxide synthases (NOS). Inducible NOS (iNOS or NOS2) is activated by inflammatory agents and cytokines, while constitutive NOS (cNOS or NOS1) provides background vasodilatation (by a cGMP-mediated mechanism) and inhibition of smooth muscle mitogenesis (12). An overactive ET-1 and/or a deficient NO state can lead to persistent proliferation of pulmonary vasculopathy with vascular injury, endothelial dysfunction, and smooth muscle proliferation.

### Right Ventricular Function

The right ventricle is a "flow generator," allowing the collection of large preload blood volumes to be oxygenated swiftly across the pulmonary capillary bed to the left ventricular chamber. Ultimately, progressive obstruction of the pulmonary blood flow can result in an increase in right ventricular afterload. Distention of the right ventricle not only limits the preload reserve but also distorts the ventricular interdependence by a leftward septal shift that in turn decreases left ventricular compliance. Increase in right ventricular afterload may also increase free wall tension, leading to hypertrophy, ischemia, and decrease in right ventricular and cardiac output (13). Signs and symptoms of right heart failure often ensue, as the thin walls of the right ventricle cannot further withstand the increasing pulmonary vascular resistance and tricuspid regurgitation.

## DIAGNOSIS AND EVALUATION

The biggest challenge for diagnosing PH is the lag time between symptom onset and confirmation of elevated pulmonary artery pressures. In 90% of patients, the mean length of time to diagnosis is 2 years, in part because symptoms of PH are usually gradual in onset and progression, and very nonspecific. Eventually, the majority of patients will develop symptoms of dyspnea (98%) and fatigue (73%), with a wide variety of other cardiac symptoms including chest pain, syncope and near-syncope, pedal edema, palpitations, skin changes, and cyanosis.

### Risk Factors for Pulmonary Hypertension

Since PH caused by a primary valvular disorder should be treated in a different manner than that caused by chronic thromboembolism, identification of the precise location of the "lesion" that is causing PH will facilitate the appropriate treatment strategies (Table 34–1) (6). In general, PAH is more likely to occur in women than in men. A careful history and physical examination is necessary to reveal other risk factors and associated conditions with PH, particularly the following:

1. A family history of PH
2. Current or remote use of anorexigens (mainly derivatives of fenfluramine [14]), amphetamines, L-tryptophan, or other illicit drugs
3. Underlying connective tissue disorders, especially CREST syndrome
4. Pre-existing liver or hematologic diseases (e.g., deep venous thrombosis, pulmonary embolism, thrombophilia, sickle cell disease)
5. Underlying left heart failure or valvular diseases
6. Chronic obstructive pulmonary disease, interstitial lung disease, or sleep apnea
7. Poorly controlled systemic hypertension (a common and often forgotten cause of elevated right ventricular systolic pressure [RVSP] in symptomatic patients)

### Clinical Evaluation

Clinical examination of PH may reveal a left parasternal lift, a loud P2 at apex, a pan-systolic murmur of tricuspid regurgitation that increases with inspiration, a diastolic murmur of pulmonary insufficiency, and a right ventricular S3. Jugular vein distension, hepatomegaly with a pulsatile liver, peripheral edema, and ascites are often indicative of advanced stages with frank right-sided heart failure (1,6).

Chest x-rays often reveal central pulmonary arterial dilatation with "pruning" (loss) of the peripheral blood vessels, clear lung fields, and a prominent right ventricular border. Chest computed tomography (CT) and perfusion-ventilation (V/Q) scans are indicated to exclude primary parenchymal or thromboembolic diseases as a cause of PH (1,6). The same pruning of the pulmonary vasculature can also be demonstrated directly in pulmonary angiograms, which is sometimes indicated to detect chronic thromboembolic causes of PH. Pulmonary angioscopy is sometimes performed in specialized centers in cases of chronic thromboembolic pulmonary hypertension to determine surgical candidacy.

**TABLE 34–1**
**SECONDARY ETIOLOGIES OF PULMONARY HYPERTENSION ACCORDING TO LESION LOCATION**

| Location | Etiologies |
|---|---|
| Pulmonary artery | Pulmonary valve stenosis<br>Pulmonary embolism and/or thrombotic disease<br>Idiopathic or familial pulmonary (arterial) hypertension<br>Collagen vascular disease<br>Congenital systemic-to-pulmonary shunts<br>HIV infection<br>Drugs (anorexigens, amphetamines, and other illicit drugs)<br>Portal hypertension |
| Pulmonary parenchyma & capillaries | Lung diseases: interstitial lung disease (e.g., idiopathic pulmonary fibrosis), sleep-disordered breathing, alveolar hypoventilation disorders, chronic obstructive pulmonary diseases<br>Miscellaneous: sarcoidosis, histiocytosis X, lymphangiomatosis<br>Hypoxia or chronic exposure to high altitude<br>Pulmonary capillary hemangiomatosis (PCH) |
| Pulmonary vein | Pulmonary venoocclusive disease (PVOD) |
| Left atrium | Mitral valve stenosis or regurgitation<br>Total anomalous pulmonary venous return (TAPVR)<br>Cor triatriatum<br>Left atrial myxoma |
| Left ventricle | Myocardial disease (cardiomyopathy)<br>Aortic valve stenosis or regurgitation |
| Aorta | Systemic hypertension |

## Echocardiographic Evaluation

The majority of PH patients have an abnormal electrocardiogram, usually presenting with evidence of right ventricular hypertrophy with strain, sometimes with right atrial enlargement (Fig. 34–2). These findings of right ventricular dysfunction and pulmonary hypertension can be confirmed by transthoracic echocardiography (15). A flattened intraventricular septum with a "D-shaped" left ventricle in the parasternal short-axis view, as well as early pulmonary valve systolic closure and an absent A-wave in M-mode, are indicative of right ventricular pressure overload. RVSP is estimated by the formula from the modified Bernoulli equation: RVSP $= [4v^2 + \text{RAP}]$, where $v$ is the tricuspid regurgitant jet velocity, and RAP is the estimated right atrial pressure based on inferior vena cava characteristics. However, RVSP has no direct relationship with the severity of tricuspid regurgitation, and can both overestimate true pulmonary artery pressures in non-PH patients and underestimate true pulmonary artery pressures in PH patients. Echocardiography is also a useful modality to detect intracardiac shunting by contrast studies, and structural assessment of the cardiac chambers. Pericardial effusion associated with pulmonary hypertension is often a poor prognostic sign.

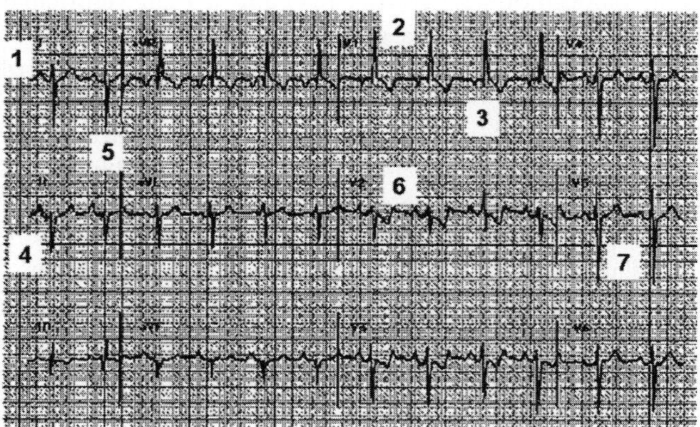


**Figure 34–2** Typical electrocardiogram for pulmonary hypertension. Key: 1, R-axis deviation; 2, tall R in V1, R/S >1; 3, qR in V1; 4, RA enlargement; 5, S1–S2–S3; 6, ST–T-wave inversion in R precordial leads; 7, tall S in V5, R/S <1.

## Hemodynamic Evaluation

Cardiac catheterization provides the definitive diagnosis of PH, with direct measurement of right heart pressures using a fluid-filled catheter (16). According to Ohm's law, change in pressure is proportional to the product of flow and resistance. In the case of PH, the gradient across the pulmonary vasculature (often referred to as "transpulmonary gradient" or TPG) should equal the flow (cardiac output) times the resistance (pulmonary vascular resistance, PVR). Translating

**TABLE 34–2**
**PULMONARY HYPERTENSION HEMODYNAMIC CLASSIFICATION**

| | Normal | Mild/Moderate PAH | Severe PAH |
|---|---|---|---|
| Catheterization | | | |
| PA mean (mm Hg) | 9–24 | 25–55 | >55 |
| TPG (mm Hg) | 2–10 | 10–15 | >15 |
| PVR (Wood) | 0.5–2 | 2–5 | >5 |
| Doppler echo | | | |
| TR velocity (m/s) | <3.4 | 2.8–4.2 | >4.2 |
| RVSP (mm Hg) | 15–57 | 36–75 | >75 |

PAH, pulmonary arterial hypertension; PA, pulmonary artery; sys, systolic; diast, diastolic; TPG, transpulmonary gradient; PVR, pulmonary vascular resistance; TR, tricuspid regurgitation; PASP, pulmonary artery systolic pressure.

into variables obtained from right heart catheterization, we have:

*Hemodynamic Calculations for Pulmonary Hypertension Evaluation:*

Mean pulmonary artery pressure (PAP) $= (2 \times \text{diastolic PAP} + \text{systolic PAP}) \div 3$

Transpulmonary gradient (TPG) $=$ mean PAP $-$ mean pulmonary capillary wedge pressure

$\therefore$ Pulmonary vascular resistance
$= (\text{TPG} \div \text{cardiac output (in Woods unit)}$, or
$= (\text{TPG} \div \text{cardiac output}) \times 80$ (in dynes-s-cm$^{-5}$)

Table 34–2 presents the hemodynamic classification of pulmonary hypertension based on catheterization and Doppler echocardiography findings. In parallel to the natural history of PH, the preclinical presentation of PH is characterized by a progressive increase in mean PAP with preserved cardiac output, leading to rising TPG and therefore PVR. However, as symptoms develop and progress to advanced stages, cardiac output deteriorates and pulmonary capillary wedge pressure increases, which may result in a relative plateau or even lowering of TPG but sustained elevation in PVR.

Cardiac catheterization has also been employed to monitor therapeutic responses in PH patients in both the acute and long-term settings. Identification of vasodilator responders was a crucial part of diagnostic work-up a decade or two ago, when calcium channel blocker therapy was the mainstay of therapy in the 10% of PH patients who were deemed "vasodilator responders" by oral nifedipine challenge. There has been a wide variation regarding the definition of a responder, and the latest guidelines advocated a >10-mm Hg decrease of mean PAP to reach <40 mm Hg in the setting of an increased or unchanged cardiac index and systemic blood pressure. Current vasodilator challenges include the use of adenosine or prostacyclin infusions, or nitric oxide inhalation if available. Generally, only 10% to 15% of idiopathic PAH patients will fulfill this criteria and will be tried on calcium channel blockers as first-line agents (17). About half of this subgroup of patients will have long-term symptomatic improvement or relief with calcium channel blocker therapy. In contrast, unfavorable responders are those with ≥20% decrease in mean arterial pressure, persistently high mean right atrial pressure, and low oxygen saturations during testing.

## TREATMENT

A summary of the findings of major randomized clinical trials of PAH and an evidence-based treatment algorithm are shown in Table 34–3 and Figure 34–3, respectively (1,18).

### General Measures

After confirming the diagnosis of PH, the general management strategy goal is to determine and treat potential underlying reversible causes, and to provide symptomatic relief as well as specific drug therapies directed at reducing pulmonary artery pressures. Symptom-limited exercise regimens should be employed if tolerated, and prophylactic vaccinations and counseling to avoid pregnancy or hormone-replacement therapy should be provided together with patient education. Patients with hypoxemia as the cause should have close monitoring of their hemoglobin levels. Anticoagulation therapy is often indicated in PH patients. The majority of patients may need symptomatic relief with diuretic therapy and oxygen for right-sided heart failure symptoms. Few studies have confirmed the potential benefits of inotropic therapy, including digoxin, dobutamine, or milrinone.

### Synthetic Prostacyclin and Prostacyclin Analogs

Prostacyclin is a potent endogenous vasodilator and an inhibitor of platelet aggregation, vascular growth, remodeling, and obliteration. This may explain why epoprostenol (Flolan), a synthetic salt of prostacyclin, can be used to acutely lower pulmonary artery pressures (as used in vasoreactivity testing) as well as to achieve long-term hemodynamic improvement for PH patients who are vasodilator nonresponders. Long-term intravenous administration of epoprostenol lowers PVR beyond the level achieved in the acute vasoreactivity tests. However, epoprostenol has to be administered in a continuous intravenous infusion, and early titration often results in unbearable side effects of nausea, headache, flushing, jaw and leg pain, and diarrhea.

**TABLE 34–3**
**RANDOMIZED CLINICAL TRIALS IN PATIENTS WITH PULMONARY ARTERIAL HYPERTENSION**

| | Epoprostenol (21) | Epoprostenol (26) | Treprostinil (22) | Bosentan (23) | Sildenafil[a] |
|---|---|---|---|---|---|
| Route | Intravenous | Intravenous | Subcutaneous | Oral | Oral |
| Sample size | 81 | 111 | 469 | 213 | 278 |
| Study population | IPAH | PAH, CTD (scleroderma) | IPAH, CTD, CHD | IPAH, CTD | IPAH |
| NYHA | III–IV | II–IV | II–IV | II–IV | II–III |
| Duration (mo) | 3 | 3 | 3 | 4 | 4 |
| Outcomes: | | | | | |
| 6MWT (m) | +47 | +94 | +16 | +44 | +45 |
| Hemodynamics | Improved | Improved | Improved | — | Improved |
| Clinical events | Reduced | No change | Reduced | Reduced | ? |
| FDA approval | Yes | Yes | Yes | Yes | Yes |
| References | Hinderliter et al., *Circulation*, 1997 | Badesch et al., *Ann Intern Med.*, 2000 | Simonneau et al., *Am J Respir Crit Care Med.*, 2002 | Rubin et al., *N Engl J Med.*, 2002 | Galìé et al., *NEJM*, 2005 |

IPAH, idiopathic pulmonary arterial hypertension; PAH, pulmonary arterial hypertension; CTD, connective tissue disorders; CHD, congenital heart diseases; 6MWT, 6-minute walk test.

The efficacy of epoprostenol has been tested in several unblinded clinical trials in idiopathic PAH and scleroderma-associated PAH; epoprostenol therapy is associated with symptomatic, functional, and hemodynamic improvement as well as a survival benefit (19–21). Continuous subcutaneous administration of another prostacyclin analog, treprostinil (Remodulin), in PAH patients also resulted in improvements in exercise capacity, hemodynamics, and clinical events (22). Other preparations of prostacyclin analogs, such as the orally active sodium beraprost and inhaled and intravenous iloprost, are available only outside the United States.

## Oral Vasodilators

Bosentan is an oral active dual $ET_A/ET_B$-receptor antagonist that has been evaluated in PAH patients. Treatment with oral bosentan resulted in improvement in exercise capacity, functional class, hemodynamics, cardiac performance by echocardiography, and clinical outcomes (23). However, concerns over liver toxicity, anemia, and fluid retention require close monitoring during the treatment period. Currently, it is used as a first-line agent in mild to moderate PH (New York Heart Association [NYHA] Class II–III) before epoprostenol infusion. Other drugs in this class, such

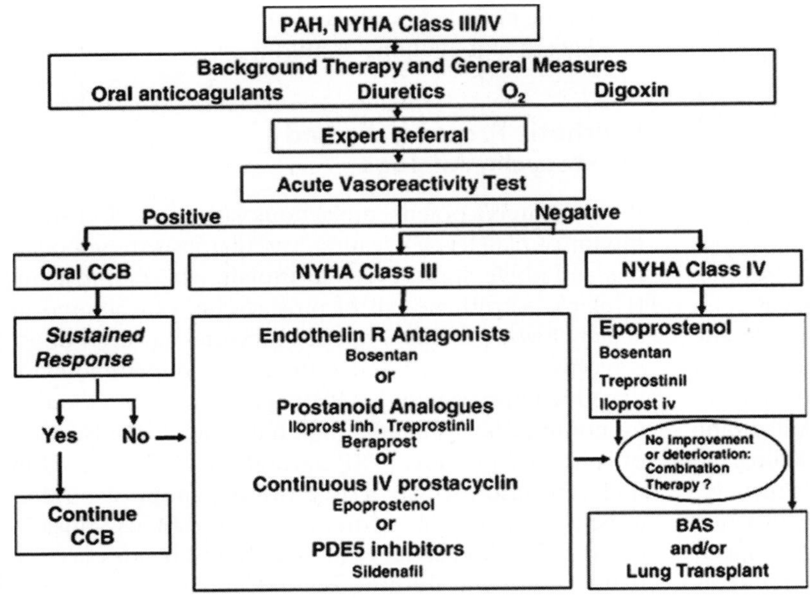


**Figure 34–3** American College of Chest Physicians/European Society of Cardiology guidelines on evidence-based treatment algorithm for pulmonary arterial hypertension (PAH). Abbreviations: CCB, calcium channel blockers; inh, inhaled; iv, continuous intravenous; PDE, phosphodiesterase; R, receptors; BAS, balloon atrial septostomy. (Reproduced from Galie N, Torbicki A, Barst R, et al. Guidelines on diagnosis and treatment of pulmonary arterial hypertension. The Task Force on Diagnosis and Treatment of Pulmonary Arterial Hypertension of the European Society of Cardiology. *Eur Heart J.* 2004;25:2243–2278.)

**TABLE 34–4**
**PROGNOSTIC VARIABLES AND SURVIVAL IN PULMONARY ARTERIAL HYPERTENSION**

| Hemodynamics (2) | Echocardiography (27) | Clinical (19) |
|---|---|---|
| Mean right atrial pressure | Pericardial effusion<br>Right atrial area | Functional class (NYHA) |
| Mean pulmonary artery pressure (mPAP) | Right ventricular end-diastolic area index | Exercise time and distance (6-minute walk test) |
| Cardiac index (CI) | Eccentricity index | B-type natriuretic peptide levels |
| Response to vasoreactivity testing:<br>PVR<br>MPAP<br>CI | Septal shift | Uric acid |

as sitaxsentan and ambrisentan, are currently undergoing active clinical investigations. Recent studies have also reported favorable effects of the orally active type 5 phosphodiesterase inhibitor, sildenafil (Viagra), in patients with PH (1) It is likely that sildenafil will be added to existing treatment regimens, either alone, in combination with ET-1 receptor antagonists, or with prostacyclin analogs.

### Surgical Therapies

In patients with chronic thromboembolic pulmonary hypertension (CTEPH), potentially curable thromboembolectomy surgery can be performed in experienced clinical centers (24). The role of balloon atrial septostomy in the treatment of PAH patients is uncertain, and is rarely performed, unless for palliation for advanced PAH patients with recurrent syncope and/or right heart failure despite all available medical treatments. Lung transplantation should be considered in a subset of eligible patients who remain in NYHA functional Class III or IV, or in those who cannot achieve a significant exercise and hemodynamic improvement after 3 months of epoprostenol therapy (24).

## PROGNOSIS

The untreated natural history of PH is one of progressive symptoms of dyspnea and right heart failure with poor survival (25). Recent clinical trials on epoprostenol indicated that long-term survival of patients with idiopathic PAH was about 65% at 3 years (19), which is far superior to that observed in the National Institute of Health PAH Registry data of <40% (2). Table 34–4 outlines the clinical, echocardiographic, and hemodynamic features that may predict prognosis in PH patients. Recent clinical trials have also suggested that improvement in NYHA functional class, 6-minute walk test distance, and fall in PVR <30% following 3 months of epoprostenol therapy may predict better prognosis (25).

## REFERENCES


1. Galie N, Torbicki A, Barst R, et al. Guidelines on diagnosis and treatment of pulmonary arterial hypertension. The Task Force on Diagnosis and Treatment of Pulmonary Arterial Hypertension of the European Society of Cardiology. *Eur Heart J.* 2004;25:2243–2278.
2. D'Alonzo GE, Barst RJ, Ayres SM, et al. Survival in patients with primary pulmonary hypertension. Results from a national prospective registry. *Ann Intern Med.* 1991;115:343–349.
3. McLaughlin VV. Classification and epidemiology of pulmonary hypertension. *Cardiol Clin.* 2004;22:327–341, v.
4. Simonneau G, Galie N, Rubin LJ, et al. Clinical classification of pulmonary hypertension. *J Am Coll Cardiol.* 2004;43:5S–12S.
5. Newman JH, Trembath RC, Morse JA, et al. Genetic basis of pulmonary arterial hypertension: current understanding and future directions. *J Am Coll Cardiol.* 2004;43:33S–39S.
6. McGoon M, Gutterman D, Steen V, et al. Screening, early detection, and diagnosis of pulmonary arterial hypertension: ACCP evidence-based clinical practice guidelines. *Chest.* 2004;126: 14S–34S.
7. Fagan KA, Badesch DB. Pulmonary hypertension associated with connective tissue disease. *Prog Cardiovasc Dis.* 2002;45:225–234.
8. Hoeper MM, Krowka MJ, Strassburg CP. Portopulmonary hypertension and hepatopulmonary syndrome. *Lancet.* 2004;363: 1461–1468.
9. Krowka MJ, Mandell MS, Ramsay MA, et al. Hepatopulmonary syndrome and portopulmonary hypertension: a report of the multicenter liver transplant database. *Liver Transpl.* 2004;10: 174–182.
10. Humbert M, Morrell NW, Archer SL, et al. Cellular and molecular pathobiology of pulmonary arterial hypertension. *J Am Coll Cardiol.* 2004;43:13S–24S.
11. Channick RN, Sitbon O, Barst RJ, et al. Endothelin receptor antagonists in pulmonary arterial hypertension. *J Am Coll Cardiol.* 2004;43:62S–67S.
12. Ghofrani HA, Pepke-Zaba J, Barbera JA, et al. Nitric oxide pathway and phosphodiesterase inhibitors in pulmonary arterial hypertension. *J Am Coll Cardiol.* 2004;43:68S–72S.
13. Chin KM, Kim NH, Rubin LJ. The right ventricle in pulmonary hypertension. *Coron Artery Dis.* 2005;16:13–18.
14. Abenhaim L, Moride Y, Brenot F, et al. Appetite-suppressant drugs and the risk of primary pulmonary hypertension. International Primary Pulmonary Hypertension Study Group. *N Engl J Med.* 1996;335:609–616.

15. Ghio S, Raineri C, Scelsi L, et al. Usefulness and limits of transthoracic echocardiography in the evaluation of patients with primary and chronic thromboembolic pulmonary hypertension. *J Am Soc Echocardiogr*. 2002;15:1374–1380.
16. Guillinta P, Peterson KL, Ben-Yehuda O. Cardiac catheterization techniques in pulmonary hypertension. *Cardiol Clin*. 2004;22: 401–415, vi.
17. Rich S, Kaufmann E, Levy PS. The effect of high doses of calcium-channel blockers on survival in primary pulmonary hypertension. *N Engl J Med*. 1992;327:76–81.
18. Galie N, Seeger W, Naeije R, et al. Comparative analysis of clinical trials and evidence-based treatment algorithm in pulmonary arterial hypertension. *J Am Coll Cardiol*. 2004;43: 81S–88S.
19. McLaughlin VV, Shillington A, Rich S. Survival in primary pulmonary hypertension: the impact of epoprostenol therapy. *Circulation*. 2002;106:1477–1482.
20. McLaughlin VV, Genthner DE, et al. Reduction in pulmonary vascular resistance with long-term epoprostenol (prostacyclin) therapy in primary pulmonary hypertension. *N Engl J Med*. 1998;338: 273–277.
21. Hinderliter AL, Willis PWt, Barst RJ, et al. Effects of long-term infusion of prostacyclin (epoprostenol) on echocardiographic measures of right ventricular structure and function in primary pulmonary hypertension. Primary Pulmonary Hypertension Study Group. *Circulation*. 1997;95:1479–1486.
22. Simonneau G, Barst RJ, Galie N, et al. Continuous subcutaneous infusion of treprostinil, a prostacyclin analogue, in patients with pulmonary arterial hypertension: a double-blind, randomized, placebo-controlled trial. *Am J Respir Crit Care Med*. 2002;165: 800–804.
23. Humbert M, Barst RJ, Robbins IM, et al. Combination of bosentan with epoprostenol in pulmonary arterial hypertension: BREATHE-2. *Eur Respir J*. 2004;24:353–359.
24. Doyle RL, McCrory D, Channick RN, Simonneau G, Conte J. Surgical treatments/interventions for pulmonary arterial hypertension: ACCP evidence-based clinical practice guidelines. *Chest*. 2004;126:63S–71S.
25. McLaughlin VV, Presberg KW, Doyle RL, et al. Prognosis of pulmonary arterial hypertension: ACCP evidence-based clinical practice guidelines. *Chest*. 2004;126:78S–92S.
26. Badesch DB, Tapson VF, McGoon MD, et al. Continuous intravenous epoprostenol for pulmonary hypertension due to the scleroderma spectrum of disease. A randomized, controlled trial. *Ann Intern Med*. 2000;132:425–434.
27. Raymond RJ, Hinderliter AL, Willis PW, et al. Echocardiographic predictors of adverse outcomes in primary pulmonary hypertension. *J Am Coll Cardiol*. 2002;39:1214–1219.

## QUESTIONS

**1.** A 45-year-old woman with a history of hypertension presented with dyspnea upon exertion. You obtained an echocardiogram showing normal left ventricular systolic and diastolic function, normal right ventricular size and function, normal valvular function, but an estimated RVSP of 56 mm Hg with 1–2+ tricuspid regurgitation. Your next step should be

a. To perform a pulmonary angiogram
b. To perform to right heart catheterization
c. To start oral bosentan therapy and follow up in 6 weeks
d. To repeat an echocardiogram in 6 months

Answer is b: Echocardiographic estimations of right ventricular systolic pressures may potentially overestimate the true pulmonary artery pressures, and should be confirmed by right heart catheterization in the setting of a clinical suspicion for pulmonary hypertension.

**2.** Routine diagnostic work-up for PAH in a patient with CREST syndrome and presenting with dyspnea upon exertion should include all of the following *except*:

a. Transthoracic echocardiography
b. Right heart catheterization
c. Pulmonary function testing with DLCO
d. Genetic testing for BNPR2 mutation

Answer is d: CREST syndrome patients have a higher probability of developing pulmonary hypertension, and should be screened, particularly with symptom onset. Echocardiography and right heart catheterization are reasonable tools to detect pulmonary hypertension, and pulmonary function testing may reveal lung parenchymal abnormalities. Genetic screening is indicated only in familial cases of pulmonary hypertension, and the incidence of BMPR2 gene mutation in patients with CREST syndrome and pulmonary hypertension is actually low.

**3.** Poor prognostic variables for PAH include all of the following *except*:

a. Septal shifting
b. Presence of pericardial effusion
c. Dilated right atrium
d. Walks 360 m in 6 minutes

Answer is d: Septal shifting, presence of pericardial effusion, and dilated right atrium are all poor prognostic signs for elevated right ventricular preload and pulmonary hypertension. In clinical trials, a distance of less than 332 m in a 6-minute walk test is considered poor functional capacity with a poor prognosis.

# Diastolic Heart Failure

35

***Oussama Wazni   Allan L. Klein***

Congestive heart failure is most often secondary to impairment of left ventricular systolic function. Diastolic heart failure is increasingly common and can be associated with significant morbidity and mortality. Clinically, it is important to distinguish these conditions, though in a given patient, combined systolic and diastolic dysfunction is frequently observed. Several pathophysiologic definitions of diastolic heart failure have been proposed:

1. Impaired ventricular filling capacity without a compensatory increase in left atrial pressure
2. Abnormal ventricular filling resulting in inadequate cardiac output with a mean pulmonary venous pressure of <12 mm Hg
3. Resistance to filling of either or both ventricles with an inappropriate shift of the pressure–volume loop.

These definitions all have an abnormal resistance to filling, causing elevated left-sided filling pressures and congestion. Diastolic dysfunction impairs filling of the ventricle by impairing relaxation (early diastole), reducing compliance (early to late diastole), or by external constraint from the pericardium. Numerous pathologic processes and disease states may produce the clinical constellation of diastolic dysfunction.

Diagnostic criteria for patients with diastolic heart failure have been proposed. The 1998 European Study Group on Diastolic Heart Failure required (a) clinical evidence of congestive heart failure, (b) normal or mild left ventricular dysfunction, and (c) the presence of impaired relaxation, filling, or compliance in order to diagnose diastolic heart failure. All three components as assessed by noninvasive testing or cardiac catheterization were necessary for a diagnosis. Vasan and Levy subsequently proposed less rigid criteria using similar inclusions but defining diastolic heart failure as definite, probable, or possible, depending on the number of elements present. Recently, there has been a debate about whether heart failure with normal systolic function is really diastolic dysfunction or whether it is related to vascular-cardiac interaction.

## PHASES OF DIASTOLE

Diastole is the period from the closure of the aortic valve to the end of mitral inflow. It is divided into two periods: (a) An isovolumic relaxation period and (b) An auxotonic period that includes rapid filling, diastasis (slow filling), and atrial systole.

### Isovolumic Relaxation Phase

The isovolumic relaxation time period occurs from the time of aortic valve closure to mitral valve opening. There is no change in left ventricular volume during this period. There is active, energy-dependent myocyte relaxation until mid-diastole. Isovolumic relaxation ends when the left ventricular pressure falls below the left atrial pressure, resulting in mitral valve opening. At this point, the rapid filling phase commences.

### Rapid Filling Phase

The auxotonic period occurs from mitral valve opening until mitral valve closure. When the left ventricular pressure falls below left atrial pressure, the mitral valve opens, resulting in the rapid filling phase. Left ventricular pressure continues to fall due to ongoing relaxation and elastic recoil. Blood acceleration occurs as a result of the development of a left atrial-to-left ventricular pressure gradient. Blood rapidly enters the left ventricle from the left atrium during the early filling period. Approximately 70% of the stroke volume received by the left ventricle is during the first third of diastole. Rapid filling ends as atrial and ventricular pressures become equal.

### Diastasis (Slow Filling) Phase

Subsequent to rapid filling, left atrial and ventricular pressures almost equalize and there is no forward driving gradient, resulting in diastasis or the slow filling. Diastasis accounts for <5% of filling.

### Atrial Filling (Contraction) Phase

Atrial contraction (atrial filling) results in a rise in left atrial pressure above ventricular pressure, forcing blood across the mitral valve and a small amount of regurgitation into the pulmonary veins. In normal hearts this accounts for 25% of ventricular end-diastolic volume, with only a small rise in mean pulmonary venous pressure. Diastole ends and systole begins with the onset of ventricular contraction, resulting in a rapid increase in left ventricular pressure that closes the mitral valve.

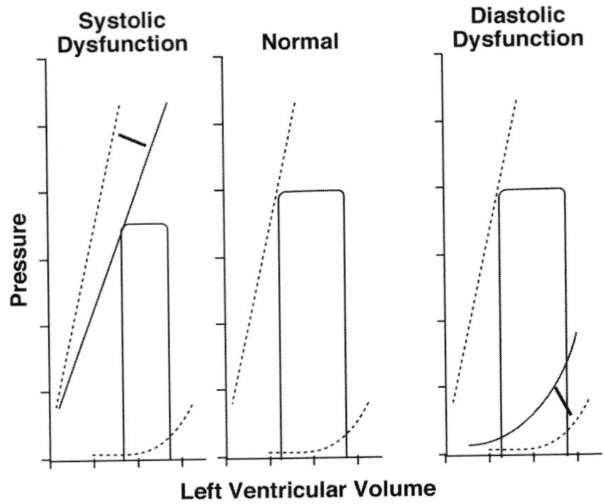


**Figure 35–1** Schematic representation of ventricular pressure–volume loops. The center panel demonstrates the normal situation. Note the exponential nature of the curve through late diastole. In systolic dysfunction **(*left*)**, the end-systolic pressure line is displayed downward and is manifest by a decreased ability of the left ventricle to generate high pressures for a given volume. Diastolic dysfunction involves an upward and leftward shift of the exponential curve, a result of elevated filling pressures for a given volume. (Adapted from Katz AM. Influence of altered inotropy and lusitropy on ventricular pressure-volume loops. *J Am Coll Cardiol.* 1988;11:438–445, with permission.)

## DETERMINANTS OF DIASTOLIC FUNCTION

Diastolic function depends on four major factors:

1. *Active myocardial relaxation.* This is mediated by intracellular ATP and calcium. Relaxation results from calcium sequestration into the sarcoplasmic reticulum by the calcium-ATPase pump after contraction. Abnormal relaxation may result from either elevated cytosolic levels of calcium in diastole or inadequate intracellular ATP levels.
2. *Passive pressure–volume relationships (i.e., left ventricular compliance).* This is determined by the viscoelastic nature of the myocardium; chamber size, shape, and wall thickness; right and left ventricular pressure–volume interaction; intrathoracic pressure; and pericardial restraint. As left ventricular volume increases during diastole, an increase in left ventricular pressure ensues. The slope of the pressure–volume curve during diastole ($dp/dV$) represents the chamber *stiffness;* and the inverse of this relation is the chamber *compliance* (Fig. 35–1).
3. *Left atrium (including atrial function), pulmonary vein, and mitral valve characteristics.*
4. *Heart rate.* As the heart rate increases, the diastolic filling period preferentially decreases with respect to the systolic ejection period.

## CLINICAL PRESENTATION

It is known that 50% of patients with heart failure have normal or near-normal left ventricular function. The presentation of heart failure may include flash pulmonary edema and hypertensive heart disease, advanced ischemic heart disease, or hypertensive hypertrophic cardiomyopathy. Patients who often do not respond to heart failure treatment include patients with aortic stenosis, hypertrophic cardiomyopathy, infiltrative cardiomyopathy, and constrictive pericarditis. Typically, elderly patients with hypertension are at highest risk for developing the clinical syndrome of diastolic heart failure. Signs and symptoms of diastolic heart failure include the following:

1. There is dyspnea on exertion and reduced exercise tolerance.
2. With disease progression, patients may have dyspnea at rest, paroxysmal nocturnal dyspnea, and orthopnea.
3. Right-sided diastolic dysfunction can cause peripheral edema, bloating, and ascites.

## PHYSICAL EXAMINATION

Physical examination cannot separate patients with diastolic heart failure from those with systolic heart failure. Most patients with diastolic heart failure have hypertension or coronary artery disease. On auscultation, an audible S4 (Stage 1 diastolic dysfunction by Doppler echocardiography, indicative of abnormal relaxation) or S3 (Stage 3 diastolic dysfunction by Doppler echocardiography, indicative of reduced compliance) can be heard. There may be pulmonary rales, jugular venous distension, and edema.

## LABORATORY EXAMINATION

### ECG

The most common abnormality is a left ventricular hypertrophy pattern. Left atrial abnormality may also be seen.

### Radiography

There are no specific findings on a chest x-ray. Pulmonary congestion with a normal cardiac silhouette suggests the presence of diastolic dysfunction.

### Echocardiography

Echocardiography is the modality of choice to assess for diastolic dysfunction. Findings on an echocardiogram include the following.

1. Normal left ventricular systolic function and isolated diastolic dysfunction. Patients with abnormal systolic function have secondary diastolic function.
2. Left ventricular hypertrophy.
3. Left atrial enlargement.
4. Evidence of impaired ventricular filling. This has four stages (Fig. 35–2):
   - *Stage I or impaired relaxation pattern.* The time from the peak early (E) wave to the baseline (the deceleration time; DT) is prolonged to >220 milliseconds. The early/atrial (E/A ratio) is <1 and the isovolumic relaxation time is >100 milliseconds. Color M-mode flow propagation slope is <40 cm/s. Tissue Doppler annulus early velocity is <8 cm/s.
   - *Stage II or pseudonormal pattern.* This is associated with a normal appearance of the transmitral inflow pattern with an E/A ratio between 1 and 2, a DT between 150 and 220 milliseconds, and an isovolumic relaxation time between 60 and 100 milliseconds. To distinguish this from normal, the pulmonary venous pattern is analyzed and shows a prolonged and increased atrial reversal time >35 cm/s and the pulmonary venous systolic-to-diastolic flow is normal or <1. Color M-mode reveals a flow propagation slope <40 cm/s. Tissue Doppler annulus early velocity is <8 cm/s.
   - *Stage III or restrictive filling pattern.* There is reduced left ventricular compliance. Elevated peak E-wave velocity and rapid deceleration are due to increased left ventricular stiffness. The E/A ratio is >2, DT <150 milliseconds, and isovolumic relaxation time is <60 milliseconds. Color M-mode reveals flow propagation slope <40 cm/s, and tissue Doppler annulus early velocity is usually <8 cm/s.
   - *Stage IV or irreversible restrictive pattern.* This stage is similar to the findings of Stage III, with no change in the Doppler pattern with preload-reducing maneuvers, and is associated with a substantially increased risk of death.

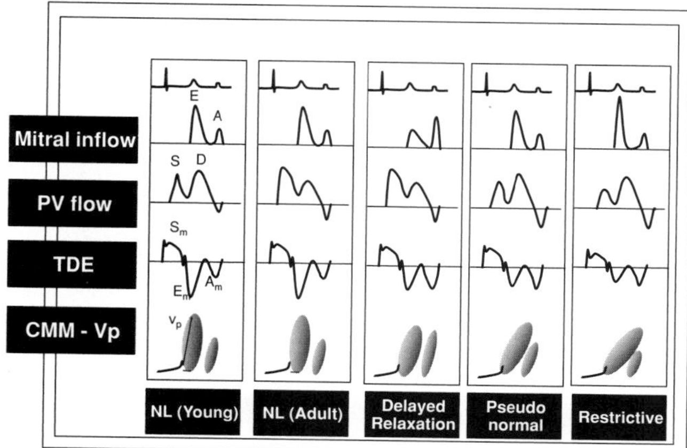


**Figure 35–2** Stage 1 or impaired relaxation pattern, Stage II or pseudonormal pattern, Stage III or restrictive filling pattern, and Stage IV or irreversible restrictive pattern. (Adapted from Garcia MJ, Thomas JD, Klein AL. New Doppler echocardiographic applications for the study of diastolic function. *J Am Coll Cardiol.* 1998;4:865–475, with permission.)

Doppler flow patterns can be used to estimate left atrial and left ventricular filling pressures. An increased E/A ratio, a shortened deceleration and isovolumic relaxation time, a decreased atrial filling fraction, a decreased pulmonary venous systolic fraction, an elevated and prolonged atrial reversal flow velocity, and increased left atrial volume may suggest an elevated mean left atrial pressure. By combining the mitral E-wave, a variable that correlates modestly with left atrial pressure and one that is associated with ventricular relaxation and is relatively preload independent (color M-mode propagation velocity or tissue Doppler echocardiography early filling velocity), closer approximations of left atrial pressure can be obtained. Algorithms for assessment of left atrial and left ventricular diastolic pressure have been proposed (Fig. 35–3).

## PROGNOSIS

Patients with congestive heart failure secondary to diastolic dysfunction generally have a better prognosis than patients with systolic dysfunction; however, they may have recurrent congestive heart failure, hospitalizations, and recurrent chest pain even with coronary revascularization. The prognosis of diastolic heart failure varies depending on the population studied, with an annual mortality rate varying at approximately 10% per year, which is lower than that of patients with systolic dysfunction (19%).

## TREATMENT OF DIASTOLIC HEART FAILURE

Treatment consists of reducing elevated filling pressures, maintaining atrial contraction, decreasing heart rate, preventing ischemia, improving relaxation, and implementing strategies to regress left ventricular hypertrophy. Treatment

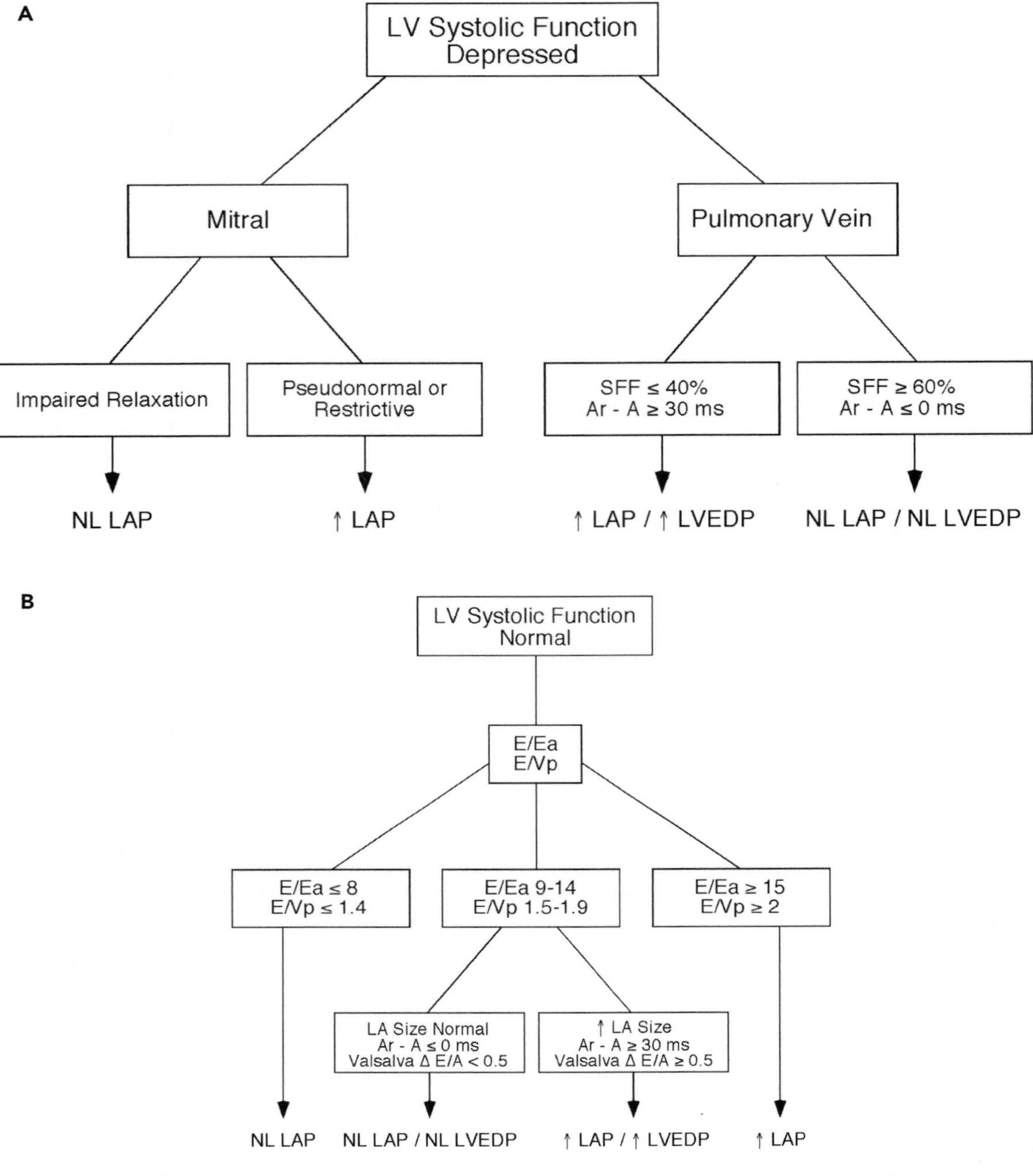


**Figure 35–3** **A:** An algorithm for assessment of left atrial (LA) pressure and left ventricular (LV)end diastolic pressure (LVEDP) in patients with depressed LV systolic function. Ar-A, difference in duration of the atrial reversal wave (pulmonary vein) and of the atrial wave of mitral inflow; NL LAP, normal left atrial pressure; SFF, systolic filling fraction; ↑LAP, increased left atrial pressure. **B:** Algorithm for estimation of LAP and LVEDP in individuals with normal LV systolic function using the new indices of diastolic function, mitral inflow E velocity (E), pulmonary vein velocity, and left atrial size. Ea, early diastolic velocity at the mitral annulus; Vp, flow propagation velocity. (Adapted from Nagueh SF, Zoghbi WA. Clinical assessment of LV diastolic filling by Doppler echocardiography. *ACC Curr J Rev.* 2001;10:45–49, with permission.)

is generally geared toward the management of the underlying pathologic condition in addition to the following:

1. Diuresis as needed to decrease central venous pressure
2. Beta-blockers to improve ventricular relaxation and enhance filling
3. ACE inhibitors, beta-blockers, calcium channel blockers, and other antihypertensives to decrease blood pressure and for afterload reduction
4. Restoration of normal sinus rhythm (NSR) in patients with atrial fibrillation and atrial flutter

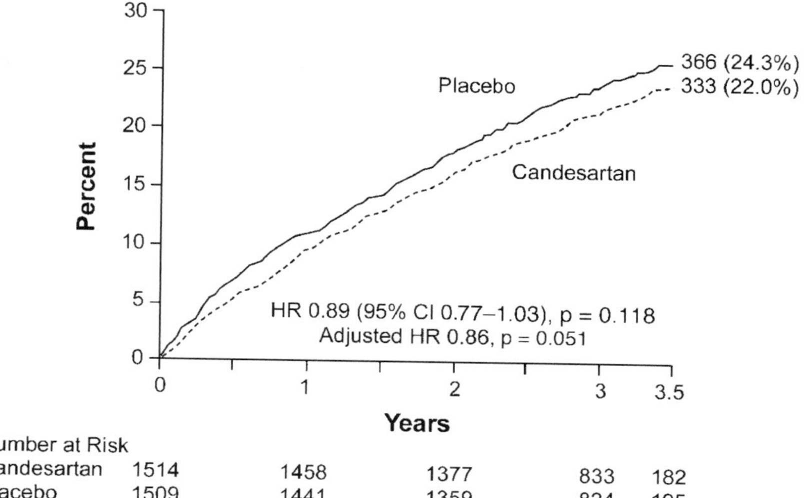


**Figure 35–4** Time to cardiovascular death or hospital admission for congestive heart failure in the CHARM study. From Yusuf, S., et al., Effects of candesartan in patients with chronic heart failure and preserved left-ventricular ejection fraction: the CHARM-Preserved Trial. *Lancet.* 2003; 362:777–781, with permission.)

A recent multicenter study (CHARM) showed that treatment with Candesartan resulted in fewer readmissions for congestive heart failure with no difference in cardiovascular death or the combined endpoint of cardiovascular death or hospitalizations (Fig. 35–4).

## RESTRICTIVE CARDIOMYOPATHIES

Restrictive cardiomyopathy is defined as a disease of the myocardium, which is characterized by"restrictive filling and reduced diastolic volume of either or both ventricles with normal or near-normal systolic function." Systolic function may be normal in the early stage of disease, whereas wall thickness may be normal or increased depending on the etiology of the disease. The disease may be "idiopathic" or associated with other disease, such as amyloidosis.

Restrictive cardiomyopathies are recognized as primary and secondary, in which the secondary forms include the specific heart muscle diseases in which the heart is affected as part of a multisystem disorder—for example, infiltrative, storage, and noninfiltrative diseases. A "working classification" of restrictive cardiomyopathy is shown Figure 35–5. Infiltrative cardiomyopathies can be further divided into *interstitial* and *storage* disorders. In interstitial diseases the infiltrates localize to the interstitium (between myocardial cells), as with cardiac amyloidosis and sarcoidosis. In storage disorders the deposits are within cells, as with hemochromatosis and glycogen storage diseases. These secondary forms of restrictive cardiomyopathies are probably more common than the primary form and display the classic restrictive hemodynamics only in their advanced form. The prototypical secondary restrictive cardiomyopathy is cardiac amyloidosis.

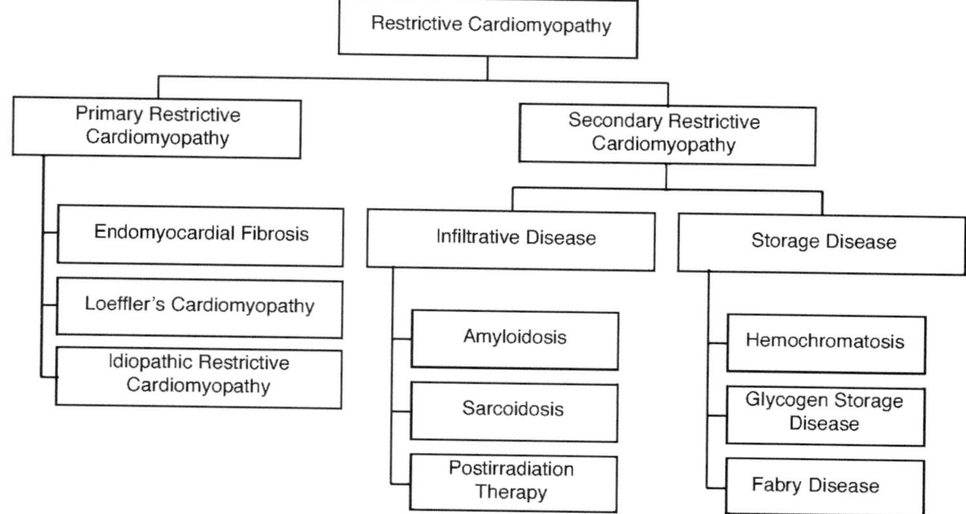


**Figure 35–5** Working classification of restrictive cardiomyopathy. (From Leung DY, Klein AL. Restrictive cardiomyopathy; diagnosis and prognostic implications. In: Otto CM. *Practice of Clinical Echocardiography*. Philadelphia: WB Saunders; 1997:474–493, with permission.)

## Primary Restrictive Cardiomyopathies

*Idiopathic restrictive cardiomyopathy* is associated with familial transmission and skeletal myopathies. There is no specific pathology on endomyocardial biopsies. The atria are disproportionately large, with normal left ventricular function. Histologic examination shows nonspecific degenerative changes seen in other cardiomyopathies, including interstitial fibrosis that may also occur in the sinoatrial and atrioventricular nodes, causing possible heart block. Most small series show a protracted clinical course in adults, with a mean survival of 4 to 14 years (mean 9 years).

*Loffler endocarditis* is associated with idiopathic hypereosinophilia. There is endocardial thickening, obliteration of the left ventricular apex, and a high incidence of thromboembolism. Steroids and hydroxyurea may be helpful in management.

*Endomyocardial fibrosis* is endemic to tropical Africa. It occurs in the left and right ventricular apices with obliteration and involvement of the subvalvular apparatus. Thromboembolism is common. Treatment is mainly palliative, although surgical debulking has been attempted, with increased surgical mortality.

## Secondary Restrictive Cardiomyopathies

*Amyloidosis* is caused by deposition of insoluble proteins in the heart consistent with the "stiff heart" syndrome. Amyloidosis can be classified by the type of protein deposited. The primary type is the most common (85% of the population). It is caused by fibrils composed of $\kappa$- or $\lambda$-immunoglobulin light chains (AL type), often associated with multiple myeloma. Cardiac amyloidosis is mostly caused by primary amyloidosis (AL type). Secondary amyloidosis (AA type) is rare, with the fibrils consisting of protein A, a nonimmunoglobulin. Familial amyloidosis results from the production of a mutant prealbumin protein (transthyretin; TTR). There are six different types that present with a cardiomyopathy, neuropathy, or nephropathy. In familial amyloidosis, cardiac involvement occurs in 28% of patients at the time of diagnosis; however, it usually presents late in the course of the disease.

Patients with cardiac amyloidosis present with diastolic heart failure and the "stiff heart syndrome" resulting from amyloid infiltration. Patients may present with various degrees of progressive biventricular heart failure, depending on the stage of disease, as shown by two-dimensional and Doppler echocardiography (Fig. 35–6). The prognosis can often be determined using Doppler echocardiography (Fig. 35–7). Treatment consists of chemotherapy and diuresis. Dose- intensive melphalan with autologous stem cell transplantation is currently being evaluated. Cardiac transplantation is generally not performed for patients with cardiac amyloidosis, because this is a systemic illness with progressive extracardiac amyloid deposition.

*Hemochromatosis* can be primary, representing a recessive genetic disease, or secondary, due to iron overload (e.g.,

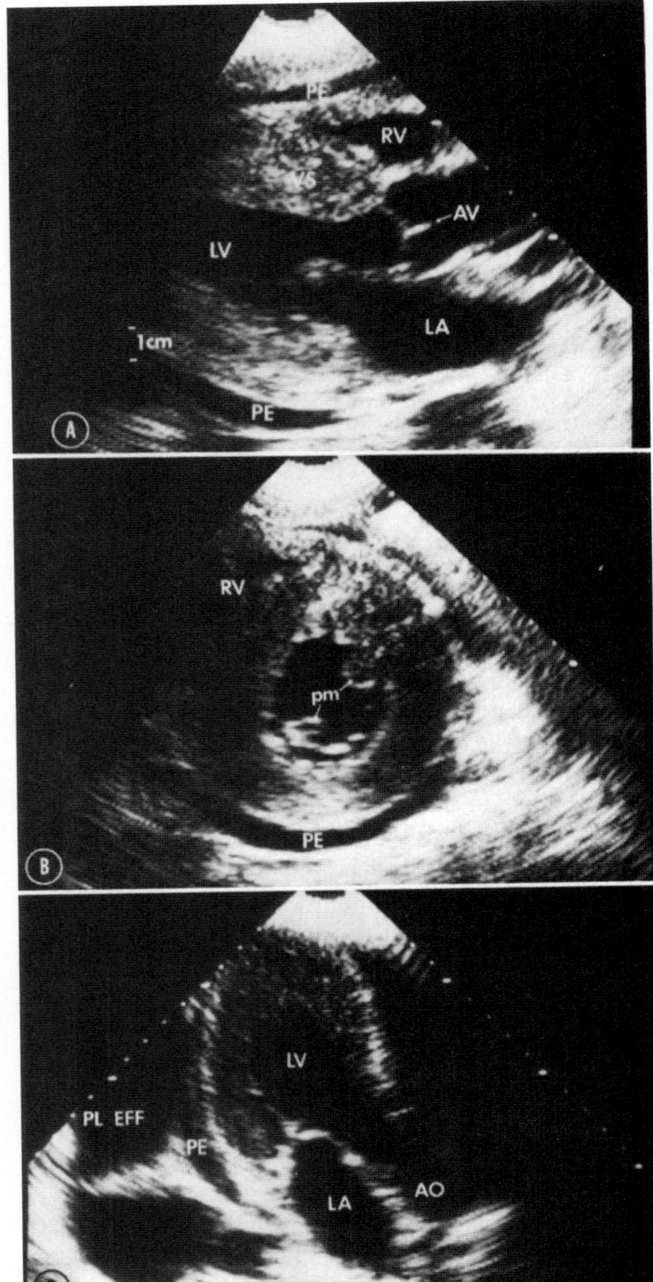


**Figure 36–6** Parasternal long **(A)** and short axis **(B)** and apical long-axis **(C)** views show typical echocardiographic features of advanced cardiac amyloidosis. Note that left ventricular size is normal with markedly thickened ventricular walls (ventricular septum = 22 mm, posterior wall = 18 mm, and right ventricular free wall = 15 mm) and its characteristic granular sparkling appearance. Small pericardial effusion (PE) and left pleural effusion (PLEFF) are also present. AO, aorta; AV, aortic valve; LA, left atrium; LV, left ventricle; PM, papillary muscle; RA, right atrium; RV, right ventricle; VS, ventricular septum. (From Klein AL, et al. Two-dimensional and Doppler echocardiographic assessment of infiltrative cardiomyopathy. *J Am Soc Echocardiogr.* 1988;1:48–59, with permission.)

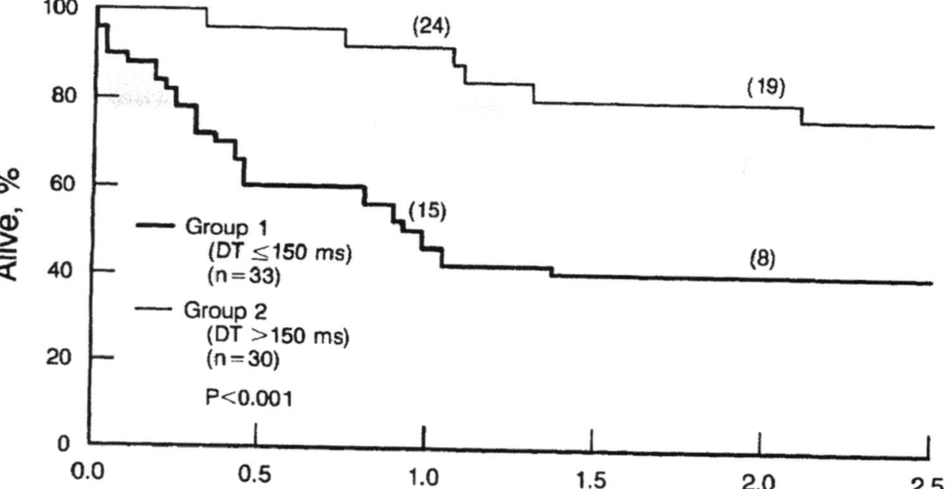


**Figure 35–7** Survival in 63 patients with cardiac amyloidosis subdivided on the basis of the deceleration time of 150 milliseconds. Patients with a shortened deceleration time of <150 milliseconds (*bold line*) had a significantly reduced survival compared with patient subgroup having deceleration time >150 msec. (From Klein AL, et al. Prognostic significance of Doppler measures of diastolic function in cardiac amyloidosis. A Doppler echocardiographic study. *Circulation*. 1991;83:808–816, with permission.)

from blood transfusions). Phlebotomy may improve cardiac symptoms.

*Storage disorders* may be caused by a number of enzymatic defects lead to accumulation of lipids or polysaccharides in the myocardium.

*Sarcoidosis:* Noncaseating granulomas involving the myocardium are found in up to 25% of patients with sarcoidosis. Most patients are asymptomatic, but rhythm and conduction disorders may predominate. VT is the most common arrhythmia. Sudden death can occur in up to 17% of patients with extensive myocardial involvement. Steroid treatment is used for patients with conduction block or arrhythmias.

## BIBLIOGRAPHY

**Asher CR, Klein AL.** Diastolic heart failure: restrictive cardiomyopathy, constrictive pericarditis, and cardiac tamponade: clinical and echocardiographic evaluation. *Cardiol Rev*. 2002;10:218–229.

**Aurigemma GP, Gaasch WH.** Diastolic heart failure. *N Engl J Med*. 2004;351:1097–1105.

European Study Group on Diastolic Heart Failure. How to diagnose diastolic heart failure. *Eur Heart J* 1998;19(7):990–1003.

**Klein AL, Asher CR.** Diseases of the pericardium, restrictive cardiomyopathy and diastolic dysfunction. In: Topol EJ, ed. *Textbook of Cardiovascular Medicine*. 2nd ed. Philadelphia: Lippincott Williams & Wilkins; 2002:595–646.

**Vasan RS, Levy D.** Defining diastolic heart failure: a call for standardized diagnostic criteria. *Circulation*. 2000;101:2118–2121.

**Yusuf S, Pfeffer MA, Swedberg K, et al.** Effects of candesartan in patients with chronic heart failure and preserved left-ventricular ejection fraction: the CHARM-Preserved Trial. *Lancet* 2003;362(9386):777–781.

**Zile MR, Brutsaert DL.** New concepts in diastolic dysfunction and diastolic heart failure: part 1, diagnosis, prognosis and measurements of diastolic function. *Circulation*. 2002;105:1387–1393.

**Zile MR, Brutasert DL.** New concepts in diastolic dysfunction and diastolic heart failure: part ii. causal mechanisms and treatment. *Circulation*. 2002;105;1503–1508.

## QUESTIONS

**1.** A 70-year-old man presents with dyspnea on exertion. Physical examination reveals a blood pressure of 160/95 mm Hg and pulmonary rales at the base. An echocardiogram reveals left ventricular hypertrophy and the following Doppler findings.

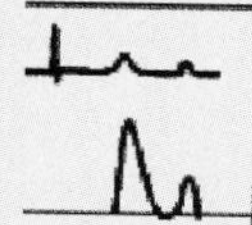

Which of the following medications would not be an initial choice?

a. Digoxin
b. Metoprolol
c. Furosemide
d. Ramipril

Answer is a: Digoxin. The figure depicts restrictive filling (Stage 3 diastolic dysfunction) in a patient with left ventricular hypertrophy and therefore digoxin is not indicated.

**2.** Which parameters are relatively preload independent?

a. Mitral inflow E wave
b. Tissue Doppler echo annular E wave
c. Color m-mode flow propagation velocity
d. b and c

Answer is d: Both tissue Doppler echocardiography annular E wave and color m-mode flow propagation are measures of relaxation and are relatively preload independent. Mitral inflow E wave is dependent on preload.

**3.** Which of the following mitral inflow patterns is associated with the worst prognosis?

a.

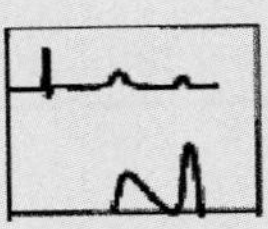

b.

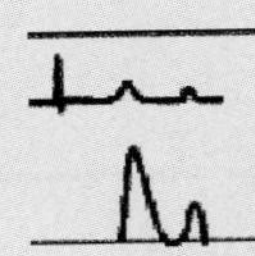

c.

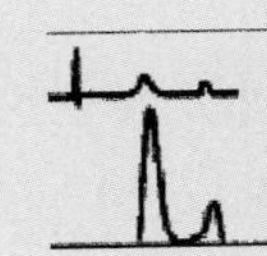

Answer is c: Restrictive pattern. Restrictive physiology has been shown to be associated with the highest mortality.

**4.** Which of the following is the most common symptom associated with diastolic heart failure?

a. Dyspnea at rest
b. Exertional dyspnea
c. Paroxysmal nocturnal dyspnea
d. Chest pain

Answer is b: Exertional dyspnea. With exertion, diastolic filling worsens and left ventricular filling pressure increases, resulting in dyspnea.

**5.** A 60-year-old obese woman is experiencing increasing dyspnea, fatigue, and leg swelling. Physical exam reveals a mildly distressed patient with visible dyspnea and 3+ bilateral leg edema. Auscultation is difficult and only distant heart sounds can be discerned. Electrocardiogram shows low voltage and a pseudoinfarct pattern. At this time, which is the best diagnostic study?

a. CT scan
b. Angiography
c. Echocardiogram with respirometry
d. MRI

Answer is c: Echocardiogram with respirometry. Echocardiography is the modality of choice for the initial assessment of cardiac amyloidosis.

36

# Chest Radiography: What the Cardiologist Needs to Know

*Ross Downey* *Richard White* *Richard A. Krasuski*

Recent advances in magnetic resonance imaging (MRI) and contrast computerized tomography (CT) have greatly expanded the ability to assess cardiovascular anatomy noninvasively. MRI, however, remains largely limited by scanner availability, and CT requires the administration of intravenous contrast with its associated risks. Chest radiography, therefore, remains a very useful part of the initial cardiovascular evaluation. With an organized approach, the cardiologist is more likely to detect the sometimes subtle findings of cardiovascular disease. The most important components of the chest radiograph with regard to cardiovascular disease include:

1. Pulmonary vascular patterns
2. Cardiomediastinal silhouette
3. Calcification patterns

Changes in each of these central components are a direct manifestation of the underlying cardiovascular disorder; and taking all three of these components into account ensures an appropriate, systematic approach to the standard chest radiograph. The following radiographs illustrate the appearance of a wide variety of cardiac abnormalities. Whenever possible, tables are included to delineate the differential diagnoses for representative chest radiographic findings. Cases are then used to illustrate use of the organized approach.

## PULMONARY VASCULAR PATTERNS

### Normal Pulmonary Physiology

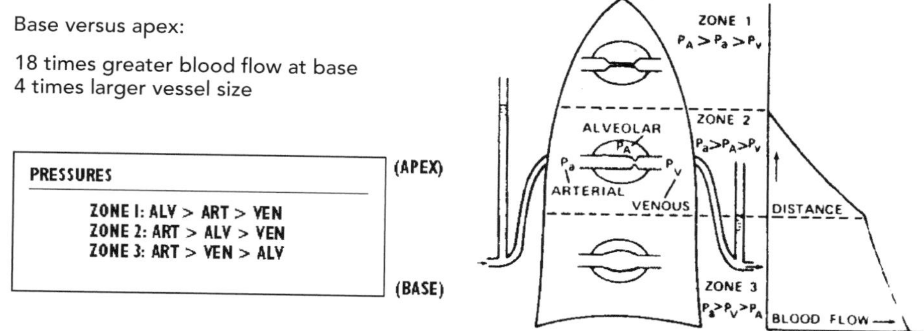


ALV, alveolar; ART, arterial; VEN, venous

*Normal Pulmonary Blood Flow Distribution*

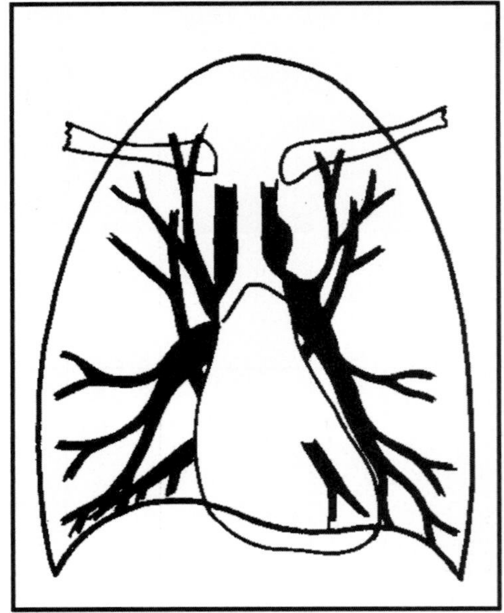

Pulmonary Artery Blood Flow

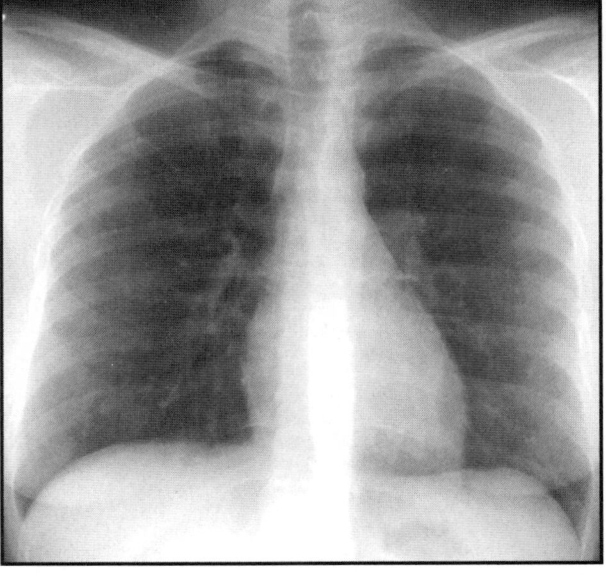

Pulmonary Venous Blood Flow

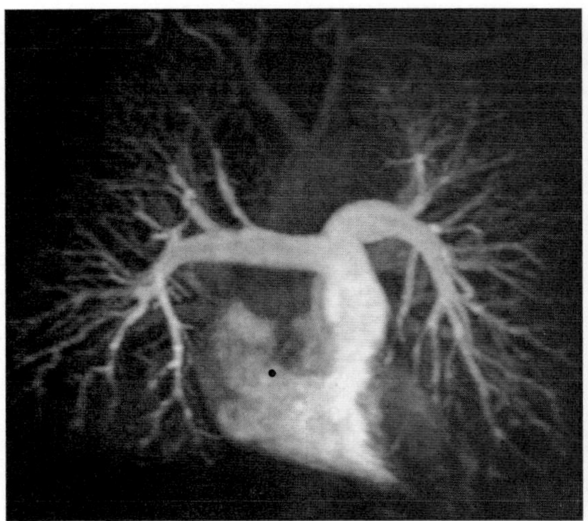

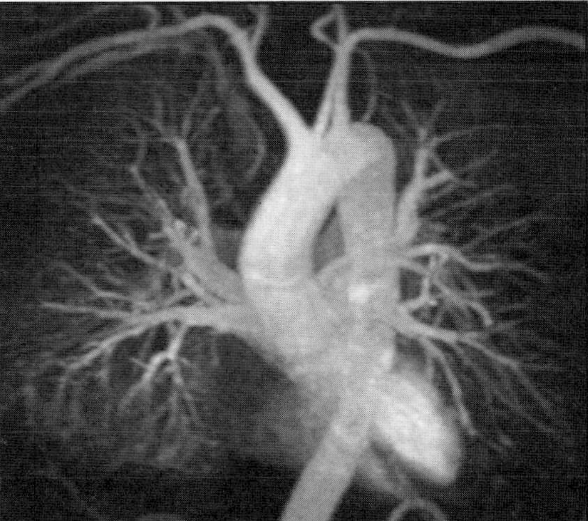

## Pulmonary Vascular Patterns in Normal and Various Cardiovascular Disease States

1. Normal
   - Pulmonary artery/pulmonic valve obstruction (no shunt or pulmonary hypertension)
   - Aorta/aortic valve obstructions (no shunt, left ventricular compromise, mitral valve disease)
   - Insignificant left-to right-shunt: $Q_p/Q_s < 1.5$
2. Increased (overcirculation)
   - Significant left-to-right shunt: $Q_p/Q_s > 1.5$ (acyanotic)
   - Atrial septal defect (ASD)
   - Ventricular septal defect (VSD)
   - Patent ductus arteriosus
   - Partial anomalous pulmonary venous return
3. Decreased (undercirculation)
   - Right-to-left shunt
   - Tetralogy of Fallot
   - Ebstein anomaly with ASD
   - Pulmonary oligemia
   - Ebstein anomaly (severe ± ASD)
4. Admixture shunt (no pulmonic stenosis or atresia/cyanotic)
   - Transposition complexes

- Truncus arteriosis
- Univentricular heart (single ventricle)
- Total anomalous pulmonary venous return: types I and II
- Tricuspid atresia + VSD

5. High-output states
   - Anemia
   - Pregnancy

## Decreased Pulmonary Blood Flow

Tetralogy of Fallot

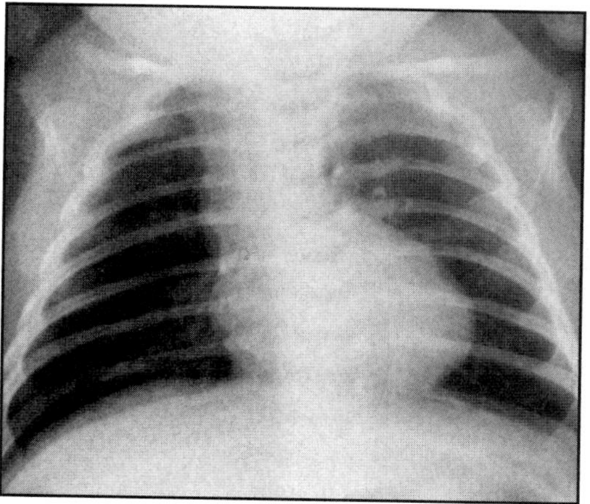

Ebstein Anomaly

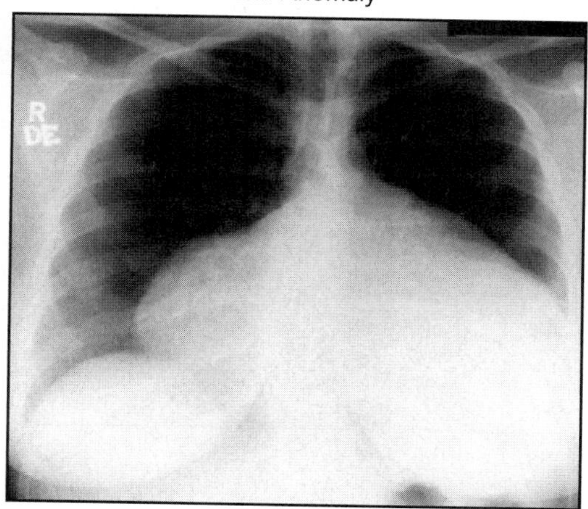


## Increased Pulmonary Blood Flow

Increased: Balanced (Overcirculation)

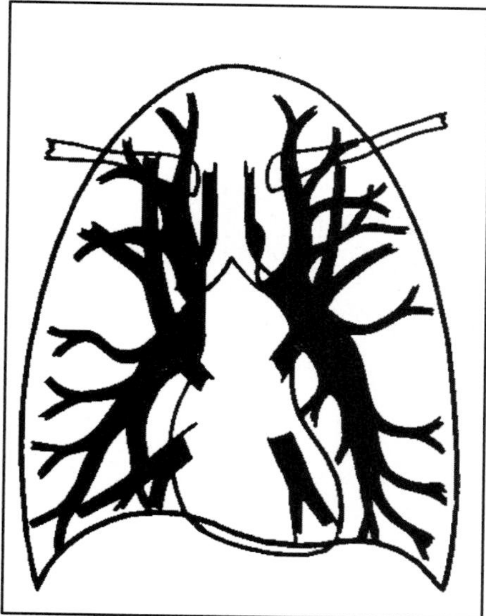

ASD (Overcirculation)

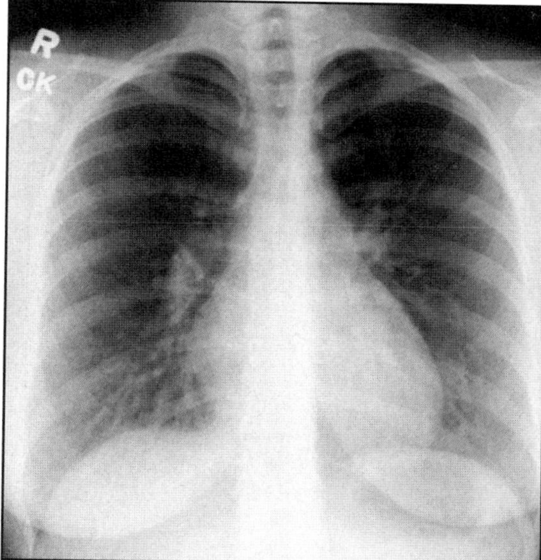

Increased: Redistributed
Pulmonary Venous Hypertension (PVH)

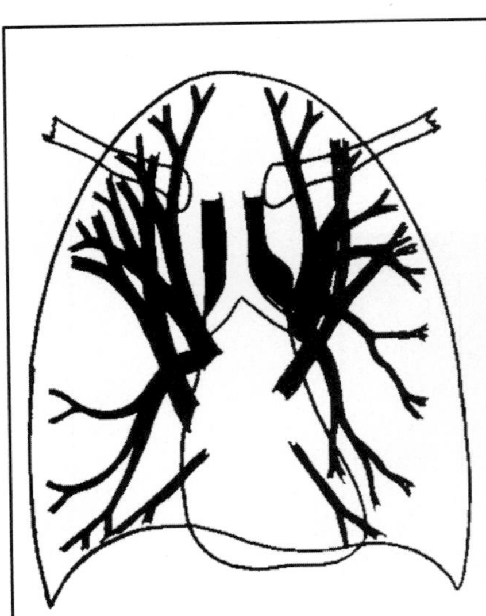

Hypertrophic Cardiomyopathy (HCM)
PVH

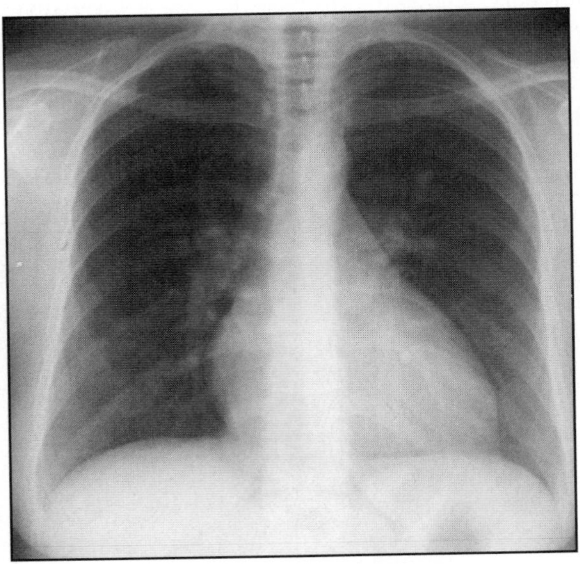

## Pulmonary Arterial Hypertension (PAH)

### *Causes of PAH*

Resistive (chronic PVH; see below)

Obstructive (primary pulmonary vascular disease)

- Idiopathic ("primary")
- Chronic thromboembolism

Obliterative (pulmonary parenchymal disease)

- Emphysema
- Pulmonary fibrosis

Increased: Central

Idiopathic "Primary" PAH

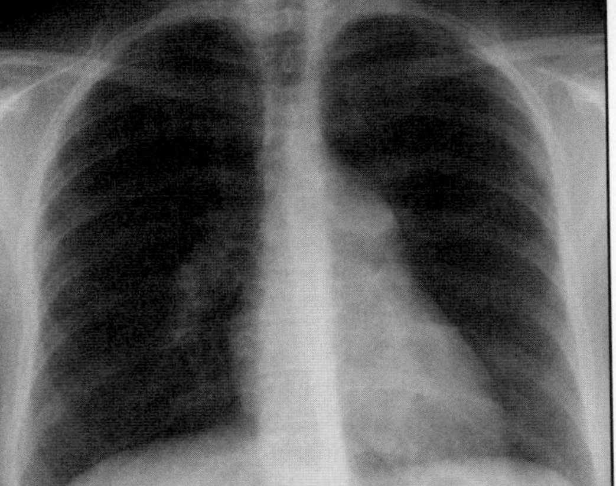

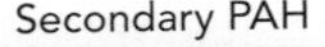

Secondary PAH

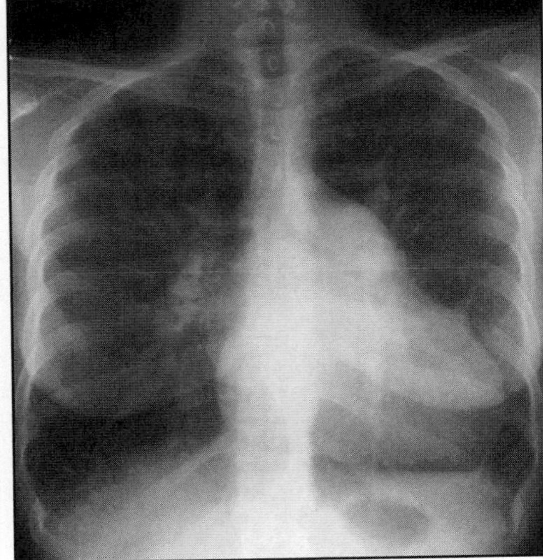

## Pulmonary Venous Hypertension (PVH)

### *Stages of PVH*

*Stage 1:* Pulmonary vascular redistribution
- PCWP: Acute, 13 to 18 mm Hg; chronic, 18 to 22 mm Hg

*Stage 2:* Redistribution + interstitial pulmonary edema
- PCWP: Acute, 18 to 25 mm Hg; chronic, 23 to 30 mm Hg

*Stage 3:* Redistribution + interstitial and alveolar pulmonary edema
- PCWP: Acute, >25 mm Hg; chronic, >30 mm Hg

Stage 1
Redistribution

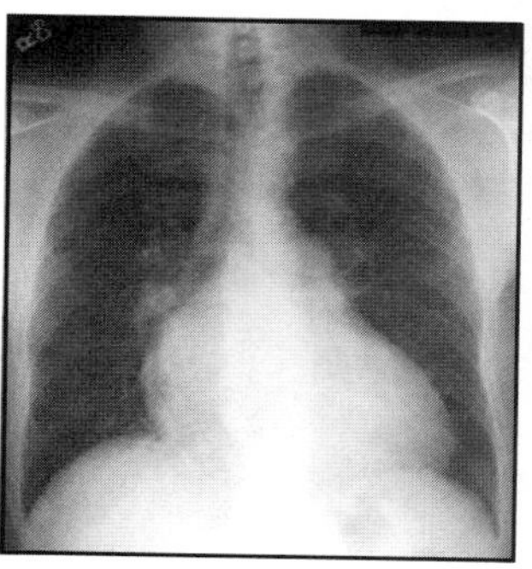

Stage 2
Kerley B Lines

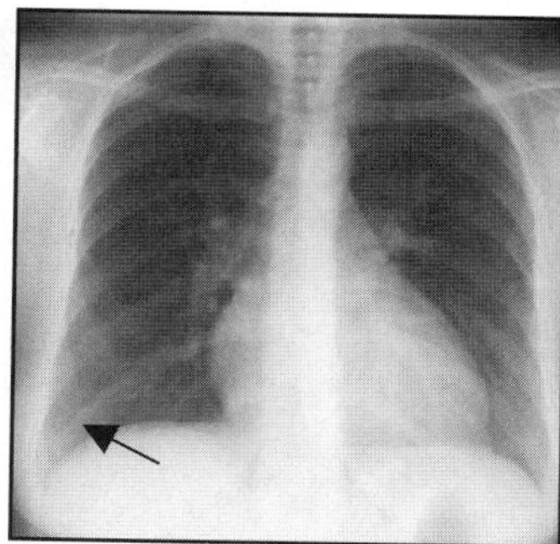

Stage 3
Alveolar Disease

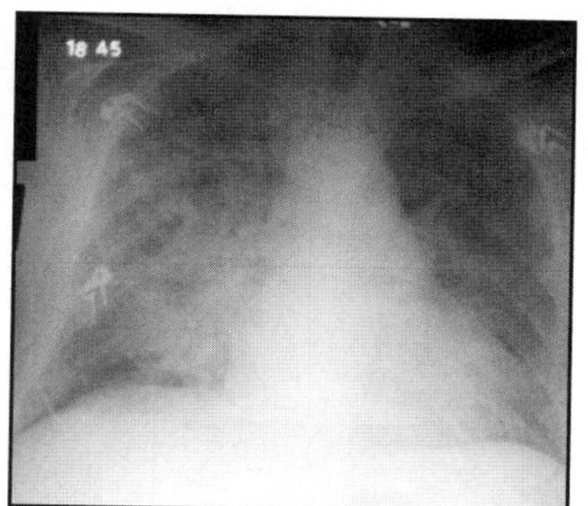


### *Causes of PVH*

- Pulmonary veno-occlusive disease
- Pulmonary vein stenosis (postradiation therapy, post–atrial fibrillation ablation)
- Left atrial/left ventricular obstruction
  - Myxoma or other tumors
- Mitral valve disease
  - Mitral stenosis
  - Mitral regurgitation
- Left ventricular compromise
  - Dilated cardiomyopathy
  - Acute or chronic myocardial ischemic disease
  - Restrictive cardiomyopathy
- Pericardial disease
  - Constrictive pericarditis

## Pulmonary Edema Patterns

- Increased hydrostatic pressure gradient
- Increased capillary permeability
- Decreased osmotic pressure gradient
- Lymphatic incompetence

PVH   Overcirculation   Increased Permeability

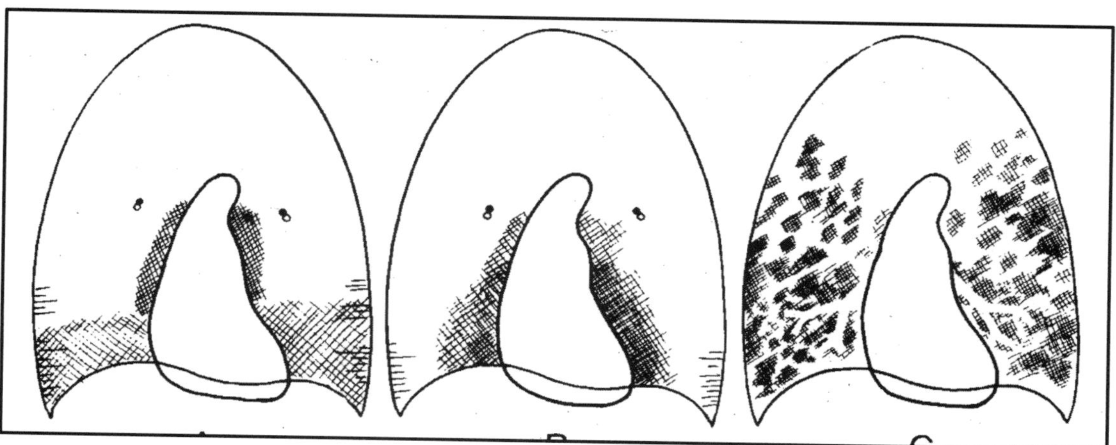

PVH

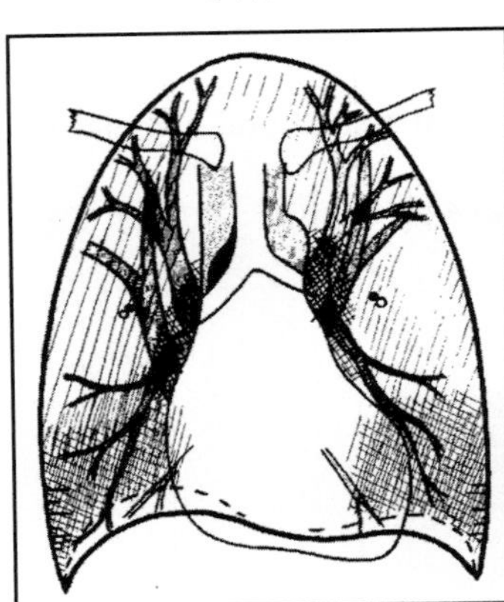

Overcirculation

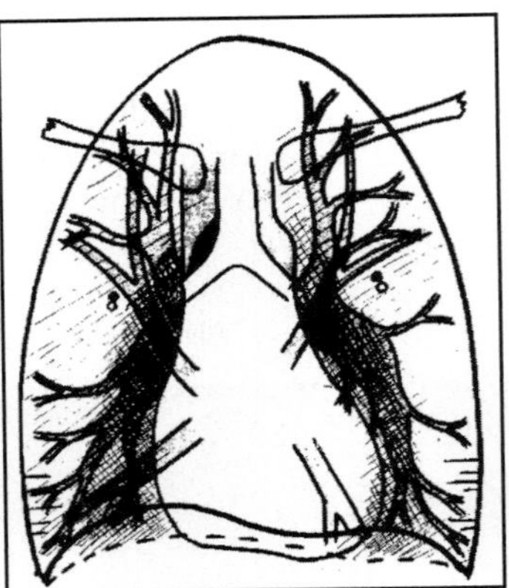

Increased Permeability

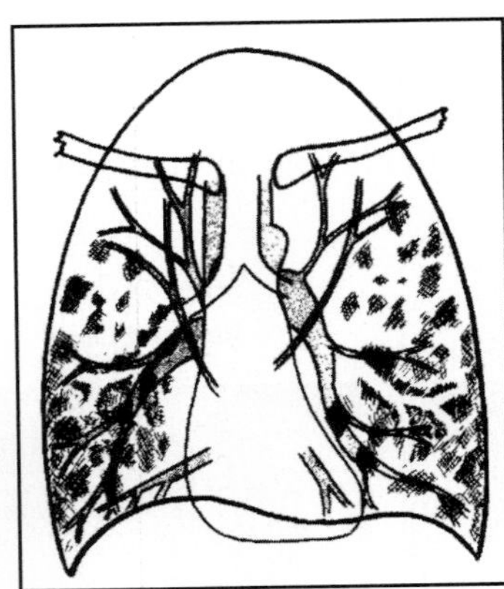

(Milne ENC, et al. *AJR, Am J Roentgenol.* 1985;144:879–894)

Healthy

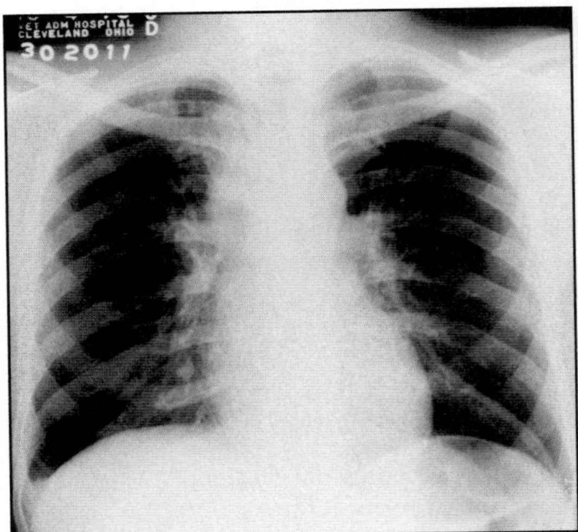


Septic

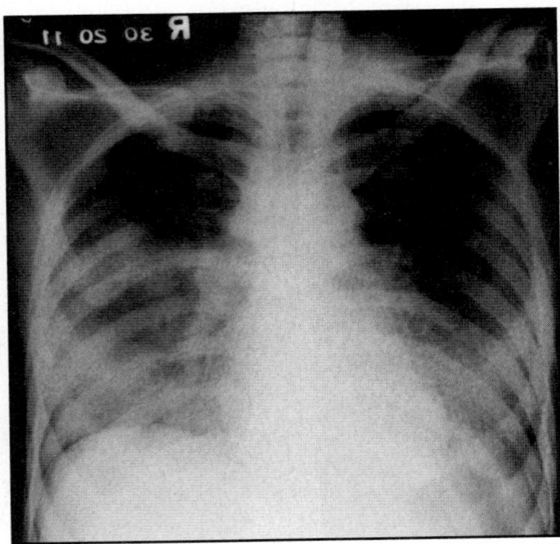


**Radiographic Features of Pulmonary Edema**

| Injury | Cardiac | Renal | Injury |
|---|---|---|---|
| Cardiac Silhouette | Often Enlarged | Enlarged | Not Enlarged |
| Pulmonary Blood Flow | Redistributed | Balanced | Normal |
| Pulmonary Blood Volume | Normal or Increased | Increased | Normal |
| Peribronchial Cuffing | Very Common | Not Common | Not Common |
| Air Bronchograms | Not Common | Not Common | Very Common |
| Lung Edema | Even | Central | Peripheral |
| Pleural Effusions | Very Common | Very Common | Not Common |

## CARDIOMEDIASTINAL SILHOUETTE PATTERNS

- Normal size
  - CT ratio <50%
- Normal landmarks
  - Central
    - Tracheobronchial tree–pulmonary artery (PA) relationship
    - Early branching to middle lobe on right
    - Right PA descends anterior to bronchus
    - Left PA passes over and descends posterior to bronchus
  - Right
    - Right chambers
    - Ascending aorta
    - Superior vena cava/azygos vein
  - Left
    - Aortic "knob" (distal arch + isthmus)
    - Descending aorta
    - Main PA
    - Descending aorta
    - Left atrium
    - Left ventricle

### Normal Cardiac Silhouette

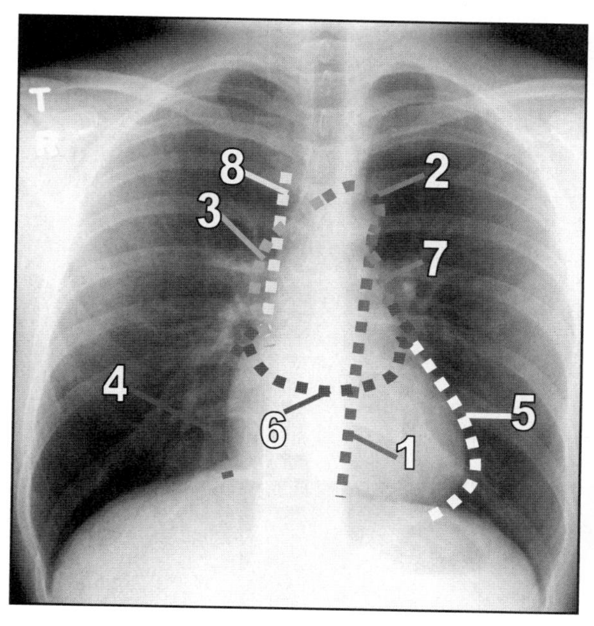


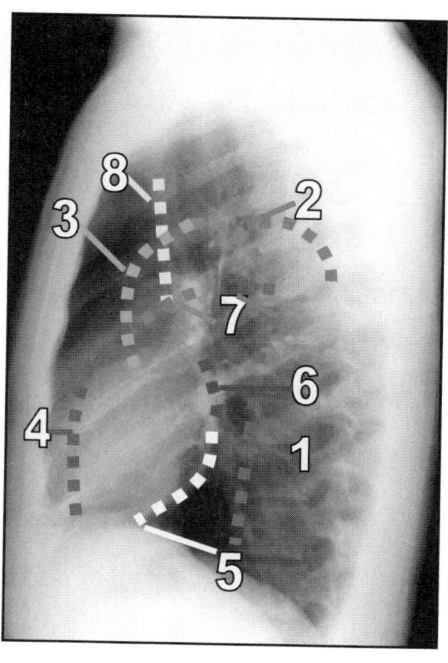


1, descending aorta; 2, aortic knob (distal arch and isthmus); 3, ascending aorta and proximal arch; 4, right ventricle; 5, left ventricle; 6, left atrium; 7, right atrium; 8, superior vena cava and azygous vein.

### Enlargement of Cardiovascular Structure: Basic Causes

| Cause | Examples |
|---|---|
| Decreased integrity of wall | Post–MI left ventricular true aneurysm |
| Volume overloading | Dilated left atrium in mitral regurgitation; dilated left ventricle in aortic insufficiency |
| Pressure overloading (differential response) | Atria dilate (dilated left atrium in mitral stenosis); ventricular hypertrophy (thick left ventricle in hypertension) |

## Pectus Excavatum

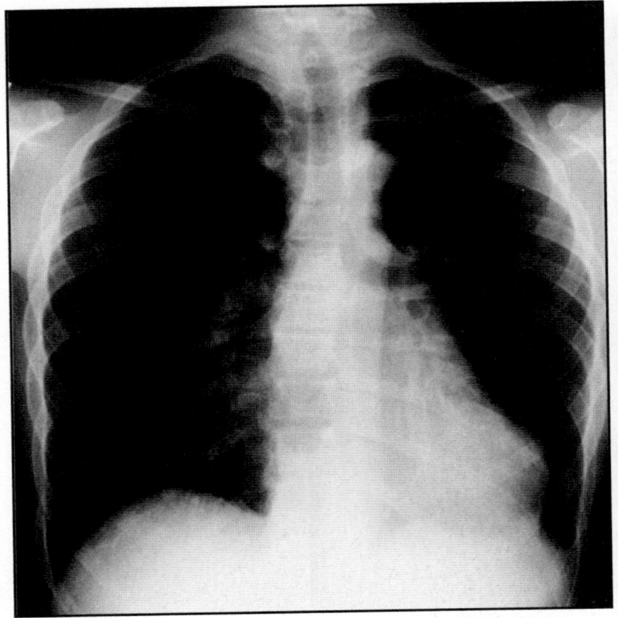

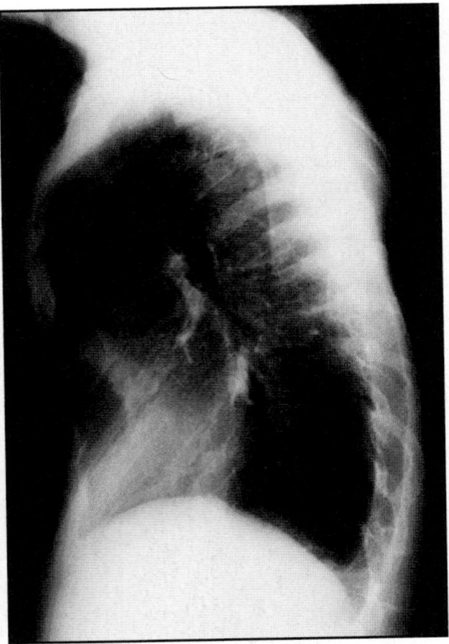

*Findings*

1. Pectus excavatum configuration of ribs

   Straight or up-sloping posterior ribs
   Sharply down-sloping anterior ribs

2. Heart usually displaced to the left; right heart border not visible

## Pericardial Cyst

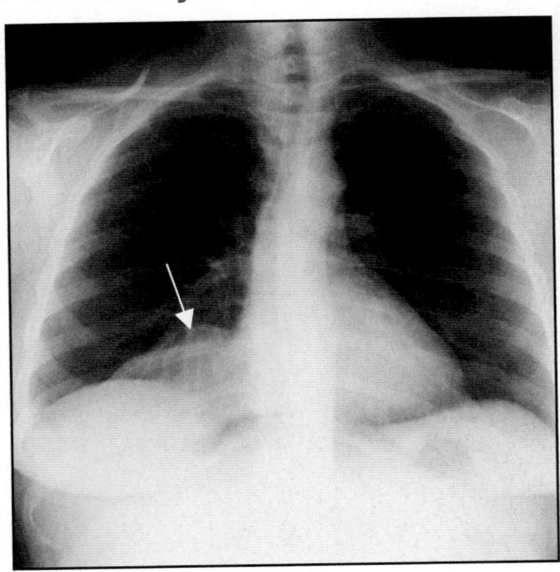

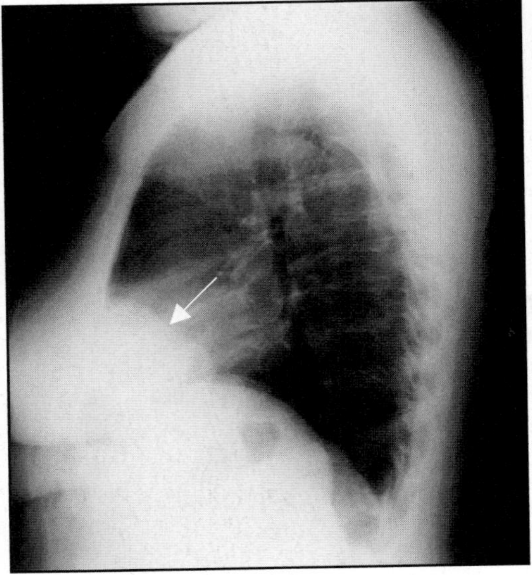

*Findings*

1. The arrows mark the pericardial cyst.

## Right Heart Failure

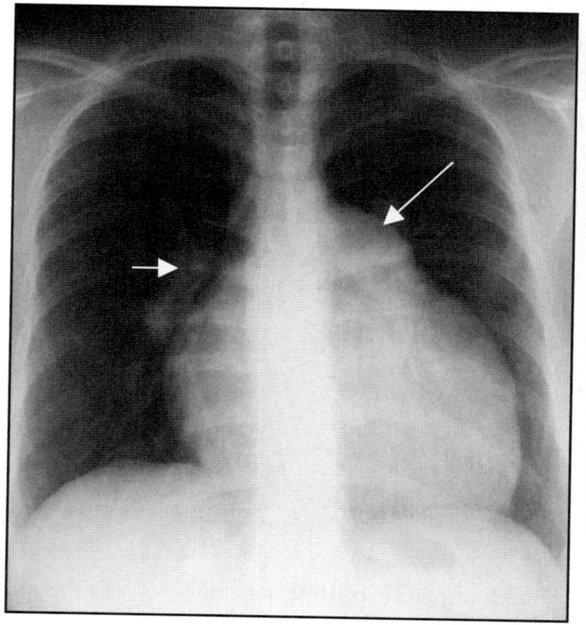

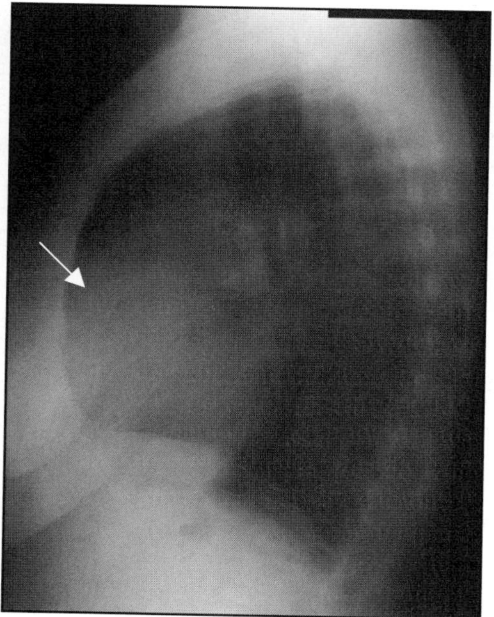

*Findings*
1. Increased right atrial size (*long arrow*)
2. Increased right ventricle size (lateral radiograph, *arrow*)
3. Increased size of pulmonary arteries centrally (*short arrow*)

## Aortic Stenosis

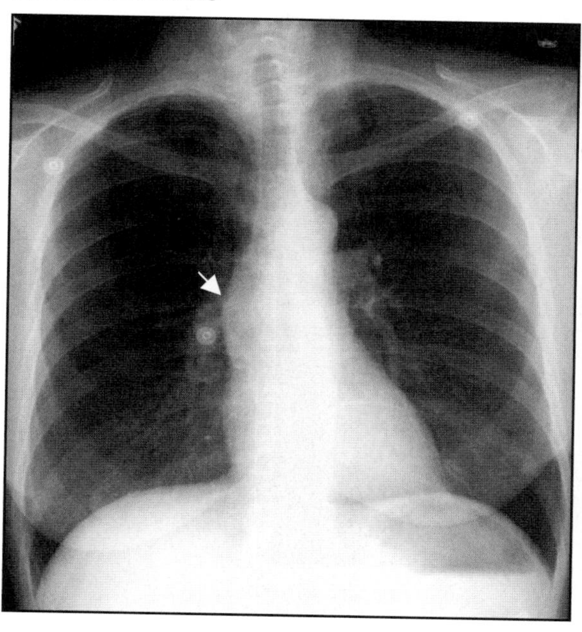

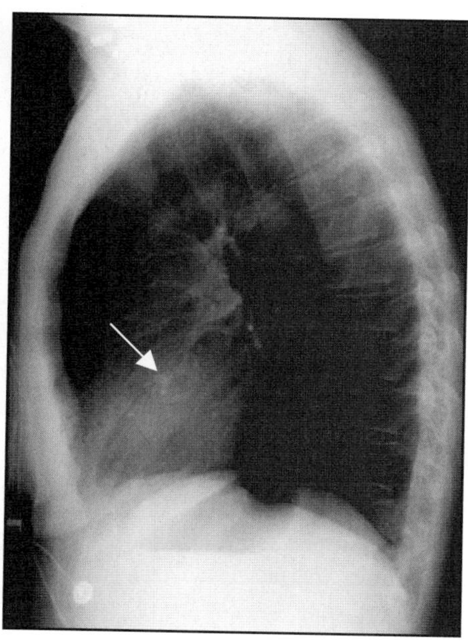

*Findings*
1. Calcified aortic valve (*long arrow*)
2. Dilated ascending aorta beyond stenotic AV (*short arrow*)
3. Normal cardiac silhouette (because only pressure and not volume overload present)

## Pseudo-Coarctation

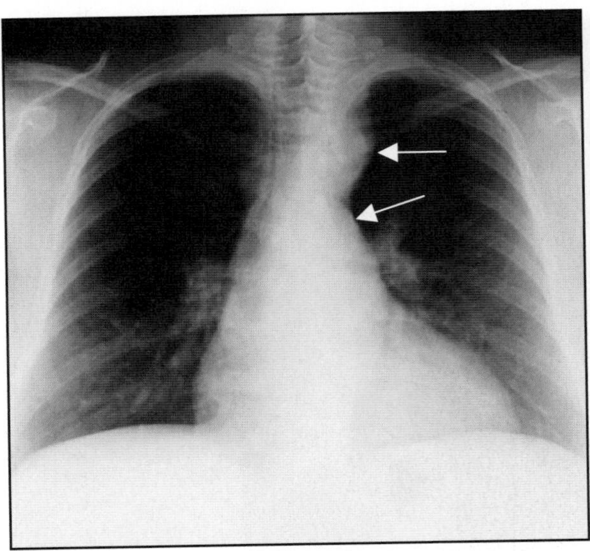

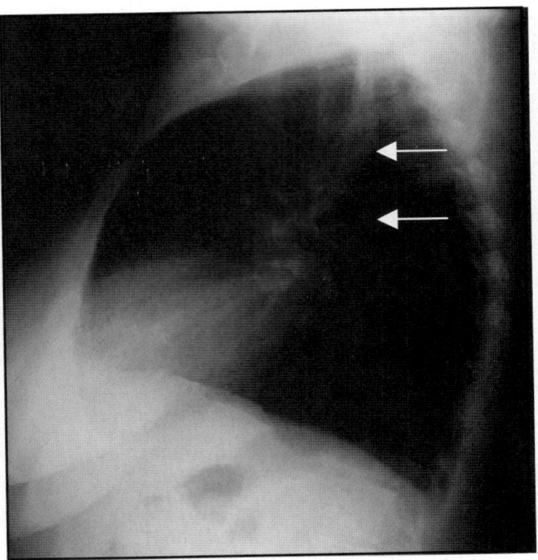

*Findings*

1. "Double left aortic arch sign" (arrows mark the "2" arches)
2. Congenital elongation of the thoracic aorta associated with "kinking" of the aorta at the relatively fixed ligamentum arteriosum as the vessel squeezes into the relatively small thorax. There is no physiologic obstruction, so there is an *absence* of collateral vessel development and subsequent rib notching.

## Coarctation

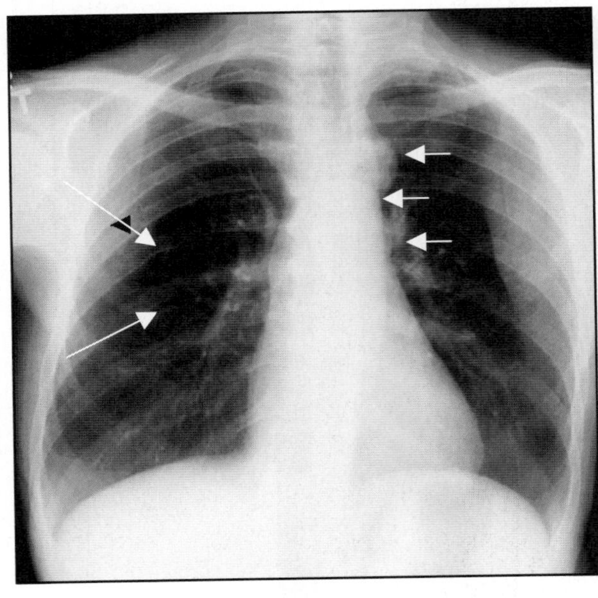

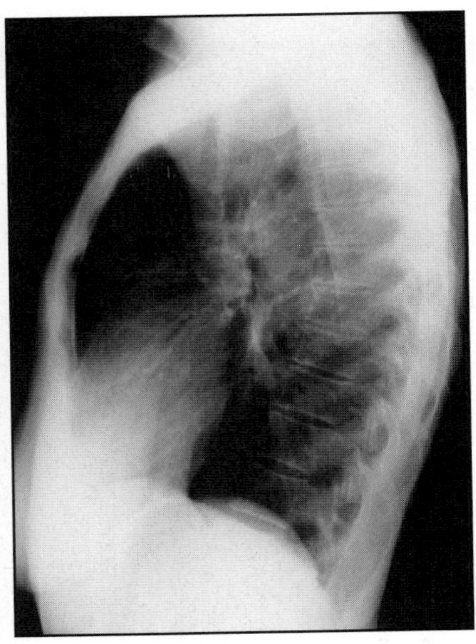

*Findings*

1. Number "3" sign (*short arrows*)
2. Rib notching (*long arrows*) on the inferior portion of the posterior ribs (third to ninth) from pressure erosion by dilated intercostals arteries that serve as collateral blood flow between the internal mammary arteries and the descending aorta

## Valvular Pulmonic Stenosis

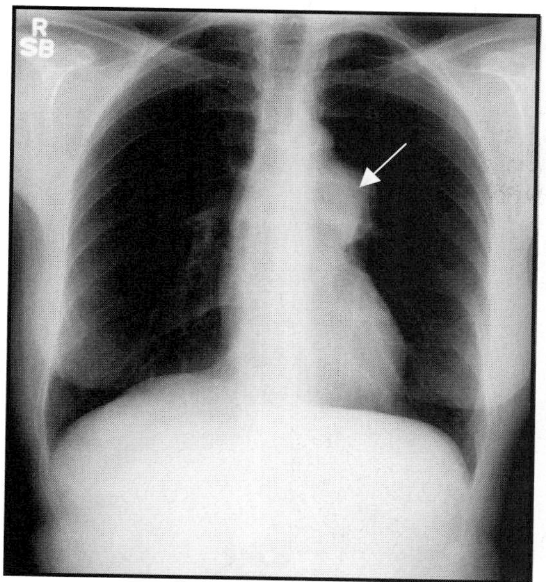


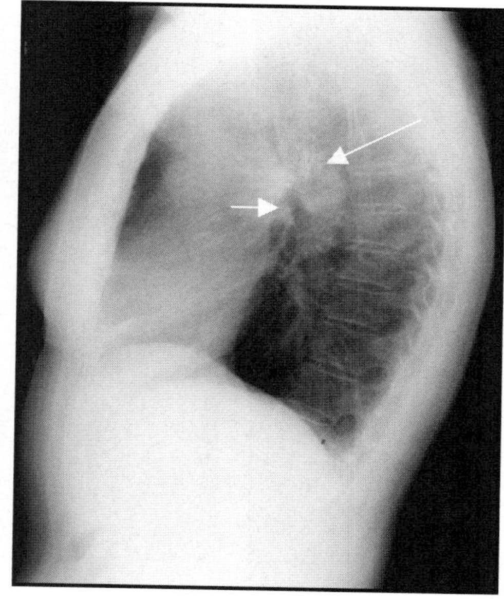

### *Findings*

1. Enlarged main pulmonary artery
2. Selective enlargement of the left PA (*long arrow*) with normal-sized right PA (*short arrow*)
3. Normal cardiac silhouette and normal to decreased pulmonary vascular markings, depending on the degree of stenosis

## Mitral Stenosis

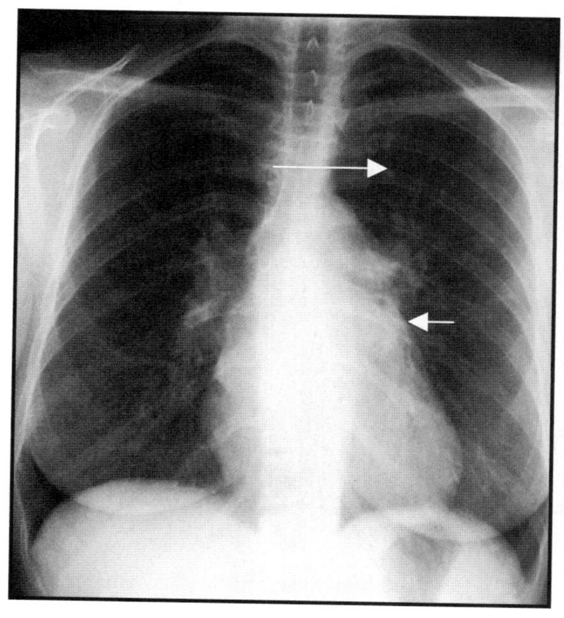

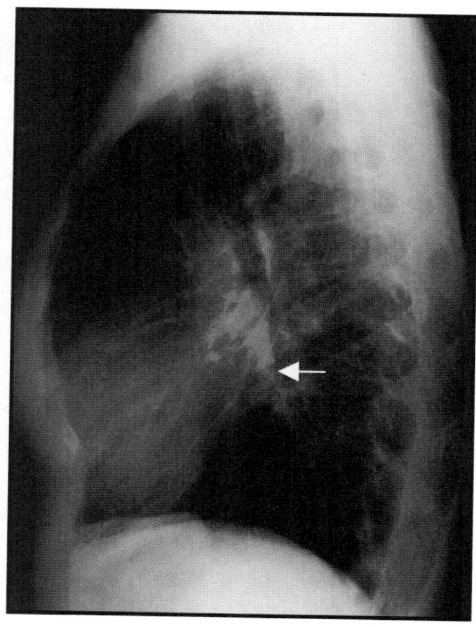

### *Findings*

1. Increased pulmonary vascularity (*long arrow*)
2. Increased left atrial size (*short arrows*)
3. Normal-size left ventricle

## Mitral Regurgitation

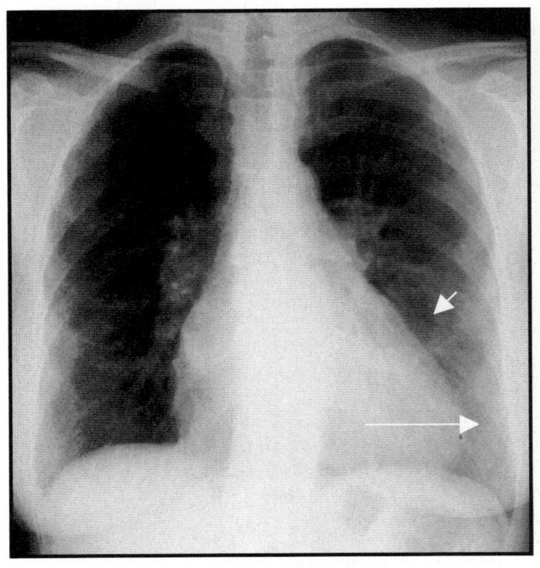

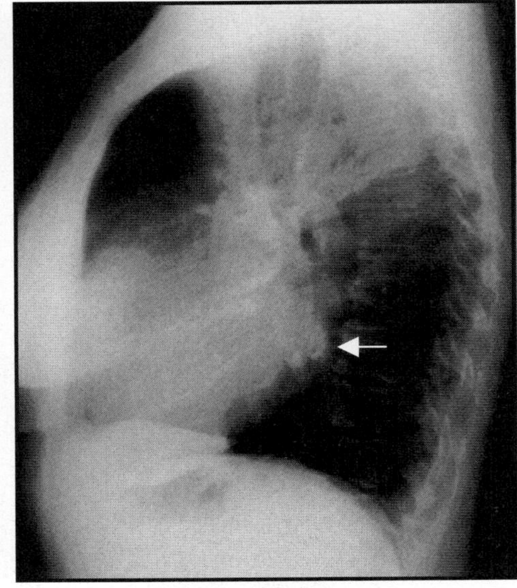

*Findings*

1. Increased pulmonary vascularity
2. Increased left atrial size (*short arrows*)
3. Increased left ventricle size secondary to volume overload (*long arrow*)

## Aortic Regurgitation

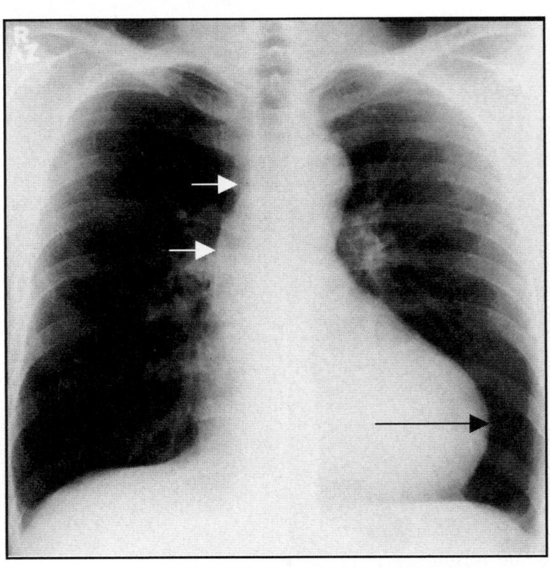

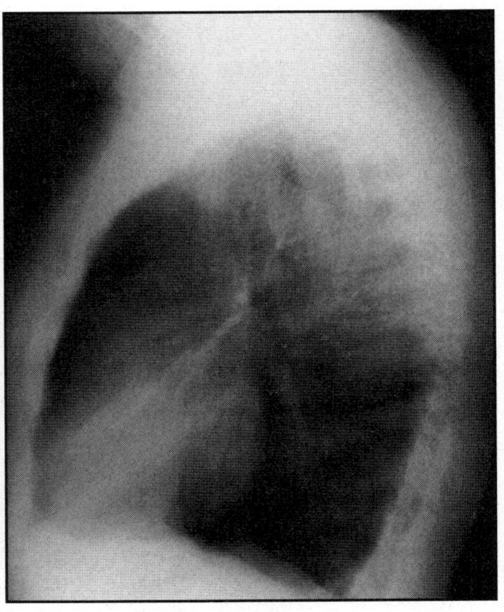

*Findings*

1. No increased pulmonary vascularity
2. Increased ascending aorta up to the arch (*short arrows*)
3. Increased left ventricle size secondary to volume overload (*black arrow*)

## CALCIFICATION PATTERNS

Paracardiac
- Pericardium
- Thoracic aorta

Cardiac
- Left atrium
- Mitral annulus
- Mitral valve
- Aortic valve
- Coronary artery

### Calcific Constrictive Pericarditis

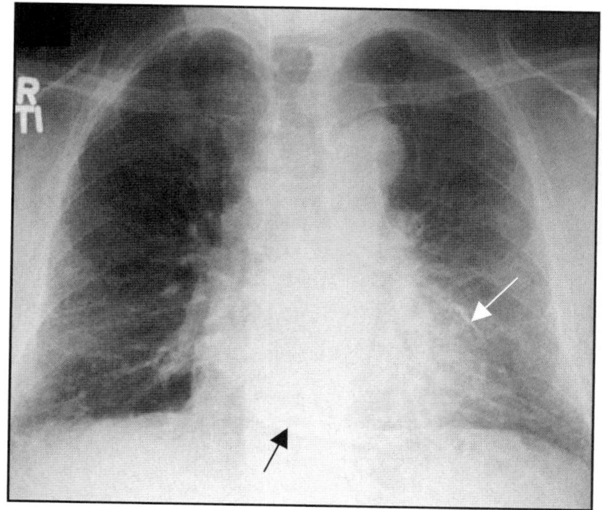


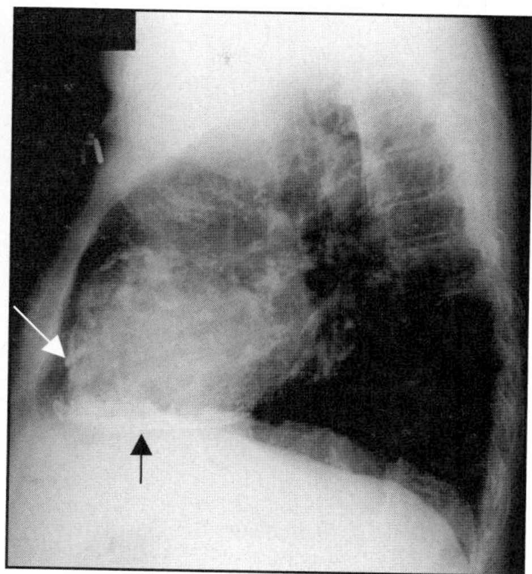

*Findings*

1. Extensive pericardial calcification (*arrows*)

### Left Atrial Wall Calcification

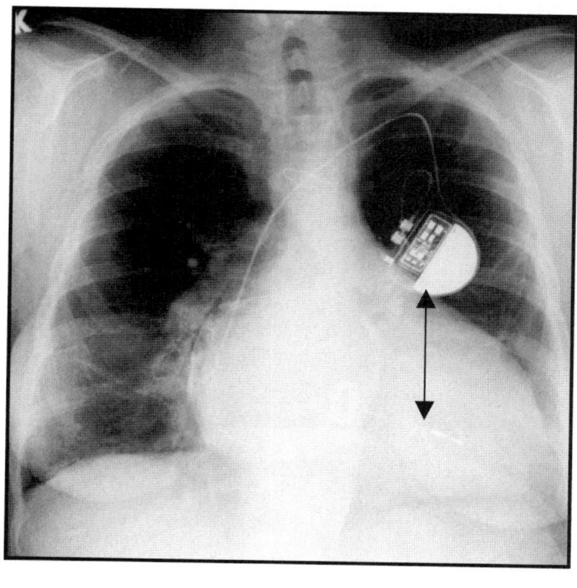

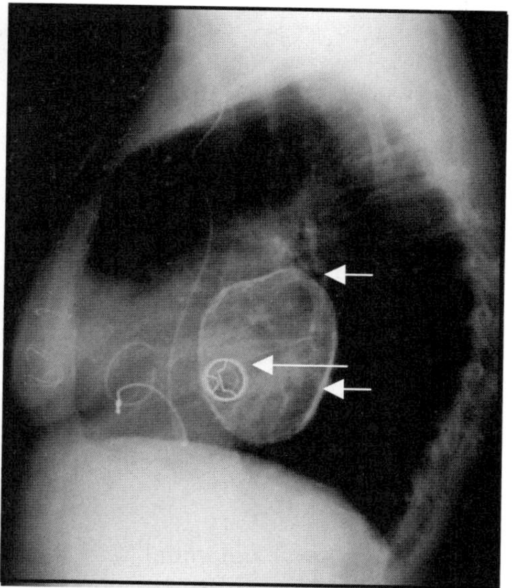

*Findings*

1. Extremely calcified left atrium (*short arrow*)
2. Bjork–Shiley valve in the mitral position (*long arrow*)
3. Single (RV)-lead pacemaker (*black arrows*)

## Mitral Annular Calcification

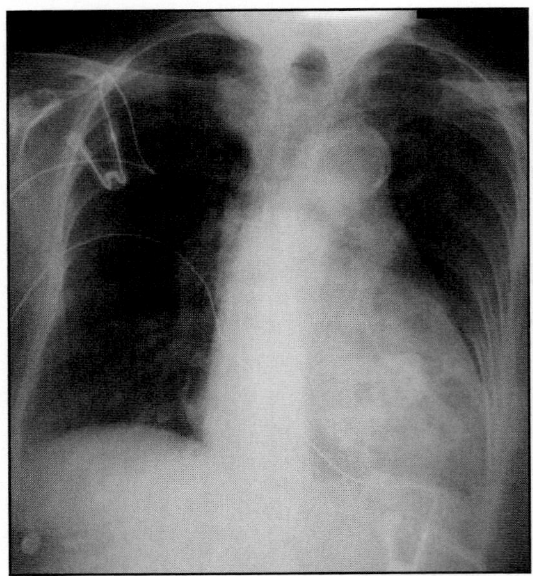

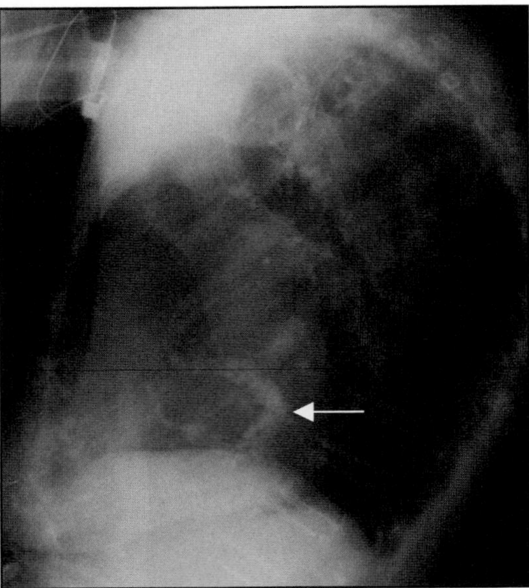

*Findings*

1. Extensive mitral annulus calcification, seen best on the lateral radiograph as a big, backward "C"

## Aortic and Mitral Valvular Calcification

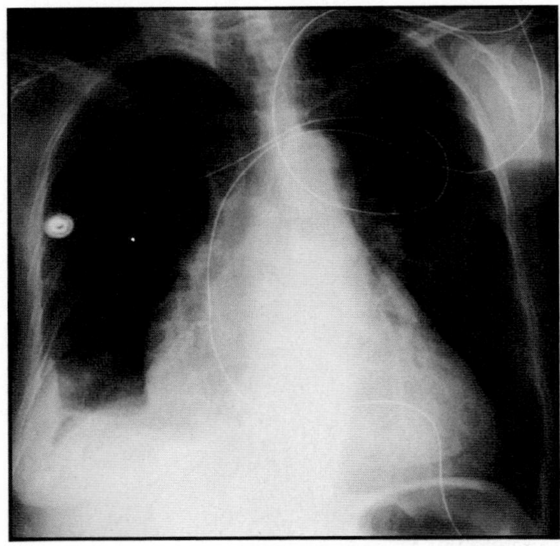

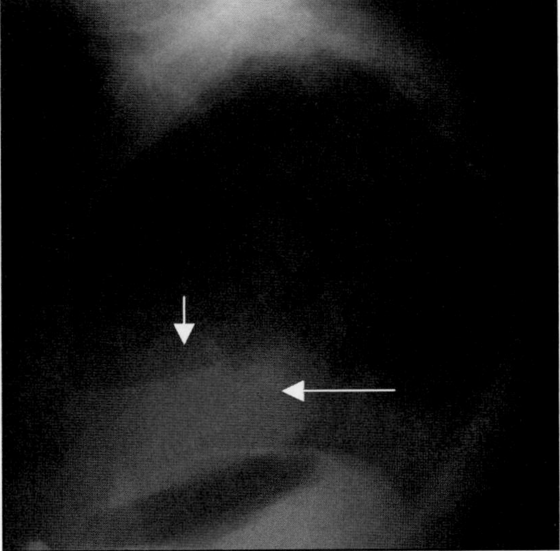

*Findings*

1. Calcification of the aortic (*short arrow*) and mitral (*long arrow*) valves, demonstrating their close proximity to one another (they share a fibrous continuity)

## Calcified Post–MI Left Ventricular True Aneurysm

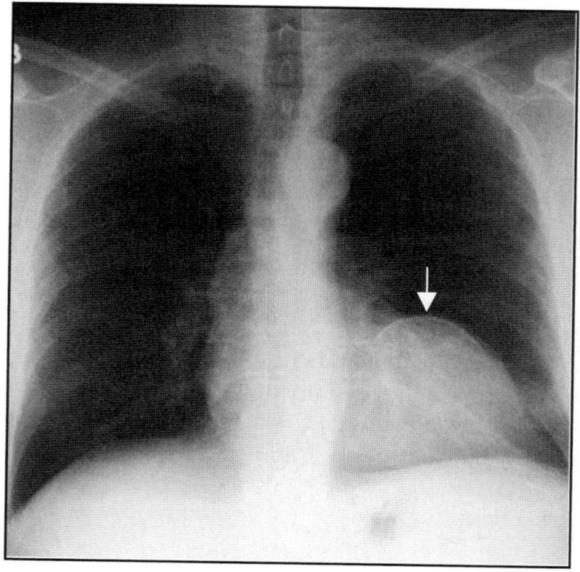

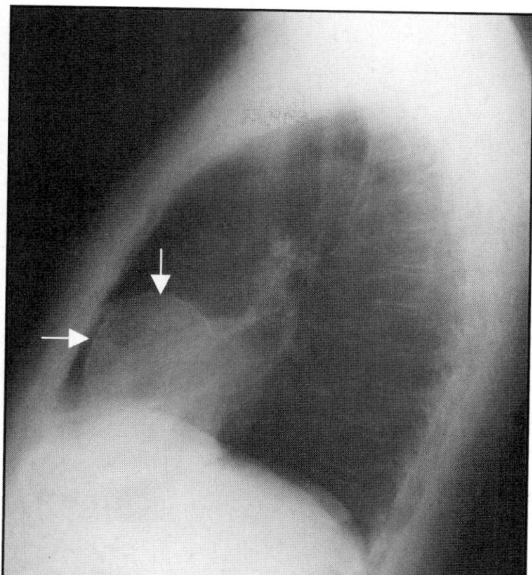

*Findings*

1. Calcified left ventricle aneurysm (*arrows*)

## Calcified Post–MI Left Ventricular Pseudo-Aneurysm

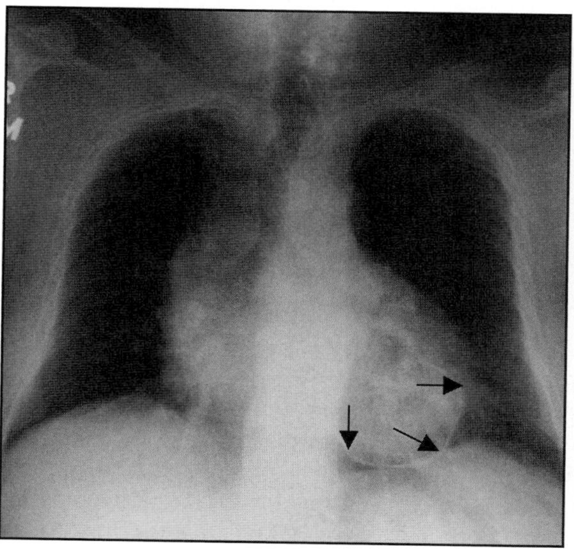

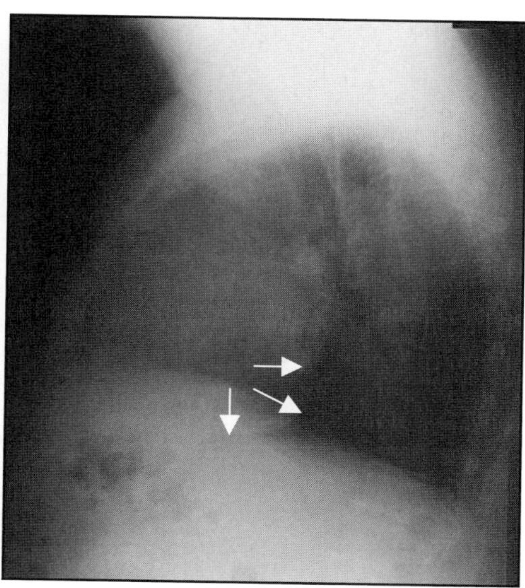

*Findings*

1. A pseudo-aneurysm is a contained rupture through all three layers (intima, media, and adventitia) of the arterial wall. This set of radiographs represents a rupture of the left ventricle following a myocardial infarction that was contained by the pericardium and became progressively calcified over time.

## Coronary Artery Calcification

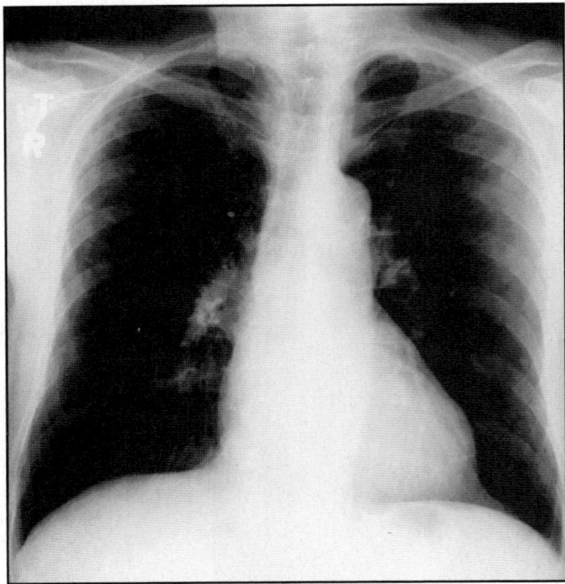

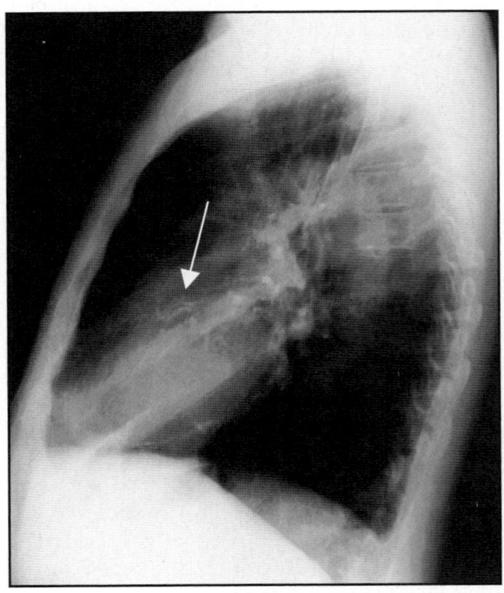

### Findings

1. Extensive coronary calcification of the left anterior descending artery (*arrow*), best seen on the lateral radiograph.

## CASES

### Case #1

Ms. G. is a 28-year-old woman who immigrated to the United States from South America approximately 4 years ago. She has been told in the past that she has a heart murmur and recently noted the onset of exertional dyspnea. Her electrocardiogram (ECG) is notable for atrial fibrillation, and examination reveals a diastolic murmur best heard at the apex. Her chest radiograph is displayed below. Her atrial fibrillation is most likely secondary to:

a. Atrial myxoma
b. Increased transmitral gradient
c. Idiopathic "primary" pulmonary hypertension
d. "Lone" atrial fibrillation
e. Advanced left ventricular dysfunction

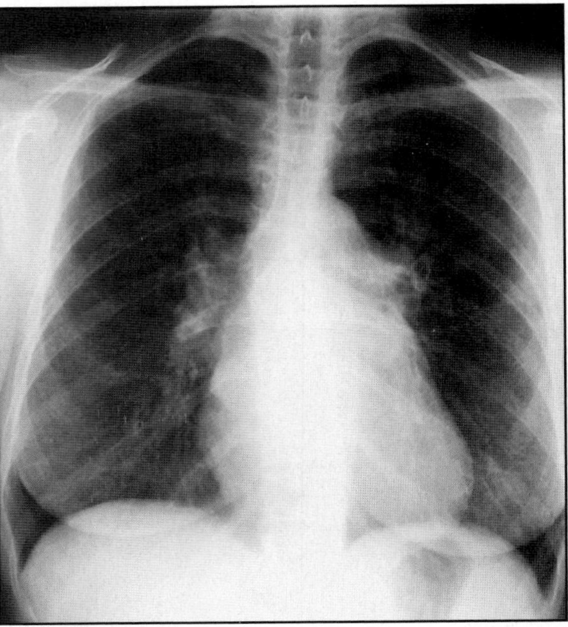

*Discussion:* Using the organized approach to radiograph interpretation, the pulmonary vascular pattern shows evidence of vascular redistribution suggestive of pulmonary venous hypertension. The left atrium is enlarged (*arrow*) and the left ventricle is normal in size, suggesting possible mitral valve pathology. No chamber calcification is present to assist in the diagnosis. The case vignette describes a classical presentation for mitral stenosis. Though persistent inflammation may contribute to atrial fibrillation in this disorder, the primary mechanism in mitral stenosis is still felt to be elevated atrial pressure resulting in stretching of the atrial myocardium.

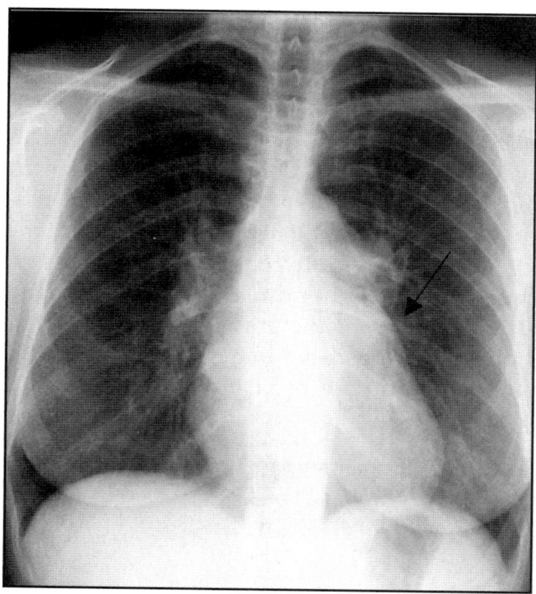

## Case #2

Mr. S. is a 38-year-old man with no prior medical history. Recently he has noticed a progressive reduction in his exercise tolerance. On examination he has a soft systolic murmur at the upper sternal border and a split second heart sound that does not appear to change with respiration. His chest radiograph is displayed below. The most likely explanation for these findings is

a. Paroxysmal atrial fibrillation
b. Undiagnosed pulmonary stenosis
c. Undiagnosed atrial septal defect
d. Undiagnosed primary pulmonary hypertension
e. Left ventricular dysfunction with mitral regurgitation

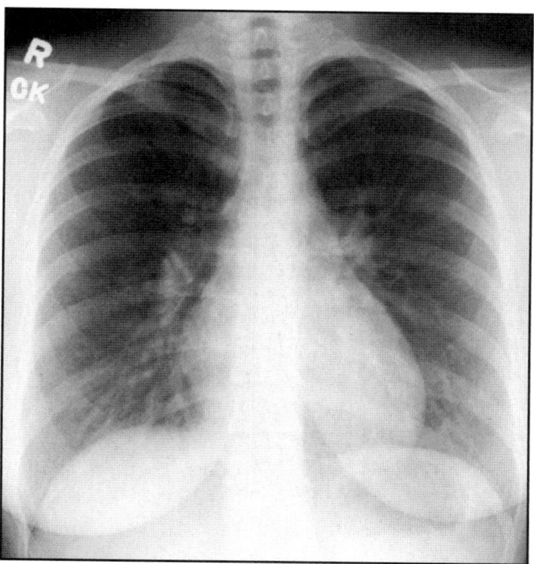


*Discussion:* Using the organized approach to radiograph interpretation, the pulmonary vascular pattern shows balanced overcirculation, and the pulmonary arteries are quite prominent. The right ventricle appears mildly enlarged. No significant calcification is present. The case vignette is notable for the physical exam, which is consistent with an atrial septal defect. Although this patient is certainly at increased risk for atrial fibrillation because of his congenital lesion, it is not the primary explanation for the findings. In pulmonic stenosis an oligemic pulmonary blood flow pattern is normally seen, and in left ventricular dysfunction with mitral regurgitation one expects to see a large left ventricle with pulmonary vascular redistribution suggestive of pulmonary venous hypertension. Primary pulmonary hypertension does not account for the physical findings in this case; additionally, a loud pulmonic closure sound would usually be present.

## Case #3

Ms. B. is a 74-year-old woman who immigrated to the United States from Southwest Asia 6 years ago. For the last 2 years she has noted progressive fatigue and lower-extremity edema. Her chest radiograph is displayed below. A right heart catheterization in this patient would be expected to show all of the following characteristics *except:*

a. Elevated pulmonary capillary wedge pressure
b. Diastolic equalization of pressures
c. Elevated right ventricular pressure
d. A significant step-up in oxygen saturations
e. Normal to decreased cardiac output

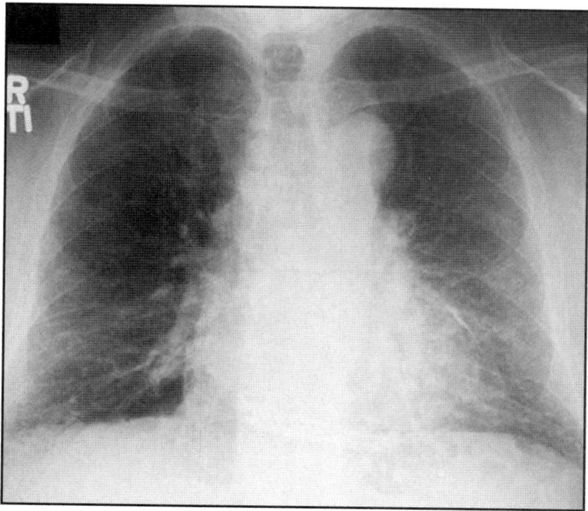


*Discussion:* Using the organized approach to radiograph interpretation, the pulmonary vascular pattern shows redistribution and pulmonary venous engorgement suggestive of elevated left heart filling pressure. There is chamber enlargement of both ventricles. The most notable feature of this radiograph, however, is the pericardial calcification, which appears circumferential. The vignette describes a case of constrictive pericarditis, possibly from old tuberculous infection. In this condition one expects elevated filling pressure and a prominent Kussmaul sign (failure of the jugular venous pressure to drop with inspiration). A pericardial knock is often present as well. A step-up in oxygen saturations (suggestive of an intracardiac shunt) would not be expected in this patient.

## Case #4

Mr. N. is a 32-year-old man with recently diagnosed hypertension that has been refractory to medical therapy. His exam is notable for a loud systolic murmur and weak peripheral pulses. His chest radiograph is shown below. The most appropriate surgical intervention for this patient is

a. Resection and end-to-end anastomosis
b. Fontan procedure
c. Glenn shunt
d. Mitral valve repair
e. Aortic valve replacement

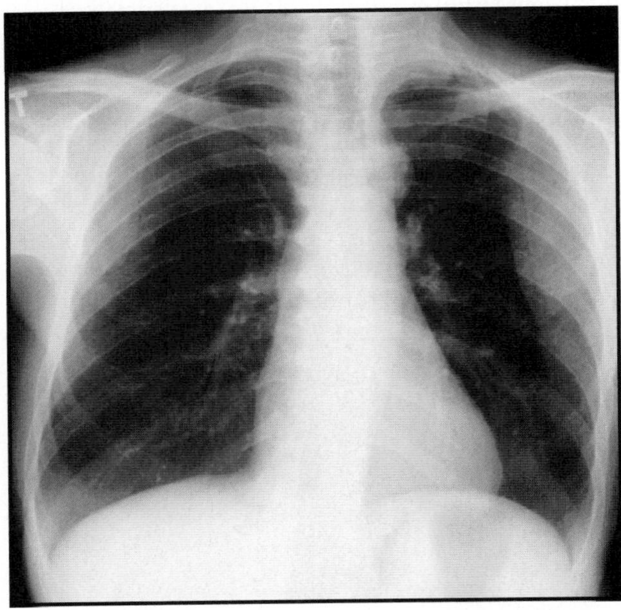

*Discussion:* Using the organized approach to radiograph interpretation, the pulmonary vascular pattern does not appear to be particularly prominent. The chambers of the heart also do not appear to be abnormal in size. There is, however, significant rib notching (*arrows*). This is due to the prominent collaterals that develop to bypass the circulation and allow adequate blood flow to reach the periphery. The presence of these collaterals combined with the case history suggests the aortic coarctation. The classical surgical correction of this abnormality is resection and end-to-end anastomosis of the aorta. Recently, percutaneous techniques have become more popular, not only for postoperative recurrence of coarctation, but also as primary therapy.

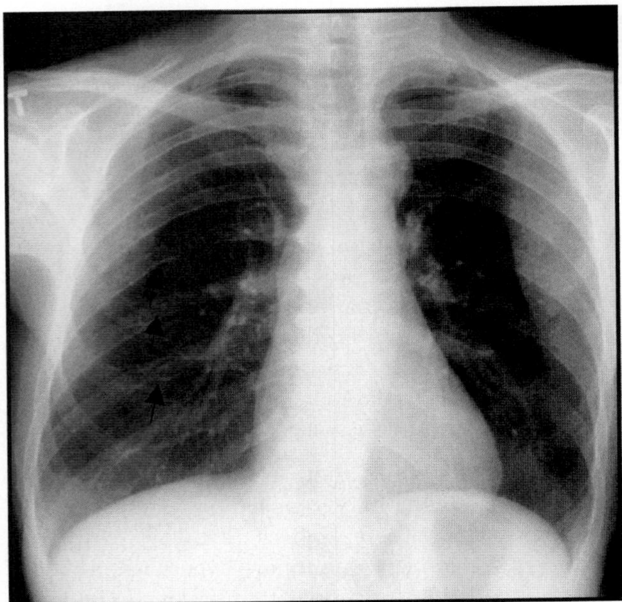

# Cardiac MRI and CT

37

***Carlos Hubbard*** ***Srikanth Sola***

Cardiac magnetic resonance imaging (MRI) and computed tomography (CT) have been recognized as established noninvasive imaging modalities with clinical utility in a wide array of cardiovascular diseases. Common indications, technical considerations, and specific clinical scenarios are reviewed, with attention to the essential knowledge base that might be expected of fellows completing a general cardiovascular medicine fellowship.

## CARDIAC MRI

Recent advances in pulse sequence design and scanner hardware have permitted MRI to become a useful tool in the noninvasive assessment of cardiovascular diseases. MRI provides high-resolution anatomic images; quantitative assessment of ventricular function as well as myocardial mechanics, perfusion, and viability; quantification of intra- and extracardiac shunts; measurements of valvular velocities and gradients; and contrast-enhanced angiography without the use of ionizing radiation or nephrotoxic contrast agents.

### Indications

#### *Evaluation of Myocardial Disease*

MRI is capable of accurately assessing cardiac function, morphology, and myocardial tissue characteristics. Various MRI techniques can be used to differentiate between ischemic and nonischemic cardiomyopathy, as well as related conditions such as restrictive heart disease and some inherited disorders of cardiac metabolism.

#### *Evaluation of Pericardial Disease*

Pericardial thickness and hyperenhancement, as well as associated functional abnormalities, can be identified in patients undergoing evaluation for acute or constrictive pericarditis.

#### *Evaluation of Congenital Heart Disease*

MRI is a useful noninvasive means to quantify ventricular size and function, evaluate valvular regurgitation, quantify $Q_p/Q_s$ ratios, and evaluate the extracardiac vasculature in patients with both simple and complex congenital heart disease.

#### *Evaluation of Cardiac Masses*

MRI is an excellent technique, providing anatomic detail and evaluating tissue characteristics of cardiac and paracardiac masses.

#### *Evaluation of the Aorta*

MRI permits visualization of the entire thoracic and abdominal aorta, including major branch vessels. It is useful for preoperative planning and postoperative follow-up. MRI may be better suited than CT for long-term follow-up in some patients because of its lack of ionizing radiation and nephrotoxic contrast.

#### *Evaluation of the Pulmonary and Peripheral Vasculature*

MRI allows accurate noninvasive assessment of the pulmonary vasculature (as in patients with congenital heart disease) and of the peripheral vasculature in patients with suspected peripheral arterial disease.

### Technical Considerations

#### *MRI Physics*

The nuclei of all atoms are composed of one or more protons; these protons have a small positive electric charge and spin at a rapid rate. This rapid spinning motion of a positively charged proton produces a small but measurable magnetic field that in a sense is similar to a tiny bar magnet. Normally, the magnetic fields of these protons are randomly oriented throughout the body. When they are placed within an MRI scanner, however, the protons within the body align themselves with the external magnetic field of the scanner, just as a compass aligns with the earth's magnetic field. By applying specific radiofrequency (RF) waves, a portion of these protons can be made to change their alignment to a more excited state. As these protons relax and return to their original alignment, they emit a signal that can be measured and used to generate a clinical image. Because hydrogen ($^1$H) is the most abundant atom in the body that is capable of generating a clinically useful image, $^1$H protons form the basis of MRI imaging.

### *Basic Imaging Sequences*

Imaging in MRI depends on using gradient coils within the scanner to send RF pulses in specific patterns to stimulate the $^1$H protons within the body. As these protons relax, they emit signals that are detected by receiver coils placed over the body, perpendicular to the main magnetic field of the scanner. Localization of the signal within the body is achieved by varying the frequency and phase encoding of the RF signals used to generate the image. Image contrast is determined by local variations in relaxation time (T1, T2, and T2*) of the different atoms that make up the tissue or organ of interest.

Pulse sequences are combinations of different types of RF pulses that can be "weighted" toward one type of relaxation versus another (e.g., T1 weighting, T2 weighting, etc.). T1-weighted images are used most commonly in cardiac imaging and provide excellent spatial resolution. T2-weighted images provide improved contrast resolution and are useful for evaluation of tissue edema after a myocardial infarction or in certain inflammatory conditions, such as Takayasu arteritis or myocarditis. T2* weighting, though rarely used, is helpful in iron overload conditions such as hemochromatosis or hemosiderosis.

The most common types of pulse sequences used in cardiac MRI are as follows.

- *Spin echo or "black blood" images.* These pulse sequences are designed so that flowing blood produces no signal, that is, they appear black (Fig. 37–1). However, because of the time required to stimulate and then saturate the signal emitted from the flowing blood, spin echo pulse sequences produce still images. These pulse sequences provide good tissue contrast and anatomic detail, making them useful for visualizing morphology. Myocardium has an intermediate signal intensity on spin echo images, whereas fat and cerebrospinal fluid have very high signal intensity (i.e., they appear bright) on spin echo images.
- *Gradient echo or "white blood" images.* These pulse sequences are fast enough to "catch" the signal coming from excited blood, so blood appears white (Fig. 37–2). Gradient echo images produce ciné images with high temporal resolution (typically 20 to 30 frames/s; up to 70 frames/s for perfusion imaging). Gradient echo sequences are useful for visualizing cardiac function as well

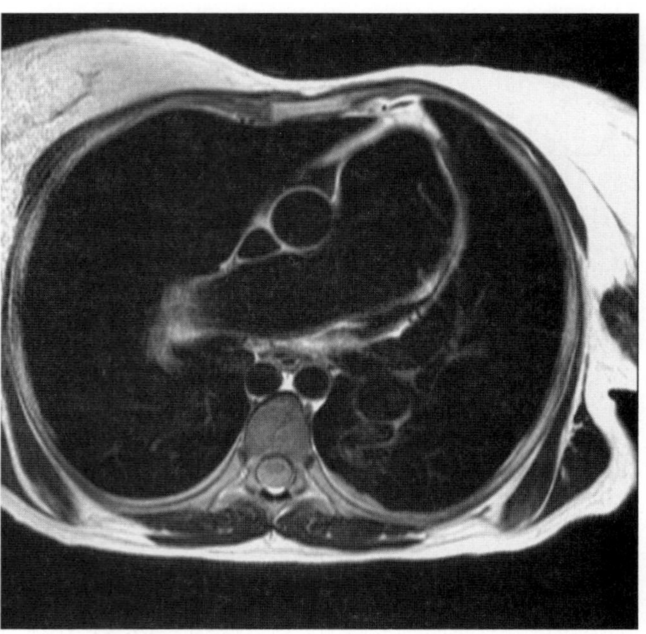

**Figure 37–1** Axial spin echo image at the level of the pulmonary artery of a patient with an ASD and Eisenmenger syndrome. Moving blood is black, whereas myocardium and fat have an intermediate and high signal intensity, respectively. Note the prominence of the main and right pulmonary arteries, suggesting pulmonary arterial hypertension.

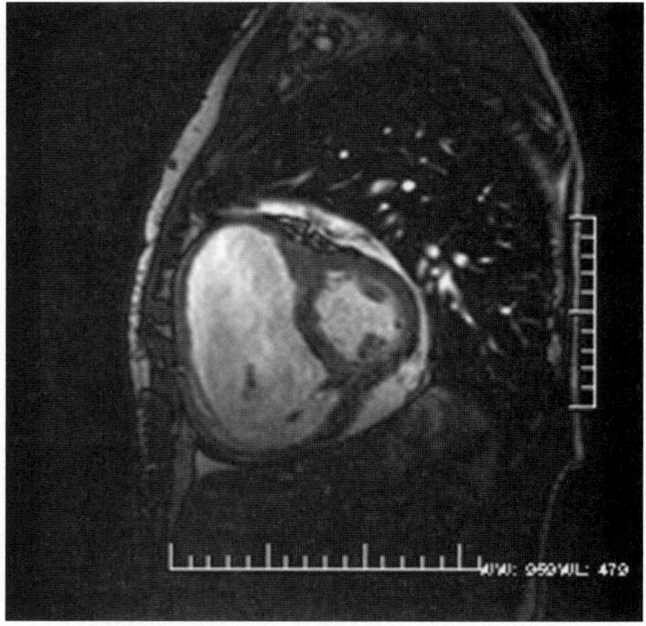

**Figure 37–2** Still frame from a gradient echo short-axis ciné loop of the same patient in Figure 37–1. Note the bright, "white blood" appearance of the blood pool within the left and right ventricular cavities. The right ventricle is severely enlarged and, on ciné images, has moderately reduced systolic function. In addition, a small pericardial effusion is present.

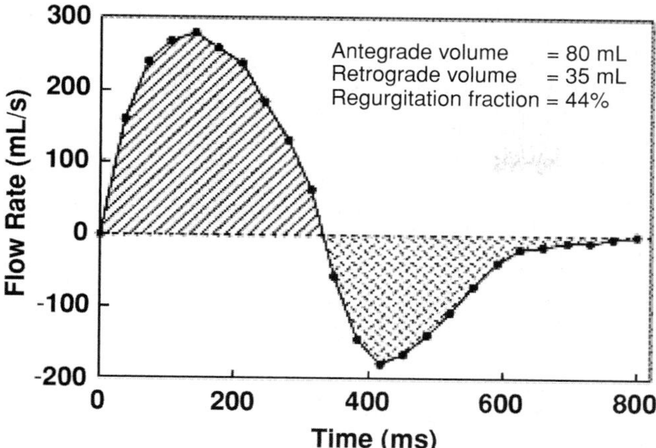


**Figure 37–3** Flow curve obtained from phase velocity images of the pulmonary artery in a patient with surgically palliated tetralogy of Fallot. Forward and regurgitant volumes as well as regurgitant fractions can be calculated, which in this case suggests moderate pulmonic insufficiency.

as turbulent flow due to valvular disease or intracardiac shunts.

- *Phase-velocity or phase-contrast imaging.* As hydrogen nuclei move through a magnetic field, they shift their particular phase (the manner in which protons rotate about a particular axis) in a way that is proportional to their velocity. Phase-contrast imaging, somewhat analogous to echo Doppler imaging, takes advantage of this change in phase with velocity to measure the velocity of blood moving through an area of interest. Since the cross-sectional area of a particular vessel (e.g., the ascending aorta) can be measured, phase-contrast imaging can be used to measure flow through a vessel (flow = velocity × area). Phase-contrast imaging is also used to calculate peak and mean velocities, as well as gradients, regurgitant volumes, and Qp/Qs ratios (Fig. 37–3).
- *Magnetic resonance angiography (MRA).* MRI contrast (most commonly gadolinium DTPA) is an extracellular agent that influences the magnetic property of adjacent tissue. Contrast appears bright (high signal intensity) on gradient echo images, and allows better visualization of the cardiac and extracardiac vasculature. Gadolinium-based contrast agents have the advantage of being non-nephrotoxic and have a very low incidence of adverse events compared with contrast dyes used in x-ray angiography or CT.
- *Perfusion imaging.* First-pass tracking of an MRI contrast bolus allows one to evaluate myocardial perfusion for ischemia/infarction under rest or stress conditions (most commonly with adenosine or dobutamine), similar to perfusion imaging protocols used in nuclear medicine.
- *Delayed hyperenhancement.* In areas where the myocardium is scarred or fibrotic, there is delayed "wash-in" and "wash-out" of MRI contrast agents. These fibrotic or scarred areas appear as bright or "hyperenhanced" areas of myocardium when "delayed" images are taken, typically 10 to 15 minutes after injection of gadolinium DPTA (Fig. 37–4). A special inversion signal given prior to the main pulse sequence is used to "null" the signal from the normal myocardium so that it can be more easily distinguished from abnormal, hyperenhanced myocardium. Specific patterns of hyperenhancement correspond with certain cardiovascular diseases, as described below.

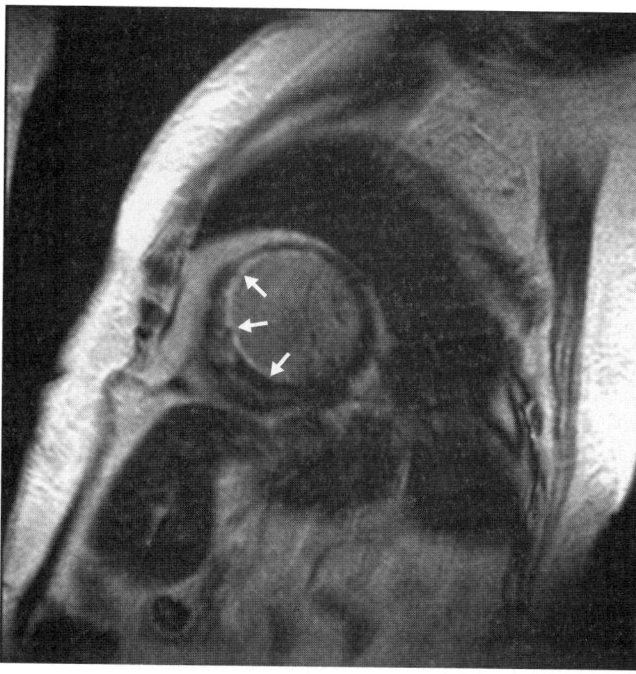

**Figure 37–4** Delayed hyperenhancement short-axis image acquired 10 minutes after the injection of gadolinium DTPA in a patient with multivessel coronary artery disease. An optimal inversion time (TI) was used in this image to "null" (darken) normal myocardium and accentuate (white) areas where gadolinium has remained in the interstitium on a "delayed basis" (delayed hyperenhancement). Note the hyperenhanced area along the subendocardial anteroseptal wall (white arrow), as well as patchy areas of hyperenhancement in the mid inferoseptal and inferolateral walls.

Most cardiac imaging is performed while the patient holds his or her breath for distinct multiple periods of 10 to 15 seconds, to minimize cardiac respiratory movement. Free-breathing acquisition can be done for those patients who are unable to hold their breath, with either a mild reduction in image quality or an increase in imaging time. Retrospective electrocardiographic (ECG) gating using MRI-compatible electrodes is used to trigger pulse sequences and to allow reconstruction of gradient echo cine loops.

Tools to monitor the patient inside the scanner include noninvasive measurement of blood pressure, heart rate, cardiac rhythm, respiration, and (when needed) oxygen saturation. Patients who require mechanical ventilation can be safely imaged using MRI-compatible ventilators.

Intravenous medications can be continued using MRI-compatible infusion pumps.

## Selected Clinical Applications

### *Heart Failure*

MRI is the "gold standard" technique for the evaluation of left and right ventricular volumes, mass, ejection fraction, and viability. Using gradient echo cine images, the ventricles can be evaluated for regional wall motion abnormalities, aneurysm or pseudoaneurysm formation, volumes, and systolic function. Other MRI techniques, such as stress perfusion imaging and delayed hyperenhancement, can be used to differentiate between ischemic and various nonischemic etiologies of heart failure, as described below.

### *Viability Assessment*

Delayed hyperenhancement imaging allows delineation of areas of acute and chronic myocardial infarction. Areas of both acute and chronic myocardial infarction appear as bright (hyperenhanced) areas of myocardium on delayed images after contrast administration. Such areas typically begin at the subendocardium and extend at a variable depth toward the epicardium, depending on the transmural extent of the infarction. These hyperenhanced areas occur within a coronary distribution, unlike other causes of abnormal hyperenhancement such as sarcoidosis or myocarditis.

Hyperenhancement in acute infarction is due to disruption of myocardial membranes, which permits the diffusion of extracellular contrast agent into the intracellular spaces. Hyperenhancement in chronic infarction is the result of decreased blood flow (delayed wash-in) and a larger volume of distribution of contrast within the collagenous scar tissue (delayed wash-out), allowing contrast to accumulate in fibrotic or scarred areas of myocardium. Areas of acute infarction appear bright on T2-weighted spin echo images due to local tissue edema, allowing one to differentiate between an acute and chronic infarct.

In patients with coronary artery disease and left ventricular dysfunction, the distinction between viable and nonviable myocardium can determine whether the patient receives revascularization. Patients with viable myocardium are more likely to have an increased left ventricular ejection fraction and improved survival after revascularization. The extent of transmural hyperenhancement by cardiac MRI has been shown to predict improvement in both myocardial contractility as well as survival after coronary revascularization in patients with ischemic cardiomyopathy, and thus is used as a measure of myocardial viability. Myocardial segments with 25% or less transmural hyperenhancement are considered viable, whereas segments with 75% or greater transmural hyperenhancement are considered nonviable. Segments with 25% to 75% of transmural hyperenhancement have an intermediate likelihood of functional recovery after revascularization. In clinical practice, the likelihood of functional recovery of these intermediate segments is often determined by the number of adjacent segments with either nonviable (75% to 100% transmural hyperenhancement) or viable (0 to 25% transmural hyperenhancement) myocardium.

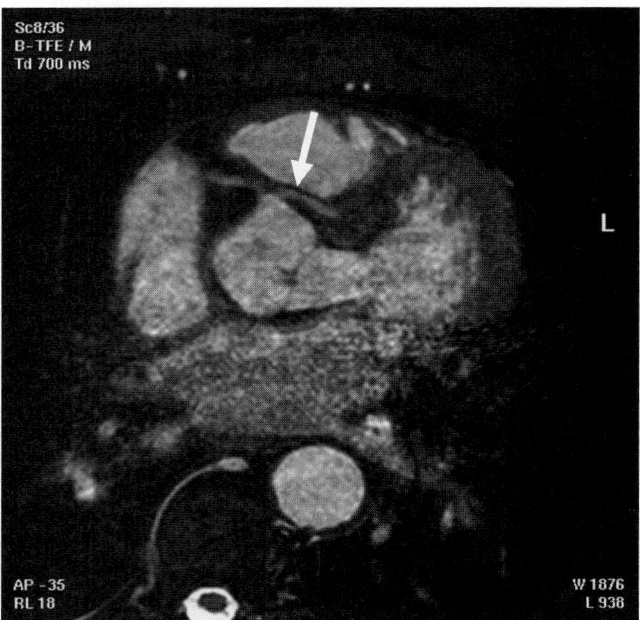


**Figure 37–5** Gradient echo axial image of an anomalous left coronary artery arising off the right sinus of Valsalva (*white arrow*) and passing between the pulmonary artery and aorta. The right coronary artery arises normally. Note the motion artifact in the lower half of the picture.

### *Coronary Artery Disease*

Visualization of the coronary arteries by MRI is technically challenging because of the small size of the coronary arteries, vessel motion during ventricular systole, and the rapid imaging time required for acquisition. Although coronary MRA is capable of accurate detection of proximal coronary artery stenoses, evaluation of small-caliber vessels and coronary stent patency is limited. However, coronary MRA is a useful tool in the assessment of anomalous origin of the coronary arteries (Fig. 37–5).

### *Myocardial Disease*

#### Dilated Cardiomyopathy

MRI can easily characterize the degree of ventricular dilatation and ventricular dysfunction in dilated cardiomyopathy. Normal perfusion and delayed hyperenhancement images support the diagnosis of a nonischemic heart failure etiology.

#### Hypertrophic Cardiomyopathy

Although hypertrophic cardiomyopathy can usually be diagnosed by echocardiography, MRI has been shown to identify those patients not initially diagnosed by echocardiography as a result of its superior ability to quantify regional left ventricular (LV) wall thickness. Asymmetric LV systolic wall thickening, subaortic poststenotic flow abnormalities due to systolic anterior motion of the anterior mitral leaflet, and related mitral regurgitation can be demonstrated on cine gradient echo images. In addition, delayed hyperenhancement images demonstrate a distinct pattern of hyperenhancement that occurs only in the hypertrophied regions in about 80% of patients. The extent of hyperenhancement is small (<10% of LV mass) but typically occurs in the middle third of the ventricular wall at the junction of the interventricular septum and the right ventricular free wall. Patients with these findings have been shown to have an increased risk of sudden cardiac death. Such findings help to distinguish hypertrophic cardiomyopathy from other, more benign conditions, such as physiologic hypertrophy of an athlete's heart.

Fabry disease, an X-linked recessive disorder of lysosomal targeting enzymes, accounts for as much as 5% of all cases of presumed hypertrophic cardiomyopathy and can be identified by marked left ventricular hypertrophy and a distinct pattern of delayed hyperenhancement in about 50%, occurring along the basal inferolateral left ventricular wall and sparing the subendocardium. Identification of these patients guides treatment, usually with intravenous $\alpha$-galactosidase replacement therapy.

#### Restrictive Cardiomyopathy

MRI can help distinguish among various etiologies of restrictive cardiomyopathy, as well as differentiate between restrictive cardiomyopathy and constrictive pericarditis.

- *Cardiac amyloidosis.* Spin echo and gradient echo images demonstrate increased thickness of the left and right ventricular myocardium, and occasionally of the atrial walls and atrioventricular valves. Systolic function is usually preserved or mildly impaired, although abnormal diastolic relaxation is evident on gradient echo ciné-tagged images. Delayed hyperenhancement images demonstrate a diffuse pattern of hyperenhancement involving most of the left and occasionally the right ventricular myocardium. Such hyperenhancement may be predominantly subendocardial, but the global pattern of myocardial hyperenhancement distinguishes amyloidosis from coronary artery disease. In addition, appropriate nulling of the myocardium with an inversion recovery prepulse on delayed hyperenhancement images may be difficult with amyloidosis, providing an additional clue to the diagnosis.
- *Cardiac sarcoidosis.* Cine gradient echo images may demonstrate normal or impaired left ventricular systolic function, oftentimes with regional wall motion abnormalities, depending on the degree of sarcoid involvement of the heart. In the early stages of sarcoidosis the myocardium may demonstrate patchy areas of high signal intensity on T2-weighted black blood images as a result of localized inflammation, along with focal, patchy areas of hyperenhancement (i.e., bright areas) that occur in a noncoronary distribution. The latter corresponds with areas of noncaseating granulomas that are the typical histologic findings of sarcoidosis. These areas of hyperenhancement are also seen in more chronic cases of cardiac sarcoidosis, along with ventricular wall thinning and aneurysms, most commonly along the basal anteroseptal wall.
- *Hemochromatosis.* These patients typically demonstrate dilated cardiomyopathy on cine gradient echo images, as well as evidence of myocardial restriction on cine-tagged images. In addition, both the myocardium and the liver appear dark on T2*-weighted spin echo images, because of loss of signal as a result of tissue iron accumulation.

#### Arrhythmogenic Right Ventricular Dysplasia/Cardiomyopathy (ARVD)

Cardiac MRI can fulfill at most one major or one minor criterion for ARVD (Table 37–1). Gradient echo cine images may demonstrate right ventricular enlargement and/or decreased right ventricular dysfunction. Right ventricular dysfunction can be diffuse, as in advanced ARVD, or limited to areas of "scalloping" or bulging of the right ventricular free wall with associated hypokinesis or dyskinesis. Both spin echo and gradient echo images may demonstrate small, saccular aneurysms that appear as nipple-shaped projections off the right ventricular free wall and right ventricular outflow tract (RVOT). Delayed hyperenhancement images demonstrate abnormal enhancement of the right ventricular free wall, indicative of fibrofatty replacement in those regions. This characteristic fibrofatty replacement is also demonstrated on special "fat saturated" spin echo images, in which signal from all fat within the field of view (e.g., epicardial fat or fatty infiltration of the RV free wall) is saturated and is no longer visible. When found at autopsy, fibrofatty replacement of the myocardium is considered a major criterion for the diagnosis of ARVD. Its significance by MRI, however, has not yet been considered for inclusion in the diagnostic criteria for ARVD.

Occasionally, findings of RVOT enlargement and/or dyskinesia, as well as small aneurysms limited to the RVOT, can be found in patients with RVOT tachycardia, a relatively more benign condition than ARVD.

### *Constrictive Pericarditis*

Characteristic findings of constrictive pericarditis by MRI include: a diastolic bounce of the interventricular septum; tubular or conical-shaped narrowing of one or both ventricles, with or without enlargement of the atria; systemic and pulmonary vein enlargement; pericardial effusion (in patients with effusive-constrictive pericarditis); and increased thickening of the pericardium. The normal pericardium is typically <2 mm in thickness and is often thickest over the right ventricular free wall. A pericardial thickness of >4 mm suggests constriction, and one >5 to 6 mm has

**TABLE 37–1**
**CRITERIA FOR DIAGNOSIS OF ARRHYTHMOGENIC RIGHT VENTRICULAR DYSPLASIA**

I. Global and/or regional dysfunction and structural alterations[a]
  Major
    Severe dilatation and reduction of right ventricular ejection fraction with no (or only mild) left ventricular impairment
    Localized right ventricular aneurysms (akinetic or dyskinetic areas with diastolic bulging)
    Severe segmental dilatation of the right ventricle
  Minor
    Mild global right ventricular dilatation and/or ejection fraction reduction with normal left ventricle
    Mild segmental dilatation of the right ventricle
    Regional right ventricular hypokinesia

II. Tissue characterization of wall
  Major
    Fibrofatty replacement of myocardium on endomyocardial biopsy

III. Repolarization abnormalities
  Minor
    Inverted T-waves in right precordial leads ($V_2$ and $V_3$) in people age >12 y, in absence of right bundle branch block

IV. Depolarization/conduction abnormalities
  Major
    Epsilon waves or localized prolongation (>110 ms) of the QRS complex in right precordial leads ($V_1$–$V_3$)
  Minor
    Late potentials (signal-averaged ECG)

V. Arrhythmias
  Minor
    Left bundle branch block type ventricular tachycardia (sustained and nonsustained) by ECG, Holter, or exercise testing
    Frequent ventricular extrasystoles (>1,000/24 h) (Holter)

VI. Family history
  Major
    Familial disease confirmed at necropsy or surgery
  Minor
    Family history of premature sudden death (<35 y) due to suspected right ventricular dysplasia
    Familial history (clinical diagnosis based on present criteria)

Arrhythmogenic right ventricular dysplasia diagnosis: two major criteria or one major and two minor criteria, or four minor criteria.
[a]Detected by echocardiography, angiography, magnetic resonance imaging, or radionuclide scintigraphy.
*Source:* From McKenna WJ, Thiene G, Nava A, et al. Diagnosis of arrhythmogenic right ventricular dysplasia/cardiomyopathy: Task Force of the Working Group Myocardial and Pericardial Disease of the European Society of Cardiology and of the Scientific Council on Cardiomyopathies of the International Society and Federation of Cardiology. *Br Heart J.* 1994;71:215–218.

a high specificity for constrictive pericarditis. However, calcification of the pericardium, a finding that sensitive for constrictive pericarditis, is better evaluated by CT because of signal loss on MRI over areas of calcified pericardium.

Two findings that make MRI particularly useful in the diagnosis of constrictive pericarditis include evaluation of ventricular interdependence and pericardial tethering. On free-breathing gradient echo cine sequences, the interventricular septum can be seen to shift toward the left ventricle during inspiration, indicative of the ventricular interdependence that occurs in this condition. The characteristic septal shift is often most prominent on the first heart beat that follows the beginning of inspiration. In addition, gradient echo "tagged" images show a tethering of the pericardium to the adjacent myocardium in constriction, rather than the normal free sliding of the pericardium over the myocardium in a healthy individual. Myocardial tagging uses special RF pulses that saturate the tissue at specific intervals creating lines of strain or "tag" lines. Cardiac motion causes deformations of these tag lines that can be analyzed to identify areas of abnormal pericardial motion or regional wall motion abnormalities.

### *Aortic Disease*

#### Aortic Dissection

Using a combination of spin echo, gradient echo, and contrast-enhanced MRA images, the thoracic and abdominal aorta can be evaluated for dissection flaps, entry and re-entry tears of the intima, involvement of aortic branch vessels, location of the true and false lumens, and associated complications (e.g., pleural effusion, cardiac tamponade, aortic regurgitation).

Compared to transesophageal echocardiography, MRI has a similar sensitivity for detection (98% to 100%) but a superior specificity (98% to 100% compared to 68% to 77%) for the diagnosis of aortic dissection. The sensitivity and specificity of MRI and CT are similar. However, the time required to obtain a complete MRI and MRA study of the aorta makes it better suited for patients who require nonemergency imaging (e.g., chronic dissection) or in the follow-up of patients after surgical repair.

#### Intramural Hematoma

Noncommunicating intramural hematomas of the aorta are thought to be a form of aortic dissection but without intimal rupture or tear. These lesions present like typical aortic dissection and on MRI appear as a smooth crescentic or circumferential area of aortic wall thickening without evidence of false lumen blood flow.

#### Aortic Aneurysm

A combination of spin echo, gradient echo, and contrast-enhanced MRA images is used to describe the size, location, and extent of a thoracic or abdominal aortic aneurysm. In addition, the rate of growth, presence of thrombus, accompanying dissection, or involvement of aortic branch vessels can also be identified. Abdominal aortic aneurysm size is best measured on spin echo or gradient echo images, as MRA can underestimate the size of the aneurysm as a result of partial filling of the aneurysm sac by thrombus. Effacement of the sinotubular junction may be seen in

**TABLE 37–2**
**CONTRAINDICATIONS TO MRI**

| Contraindications | Concern |
|---|---|
| **Absolute Contraindications** | |
| Cerebral aneurysm clips | May become displaced by the strong external magnetic field of the scanner, causing severe local injury. Aneurysm clips that are "nonferromagnetic" or "weakly ferromagnetic" are safe to image. |
| Implanted neural stimulator; cochlear implant; implanted insulin or other drug pump | Most implantable devices employ a strong internal magnet or utilize electronic circuitry that can be damaged by the strong external magnetic field the scanner. |
| Cardiac pacemaker or defibrillator | Pacemakers/defibrillators are important contraindications to MRI imaging because of the potential for device malfunction. Small studies suggest that some non–pacer-dependent patients with pacemakers can be imaged, although the devices must be interrogated and potentially reprogrammed before and after imaging. MRI-compatible devices are in development. |
| Ocular foreign body; metal shrapnel or bullet fragment | Metallic foreign objects within the body can become displaced by the strong external magnetic field of the scanner, causing severe local tissue injury. |
| Temporary pacemaker wires or pulmonary artery catheters | Contain metallic tips that may become heated during MRI imaging, causing local tissue damage. |
| **Relative Contraindications** | |
| Intravascular stents, coils, and filters | Initial concerns that these objects may migrate after early exposure to MRI magnetic fields have been largely unfounded. Coronary stents have been safely imaged as early as several hours after implantation. However, most manufacturers recommend waiting 6 weeks after implantation so that these objects can endothelialized by the vessel wall. |
| Hearing aids | Same concerns as for cochlear implants; must be removed prior to entering the scanner. |
| Pregnancy | Considerable evidence suggests that exposure to MRI is safe. However, exposure during the first trimester, particularly to MRI contrast agents, should be avoided. |
| Claustrophobia | Some claustrophobic patients may have difficulty within the confines of an MRI scanner. Oral anxiolytics (e.g., alprazolam) may be useful in such patients. |

aneurysms of the ascending aorta and indicate the presence of cystic medial necrosis, conferring a higher risk of aortic rupture. Mycotic aneurysms of the aorta or its branch vessels can be identified by their typical saccular appearance, as well as increased signal intensity of the aneurysm wall on T2-weighted spin echo due to the presence of localized inflammation.

### Limitations of Cardiac MRI

Despite its increasing versatility and robustness, important limitations still remain in cardiac MRI imaging. The electromagnetic forces created by the MRI scanner can induce important thermal and nonthermal effects in some patients. Therefore, the presence of patient contraindications to MRI imaging must be identified before the patient enters the scanner (Table 37–2). Nonferromagnetic metallic devices, such as mechanical heart valves, sternal wires, and retained pacing wires after cardiac surgery, are safe to image, although they are often a source of image artifact. Internal orthopedic prostheses (e.g., artificial hip joints) are safe to image.

Patient cooperation is critical to successful cardiac imaging. Patient movement during image acquisition can result in degraded image quality, and uncooperative patients may require oral or intravenous sedation to prevent unwanted motion artifacts. Multiple breath holds of 10 to 15 seconds each are often utilized in adults to limit cardiac motion due to respiration. Children and adult patients who are unable to hold their breath can still be imaged successfully, although acquisition times are often increased to preserve image quality. Arrhythmias are problematic due to image degradation and make flow quantification by phase velocity imaging unreliable.

Cost and availability are important limitations to the widespread use of cardiac MRI, although this will become less of an issue as the cost of MRI scanners decreases over time. MRI scanners are not portable, and acquisition times can vary between 15 and 60 minutes, making imaging of unstable patients difficult.

## CARDIAC CT

Technological advances have revolutionized the use of multidetector CT (MDCT) in cardiac imaging. Improvements in gantry rotation, increased detector rows, image acquisition protocols, and postprocessing algorithms have lead to vastly improved spatial and temporal resolution.

## Indications

There is considerable overlap in many of the clinical indications for cardiac MRI and cardiac CT. For example, both can be useful in the evaluation of patients with diseases of the aorta. CT, however, may be preferred when emergency imaging is required, whereas MRI may be better suited for long-term follow-up because of its lack of ionizing radiation. Unlike MRI, CT offers limited assessment of myocardial function because of the low number of frames/second acquired (usually 10 frames/s, compared with 20 to 30 frames/s with MRI). However, CT is clearly superior to MRI in the assessment of coronary artery stenoses and anomalous coronary arteries.

## Technical Considerations

### *CT Physics*

Data acquisition in CT depends on the measurement of transmitted x-rays after they pass through an object. An x-ray source is used to produce a collimated, fan-shaped x-ray beam. As this x-ray beam passes through a patient, some of the photons are absorbed or scattered, thereby reducing x-ray transmission to a set of x-ray detectors on the opposite side. This process, known as attenuation, depends on the atomic composition and density of the objects through which the photons pass, as well as the energy of the photons themselves. Objects with a relatively high attenuation, such as bone or metal, absorb most of the transmitted photons from the x-ray beam, whereas low-attenuation tissues such as lung allow most of these photons to pass through to the x-ray detectors.

X-ray detectors opposite to the x-ray source receive the attenuated signal and digitize the information so that a set of attenuation values can be calculated. To create images from the x-ray measurements, specific mathematical reconstruction algorithms—most commonly filtered back-projection or convolution—are followed. The raw data are "filtered" or preprocessed to minimize beam hardening and scattered radiation, after which "back-projection" is performed to create a set of axial images with specific density values from the raw data as the x-ray tube rotates around the patient.

CT densities are expressed as Hounsfield units (HU), which range in value from −1,024 to +3,071 HU. Although this full range of density values could be displayed as a gray scale from black (lowest) to white (highest), the human eye is incapable of distinguishing between small changes in densities within this scale. The image display is therefore adjusted using "window levels" and "widths" to optimize contrast. The window level (or center) indicates which density value is in the middle of the displayed gray scale. In effect, window level determines which attenuation values or tissue types are visualized. The window width determines which density values around the window level are within the gray-scale display. Objects with a CT density above the window width are displayed as white; objects below the window width are displayed as black. In effect, the window width determines the image contrast.

The density of water is defined as 0 HU. The value of nonenhanced (i.e., no contrast) tissues, such as muscle and blood, range from −100 HU to +200 HU. Fat tissue has somewhat lower density values, whereas bone and calcium have higher density. Contrast-enhanced arterial blood, such as the coronary arteries, has a density level of +200 HU to +400 HU. For cardiac imaging, the window level is usually set between +250 HU and +300 HU, with a window width of +600 HU to +1,000 HU, depending on the vendor and study indication.

### *Electron-Beam CT*

Electron-beam CT (EBCT) scanners, although decreasing in popularity, were the first technique developed to evaluate coronary calcium scoring. EBCT images are generated by scanning an electron beam at four tungsten coils positioned below the patient. Because there is no mechanical motion within the gantry, temporal resolution is excellent (50 to 100 milliseconds). Although it is still used in a limited number of practices, EBCT scanners have largely been replaced by more advanced multidetector CT (MDCT) imaging.

### *Multidetector CT*

MDCT scanners utilize an x-ray tube mounted opposite a series of detectors; the assembly then rotates on a gantry around the patient. The x-rays form a "cone beam" flowing from the source on one side to the detectors on the opposite side of the rotating gantry. This type of scanner is the most common type of CT scanner used today. In most CT imaging, including cardiac imaging, the patient is moved at a fixed speed, or pitch, through the constantly rotating gantry (spiral acquisition). The use of multiple detector rows allows for the acquisition of multiple simultaneous parallel slices per gantry rotation, which occurs at speeds between 300 and 400 milliseconds per rotation. Current 64-slice MDCT scanners can acquire the entire cardiac image during a single breath hold of 8 to 10 seconds.

Image acquisition must be gated to the cardiac cycle, which is measured by the patient's ECG tracing. Most current scanners use retrospective ECG gating, in which data are collected during the entire cardiac cycle, but the ECG signal is used to trigger image reconstruction in late diastole.

In cardiac CT, an additional data reconstruction technique known as multisegment reconstruction may be performed. This technique utilizes data from more than one cardiac cycle to construct a clinically useful image. Multisegment reconstruction improves temporal resolution (the time required to acquire one image), at the cost of a slight increase in radiation exposure, because sampling occurs during more than one cardiac cycle.

### *Patient Selection and Preparation*

Appropriate patient selection is an important part of maximizing the clinical utility of any diagnostic test. Coronary CT angiography (CTA) of the coronary arteries, the most popular application for cardiac CT, is best suited for patients with a low to intermediate risk of coronary artery disease. To avoid unnecessary contrast and radiation exposure, high-risk patients are better served by cardiac catheterization. In addition, patients with a high likelihood of significant coronary calcification (e.g., a patient with renal failure on dialysis), patients with coronary stents, or those with ongoing cardiac arrhythmias are not well suited for coronary CTA.

Unlike cardiac MRI, cardiac catheterization, or other imaging modalities, the image acquisition from cardiac CT cannot be immediately repeated, because of the contrast and radiation dose just delivered. Appropriate patient preparation will increase patient comfort and maximize the quality of the resulting images. Each step of the scan should be explained to the patient, and breath holds should be practiced before the actual scan. Heart rate should be slowed to a target heart rate of 50 to 60 beats/min prior to the scan—typically with oral atenolol or metoprolol (50 to 100 mg 1 hour prior to the scan) and intravenous metoprolol (5 mg IV every 5 minutes up to a maximum dose of 50 mg) as tolerated. Calcium channel blockers have been used to slow the heart rate in patients who are unable to tolerate beta-blockers as a result of bronchospastic disease, although with relatively decreased efficacy. Finally, in patients undergoing coronary CTA, a sublingual nitroglycerin spray or tablet is given immediately before the scan, to dilate the coronary arteries.

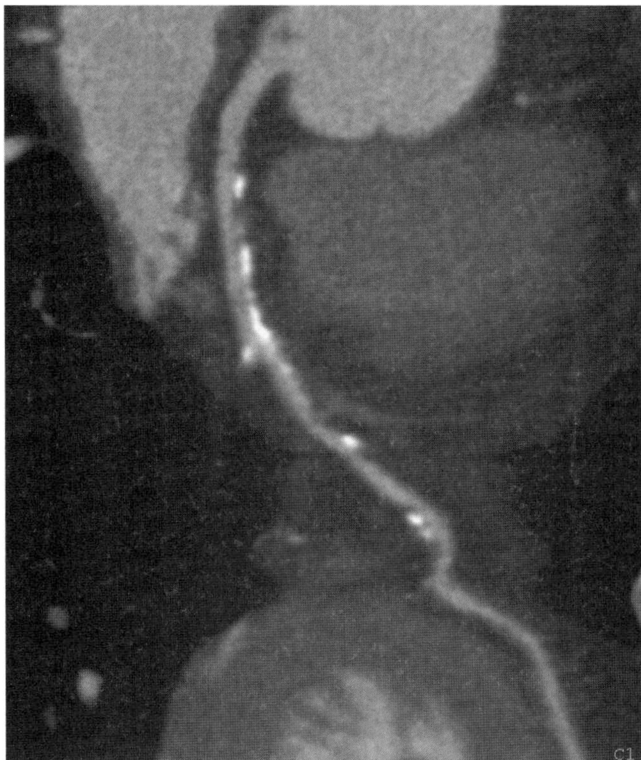


**Figure 37–6** Multiplanar reformation (MPR) MDCT image of the left anterior descending (LAD) artery. The vessel is viewed from the beginning of the left coronary artery ostium, through the left main, to the distal LAD. The bifurcation of the left circumflex and diagonal arteries are not shown in this view. Note the calcified and noncalcified plaque in the proximal and mid-portion of the vessel, causing mild stenosis.

## Selected Clinical Applications

### *Coronary Artery Disease*

With coronary CTA, both stenoses of the vessel lumen as well as abnormalities of the vessel wall can be visualized. Images are often interpreted in traditional orthogonal planes (axial, sagittal, and coronal) as well as oblique planes that follow the axis of the coronary arteries or heart (e.g., horizontal long axis). Multiplanar reformation, or MPR, is a reconstruction technique that uses straight or curved thin images from a three-dimensional volume of images to create a two-dimensional representation of a vessel. This technique is useful for following tortuous coronary artery segments and for visualizing an entire vessel simultaneously (Fig. 37–6). Maximum-intensity projections, or MIPs, select the brightest voxel (3-dimensional pixel) from a three-dimensional stack of images and displays them as one projection (Fig. 38–7). MIPs form the basis of angiographic images in cardiac catheterization.

Coronary artery stenoses identified by CT can be classified as calcified or noncalcified plaque. Noncalcified plaques are of low to intermediate attenuation and appear as defects in the vessel wall as outlined by contrast. Calcified

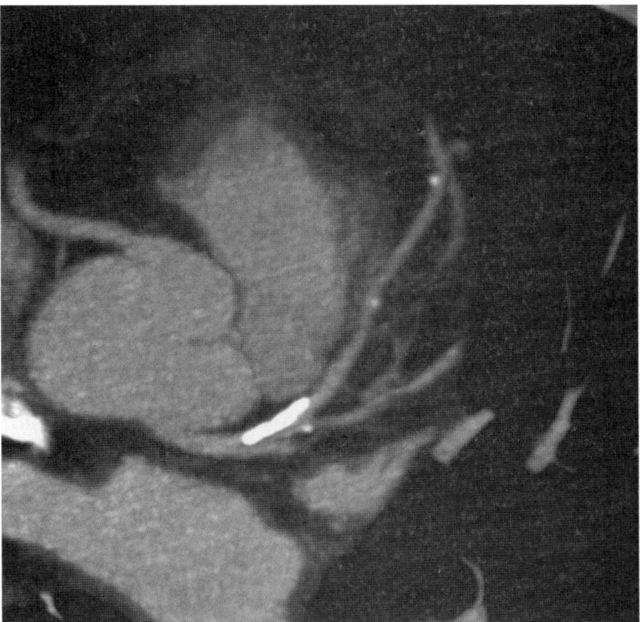

**Figure 37–7** Maximum intensity projection (MIP) of an oblique axial MDCT image of the LAD. Note the calcified plaque in the proximal portion of the vessel. It is not possible to accurately quantify the degree of stenosis behind the calcified plaque.

plaques appear as high attenuation (i.e., bright) lesions that are associated with calcium blooming artifacts—the false appearance that the degree of stenosis is more severe than actuality due to attenuation of the x-ray photons by calcium. When vessel or plaque calcification is significant, it is often not possible to quantify the degree of vessel stenosis, as the x-ray attenuation precludes assessment of the full vessel lumen (see Fig. 37–7).

Coronary stenoses are classified as mild (<50% diameter stenosis), moderate (50% to 70% stenosis), or severe (>70% stenosis). Spatial resolution of the current generation of 64-slice CT scanners is approximately 0.4 × 0.4 × 0.4 mm or less. In comparison, coronary angiography by cardiac catheterization provides a spatial resolution of 0.2 mm or less. Despite this limitation, current scanners have >90% sensitivity and specificity for the detection of >70% coronary artery stenosis compared with cardiac catheterization. The negative predictive value of a normal coronary CTA is typically >98%.

Despite its utility in evaluating low- to intermediate-risk patients for coronary artery disease, coronary CTA remains an evolving field with several important limitations. Although contrast within a stent may suggest stent patency, in-stent restenosis cannot be reliably quantified because beam-hardening artifact obscures the vessel lumen. Coronary artery bypass grafts can be evaluated for patency; however, the distal anastomosis often cannot be visualized due to a combination of small vessel size and calcium artifacts. Although these factors will improve as CT technology progresses, artifacts due to coronary artery calcification will likely remain an important limitation.

### *Coronary Calcium Scoring*

Coronary artery calcification is a reliable, albeit somewhat limited, sign of coronary atherosclerosis. The prevalence and extent of coronary calcium increases with age in both men and women, although the onset of calcification seems to be delayed by about 10 years in women compared with men. Men in general have higher calcium scores than women. Individuals of either gender with diabetes or renal insufficiency have an increased extent of coronary calcification.

Coronary calcium scoring uses noncontrast EBCT or MDCT to quantify the degree of calcification of the coronary arteries. Several algorithms to quantify calcium are available. The most commonly used method, the Agatston score, assigns a calcium score based on the maximal HU number and the area of calcium deposits. Only areas of calcification $\geq 1$ mm$^2$ and >130 HU are included in this algorithm. Other methods quantify the volume or mass of coronary calcium.

Coronary calcium scoring has been used for the assessment of long-term cardiac risk. However, it adds only incremental value to current standards of risk assessment and should not be used in isolation. Coronary plaque calcification does not correlate well with the degree of histopathologic stenosis, and the typical plaque rupture that leads to acute coronary syndromes do not always occur at the site of calcification. The test is most useful in intermediate-risk populations, in whom a normal or abnormal score result may reclassify individuals to a lower or higher risk group, respectively. Some centers use calcium scoring prior to coronary CTA in elderly patients; patients with a calcium score >800 are thought to have excessive calcification and the coronary CTA study is aborted, saving the patient unnecessary contrast and radiation exposure.

### *Pulmonary Vein Assessment*

Pulmonary vein ablation/isolation is an increasingly common treatment for the management of patients with atrial fibrillation. Cardiac CT is useful in preprocedure planning to delineate the number and location of pulmonary veins, as well as to evaluate the patient postprocedure for the development of pulmonary venous stenosis, a known complication of the procedure. The latter is often detected early as pulmonary vein wall thickening and mediastinal lymph node enlargement; later stages show narrowing or obstruction of the venous lumen. In addition, some centers incorporate the anatomic data provided by cardiac CT into procedural left atrial electrophysiologic maps.

### *Aortic Disease*

As with MRI, CT is well suited for the evaluation of aortic anatomy and pathology. Cardiac CT is the test of choice when acute aortic dissection, transection, intramural hematomas, or penetrating ulcers are suspected. In addition, the location of internal mammary artery grafts can be identified prior to thoracic surgery, an important factor to consider in patients undergoing sternotomy for repeat coronary artery bypass grafting (CABG). Motion artifacts of the aorta are uncommon because of its relative immobility, and most studies can be adequately imaged using older 16-slice scanners and 3-mm-thick slices. Images of the entire thoracic and abdominal aorta can be acquired in a single breath hold.

## Limitations of Cardiac CT

### *Image Quality*

A number of factors influence image quality by cardiac CT. Characteristics related to the MDCT scanner include detector row number and type, detector width, gantry rotation time, and tube output. Tube output can be varied according to the patient's body habitus (higher output for larger patients) or the clinical condition (e.g., lower output for evaluation of prosthetic valve motion). Other factors that affect image quality are determined by the patient or by clinical conditions at the time of image acquisition (Table 37–3). Finally, streak artifacts can occur as a result of the presence of metallic objects within the thorax (e.g., bypass graft clips, pacemaker wires) or an excess of contrast dye in the right atrium or ventricle. The latter can be minimized by the use of a saline flush immediately following contrast bolus injection so that contrast is cleared from the right side of the heart.

**TABLE 37–3**
**FACTORS INFLUENCING CARDIAC CT IMAGE QUALITY**

| Factor | Concern |
|---|---|
| Patient size | Higher degree of x-ray beam attenuation in obese patients causes degraded image quality. Tube output can be increased to compensate, but results in a higher radiation dose exposure. |
| Patient motion | Failure to hold breath appropriately or patient movement during image acquisition leads to motion artifacts. Breath-hold training and practice prior to the actual image acquisition significantly increases patient cooperation. Inform patients to expect to experience a hot sensation during contrast injection. |
| Heart rate | Heart rates >70 beats/min during image acquisition reduces the amount of time spent in diastole (when there is minimal coronary artery motion), resulting in degraded image quality. Oral and intravenous beta-blockade prior to image acquisition should be employed whenever possible. |
| Cardiac rhythm | Cardiac arrhythmia, PACs, or PVCs result in degraded image quality as a result of inappropriate ECG triggering. |
| Coronary calcification | "Blooming artifact" due to coronary calcium obscures the vessel lumen, rendering stenosis quantification unreliable. |

### *Radiation Exposure*

Cardiac CT uses ionizing radiation to image the heart, resulting in a predictable amount of radiation exposure to the patient that depends in part on the type of protocol used (Table 37–4). The effective radiation dose is higher in women and obese patients because of their increased body fat. The radiation dose is also higher in patients with faster heart rates, which negates the benefits in radiation dose reduction when dose modulation is used.

"Dose modulation," or ECG-controlled tube current modulation, is a technique that limits radiation exposure while still providing adequate image quality. This technique uses ECG triggering to adjust the scanner's tube current so that it is highest during ventricular diastole (when cardiac motion is minimized) and lowest during systole. Dose modulation can reduce the effective radiation dose by 35% to 45% when used appropriately. This reduction in exposure is maximized at slower heart rates because of the relative increase in the duration of diastole and overall shorter scan time. The resulting systolic images are acquired during periods of reduced tube output, resulting in low-resolution images. This proves acceptable, as systolic frames are typically used only in reconstruction of ciné loops.

In general, CT scanning should be avoided in pregnant women because of the risk of teratogenicity and potential increase in childhood malignancy. Breast feeding is a relative contraindication to contrast exposure.

### *Contrast Exposure*

The iodinated contrast agents used in cardiac CT imaging carry a 2% to 4% risk of contrast allergy and a variable risk of renal dysfunction after contrast exposure. Most cardiac

**TABLE 37–4**
**RELATIVE RADIATION EXPOSURE DUE TO MEDICAL PROCEDURES**

| Diagnostic Procedure | Typical Effective Dose (mSv) | Equivalent Period of Natural Background Radiation |
|---|---|---|
| Natural background radiation | 3 to 4 (range 1.5 to 7.5) | 1 y |
| Chest x-ray (PA and lateral) | 0.04 | 6 d |
| Transatlantic flight | 0.03 | 5 d |
| Lung ventilation (81 mKR) | 0.1 | 2 to 4 wk |
| Lung perfusion study (99m-Tc) | 1 | 4 to 6 mo |
| Calcium scoring | 0.8 to 2 | 3 to 6 mo |
| CT head | 2 | 8 mo |
| Cardiac catheterization (diagnostic) | 3 to 4 | 1 y |
| 64-slice MDCT (with dose modulation) | 8 to 12 | 2 to 3 y |
| Myocardial perfusion (201 Tl) | 15 to 18 | 4 to 5 y |
| CT abdomen/pelvis | 10 to 20 | 3 to 6 y |
| Cardiac PET | 14 to 20 | 4 to 6 y |

studies currently require between 80 and 100 cc of contrast dye, followed by 30 to 50 cc of a saline flush. In general, the risk of contrast nephropathy is negligible in patients with a serum creatinine ≤1.8 mg/dL and no predisposing factors to renal dysfunction. Factors that increase the risk of contrast nephropathy include increasing age, elevated serum creatinine level or a history of renal dysfunction, volume depletion, heart failure, and diabetes. Because of the presence of multiple co-morbidities in patients undergoing cardiac CT studies, most centers use low-osmolar nonionic dye. Patients with a history of contrast dye allergy should be premedicated with steroids and diphenhydramine several hours prior to their study.

Gadolinium DPTA (an MRI contrast agent) can be substituted for traditional CT contrast agents in those patients who require imaging by CT but who have significant renal dysfunction or a history of anaphylaxis with ionic contrast dye. The disadvantages are a reduction in contrast attenuation and the higher cost of gadolinium.

## EVALUATION OF CARDIAC MASSES BY CT AND MRI

CT and MR are able to visualize not only cardiac anatomy but also the surrounding mediastinal, pulmonary, and chest wall structures. The wide field of view, coupled with high spatial resolution, make these imaging modalities useful techniques in the evaluation of cardiac and paracardiac masses.

Both benign and, to a lesser extent, malignant masses have various anatomic and tissue characteristics by CT and MR that help to narrow the differential diagnosis of a cardiac mass (Table 37–5). Findings suggestive of malignancy

**TABLE 38–5**
**EVALUATION OF CARDIAC MASSES BY MRI AND CT**

| Mass | Location | MRI | CT |
|---|---|---|---|
| Myxomas | Left atrial cavity, attached to the interatrial septum at the border of the fossa ovalis (85%); posterior and atrial walls; atrial appendage | Variable composition of water-laden myxomatous tissue, fibrous tissue and calcification T2-W higher signal than myocardium | Calcifications evident |
| Lipomas | 50% subendocardial, 25% subepicardial, 25% wall of cardiac chamber extending intracavitary | T1-W high signal intensity similar to subcutaneous fat; T2-W moderate signal intensity | Density of lipoma is similar to mediastinal fat |
| Thrombus | Posterolateral wall or left atrial cavity; left atrial appendage; apex of impaired left ventricle | T1-W fresh thrombus has higher signal intensity than myocardium; older thrombus may have increased signal on T1-W with decreased signal intensity on T2-W | Fresh thrombus has lower density, older thrombus may have calcifications |
| Angiosarcomas | Right sided, especially right atrium; pericardium with hemopericardium | Heterogenous mass with hemorrhagic areas appearing as hyperintense on T1-W | Hypodense nodular mass with inhomogeneous enhancement postcontrast |
| Rhabdomyomas | Myocardium or ventricles (right = left), large and may obstruct a valve or chamber; multiple sites involved in most cases and atria involved in 30% cases | Indeterminate signal on T1-W; slightly hyperintense on T2-W | Intracavitary low-attenuation mass postcontrast |
| Fibromas | Myocardium, particularly the anterior free wall and interventricular septum causing conduction abnormalities | Indeterminate signal on T1-W compared to skeletal muscle; lower signal intensity than myocardium on T2-W | Calcified areas of necrosis |
| Metastases | Nodular deposits or localized or diffuse pericardial thickening with hemorrhagic or serosanguinous pericardial effusion | Nonspecific | Nonspecific |
| Pericardial cyst | Typically right cardiophrenic angle | Simple fluid characteristics with intermediate signal intensity on T1-W and high signal intensity on T2-W | Well-circumscribed, low-attenuation, nonenhancing mass adjacent to pericardium |

T1-W, T1-weighted spin echo images; T2-W, T2-weighted spin echo images.

include right ventricular or right atrial involvement, infiltration into surrounding structures (e.g., penetration through the pericardium), irregular borders, pulmonary or mediastinal involvement, and hemopericardium. Findings suggestive of a benign tumor are left-sided involvement along the interatrial septum, smooth borders, and lack of pericardial effusion. Contrast perfusion through the mass can be used to identify vascular tumors, both benign and malignant, and to differentiate tumors from thrombus.

## BIBLIOGRAPHY

### MRI

**Bogaert J, Dymarkowski S, Taylor AM.** *Clinical Cardiac MRI.* New York: Springer-Verlag; 2005.

**Lardo, A, Fayad ZA, Chronos NAF, Fuster V.** *Cardiovascular Magnetic Resonance: Established and Emerging Applications.* London: Taylor & Francis; 2003.

**Lima JA, Desai M.** Cardiovascular magnetic resonance imaging: current and emerging applications. *J Am Coll Cardiol.* 2004;44: 1164–1171.

**McKenna WJ, Thiene G, Nava A, et al.** Diagnosis of arrhythmogenic right ventricular dysplasia/cardiomyopathy: Task Force of the Working Group Myocardial and Pericardial Disease of the European Society of Cardiology and of the Scientific Council on Cardiomyopathies of the International Society and Federation of Cardiology. *Br Heart J.* 1994;71:215–218.

**Nagel E, van Rossum AC, Fleck E.** *Cardiovascular Magnetic Resonance.* Darmstadt, Germany: Steinkopff-Verlag; 2004.

### CT

**de Feyter PJ, Krestin GP.** *Computed Tomography of the Coronary Arteries.* London: Taylor & Francis; 2005.

**Gerber TC, Kuzo RS, Morin RL.** Techniques and parameters for estimating radiation exposure and dose in cardiac computed tomography. *Int J Cardiovasc Imaging.* 2005;21:165–176.

**Rumberger, JA.** Clinical use of coronary calcium scanning with computed tomography. *Cardiol Clin.* 2003;21:535–547.

**Schoenhagen P, Stillman AE, Halliburton SS, White RD.** CT of the heart: principles, advances, clinical uses. *Cleveland Clinic J Med.* 2005;72:127–138.

**Stanford W.** Advances in cardiovascular CT imaging: CT clinical imaging. *Int J Cardiovasc Imaging.* 2005;21:29–37.

## QUESTIONS

**1.** A 51-year-old man presents to your clinic for evaluation of progressive exertional dyspnea over the last 6 months. On physical examination, his heart rate is 85 beats/min, his respiratory rate is 22, and his blood pressure is 108/65 mm Hg. His jugular venous pulse is visible 8 cm above the sternal angle at 45 degrees. The PMI is sustained but normal in location. He has an S4 gallop and 1+ bilateral pedal edema. A PA and lateral chest x-ray are unremarkable. A transthoracic echocardiogram reveals normal left and right ventricular systolic function with mild left ventricular hypertrophy and abnormal diastolic function. A cardiac MRI with gadolinium contrast is obtained.

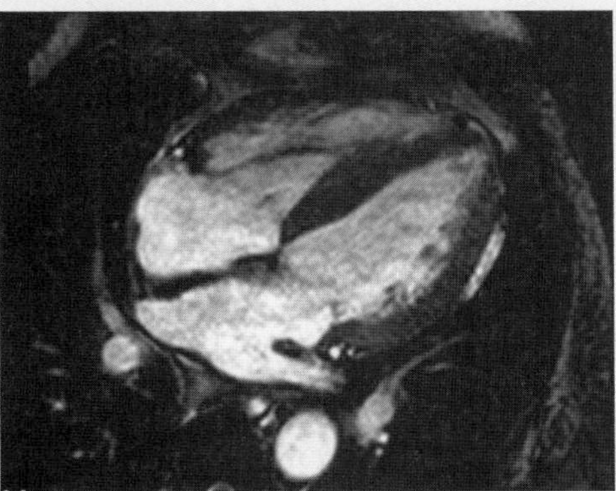

Still frame gradient echo image, four-chamber view.

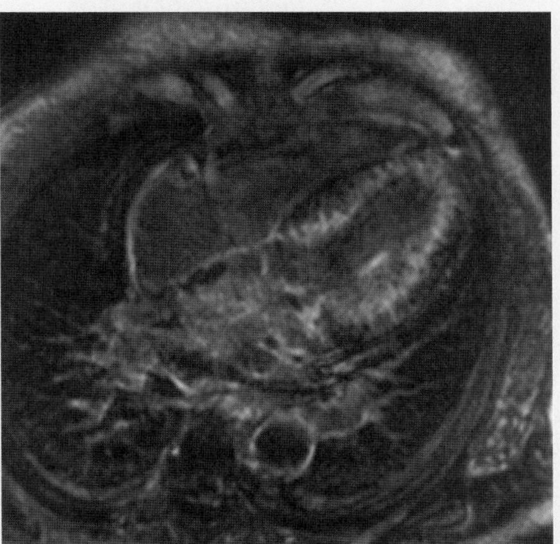

Corresponding delayed hyperenhanced image, four-chamber view.

Based on these images, the next most appropriate clinical step is

a. Endomyocardial biopsy
b. Fat pad biopsy
c. Initiate corticosteroid therapy
d. Surgical pericardial stripping

Answer is b: Fat pad biopsy. Although the mildly thickened ventricular myocardium is consistent with several different etiologies of cardiomyopathy, the diffuse pattern of hyperenhancement throughout the left ventricle on delayed hyperenhanced black blood MRI images (second figure above) is typical of cardiac amyloidosis. Cardiac sarcoidosis, which might be an indication to begin corticosteroid or other immunosuppressive therapy, typically demonstrates patchy areas of hyperenhancement, along with ventricular wall thinning and aneurysms, most commonly along the basal anteroseptal wall. Ciné gradient echo images in sarcoidosis may demonstrate normal or impaired left ventricular systolic function, often with regional wall motion abnormalities.

Fat pad biopsy is often preferred over endomyocardial biopsy for evaluation of amyloidosis because of its less invasive nature and higher sensitivity. Although there may be a role for immunosuppressive therapy in specific subtypes of amyloidosis, histologic diagnosis should be confirmed before therapy is initiated. There is no thickening of the pericardium, conical deformity of the ventricles, or atrial enlargement on these images to suggest constrictive pericarditis, making pericardial stripping inappropriate.

**2.** You are asked to see a 58-year-old woman in the emergency room who has presented with intermittent retrosternal chest pain without radiation lasting for less than 1 minute and a single episode of rest pain lasting 10 minutes today. She states she has been having these symptoms since shoveling snow 1 week prior to presentation. Her past medical history is significant for gastroesophageal reflux, for which she takes an over-the-counter $H_2$ blocker infrequently. She takes no other medications. She was told at a health screening fair a few months ago that her cholesterol levels were high, but she has not seen her family physician about it. Physical examination is unremarkable. ECG reveals normal sinus rhythm with no ischemic changes. Initial laboratory evaluation, including a portable chest x-ray and cardiac enzymes, are within normal limits. A cardiac CTA is obtained to further evaluate the etiology of her chest pain.

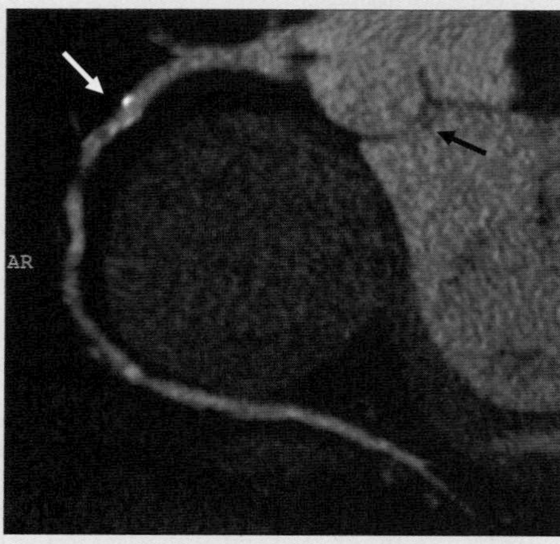


Curved multiplanar reformatted (MPR) image of the aortic valve (*black arrow*) and right coronary artery (*white arrow*).

Based on this image, the next most appropriate step is

a. Begin therapy with an angiotensin-converting enzyme (ACE) inhibitor, beta-blocker, and diuretic,
b. Begin therapy with a proton pump inhibitor.
c. Obtain a transthoracic echocardiogram to evaluate for aortic stenosis.
d. Refer the patient for a nuclear stress study.
e. Refer the patient for cardiac catheterization.

Answer is e: Refer the patient for cardiac catheterization. The curved MPR image reveals a noncalcified atherosclerotic plaque in the mid-RCA associated with severe luminal stenosis, which can be compared to her corresponding coronary angiogram (see image below). The low attenuation characteristics of this lesion on coronary CTA suggest that it is a noncalcified plaque, unlike the higher-attenuation calcified plaque that occurs more proximally. Current CT technology does not allow precise quantification of coronary stenoses as is done with invasive angiography. Therefore, most lesions are graded as mild (<50%), moderate (50% to 70%), or severe (>70%) stenoses. There is no evidence of heart failure that would suggest therapy with ACE inhibitors, beta-blockers, and diuretics. The aortic valve leaflets appear thin and noncalcified, making aortic stenosis less likely. Ciné CT images of the ventricles and aortic valve could be reconstructed, if desired, to assess ventricular function and leaflet mobility. Additional noninvasive testing is not indicated in this patient because of the abnormalities seen on coronary CTA.

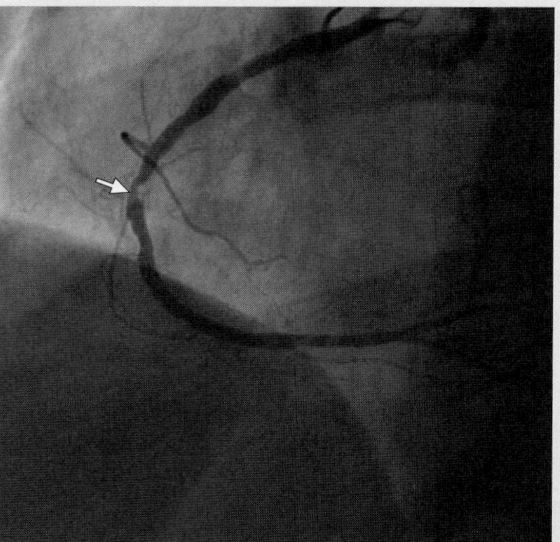

Left anterior oblique cranial projection of the right coronary artery reveals a 60% to 70% stenosis in the mid-portion of the vessel (*white arrow*).

**3.** A 42-year-old man with diabetes and a family history of coronary artery disease undergoes coronary CTA after an equivocal exercise stress test. The following MPR image is obtained of the left main and left anterior descending (LAD) arteries.

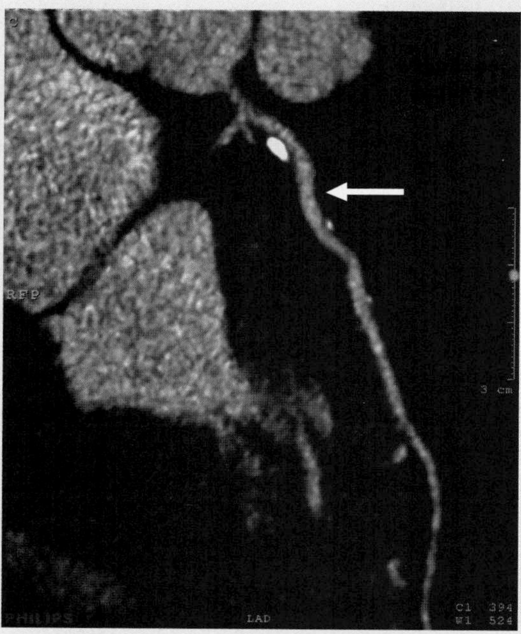


Curved MPR image of the LAD (*white arrow*).

Which of the following statements is *true* regarding the calcified plaque seen in the proximal LAD in this image?

a. Additional postprocessing should be performed to remove the calcium blooming artifact.
b. Coronary calcification may occur in the presence of atherosclerosis but is a nonspecific finding.
c. Coronary calcification tends to overestimate coronary artery stenosis due to blooming artifact.
d. The degree of coronary calcification correlates well with the severity of stenosis in the underlying vessel.

Answer is c: Coronary calcification tends to overestimate coronary artery stenosis due to blooming artifact. This is due to attenuation (absorption) of the x-ray photons by deposits of calcium, which is relatively dense compared to its surrounding tissues. Currently, this artifact cannot be removed by postprocessing techniques. The presence of coronary calcification does correlate with an individual's overall atherosclerotic disease burden, but it does not predict the severity of stenosis of the underlying vessel. Calcification within an artery is a specific sign of atherosclerosis.

**4.** A 60-year-old man with a history of hypertension and dyslipidemia presents to the hospital in acute pulmonary edema approximately 72 hours after probable onset of an anterior myocardial infarction. The patient is stabilized and a cardiac catheterization is performed, which demonstrates a diffusely calcified 90% lesion of the ostial-proximal LAD that is not amenable to percutaneous intervention. The RCA and LCX arteries demonstrate mild to moderate diffuse disease. A transthoracic echocardiogram demonstrates a left ventricular ejection fraction of approximately 15%. He is referred for coronary artery bypass surgery and a cardiac MRI is obtained to assess for myocardial viability.

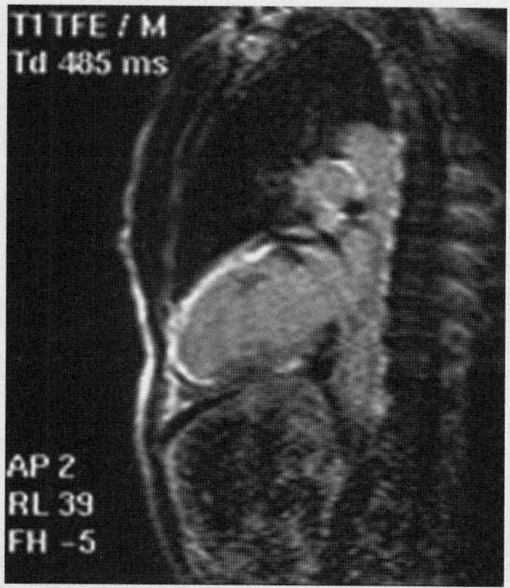


Delayed hyperenhanced image obtained 15 to 20 minutes after gadolinium DTPA, two-chamber view.

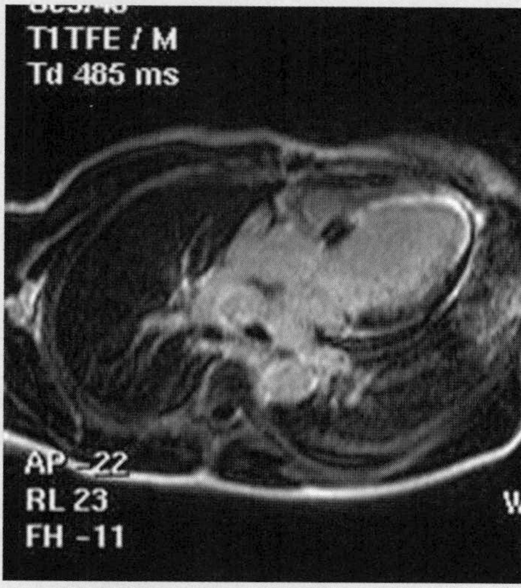


Delayed hyperenhanced image obtained 15 to 20 minutes after gadolinium DTPA, three-chamber view.

All of the following would be appropriate *except*:

a. Surgical revascularization of the left anterior descending artery
b. Medical therapy with an ACE inhibitor, beta-blocker, and diuretic

c. Medical therapy with aspirin and a statin
d. Consideration for implantation of a defibrillator

Answer is a: Surgical revascularization of the left anterior descending artery. Delayed hyperenhancement images demonstrate transmural scarring from the proximal to distal anterior and anteroseptal walls, as well as the apex and inferoapical segments. The transmural extent of hyperenhancement suggests a poor likelihood of recovery of myocardial function after revascularization (whether surgical or percutaneous), consistent with nonviable myocardium. Surgical revascularization would be high risk given his low ejection fraction, and unlikely to improve his long-term survival or ventricular function because of the nonviable myocardium in the infarct-related territory. The other choices would be indicated given the clinical scenario.

**5.** A 32-year-old woman is referred to your office for evaluation of occasional palpitations and increasing exertional dyspnea. She denies any history of fever, syncope, or neurologic deficits. Physical examination is unremarkable. A transthoracic echocardiogram demonstrates a poorly defined left ventricular mass, and a cardiac MRI is obtained for further evaluation of the lesion.

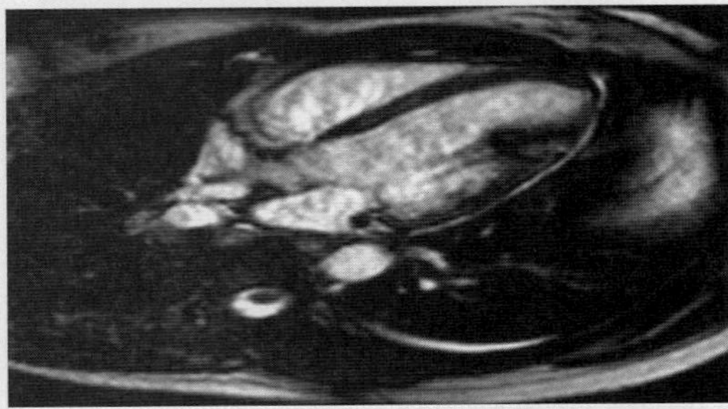

Still frame gradient echo image, three-chamber view.

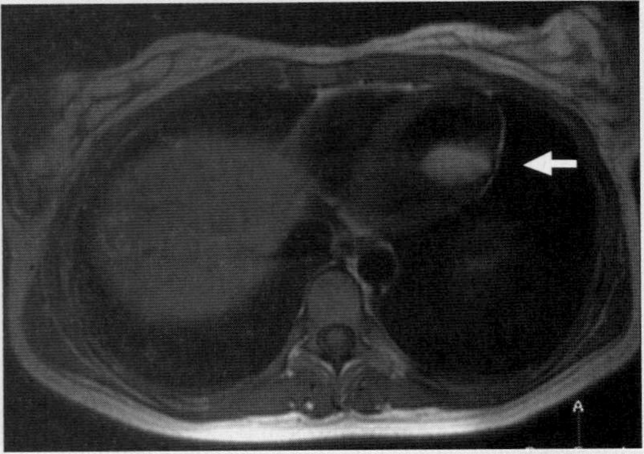

Black blood (turbo spin echo) axial image depicting an intracardiac mass (*white arrow*).

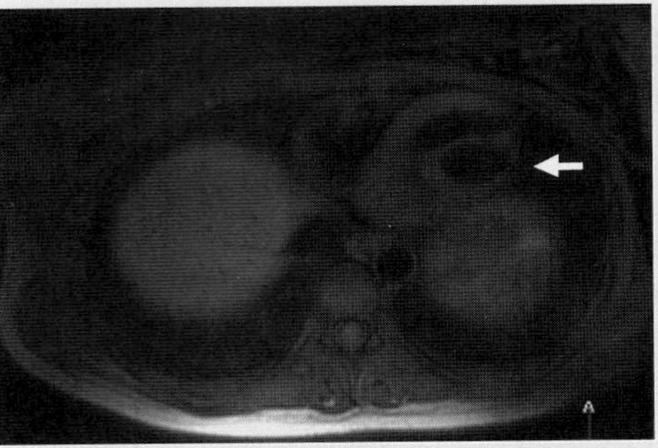

Corresponding fat saturated black blood (T2-weighted STIR) axial image.

Both echo and MRI demonstrate normal systolic function and no valvular abnormalities. No other lesions are noted on the cardiac MRI study. A CT scan of the chest, abdomen, and pelvis are otherwise normal. Given the signal characteristics on the above image, this lesion most likely represents:

a. Fibroma
b. Lipoma
c. Mxyoma
d. Thrombus
e. Papillary fibroelastoma

Answer is b: Lipoma. In the first and second images, an encapsulated mass is visible in the posterolateral wall of the left ventricle. In the third image, the mass has similar signal intensity as the nearby subcutaneous fat, suggesting a possible fatty nature. This is confirmed on the subsequent fat-saturated black blood axial image, in which a special pulse is given prior to acquisition of the image to suppress signal arising from fatty tissue. The mass now appears black due to loss of signal, as does the nearby subcutaneous fat, confirming the fatty nature of the mass.

The fatty content of the mass and the normal left ventricular systolic function are not consistent with a left ventricular thrombus. Papillary fibroelastomas do occur on the endocardium but most often (50%) occur on the aortic valve. They are not usually encapsulated and often demonstrate a "frondlike" appearance (similar to pompoms used by cheerleaders) and frequently have a stalk. Myxomas are most often located in the atria and are not characterized by this degree of fat content. Many myxomas have patchy, dark areas of low signal intensity on MRI because of calcification within the tumor.

# Aorta/Peripheral Vascular Disease

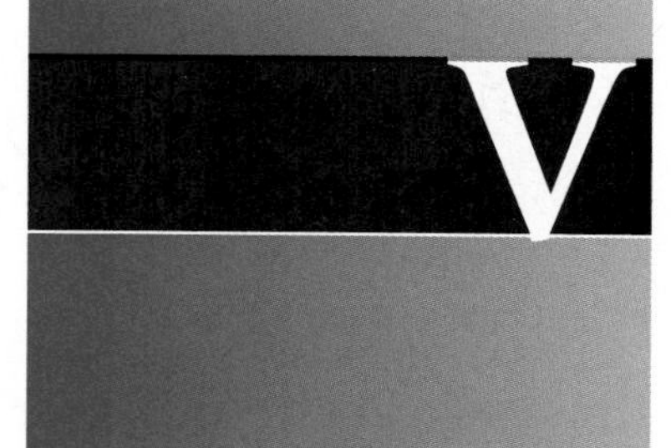

# Diseases of the Aorta

38

***Soufian Almahameed*** ***Gian M. Novaro***

Diseases of the aorta account for significant cardiovascular morbidity and mortality. The incidence of these diseases is expected to rise with the increasing age of the population. Diagnostic evaluation of aortic disorders has improved in the last decade, allowing for earlier diagnosis and therapeutic intervention. This review summarizes the major disease entities affecting the aorta.

## ANATOMY OF THE AORTA

The aorta is the main conduit of blood in the body. It is an elastic artery composed of three layers:

1. The intima, which includes the single-layered endothelium.
2. The media, which is the thickest layer of the aortic wall. It is composed of sheets of elastic tissue and collagen, which provide the aorta its tensile strength and distensibility. Smooth muscle cells and ground substance are also present. The components of the media are organized into functional units known as lamellae.
3. The adventitia, which is composed of loose connective tissue and contains the vasa vasorum, which provides the blood supply to the aortic wall. Elastin, collagen, and fibroblasts are also present.

Anatomically, the aorta is divided into two main subcomponents:

1. The thoracic aorta consists of the aortic root (from the aortic annulus, including the sinuses of Valsalva, up to the level just above the sinotubular junction); the ascending aorta (average diameter 3 cm); the arch; and the descending thoracic aorta (average diameter 2.5 cm—begins after the origin of the left subclavian artery).
2. The abdominal aorta, which is the part of the descending aorta after it passes through the diaphragm. The abdominal aorta (average diameter 2.0 cm) is further classified as either suprarenal or infrarenal.

## PATHOLOGIC PROCESSES

### Cystic Medial Degeneration

Cystic medial degeneration is an important predisposing factor to diseases of the aorta, particularly the ascending aorta. It is characterized by smooth muscle cell necrosis and apoptosis plus degeneration of elastic fibers within the media of the aortic wall. Cystic spaces form in these areas of degeneration. This degenerative process also extends to the elastic components of the adventitial layer. The weakened aortic wall is prone to aneurysm formation and dissection. This degenerative process, which may be determined genetically, is seen classically in connective tissue diseases such as Marfan syndrome and Ehlers–Danlos. However, various degrees of degeneration can be seen in patients without these disorders, occurring as an idiopathic variant, in familial syndromes, or as an acquired form. Hypertension and advancing age are associated with the latter. Varying degrees of cystic medial degeneration can also be seen in genetically predisposed aortas in association with congenital abnormalities including bicuspid or unicuspid aortic valve, aortic coarctation, Turner syndrome, and Noonan syndrome.

### Atherosclerosis

Atherosclerosis appears to play a significant role in diseases of the aortic arch, descending thoracic, and abdominal aorta. Atherosclerosis can result in weakening of the aortic wall, making it prone to aneurysm formation or dissection.

The development of aortic atherosclerosis is associated with the traditional cardiac risk factors of smoking, hypertension, hyperglycemia, and atherogenic lipoproteins. Atherosclerosis can also result in formation of complex atheromatous plaques, which are prone to embolization, resulting in cerebral and peripheral arterial events.

### Inflammatory Disorders

Inflammatory disorders represent a third broad category in the etiology of aortic diseases. These can occur in isolation, or in the context of systemic disorders.

### Trauma

Aortic injury from trauma usually occurs as a result of deceleration injuries. It frequently occurs at the level of the left subclavian artery. If the patient survives, injury can progress to form a chronic pseudo-aneurysm.

## AORTIC DISSECTION

Aortic dissection comprises one of the more ominous acute aortic syndromes (also known as acute thoracic pain syndromes), which include the dissection variants of penetrating aortic ulcers, intramural hematomas, and symptomatic aneurysms. It involves tearing of the aortic wall, resulting in the formation of an aortic false lumen, which courses along with a true lumen.

The hallmark of aortic dissection is an intimal tear, which permits access of pulsatile high-pressure blood into the aortic media, separating it from the basal layers (Fig. 38–1). Typically, the so-called intimal flap is usually an intimal-medial flap.

The initiating event of dissection may be a tear in the intima. Alternatively, primary rupture of the vasa vasorum may result in an intramural hematoma, which leads secondarily to an intimal tear as blood vents from the intramural space (Fig. 38–2). Regardless of the initiating event, the force of blood flow propagates the dissection antegrade (and less commonly retrograde) a variable extent along the vessel, cleaving the aortic wall usually along the outer one third of the medial layer.

### Classification

Dissections are classified by their location of origin and how far along they extend in the aorta. There are two important classification systems: the DeBakey system and the Stanford system (Table 38–1; Fig. 38–3). Dissections are also classified by their duration. Acute dissections are those of less than 2 weeks' duration after symptom onset; chronic are those that have been present for more than 2 weeks.

### Clinical Presentation

Dissections typically present between the fifth and seventh decades of life, with a male preponderance. Patients typically present with the acute onset of pain, present in 96% of cases. Pain is often most severe at its onset, and described as a "tearing," "ripping," or "stabbing" sensation. Often the pain is migratory, a crucial component of the history, reflecting propagation of the dissection. Involvement of the ascending aorta results in anterior chest or neck pain, with intra-/subscapular pain with involvement of the descending thoracic aorta, and lower back with left flank pain with the thoracoabdominal aorta.

Hypertension upon presentation is common, more so in distal dissection, although hypotension can be seen if complications have developed, particularly in proximal dissections. The dissection may compromise flow to the great vessels, and pulse deficits (these can be transient, as the dissection flap can oscillate) may be present. Actual blood pressure may not be appreciated if the arm utilized has compromise of the brachial vasculature (pseudohypotension).

If the dissection involves the aortic root, commissural involvement of the aortic valve can lead to aortic insufficiency. Dilatation of the root and aortic annulus, without

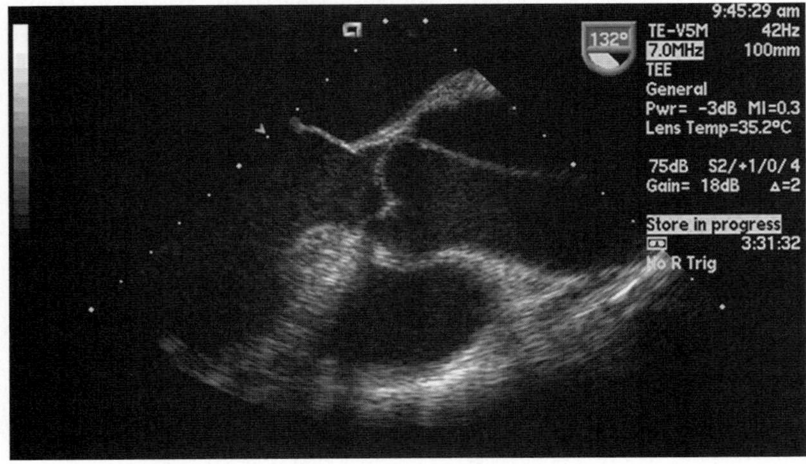


**Figure 38–1** Transesophageal echocardiography in a long-axis view that shows a large dissection flap in the ascending aorta extending from the level of the aortic sinuses.

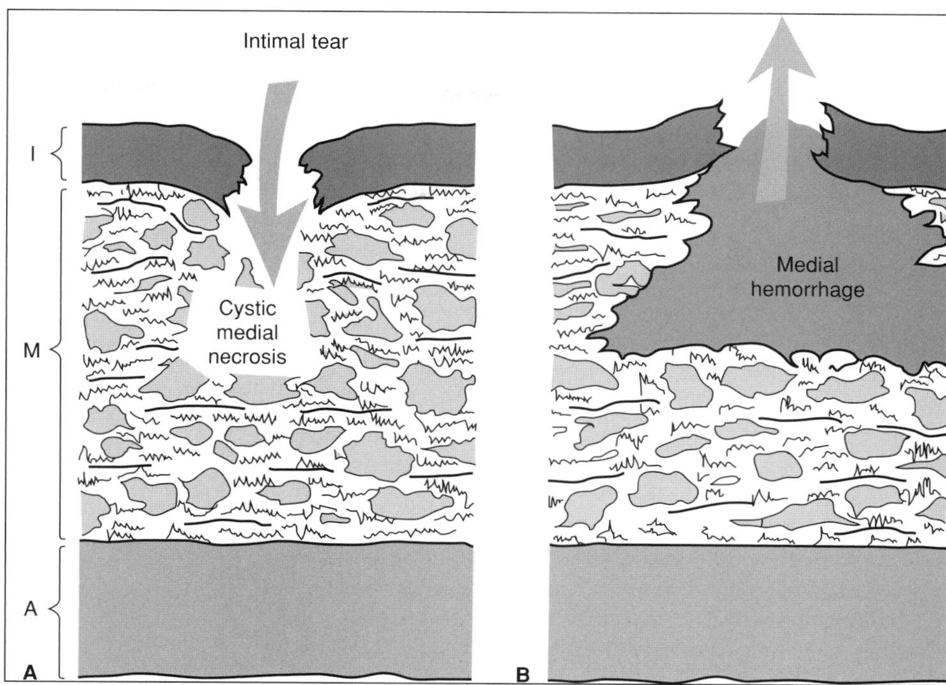


**Figure 38–2** Schematic representing the initiating event of aortic dissection. Panel **(A)** shows a tear in the intima. Panel **(B)** shows primary rupture of the vasa vasorum, secondarily leading to an intimal tear as blood vents from the intramural space.

leaflet involvement, can also lead to aortic valve insufficiency. A diastolic murmur will be evident in these cases.

Dissections can involve the ostia of the coronary arteries, resulting in acute myocardial ischemia and infarction (2% to 3% of cases). The right coronary artery ostium is more commonly affected than the left main. The dissection can extend proximally into the pericardial space, resulting in pericardial effusion and tamponade, a common mechanism of syncope and hypotension in dissection. A pericardial friction rub can be a clue to the presence of hemopericardium. Rupture in to the pericardial space represents the most common mode of death in patients with aortic dissection. Acute lower-extremity, renal, or mesenteric ischemia can be seen in descending aortic dissections. Focal neurologic deficits can occur with involvement of the great vessels. Compromise of spinal artery perfusion may result in paraparesis.

Although chest pain and pulse deficits are classically described, it is important to recognize that <20% of patients present with these findings. Therefore, a high clinical suspicion for dissection is paramount.

**TABLE 38–1**
**CLASSIFICATION OF AORTIC DISSECTIONS**

| Classification System | Extent of Aortic Involvement |
|---|---|
| DeBakey | |
| Type I | Originates in ascending aorta, propagates to involve the descending aorta |
| Type II | Confined to ascending aorta |
| Type IIIa | Confined to descending thoracic aorta |
| Type IIIb | Involves the descending aorta, extending to abdominal aorta |
| Stanford | |
| Type A | Involves the ascending aorta |
| Type B | Restricted to the descending aorta |

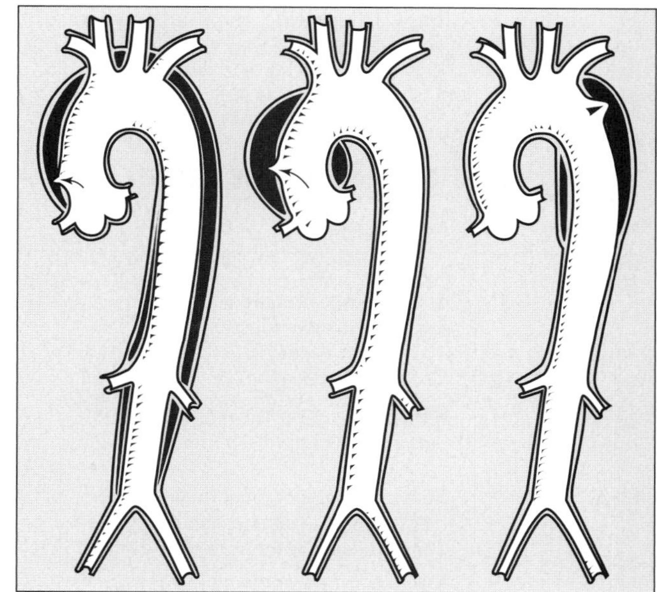

**Figure 38–3** Diagram showing the types of aortic dissection by the DeBakey classification. Shown are types I, II, and IIIa, from left to right.

## Diagnostic Testing

The chest x-ray can be normal in cases of dissection. A well-recognized finding is mediastinal widening, present in about 60% of cases. Rupture into the pleural or pericardial space manifests as pleural effusions or an enlarged cardiac silhouette (the latter may also be present, as a result of chronic aortic insufficiency). The electrocardiogram may be normal, but it often shows nonspecific ST–T-wave changes. Involvement of the coronary artery ostia may result in ST-segment elevation, representing an acute myocardial injury pattern. Transthoracic echocardiography can on occasion identify a proximal or even distal dissection flap. Even if a flap is not seen, the presence of aortic dilatation, aortic insufficiency, and/or an unexplained pericardial effusion can be important clues in the diagnostic consideration of a patient with chest pain.

More definitive diagnostic modalities include transesophageal echocardiography (TEE), computed tomography (CT), and magnetic resonance angiography (MRA). Each has relative advantages and disadvantages, but all have excellent sensitivity and specificity (Table 38–2).

Angiography is less commonly utilized for the primary diagnosis of aortic dissection. The choice of test is often dependent on expedited availability and expertise at the center where the patient is evaluated. An important caveat is that in most patients, more than one test may be required. If the clinical suspicion is high enough and the initial test is negative or equivocal, then consideration should be given to performing another confirmatory test.

## Management

Anti-impulse medical therapy should be initiated as soon as the diagnosis of dissection is considered, even while awaiting confirmatory diagnostic testing. In patients who are hypertensive, intravenous beta-blockade and sodium nitroprusside are the treatment agents of choice. Beta-blockade should be initiated prior to sodium nitroprusside to avoid a rise in cardiac contractility and *dp*/*dt* associated with the isolated use of vasodilators. In the absence of hypertension, beta-blockers can be used alone. For patients with ascending aortic dissections, these are temporizing agents while preparing for definitive surgical therapy. For patients with descending dissections, these agents are first-line therapy, before longer-acting oral agents are initiated. Intravenous nondihydropyridine calcium antagonists such as verapamil and diltiazem are alternatives for those who cannot tolerate beta-blockers.

Dissections that involve the ascending aorta (proximal, type A) require urgent surgical therapy, as there is a very high early mortality rate (approaching 1% to 2% per hour for the first 24 to 48 hours).

An important management point arises with patients who have pericardial effusion or tamponade in association with a proximal dissection. These patients should not undergo percutaneous pericardiocentesis, unless they are in absolute extremis. The evacuation of pericardial blood by such a route has been associated with aortic rupture and increased mortality, perhaps secondary to dissection extension and/or aortic rupture as blood pressure and *dp*/*dt* increase after tamponade resolution. Pericardial access should be obtained in the operating room, with the institution of cardiopulmonary bypass.

Dissections that involve the descending aorta (distal, type B) should be initially treated medically. Data suggest that medical therapy is the preferred initial treatment, with surgery guided by a complication-specific approach. This is because acute aortic surgery is associated with a high mortality and paraplegia rate (inadequate protection of the spinal arteries). Surgery should be considered for

**TABLE 38–2**
**COMPARISON OF IMAGING MODALITIES FOR AORTIC DISSECTION**

| Modality | Advantages | Disadvantages |
|---|---|---|
| TEE | Portability<br>Assess valvular function<br>Assess ventricular function<br>No contrast agent | "Blind spot": ascending aorta at level bronchi crosses esophagus<br>Difficulty in assessing the great vessels<br>Difficulty in diagnosing intramural hematoma<br>Invasive procedure |
| Spiral CT | Assess great vessels and branch vessels | Lack of valvular and ventricular function assessment<br>Lack of portability<br>IV contrast agent required |
| MRA | Detailed resolution of aorta (i.e., intramural hematoma) in addition to assessing branch vessels<br>Contrast agent without nephrotoxicity | Lack of portability<br>Access to scanners<br>Cost |
| Angiography | Assess coronary anatomy (controversial whether this should be done prior to surgery for dissection) | Invasive<br>Risk and difficulty in accessing true lumen<br>Contrast agent required |

TEE, transesophageal echocardiography; CT, computed tomography; MRA, magnetic resonance angiography.

the following indications: evidence of organ ischemia secondary to compromise of the branch vessels; persistent pain; aneurysm formation particularly if saccular; and retrograde dissection to a proximal extent. Alternatively, aortic fenestration, surgical or percutaneous, can also be considered for organ or limb malperfusion in carefully selected patients.

Distal (type B) dissections in Marfan syndrome patients carry a poor prognosis and have thus led to recommendations of early aortic surgery.

### Aortic Dissection in the Young

Dissections occurring in younger patients (<40 years old) typically occur in the context of connective tissue disorders such as Marfan syndrome, congenital bicuspid aortic valve, patients with prior aortic surgery, or women in the peripartum period. During late pregnancy, it is thought that hormonal changes and a loosening in the ground substance of connective tissue can lead to a heightened risk of dissection.

### Chronic Aortic Dissection

Chronic dissection patients (present for >2 weeks) have survived the period of increased mortality. They can often be managed medically, even in the presence of a proximal dissection. However, their aortas often dilate and are at higher risk for aneurysm formation because of the thinned aortic wall as a result of dissection.

A complication-specific approach can be used for chronic dissection patients to guide elective surgical therapy: recurrent pain; aneurysm formation, particularly if saccular; and retrograde dissection extension to a proximal extent. Serial follow-up imaging (usually with CT or MRA), initially at shorter intervals, is vital in these patients because of their weakened aortic walls.

### Iatrogenic Aortic Dissection

Special mention should be afforded to iatrogenic dissections. Angiographic catheters and guidewires can disrupt the intima and result in dissections anywhere along the aorta's course. These typically result in retrograde dissections, and the false lumens generally thrombose spontaneously. They can often be managed medically unless the dissection is extensive (Fig. 38–4).

Dissections can also occur during aortic cross clamping or cannulation during cardiac surgery. Such dissections are usually diagnosed and treated urgently and successfully at the time of surgery.

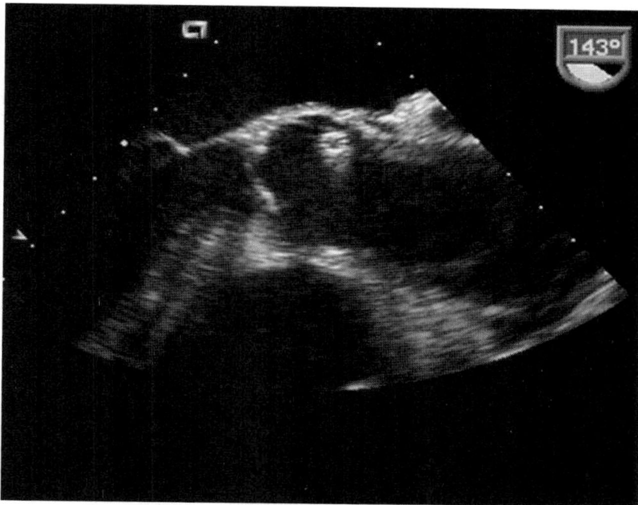


**Figure 38–4** Transesophageal echocardiography in a long-axis view demonstrating a case of iatrogenic dissection. A bare metal stent is entrapped in the left main trunk and has caused a retrograde dissection to the aortic sinuses with antegrade propagation distally to the descending thoracic aorta (not shown).

## INTRAMURAL HEMATOMA AND PENETRATING AORTIC ULCER

Intramural hematoma and penetrating aortic ulcer are two aortic dissection variants that vary from classic dissection by the absence of an intimal flap. Recent advances in diagnostic imaging modalities have led to an increased awareness and better understanding of these entities.

### Intramural Hematoma

Intramural hematoma consists of a noncommunicating blood collection in the aortic wall. Unlike a true dissection, there is no loss of intimal continuity, no entry tear, and thus no intimal flap. The pathophysiology may be related to rupture of the aortic vasa vasorum.

By transesophageal echocardiography, intramural hematoma is characterized by absence of a dissection flap, a regional crescent-shaped thickening of the aortic wall usually >0.7 cm, and central displacement of intimal calcium (Fig. 38–5). At times, intramural echolucencies representing noncommunicating pockets of fresh blood can be seen. Distinguishing intramural hematoma from severe atheroma, a thrombosed false lumen, or aneurysm with mural thrombus can be difficult. Angiography is of limited diagnostic accuracy in the evaluation of hematomas, as it fails to image the aortic wall. If the clinical history is concerning, a negative TEE should not represent the final diagnostic evaluation. CT and MRA represent highly accurate imaging modalities that are frequently used as an initial or complementary study in the evaluation of hematomas.

Intramural hematomas can communicate with the adventitial space, lead to rupture, or progress to overt dissection with an intimal tear. However they may also have a more benign course, and gradually resolve with medical therapy and blood pressure control.

### Penetrating Aortic Ulcer

Penetrating aortic ulcer exists when an atheromatous plaque erodes inward into the aortic media. The advanced

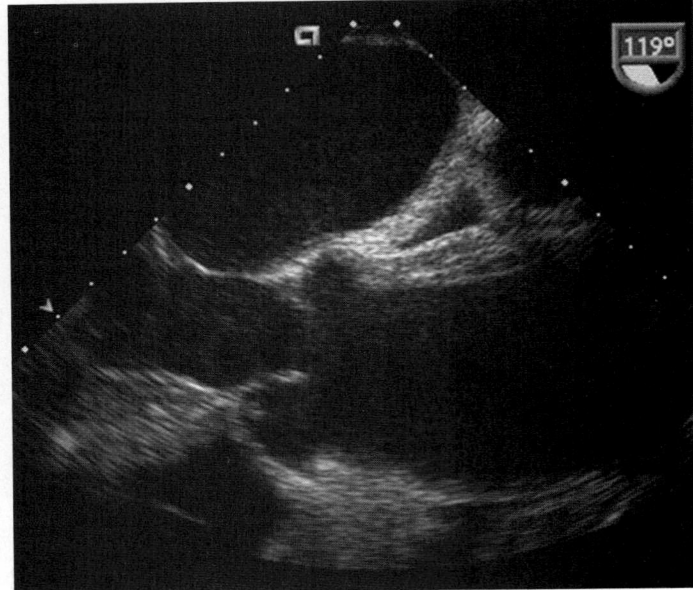

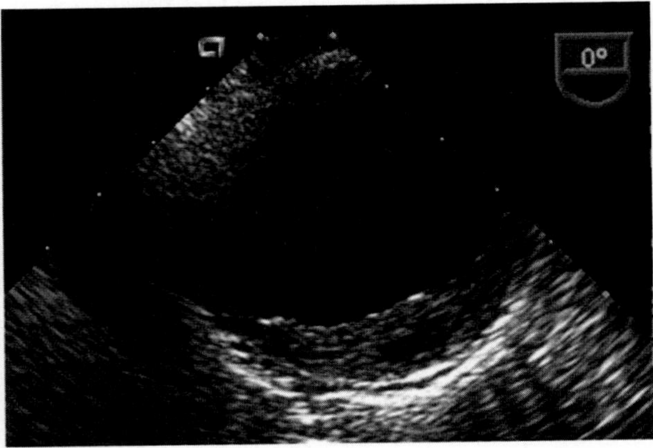

**Figure 38–5** Transesophageal echocardiography in both long- and short-axis views showing an intramural hematoma, characterized by no dissection flap, a crescent-shaped thickening of the aortic wall, central displacement of intimal calcium, and echolucent intramural pockets representing intramural blood.

atherosclerotic disease prevents the erosion from extending longitudinally along the vessel as in classic dissection. The ulcer is apparent on imaging modalities as an ulcer crater or contrast-filled outpouching. Depending on how far into the aortic wall the plaque erosion occurs, there may be formation of an intramural hematoma, saccular aneurysm, pseudo-aneurysm, or even complete aortic rupture (Fig. 38–6).

## Clinical Presentation

Patients with these acute aortic syndromes often present with the same chest and/or back pain as do patients with classic dissection. They may be associated with a higher incidence of rupture than seen for classic dissections. Compared to intramural hematomas, patients with penetrating ulcers are usually older and tend to have more atherosclerotic burden. Isolated intramural hematomas tend to occur more often in the ascending aorta, whereas intramural hematomas associated with penetrating aortic ulcers are more commonly located in the descending aorta, where atherosclerosis is more common.

## Management

As in aortic dissection, anti-impulse medical therapy should be initiated as soon as the diagnosis of a dissection variant is considered. Intravenous beta-blockade and, if needed for blood pressure control, sodium nitroprusside are the treatment agents of choice.

For the dissection variants involving the ascending aorta, prompt surgical intervention is considered the

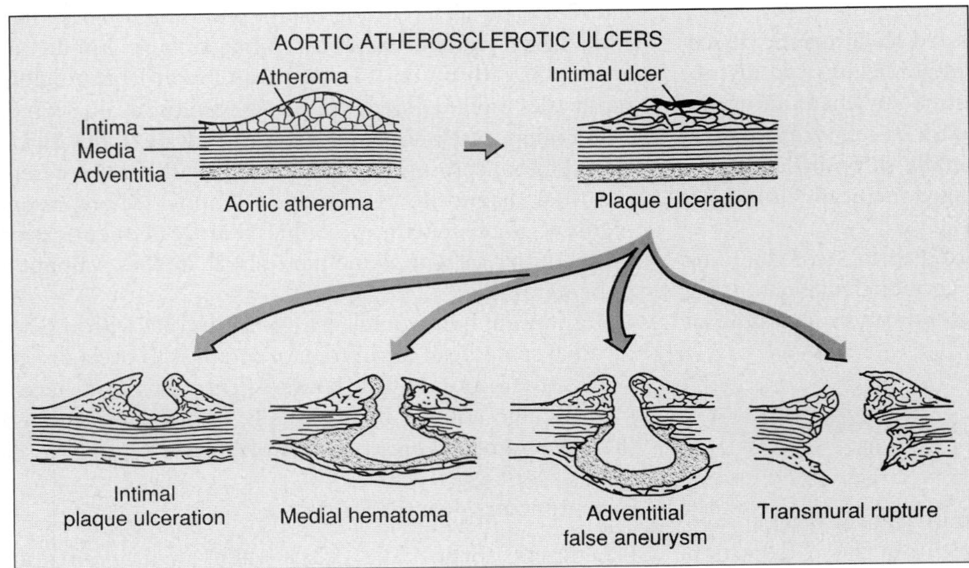


**Figure 38–6** Schematic of a penetrating aortic ulcer and the progression to the various aortic wall complications.

treatment of choice. However, some data suggest that select patients with intramural hematomas in the ascending aorta can be managed medically. Recent data suggest that penetrating ulcerlike findings in an area of intramural hematoma can identify high-risk individuals. Symptoms of sustained or recurrent pain or findings of an increasing pleural effusion are suggestive of disease progression and favor surgical intervention. Guidelines and management strategies for this patient population are still evolving.

For the dissection variants that involve the descending aorta, especially intramural hematomas without penetrating ulcers, medical therapy is the preferred initial treatment. However, some have argued that there should be a lower threshold for surgical intervention than for classic distal dissection, particularly when clinical signs of instability are present. The presence of a severely bulging hematoma or a deeply penetrating ulcer may warrant surgical repair. The development of a saccular aneurysm or pseudo-aneurysm should merit consideration for surgical repair. For those treated medically, serial imaging studies are warranted to assess for progression or increase in aortic diameter, in which case surgical repair or stent-graft placement may be considered.

## AORTIC ANEURYSM

An aortic aneurysm is present when there is dilatation of the aorta, typically at least 1.5 times its normal reference dimension for an adjacent segment. This dilatation may involve the entire circumference of the aortic wall (fusiform) or a localized protrusion of one of the walls (saccular). Ectasia is characterized by dilatation <1.5 times the normal reference dimension.

### Thoracic Aortic Aneurysm

The incidence of thoracic aortic aneurysm (TAA) is estimated at 5.9 cases per 100,000 patient years. Leading etiologies include congenital bicuspid aortic valve; Marfan syndrome (Fig. 38–7); idiopathic annuloaortic ectasia; familial thoracic aortic aneurysm syndrome; inflammatory aortitis; acquired due to increased age and hypertension; syphilis; and trauma.

Descending TAA may extend distally and involve the abdominal aorta creating a thoracoabdominal aneurysm. Patients are often asymptomatic at time of presentation, and the TAA may be diagnosed by an imaging modality ordered for other clinical indications. Physical findings may likewise be absent. When signs and symptoms do manifest, they are often the result of mass effect. The enlarging aorta may compress nearby structures such as the superior vena cava, the trachea, esophagus, and recurrent laryngeal nerve. This may result in superior vena cava syndrome, stridor, dysphagia, and hoarseness, respectively.

Progressive dilatation of the aortic root can lead to aortic insufficiency, which can produce symptoms of congestive

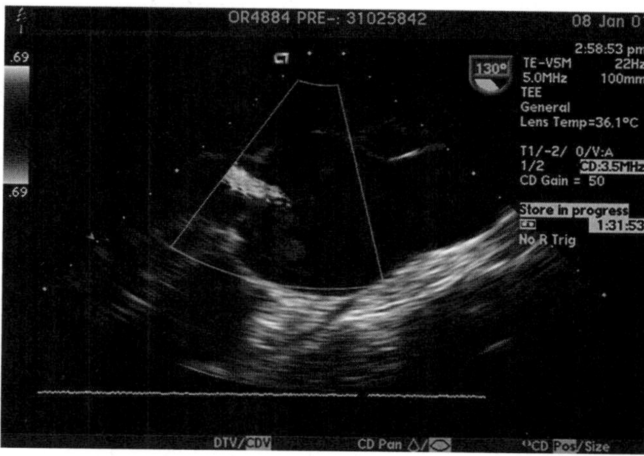


**Figure 38–7** Transesophageal echocardiography in a long-axis view illustrating an ascending thoracic aortic aneurysm, with predominant dilatation at the level of the sinuses, in a patient with Marfan syndrome.

heart failure. Enlargement of the aortic sinuses can lead to narrowing of the coronary artery ostia, which can lead to myocardial ischemia and even infarction.

Blood flow can be static in large aneurysms, predisposing to thrombus formation and distal embolization.

#### *Noninvasive Imaging*

- TAA are often noted incidentally on chest x-ray as mediastinal widening or a prominent aortic knob.
- Transthoracic echocardiography is the most common modality to initially diagnose and monitor dilatation of the aortic root.
- CT scanning and MRA are the preferred techniques to accurately define the entire thoracic aorta and its branch vessels, and precisely measure TAA.

Because the thoracic aorta may be tortuous, care must be given to not measure off-axis axial cuts, as these can overestimate the true cross section as compared to the actual orthogonal diameter.

#### *Medical Treatment*

There are data that beta-adrenergic blockade can slow the rate of thoracic aneurysm expansion in patients with Marfan syndrome, resulting in improved survival. Although the data are extrapolated to those without Marfan syndrome, it seems reasonable to recommend such therapy while TAA patients are being followed medically.

Recognizing that patients treated with beta-adrenergic blockade can still manifest aortic dilatation is important, as serial evaluation and imaging is required.

#### *Marfan Syndrome, Thoracic Aortic Aneurysms, and Pregnancy*

- Women with Marfan syndrome have an increased risk of aortic dissection during pregnancy, particularly during the third trimester.

- The risk of dissection greatly increases if the aortic root diameter is >4.0 cm or if there is evidence of rapid aortic root dilatation during pregnancy.
- If elective surgical repair is not performed prepartum, beta-adrenergic blockade should be used during pregnancy.
- Close echocardiographic follow-up and Caesarean delivery should be considered if the aortic root size exceeds 4.0 cm or rapid aortic dilatation is evident.

### Indications for Surgical Treatment

Dissection and rupture are the feared complications of TAA, and prevention of these conditions is the purpose for elective surgical aortic repair. Size is clearly a risk factor for dissection and rupture. In one series, the annual rate of dissection or rupture was 2% for TAAs <5 cm, 3% for TAAs between 5.0 and 5.9 cm, and 7% for TAAs >6 cm. Therefore, prophylactic surgical intervention should be considered before a TAA reaches a size that predisposes to aortic instability.

Although the optimal timing of prophylactic surgery remains uncertain, recommendations for surgical repair are 5.5 to 6.0 cm for an ascending TAA and 6.0 to 6.5 cm for a descending TAA. Patients with Marfan syndrome, bicuspid aortic valve, or family history of premature aortic instability should be considered for earlier repair (perhaps at 5.0 cm and 5.5 to 6.0 cm for ascending and descending TAAs, respectively).

Rapid enlargement of the aorta (>0.5 to 1.0 cm/year) or symptom development has also been advocated as indications for surgery. The decision for operative repair must of course take into account the patient's medical comorbidities, and a risk/benefit ratio must be individualized for each patient. Patients who are otherwise low medical risk may be considered for intervention at smaller aortic sizes.

## Abdominal Aortic Aneurysm

- The incidence of abdominal aortic aneurysm (AAA) is estimated at 36.5 per 100,000 person years.
- AAA represents the most common form of arterial aneurysm.
- The majority of AAAs are infrarenal in location (75%).
- Atherosclerosis is the dominant risk factor in the development of an AAA. Additional risk factors associated with AAAs are male gender (AAA is 4 to 5 times more common in men), increasing age, smoking, and hypertension.
- There is a clear familial predisposition to AAA, with relatives of affected patients having a 30% increased risk for the development of an AAA.

Asymptomatic AAA is often diagnosed on physical examination by abdominal palpation. The most common symptom is pain, and is usually steady. The pain may be localized abdominal pain, or may radiate to the back, flank, or groin. Sudden onset of severe abdominal and back pain suggests rupture, representing a surgical emergency. Up to only a third of patients with rupture will present with the classic triad of pain, pulsatile abdominal mass, and hypotension. Atheroemboli may be the first manifestation of an AAA.

### Noninvasive Imaging

Ultrasonography, CT scanning, aortography, and MRA have all been used in the initial diagnosis, sizing, and monitoring of AAA. Ultrasonography represents the most practical method of screening and serial monitoring, while CT scanning and MRA remain superior in accurately detailing the morphology and extent of the AAA.

At initial diagnosis, the rate of dilatation cannot be determined and thus the next serial study should be performed in 6 months. In general, for AAAs <4.0 cm, yearly surveillance imaging is recommended; for AAAs 4.0 to 5.0 cm, imaging every 6 to 12 months; and for AAAs >5.0 cm, imaging every 3 to 6 months.

Baseline AAA size is the best predictor of rate of dilatation. Larger aneurysms expand at higher rates than smaller ones.

### Medical Treatment

Beta-adrenergic blockade with careful control of hypertension appears to have impact on delaying the rate of AAA expansion.

Smoking should be discontinued, as rupture risk is greater among active smokers.

### Indications for Surgical Treatment

Mortality from an AAA is primarily related to rupture. As with thoracic aneurysms, increasing size is the harbinger of rupture risk. Aneurysms <4 cm in size have a 0 to 2% risk of rupture over 2 years, whereas those that are >5 cm in size have a 22% risk of rupture over 2 years, with those >6 cm showing the sharpest rise in risk. As such, an aortic diameter of 5.0 to 5.5 cm is recommended as an indication for prophylactic surgery in asymptomatic AAA patients. Although AAAs are less common in women, when they are present they are at greater risk of rupture and at smaller aortic diameters than in men. Thus, it is recommended that women undergo prophylactic AAA repair at 4.5 to 5.0 cm.

Aneurysms that expand rapidly (>0.5 to 1.0 cm/year) are also associated with an increased risk of rupture, and are thus considered for elective surgical repair.

Inflammatory AAA is present in up to 10% of cases. There appears to be a familial tendency for these, and they often occur in the context of smoking. Patients will present with constitutional symptoms and have an elevated sedimentation rate in addition to the classic symptoms of pain. CT scanning or MRA can identify the inflammatory component. Treatment is aortic surgery.

### *Endovascular Stent-Graft Repair*

A relatively recent therapeutic option for AAA repair is the percutaneous placement of an endovascular stent-graft. The endovascular stent-graft is placed within the aneurysmal segment of the aorta, bridging the normal segments and excluding the aneurysm. However, just over half of all AAA possess anatomy favorable for stent-graft placement.

Data are still forthcoming on the long-term success of endovascular stent-grafting. Nonetheless, the procedure remains an attractive alternative to conventional surgical repair, but is usually limited to patients with significant comorbid medical conditions who are at high surgical risk.

## ATHEROMATOUS AORTIC DISEASE

- Atherosclerotic plaques in the aorta can give rise to cerebral and peripheral embolic events (Fig. 38–8).
- TEE, in particular, has been a valuable imaging modality in assessing the presence and extent of these plaques.
- Plaques >4 mm in thickness, or those with mobile components, appear to be strongly associated with subsequent embolic events.

Treatment strategies for patients with such plaques have not been evaluated in sufficient numbers in a prospective randomized fashion. However, there is the suggestion that lipid-lowering therapy and anticoagulation with warfarin may benefit some patients.

Earlier reports of a potential association between warfarin and the cholesterol embolization syndrome have produced some reluctance to use such anticoagulant therapy in these patients, and further study is thus needed. The potential role of aortic replacement or removal of atheroma remains to be defined.

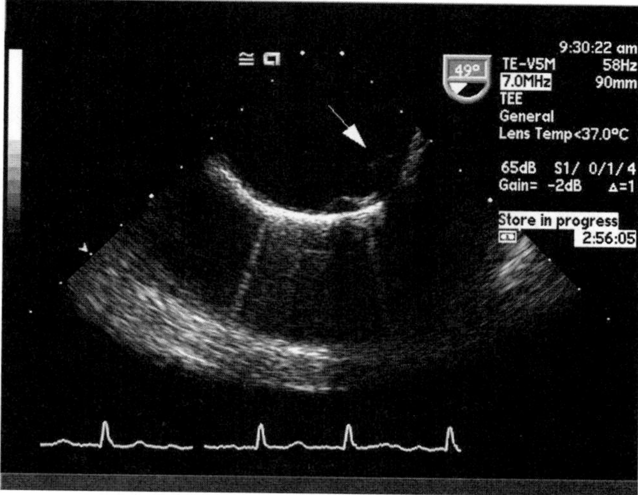


**Figure 38–8** Transesophageal echocardiography in a short-axis view identifying a protruding thick (>4-mm) atheroma in the descending thoracic aorta.

It has become increasingly common for cardiac surgeons to assess the aorta before the institution of cardiopulmonary bypass. The presence of significant plaque may alter the cross-clamp site or may even lead to endarterectomy or aortic replacement at the time of surgery.

### Cholesterol Embolization Syndrome

The cholesterol embolization syndrome can be seen in patients undergoing diagnostic angiography, but can also occur spontaneously. There is a reported association between warfarin anticoagulation and these events.

The syndrome represents a showering of emboli, typically from the descending aorta. Patients most often present with the skin findings of livedo reticularis and blue toes, in the presence of palpable pulses. Renal insufficiency may occur, and may not be reversible. Transient eosinophilia is often present, and treatment is supportive.

If the atheroma arose from an AAA, then surgical intervention can help prevent future events.

## INFLAMMATORY AORTITIS

### Giant-Cell Arteritis

Giant-cell arteritis is an inflammatory disease that affects the temporal arteries, producing local tenderness and headaches. Patients affected are typically over the age of 55 years, and women are affected twice as frequently as men.

The most devastating consequence is blindness. Although temporal arteritis is the hallmark of this disorder, there may be involvement of the thoracic aorta and the great vessels. This can lead to branch vessel occlusion, aneurysm formation, or even dissection.

Corticosteroid treatment is the mainstay of therapy. With the development of advanced aortic involvement, surgical treatment may be required.

### Takayasu Arteritis

Takayasu arteritis is an inflammatory disorder of the aorta that typically affects women under age 40 years. Its prevalence is greater in Asian and African populations than in those of European or North American descent.

A subacute inflammatory illness phase is manifested by constitutional symptoms. Later, there is occlusive inflammation of the aorta and branch vessels, with segmental narrowing apparent. Symptoms of arterial insufficiency will be present, depending on the vessels involved. Acquired coarctation can occur, leading to hypertension, as can aneurysm formation.

Treatment is corticosteroids. For occlusive lesions that do not respond to steroids, surgical bypass is warranted.

### Syphilitic Aortitis

Syphilitic aortitis represents a manifestation of tertiary syphilis, which may occur 10 to 30 years after the initial infection. This inflammation results in a weakening of the vessel wall and can lead to aneurysm formation, usually saccular.

Syphilitic aortitis most commonly affects the ascending aorta, and hence can result in aortic insufficiency. The arch may also be affected. Involvement of the descending aorta occurs less often.

### Other Inflammatory Aortitis

Aortitis can also be seen in other systemic inflammatory diseases, such as reactive arthritis, ankylosing spondylitis, rheumatoid arthritis, Wegener granulomatosis, and enteropathic arthropathies.

A common genetic underpinning of these conditions is the HLA-B27 genotype, which should be considered in cases of lone aortic regurgitation, ascending aortic dilatation, and conduction system disease.

Treatment involves addressing the underlying disorder, with surgery as needed for aneurysmal or aortic valvular complications.

### Mycotic Aneurysms

Bacteremia (from endocarditis, trauma, intravenous drug abuse) can result in infection within the weakened aneurysmal arterial wall. Persistent fevers after treatment of the inciting event should raise concern for an infected aneurysm.

Mycotic aneurysms more commonly involve the abdominal aorta. Atheromatous plaques can also become infected (bacterial aortitis), serving as a nidus for infection requiring prolonged antibiotic therapy.

## ESSENTIAL FACTS

### Aortic Dissection

- The hallmark of aortic dissection is an intimal flap.
- Increasing aortic size and aneurysm formation is a harbinger of aortic dissection.
- Proximal (ascending) aortic dissections are treated with surgery.
- In cases of cardiac tamponade, evacuation of hematoma should be performed in the operating room under cardiopulmonary bypass support.
- Distal (descending) aortic dissections are treated medically, with surgery guided by a complication-specific approach.
- Congenital bicuspid aortic valve, Marfan syndrome, prior aortic surgery, and the peripartum period represent risk factors for aortic dissection in the young.
- A negative surface echocardiogram, absence of pulse deficits, or a normal mediastinum on chest x-ray does not exclude the presence of aortic dissection.
- Anti-impulse medical therapy with intravenous beta-blockade followed by sodium nitroprusside is the mainstay of medical treatment.

### Intramural Hematoma and Penetrating Aortic Ulcer

- Penetrating aortic ulcers arise more commonly in areas of atheromatous disease such as the thoracoabdominal aorta.
- Penetrating aortic ulcers that involve the ascending aorta are treated surgically.
- Intramural hematomas that involve the ascending aorta are generally treated surgically, although recent publications have raised some controversy and suggest that medical management may be an option.
- Neither of the aortic dissection variants involves an intimal dissection flap.

### Aortic Aneurysm

- Indications for surgery:

  Symptoms
  Inflammatory or infectious
  Rapidly expanding 0.5 to 1.0 cm/year, even if asymptomatic
  >5.5 to 6.0 cm diameter for ascending thoracic
  >6.0 to 6.5 cm diameter for descending thoracic
  >5.0 to 5.5 cm diameter for abdominal

- Earlier surgical intervention is recommended in Marfan syndrome and congenital bicuspid aortic valve patients.
- Beta-adrenergic blockade may slow the progression of aortic dilatation.

### Atheromatous Aortic Disease

- Mobile and thick atheromatous plaques (>4 mm) identified by TEE are associated with embolic events.

## BIBLIOGRAPHY

**Coady MA, Rizzo JA, Elefteriades JA.** Developing surgical intervention criteria for thoracic aortic aneurysms. *Cardiol Clin.* 1999;17:827–839.

**Coady MA, Rizzo JA, Elefteriades JA.** Pathologic variants of thoracic aortic dissections. Penetrating atherosclerotic ulcers and intramural hematomas. *Cardiol Clin.* 1999;17:637–657.

**Coady MA, Rizzo JA, Goldstein LJ, Elefteriades JA.** Natural history, pathogenesis, and etiology of thoracic aortic aneurysms and dissections. *Cardiol Clin.* 1999;17:615–635.

**Daily PO, Trueblood HW, Stinson EB, et al.** Management of acute aortic dissections. *Ann Thorac Surg.* 1970;10:237–247.

**Hagan PG, Nienaber CA, Isselbacher EM, et al.** The International Registry of Acute Aortic Dissection (IRAD): new insights into an old disease. *JAMA.* 2000;283:897–903.

**Isselbacher EM.** Thoracic and abdominal aortic aneurysms. *Circulation.* 2005;111:816–828.
**Isselbacher EM, Eagle KA, DeSanctis RW.** Diseases of the aorta. In: Braunwald E, ed. *Heart Disease; A Textbook of Cardiovascular Medicine.* 5th ed. Philadelphia: WB Saunders; 1997:1546–1581.
**James KB, Healy BP.** Heart disease arising during or secondary to pregnancy. *Cardiovasc Clin.* 1989;19:81–96.
**Johnston KW, Rutherford RB, Tilson MD, et al.** Suggested standards for reporting on arterial aneurysms. *J Vasc Surg.* 1991;13:452–458.
**Milewicz DM, Dietz HC, Miller DC.** Treatment of aortic disease in patients with Marfan syndrome. *Circulation.* 2005;111:150–157.
**Pyertiz RE, McKusick VA.** The Marfan syndrome: diagnosis and management. *N Engl J Med.* 1979;300:772–777.
**Schoen FJ, Cotran RS.** Blood vessels. In: Kumar V, Collins T, Robbins S, Cotran RS, eds. *Robbins Pathologic Basis of Disease.* 6th ed. Philadelphia: WB Saunders; 1999:493–554.
**Spittell PC.** Diseases of the aorta. In: Topol EJ, ed. *Comprehensive Cardiovascular Medicine.* Philadelphia: Lippincott-Raven; 1998:3031–3051.

## QUESTIONS

1. A 70-year-old man presents with the sudden onset of tearing chest pain. On presentation, he has a heart rate of 130 beats/min with a systolic blood pressure of 80 mm Hg. A bedside TEE demonstrates the presence of a proximal aortic dissection. A pericardial effusion with partial diastolic collapse of the right ventricle is also present. Significant respiratory variation is noted across mitral and tricuspid Doppler inflows. Appropriate treatment is
   a. Immediate percutaneous pericardiocentesis to relieve the tamponade, followed by surgery to replace the ascending aorta
   b. to proceed immediately to the operating room
   c. Emergency angiography to define coronary anatomy, followed by surgery
   d. Intra-aortic balloon pump to stabilize the hemodynamics, followed by surgery

Answer is b: This patient should be taken to the operating room immediately. Percutaneous drainage has been associated with increased mortality in this setting. Given the hemodynamic status, there is no time to proceed with angiography first. Balloon pumps are contraindicated with aortic dissection.

2. A 60-year-old hypertensive man presents with tearing back pain. MRI confirms the presence of a descending thoracic dissection originating beyond the left subclavian artery. Appropriate initial treatment includes:
   a. Immediate surgery to replace the descending aorta
   b. Intravenous nitroprusside followed by immediate surgery
   c. Intravenous nitroprusside alone; surgery for persistent pain, or for involvement of renal or mesenteric arteries
   d. Intravenous beta-blockade and nitroprusside; surgery for persistent pain, or for involvement of renal or mesenteric arteries

Answer is d: Initial therapy for descending aortic dissection is medical, with surgery reserved for special circumstances. The goal of treatment is reduction in blood pressure, as well as reduction in *dp*/*dt*. Both beta-blockade, started immediately, and nitroprusside should be used.

3. A 56-year-old man presents for screening physical examination. He is asymptomatic. Vital signs reveal a heart rate of 80 beats/min with a blood pressure of 160/90 mm Hg. His exam is remarkable only for a pulsatile mass in the abdomen. Ultrasound reveals the presence of a 3.9-cm AAA. Appropriate management includes:
   a. Immediate referral for surgery
   b. Start a beta-blocker and repeat ultrasound in 6 months
   c. Refer for stenting of the AAA

Answer is b: Asymptomatic aneurysms of 3.9 cm have a very small risk of rupture. The patient should be followed by serial examination to assess size and rate of expansion. Control of his hypertension with beta-blockers may delay the growth of the aneurysm. There are no data as of yet that endovascular stent-grafts will lower the threshold for intervention for these aneurysms.

4. A 76-year-old woman with hypertension presents with severe chest pain. Her blood pressure is 200/110 mm Hg. Electrocardiogram reveals nonspecific ST–T changes. Chest x-ray is unremarkable. CT scan demonstrates the presence of a penetrating ulcer in the ascending aorta. No dissection flap is seen. Appropriate management includes:
   a. Start intravenous beta-blocker and nitroprusside while plans are being made for surgery
   b. Intravenous beta-blocker and nitroprusside, with surgery only if complications develop
   c. Intravenous nitroprusside alone, with surgery only if complications develop

Answer is a: Penetrating aortic ulcers involving the ascending aorta are generally treated like dissections, with prompt referral for surgery.

5. A 23-year-old patient with Marfan syndrome presents for routine evaluation. He is

asymptomatic. Work-up includes a CT scan, which reveals the presence of a 4.2-cm ascending aorta. Appropriate management includes:

a. Refer for surgery
b. Start on beta-blocker and re-image in 6 to 12 months
c. Re-image in 6 to 12 months

Answer is b: The patient's aorta has not yet reached a size that would be considered for surgery in the absence of symptoms. There are data that beta-blockers can slow the rate of expansion of these aneurysms and improve survival.

**6.** The same patient returns for follow-up in 12 months. The aorta now measures 5.0 cm in size. He remains asymptomatic. Appropriate management includes:

a. Refer for surgery
b. Continue beta-blocker, reassess in 6 months
c. Reassess in 3 months

Answer is a: There has been rapid growth in the size of the aneurysm (0.8 cm in 1 year). The patient should be referred for surgery.

**7.** Which of the following disorders is associated with involvement of the aorta?

a. Marfan syndrome
b. Giant-cell arteritis
c. Ankylosing spondylitis
d. Syphilis
e. All of the above can have aortic involvement.

Answer is e: All of the above can include involvement of the aorta.

**8.** Which of the following statements regarding transesophageal findings of aortic atheroma is *not* true?

a. Plaques >2 mm in the ascending aorta are associated with increased risk of stroke.
b. Plaques >4 mm in the ascending aorta are associated with increased risk of stroke.
c. Mobile components are associated with an increased risk of stroke.
d. Limited data suggest that these patients may benefit from anticoagulation therapy with warfarin.

Answer is a: Plaques >4 mm have been associated with cerebral embolic events. The role of anticoagulation needs to be more clearly defined, but there are some data to support its use.

# Venous Thromboembolism

# 39

***Raghu Kolluri John R. Bartholomew***

Venous thromboembolism (VTE) is a common disease that includes both pulmonary embolism (PE) and deep vein thrombosis (DVT). It is the third most frequently occurring cardiovascular condition after ischemic heart disease and cerebrovascular accidents in the United States. Approximately 2 million people develop DVT and 600,000 develop PE each year, and death from VTE has been estimated to occur in as many as 60,000 to 200,000 Americans annually (1). VTE is more common in Caucasians and African Americans than in Hispanics or Asian-Pacific islanders.

## ESSENTIAL FACTS ABOUT VTE

It is important to recognize the natural history of VTE to more fully appreciate its short-term mortality and long-term morbidity.

### Facts about Pulmonary Embolism

- Approximately 10% of symptomatic PEs are fatal within the first hour.
- The highest risk for a postoperative PE occurs 3 to 7 days following surgery.
- Patients with an acute PE who have right ventricular dysfunction documented by a transthoracic echocardiogram have higher in-hospital mortality (14%) and short-term mortality (20%) rate at 3 months (2).
- Chronic thromboembolic pulmonary hypertension (CTPH) develops in as many as 3.8% of all PE patients by 2 years after the initial event.

### Facts about Deep Vein Thrombosis

- Approximately 40% to 50% of all patients with an acute symptomatic DVT (proximal to the popliteal vein), but who are asymptomatic for a PE, have a high-probability ventilation perfusion scan.
- The most common long-term complication of DVT is postthrombotic syndrome (PTS), characterized by chronic leg swelling, pain, and nonhealing venous stasis ulcers, which occurs in 20% to 50% of patients after a documented DVT.

## RISK FACTORS FOR VENOUS THROMBOEMBOLISM

Risk factors for the development of VTE can be divided into acquired and hereditary causes. The most common acquired and hereditary risk factors (referred to as hypercoagulable states or thrombophilia) are shown in Tables 39–1 and 39–2.

As many as 20% of Caucasian patients presenting with an idiopathic DVT are heterozygous for the factor V Leiden mutation, while 6% are heterozygous for the prothrombin G20210A mutation (3) Both of these disorders are rare in Africans and Asians (4,5). Other, less common hereditary hypercoagulable states include: dysfibrinogenemia, plasminogen-activating inhibitor type 1 (PAI-1), tissue plasminogen-activator (t-PA) antigen or deficiency, plasminogen deficiency, and tissue factor pathway inhibitor (TFPI) deficiency.

## DEEP VEIN THROMBOSIS: CLINICAL PRESENTATION AND DIAGNOSIS

Although VTE is considered to be one disease entity, the clinical presentation and diagnosis for DVT and PE are different.

**TABLE 39–1**
**ACQUIRED RISK FACTORS FOR VENOUS THROMBOEMBOLISM**

| |
|---|
| Older age |
| MI, CHF, stroke |
| Prolonged immobilization |
| Long-distance travel (airplane/car rides) |
| Surgery or trauma |
| Obesity |
| Malignancy |
| Pregnancy, oral contraceptives, or hormone replacement therapy |
| Previous VTE |
| Pacemaker wires, CVP catheters |
| Varicose veins |
| Antiphospholipid antibody syndrome |
| Heparin-induced thrombocytopenia |
| Nephrotic syndrome |

The characteristic symptoms for an acute DVT include leg or arm pain, swelling, increased skin temperature, and discoloration (erythrocyanosis), although these findings may be absent and PE the presenting complaint. Unfortunately, the clinical examination is often unreliable and the diagnosis is only confirmed in 20% to 40% of patients presenting with typical signs and symptoms (6). This is due in part to the varied differential diagnosis for DVT, which includes:

- Cellulitis
- Arthritis, synovitis, myositis
- Lymphedema
- Arterial insufficiency
- Muscle ache or tear
- Baker cyst
- Chronic venous insufficiency
- Systemic causes of edema (congestive heart failure [CHF], nephrotic syndrome, liver dysfunction, hypoalbuminemia)

Clinical models have been developed to help diagnose an acute DVT. Wells et al. stratified outpatients presenting with a suspected DVT into low, intermediate, or high pretest probability categories based on a number of clinical "points" (7). According to their model, 3% of low, 17% of moderate, and 75% of high pretest probability patients were diagnosed with a DVT. Although it is not widely used, this model may be a helpful objective assessment tool for clinicians (Table 39–3).

**TABLE 39–2**
**HEREDITARY RISK FACTORS FOR VENOUS THROMBOEMBOLISM**

| |
|---|
| Activated protein C resistance due to factor V Leiden mutation |
| Prothrombin gene mutation (G20210A) |
| Antithrombin deficiency |
| Protein C and S deficiency |
| Elevated factor VIII levels |
| Increased levels of homocysteine |

**TABLE 39–3**
**CLINICAL FEATURE SCORE ACCORDING TO WELLS ET AL. CRITERIA**

| | Points |
|---|---|
| Active cancer | 1 |
| Paralysis, paresis, or recent cast | 1 |
| Recent immobilization for >3 d or major surgery <4 wk | 1 |
| Local tenderness along the deep veins | 1 |
| Swelling of entire leg | 1 |
| Calf swelling by >3 cm when compared with the asymptomatic leg | 1 |
| Pitting edema | 1 |
| Collateral veins | 1 |
| Alternative diagnosis likely | −2 |

Risk score: low, <0 points; moderate, 1–2 points; high, >3 points.
*Source:* Adapted from Wells PS, Anderson DR, Bormanis J, et al. Value of assessment of pretest probability of deep-vein thrombosis in clinical management. *Lancet.* 1997;350:1795–878.

## OBJECTIVE TESTING FOR DEEP VEIN THROMBOSIS

DVT can be confirmed using invasive and noninvasive studies as well as laboratory tests. These tests include:

- D-dimer assay
- Duplex ultrasonography
- Venography
- Computed axial tomography (CT)
- Magnetic resonance venography (MRV)
- (99m)-Tc-apcitide scintigraphy (AcuTect)
- Impedance plethysmography (IPG)

The more commonly used diagnostic tests include a D-dimer assay and duplex ultrasonography.

### D-Dimer

D-dimer is a specific fragment of a fibrin clot whose presence indicates degradation of fibrin and serves as an indirect indicator for thrombotic activity. An elevated D-dimer level, however, is not specific for VTE and can be seen in a variety of conditions, including pregnancy, infection, disseminated intravascular coagulation (DIC), hemorrhage, malignancy, liver disease, surgery, trauma, cardiac or renal failure, acute coronary syndrome, and acute nonlacunar stroke. D-dimer assay has been utilized to a great extent in the outpatient setting and emergency departments to rule out VTE, because of its high negative predictive value. It is important to remember that not all D-dimer assays are alike and that D-dimer can be measured using a number of different methods, including: (a) enzyme-linked immunosorbent assay (ELISA), (b) qualitative rapid ELISA, (c) quantitative rapid ELISA, (d) quantitative latex agglutination, and (e) the whole blood agglutination method. A recent analysis found that the ELISA and quantitative rapid ELISA tests were superior to other methods (8). In this study, a negative result of a quantitative rapid ELISA D-dimer was similar to that of a negative venous ultrasound or a normal ventilation perfusion scan in excluding patients suspected of having an acute VTE.

Most physicians feel that anticoagulation can be withheld from patients suspected of acute VTE in the outpatient setting if the D-dimer assay is negative. It is extremely important, however, for clinicians to know the sensitivity and specificity of their hospital's D-dimer assay before making such a decision. If the clinician's suspicion of VTE remains high despite a negative D-dimer assay, further imaging studies are recommended.

## Duplex Ultrasonography

Duplex ultrasonography is a readily available, noninvasive modality that can be performed routinely in the hospital or outpatient setting, and at bedside for a critically ill patient. It has replaced venography as the diagnostic method of choice for acute DVT and is the most accurate noninvasive test. Duplex ultrasonography allows for direct visualization of the venous system, and the essential diagnostic feature to confirm acute DVT is an inability to compress the vein. The other ultrasound findings that may help in the diagnosis of acute DVT are listed in Table 39–4.

Physicians must recognize that duplex ultrasonography is very operator dependent. Its sensitivity is approximately 95% and its specificity 96% in *symptomatic* patients with a proximal DVT, but it is less reliable in *asymptomatic* patients, those with thrombus above the inguinal ligament, or those with calf vein thrombosis. The sensitivity and specificity for isolated calf vein thrombosis approaches 60% to 70% (9).

**TABLE 39–4**
**ULTRASOUND CHARACTERISTICS OF ACUTE DVT**

Inability to compress the vein
Low echogenicity (of thrombus)
Dilated veins
Free floater
Absence of collateral vessels
Filling defects found on color Doppler
Absence of Doppler flow

In a recent study involving 375 patients, the validity of withholding anticoagulation in patients with a negative ultrasound and a low clinical suspicion for DVT was examined (10). Only three patients who had anticoagulation withheld developed a new VTE event. Two patients developed an isolated calf vein DVT and one patient a proximal DVT (total of 0.8%). No patient developed a PE at the 3-month follow-up.

Duplex ultrasonography may also be useful in patients suspected of an acute PE. If the arms or legs are positive for an acute DVT, further confirmatory studies may be unnecessary in most patients, assuming they would not change the management of the patient.

## Venography

The venogram is still considered the reference standard for the objective diagnosis of DVT. An intraluminal-filling defect must be seen in at least two different projections for confirmation. Venograms should be considered in the appropriate clinical setting, or when other tests are nondiagnostic. Despite its clinical utility, complications such as contrast allergy and post-procedural acute DVT should not be overlooked. The latter complication has been reported to occur in approximately 1% to 2% of all patients.

## Other Diagnostic Testing Options

CT venography of the legs can be performed in conjunction with a spiral CT of the chest used to rule out PE. No additional contrast is needed, and imaging of the more proximal leg veins (iliacs), pelvic veins, and the inferior vena cava (IVC) is possible. As multidetector CT scanners with the ability to image both the pulmonary vessels and the legs are necessary, the unavailability of CT scanners with this potential at many hospitals may be a limiting factor.

Magnetic resonance venography (MRV) imaging can also be utilized to diagnose DVT. Its sensitivity and specificity has been reported to be >95% when compared to standard venography for the diagnosis of a proximal DVT, although outcome data are lacking. It has several advantages, including: (a) detecting pelvic, iliac, and IVC thrombosis; (b) no need for ionizing radiation; and (c) an ability to differentiate acute versus chronic DVT. Potential drawbacks include lack of availability, high cost, reader expertise, difficulty with morbidly obese patients, and the presence of metallic objects (stents or other hardware) in the area of interest. The MRV modality may be beneficial in pregnancy when there is a high clinical suspicion for an IVC, pelvic, or iliac vein DVT that is not detectable with duplex ultrasonography, or for patients with an allergy to contrast dye.

Impedance plethysmography (IPG) has largely been replaced by duplex ultrasonography at almost all hospitals in the United States.

The (99m)-Tc-apcitide scintigraphy (AcuTect), a nuclear medicine scan, may also be helpful in the diagnosis of acute DVT. This test uses a synthetic peptide genetically engineered to bind to the GP IIb/IIIa receptors of platelets (upregulation of platelets is the initial step of thrombus formation in the veins). When compared with contrast venography, it has a sensitivity of 90.6% and specificity of 83.9% (11). Although it is not widely available, it can be used when there is a diagnostic dilemma regarding the age of the thrombus (acute versus chronic) or in patients with renal failure or an allergy to contrast dye.

## PULMONARY EMBOLISM: CLINICAL PRESENTATION AND DIAGNOSIS

Autopsy studies continue to demonstrate that most fatal cases of PE are unrecognized or not diagnosed (12). Patients presenting with PE often have nonspecific signs and symptoms, making the diagnosis more difficult and frequently overlooked. In a review of the most common signs and symptoms of patients presenting with an acute PE without underlying cardiopulmonary disease, dyspnea was most common, followed by pleuritic chest pain. These manifestations are valuable clues to the diagnosis in this patient population. However, in the individual with heart or lung disease, they may be mistaken for symptoms of the underlying disease process. Other signs and symptoms of an acute PE include cough, leg swelling, thrombophlebitis, hemoptysis, palpitations, wheezing, anginalike pain, apprehension, and fever (13).

Patients may present with a massive or submassive PE, or they may be entirely asymptomatic. Patients who have a massive PE (systolic arterial pressure under 80 mm Hg) present with circulatory collapse and shock or syncope. Fortunately, this is not a common manifestation, representing approximately 8% of all patients (14). Acute shortness of breath, with tachycardia, chest pain, tachypnea, and cyanosis,may be the result of a submassive PE (pulmonary hypertension or right ventricular dysfunction without arterial hypotension or shock). Patients with acute PE may also be entirely asymptomatic, especially in the postoperative period. Because of the wide variety of clinical presentations, both noninvasive and invasive diagnostic methods may be necessary to confirm the diagnosis. The differential diagnosis of PE includes:

- Unstable angina, myocardial infarction (MI)
- Pneumonia
- Chronic obstructive pulmonary disease (COPD), bronchitis
- Congestive heart failure
- Pericarditis
- Pneumothorax
- Costochondritis

**TABLE 39–5**
**WELLS ET AL. CLINICAL PREDICTION FOR PE**

| | Points |
|---|---|
| Major criteria | |
| Clinical symptoms of DVT | 3 |
| Other diagnosis less likely than PE | 3 |
| Minor criteria | |
| Heart rate greater than 100 beats/min | 1.5 |
| Immobilization or surgery within past 4 wk | 1.5 |
| Previous DVT or PE | 1.5 |
| Hemoptysis | 1.5 |
| Malignancy | 1 |

*Source:* Adapted from Wells PS, Anderson DR, Rodger M, et al. Derivation of a simple clinical model to categorize patients probability of pulmonary embolism: increasing the models utility with the SimpliRED D-dimer. *Thromb Haemost.* 2000;83:416–420.

Wells et al. stratified the clinical features of PE into "points" (similar to their DVT criteria), and their model may be useful as an objective tool to assess the pretest probability of an acute PE (Table 39–5) (15). In their model, the probability of an acute PE with >6 points (high risk) was 78.4%; while that for 2 to 6 points (moderate risk) was 27.8% and for <2 points (low risk) it was 3.4%.

## OBJECTIVE TESTING FOR PULMONARY EMBOLISM

Traditional tests used to assist a physician faced with the presumptive diagnosis of an acute PE include a chest x-ray, electrocardiogram (ECG) and arterial blood gas.

The chest x-ray may be more helpful to rule out pneumonia, a pneumothorax, or a malignancy. The most common x-ray features of acute PE are consolidation, a pleural effusion, atelectasis, Hampton hump (wedge-shaped opacity along the pleural surface), Westermark sign (oligemia), and Palla sign (an enlarged right descending pulmonary artery) (16). These latter three classic radiographic findings are rarely seen, however.

An ECG may exclude cardiac causes that mimic PE, such as a MI or pericarditis. ECG findings suggestive of a PE include sinus tachycardia, new-onset atrial fibrillation or flutter, right bundle branch block, right-axis deviation, and nonspecific ST–T-wave changes. The classic finding of $S_1Q_3T_3$ indicates acute cor pulmonale but is seen in <10% of all patients (16). Evidence of acute right ventricular myocardial injury may also be seen, manifest as ST-segment elevation isolated to lead $V_1$ and, at times, extending to lead $V_2$.

PE must not be excluded based on either a normal arterial blood gas or a normal alveolar-arterial gradient (A-a gradient). In several studies, up to 20% of patients had normal oxygen levels and A-a gradients despite angiographically proven PE (17).

### Ventilation Perfusion Scan

The ventilation/perfusion (V/Q) scan has long been considered one of the most useful aids to diagnose acute PE. The PIOPED trial (prospective investigation of pulmonary embolism diagnosis) combined low, intermediate or high preclinical suspicion with a normal, low-, intermediate-, or high-probability V/Q scan (18). A normal V/Q scan effectively excluded the diagnosis of an acute PE, whereas if the clinical suspicion and the perfusion scan showed high probabilities, the diagnosis was very likely. V/Q scans interpreted as low or intermediate probability were considered nondiagnostic and required further testing to confirm or exclude an acute PE.

In the PIOPED trial, 88% of patients with a high clinical suspicion and high-probability V/Q scan had acute PE confirmed by pulmonary angiography. Among patients with a low-probability V/Q scan, angiographically proven PE was identified in 40% and 4% of patients with a high and low preclinical suspicion, respectively.

Unfortunately, in as many as 75% to 80% of all PIOPED patients, no definitive diagnosis could be made because studies were interpreted either as low or intermediate probability.

The V/Q scan remains a valuable tool in the diagnosis of acute PE. It is most helpful in patients with a normal chest x-ray, but it is being utilized less often at many institutions because, as outlined above, many scans are considered nondiagnostic.

### Spiral (Helical) Computed Tomography

Over the last decade, spiral CT has been used increasingly to diagnose acute PE. Several reports suggest that spiral CT is both highly sensitive and specific for the diagnosis of a central PE (main, lobar, or segmental pulmonary arteries) but insensitive to the diagnosis of a subsegmental event, with a potential to miss smaller emboli. Spiral CT is also of value in excluding other diseases, including an aortic dissection or malignancy.

Van Strijen et al. followed for 3 months a cohort of 246 patients who had a negative *single-detector* spiral CT performed to exclude the diagnosis of acute PE. A positive CT scan led to treatment, but if the CT scan was normal or inconclusive, serial duplex ultrasounds were performed to rule out a DVT beginning on the same day and repeated on days 4 and 7. Only two patients were subsequently diagnosed with an acute DVT by duplex scan, whereas one individual was found to have a non-fatal PE. In this study, no patient died of a fatal PE, and VTE occurred in only 0.4% of the subset of patients who presented with a normal scan (19).

In another large prospective multicenter trial, a combination of clinical assessment, D-dimer assay, duplex ultrasonography, and spiral CT was assessed in 685 patients. Anticoagulation was withheld based on negative results. There were seven episodes of VTE (1%), of which two had fatal PE, three had nonfatal PE and two had calf vein DVTs at the three-month follow-up (20).

There are no prospective studies that demonstrate the safety of excluding PE (and withholding anticoagulation) based *solely* on a negative spiral CT. However, Perrier et al. have advised that anticoagulation can be safely withheld if a normal CT is combined with a negative duplex scan and a low clinical suspicion (21).

Most of the data on CT imaging for diagnosing acute PE is derived from *single-detector* CT scanners that obtain 5-mm reconstructions. With the advent of multidetector row CT scanners, it is now possible to perform 1-mm reconstructions. These will likely lead to improved diagnostic accuracy for detecting smaller segmental and subsegmental PEs and may eliminate the need to perform additional diagnostic studies in individuals with a normal or nondiagnostic CT scan.

### Pulmonary Angiography

Pulmonary angiography remains the reference standard for which most studies are compared in the diagnosis of PE, despite the fact that it is not universally available, is invasive, and is costly. The definitive diagnosis of acute PE requires the presence of an intraluminal-filling defect in at least two views or demonstration of an occluded pulmonary artery. It is not without complications, and morbidity of 5% and mortality of 0.5% was reported in the PIOPED trial (18).

### Cardiospecific Biomarkers in Pulmonary Embolism

Cardiospecific biomarkers, cardiac troponin-I (cTn-I) and -T (cTn-T), and brain natriuretic peptide (BNP), have become useful in the diagnosis and management strategy of patients with an acute PE. Plasma troponin levels and BNP correlate with the presence of right ventricular dysfunction and appear to be independent risk factors for poor or fatal results. Kucher et al. reported that patients with normal troponin and BNP levels had a better prognosis compared to those with elevated levels and they found a negative predictive value of 97% to 100% (22). Elevated levels of these cardiospecific markers may be of particular value in identifying patients who are hemodynamically stable at presentation, but who may carry a higher risk for a poor outcome because of right ventricular dysfunction.

## TREATMENT OF VENOUS THROMBOEMBOLISM

The goals of treatment for VTE are to prevent extension, propagation, or embolization and recurrence of thrombosis. Treatment is also aimed at preserving valve function and preventing postthrombotic syndrome in patients with DVT and to prevent CTPH and right ventricular dysfunction in individuals with PE. Initial inpatient management should begin with a weight-adjusted unfractionated heparin (UFH), a weight-based low-molecular-weight heparin (LMWH) preparation, or the synthetic pentasaccharide, Fondaparinux. A vitamin K antagonist (VKA) should be started as soon as possible, overlapping for a minimum of 4 to 5 days with one of the above-listed anticoagulants until the international normalized ratio (INR) is stable and >2.0.

## Unfractionated Heparin

Unfractionated heparin is generally administered intravenously, although it can also be effective when given subcutaneously. Dosing is generally determined from a weight-based nomogram, and a bolus of 80 U/kg followed by 18 U/kg/h is commonly recommended for most adult patients. Subsequent dose adjustments are made based on the results of either an aPTT or an anti-Xa assay using an amidolytic assay.

Heparin has a number of drawbacks. It has a variable anticoagulant response among patients, a relatively short half-life, and adverse effects of bleeding, osteoporosis, and heparin-induced thrombocytopenia (HIT). HIT is reported to occur in as many as 3% to 5% of all patients receiving UFH but occurs much less frequently in patients on the LMWH preparations. It can result in significant morbidity and mortality, with loss of limb, stroke, MI, DVT, or PE. Treatment revolves around immediate cessation of UFH or LMWH and replacement with an alternative antithrombotic agent. Currently, two agents are approved by the U.S. Food and Drug Administration (FDA) for HIT: argatroban, a small synthetic molecule; and a hirudin derivative (lepirudin).

## Low-Molecular-Weight Heparin

Depolymerization of UFH by chemical or enzymatic cleavage of its polysaccharide chains yields a mixture of heparin fragments known as LMWH that have a mean molecular weight of approximately 5,000 daltons. This reduction in molecular weight leads to more predictable pharmacokinetics and a greater bioavailability than with UFH. The LMWHs have become the standard of care for the management of VTE in many hospitals in the United States. Advantages of the LMWHs include:

- Once- or twice-daily subcutaneous injections
- Easy administration
- Dose by a weight-adjusted regimen
- No monitoring necessary (for most patients)
- Outpatient administration
- Lower incidence of HIT
- Less osteoclast activation and lower incidence of osteoporosis

Although laboratory monitoring is generally not necessary, it is recommended in patients who are morbidly obese or who have significant renal disease, and in pediatric or pregnant patients. In these populations, a 4-hour postinjection anti-Xa level using LMWH as the standard is recommended. Therapeutic levels are 0.6 to 1.0 IU/mL for twice-daily injections and 1.0 to 2.0 IU/mL for once-a-day administration (23).

The introduction of LMWH has dramatically altered the management of DVT; however, it has had less of an impact on the acute management of PE in the United States. Two landmark clinical trials and a recent meta-analysis have demonstrated that subcutaneous injection of LMWH is as safe and effective in the outpatient treatment of acute DVT as UFH given in a hospital setting (24). Meta-analyses comparing LMWH to UFH found similar rates of major bleeding and recurrent VTE (25).

Although the LMWHs are not approved in the United States for outpatient treatment of acute PE, several clinical trials have demonstrated their safety. A meta-analysis comparing UFH with LMWH in the inpatient treatment of hemodynamically stable PE patients demonstrated similar incidences of recurrent VTE, bleeding, and death (26).

## Fondaparinux

Fondaparinux (Arixtra), is the only synthetic pentasaccharide that has been approved by the FDA for the inpatient treatment of acute DVT and PE. It is administered subcutaneously once daily and is almost 100% bioavailable. Dosing is weight-based; 5 mg is recommended for individuals weighing <50 kg, 7.5 mg for those who weigh 50 to 100 kg, and 10 mg for individuals who weigh >100 kg. Fondaparinux does not require dose adjustment or monitoring, but caution should be exercised while using this drug because of its long half-life and the lack of an antidote. Warfarin should be started concurrently and continued for at least 5 days, until a therapeutic INR is attained. Fondaparinux is contraindicated in patients with renal insufficiency defined as a creatinine clearance <30 mL/min.

## Vitamin K Antagonists

Warfarin is the only vitamin K antagonist (VKA) available for long-term management of VTE in the United States. Despite its use for many decades, two areas often remain confusing and controversial to physicians. One is the optimal dose for initiating therapy; the other revolves around duration of anticoagulation. Two trials compared different initiating doses of warfarin (5 mg versus 10 mg). Both studies reported that 5 mg reduced the likelihood of excessive early anticoagulation, avoided rapid drops in the level of protein C, and did not appear to prolong the time required to achieve a therapeutic INR (27,28). In contrast, a more recent study performed in the outpatient setting demonstrated that higher initial doses (10 mg) of warfarin were superior to lower doses (5 mg) (29). In this study, patients reached a target INR on average 1.4 days earlier, without an increase in recurrent events or major bleeding. In general, the dose should be tailored to each individual patient. Lower doses are often recommended for elderly patients, and for those who have co-morbid conditions such as recent surgery, hypertension, stroke, CHF, renal or liver disease, anemia, diabetes, cancer, or a history of bleeding.

There is controversy about the optimal length of treatment. Most patients require a minimum of 3 to 6 months of therapy if an underlying precipitating event (surgery, trauma, medical condition) has been identified, whereas longer therapy is recommended if no underlying cause can be found.

Two studies have demonstrated the benefits of long-term anticoagulation in patients with an idiopathic DVT. The prevention of recurrent venous thromboembolism (PREVENT) trial compared patients treated with low-intensity warfarin (INR of 1.5 to 2.0) to placebo following 6 months of standard VKA therapy. This trial showed a 64% reduction in recurrent VTE in the low-intensity warfarin group when compared to those on placebo. Patients were followed on average for 4.3 years, and there was no significant difference in bleeding between the two groups (30).

The second trial, Extended Low-Intensity Anticoagulation for Thromboembolism (ELATE) trial, compared long-term low-intensity warfarin (INR 1.5 to 1.9) to the conventional dose maintaining an INR between 2.0 to 3.0. These authors found conventional-dose warfarin better than low-intensity warfarin in preventing recurrences of VTE, without a significant increase the risk of bleeding (31).

The latest American College of Chest Physicians (ACCP) guidelines recommend at least 6 to12 months of therapy for patients with an idiopathic DVT and suggest that indefinite therapy be considered (32).

Patients with the antiphospholipid antibody syndrome, who are homozygous for factor V Leiden, or individuals with two or more hereditary thrombophilia conditions should also be considered for long-term anticoagulation. For patients with VTE and cancer, LMWH is recommended for the first 3 to 6 months of treatment. This patient population should receive indefinite anticoagulation or until the cancer is deemed cured (32).

### Thrombolytic Therapy for Venous Thromboembolism

Thrombolytic therapy for the initial treatment of VTE has been used for over a quarter of a century. It has been promoted for the treatment of both DVT and PE. Currently there are three agents available in the United States: streptokinase, rt-PA, and reteplase.

The goal of thrombolytic therapy for an acute DVT is to produce rapid clot lysis, with the intent of preserving valvular function and preventing the PTS. Earlier data pooled from six randomized DVT trials comparing streptokinase to heparin demonstrated that thrombus resolution was achieved 3.7 times more often among individuals treated with streptokinase. These studies also showed that major bleeding was approximately three times more frequent in the streptokinase groups (33). More recent reports utilizing urokinase and recombinant tissue–type plasminogen activator (t-PA) have reported similar findings (34).

Thrombolytic therapy for DVT is best performed using a catheter-directed infusion. It should be initiated within the first 2 weeks of an acute event and should be reserved for younger individuals with an extensive ileofemoral DVT, or patients with a limb-threatening circulatory compromise as in phlegmasia cerulea dolens, or individuals with effort vein thrombosis of the upper extremity (Paget–von Schroetter syndrome). It may also be beneficial in patients with an occluded central venous catheter, in hopes of preserving its function.

One of the more controversial areas is the use of thrombolytic therapy for acute PE. Most clinicians favor the use of these agents over pulmonary thromboembolectomy for patients with a massive PE. Thrombolysis accelerates resolution of emboli, improving right ventricular function, pulmonary perfusion and the hemodynamic status of the patient.

In a meta-analysis of nine trials using thrombolytic therapy for acute PE, Anderson et al. found more rapid resolution of the radiographic appearance and hemodynamic abnormalities when compared to heparin. There was no difference, in the clinically relevant outcomes of death or the rate of resolution of symptoms in the two groups, but there was a 1% to 2% increased risk of intracranial hemorrhage in the thrombolysis group (32).

Thrombolytic therapy has also been recommended for hemodynamically stable patients who have echocardiographic evidence for right ventricular dysfunction. In this setting, the goal of therapy is rapid reversal of right-sided heart dysfunction, to reduce the potential for death and recurrent pulmonary emboli.

To date, most studies demonstrate a favorable outcome for patients who are hemodynamically stable and who are promptly diagnosed and treated for acute PE with UFH, LMWH, or Fondaparinux. Thrombolytic therapy should be reserved for those individuals with a massive pulmonary embolism and hemodynamic instability. Although the risk for major bleeding has improved with physician experience, and the intracranial bleeding rate is small, the ACCP guidelines do not recommend thrombolytic therapy for patients with smaller emboli or for individuals with PE-associated right ventricular dysfunction (32).

## MECHANICAL AND SURGICAL APPROACHES TO TREATING VENOUS THROMBOEMBOLISM

Other therapeutic options for the management of acute VTE have been tried, including mechanical and surgical approaches. Open surgical thrombectomy had previously fallen out of favor; however, with newer surgical techniques it has regained a role in the management of DVT.

Percutaneous mechanical thrombectomy using rotational or hydrodynamic (rheolytic) devices may provide another option for patients with DVT. These devices may be beneficial in individuals who are not candidates for thrombolytic therapy or in patients who may not tolerate traditional doses of thrombolytic therapy, but who have considerable clot burden. Angioplasty and stenting have also been used, and may be of help in treating individuals with left common iliac vein stenosis, known as the May–Thurner syndrome. For most of these devices, only small case studies have been reported; therefore, the experience has been insufficient to recommend their routine use.

Percutaneous embolectomy and surgical embolectomy are other available options for a patient with PE who is not a candidate for thrombolytic therapy. The percutaneous devices remove, fragment, or aspirate emboli, offering rapid relief of central thrombus. Surgical embolectomy, generally considered for select patients with CPTH, may be life saving for a patient presenting with hemodynamic instability.

### Vena Caval Interruption (IVC Filters)

Absolute indications for IVC filter placement are (a) a contradiction to anticoagulation, (b) recurrent thromboembolic disease despite adequate anticoagulation therapy, (c) complication of anticoagulation therapy, and (d) for patients who require pulmonary embolectomy.

There are a number of relative indications for IVC filter placement, including: free-floating thrombus, PE in the setting of cor pulmonale, ataxia, or patients with a recent VTE who require urgent surgery.

Recurrent clinically symptomatic PE after IVC filter placement has been reported in approximately in 2% to 5% of cases (35). The source of PE could be *de novo* thrombus forming within the filter, or propagation of a preexisting thrombus through the filter, or thrombus that originates from the arm or neck veins. Current recommendations advise that patients with IVC filters receive long-term anticoagulation once it becomes safe to do so. In one study of 400 patients who received either an IVC filter or standard anticoagulation for treatment of VTE, a statistically higher DVT recurrence rate was identified in the filter population (36).

In addition to the increased risk for recurrent VTE, IVC filters can lead to thrombosis at the venous access site, filter migration, or penetration and obstruction of the vena cava. Therefore, it is prudent to adhere strictly to the appropriate criteria when evaluating patients for IVC filter placement.

Although they are not yet FDA approved, the introduction of retrievable IVC filters may help to alleviate or eliminate many of these issues.

## THROMBOPROPHYLAXIS

Although thromboprophylaxis should be provided to all hospitalized patients, all physicians do not universally practice this policy, largely because it is either overlooked or not even considered. Individuals who are considered at greatest risk are those over 40 years of age, patients who are immobilized or who have an underlying medical condition (MI, stroke), trauma, or recent surgical procedure (hip fracture, total knee or hip replacement, neurosurgery).

There are two major forms of prophylaxis, mechanical and pharmacologic. Those who require surgery but cannot receive prophylactic anticoagulation should be prescribed mechanical modalities such as graduated compression stockings or intermittent pneumatic compression devices. Pharmacologic prophylaxis can be achieved by a number of agents, including UFH, LMWH, Fondaparinux, or a VKA. In high-risk populations such as those with hip fracture, or hip or knee replacement, a combination of mechanical and pharmacologic therapies should be used.

More specific indications for certain high-risk clinical situations are listed below. These recommendations are based on the most recent ACCP guidelines (37).

- Hip fracture surgery—Fondaparinux
- Total hip/knee arthroplasty—LMWH, Fondaparinux, or warfarin with an INR target of 2.0–3.0
- Neurosurgery—Intermittent pneumatic compression devices with or without graduated compression stockings, postoperative use of UFH or LMWH when acceptable
- Medical conditions—LMWH or UFH
- High-risk general surgery/gynecologic surgery—LMWH or UFH and intermittent pneumatic compression $\pm$ graduated compression stockings

Prophylaxis should continue until the patient starts ambulating, and/or the physician is comfortable that the individual is no longer at risk to develop a VTE. In select surgical procedures, extended prophylaxis is recommended. For example, extended prophylaxis for up to 28 to 35 days is recommended for patients who have had a hip fracture or who undergo total hip replacement surgery (37). Patients undergoing high-risk general surgery or gynecologic surgery (especially cancer surgery) should also receive extended prophylaxis (4 to 6 weeks is recommended) (37).

## REFERENCES


1. Hirsh J, Hoak J. Management of deep vein thrombosis and pulmonary embolism. A statement for healthcare professionals. Council on Thrombosis (in consultation with the Council on Cardiovascular Radiology), American Heart Association. *Circulation.* 1996;93:2212–2245.
2. Goldhaber SZ, Visani L, De Rosa M. Acute pulmonary embolism: clinical outcomes in the International Cooperative Pulmonary Embolism Registry (ICOPER). *Lancet* 1999;353:1386–1389.
3. Bauer KA. The thrombophilias: well-defined risk factors with uncertain therapeutic implications. *Ann Intern Med.* 2001;135:367–373.
4. Thomas RH. Hypercoagulability syndromes. *Arch Intern Med.* 2001;161:2433–2439.
5. Seligsohn U, Lubetsky A. Genetic susceptibility to venous thrombosis. *N Engl J Med.* 2001;344:1222–1231.

6. Kahn SR. The clinical diagnosis of deep venous thrombosis: integrating incidence, risk factors, and symptoms and signs. *Arch Intern Med.* 1998;158:2315–2323.
7. Wells PS, Anderson DR, Bormanis J, et al. Value of assessment of pretest probability of deep-vein thrombosis in clinical management. *Lancet.* 1997;350:1795–1798.
8. Stein PD, Hull RD, Patel KC, et al. D-dimer for the exclusion of acute venous thrombosis and pulmonary embolism: a systematic review. *Ann Intern Med.* 2004;140:589–602.
9. Kearon C, Ginsberg JS, Hirsh J. The role of venous ultrasonography in the diagnosis of suspected deep venous thrombosis and pulmonary embolism. *Ann Intern Med.* 1998;129:1044–1049.
10. Stevens SM, Elliott CG, Chan KJ, et al. Withholding anticoagulation after a negative result on duplex ultrasonography for suspected symptomatic deep venous thrombosis. *Ann Intern Med.* 2004;140:985–991.
11. Taillefer R, Edell S, Innes G, Lister-James J. Acute thromboscintigraphy with (99m)Tc-apcitide: results of the phase 3 multicenter clinical trial comparing 99mTc-apcitide scintigraphy with contrast venography for imaging acute DVT. Multicenter Trial Investigators. *J Nucl Med.* 2000;41:1214–1223.
12. Ryu JH, Olson EJ, Pellikka PA. Clinical recognition of pulmonary embolism: problem of unrecognized and asymptomatic cases. *Mayo Clin Proc.* 1998;73:873–879.
13. Walsh PN, Stengle JM, Sherry S. The urokinase-pulmonary embolism trial. *Circulation.* 1969;39:153–156.
14. Stein PD, Terrin ML, Hales CA, et al. Clinical, laboratory, roentgenographic, and electrocardiographic findings in patients with acute pulmonary embolism and no pre-existing cardiac or pulmonary disease. *Chest.* 1991;100:598–603.
15. Wells PS, Anderson DR, Rodger M, et al. Derivation of a simple clinical model to categorize patients probability of pulmonary embolism: increasing the models utility with the SimpliRED D-dimer. *Thromb Haemost.* 2000;83:416–420.
16. The urokinase Pulmonary Embolism Trial. A national cooperative study. *Circulation.* 1973;47:II1–II108.
17. Stein PD, Goldhaber SZ, Henry JW. Alveolar-arterial oxygen gradient in the assessment of acute pulmonary embolism. *Chest.* 1995; 107:139–143.
18. Value of the ventilation/perfusion scan in acute pulmonary embolism. Results of the Prospective Investigation Of Pulmonary Embolism Diagnosis (PIOPED). The PIOPED Investigators. *JAMA.* 1990;263:2753–2759.
19. van Strijen MJ, de Monye W, Schiereck J, et al. Single-detector helical computed tomography as the primary diagnostic test in suspected pulmonary embolism: a multicenter clinical management study of 510 patients. *Ann Intern Med.* 2003;138:307–314.
20. Perrier A, Roy PM, Aujesky D, et al. Diagnosing pulmonary embolism in outpatients with clinical assessment, D-dimer measurement, venous ultrasound, and helical computed tomography: a multicenter management study. *Am J Med.* 2004;116:291–299.
21. Perrier A, Bounameaux H. Validation of helical computed tomography for suspected pulmonary embolism: a near miss? *J Thromb Haemost.* 3 vol; 2005:14–16.
22. Kucher N, Goldhaber SZ. Cardiac biomarkers for risk stratification of patients with acute pulmonary embolism. *Circulation.* 2003;108:2191–2194.
23. Hirsh J, Lee AY. How we diagnose and treat deep vein thrombosis. *Blood.* 2002;99:3102–3110.
24. van Dongen CJ, van den Belt AG, Prins MH, Lensing AW. Fixed dose subcutaneous low molecular weight heparins versus adjusted dose unfractionated heparin for venous thromboembolism. *Cochrane Database Syst Rev.* 2004:CD001100.
25. Dolovich LR, Ginsberg JS, Douketis JD, et al. A meta-analysis comparing low-molecular-weight heparins with unfractionated heparin in the treatment of venous thromboembolism: examining some unanswered questions regarding location of treatment, product type, and dosing frequency. *Arch Intern Med.* 2000;160: 181–188.
26. Quinlan DJ, McQuillan A, Eikelboom JW. Low-molecular-weight heparin compared with intravenous unfractionated heparin for treatment of pulmonary embolism: a meta-analysis of randomized, controlled trials. *Ann Intern Med.* 2004;140:175–183.
27. Harrison L, Johnston M, Massicotte MP, et al. Comparison of 5-mg and 10-mg loading doses in initiation of warfarin therapy. *Ann Intern Med.* 1997;126:133–136.
28. Crowther MA, Ginsberg JB, Kearon C, et al. A randomized trial comparing 5-mg and 10-mg warfarin loading doses. *Arch Intern Med.* 1999;159:46–48.
29. Kovacs MJ, Rodger M, Anderson DR, et al. Comparison of 10-mg and 5-mg warfarin initiation nomograms together with low-molecular-weight heparin for outpatient treatment of acute venous thromboembolism. A randomized, double-blind, controlled trial. *Ann Intern Med.* 2003;138:714–719.
30. Ridker PM, Goldhaber SZ, Danielson E, et al. Long-term, low-intensity warfarin therapy for the prevention of recurrent venous thromboembolism. *N Engl J Med.* 2003;348:1425–1434.
31. Kearon C, Ginsberg JS, Kovacs MJ, et al. Comparison of low-intensity warfarin therapy with conventional-intensity warfarin therapy for long-term prevention of recurrent venous thromboembolism. *N Engl J Med.* 2003;349:631–639.
32. Buller HR, Agnelli G, Hull RD, et al. Antithrombotic therapy for venous thromboembolic disease: the Seventh ACCP Conference on Antithrombotic and Thrombolytic Therapy. *Chest.* 2004;126:401S–428S.
33. Goldhaber SZ, Meyerovitz MF, Green D, et al. Randomized controlled trial of tissue plasminogen activator in proximal deep venous thrombosis. *Am J Med.* 1990;88:235–240.
34. Ouriel K, Gray B, Clair DG, Olin J. Complications associated with the use of urokinase and recombinant tissue plasminogen activator for catheter-directed peripheral arterial and venous thrombolysis. *J Vasc Interv Radiol.* 2000;11:295–298.
35. Kinney TB. Update on inferior vena cava filters. *J Vasc Interv Radiol.* 2003;14:425–440.
36. Decousus H, Leizorovicz A, Parent F, et al. A clinical trial of vena caval filters in the prevention of pulmonary embolism in patients with proximal deep-vein thrombosis. Prevention du Risque d'Embolie Pulmonaire par Interruption Cave Study Group. *N Engl J Med.* 1998;338:409–415.
37. Geerts WH, Pineo GF, Heit JA, et al. Prevention of venous thromboembolism: the Seventh ACCP Conference on Antithrombotic and Thrombolytic Therapy. *Chest.* 2004;126:338S–400S.

# Congenital Heart Disease

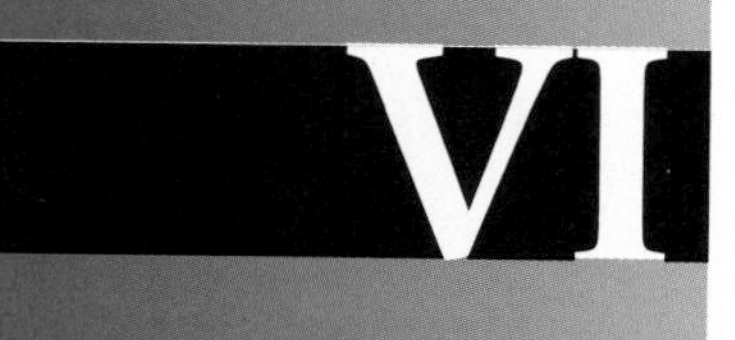

# 40 Congenital Heart Disease in the Adult

*Richard A. Krasuski*

Adults with congenital heart disease (CHD) are a rapidly growing population of patients, owing to advances in the diagnosis and treatment of children with CHD. Most children with congenital heart disease are now expected to survive to adulthood, either with or without the aid of surgical correction or palliation (Table 40–1). According to recent estimates, there are now nearly three quarters of a million adults with CHD, and these numbers should continue to rise with further advancements in diagnosis and treatment. Although ideally served by cardiologists with advanced training in adult CHD, most of these patients receive the majority of their care from primary care physicians and general cardiologists, even though very few cardiology training programs have a formalized adult CHD curriculum. Being aware of the often unique clinical presentations, and having a general understanding of the anatomy and the pathophysiologic consequences of congenital disease is vital to facilitating the timing of percutaneous, electrophysiologic, and surgical interventions.

## GENERAL CONCEPTS

An organized approach to diagnosis and management is especially important for patients with CHD, and the critical first step is gathering historical data. Reviewing the pediatric records, if available, is essential in understanding the complexities of the cardiac and vascular anatomy and to define the outcomes of previous diagnostic studies and surgeries. Surgical procedures have changed considerably over the last several decades, and anatomic presumptions based on current practice may not apply.

Certain signs and symptoms should prompt an extensive evaluation of adults with CHD, particularly syncope and progressive exertional dyspnea. Arrhythmias are not uncommon in adults with CHD, and often originate near the myocardial scars of previous surgeries. Supraventricular arrhythmias, such as atrial flutter or fibrillation, are often poorly tolerated because of a dependence on atrial mechanical function. Ventricular arrhythmias, which can result in sudden death, appear to be more common in certain populations, such as corrected tetralogy of Fallot with a widened QRS interval on a surface electrocardiogram (ECG).

Hemodynamic derangements can be quite subtle, such as pulmonic regurgitation following a patch outflow repair of tetralogy of Fallot. Because the pulmonic insufficiency has a low pressure gradient, it can be missed during auscultation and routine echocardiography, and can eventually result in right ventricle enlargement and increased risk of sudden death.

Diagnostic imaging is a critical adjunct, and less invasive modalities such as echocardiography are an important first step (see Chapter 41). Limitations of echocardiography include difficult windows due to excessive scar tissue from previous surgeries, concomitant lung disease, and obesity. Subsequent computerized tomography scanning (CT) or magnetic resonance imaging (MRI) may add substantially to the anatomic description, especially in patients with unclear great vessel or pulmonary vascular anatomy. The use of MRI has expanded with more widely available scanners and simplified scanning protocols. It is important to remember, however, that CT scanning is complicated by the need for intravenous contrast, and MRI is generally not compatible with current implantable cardiac devices.

Diagnostic cardiac catheterization, though generally performed later in the diagnostic workup of CHD patients than in the past, remains the "gold standard" for pressure measurement, cardiac output calculation, and vascular

**TABLE 40–1**
**CONGENITAL HEART DISEASE: SURVIVAL TO ADULTHOOD**

| Survival to Adulthood Without Surgery | |
|---|---|
| Mild–moderate stenoses | Corrected transposition |
| Coarctation of the aorta | Simple shunt lesions |
| Aortic stenosis and subaortic stenosis | Partial anomalous pulmonary veins |
| PS and peripheral PS | Pulmonary AV fistulae |
| Regurgitant lesions | ASD, VSD |
| Aortic insufficiency | Restrictive PDA |
| Pulmonic insufficiency | Tetralogy of Fallot |
| Ebstein anomaly | Coronary anomalies |
| Dextrocardia | |
| **Surgery Required for Survival to Adulthood** | |
| Cyanotic lesions | Severe obstructive lesions |
| Tetralogy of Fallot | Aortic stenosis |
| Truncus arteriosus | PS |
| Transposition of the GV | Aortic coarctation |
| Tricuspid atresia | Supra and subvalvular AS |
| AV canal defect | Cor triatriatum |
| Unrestricted VSD | |

PS, pulmonic stenosis; AV, atrioventricular; ASD, atrial septal defect; VSD, ventricular septal defect; PDA, patent ductus arteriosus; GV, great veins; AS, aortic stenosis.

resistance determination. The relative size of shunts lesions can be assessed using oximetry and the hemodynamic consequences of additional blood flow can be assessed. Most important, cardiac catheterization affords the opportunity to intervene and palliate or repair anatomic defects or to clarify the suitability of further surgical intervention.

Anatomic shunting can be quantified in the catheterization laboratory by examining the blood oxygen saturations in the respective chambers. The mixed venous (MV) saturation is the saturation of blood returning to the right atrium (RA) with contributions from the inferior vena cava (IVC), superior vena cava (SVC), and coronary sinus (CS). IVC saturation is normally higher than the SVC due to high renal blood flow and less oxygen extraction by the kidney. The CS saturation is very low, but its volume of contribution is negligible and usually ignored. To normalize the MV saturation, three times the SVC saturation is added to the IVC saturation and the sum is divided by 4.

Because so much mixing of blood with differing saturations occurs in the RA, an 11% increase in oxygen step-up (saturation increase from a chamber to its successive chamber) is required to diagnose a shunt lesion between the SVC and the RA. A 7% increase is necessary to detect a shunt between the RA and right ventricle (RV) and a 5% increase to detect a shunt between the RV and pulmonary artery (PA). A quick and simple measure of the overall size of a left-to-right shunt ratio can be obtained by using the formula (aortic saturation − MV saturation)/(PV saturation − PA saturation). The PV saturation can be assumed to be 95% if not measured directly.

In general, a "significant shunt" is present when the shunt ratio is $\geq$1.5:1.0. This simplified definition may not apply to older adults, however. As pulmonary hypertension develops and RV compliance falls, a left-to-right shunt that was 3:1 for 30 years may become $<$1.5:1 as a result of the gradual reversing of the shunt. In fact, the left-to-right shunt may totally reverse at some point, and result in arterial desaturation, the so-called Eisenmenger syndrome. The significance of a shunt in the adult must, therefore, be examined in the context of the other hemodynamics, chamber sizes, and the history of the defect over time.

Pulmonary hypertension is a frequent complication of certain congenital heart diseases. It can be secondary to pulmonary venous hypertension from elevated left-sided filling pressures, or the result of systemic-to-pulmonary artery shunting. For unclear reasons, shunts proximal to the tricuspid valve (atrial septal defects or partial anomalous pulmonary venous return) infrequently result in pulmonary hypertension ($\sim$15% of cases) despite high pulmonary blood flow. The development of pulmonary hypertension from shunts distal to the tricuspid valve, however, is very dependent on pulmonary blood flow. For example, a large unrestricted ventricular septal defect may not result in pulmonary hypertension if the pulmonary circuit is protected by concomitant pulmonary valvular or subvalvular obstruction.

To help differentiate the cause of pulmonary hypertension, the pulmonary vascular resistance should be determined: (mean PA pressure − mean pulmonary capillary wedge pressure [mm Hg])/(pulmonary blood flow [L/min]). Higher resistances ($>$7 Wood units or a ratio of the pulmonary-to-systemic vascular resistance of $>$0.5) have also been associated with considerably higher perioperative mortality. In addition, assessment of pulmonary vascular reactivity with endothelium-dependent vasodilators, such as inhaled nitric oxide or intravenous adenosine, may provide additional prognostic information in these patients by confirming whether any of the observed pulmonary hypertension has a vasoconstrictor component.

## TYPES OF CONGENITAL LESIONS

Congenital heart lesions can be divided into three general categories (by descending incidence): simple shunt lesions, obstructive lesions, and complex lesions—acyanotic and cyanotic. The most frequently encountered abnormalities in these categories are mentioned below.

### Shunt Lesions

Intracardiac shunts are the most common form of congenital heart lesion and are frequently diagnosed in otherwise healthy adults. They are associated with increased pulmonary blood flow, which can lead to right heart chamber enlargement and arrhythmias, as well as pulmonary hypertension. The surgical correction of many of these lesions has been determined to be safe and efficacious. Recently, percutaneous device closures have been increasingly utilized in order to avoid the morbidity and mortality of surgery. There are three main types of shunt lesions to be aware of: atrial septal defect (ASD), ventricular septal defect (VSD), and patent ductus arteriosus (PDA).

### *Atrial Septal Defect*

The ASD is the most common congenital heart defect encountered in adults (excluding mitral valve prolapse and bicuspid aortic valve), accounting for up to 15% of all adult CHD. It results from the failure of proper embryologic development of the atrial septum. There are many different types of ASD, the most common of which is the secundum ASD, in which the defect lies in the middle of the atrial septum.

The secundum ASD is often mistaken for other abnormalities or overlooked because the symptoms associated with it, typically fatigue and breathlessness, can be subtle and nonspecific. Physical examination findings, such as a fixed split second heart sound (due to loss of differential effects on right- and left-sided filling pressures from a drop in intrathoracic pressure that normally occurs during inspiration) and a pulmonic outflow murmur (the result of increased pulmonary blood volume from shunting), can also be overlooked. The flow of blood across the defect (shunt) is determined by the size of the defect and the compliance of the atria. ASD should be suspected whenever right heart enlargement is present without another good explanation. Occasionally patients can present late in life with ASD-related symptoms when the left atrial pressure rises because of a stiff left ventricle and diastolic dysfunction (usually the result of long-standing hypertension or coronary artery disease).

The larger the left-to-right shunt in patients with ASD, the greater is the risk for long-term complications such as atrial fibrillation and pulmonary hypertension. The latter condition effects up to 15% of adults with ASD, and if uncorrected can result in Eisenmenger syndrome. In Eisenmenger syndrome the right-sided pressure increases to the point that shunting is reversed (becoming right to left) and systemic oxygenation decreases. Patients with this complication will not improve their oxygen saturation when oxygen is administered to them (the telltale sign of a right-to-left shunt). Multiple complications eventually ensue, and until recently this condition was considered irreversible. Another condition associated with ASD is stroke, which presumably results from paradoxical embolization (blood clots forming in the extremities and reaching the cerebral circulation by passing through the ASD).

Indications to repair an ASD have historically included evidence of right heart volume overload (resulting from the ASD) or the presence of a hemodynamically significant defect (classically, a Qp/Qs of 1.5:1). The timing of closure of an ASD appears important. Closure after the age of 40 years is associated with an increased incidence of arrhythmias (i.e., atrial fibrillation) compared with closure before age 40. Epidemiologic evidence also suggests that long-term survival is worse with unrepaired defects.

Other, less common variations of ASD include sinus venosus ASD, in which there is abnormal fusion of the vena cava (superior or inferior) to the left atrium. This defect is almost always associated with partial anomalous return of the pulmonary veins (right superior or both right pulmonary veins drain into the right atrium). Because of its location, this defect can be missed on transthoracic echocardiography and usually requires either transesophageal echo or advanced radiographic imaging to make the diagnosis. Primum ASD involves the lower portion of the atrial septum and typically affects the ventricular septum as well (the AV canal defect). Both AV valves are structurally abnormal and the mitral valve is typically cleft. This defect is commonly seen in patients with trisomy 21 (Down syndrome). The least common ASD involves unroofing of coronary sinus roof, which results in shunting into the left atrium. At this time, only secundum ASD has been successfully occluded through percutaneous methods. Important differences in clinical findings among the various types of ASD are listed in Table 40–2.

### *Ventricular Septal Defect*

VSD is the most common congenital heart defect seen in children. Defects can occur at various locations in the septum but most commonly occur in either the membranous or muscular portions. Small defects often close spontaneously during childhood. One type of defect, outflow or supracristal VSD, can be occluded by one of the aortic leaflets prolapsing into it. This can result in the development of rather significant aortic insufficiency.

Small VSDs produce a very loud systolic murmur and frequently a palpable thrill at the left sternal border, but patients with small defects are asymptomatic and require little more than antibiotics for endocarditis prophylaxis. Larger defects have less conspicuous murmurs and are more likely to present during childhood with heart failure. VSD is also the most frequent cause of Eisenmenger syndrome.

### *Patent Ductus Arteriosus*

PDA is the second most common congenital heart defect seen in adults (~10% to 15% of all CHD in adults). It has been associated with maternal rubella. PDA is present as an isolated lesion in most adults, unlike in children, where it is frequently seen with more complex heart defects. The ductus connects the descending aorta at the level of the subclavian artery to the left pulmonary artery. Patients with PDA have a continuous murmur (systole and diastole) that is often described as a "machinery murmur" heard best under the left clavicle and accompanied by a widened pulse pressure. As in VSD, patients with a large uncorrected PDA

**TABLE 40–2**
**UNIQUE FEATURES OF THE ATRIAL SEPTAL DEFECTS (ASDs)**

| | Secundum ASD | Primum ASD | Sinus Venosus ASD |
|---|---|---|---|
| Unique anatomic features | Partial anomalous pulmonary venous return (only ~20% | 1. Mitral valve involvement<br>2. ± VSD | Partial anomalous pulmonary venous return |
| Physical exam findings | 1. Fixed split S2<br>2. Pulmonic outflow murmur | 1. Same as secundum ASD<br>2. Murmurs of MR ± VSD | Same as secundum ASD |
| ECG | 1. RSR′ pattern<br>2. Incomplete RBBB<br>3. ± right axis | 1. RBBB<br>2. Left axis<br>3. ±1° AV block | 1. Same as secundum<br>2. ± Leftward-shifted P-wave axis (inverted P in lead III) |

ASD, atrial septal defect; VSD, ventricular septal defect; ECG, electrocardiogram; RBBB, right bundle branch block; AV, atrioventricular.

can develop pulmonary hypertension. Most experts believe that any PDA should be occluded to prevent endarteritis and to remove any excess flow from the pulmonary circuit, which could result in volume overload over time. Defects can be ligated surgically or closed percutaneously (device closure or coils), depending on size.

## Stenotic Lesions

### *Pulmonary Stenosis*

Pulmonic stenosis (PS) is the most common congenital valve lesion to necessitate therapy in adults. It is occasionally associated with the Noonan syndrome, in which the valve is usually dysplastic. Gradients across the pulmonary outflow tract can involve the valvular level, but may also involve the infundibulum (right ventricular outflow tract) and/or the peripheral pulmonary arteries. Careful tracking of the gradient is critical for decision making. Generally, an intervention is warranted when the transvalvular gradient exceeds 50 mm Hg (moderate or greater PS), though patients with lesser gradients may benefit if it can be clearly shown that exertional symptoms (typically exertional dyspnea) accompany elevated gradients during provocation. Percutaneous balloon valvuloplasty has proven to be safe and effective in adults and is the therapy of choice in patients with significant stenosis.

### *Coarctation of the Aorta*

Aortic coarctation (CoA) is a common congenital heart defect, accounting for ~8% of all congenital defects. It likely results from extraneous ductal tissue that contracts following birth. Anatomically, it can occur before, at the level of, or after the ductus arteriosus; though adults with previously undiagnosed CoA almost always have postductal lesions. The most common presentation in adults is fortuitous discovery during secondary workup for systemic hypertension. Lower-extremity and renal hypoperfusion leads to a hyperrenin state that may not abate even after coarctation repair. In most patients there is upper-extremity hypertension and the development of collateral vessels around the coarctation to the lower extremity. These collateral channels result in a continuous murmur heard in the back, and involvement of the intercostal arteries leads to the familiar rib notching noted on chest radiographs. An associated bicuspid aortic valve is present in up to 85% of coarctation, and a significant aortic gradient is particularly important to exclude when deciding on definitive therapy. Also not to be forgotten is an association with berry aneurysms in the circle of Willis, which can be seen in up to 10% of patients and may lead to central nervous system bleeding.

Echocardiography with a focus on the descending aorta is an excellent noninvasive tool for making the clinical diagnosis in patients with suspicious clinical findings. A resting peak systolic velocity ≥3.2 m/s or a diastolic velocity of ≥1.0 m/s is suggestive of significant coarctation. Symptomatic patients with a peak gradient >30 mm Hg on invasive measurement, or a similar gradient in asymptomatic patients with upper-extremity hypertension that becomes severe with exercise or is associated with left ventricular hypertrophy, should be considered for therapy. Other evolving indications for treatment include the presence of aortic aneurysms and symptomatic aneurysms of the circle of Willis. Young women who wish to bear children are also at risk, as there may be inadequate placental flow should they become pregnant.

Surgery has previously been the mainstay in the approach to a native CoA, with available options including resection and end-to-end anastomosis, prosthetic patch aortoplasty, and interposition (tube bypass) grafting. Angioplasty and stenting is now considered the procedure of choice in patients with recoarctation following surgery and is experiencing an expanding role in primary treatment.

## Complex Lesions (acyanotic)

### *Transposition of the Great Arteries*

Transposition of the great arteries (TGA) refers to an abnormality in the embryologic separation of the great vessels that results in the aorta emanating from the right ventricle and the pulmonary artery coming off the left ventricle. Two varieties are most commonly seen in adults. The first type is the surgically corrected patient, most often following a Senning or Mustard procedure in which blood is baffled from the vena cavae to the left atrium and from the pulmonary veins to the right atrium. The primary long-term concern in these patients is that the right ventricle is ill-prepared to serve as a systemic ventricle. It can weaken and fail over time (usually when patients enter their 30s and 40s), and these patients typically also develop significant systemic atrioventricular (tricuspid valve in the mitral position) regurgitation. The other type of TGA is the so-called congenitally repaired lesion. In this case the ventricles are also inverted. This variation results in a circulation in which the circulation goes from vena cavae to right atrium to left ventricle to pulmonary artery to pulmonary veins to left atrium to right ventricle to aorta. Again the problem remains a right ventricle pumping into the systemic circulation. Both these conditions are also associated with about a 1-in-3 lifetime prevalence of complete heart block. Surgical repair for systemic atrioventricular valve regurgitation is generally ineffective, and cardiac transplantation is often considered if symptoms of heart failure are severe and refractory.

## Complex Lesions (cyanotic)

### *Tetralogy of Fallot*

Tetralogy of Fallot (TOF), a conotruncal abnormality, is the constellation of four findings: an aorta that overrides the right ventricular outflow tract, right ventricular outflow obstruction, a large subaortic VSD, and hypertrophy of the right ventricle. The frequent coexistence of an ASD can make for a "pentalogy." Occasionally, unrepaired patients with TOF can present in adulthood, owing to a remarkable balance between the pulmonic obstruction and the VSD that limits cyanosis.

Early palliation with a systemic-to-arterial shunt (i.e., a Blalock–Taussig procedure, which connects the subclavian artery and pulmonary artery) facilitates growth of the pulmonary arteries and is a precursor to definitive surgical repair in the young child. Definitive repair (particularly if the pulmonic valve is found to be atretic) often requires compete removal of the pulmonic valve and therefore results in wide-open pulmonic regurgitation. Though this may be tolerated for several years, the right ventricle eventually succumbs to volume overload and progressively increases in size. Surgical repair of this condition involves implanting either a pulmonic valve bioprosthesis or homograft, and is indicated if progressive decline in exercise tolerance, decrement in right ventricular function, or severe widening of the QRS complex on ECG can be demonstrated.

### *Ebstein Anomaly*

Ebstein anomaly is the result of inferior displacement of the tricuspid valve into the right ventricle, which results in "atrialization" of the right ventricle. As a result, the right ventricle is very small and not infrequently hypocontractile. The posterior and septal leaflets of the tricuspid valve are often small and inadequate, and the anterior leaflet is very large and redundant, resembling a "sail." The latter feature results in the characteristic "sail sound," which occurs during closure of the tricuspid valve, followed by the tricuspid regurgitation murmur (if present). The ECG of Ebstein patients shows very tall P waves (Himalayan P waves), which are a characteristic finding. Also, about 25% of Ebstein patients have accessory pathways for atrioventricular conduction (Wolf–Parkinson–White syndrome), which are frequently multiple. About 50% of patients also have either an ASD or patent foramen ovale (PFO), and right-to-left shunting through these defects results in cyanosis. Surgery involves complex repair of the tricuspid valve in addition to closure of the atrial communication, and should be limited to centers with extensive experience in this area. Indications for surgery include significant cyanosis, severe tricuspid regurgitation and right heart enlargement (often defined as a cardiothoracic ratio >60%), or the development of symptomatic right heart failure.

### *Eisenmenger Syndrome*

As mentioned above, Eisenmenger physiology refers to the condition in which an intracardiac shunt has resulted in extensive pulmonary vascular disease and pulmonary hypertension that is so severe that the shunt has now reversed. The physical exam of these patients is notable for cyanosis (which often worsens during exercise) and clubbing. If differential clubbing is seen (usually clubbing of the feet and left arm and not the right arm), then the clinical diagnosis is Eisenmenger physiology in the context of PDA. Because pulmonary and systemic pressures differ only slightly, a murmur across the lesion is generally not heard.

In general, patients with Eisenmenger syndrome have much better long-term survival than comparable patients with idiopathic (primary) pulmonary hypertension. Rapid deterioration can be seen during atrial or ventricular arrhythmias or with complications such as pulmonary embolism or infection, or generally any condition that results in even transient hypotension. Patients with Eisenmenger syndrome are also at increased risk of developing hemoptysis, which in some cases can be life threatening.

There are a number of complications that result from long-standing hypoxia, including significant erythrocytosis (elevated red blood cell count). Symptoms of hyperviscosity (changes in mental status, fatigue, and headache) are quite rare, and phlebotomy should be performed only to relieve these symptoms. If phlebotomy is attempted, it should be accompanied by at least equal fluid replacement. Repeated phlebotomy can result in iron deficiency and actually increases the risk of hyperviscosity. Patients with

Eisenmenger syndrome often develop proteinuria and a decreased glomerular filtration rate (GFR). Because of the low GFR and the high turnover of red blood cells, elevated uric acid levels are frequently seen and can result in acute renal failure, particular after administration of contrast dye if the patient is not adequately hydrated.

## GENERAL MANAGEMENT STRATEGIES

Although adult patients with CHD can be intimidating at first presentation, sticking to basic concepts can be helpful in choosing appropriate management strategies. Nearly all patients should be offered antibiotics for endocarditis prophylaxis, with the exception of patients with an isolated secundum ASD or those at least 6 months following the successful correction (no residual shunt) of a secundum ASD, VSD, or PDA. Patients with intracardiac shunts should be counseled to avoid high-risk activities such as SCUBA diving and have filtering devices placed on all intravenous lines whenever hospitalized, to prevent the risk of paradoxical embolization. Noncardiac surgery should be considered on a patient-by-patient basis only after the risks and benefits have been carefully considered, particularly for patients with Eisenmenger syndrome. For illustrative cases of CHD patients, refer to Chapter 41.

## BIBLIOGRAPHY


Berman EB, Barst RJ. Eisenmenger's syndrome: current management. *Prog Cardiovasc Dis*. 2002;45(2):129–138.

Gatzoulis MA, Webb GD, Daubeney PEF, eds. Diagnosis and Management of Adult Congenital Heart Disease. New York: Churchill Livingstone; 2003.

Gatzoulis MA, Balaji S, Webber SA, Siu SC, Hokanson JS, Poile C, et al. Risk factors for arrhythmia and sudden cardiac death late after repair of tetralogy of Fallot: a multicentre study. *Lancet*. 2000;356(9234):975–981.

Goo HW, Park IS, Ko JK, Kim YH, Seo DM, Yun TJ, et al. CT of congenital heart disease: normal anatomy and typical pathologic conditions. *Radiographics*. 2003;23 Spec No:S147–S165.

Haselgrove JC, Simonetti O. MRI for physiology and function: technical advances in MRI of congenital heart disease. *Semin Roentgenol*. 1998;33(3):293–301.

Krasuski RA, Bashore TM. The emerging role of percutaneous intervention in adults with congenital heart disease. *Rev Cardiovasc Med*. 2005;6(1):11–22.

Perloff JG, ed. Clinical Recognition of Congenital Heart Disease. 5th ed. Philadelphia: Saunders; 2003.

Warnes CA, Liberthson R, Danielson GK, Dore A, Harris L, Hoffman JI, et al. Task force 1: the changing profile of congenital heart disease in adult life. *J Am Coll Cardiol*. 2001;37(5):1170–1175.

# 41

# Essential Echocardiographic Images in Adult Congenital Heart Disease

***Ellen Mayer Sabik***

Congenital heart disease is by definition an abnormality in cardiac structure that is present at birth, even if it is not diagnosed until later in life. These defects are usually the result of altered embryonic development of a normal structure or failure of development. Four categories of etiologic agents may be responsible for this abnormal development, and these are the same influences that may cause cancers. They include hereditary and chromosomal defects (Table 41–1), viruses (rubella with patent ductus arteriosus [PDA]), chemicals (thalidomide with truncus arteriosus or tetralogy of Fallot), and radiation (x-irradiation with ventricular septal defects). Although these agents cause certain known defects, most defects have no specific cause and the etiology may in fact be multifactorial. The incidence of congenital heart disease (excluding bicuspid aortic valve and myxomatous mitral valve disease with mitral valve prolapse [MVP]) is approximately 0.5% to 0.8% of live births. Congenital cardiac malformations are much more common in stillbirths than in live births. Some congenital lesions have a high rate of survival without surgery and may be seen in the unoperated adult with different relative frequencies (Table 41–2). Other lesions, with worse prognosis, are usually not seen in adults. However, as both diagnosis and treatment (both medical and surgical) improve, more of these patients are surviving into adulthood and are more likely be seen in a cardiology office as adults. Thus, all cardiologists should be familiar with the lesions discussed in this chapter.

## ATRIAL SEPTAL DEFECTS

Atrial septal defect (ASD) accounts for 22% of adult congenital defects. Excluding bicuspid aortic valves and MVP, ASDs are the most common form of adult congenital heart disease. They make up 10% of all congenital heart defects and demonstrate a female-to-male preponderance of 3:2.

Diagnosis of ASD is aided by the following features:

- On auscultation, a wide fixed split $S_2$ with a pulmonary flow murmur is heard.
- On electrocardiogram (ECG), ostium primum ASD shows marked left-axis or right bundle branch block

**TABLE 41–1**
**CHROMOSOMAL ANOMALIES AND THEIR CONGENITAL SYNDROMES ASSOCIATED WITH HEART DEFECTS**

| | Common Associated Lesions | | |
|---|---|---|---|
| **Anomaly** | **#1** | **#2** | **#3** |
| Trisomy 13 | VSD | PDA | Dextrocardia |
| Trisomy 18 | VSD | PDA | PS |
| Trisomy 21 | VSD | AV canal | ASD |
| Turner syndrome (45, X) | Coarctation | AS | ASD |
| Noonan syndrome | PS | ASD | |

VSD, ventricular septal defect; PDA, patent ductus arteriosus; PS, pulmonic stenosis; AV, atrioventricular; AS, asaortic stenosis; ASD, atrial septal defect.

(RBBB) with signs of right ventricular enlargement. There may be first-degree atrioventricular (AV) block. Ostium secundum ASD is marked by RSR or rSR in $V_1$, QRS less than 0.11 seconds, right axis deviation, right ventricular hypertrophy (RVH), and possibly first-degree AV block and right atrial enlargement (RAE).

- Shunt can be visualized by echocardiography with color Doppler and agitated saline contrast.
- Shunt at the atrial level is a potential source of paradoxical embolus.

The locations of types of ASD are shown in Figure 41–1. The four types of ASD are

- Primum ASD
- Secundum ASD
- Sinus venosus
- Unroofed coronary sinus

## Primum Atrial Septal Defect

Primum ASD accounts for 20% of cases of ASD (Fig. 41–2A–C) and is part of an AV canal defect in which embryonic endocardial cushions fail to meet normally and partition the heart (Figs. 41–3 and 41–4).

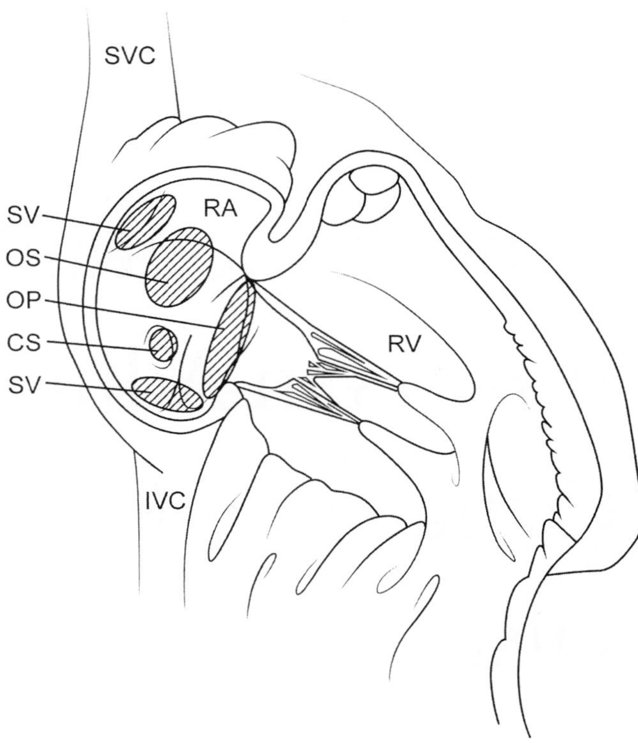


**Figure 41–1** Location of types of ASD. SV, sinus venosus ASD; OP, ostium primum ASD; OS, ostium secundum ASD; CS, coronary sinus ASD.

A complete AV canal defect consists of four components:

- Inlet VSD
- Primum ASD
- Cleft mitral valve
- Widened anteroseptal tricuspid commissure

A partial AV canal defect is as above without the VSD.

## Secundum Atrial Septal Defect

Secundum ASD is an ASD at the fossa ovalis (Fig. 41–5A–D). It is the most common form of ASD (75%

**TABLE 41–2**
**CONGENITAL HEART DEFECTS IN THE UNOPERATED ADULT**

| Most Common | Less Common | Rare |
|---|---|---|
| ■ Bicuspid aortic valve<br>■ Pulmonic stenosis<br>■ Coarctation of aorta<br>■ Atrial septal defect | ■ Ventricular septal defect<br>■ Discrete subaortic stenosis<br>■ Patent ductus arteriosus<br>■ Ebsteins anomaly<br>■ Tetralogy of Fallot<br>■ Coronary arteriovenous fistula<br>■ Sinus of Valsalva aneurysm<br>■ Corrected transposition of great arteries | ■ Complete transposition<br>■ Double-outlet right ventricle<br>■ Truncus arteriosus<br>■ Tricuspid atresia<br>■ Univentricular heart |

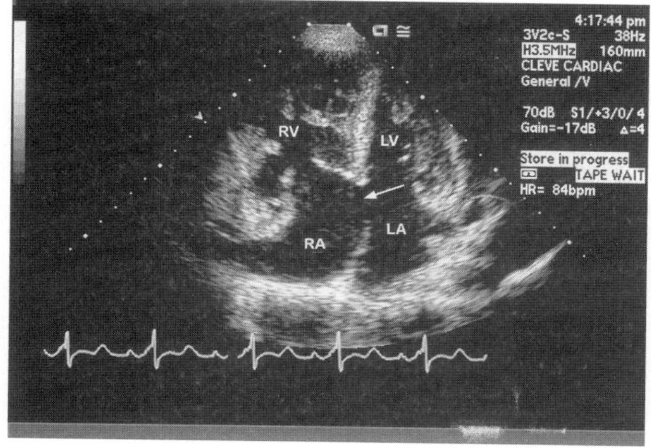


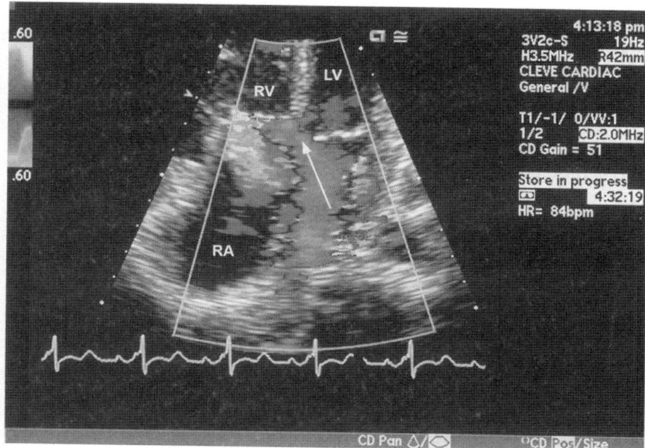


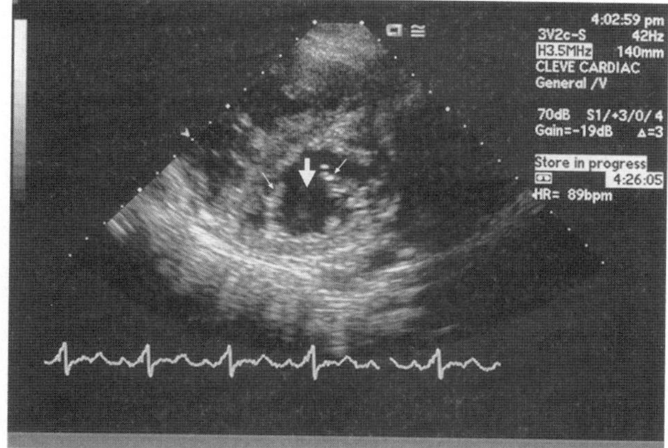


**Figure 41–2** **A:** Apical four-chamber view of a patient with AV canal defect. Note the primum ASD (*arrow*) and the dilated right side. **B:** Magnified apical four-chamber view with color Doppler demonstrating the left-to-right flow (*arrow*) across the primum ASD. **C:** Parasternal short axis-view demonstrating the cleft anterior mitral leaflet with a gap (*arrow*) representing the cleft in the AML.

of cases). The following features distinguish a secundum ASD:

- Left-to-right shunt, because the right ventricle is thin walled and fills more easily than the left ventricle and pulmonary vascular resistance is lower than systemic.

Partial AV Canal
Complete AV Canal
ASD
VSD

**Figure 41–3** Apical four-chamber view of partial AV canal defect **(left)** and complete AV canal defect **(right).** The partial AV canal defect has a primum ASD, cleft mitral valve, and widened anteroseptal tricuspid commissure. The complete AV canal defect has all of these and a VSD.

- Pulmonary blood flow is often two to four times normal.
- Dilated right side due to right atrial (RA) and right ventricular (RV) volume overload.
- The pulmonary artery (PA) is often dilated.

## Sinus Venosus Atrial Septal Defect

Sinus venosus ASD accounts for 5% of ASD (Fig. 41–6). The following are typical features:

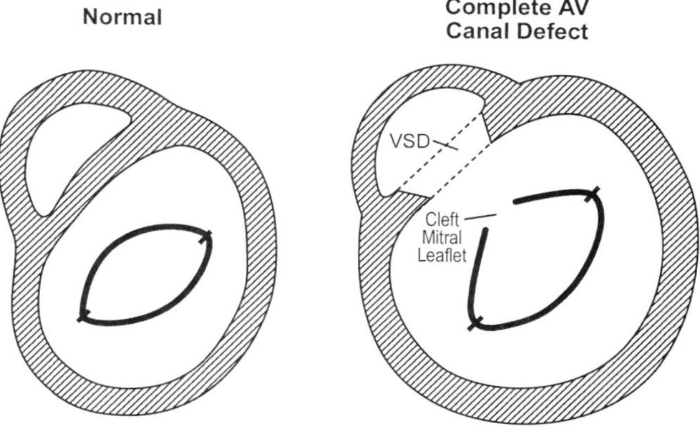


**Figure 41–4** Parasternal short-axis view showing complete AV canal defect **(right)** compared to a normal heart **(left).** Note the cleft anterior mitral leaflet and VSD in the complete AV canal defect.

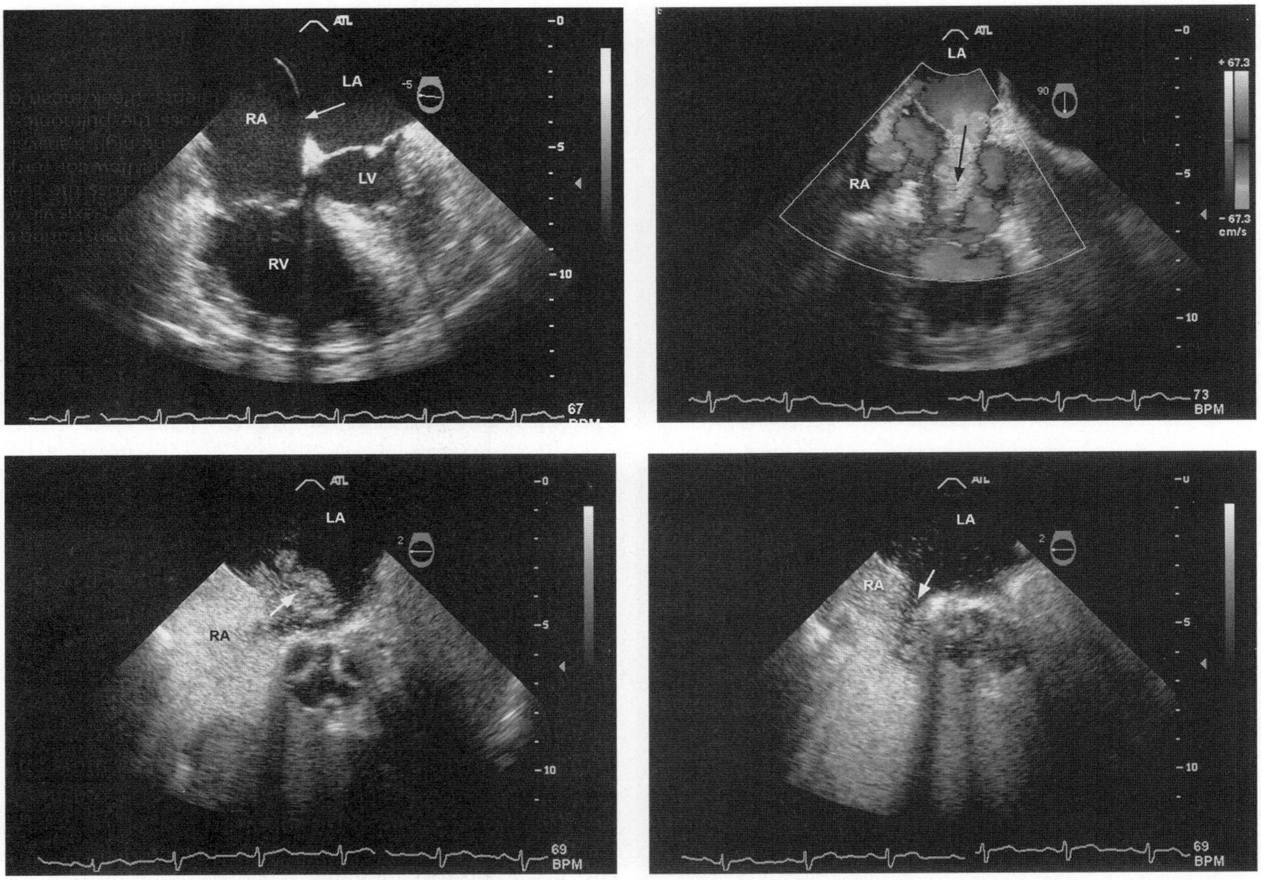

**Figure 41–5** **A:** Four-chamber midesophageal view of a transesophageal echocardiogram demonstrating a secundum ASD (*arrow*). **B:** Transesophageal echocardiogram with color Doppler demonstrating the left-to-right flow across the secundum ASD. Note that although there is one larger shunt, there are multiple defects with shunting through the atrial septum. **C:** Transesophageal echocardiogram with agitated saline contrast demonstrating the intermittent right-to-left shunting across the secundum ASD. **D:** Transesophageal echocardiogram with agitated saline contrast demonstrating the intermittent left-to-right shunting across the secundum ASD and the unopacified blood from the left side of the heart (specifically the LA) displacing the contrast within the RA. The combination of this image and the prior image demonstrates the bidirectional shunting across this ASD.

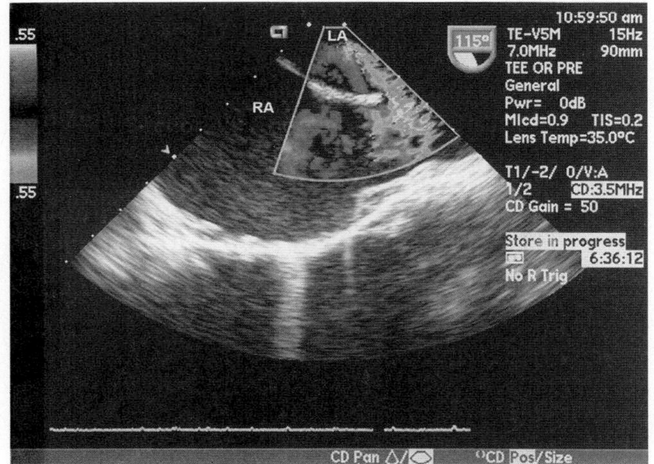


**Figure 41–6** Bicaval TEE view with color Doppler demonstrating a sinus venosus ASD with left-to-right shunting. This ASD is located near the connection between the SVC and the RA.

- Defect near the junction of the superior vena cava (SVC) or the inferior vena cava (IVC) with the right atrium (posterior to fossa ovalis).
- Often difficult to detect (typically requires transesophageal echocardiography [TEE]).
- If unexplained right-sided dilatation is seen on the echocardiogram, echocardiography should be performed with agitated saline contrast to look for a shunt, with follow-up TEE if needed.
- Superior sinus venosus ASD is almost always associated with partial anomalous pulmonary venous return: right PV to either SVC or high RA.

## Coronary Sinus Atrial Septal Defect

Coronary sinus atrial septal defect is very rare. A distinguishing feature is that the roof of the coronary sinus is absent.

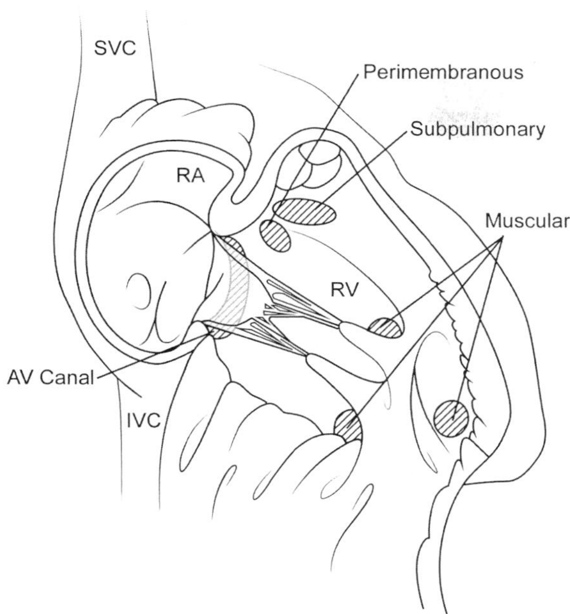


Figure 41–7 Locations of types of VSD: membranous, muscular (may be multiple), supracristal, or "subpulmonic" AV canal defects.

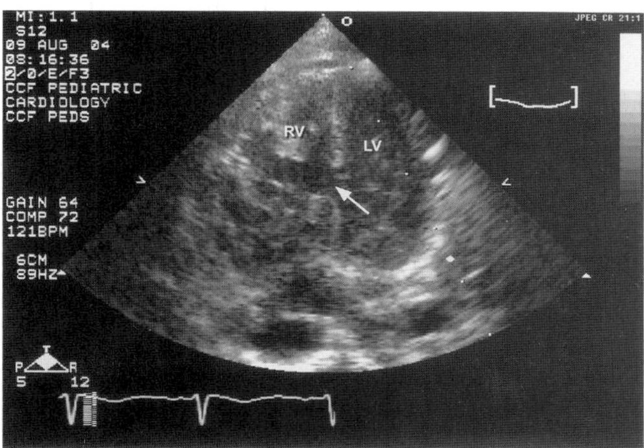


Figure 41–9 Apical four-chamber view demonstrating a large muscular VSD in the mid-septum. Note the dilated right side as a result of long-term left-to-right shunting and right-sided volume overload.

## VENTRICULAR SEPTAL DEFECT

Ventricular septal defect (VSD) is the most common form of congenital abnormality at birth but accounts for only 10% cases of congenital heart disease in adults (Fig. 41–7). Distinguishing features include the following:

- At least 50% to 80% of VSDs close spontaneously.
- Perimembranous VSD is the most common form of VSD.
- VSD carries a risk of endocarditis.
- Perimembranous VSD is often associated with a ventricular septal aneurysm formed by septal leaflet of tricuspid valve closing defect (the defect may be larger than appears).
- Restrictive VSDs have high-velocity jets with a large pressure difference between the right and left ventricles (larger defects are associated with a low-velocity jet). Recall the modified Bernoulli equation: $\Delta P = 4V^2$.

Types of VSDs include the following:

- Membranous VSD: accounts for 80% of cases of congenital VSD; has the highest rate of spontaneous closure (Fig. 41–8A,B)
- Muscular VSD: accounts for 10% of VSD and may be multiple (Fig. 41–9)

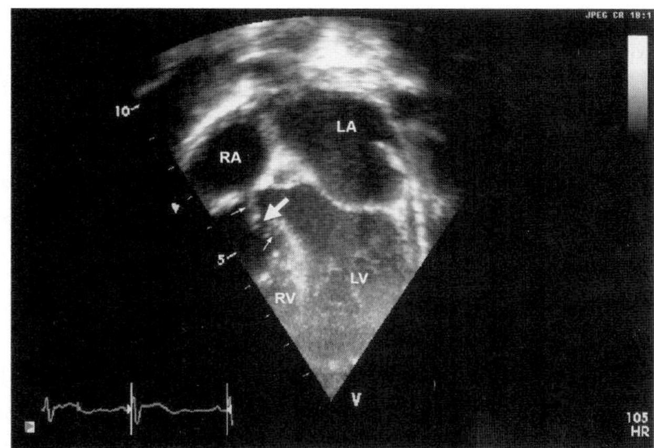


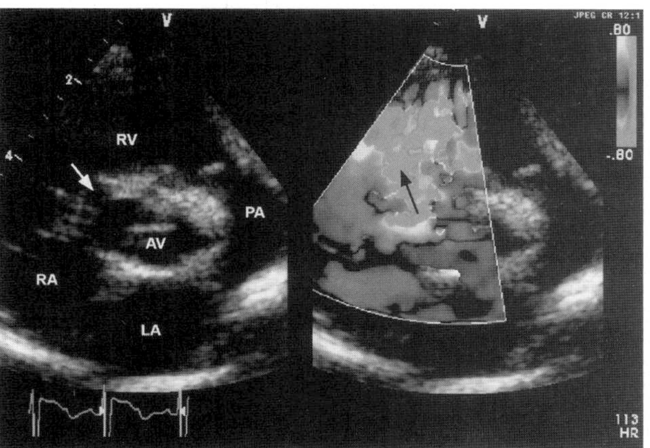


Figure 41–8 A: Inverted apical four-chamber view (pediatric convention) demonstrating a perimembranous VSD with a ventricular septal aneurysm formed as the septal leaflet of the TV attempts to close the defect. The big arrow denotes the VSD and the region enclosed by the smaller arrows demonstrates the extent of the ventricular septal aneurysm. B: Parasternal short-axis views (two-dimensional images on the left and color Doppler images on the right) demonstrate a perimembranous VSD with a two-dimensional defect noted near the RV inflow region near the tricuspid valve, with left-to-right shunting seen in that location.

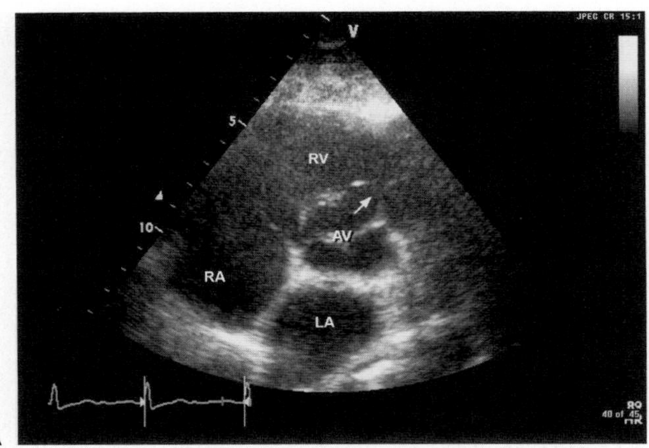


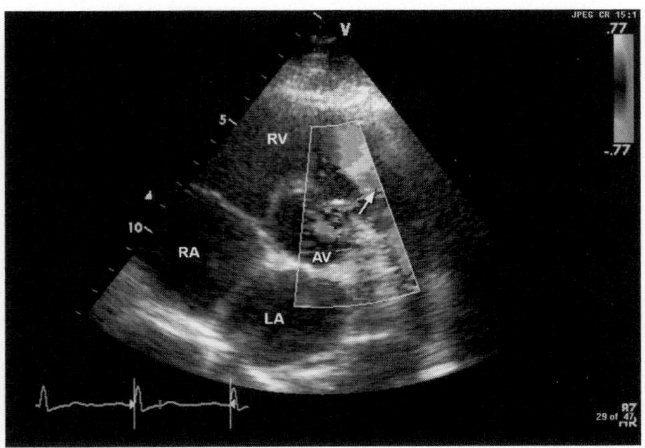


**Figure 41–10** **A:** Parasternal short-axis view demonstrating the two-dimensional defect of a supracristal VSD located near the RVOT. **B:** Parasternal short-axis view with color Doppler demonstrating a fine jet of left-to-right flow through the supracristal VSD.

- Supracristal VSD: accounts for 5% of VSD (Fig. 41–10A,B), involves LVOT/RVOT, and carries a high incidence of aortic insufficiency (AI) due to prolapse of right coronary cusp (RCC) or left coronary cusp (LCC) into the VSD
- AV canal defect: discussed in relation to ASD

## BICUSPID AORTIC VALVE

Bicuspid aortic valve occurs in 1% to 2% of the general population. The most common form is a fusion of the RCC and the LCC. Congenital abnormalities of aortic cusp anatomy are shown in Figure 41–11A–G. Characteristics of bicuspid aortic valve include the following:

- The mechanism of aortic insufficiency (AI) is prolapse of the conjoined cusp.
- The long-axis view shows asymmetric closure of the AV with doming leaflets.
- It may be associated with coarctation of the aorta. At least 50% of patients with coarctation have bicuspid AV; fewer with bicuspid valves have coarctation.
- Early (typically ages 30s to 40s), affected individuals have problems with AI. RCC and LCC fusion produces a posteriorly directed jet.
- Later (typically, ages 50s to 60s), they have problems with aortic stenosis (AS).
- AI may be amenable to valve repair.

*Helpful hint:* To identify and name cusps, look for the interatrial septum. The leaflet closest to the interatrial septum is the noncoronary cusp (NCC). The LCC is always at the right of the screen.

## SUBAORTIC AORTIC STENOSIS

Subaortic aortic stenoses, or subaortic membrane, is shown in Figure 41–12A,B and involves the following features:

- The membrane is usually 1 to a few millimeters below the AV.
- It may be associated with perimembranous VSD, coarctation of the aorta, or valvular AS.
- Eccentric turbulent flow through the AV often traumatizes and causes scarring, leading to development of AI.
- Patients at risk for endocarditis need antibiotic prophylaxis.
- Patients can develop LVH in response to high gradients.
- A small percentage of membranes grow back postresection.
- Surgical excision is appropriate for patients with symptoms, LVH with strain, or significant outflow gradients. It may or may not be appropriate for patients who are asymptomatic with low gradient. Resection may prevent trauma to the AV and help prevent the development of AI.

## PATENT DUCTUS ARTERIOSUS

In the fetus, the ductus diverts blood flow from the nonfunctioning pulmonary circuit into the aorta and back to the placenta. It normally closes within 24 to 48 hours of birth. Patent ductus arteriosus is found in 2% of adults with congenital heart disease (Figs. 41–13A,B and 41–14A,B). It is distinguished by the following:

- It is usually isolated, but it can occur with complex lesions, coarctations, or VSD.
- When the ductus remains patent after birth, there is left-to-right shunting through the ductus arteriosis. Therefore, there is an abnormal persistent fetal connection between the left pulmonary artery (PA) and the descending aorta.
- Auscultation reveals a machinery-type murmur.
- Applying a modified Bernoulli equation, one can use the peak systolic velocity of the PDA jet to determine the systolic gradient between the aorta and the PA.

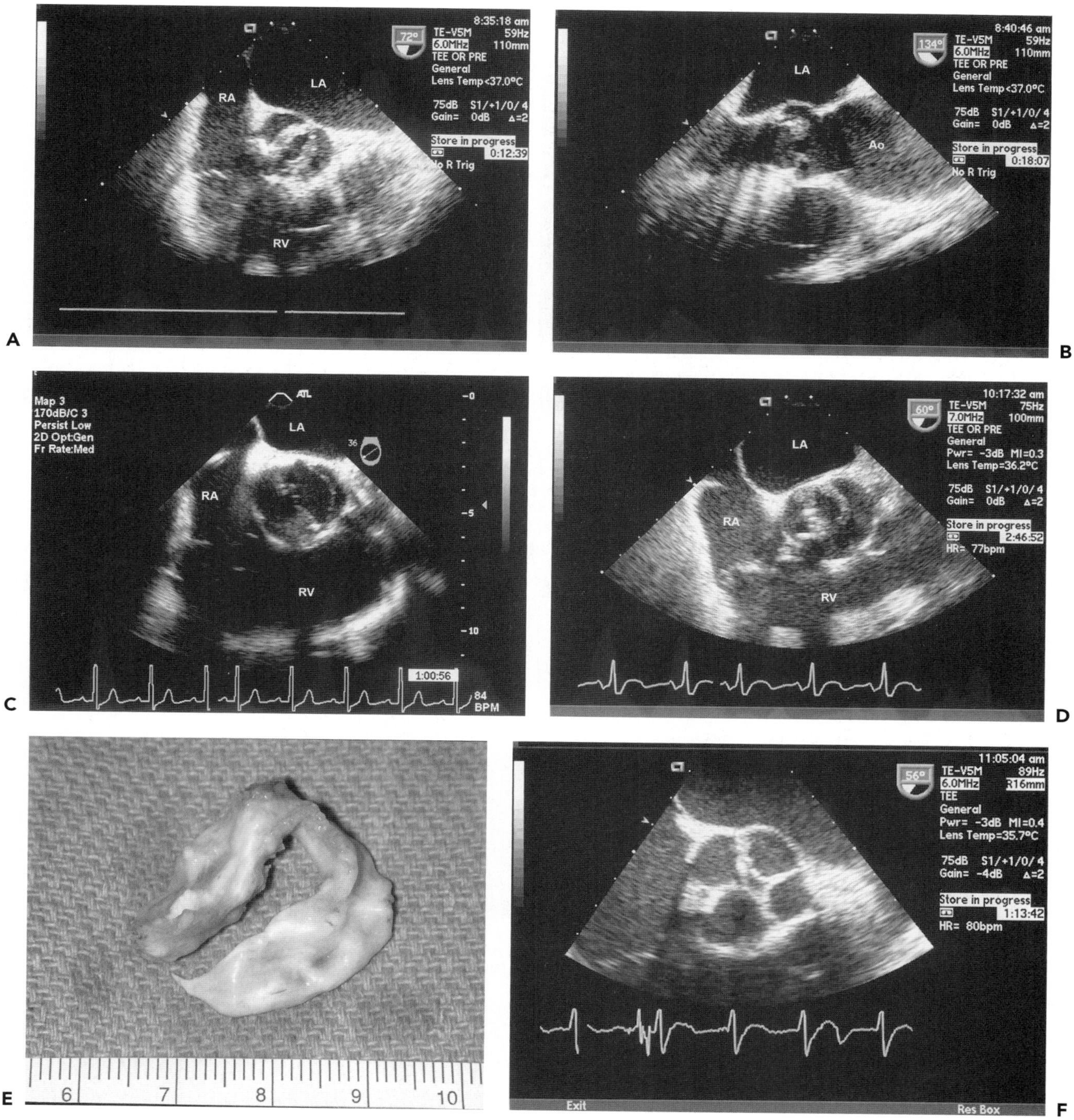

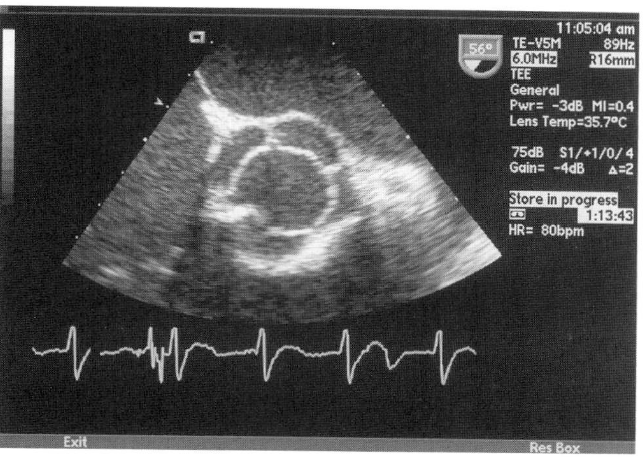


G

**Figure 41–11** **A:** Mid-esophageal short-axis view of the aortic valve demonstrating a bicuspid aortic valve with fusion of the right coronary cusp and the left coronary cusp. The leaflets are somewhat thickened and there is a combination of aortic regurgitation as well as a component of stenosis. **B:** Long-axis mid-esophageal view demonstrating doming of a bicuspid aortic valve. Because of the significant leaflet doming, it is very important to obtain an on-axis, short-axis view. Off-axis images may cause overestimation of a planimetered aortic valve area (therefore underestimateing the degree of aortic stenosis). **C:** Mid-esophageal short-axis view of the aortic valve demonstrating a bicuspid aortic valve with noncoronary cusp and right coronary cusp fusion. **D:** Mid-esophageal short-axis view of the aortic valve demonstrating a unicuspid aortic valve. Note the eccentric opening with a single commissure at the 11:00 position. **E:** Gross pathologic specimen of a unicuspid aortic valve. **F:** Magnified mid-esophageal short-axis view of the aortic valve demonstrating a quadricuspid valve in diastole. **G:** Magnified mid-esophageal short-axis view of the aortic valve demonstrating a quadricuspid valve in systole. Note the presence of four separate cusps.

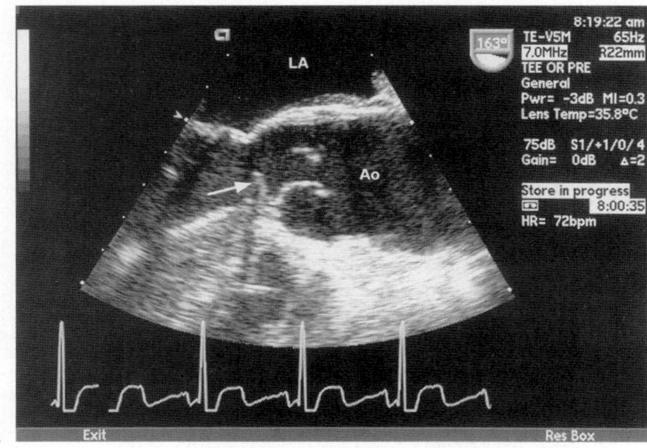


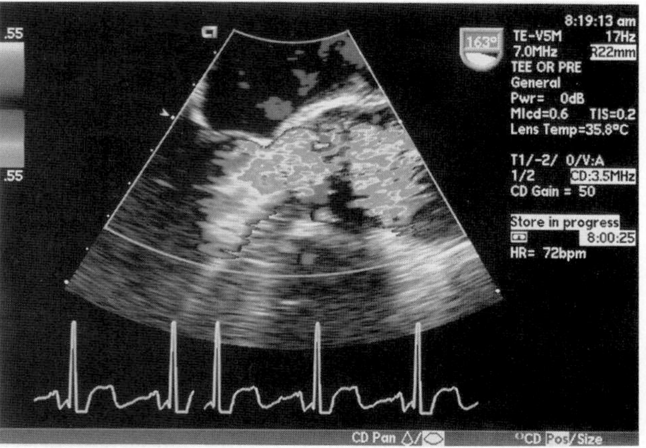


**Figure 41–12** **A:** Magnified mid-esophageal long-axis view of the aortic valve and LVOT demonstrating a subaortic membrane 1 mm beneath the aortic valve. **B:** Magnified long-axis view of the aortic valve and LVOT with color Doppler demonstrating a subaortic membrane with the color disturbance/acceleration occurring in the LVOT at the site of the membrane. It is important to note that the color acceleration occurs *before* the aortic valve, which should alert the cardiologist to the presence of a membrane (by TTE or TEE), even if the membrane is not seen by two-dimensional imaging alone).

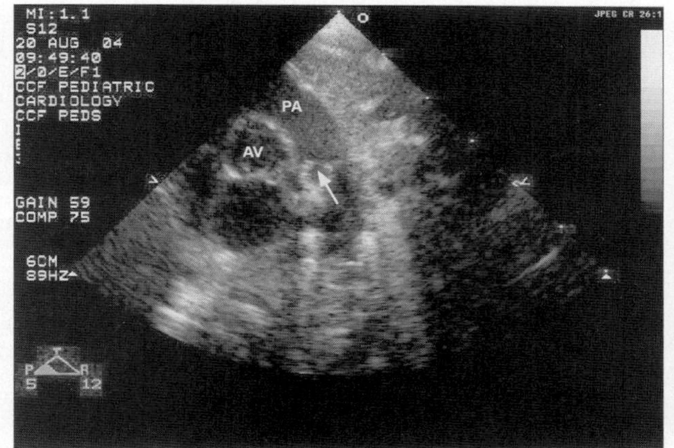


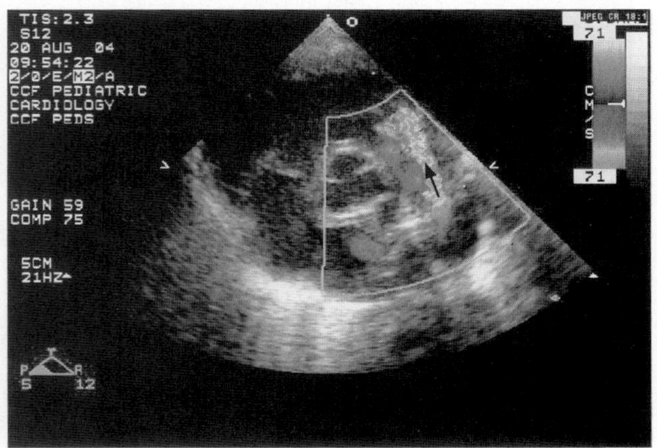


**Figure 41–13** **A:** Parasternal short-axis view demonstrating the opening of a patent ductus arteriosus into the PA (*arrow*). **B:** Parasternal short-axis view with color Doppler demonstrating flow from the descending aorta into the PA (*arrow*).

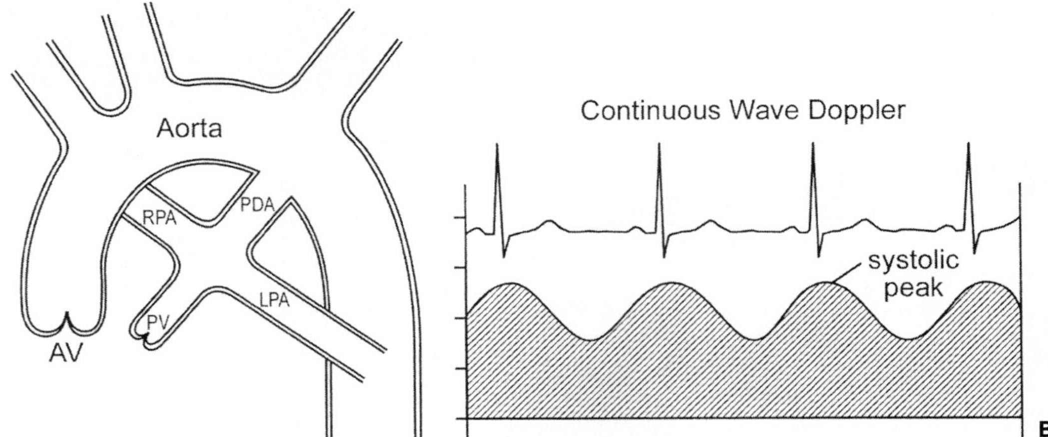


**Figure 41–14** **A:** Diagram of patent ductus arteriosus. Aortic arch view with great vessels arising superiorly off the aorta, with the patent ductus arising from the aorta across from the origin of the subclavian artery, with flow into the pulmonary artery. **B:** Continuous-wave Doppler pattern of flow in PDA.

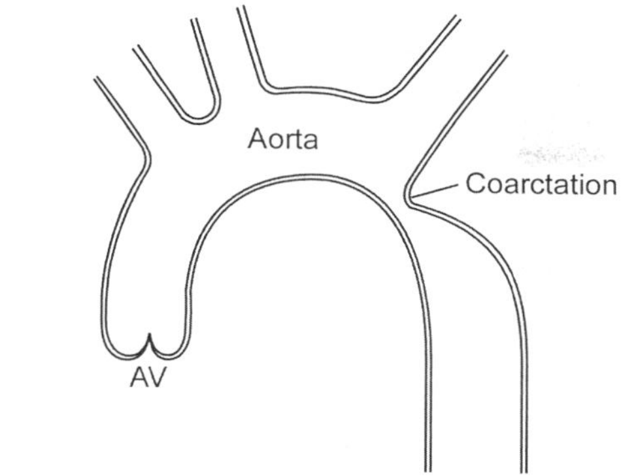


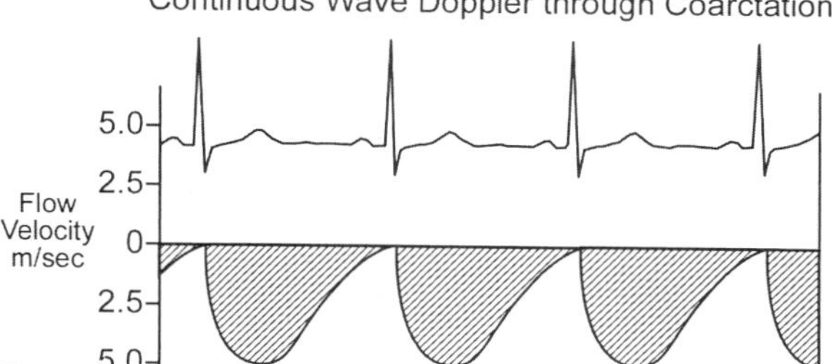


**Figure 41–15** **A:** Diagram of coarctation of the aorta. Aortic arch view showing narrowing immediately distal to the take-off of the subclavian artery. **B:** Continuous-wave Doppler in the proximal descending aorta across the coarctation, with classic "sawtooth" flow pattern.

- If PDA is left untreated, patients may develop congestive heart failure (CHF) from chronic left heart volume overload. Rarely, they can develop endocarditis and therefore need antibiotic prophylaxis. Typically, antibiotic prophylaxis is continued for 6 months after surgical or percutaneous closure.

## COARCTATION OF THE AORTA

Coarctation of the aorta in adults involves a discrete ridge or focal narrowing of the descending aorta opposite the ligamentum arteriosus of the ductus arteriosus (Fig. 41–15A). Characteristics of this condition include the following:

- Clinical presentation includes hypertension, a decrease in femoral pulses, and left ventricular hypertrophy.
- 50% of adults with coarctation have bicuspid aortic valves.
- Continuous-wave Doppler through the proximal descending aorta displays high peak velocity in systole and a gradient that persists into diastole (Fig. 41–15B).
- Alternative imaging modalities may be needed to define the anatomy of coarctation exactly.
- Chest radiography shows rib notching due to development of collaterals (intercostal arteries) (Fig. 41–16).

Coarctation of the aorta is further illustrated in Figure 41–17A–D.

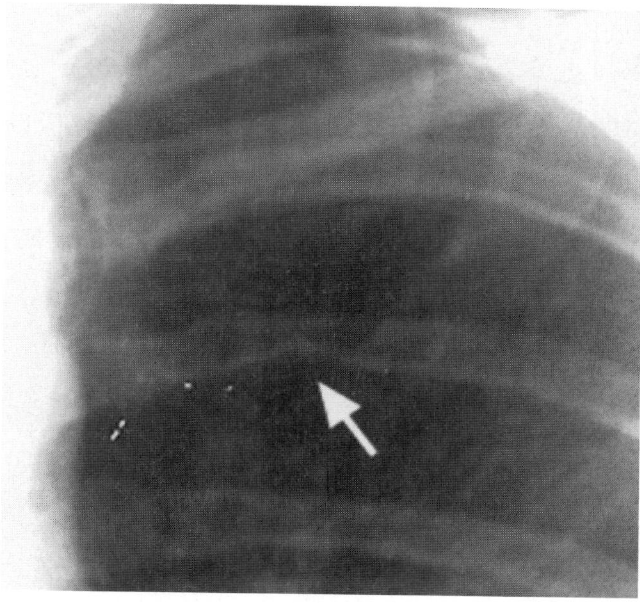

**Figure 41–16** Chest radiograph demonstrating rib notching (*arrow*) that is characteristic of coarctation of the aorta, resulting from the markedly increased blood flow through the intercostal arteries.

## PULMONIC STENOSIS

Pulmonic stenosis (PS) can be valvular, subvalvular (infundibular), or supravalvular (Fig. 41–18A–C). The following features distinguish PS:

- ECG findings may be normal in mild cases.
- Right-axis deviation and RVH are seen on ECG in moderate cases.
- The degree of RVH correlates with the severity of the PS.
- On chest radiograph, the heart size is usually normal but the main PA is prominent.
- Pulmonary vascular marking are usually normal but may be decreased in severe cases.
- Balloon valvuloplasty is often the procedure of choice for treatment (with RV pressure ≥50 mm Hg). Surgery is often reserved for cases of failed percutaneous intervention.
- Subacute bacterial endocarditis (SBE) prophylaxis is necessary, even after relief of stenosis.

## TETRALOGY OF FALLOT

The four elements of tetralogy of Fallot are

1. VSD (large and nonrestrictive)
2. Overriding aorta
3. Infundibular PS
4. RVH

Defects in this condition result from abnormal conotruncal septation (anterior deviation of the infundibular septum).

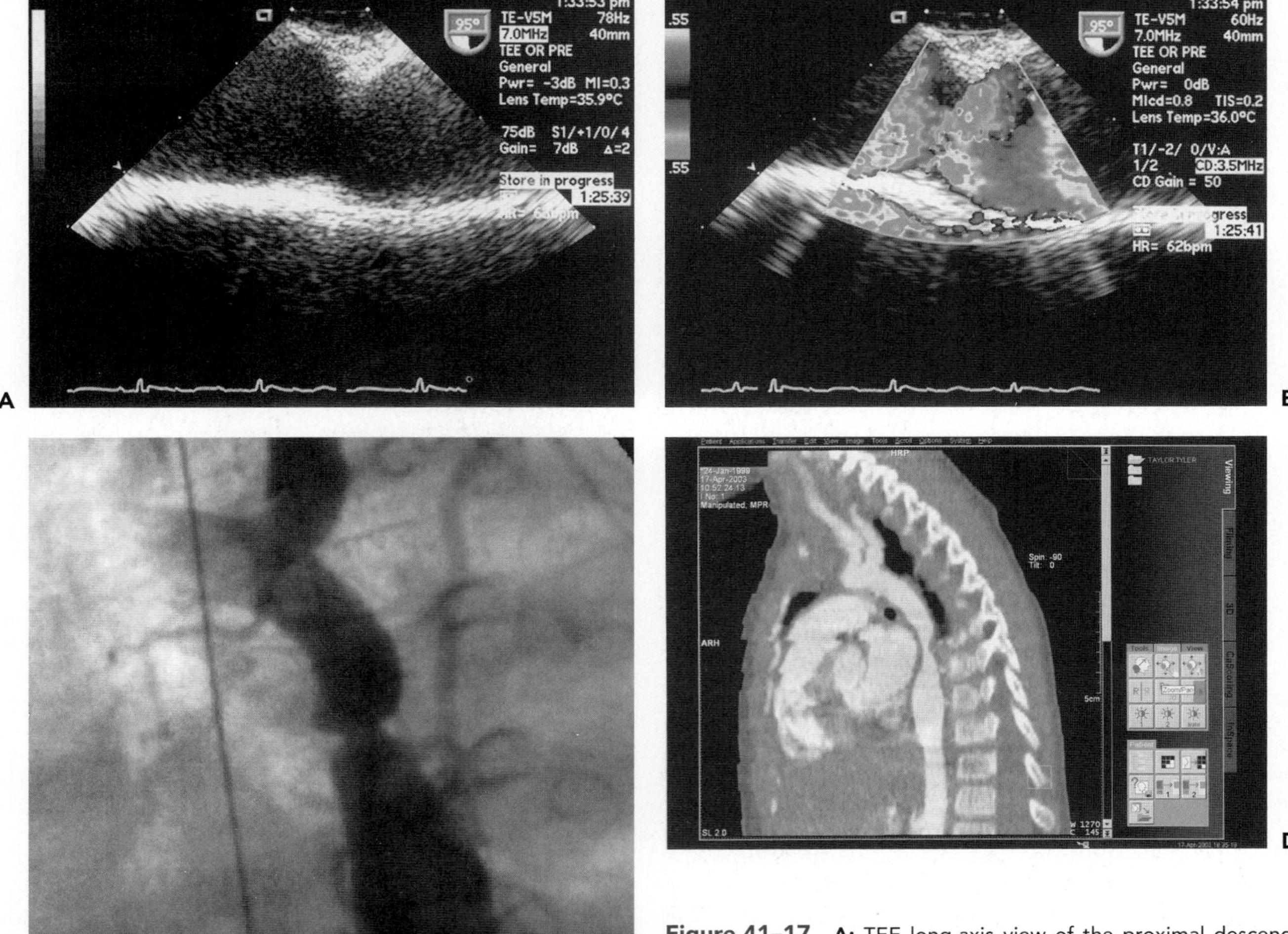


**Figure 41–17** **A:** TEE long-axis view of the proximal descending aorta demonstrating the coarctation narrowing. **B:** TEE long-axis view of the proximal descending aorta with color Doppler demonstrating flow acceleration across the coarctation narrowing. **C:** Aortography demonstrating aortic coarctation narrowing in the descending aorta. **D:** MRI sagittal view of the thoracic aorta demonstrating coarctation narrowing.

About 15% of patients also have ASD, making the condition "pentology" of Fallot. Other associated defects may include valvular PS (50% to 60%), right aortic arch (25%), muscular VSD (2%), and coronary anomalies (5%).

Early in life, mild PS may be present with no significant shunting, known as "pink tetralogy." As subvalvular PS increases with time, pulmonary blood flow decreases and patients develop significant right-to-left shunting, causing cyanosis, or "blue tetralogy."

Tetralogy of Fallot is illustrated in Figure 41–19A–D.

## EBSTEIN'S ANOMALY OF THE TRICUSPID VALVE

Ebstein's anomaly of the tricuspid valve is characterized by apical displacement of the tricuspid valve (TV) into the right ventricle (RV) (Fig. 41–20). The following features distinguish this condition:

- TV tissue is dysplastic, with portions of the septal and inferior cusps adherent to RV away from the AV junction.
- Clinical manifestations are variable, depending on associated manifestations.
- Patent foramen ovale (PFO) or secundum ASD is present in >50% cases.
- A common important associated defect is pulmonic stenosis or atresia.
- Other associations include primum atrial septal defect (ASD) and VSD or congenitally corrected transposition.
- Wolf–Parkinson–White syndrome (WPW) is found in 10% to 15% of patients with Ebstein anomaly.
- ECG commonly shows RBBB or WPW. Most common is giant P waves and prolonged P–R interval with variable degrees of RBBB.

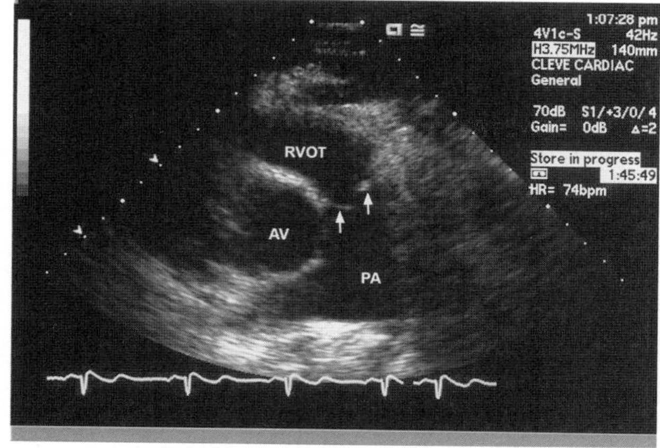


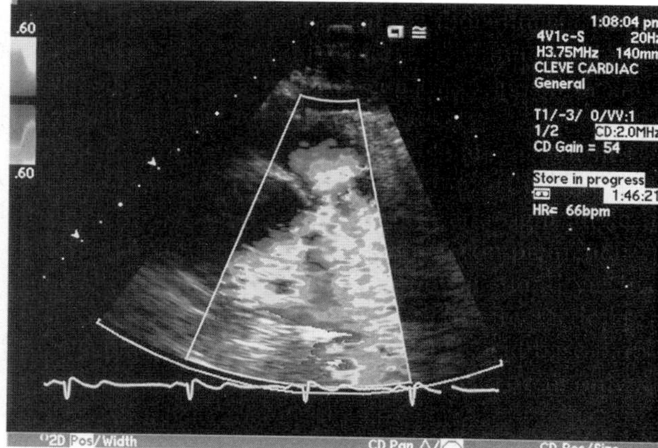


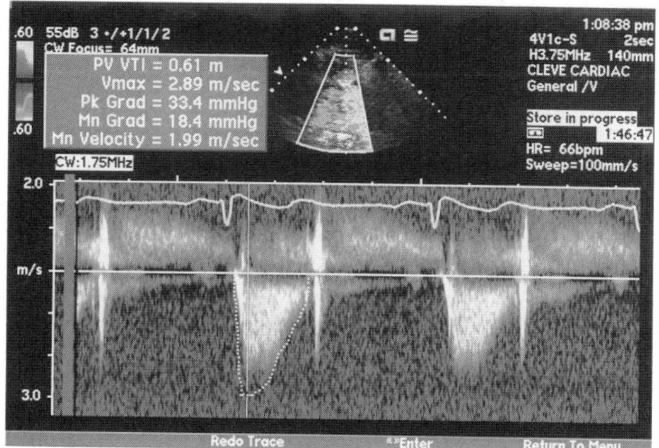


**Figure 41–18** **A:** Parasternal short-axis view demonstrating doming of the stenotic pulmonic valve. **B:** Parasternal short-axis view with color Doppler demonstrating flow acceleration across the stenotic pulmonic valve. There is a relatively large proximal flow convergence zone proximal to the pulmonic valve, due to the high transvalvular gradient. **C:** Continuous-wave Doppler across the pulmonic valve with traced peak and mean pressure gradients. (Peak/mean gradients are 33/18 mm Hg.)

- The presence of WPW increases the risk of paroxysmal supraventricular tachycardia.
- Chest radiography shows a large RA and small RV with decreased pulmonary vascularity if a large right-to-left shunt is present.

## TRANSPOSITION OF THE GREAT ARTERIES

Transposition of the great arteries (D-TGA) is defined as "ventriculoarterial discordance," with the aorta connected to the right ventricle and the pulmonary artery connected to the left ventricle (Fig. 41–21A,B). It is caused by abnormal conotruncal septation in development, with "D-transposition" denoting that the direction of septal rotation is in a dextro, or rightward, direction (Fig. 41–22).

TGA may or may not have associated lesions. There must be mixing of venous and systemic blood at some level for survival (ASD, VSD, or PDA). Otherwise, the pulmonic circulation and the systemic circulation would be two separate and parallel circuits, which is not compatible with life. Common associated defects include ASD, perimembranous VSD, coarctation of the aorta, pulmonic stenosis, and PDA. Further features of this condition include the following:

- The aorta is anterior and to the right of the PA, because the aorta arises from the RV. The two great arteries run parallel (Fig. 41–23).
- There is fibrous continuity between the anterior mitral leaflet and the pulmonic valve compared to the normal relationship with continuity between the anterior mitral leaflet and the aortic valve.

## CONGENITALLY CORRECTED TRANSPOSITION OF THE GREAT ARTERIES

Congenitally corrected transposition of the great arteries is defined as levotransposition, or L-transposition, in which the great arteries are transposed and the ventricles are inverted as well (Fig. 41–24A,B). There is a "double switch" that allows a physiologically appropriate flow of blood. Atria are in normal position and are connected to the "opposite ventricle." Systemic venous return is pumped to the lungs by the morphologic left ventricle and pulmonary venous return is pumped to the aorta by the morphologic

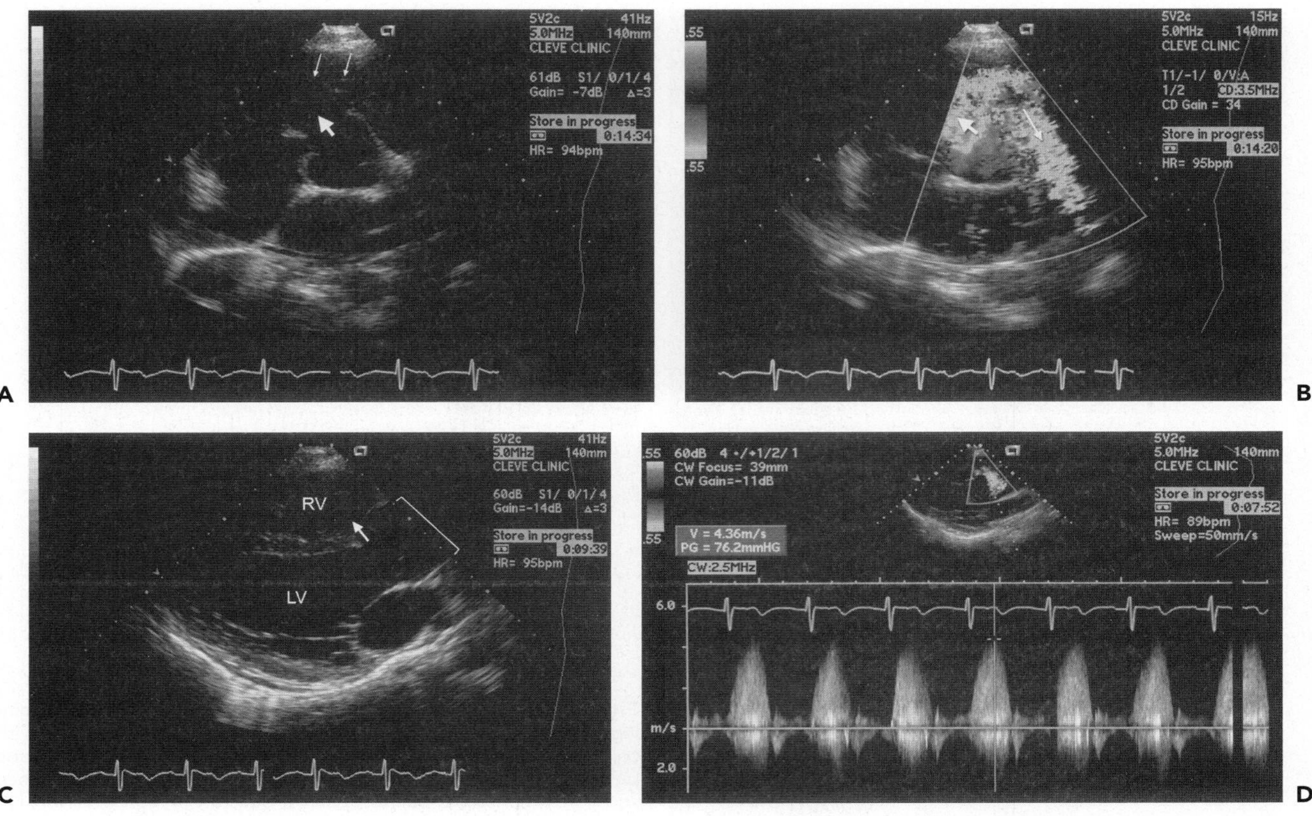


**Figure 41–19** **A:** Parasternal short-axis view demonstrating a large, nonrestrictive VSD (*thick arrow*) and infundibular PS (*thin arrows*) with hypertrophy of the RVOT. **B:** Parasternal short-axis view with color Doppler showing a large VSD with significant left-to-right shunting (*thick arrow*) and the color acceleration/high-velocity flow associated with subpulmonic PS (*long thin arrow*). **C:** Parasternal long-axis view demonstrating a large perimembranous VSD and an overriding aorta. **D:** Continuous-wave Doppler through the RVOT/pulmonic valve demonstrating the high pressure gradients of the infundibular PS. The peak gradient across the stenosis is 76 mm Hg.

right ventricle. Echocardiographic features include the following (Fig. 41–25A–C):

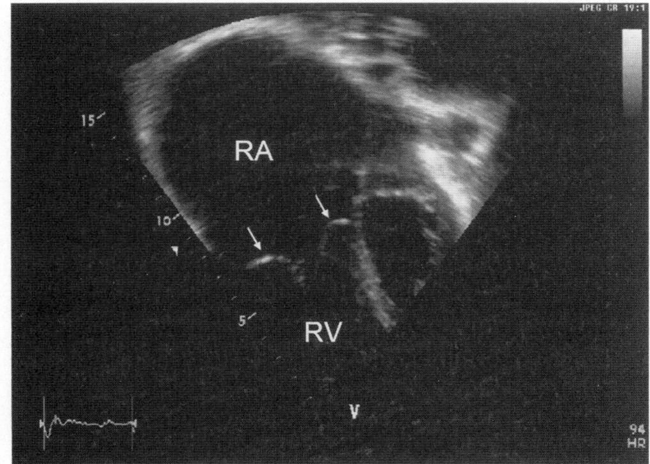


**Figure 41–20** Apical four-chamber view (pediatric view) demonstrating apical displacement of the tricuspid valve with apical tethering of the leaflets causing severe TR. Note the severe right atrial dilatation.

- The tricuspid valve is the apically displaced AV valve with respect to the mitral valve.
- The morphologic RV is identified by the presence of a moderator band and the presence of trabeculations. Recall that AV valves always feed the appropriate ventricle (i.e., TV always feeds the RV).
- The LV is identified by its smooth walls, absence of moderator band, and continuity between the AV and semilunar valves.
- There is discontinuity between the left-sided AV valve and the semilunar valve (aortic).
- The pulmonary artery and aorta run parallel (as opposed to normal orthogonal position). The aorta lies anterior to the PA.

Several associated lesions can be found in patients with congenitally corrected transposition of the great arteries. Abnormalities of left-sided tricuspid valve occur in 90% of patients. Ebstein-type abnormality is the most common of these, with apical displacement of the valve and the septal leaflet typically being most deformed. VSD occurs in 70% of patients, most commonly perimembranous. Pulmonic

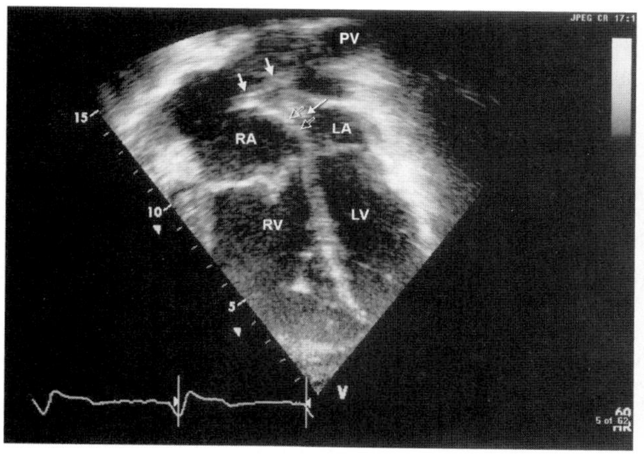


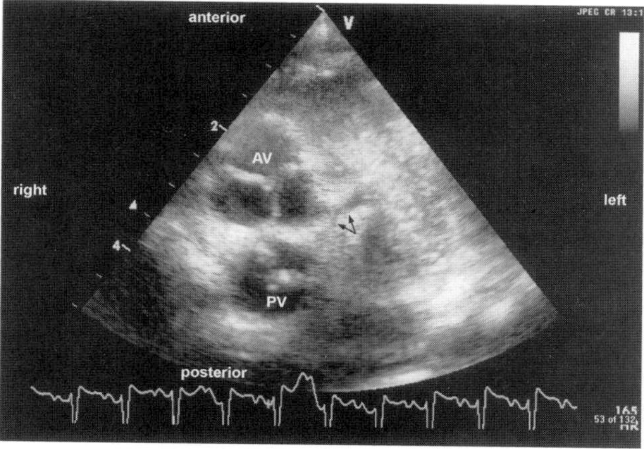


**Figure 41–21** **A:** Apical four-chamber view with baffles (*arrows*) at the atrial level directing blood from the pulmonary veins to the RA and caval flow directed to the left atrium. Note that the pacemaker wire is within the left atrium (a clue to the presence of D transposition). **B:** Parasternal short-axis view of both the aortic and pulmonic valves showing the parallel course of the great vessels in D transposition of the great arteries. In D transposition, the aorta (with the left coronary artery marked by *arrows*) is located anterior and to the right of the pulmonary artery.

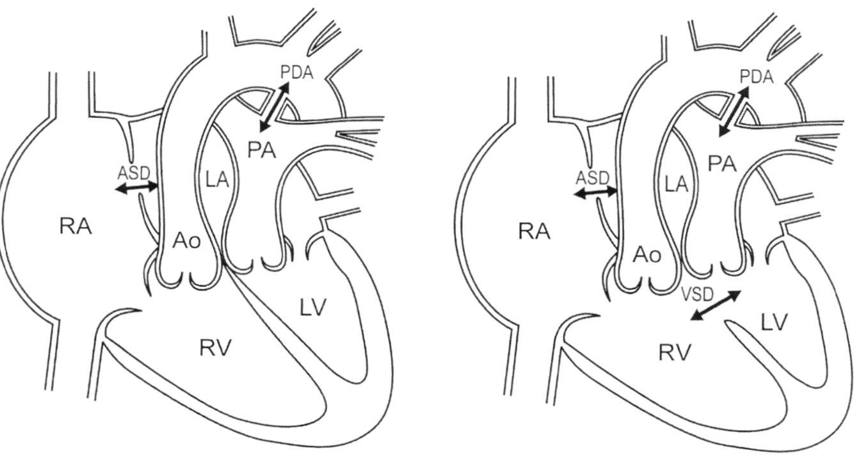


**Figure 41–22** Diagram of D transposition both with and without VSD.

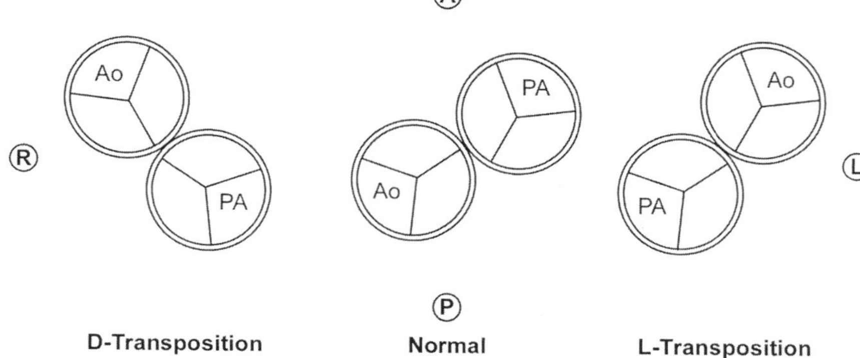


**Figure 41–23** Relative position of great arteries in TGA. Normal position of great arteries **(center):** the pulmonary artery wraps anteriorly around the aorta. D transposition **(left):** great arteries run parallel, with the aorta anterior and to the right of the pulmonary artery. L transposition **(right):** great arteries run parallel with the aorta anterior and to the left of the pulmonary artery.

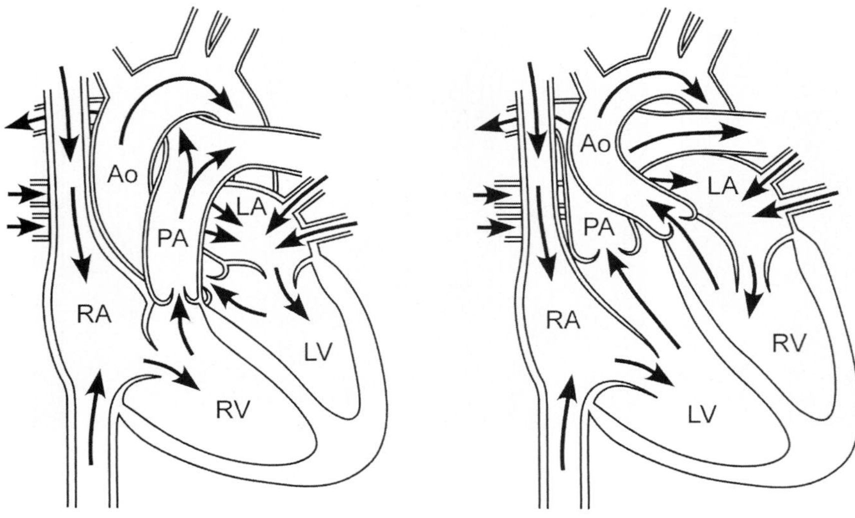


**Figure 41–24** Normal blood flow versus blood flow and anatomy in congenitally corrected transposition. In congenitally corrected transposition **(right),** systemic venous return ⟶ RA ⟶ LV ⟶ PA ⟶ lungs. Pulmonary venous return ⟶ LA ⟶ RV ⟶ Aorta ⟶ body.

outflow obstruction (i.e., LVOT obstruction) occurs in 40% of patients, sometimes in conjunction with VSD. Patients have an increased risk of acquired complete heart block due to the abnormally placed AV node.

On chest radiograph, because the aorta is anterior and to the left, the left heart border is straightened. The left PA is not well defined. If there is PS, there may be decreased lung markings; and if there is a VSD, there may be increased lung markings.

On ECG, typically one can see left-axis deviation. A variety of AV node conduction abnormalities may be seen and over time progress to complete heart block.

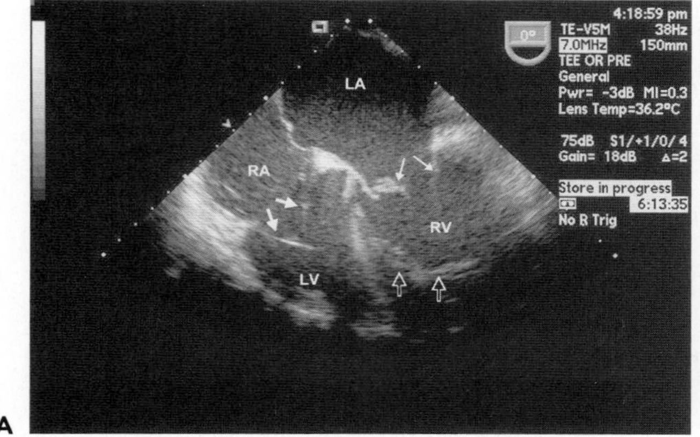


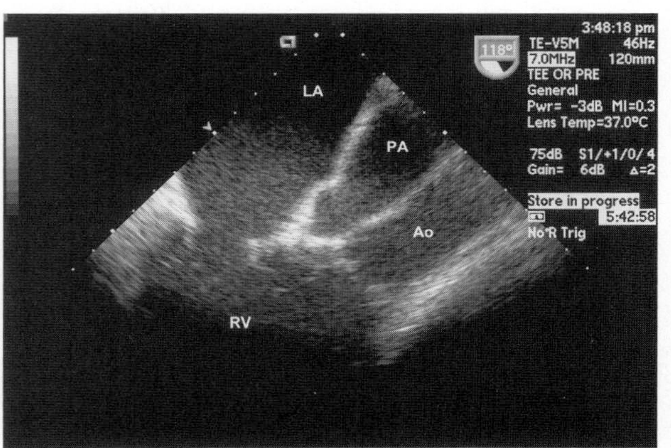


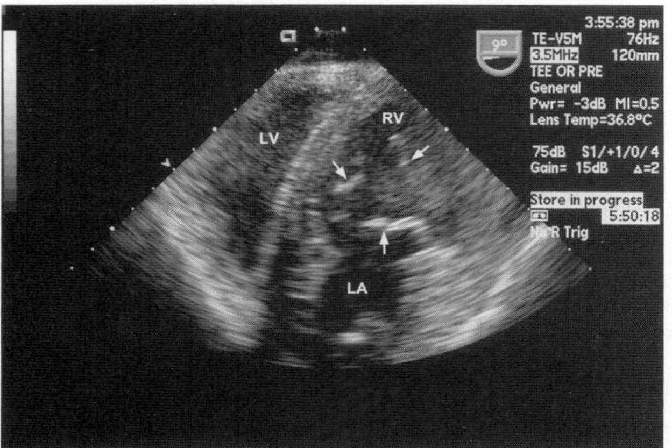


**Figure 41–25** **A:** Apical four-chamber view of a patient with congenitally corrected transposition of the great arteries with an apically placed tricuspid valve on the left side of the heart with the systemic RV. Note the location of the moderator band within the systemic ventricle. The LV pumps blood to the lungs. **B:** Transesophageal echocardiogram demonstrating the parallel course of the great arteries with the anterior mitral leaflet contiguous with the pulmonic valve with a separation between the atrial mitral leaflet and the aortic valve. **C:** Deep transgastric view demonstrating the systemic RV with the left-sided tricuspid valve (*arrows*).

**TABLE 41–3**
**PALLIATIVE AND CORRECTIVE OPERATIONS FOR CONGENITAL HEART LESIONS**

| Name of Operation | Palliative vs. Corrective | Anatomy/Description | Goal/Outcome |
|---|---|---|---|
| Blalock–Taussing shunt (classic) (1944) | P | Shunt from subclavian artery to pulmonary artery | ↑ pulmonary blood flow |
| Modified Blalock–Tassing shunt | P | Gortex interposition graft from subclavian artery to pulmonary artery | ↑ pulmonary blood flow |
| Potts shunt (1946) | P | Anastomosis of descending aorta & left pulmonary artery | ↑ pulmonary blood flow |
| Waterston shunt (1960) | P | Anastomosis of ascending aorta to right pulmonary artery | ↑ pulmonary blood flow |
| Central shunt | P | Gortex graft from ascending aorta to pulmonary artery | ↑ pulmonary blood flow |
| Glenn shunt (1954) | P | Shunt from SVC to right pulmonary artery | Provides low-pressure flow to pulmonary artery |
| Pulmonary artery band | P | Band around main pulmonary artery | ↓ pulmonary blood flow |
| Fontan operation | C | Separate systemic & pulmonary circulations by creating cavopulmonary connection | ■ Directs systemic venous blood to lungs<br>■ Allows ventricle(s) to pump pulmonary venous blood to body<br>■ ↓ Volume load from single ventricle |
| Jatene (1975) | C | Arterial switch for transposition | |
| Mustard (1964) | C | Pericardial baffle to redirect pulmonary venous return toward tricuspid valve & systemic return toward MV | Atrial-level correction for transposition |
| Sennig (1959) | C | | Atrial-level connection/inversion for D transposition |
| Rastelli (1969) | C | Connecting LV with aorta & RV with PA | Providing corrected circulation—LV pumping to systemic circulation & RV-to-pulmonary circulation |

LV, left ventricle; RV, right ventricle; PA, pulmonary artery; SVC, superior vena cava; MV, mitral valve;

## OPERATIONS FOR CONGENITAL HEART DISEASE

Surgical techniques to treat congenital heart disease have evolved over the last 50 years. Early techniques were predominantly palliative, providing temporary relief of symptoms or of a clinical condition. Over time, with improvement in diagnostic as well as surgical capabilities, corrective techniques were developed. Corrective operations can achieve "normal anatomy," "normal hemodynamics," and/or normal physiology. Some surgical approaches may require staged procedures. The trend has been toward performing corrective procedures earlier, with fewer palliative procedures being performed. Many acronyms are used to describe the various surgical techniques (Table 41–3). As more of these surgical techniques are performed, more of these patients will survive into adulthood and will transition to the care of specialists in adult cardiology. Having a basic knowledge of simple congenital heart disease as well as of classic postoperative conditions will be useful for all cardiologists.

## BIBLIOGRAPHY


**Child SJ.** Echocardiographic evaluation with postoperative congenital heart disease. In: Otto CM, ed. *The Practice of Clinical Echo.* Philadelphia: WB Saunders; 1997:719–752.

**King ME.** Echocardiographic evaluation of the adult with unoperated congenital heart disease. In: Otto CM, ed. *The Practice of Clinical Echo.* Philadelphia: WB Saunders; 1997:697–728.

**Marelli AJ, Moodie DS.** Adult congenital heart disease. In Topol EJ, ed. *Textbook of Cardiovascular Medicine.* Lippincott Williams & Wilkins; 2002:707–731.

**Moore JD, Moodie DS.** Adult congenital heart disease. In: Marso SP, Griffin BP, Topol EJ, eds. *Manual of Cardiovascular Medicine.* Philadelphia: Lippincott Williams & Wilkins; 2000:387–407.


## QUESTIONS

1. A cleft mitral valve is associated with which of the following conditions?
   a. Secundum ASD
   b. Primum ASD
   c. Coarctation of the aorta
   d. Sinus venosus ASD
   e. Tetralogy of Fallot

Answer is b: A cleft mitral valve is part of an atrioventricular canal defect, which is due to failure of the embryonic endocardial cushions to meet and partition the heart normally. A complete endocardial cushion defect has four components: primum ASD, cleft mitral valve, inlet VSD, and a widened anteroseptal tricuspid commissure. A partial AV canal defect does not have the VSD.

**2.** All of the following regarding bicuspid aortic valves are true *except:*

a. May be associated with coarctation of the aorta
b. Often associated with posteriorly directed jets of AI
c. Commonly seen with congenitally corrected transposition of the great vessels
d. May be amenable to aortic valve repair
e. Most common type involves fusion of the RCC and LCC

Answer is c: The most common form is fusion of the RCC and LCC, and the mechanism of AI in those patients is prolapse of the conjoined cusp. The conjoined cusp in the case of RCC and LCC fusion is anterior, and thus the AI is directed posteriorly. At least 50% of patients with coarctation of the aorta have a bicuspid valve. A bicuspid aortic valve with severe aortic insufficiency can often be surgically repaired, depending on the expertise of the surgical center.

**3.** A sinus venosus ASD is most often associated with which of the following?

a. Coarctation of the aorta
b. Marfan syndrome
c. Partial anomalous pulmonary venous drainage
d. Tetralogy of Fallot

Answer is c: A sinus venosus ASD is a defect located near the junction of the IVC or SVC and the RA. It is typically difficult to see by surface echocardiogram, often requiring a TEE for diagnosis. It is usually associated with drainage of the right pulmonary veins to the RA.

**4.** All of the following regarding Ebstein's anomaly are true *except:*

a. A portion of the RV is atrialized.
b. TV leaflets are dysplastic and adherent to the RV.
c. Common important associated defects include pulmonic stenosis or atresia.
d. A PFO or secundum ASD is associated in >50% of cases.
e. A common associated defect is coarctation of the aorta.

Answer is e: Ebstein's anomaly of the tricuspid valve is characterized by apical displacement of the tricuspid valve into the RV. As a result, a portion of the RV becomes atrialized. TV tissue is dysplastic, with portions of the septal and inferior leaflets becoming adherent to the RV. Clinical manifestations depend on associated conditions. An important associated defect is pulmonic stenosis or atresia. Other associations include primum ASD and VSD, and congenitally corrected transposition of the great vessels.

**5.** Complications associated with a subaortic membrane include all of the following *except:*

a. Aortic insufficiency
b. Endocarditis—require antibiotic prophylaxis
c. Left ventricular hypertrophy
d. Atrial arrhythmias
e. May recur postresection

Answer is d: The presence of a subaortic membrane puts a patient at increased risk of endocarditis, due to the turbulent flow caused by the membrane, so antibiotic prophylaxis is recommended. In addition, the turbulent, high-velocity jets produced by the membrane damage the aortic valve over time, and patients often develop AI that requires surgery. The subaortic membrane is a fixed obstruction, which requires the left ventricle to develop high intracavitary pressures for ejection. As the LV pumps against the fixed obstruction, LVH develops (similar to what is seen with valvular AS). Subaortic membranes are known to recur occasionally postresection, although the frequency with which this occurs is unknown.

# 42 Genetics in Cardiovascular Medicine

***Brian K. Jefferson*** ***Eric J. Topol***

The sequencing of the human genome is one of the greatest achievements in science and medicine. That many diseases are heritable has been understood for hundreds of years, but tools giving us the ability to diagnose and treat patients with inherited disorders based on their underlying gene sequence were only recently developed. Many of the tools that have afforded us the ability to diagnose these conditions have also contributed to the development of novel treatment strategies. The advent of these new molecular techniques has pioneered a frontier of cardiovascular medicine, one in which we can apply the fundamental concepts of genetic screening to diagnose and identify the underlying pathology of many diseases, and develop treatments for the diseases themselves. Over the last quarter of a century, these techniques have allowed us to further understand the pathogenesis of inherited disorders such as Marfan syndrome, hypertropic cardiomyopathy, and long-QT syndrome. New treatments for acute coronary syndromes such as recombinant tissue plasminogen activator and the monoclonal glycoprotein IIb/IIIa antibodies would not have been possible without these developments. Therapies for treating cardiomyopathy with stem cell therapy, and large gene association studies to elaborate the causes of complex diseases such as atherosclerosis, are well underway. Although a comprehensive review of genetics is beyond the scope of this book, this chapter will familiarize Cardiology Board examinees with basic genetic concepts, methodology, and terminology. The chapter will also highlight several specific genetic diseases along with key points that will be testable on the cardiovascular Boards.

## DNA AND GENES

Almost every cell in the human body contains the entire genetic blueprint for that individual. This information, known as the genome, is contained on the chromosomes located in the nucleus of the cell. Each human cell contains 23 pairs of chromosomes, one of each pair coming from each parent. The timing and sequence with which this information is copied and synthesized into protein products is a complex regulated series of events that is ultimately the determinant of the properties of each cell and the subsequent individual.

The material that composes each chromosome is deoxyribonucleic acid (DNA). DNA is composed of two long strands of polynucleotide sugars wrapped clockwise around each other into a double helix. Each strand is composed of long polymers of nucleotide subunits. Each subunit is composed of deoxyribose with a phosphate group attached to the 5′-carbon position and a nucleic acid base attached to the 1′-carbon position. The units are linked via a phosphodiester bond between the 5′ position and the 3′ position of the adjacent subunit.

The four nucleic acid bases in DNA are the purines (adenine and guanine) and the pyrimidines (thymine and cytosine). These nucleic acids project at a right angle from each sugar on the subunit and form a complementary pair with the nucleic acid on the opposite strand via hydrogen bonding. The stereochemistry of this interaction results in specific rules governing the nucleic acid base pairs between the strands. As a result, bonding can occur only when adenine on one strand pairs with thymine on the opposite strand, or when guanine pairs with cytosine. Two important consequences arising from the structure of DNA are that (a) each strand has a polarity (5′→3′ or 3′→5′) depending on the open position on the sugar, and (b) each strand forms a perfect reverse copy (sense or antisense) of the opposite strand as they wrap around each other and align in antiparallel fashion.

The base pairs that encode the gene are arranged in multiple discrete packets of information interspersed on the chromosome in a large amount of base-pair "filler" that contains no known specific information. Each gene contains the specific sequence of bases that is required to encode one protein. Overall, the entire genome is made of $3 \times 10^9$ base pairs. Of this large number of base pairs, there are <26,000 genes.

A gene contains a portion of DNA sequence that will eventually be discarded from the final protein, an intron, and the portion that ultimately encodes the final protein, an exon. In addition to the introns and exons, the DNA sequence around the gene itself is composed of regulatory regions that control the timing and quantity of each gene product. These regulatory sequences, called promoters, silencers, and enhancers, are modulated by transcription factors. Transcription factors are a group of proteins that, depending on the regulatory sequence, can turn on, turn off, increase, or decrease the amount of each gene's expression. The complex interaction of transcription factors and the external cellular environment gives rise to the specific genetic profile of each cell and organism.

## DNA TRANSCRIPTION AND PROTEIN TRANSLATION

The process of making a protein from the DNA gene sequence is called translation. Translation begins with transcription, a series of complex events in the nucleus that involves making a single-stranded RNA copy of the DNA gene sequence by a specialized protein, RNA polymerase. RNA is similar to DNA, with two exceptions. First, it is ribose rather than deoxyribose sugars that form its phosphate sugar backbone. Second, the same base-pairing rules governing the parent DNA strand apply, except that uracil is substituted for thiamine in the RNA copy. Thus, the RNA transcript is an exact reverse or antisense copy of the sense-oriented gene sequence and contains both the exons and introns from the parent DNA. The RNA subsequently undergoes further processing, which involves removing the intronic sequences and splicing together the exons to form the final messenger RNA copy (mRNA). The ends of the mRNA are subsequently modified further through capping the 5′ end, adding a polyadenylated tail, and exporting the mRNA transcript into the cytoplasm for translation into the protein.

Protein translation is the process of synthesizing the amino acid sequence of the protein from the nucleotide base sequence of the mRNA. In the cellular cytoplasm, the single-stranded mRNA is bound to a complex group of ribonucleoprotein structures called ribosomes, in which the process of decoding the mRNA and synthesizing protein takes place. Ribosomes bind to and read the mRNA sequence like a ticker-tape, adding amino acids to the growing protein chain based on the sequence or coding of the nucleotides of the mRNA. Each three-base sequence, or triplet, of nucleotides from the mRNA forms a codon that is paired on the ribosome with a specific transfer RNA (tRNA). The tRNA interprets the codon and adds the appropriate amino acid to the growing peptide chain. Because RNA is composed of four nucleotides, there are 64 possible codon triplets. Because only 20 amino acids are commonly found in human proteins, some amino acids can be specified by more then one codon triplet. In addition to the codons that specify each amino acid, other specific codons initiate and terminate the protein synthesis. The rule that governs which codon is translated into which amino acid is known as the genetic code (Fig. 42–1). The genetic code is similar if not identical in almost all species. This conservation of the genetic code and even much of the genetic machinery in the cell forms the basis of many of the powerful molecular technologies, such as recombinant protein synthesis and targeted gene therapies.

## GENETIC TOOLS AND METHODOLOGIES

Because of the extreme complexity of the human genome, it was historically difficult to study the structure and effects of a single gene in an organism. Fortunately, advances in molecular biology over the last 25 years have greatly simplified the complexity of the genome, even allowing us to isolate and manipulate genes themselves. Tools are now available in the laboratory to excise a portion of the DNA sequence from a gene, determine its underlying nucleotide sequence, and copy or clone it in large quantities. DNA isolated from a gene can be altered and reintroduced into bacteria, viruses, and cultured eukaryotic cells to examine the effect of this engineering on the gene's protein product. Further, the effect of the gene on an organism can be observed by placing the engineered DNA into the germline cells of an animal so that the manipulated gene is inherited into every cell of an organism and its offspring.

Cutting DNA is accomplished with specific bacterial proteins called restriction nucleases. Restriction nucleases are bacterial proteins that protect bacteria from foreign DNA by cleaving DNA at specific nucleotide sequences. Native bacterial DNA is methylated, however, which prevents it from being cut by the restriction nucleases. Once DNA is cut into fragments using these enzymes, the cut fragments can be inserted into the DNA from bacterial plasmids or viral vectors. Such pasting together of DNA is accomplished using proteins—ligases—that join the DNA fragments. Restriction nucleases cleave DNA at specific sequences, which

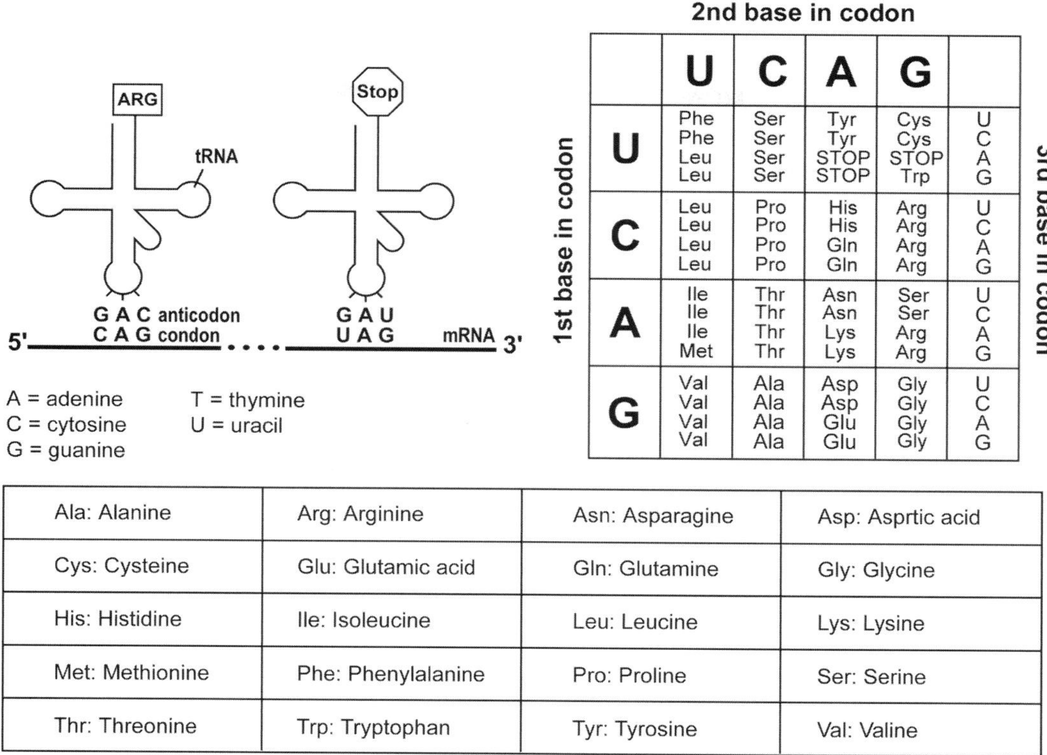


| 1st base | U | C | A | G | 3rd base |
|---|---|---|---|---|---|
| U | Phe | Ser | Tyr | Cys | U |
| | Phe | Ser | Tyr | Cys | C |
| | Leu | Ser | STOP | STOP | A |
| | Leu | Ser | STOP | Trp | G |
| C | Leu | Pro | His | Arg | U |
| | Leu | Pro | His | Arg | C |
| | Leu | Pro | Gln | Arg | A |
| | Leu | Pro | Gln | Arg | G |
| A | Ile | Thr | Asn | Ser | U |
| | Ile | Thr | Asn | Ser | C |
| | Ile | Thr | Lys | Arg | A |
| | Met | Thr | Lys | Arg | G |
| G | Val | Ala | Asp | Gly | U |
| | Val | Ala | Asp | Gly | C |
| | Val | Ala | Glu | Gly | A |
| | Val | Ala | Glu | Gly | G |

| | | | |
|---|---|---|---|
| Ala: Alanine | Arg: Arginine | Asn: Asparagine | Asp: Asprtic acid |
| Cys: Cysteine | Glu: Glutamic acid | Gln: Glutamine | Gly: Glycine |
| His: Histidine | Ile: Isoleucine | Leu: Leucine | Lys: Lysine |
| Met: Methionine | Phe: Phenylalanine | Pro: Proline | Ser: Serine |
| Thr: Threonine | Trp: Tryptophan | Tyr: Tyrosine | Val: Valine |

**Figure 42–1** The genetic code.

are often palindromic. Thus, by cutting the target DNA and a DNA vector with the same enzyme, it is possible to insert the DNA into the vector. The vector and inserted DNA can then be reintroduced or transfected back into cells that are made temporarily permeable to the vector. Ultimately, these transformed cells can be used to make large quantities of DNA, protein product, or to screen another DNA library for genes of interest. This ability to clone, sequence, and manipulate DNA has been made simple and efficient in large part by the development of the technique called polymerase chain reaction (PCR).

## POLYMERASE CHAIN REACTION

PCR is a molecular technique that results in a selective and geometric amplification of DNA of interest to the order of $2^{30}$ to $2^{50}$ times. The result is a millionfold or higher selective amplification that can yield microgram quantities of a DNA sequence in a short time. The PCR reaction attained convenient efficacy with the development of several key molecular tools and techniques. First, the discovery of a heat-stable DNA polymerase from a thermophilic bacteria, *Thermophilus aquaticus*, made available a DNA replication protein that could tolerate the high temperatures required to denature DNA from a double-stranded to a single-stranded form. Second, synthetic oligonucleotides of any sequence can now be produced rapidly and efficiently. Lastly, cheap technology is available to any laboratory to automate the entire process using a small amount of counter space.

The PCR reaction mixture consists simply of a double-stranded DNA sequence, *taq* polymerase, short oligonucleotide primers of 10 to 100 bases, and a mixture of four types of deoxynucleotide triphosphates for building blocks to construct the DNA copies (Fig. 42–2). Each round of amplification involves three rigid thermally controlled steps that lead to amplification of the template DNA sequence. In the first step, the mixture is heated to a temperature sufficient to cause denaturing of the double-stranded DNA template. Next, the mixture is cooled, which allows the denatured strands to aneal to the complementary sequence of DNA primers. Then, with reheating of the mixture, the heat-stable polymerase polymerizes the sequence in between the DNA primers. This sequence is then repeated over and over, allowing the newly synthesized DNA to serve as a further template in the next round of PCR and a doubling of the DNA template from the previous round.

PCR is quite powerful and allows for the detection of a single gene from small amounts of DNA template. In addition, by using specific primers, mutations in the DNA sequence can be detected and identified, thus providing a powerful clinical diagnostic tool.

The ease of synthesizing, sequencing, and modifying DNA using these new molecular techniques confers great power to investigators. Purified DNA can be deliberately

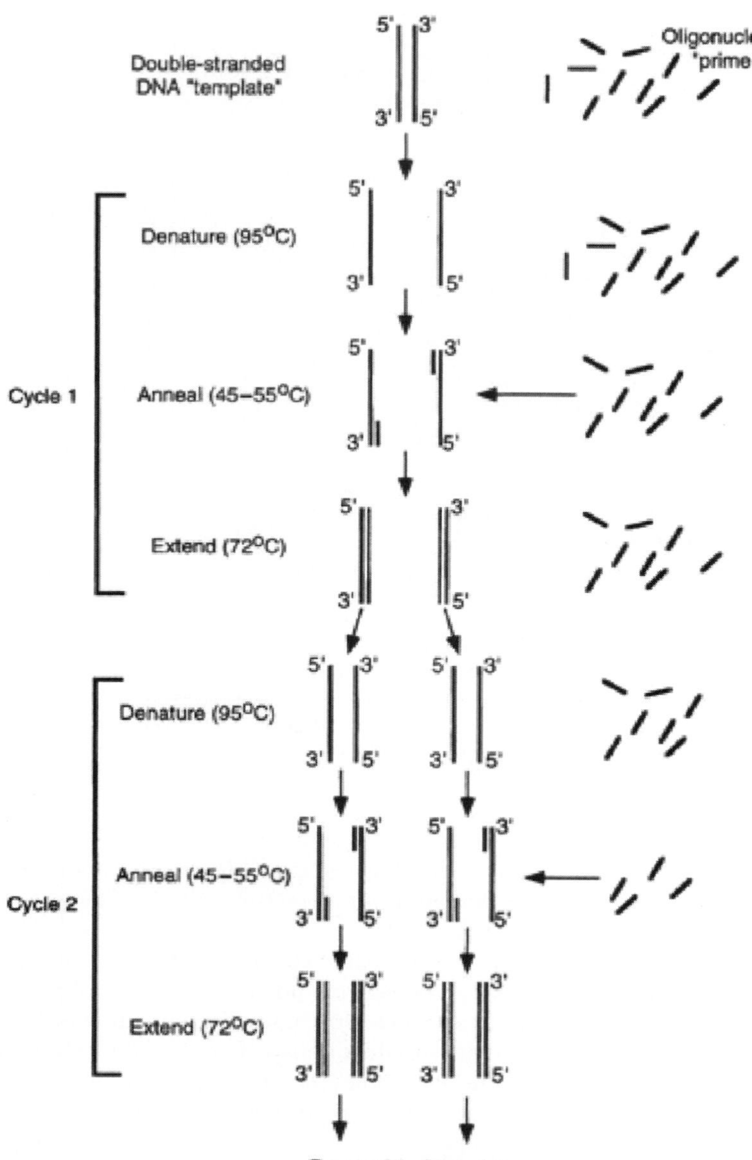


**Figure 42–2** Polymerase chain reaction for amplification of DNA. The schematic shows two complete cycles of polymerase chain reaction. The procedure is repeated, each time doubling the target sequence, and achieving over a million-fold selective amplification of the DNA sequence flanked by the primers. (Reproduced with permission from *The Textbook of Cardiovascular Medicine*, 2nd ed.)

modified or mutated to create novel genes that do not occur in nature. These genetically engineered products provide the potential to generate useful new biologic entities, such as modified live virus, purified peptide vaccines, altered proteins customized for specific therapeutic uses, and altered combinations of regulatory and structural genes that will allow for the generation of new functions by particular gene systems.

## GENETIC ENGINEERING AND DNA MANIPULATION

Once identified and sequenced, knowledge of the gene structure facilitates the study of gene regulation in many ways. DNA probes for molecular hybridization assays can be made from the cloned sequence, which can be used to screen large libraries constructed from any organism's DNA to identify genes of similar phylogeny. The identified gene candidates provide the DNA substrate required to determine the exact nucleotide sequence. Previously, identification of a gene sequence required the purification of large amounts of protein to determine the amino acid sequence. This tedious and time-consuming process was necessary to synthesize enough protein to obtain the sequence. However, current DNA manipulation and sequencing techniques have become so reliable and efficient that it is often easier to clone the gene encoding a protein of interest to determine its DNA sequence. Using the genetic code, the DNA sequence from a gene can exactly predict the amino acid sequence of its protein product. Also, the sequence can be compared with genes from subjects with a disease. Use of this method to compare the normal gene sequence with one known to be abnormal has facilitated the elucidation of the molecular mechanisms underlying various genetic disorders. In this manner, it is possible to identify and screen for specific mutations responsible for various forms of disease.

The conservation of the genetic code and the ease of placing native or manipulated gene sequences into cells allows for the synthesis of large amounts of protein product. Customized regions of synthesized proteins can be used for therapeutic purposes. Examples include the small peptide fragments containing the RGD sequence from the glycoprotein IIb-IIIa receptor, tirofiban, and the fibrinolytic agent, rTPA. The synthesized protein can also be used as an immunogen to synthesize specific therapeutic monoclonal antibodies such as abciximab, the monoclonal glycoprotein IIb-IIIa receptor inhibitor.

## USE OF TRANSGENIC AND KNOCKOUT MICE TO DEFINE GENE FUNCTION

Analysis of the role of genes and gene mutations in living systems has been made possible by the development of methods that allow the production of organisms that are genetically altered at the locus of interest. Using these techniques, genetically altered animals containing a cloned or manipulated DNA sequence can be produced quickly and in large numbers, providing an in vivo model of gene function.

To create a transgenic mouse, exogenous DNA from a gene is injected into a fertilized mouse oocyte pronucleus and reimplanted in a pseudo-pregnant mouse. The gene of interest, or transgene, can be put under the control of a promoter that overstimulates expression of the exogenous gene in every tissue, allowing for assessment of the effect of widespread overexpression of the gene. Conversely, using tissue-specific promoters, transgenic mice can be developed that contain the manipulated sequence only in specific organs and tissues.

Whereas a transgenic model facilitates studying the expression of specific genetic elements, the technique of producing a knockout animal allows us to study the effect of the complete lack of a gene product. To create a knockout animal model, a genetic locus is altered by homologous recombination between the locus and a vector carrying an altered version of that gene. This alteration is accomplished by synthesizing a nonfunctional copy of the gene of interest, with enough DNA to facilitate homologous recombination between the native gene in an embryonic stem cell and the mutated genetic sequence. Thus, the nonfunctional gene replaces the normal gene in the recipient cell. Selection of the cells that undergo recombination is accomplished using a selective marker in the altered gene. The cells with the knockout gene are introduced into the blastocyst of a developing mouse embryo. As these chimeric mice develop, some of the cells that are derived from the altered stem cell will contain the nonfunctional gene. If the germline cells from the mouse contain the altered gene, then some of the subsequent generations of offspring will carry the nonfunctional allele in all of their cells. These heterozygous mice can be further inbred to produce mice that are homozygous for the mutated gene. As these homozygous knockout mice develop, the biologic role of the gene can be studied by observing the result of lack of the gene product. Use of these techniques has further elaborated the understanding of the role of genes and their mutations in cardiovascular health and disease. Effective animal models for complex cardiovascular diseases such as coronary atherosclerosis, myocardial infarction, and dilated cardiomyopathy have been developed.

## GENETICS AND HUMAN CARDIOVASCULAR DISEASE

Just as genes and their interaction with the environment control the normal function and behavior in our body, abnormal physiologic states and diseases can also result from these interactions. Mutations are changes in the structure of an individual gene that can cause changes in the proteins they encode. Depending on the role that a particular protein may play in development and normal physiology, mutations leading to quantitative or qualitative defects in a protein's function can create a wide array of disease states. Hereditary disease can generally be classified into one of three main categories: (a) chromosomal abnormalities, (b) monogeneic or single-gene disorders, or (c) polygenic disorders or complex traits that are the results of interactions among multiple genes. Most of the diseases we encounter and treat in cardiovascular medicine fall into the latter category.

Because of the complex interaction between our inherited genetic blueprint and the environment, a disease may present differently in any given individual. A genotype is defined as the genetic constitution of an individual and refers to what version of a gene (allele) is present in an individual at a specific location or locus on a chromosome. The phenotype is defined as the externally observed characteristics of an individual due to the presence of a particular allele. Genetic heterogeneity refers to the observation that different mutations in the same gene or different genes can cause the same phenotype.

An individual inherits two alleles of each gene, one from each parent. When both inherited copies of the gene are the same, the individual is homozygous for that allele. When an individual has one mutant and one normal copy, then he or she is heterozygous for that allele. Monogenic disorders typically exhibit classic Mendelian patterns of inheritance. The allele is described as dominant if an individual

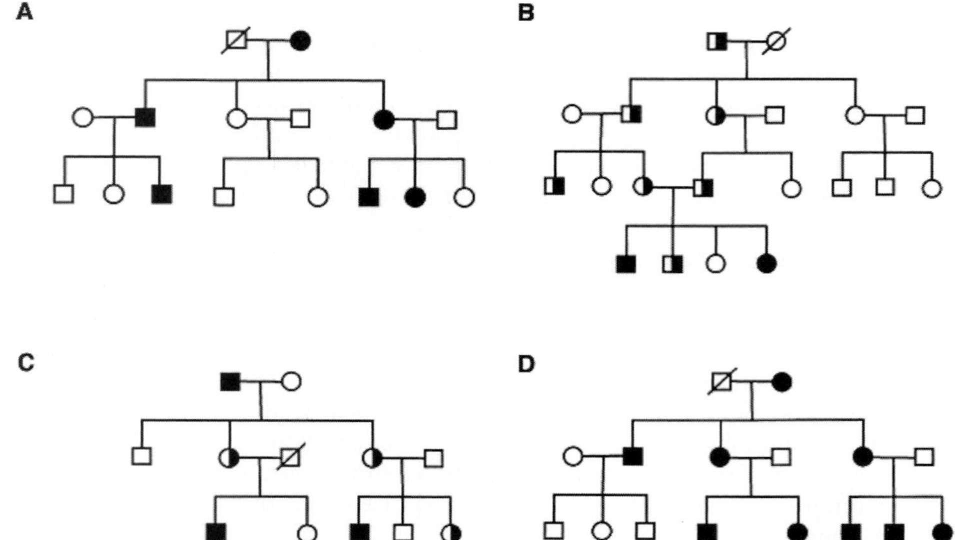


**Figure 42–3** Inheritance patterns of genetic disease. **A:** Autosomal dominant inheritance. **B:** Autosomal recessive inheritance. **C:** X-linked recessive inheritance. **D:** Mitochondrial inheritance. Affected individuals are shown as filled circles (female subjects) or squares (male subjects), and unaffected individuals as empty symbols. Heterozygous carriers in **(B)** and **(C)** are shown as half-filled symbols. (Reproduced with permission from *The Textbook of Cardiovascular Medicine*, 2nd ed.)

has the mutant phenotype despite heterozygosity for the allele. If it takes both mutant alleles to manifest the phenotype, the allele is recessive. Alleles can be inherited on both nonsex chromosomes, or autosomes, and on the X and Y chromosomes. An individual who inherits an autosomal dominant allele has a 50% chance of manifesting the disease; an individual with two heterozygous parents has a 25% chance of inheriting the disease. With X-linked inheritance, generally only males display the disease phenotype (Fig. 42–3).

Locating genes associated with a specific disease state is often a difficult and arduous process. Traditionally, functional cloning has been used to identify and isolate specific genes associated with a particular disorder. In this approach, *a priori* knowledge of an abnormal gene product leads to identification of the mutant gene. Using various microbiologic techniques allows the gene to be cloned, replicated, and studied to characterize the changes associated in carriers of the normal protein and mutation. In most disorders, however, there is no clue as to what the defective gene product is, so an alternative approach known as positional cloning must be employed. This strategy involves mapping the disease phenotype to a particular location on a chromosome and identifying candidate genes and mutations responsible for the phenotype (Fig. 42–4).

The completion of the human genome sequence has shown that only about 2% of the genome actually encodes for functional proteins, with the remainder representing blocks of nucleotides with no known function. Surprisingly, genomes are very well conserved among species. In humans, only about 0.1% of the entire genome, or about 3 million base pairs, represents the variability in individuals in health and disease. The mapping of these small differences, accounting for important regions in the genome, has been catalyzed by the development of powerful new molecular analytical techniques, giving us the ability to rapidly process and analyze large samples of DNA. Two of these molecular analysis techniques are single-nucleotide polymorphism studies and genome-wide scanning.

Single-nucleotide polymorphisms (SNPs) are single-base substitutions resulting from mutation of one nucleotide for another in a DNA sequence. There are >10 million SNPs in the human genome, but only a fraction of these are associated with important functional significance and generation of complex traits. Given the complexity of the human genome, SNPs serve as signal points to help simplify and identify target areas that may contribute to the primary mechanisms leading to the disease state.

Genetic association studies using SNPs provide an analysis of statistically significant relationships between the SNP and the phenotypic differences observed in a population of individuals. The power of a genetic association study is related directly to the number and quality of the SNPs used to screen a population for phenotypic variability. For this reason, large databases of SNPs have been developed along with improved methods to screen immense numbers of SNP candidates. The observed association between a SNP and particular phenotype may be due to a primary effect on the gene product or may result from linkage with nearby genes. For complex diseases such as coronary artery disease, hypertension, or myocardial infarction, a single SNP is not likely to determine susceptibility. Instead, haplotypes, a block of SNPs, combine to exert a biologic vulnerability to the condition. and have validity across populations of ethnic diversity are more useful. There are now several SNPs and haplotypes with clear association and independent replication to complex diseases such as myocardial infarction and coronary disease, such as polymorphisms in the 5-lipoxygenase-activating protein gene.

In addition to high-throughput SNP studies, genome-wide scanning has illuminated other specific genes and

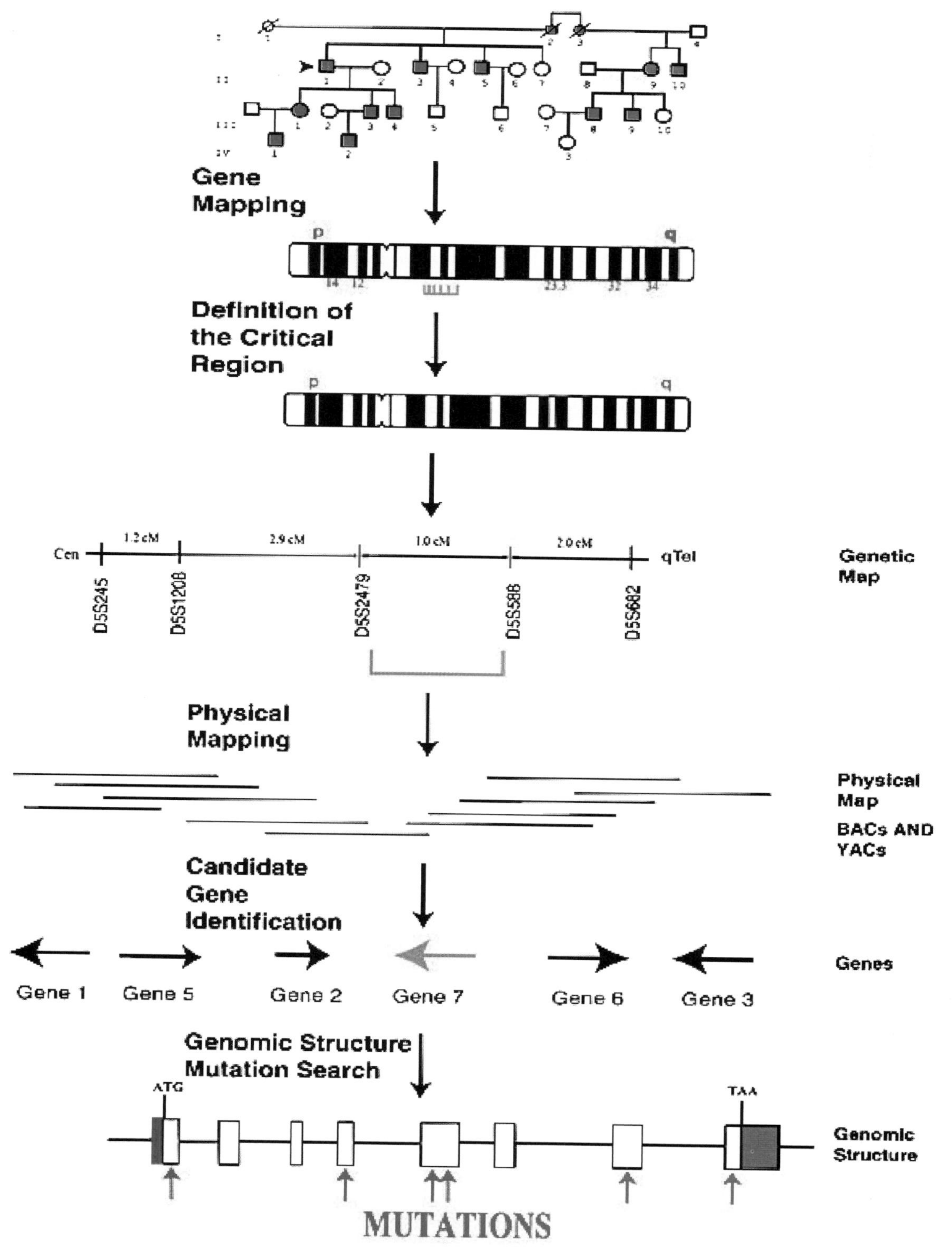


**Figure 42–4** Positional cloning. The major steps are shown in the figure. Bacterial artificial chromosomes (BAC) and yeast artificial chromosomes (YAC) are vectors that are able to clone large segments of DNA. (Reproduced with permission from *The Textbook of Cardiovascular Medicine*, 2nd ed.)

markers for complex cardiovascular disorders. In SNP association studies, a gene candidate is identified and evaluated for association with a particular phenotype. In traditional genome-wide scans, microsatellites (short tandem repeat markers) evenly spaced every 10 cM (centimorgans) across the genome are evaluated to search for a linkage peak of shared alleles in patients with a phenotype of interest. Sections of DNA delineated by these markers may vary among a particular phenotype and thus serve as signals for signs of genetic variation. This variability can be used to determine regions of DNA that may be in proximity to the gene or genes associated with a particular phenotype. As with SNP association studies, there are limitations to this approach. The sections of DNA are large, and a region of interest may contain multiple genes that may or may not have significance. Further fine mapping and analysis of the region of interest must occur to identify the specific locus responsible for the observed phenotype.

These molecular methods are shedding light on complex cardiovascular diseases. Eventually, the map of the human genome will be used to help identify patients with an underlying genetic predisposition for a particular cardiovascular disease. Pharmacogenomics will eventually allow specific pharmacotherapies to be targeted to particular individuals known to be responsive to medical therapies based on their underlying DNA sequence.

In the coming years, a greater emphasis will be placed on these methodologies in the cardiovascular Boards. For now, the main questions of genetics in cardiovascular disease will focus on specific cardiovascular diseases in which either (a) the underlying defect and its phenotypic result is known, such as for Marfan syndrome, or (b) the defect is associated with common disorders such as venous thrombosis, or (c) where underlying risk of the disease can be determined by the underlying DNA sequence, such as long-QT syndrome and hypertrophic cardiomyopathy. The next sections highlight several genetic disorders that are likely to appear on the cardiovascular Boards.

## HYPERTROPHIC CARDIOMYOPATHY

Hypertrophic cardiomyopathy (HCM) is a common autosomal dominant genetic disorder affecting roughly one in 500 individuals in the general population. HCM was first described in 1958 by Donald Teare, who described a unique asymmetric thickening of the left ventricular wall in a series of young adults as a benign muscular hamartoma of the heart. In the classical form originally described by Teare, HCM is pathologically characterized by asymmetric hypertrophy of the ventricular septum below the aortic valve, leading to variable degrees of left ventricular outflow obstruction (Fig. 42–5). However, since the initial description, other forms of HCM have been recognized.

The most common form of HCM, occurring in >30% of cases, involves severe concentric thickening of the left ventricular cavity. The large degree of hypertrophy results in diminished ventricular cavity size and abnormal diastolic function, which leads to classic heart failure symptoms. Other forms of HCM, all of which are characterized macroscopically by global or regional left ventricular hypertrophy, have also been described. Underlying the macroscopic pathology is the histologic triad of extensive myocyte hypertrophy, myocyte disarray, and interstitial fibrosis. Some other inherited diseases have also been described that mimic HCM, including the X-linked recessive glycogen storage disorder, Fabry disease, which can simulate HCM on echocardiogram.

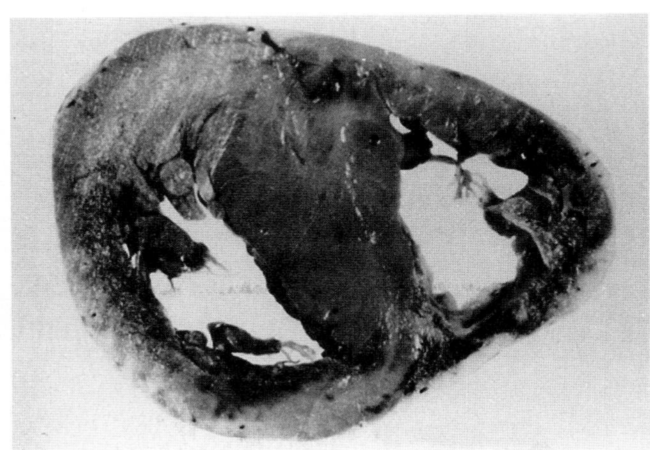

**Figure 42–5** Myocardial section demonstrating the classical appearance described by Tear of severe asymmetric septal hypertrophy in a patient with hypertrophic cardiomyopathy. (From Teare D. Asymmetrical hypertrophy of the heart in young adults. *Br Heart J.* 1958;20:1–8, with permission.)

All of the mutations leading to HCM are in the cardiac muscle proteins, and the disease is best described as a disease of the cardiac sarcomere (Fig. 42–6). Although multiple mutations may lead to HCM, the most common causes are mutations in the cardiac $\beta$-myosin heavy chain, myosin-binding protein C, and cardiac troponins T and I (Table 42–1). HCM is a genetically heterogeneous disorder, having both variability of loci and alleles. For example, mutations in the troponin T gene are associated with a higher incidence of sudden cardiac death and less clinical degree of hypertrophy, different mutations in cardiac $\beta$-myosin heavy chain display early onset of marked hypertrophy and a variable clinical course, whereas mutations in myosin-binding protein C are associated with late-onset hypertrophic changes and a favorable clinical course (Fig. 42–7). Given these facts, some centers now routinely screen family members of HCM patients for particular mutations. However, individuals in the same family or with the same mutation can display phenotypic variability, suggesting extrinsic influences on the disease course and pathogenesis. Consequently, there is no formal recommendation for the use of genetic screening in HCM.

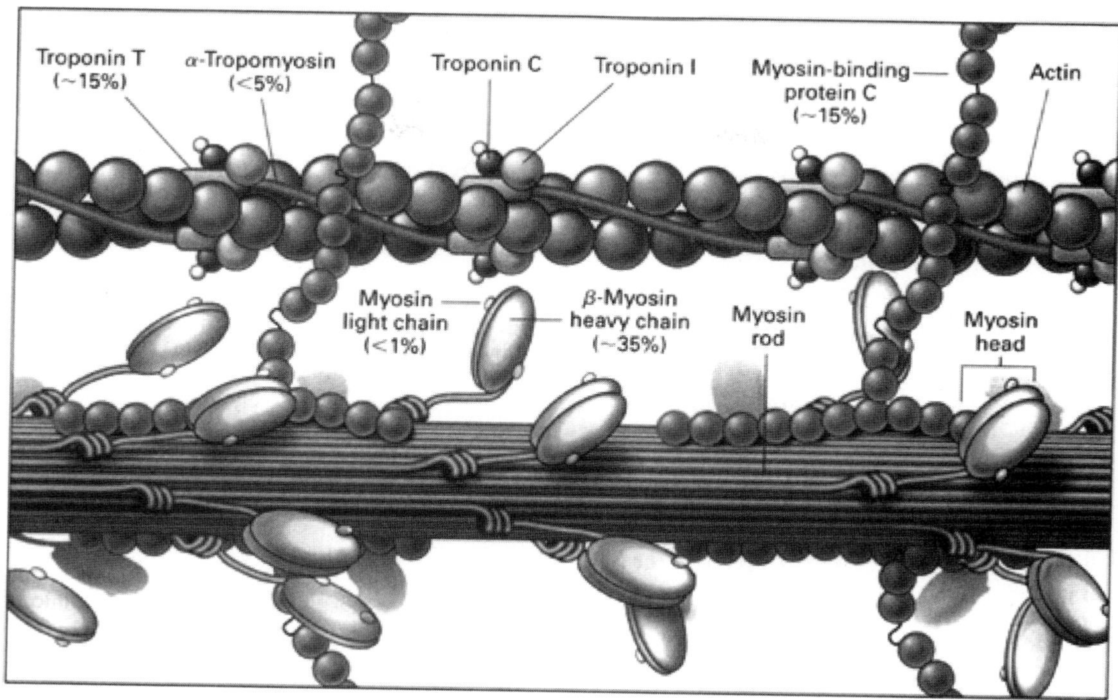


**Figure 42–6** Kaplan–Meier survival curves representing the genetic heterogeneity of hypertrophic cardiomyopathy. The survival of patients with a "benign" β-myosin heavy-chain mutation Val606Met is much longer than that of patients with either troponin T mutations (Intron 15 G1-A, Ile79Asn, D Glu160, and Arg92Gln) or a "malignant" β-myosin heavy-chain mutation, Arg403Gln. (From Watkins H, McKenna WJ, Thierfelder L, et al. Mutations in the genes for cardiac troponin T and alpha-tropomyosin in hypertrophic cardiomyopathy. *N Engl J Med.* 1995;332:1058–1064.)

## MARFAN SYNDROME

Marfan syndrome is an inherited disease that affects the connective tissues of the body, including the skeleton, eyes, and cardiovascular system. Marfan syndrome occurs in all races and ethnic groups with an overall frequency of approximately one per 5,000 to 10,000. Marfan syndrome arises from a mutation in a component of the extracellular matrix structural glycoprotein called fibrillin-1. Fibrillin occurs in two forms, encoded by the FBN1 and FBN2 genes. Marfan syndrome is associated with mutations in the FBN1 gene, located on chromosome 15. Mutations in the FBN2 gene give rise to congenital contractural arachnodactly. The FBN1 gene encodes the protein fibrillin-1, which in polymeric form is one of the main components of microfibrils. The presence of one mutant allele gives rise to a dominant negative mutation whereby the microfibrils contain all mutant monomers. Microfibrils perform many functions in the body. In conjunction with elastin, they form the elastic fibers that are prominent in ligaments and the aorta. They also form the ocular zonules, which hold the lens to the ciliary body in the eye. Defects in these tissues are responsible for some of the main phenotypic manifestations of Marfan syndrome (Figs. 42–8 and 42–9).

There are >500 mutations that have been described in the FBN gene. About 75% of the cases are familial and transmitted in an autosomal dominant inheritance pattern. The remainder of cases are sporadic and arise through *de novo* mutation. Because of high clinical variability, age of onset, and a high rate of new mutations, genetic analysis and diagnosis are difficult outside of families with the classical phenotypes. Despite an understanding of the underlying genetic pathology, diagnosis still relies somewhat on an experienced clinician's evaluation.

**TABLE 42–1**
**CHROMOSOMAL LOCI AND PROTEIN PRODUCTS ASSOCIATED WITH AUTOSOMAL DOMINANT HYPERTROPHIC CARDIOMYOPATHY**

| Locus | Protein |
|---|---|
| 14q11 | β-Myosin heavy chain |
| 1q32 | Troponin T |
| 12q23 | Troponin I |
| 15q2 | α-Tropomyosin |
| 11p11 | Myosin-binding protein C |
| 3p21 | Myosin essential light chain |
| 2q31 | Myosin regulatory light chain |
| 2q31 | Titin |

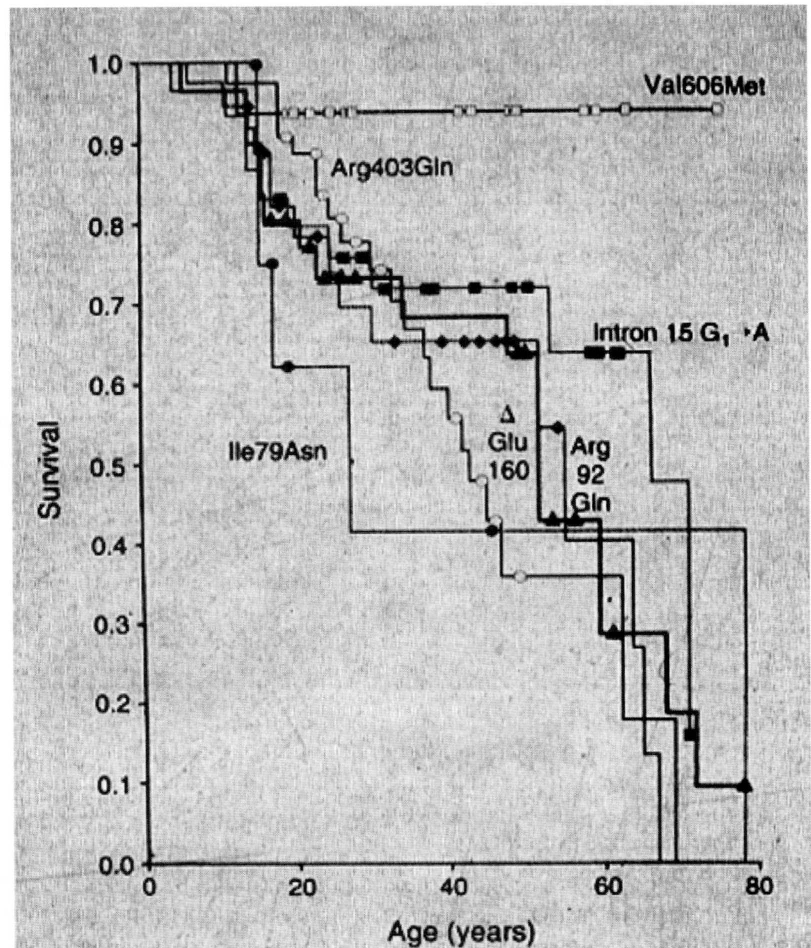


**Figure 42–7** HCM is a disease of the cardiac sarcomere. Structure of the human sarcomere. Cardiac contraction occurs as a consequence of actin–myosin interaction. This is initiated by the binding of calcium to the troponin complex (C, I, and T) and $\alpha$-tropomyosin. Actin then stimulates adenosinetriphosphatase activity in the globular myosin head, resulting in the generation of contractile force. Cardiac myosin-binding protein C binds to myosin and modulates contraction. The estimated frequency of sarcomeric protein gene mutations that cause hypertrophic cardiomyopathy is shown. (From Spirito P, Seidman CE, McKenna WJ, et al. The management of hypertrophic cardiomyopathy. *N Engl J Med.* 1997;336:775–785, with permission.)

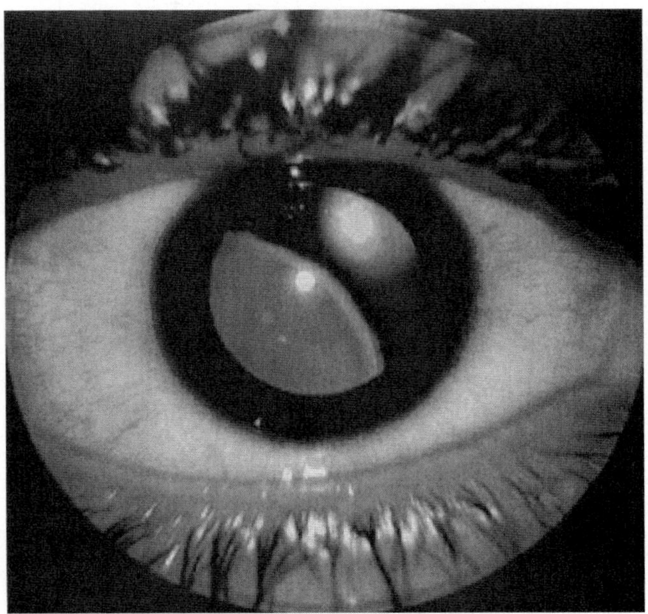

**Figure 42–8** Ectopia lentis: the dislocation of the lens associated with Marfan syndrome.

The criteria for clinical diagnosis of Marfan syndrome are based on a constellation of the specific clinical manifestations found in patients with Marfan syndrome. Criteria that are highly specific for Marfan syndrome are known as major criteria, whereas less specific criteria for Marfan are called minor criteria. Subjects in families with a history of Marfan syndrome are required to have one major criterion and involvement of a second organ system. A patient with no family history is required to have at least two of the major manifestations and involvement of a third organ system. The presence of a known mutation in the FBN1 gene confers the same diagnostic criteria as having a known first-degree relative with the disease (Table 42–2).

Routine screening for aortic root dilatation and improvement in surgical outcomes have markedly improved prognosis for patients with Marfan syndrome, and most patients can expect to survive to advanced years.

## DILATED CARDIOMYOPATHY

Idiopathic dilated cardiomyopathy (DCM) is the most common cause of congestive heart failure (CHF) in young

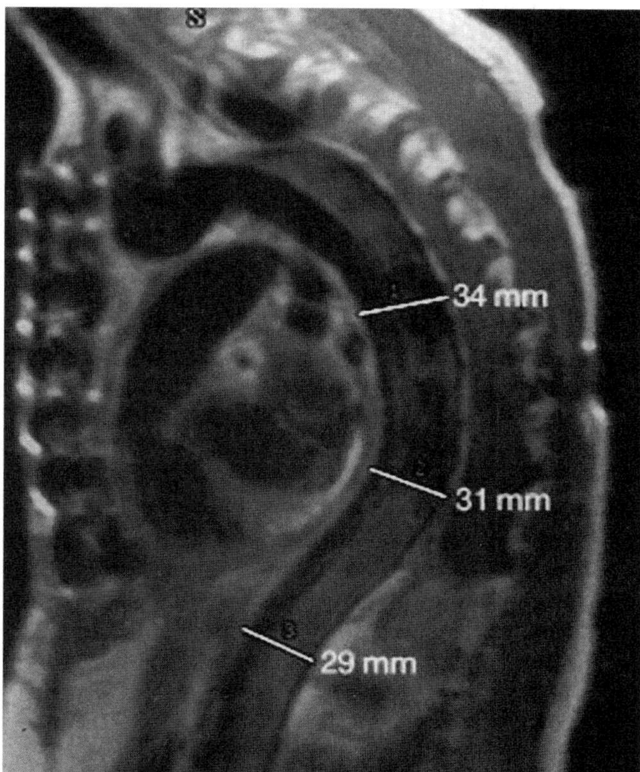


**Figure 42–9** Magnetic resonance scan of the thoracic aorta from a patient with Marfan syndrome. There is dilation of the descending aorta, with an average diameter of approximately 3 cm.

patients in Western society. It is a clinically and genetically heterogeneous disorder that is characterized phenotypically by both increased ventricular chamber size and reduced contractile cardiac reserve in the absence of coronary, valvular, or pericardial diseases (Fig. 42–10). The enlargement and decline of cardiac function are generally accompanied by various forms of CHF symptomatology. Mortality generally results from either sudden cardiac death or pump failure. The clinical course varies in severity, but is overall associated with a 50% mortality within 5 years in the absence of transplantation. The overall prevalence is 40 to 50 per 100,000 persons and may be underestimated, as many asymptomatic patients often go undetected. Up to 35% of patients may have a familial form of the disease. Inheritance patterns of familial DCM (FDCM) are variable and include autosomal dominant, autosomal recessive, X-linked, and mitochondrial inheritance. Mitochondrial inheritance is seen mostly in the childhood forms of FDCM.

The X-linked forms of DCM include X-linked DCM and Barth syndrome. X-linked DCM generally occurs in males in adolescence or early adulthood and is characterized by a rapidly progressive decline in cardiac function. Female heterozygotes typically possess a mild form of the disease, with onset in middle age. X-linked DCM is caused by mutations in the dytrophin gene. There is sometimes a serum hyper-CKemia without any frank skeletal muscle disease. Interestingly, mutations in the dystrophin gene are also associated with the inherited muscular dystrophies such as Duchene and Becker, which often have a cardiomyopathy component associated with the disease. Barth syndrome generally presents in male infants as CHF, neutropenia, and 3-methylglutaconic aciduria. The genetic defect is in the G4.5 gene, which encodes the protein tafazzin, whose protein products are homologous to phospholipid acyltransferases. Mutations in the G4.5 gene are also associated with DCM, HCM, and left ventricular noncompaction.

The autosomal inherited forms of DCM can generally be grouped as either FDCM or DCM with conduction system disease. Clinically, both disorders are genetically heterogeneous. Dilated cardiomyopathy associated with conduction system disease generally presents in patients earlier in life along with mild conduction disease that can progress in severity over time. Although several loci have been mapped in this disorder, the only identified gene product is lamin A/C, located on chromosome 1. Mutations in the lamin A/C gene have also been associated with Emery–Dryfuss muscular dystrophy.

Mutations in $>10$ loci have been mapped in pure autosomal dominant cardiomyopathy. Several of these genes have been identified, including: actin, desmin, d-sarcoglycan, b-sarcoglycan, cardiac troponin T, $\beta$-myosin heavy chain, and $\alpha$-tropomyosin. The underlying common molecular pathways of most of these mutations are in myocardial proteins, leading to abnormalities in contractile force transmission and resulting in cardiac dysfunction (Table 42–3).

## LONG-QT SYNDROME

Long-QT syndrome (LQTS) is characterized by the appearance of prolongation of the QT interval on the surface electrocardiogram (ECG), polymorphic ventricular tachycardia (torsades de pointes), and a high risk for sudden cardiac death. Traditionally, the congenital form of the disease is classified into two forms: (a) Romano–Ward syndrome (RWS), an autosomal dominant disease that is not associated with auditory deficiency; and (b) Jervell–Lange–Nielsen (JLN) disease, an autosomal recessive disease associated with congenital sensorineural hearing loss. More recently, the molecular pathogenesis of LQTS has been elucidated. LQTS is a genetically heterogeneous disorder with seven distinct genotypes distinguished by mutations in at least six different ion channel genes and an anchoring protein (Table 42–4).

The most common form of the LQTS, accounting for almost 50% of patients, is LQT1. The gene responsible, KCNQ1, is found on chromosome 11 and encodes the $\alpha$-subunit of a potassium pore-forming ion channel. Coexpression of KCNQ1 with the $\beta$-subunit gene, KCNE1, forms the slowly activating component of the delayed rectifier potassium current $I_{Ks}$. The KCNQ1 gene consists of 16 exons

**TABLE 42–2**
**DIAGNOSTIC CRITERIA FOR MARFAN SYNDROME[a]**

| System | Major Criteria | Minor Criteria |
|---|---|---|
| Cardiovascular system | Dilation of the ascending aorta involving at least the sinuses of valsalva<br>*or*<br>Ascending aortic dissection | Mitral valve prolapse<br>Dilatation of the mPA without cause before the age of 40 y<br>Dilitation or dissection of the descending thoracic aorta or abdominal aorta before the age of 50 y<br>Calcification of the mitral annulus before the age of 40 y |
| Ocular | Ectopia lentis | Flat cornea measured by keratometry<br>Increased axial globe length<br>Retinal detachment |
| Dura | Lubosacral dural ectasia | None |
| Skeletal | Presence of at least four of the following manifestations:<br>■ Pectus carinatum<br>■ Pectus excavatum requiring surgery<br>■ Reduced upper-to-lower segment ratio or arm span-to-height ratio >1.05<br>■ Wrist and thumb signs<br>■ Scoliosis >20° or spondylotheis<br>■ Reduced extension at the elbows <170°<br>■ Pes planus<br>■ Protrusion acetabulae | Pectus excavatum of moderate severity<br>Joint hypermobility<br>Highly arched palate<br>Characterisitic facies |
| Family/genetic history | First-degree relative with clinical diagnosis of Marfan syndrome<br>Mutation in the FBN1 gene known to cause Marfan syndrome | None |
| Pulmonary system | None | Spontaneous pneumothorax<br>Apical blebs on radiography |
| Skin and integument | None | Striae atrophicae<br>Incisional hernia |

[a]For index cases, at least two major criteria and one other organ system are required for diagnosis.

spanning over 400 kilobases (kb), with the translated protein forming six transmembrane segments. LQT2 is caused by mutations in the KCNH2/HERG gene on chromosome 7. This gene encodes a potassium channel subunit forming $I_{Kr}$, the rapidly activating component of the delayed rectifier potassium current. Other forms of the disease include LQT3, resulting from a mutation in the gene for SCN5A that encodes the cardiac sodium channel; and LQT4, mapped to the gene ANKB encoding ankyrin-B. Other characterized forms of LQTS are listed in Table 42–4.

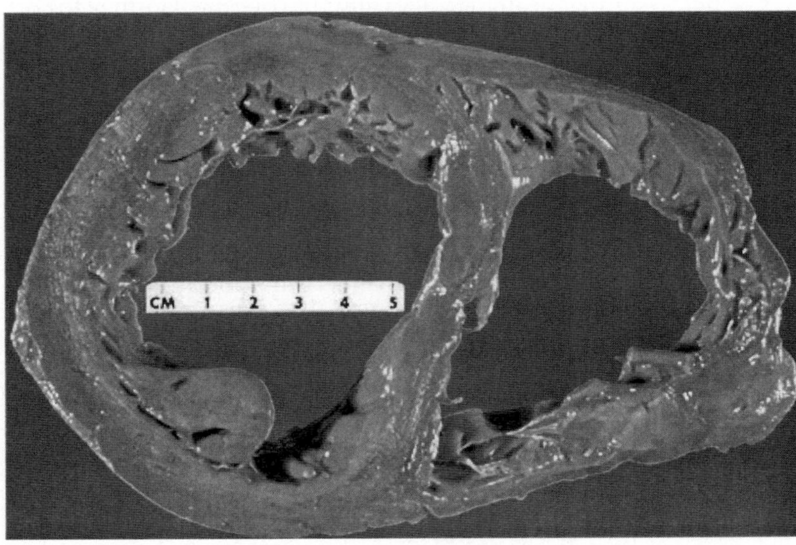


**Figure 42–10** Dilated cardiomyopathy. The cardiomegaly, globular shape of the heart, dilated ventricular chambers, and flattened trabeculae, which are characteristic of this disease, are all evident in this photograph. No significant endocardial fibrosis is present. (Reproduced with permission from *The Textbook of Cardiovascular Medicine*, 2nd ed.)

**TABLE 42–3**

**INHERITANCE PATTERNS OF DILATED CARDIOMYOPATHY[a]**

| Locus | Protein |
|---|---|
| 15q14 | Actin |
| 2q35 | Desmin |
| 5q33 | δ-Sarcoglycan |
| 1q32 | Troponin T |
| 14q11 | β-Myosin heavy chain |
| 15q2 | α-Tropomyosin |
| Mitochondrial DNA | Mitochondrial respiratory chain |

[a]Dilated cardiomyopathy has multiple inheritance patterns and is a genetically heterogeneous disorder involving multiple loci and protein products. The mutations effect proteins involved in cardiac myocyte force transmission.

Clinically, the RWS phenotype is associated with heterozygosity in one of the genes responsible for LQTS. JLN is associated with homozygosity in KCNQ1 or heterozygosity in two alleles of the other genes associated with LQTS. Just as with other conditions, severity of disease is variable with each different mutation. Patients with LQT1 and LQT2 have a higher risk of cardiac events than patients with LQT3, but respond well to beta-blockade. Patients with LQT3 have the highest mortality rate, and implantable cardioverter-defibrillator (ICD) implantation is often recommended.

Phenotypic findings on the surface ECG are also characteristic of the underlying genotype. LQT1 patients generally exhibit symptoms with a higher heart rate and have a broad-based T-wave morphology. LQTS2 patients commonly develop symptoms with auditory stimulation, and the T waves are of low voltage and are often bifurcated or notched. In contrast, patients with LQT3 experience events during sleep, and the ECG shows a late-appearing T wave with a long isoelectric segment.

## INHERITED THROMBOPHILIAS

The incidence of venous thromboembolism is approximately three to five per 1,000 individuals per year, making it the second most common cardiovascular disorder. Virchow's original description of thrombosis included the three components required to initiate vascular thrombosis. This classic triad was composed of (a) damage to the vessel wall, (b) decrease in blood flow—stasis, and (c) a shift toward thrombosis or hypercoagulability. Whereas the first two components of the triad are generally acquired, the last has a significant inherited component, with at least one defect predisposing to thrombosis found in >70% of thrombosis patients. Of these patients, >30% have at least one symptomatic relative. For several decades, inherited ATIII was the only known genetic cause of thrombophilia, but in the early 1980s quantitative deficiencies of protein C and protein S were shown to be associated with venous thromboembolism. However, with a prevalence of only 2.5% and 1.5% in patients with venous thrombosis, respectively, these disorders remained relatively uncommon.

The most significant inherited factor predisposing to venous thrombosis is a mutation in the gene encoding factor V. The original observation of this phenotype by Dahlback showed that addition of activated protein C (APC) to plasma of a thrombotic patient resulted in abnormal coagulation. This phenomenon was subsequently found to be inherited in an autosomal dominant pattern, with a prevalence of almost 50% in patients with a history of thrombophilic disease. The mutation underlying this phenomenon, known as factor V Leiden, involves the loss of an APC cleavage site within the factor V protein. This mutation results from a guanine → adenine base substitution at position 1,691, which causes an arganine-to-glutamine amino acid change at position 506. APC cleavage at this site is necessary for inactivation of factor V, and the site is abolished in the mutant protein. Factor V Leiden is associated with an almost 10-fold increase of venous thromboembolism in heterozygote carriers of the allele and a >80-fold increase in homozygotes. In patients with recurrent thromboembolism, the mutation is found in 40% to 60% of patients. There is an ethnic predisposition for carriers of factor V Leiden, with high frequencies in European populations and low frequencies in those of Asian and African descent.

Another common mutation associated with inherited thrombophilia is a single-base substitution in the prothrombin gene, located on chromosome 11. This mutation is found in 18% of patients with recurrent venous thrombosis and results from a single nucleotide mutation (G → A) at position 20,210, located in the 3′-untranslated region of the gene. Carriers of this mutation have elevated prothrombin levels and a >threefold increase in incidence of venous thromboembolism. Similar to factor V Leiden, the defect is more common in Caucasian populations (2%) than in those of either Asian or African descent.

Elevations of homocysteine are associated with both arterial and venous thrombosis. High homocysteine levels cause an increase in endothelial tissue factor activity and activation of protein C and factor V. Intermediate

**TABLE 42–4**

**LONG-QT SYNDROME IS ASSOCIATED WITH MUTATIONS IN AT LEAST SIX DIFFERENT ION CHANNEL GENES AND AN ANCHORING PROTEIN**

| Syndrome | Locus | Ion Channel | Gene |
|---|---|---|---|
| LQT1 | 11p15 | $I_{Ka}$ | KCNQ1, KvLQT1 |
| LQT2 | 7q35 | $I_{Kr}$ | KCNH2, HERG |
| LQT3 | 3p21 | $I_{NA}$ | SCN5A |
| LQT4 | 4q25 | — | ANKB, ANK2 |
| LQT5 | 21q22 | $I_{Ka}$ | KCNE1, minK |
| LQT6 | 21q22 | $I_{Kr}$ | KCNE2, MiRP1 |
| LQT7 | 17q23 | $I_{KI}$ | KCNJ2, Kir 2.1 |

**TABLE 42–5**
**CLASSIFICATION OF FAMILIAL DYSLIPIDEMIAS**

| Genetic Disorder | Molecular Defect | Lipoproteins Elevated | Lipoprotein Phenotype | Genetic Transmission | Estimated Incidence |
|---|---|---|---|---|---|
| Familial chylomicronemia syndrome | LPL deficiency, apolipoprotein C-II deficiency | Chylomicrons | Type I | Autosomal recessive | Rare |
| Familial dysbetalipoproteinemia | Abnormal apolipoprotein E | Chylomicron and VLDL remnants | Type III | Autosomal recessive or autosomal codominant | 1/5,000 |
| Familial combined hyperlipidemia | Unknown | VLDL and LDL | Type IIb, sometimes IIa or IV, rarely V | Autosomal dominant | 1/200 |
| Familial hypertriglyceridemia | Unknown | VLDL, occasionally chylomicrons | Type IV, occasionally V | Autosomal dominant | 1/500 |
| Familial hepatic lipase deficiency | Hepatic lipase | VLDL remnants | Type III deficiency | Autosomal recessive | Rare |
| Familial hypercholesterolemia | LDL receptor | LDL | Type IIa | Autosomal codominant | 1/500 |
| Familial defective apolipoprotein B-100 | Abnormal apolipoprotein B-100 | LDL | Type IIa | Autosomal codominant | 1/700 |

LDL, low-density lipoprotein; LPL, lipoprotein lipase; VLDL, very-low-density lipoprotein.
Reproduced with permission from *Textbook of Cardiovascular Medicine*, 2nd ed.

homocyteinuria is inherited as an autosomal recessive disorder and is associated with up to a threefold increase in cardiovascular disease.

## FAMILIAL HYPERLIPIDEMIA

Traditionally, the classification of primary disorders of lipoprotein metabolism was based on which lipoprotein fraction was elevated. More recently, classification systems based on the molecular etiology of the dyslipidemia or on the level of elevation in the triglyceride fraction have become more useful and practical (Table 42–5).

Marked elevations of triglycerides levels, >1,000 mg/dL, are associated with the familial chylomicronemia (FC) syndrome and type V hyperlipoproteinemia. FC usually presents in childhood with acute pancreatitis and a triglyceride level >1,000 mg/dL. Affected children have eruptive xanthomas, lipemia retinalis, hepatosplenomegaly, and pancreatitis. The disorder itself is not associated with premature atherosclerotic disease. FC is autosomal recessive and is associated with two underlying genetic defects, mutation in either lipoprotein lipase (LPL) or apolipoprotein C-II. Defects in either of these genes result in a functional deficiency of LPL, with inability to hydrolyze tryglycerides from chylomicrons, causing hyperchylomicronemia. Heterozygotes have normal or near-normal levels of TG. FC is rare, with lipoprotein lipase deficiency the more common of the two mutations. Type V hyperlipoproteinemia is more common than familial chylomicronemia and is associated clinically with TG levels >1,000 mg/dL in the absence of one of the mutations causing FC. The molecular mechanism responsible for the disorder is unknown.

Familial dysbetalipoproteinemia is associated with modest to severe elevations in serum TG levels and clinically with premature atherosclerosis, xanthomas (tuberoeruptive and palmar), and hyperlipidemia. Peripheral vascular disease is also common. In contrast to lipoprotein lipase deficiency, patients generally have both hypertriglyceridemia and hypercholesterolemia, with elevations of both fractions to similar levels. High-density lipoprotein (HDL) is usually in the normal range. The underlying molecular defect is a mutation in the gene that encodes apolipoprotiein E (ApoE). ApoE is present on both chylomicron and very-low-density lipoprotein (VLDL) remnants and facilitates hepatic clearance by the liver. Mutation in Apo-E causes accumulation of chylomicrons and VLDL remnants in the circulation. The most common form of familial dysbetalipoproteinemia is associated with a common polymorphism of ApoE. The normal form of ApoE is ApoE3. The ApoE2 polymorphism has a gene frequency of 7% and results in a single amino acid change from the ApoE protein. ApoE2 results in defective binding to the LDL receptor, leading to dyslipidemia. Homozygosity of ApoE2 causes the most common form of familial dysbetalipoproteinemia, but other mutations associated with the disorder have been described in the ApoE gene. Interestingly, another polymorphism in the ApoE gene, ApoE4, is associated with coronary heart disease and Alzheimer disease but not familial dysbetaproteinemia.

Familial combined hyperlipidemia is the most common hereditary primary lipid disorder in humans. This form of hyperlipidemia is associated with premature atherosclerotic disease, and the disorder is usually associated with mixed dyslipidemia characterized by moderate elevations of triglycerides, increased total cholesterol, high LDL, and low HDL. It is often associated with obesity and insulin resistance, and usually a first-degree relative has the condition. FCL is inherited in an autosomal dominant pattern, with full expression increasing at onset of maturity. FCL is often associated with high levels of ApoB, which gives rise to highly atherogenic, small dense LDL particles. The underlying molecular defect that causes FCL is unknown.

Familial hypercholesterolemia is associated with normal triglyceride levels and is caused by mutations in the gene for the LDL receptor that result in the inability to bind and internalize LDL, thus leading to a high LDL level. It is a genetically heterogenous disorder, with >200 mutations of differing severity described in the LDL receptor. FH has an autosomal codominant inheritance pattern in which heterozygote carriers of the mutation possess an elevated level of cholesterol and homozygotes have more severe hypercholesterolemia. Carriers of the mutant allele are found in about one in 500 individuals in the North American population. The disorder is characterized by an elevated LDL fraction, generally between 200 and 400 mg/dL. Physical findings include tendonous xanthomas and xanthelasma. Another inherited dyslipidemia, which clinically resembles FHC, is familial defective apolipoprotein B-100.

## BIBLIOGRAPHY


**Antzelevitch C.** Molecular genetics of arrhythmias and cardiovascular conditions associated with arrhythmias. *J Cardiovasc Electrophysiol.* 2003;14(11):1259–1272.

**Bashyam MD, Savithri GR, Kumar MS, et al.** Molecular genetics of familial hypertrophic cardiomyopathy (FHC). *J Hum Genet.* 2003; 48(2):55–64.

**Hughes SE, McKenna WJ.** New insights into the pathology of inherited cardiomyopathy *Heart.* 2005;91(2):257–264.

**Jefferson, BK, Topol ET.** Molecular mechanisms of myocardial infarction.

**Leiden J.** Principles of cardiovascular molecular biology and genetics. In: Braunwald E, Zipes DP, Libby P, eds. *A Textbook of Cardiovascular Medicine.* Philadelphia: WB Saunders; 2001:1955–1976.

**Lieb ME, Taubman MB.** General techniques in molecular cardiology. In: Topol EJ, ed. *Textbook of Cardiovascular Medicine.* Philadelphia: Lippincott Williams & Wilkins; 2002:1951–196.

**Marz W, Nauck M, Wieland H.** The molecular mechanisms of inherited thrombophilia. *Z Kardiol.* 2000;89(7):575–586.

**Pecheniuk NM, Walsh TP, Marsh NA.** DNA technology for the detection of common genetic variants that predispose to thrombophilia. *Blood Coagul Fibrinol.* 2000;11(8):683–700.

**Pyeritz R.** Principles of cardiovascular molecular biology and genetics. In: Braunwald E, Zipes DP, Libby P, ed. *A Textbook of Cardiovascular Medicine.* Philadelphia: WB Saunders; 2001:1977–2018.

**Rader D.** Lipid disorders. In: Topol EJ, ed. *Textbook of Cardiovascular Medicine.* Philadelphia: Lippincott Williams and Wilkins; 2002: 43–74.

**Towbin JA, Bowles NE.** The failing heart. *Nature.* 2002;415(6868): 227–233.

**Wang Q, Bond M, Elston R, Tian Xiao-Li.** Molecular genetics. In: Topol EJ, ed. *Textbook of Cardiovascular Medicine.* Philadelphia: Lippincott Williams & Wilkins; 2002.

**Wang Q, Pyeritz R, Seidman C, Basson C.** Genetic studies of myocardial and vascular disease. In: Topol EJ, ed. *Textbook of Cardiovascular Medicine.* Philadelphia: Lippincott Williams & Wilkins; 2002:1967–1990.


## QUESTIONS

**1.** Match each of the following terms with the appropriate description.

(1) The process of making a protein from the DNA gene sequence

(2) A series of complex events in the nucleus that involves making a single-stranded RNA copy of the DNA gene sequence

(3) Uracil base-pairs with adenosine

(4) Portion of the gene sequence that eventually be discarded

(5) Portion of the gene sequence that ultimately encodes the final protein

a. DNA
b. RNA
c. Transcription
d. Translation
e. Exon
f. Intron

Answers: (1) d; (2) c; (3) b; (4) f; (5) e. See text for discussion.

**2.** What percentage of dilated cardiomyopathies are directly inherited

a. 5%
b. 10%
c. 35%
d. 50%
e. 75%

Answer is c: The prevalence of dilated cardiomyopathy is approximately 40 to 50 per 100,000. Most cases of dilated cardiomyopathy are idiopathic. However, up to 35% of patients are thought to have a familial component to their disease. Inheritance patterns of dilated cardiomyopathy are variable and include autosomal dominant, autosomal recessive, X-linked, and mitochondrial forms of disease.

**3.** A 23-year-old woman taking an oral contraceptive presents with an acute pulmonary saddle embolus. A mutation in the gene of which coagulation factor is most likely to be found via genetic screening?

a. Prothrombin
b. Protein C

c. Thrombin
d. Factor VII
e. Factor V

Answer is e: Mutations in of many genes that encode proteins in the coagulation pathway have been associated with hypercoaguability. The most significant mutation that increases the risk of venous thrombosis is a point mutation in the gene for factor V, which leads to an arganine-to-glutamine amino acid substitution in the factor V protein. This mutation, known as factor V Leiden, results in the loss of the activated protein C cleavage site in the factor V protein. Heterozygotes with the factor V Leiden mutation have a 10-fold increase in risk for venous thrombosis, whereas homozygotes have up to an 80-fold increase in risk. It is generally regarded that oral contraceptives increase the risk of thrombotic complications in patients with inherited thrombophilia.

**4.** Match the following genes/protieins with their associated diseases:

(1) KCNQ1
(2) Myosin-binding protein C
(3) Actin
(4) Dystrophin

a. Hypertrophic cardiomyopathy
b. Duchene muscular dystophy
c. Dilated cardiomyopathy
d. Long-QT syndrome

Answers: (1) d; (2) a; (3) c; (4) b. See text for discussion.

**5.** A 35-year-old man presents with the acute onset of 10/10 tearing chest pain. Physical exam reveals a tall slender male in moderate discomfort. Closer exam reveals a high arched palate, with long thin fingers. Cardiovascular exam is notable for pectus excavatum, and a II/VI short diastolic murmer. His father died at age 38 years of unknown cause.

Genetic analysis most likely will reveal mutations in which of the following genes?

a. Apo E
b. $\beta$-Myosin heavy chain
c. Dystrophin
d. Fibrillin-1
e. Troponic C

Answer is d: The patient presents with clinical features of Marfan syndrome and an acute aortic dissection. Marfan syndrome arises from mutations in the gene encoding a matrix glycoprotein, fibrillin-1. Many different mutations have been described that may lead to Marfan syndrome.

# Hypertension/ Pulmonary Disease

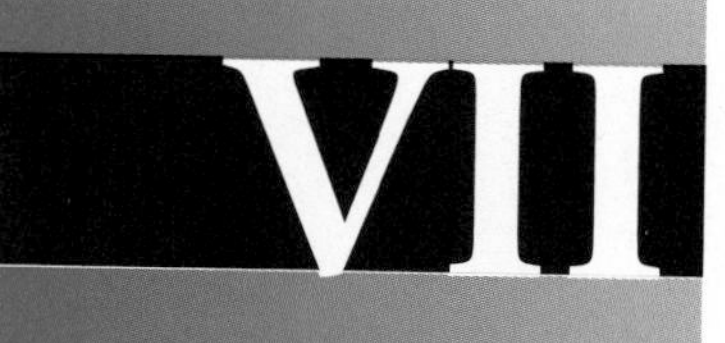

# Hallmarks of Essential and Secondary Hypertension

43

*Martin J. Schreiber, Jr.*    *Joseph V. Nally, Jr.*

## PATHOGENESIS OF HYPERTENSION

A number of pathophysiologic factors have been implicated in the development of essential hypertension, making selective mechanistically based antihypertensive therapy in any one patient difficult (1). In a broad sense, increased sympathetic nervous system activity, autonomic imbalance (increased sympathetic tone, abnormally reduced parasympathetic tone), vascular remodeling, arterial stiffness, and endothelial dysfunction contribute to both the development and maintenance of essential hypertension. Increased sympathetic activity may stem from alterations in baroflex and chemoreflex pathways, both peripherally and centrally. The renin–angiotensin system plays a major role in vascular remodeling (alterations in structure, mechanical properties, and function of small arteries) and critical target organ damage (TOD) (myocardial fibrosis, renal injury). In addition, arterial stiffness—a primary contributor to increased vascular resistance, especially with advancing age—results from continued collagen deposition, smooth muscle hypertrophy, and changes in the elastin media fibers. Although intact vascular endothelium is critical to maintaining vascular tone (relaxation and contraction), we now know that multiple insults (decreased nitric oxide synthesis, increased endothelin, estrogen deficiency, high dietary salt intake, diabetes mellitus, tobacco use, and increased homocysteine) can damage vascular endothelium and contribute to important clinical findings. These vascular factors or conditions disrupt normal endothelial function, initiating the cascade of cardiovascular events that results in atherosclerosis, thrombosis, and heart failure.

Renal microvascular disease remains a viable theory as being responsible for the development of hypertension (2). Renal vasoconstriction resulting from the renin–angiotensin–aldosterone system (RAAS) activation, increased sodium reabsorption, and primary microvascular injury may all lead to renal ischemia (particularly in the outer medullary section). Local production of angiotensin-II plus reactive oxygen species at sites of renal injury potentially result in structural alterations and hemodynamic events that cause hypertension (3).

Hyperuricemia in humans is associated with renal vasoconstriction, activation of the RAAS, cardiovascular disease (CVD) risk, and hypertension. Theoretically, uric acid stimulates renal afferent arteriopathy and tubular interstitial disease, resulting in hypertension. As previously reported, renal lesions and hypertension could be prevented or reversed in a rodent model by decreasing uric acid levels coupled with use of angiotensin-converting enzyme (ACE) inhibition, but not hydrochlorothiazide (HCTZ) (4). Continued studies leveraging these observations in humans warrant further investigation. Moving forward, medication selection may be directed as much to specific detrimental microvascular effects as to the actual lowering of blood pressure (BP) to target levels.

## GENETICS OF HYPERTENSION

Hypertension results from a complex interaction of genetic, environmental, and demographic factors. Variation in BP results from the contributions of many different genes (it is polygenic) (5). In most patients with essential hypertension, genetic profiling is not currently beneficial in the diagnostic evaluation. Variations in BP appear to be polygenic in character. Although the majority of cases of essential hypertension are considered polygenic and are characterized by a complex mode of inheritance, there are rare cases of simple Mendelian forms of high BP in which a single gene defect may be largely responsible for the hypertensive phenotype. Improved techniques of genetic analysis (i.e., genetic-wide linkage analysis) have aided in the search for genes that contribute to the development of primary hypertension. Genetic causes of hypertension, though uncommon in the general population, may be more frequent in selective hypertensive populations, particularly patients with resistant hypertension. Genome scans have identified regions of specific human chromosomes that influence BP, which are called the blood pressure quantitative trait loci (QTL) (i.e., chromosome 6.2).

From the clinical perspective, a family with a history of hypertension can be a surrogate marker for undefined, genetically-linked risk factors shared by the family. Risk factors such as obesity, dyslipidemia, and insulin resistance are predictive of future hypertension. Having a single first-degree relative with hypertension is only a weak predictor of hypertension, whereas a finding of two or more relatives with hypertension at an early age (before age 55 years) identifies a smaller subset of families who are at much higher risk for the future development of hypertension (6).

Wilk et al. reported findings to support a link between the quantitative trait age at hypertensive diagnosis and the qualitatively defined early-onset trait in African Americans (7) Several genes with specific salt interactions have been identified, for example, ones for glucocorticoid remedial hypertension, and apparent mineralocorticoid excess (8). In addition, the $\alpha$-adducin gene is associated with an increased risk of renal tubular absorption of sodium, and angiotensinogen gene polymorphism (A-to-G substitution and methionine-to-threonine amino acid substitution) has been linked to an increase in plasma levels of angiotensinogen (9).

Patients with specific gene patterns may respond preferentially to one class of drugs more than another. Patients with the $\alpha$-adducin gene respond best to thiazide diuretics; those with (Met235 thr) angiotensinogen to ACE inhibitor, and calcium channel blocker (CCB) and specific G-protein genes impart response to beta-blockers and diuretics (10).

A number of syndromes represent genetic mutations of hypertension single-gene forms, including glucocorticoid remedial hypertension (chimeric gene formation; autosomal dominant), 11-$\beta$-hydroxylase (mutation in gene encoding), 17-$\alpha$-hydroxylase deficiency, Liddle syndrome (mutation in the sodium channel gene), hypertension exacerbated by pregnancy, syndrome of apparent mineralocorticoid excess, and pseudo-hypoaldosteronism (11). Also, human atrial natriuretic peptide (hANP) is an attractive gene for linking specific population groups to an associated increased risk for hypertension. More recently, polymorphisms of the angiotensinogen gene have been detected in hypertensive patients and in children of hypertensive parents.

The continued advances in molecular biology and newer technologies make likely the possibility of gene expression profiling being applied to hypertensive research, diagnosis, and treatment selection in the future (12).

## SIGNIFICANCE OF SYSTOLIC, DIASTOLIC, AND PULSE PRESSURE

A shift in diagnostic emphasis from diastolic BP to systolic BP has occurred over the last decade (13–15). A reanalysis of the Framingham Heart Study with longer follow-up data and more extensive cardiovascular data tracking showed that at all levels of systolic pressure (even within a normal range), the height of the systolic BP accurately predicted coronary heart disease (CHD) (16). In addition, these data also suggest that the pulse pressure (systolic BP—diastolic BP) is a major independent predictor of CHD. A wide pulse pressure is a marker for large artery stiffness and for vascular aging (arteriosclerosis). Elevated coronary arterial calcification scores are associated with arterial stiffness and increased pulse pressure (17). Age is a determinant of the importance of pulse pressure in hypertension. A growing body of evidence supports pulse pressure readings as an important predictor in patients >65 years of age (18,19). Furthermore, pulse pressure may be a strong predictor of CV risk in the presence of compromised ventricular function with normal or low systolic BP (20).

Therefore, systolic BP, diastolic BP, and pulse pressure are important in staging hypertension at different ages. Earlier generations of physicians favored the importance of diastolic BP over systolic, in part because hypertension was apparently a young person's disease. With the aging of the population, hypertension has become a disease of older patients specifically reflected by isolated systolic hypertension (ISH). As arteries stiffen and pulse wave amplification decreases with aging, a general shift in elevation occurs from diastolic BP to systolic BP, and eventually in some, to pulse pressure as predictors of CV risk (21).

There are patients in whom pulse pressure does not represent arterial stiffness (discrepancy between central and brachial pulse pressure, mild arterial stiffness, increased cardiac output, variable heart rate, and vasodilation). Moreover, pulse pressure cannot replace systolic BP as a single measure of CHD risk. Systolic BP and diastolic BP together are frequently superior to systolic BP alone in predicting CV risk. From a practical standpoint, physicians should first measure systolic BP (especially in healthy middle-aged and elderly cohorts), and then adjust risk upward for pulse pressure if there is a discordantly low diastolic BP (post–myocardial infarction, heart failure, end-stage renal disease (ESRD), etc.). Only when there is a discordantly low diastolic BP does pulse pressure embellish systolic BP in predicting CV risk.

## EVALUATION OF HYPERTENSION

A complete history, physical examination, basic serum chemistries, urinalysis, and electrocardiogram (ECG) are recommended for the initial evaluation of a hypertensive patient. Urinalysis is especially important because of the impact that renal disease has on both treatment selection and target goals for BP lowering.

The patient's history should include a detailed family history, notation of early cerebrovascular hemorrhagic stroke (if <60 years old), nonprescription medications (nonsteroidal anti-inflammatory drugs, diet pills, decongestants, appetite suppressants, herbal therapy), birth control pills, alcohol/street drugs, and sleep history. The physician should always be alert to history or physical exam findings that suggest a secondary cause for the hypertension.

The physical examination should include two or more BP measurements separated by 2 minutes, with the patient either supine or seated, and after standing for at least 2 minutes, in accordance with recommended techniques. BP should be verified in the contralateral arms; if values are different, the higher value should be used. Measurements of height, weight, and waist circumference should be obtained. Special attention should be directed to the funduscopic examination, the presence or absence of carotid bruits or distended neck veins, thyroid enlargements; and examination of the heart, lungs, abdomen, and extremities. Particular attention should be directed to peripheral pulses, presence of abdominal bruits, and presence or absence of edema. A neurologic assessment should also be performed.

The presence of significant arteriosclerosis or arteriovenous nicking on funduscopic examination indicates in most cases that the BP has been elevated for >6 months. Arteriolar changes are the most common manifestation of hypertensive retinopathy. The mean ratio of arteriole-to-venular diameter in nonhypertensive patients is 0.84. This ratio progressively decreases with increased mean arterial BP. Arteriovenous (AV) nicking can be detected where branch retinal arteries cross over veins. The thickened arteriole wall compresses the thin-walled vein, causing a tapering or "nicked" appearance.

A basic laboratory evaluation should include a urinalysis, microalbuminuria measurement, complete blood count, blood chemistry (potassium, sodium, creatinine, fasting glucose, uric acid), a full fasting lipid profile, and an ECG. An elevated uric acid value may predict the development of hypertension, is frequently present in patients with hypertension, and the degree of elevation also correlates with the degree of BP elevation. Uric acid may also have a pathogenic role in progressive renal disease.

Ambulatory blood pressure monitoring (ABPM), an echocardiogram, and assessment of plasma renin activity are not indicated for routine evaluation of most hypertensive patients at the first visit. ABPM may be useful in separating those patients who require antihypertensive therapy from those who can be managed by lifestyle modifications. Higher ambulatory systolic or diastolic BP predicts CV events even after adjustment for classic risk factors (22). In select situations (e.g., "white coat" hypertension, nocturnal hypotension with treatment), ABPM may be helpful.

## REFRACTORY HYPERTENSION

Refractory hypertension is defined as the persistence of BP >140/90 mm Hg while being treated with a rational triple-drug therapy, optimally including a diuretic. Refractory hypertension falls into two broad categories: apparent resistance and true resistance (Table 43–1) (23).

Refractory hypertension is present in approximately 10% of patients in a primary care setting and in more than 30% of patients seen in subspecialty clinics. Patient noncompliance and suboptimal therapeutic regimens are the major causes for apparent refractory hypertension (Fig. 43–1) (24). More intensive therapy with emphasis on targeted volume control using diuretic therapy can achieve goal BP levels in a significant percentage of patients with apparent resistant hypertension (25).

Awareness of the association among sleep-disordered breathing, sleep apnea, and hypertension has increased over the past few years (26). Both hypoxia and $CO_2$ retention excite central and peripheral chemoreceptors

**TABLE 43–1**
**CAUSES OF REFRACTORY HYPERTENSION**

| Apparent Resistance | True Resistance |
|---|---|
| Cuff-related artifacts | Excess plasma volume |
| Pseudo-hypertension | Associated conditions[a] |
| Nonadherence to therapy | Drug-related causes[b] |
| Prescription errors | Secondary hypertension |

[a]Obesity, insulin resistance, ethanol excess, sleep apnea.
[b]Drug–drug interactions and specific drugs that may produce refractory hypertension include: nonsteroidal anti-inflammatory drugs (NSAIDs), sympathomimetic drugs (decongestants, appetite suppressants), corticosteroids, chlorpromazine, over-the-counter dietary substances (i.e., ephedra, rehung, bitter orange), tricyclic antidepressants, cocaine, amphetamines, cyclosporine, tacrolimus, erythropoietin, anabolic steroids, monamine oxidase inhibitors, oral contraceptives, licorice, and some chewing tobaccos.

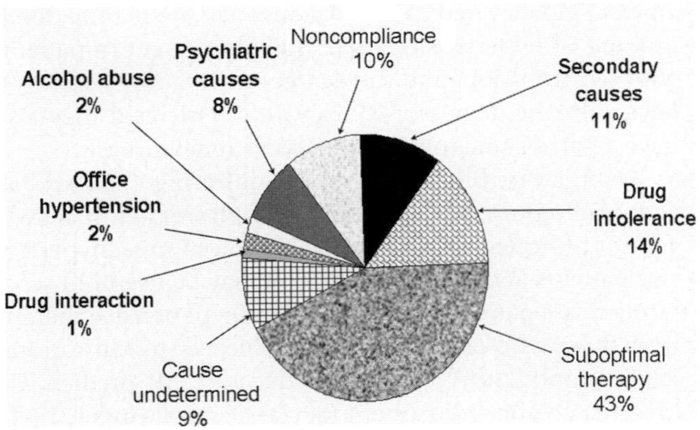


**Figure 43–1** Of 436 patients treated at a hypertension clinic, 92 (21%) had refractory hypertension. In 83 patients a cause was identified, the most frequent being suboptimal therapy. Blood pressure was brought under control or improved in 58 patients. (Data from Yakovlevitch M, Black HR. Resistant hypertension in a tertiary care clinic. *Arch Intern Med*. 1991;151:1786–1792.)

activating the renin–angiotensin system, which can lead to vasoconstriction and increased BP. Typically, the onset of sleep is associated with a significant decrease in BP of 10% to 20% in normotensive individuals. Patients with disrupted sleep patterns do not experience a nocturnal dip in BP. When treated with cPAP, the nocturnal dip in BP is restored (Fig. 43–2) (27).

## CLINICAL APPROACHES TO HYPERTENSION

Hypertension prevalence is increasing in the United States, occurring in 31% of the adult population and in more than two thirds of individuals >65 years of age. Recent data support the contention that hypertension control rates remain low, as only 34% of patients achieve a target BP of <140/90 mm Hg. Hypertension prevalence is highest among non-Hispanic blacks and women, and increases with age and elevated body mass index (BMI) (28).

Over the last 5 years, several landmark clinical trials have assessed the impact of different therapeutic agents on outcome in the presence of hypertension. These studies highlight the importance of treatment selection in the individual hypertension patient (29). These trial findings, coupled with the recommendations of the Seventh Report of the Joint National Committee on the Prevention, Detection, Evaluation and Treatment of High Blood Pressure (JNC VII) (30,31), underscore the importance of recognizing up-to-date BP classification, selecting the appropriate agents for the clinical setting, and achieving effective target BP lowering.

The new classification of BP for adults 18 years of age or older in JNC VII defines a prehypertension category that precedes stages I and II (Table 43–2) (32). When considering the number of patients with a BP of 120 to 139/80

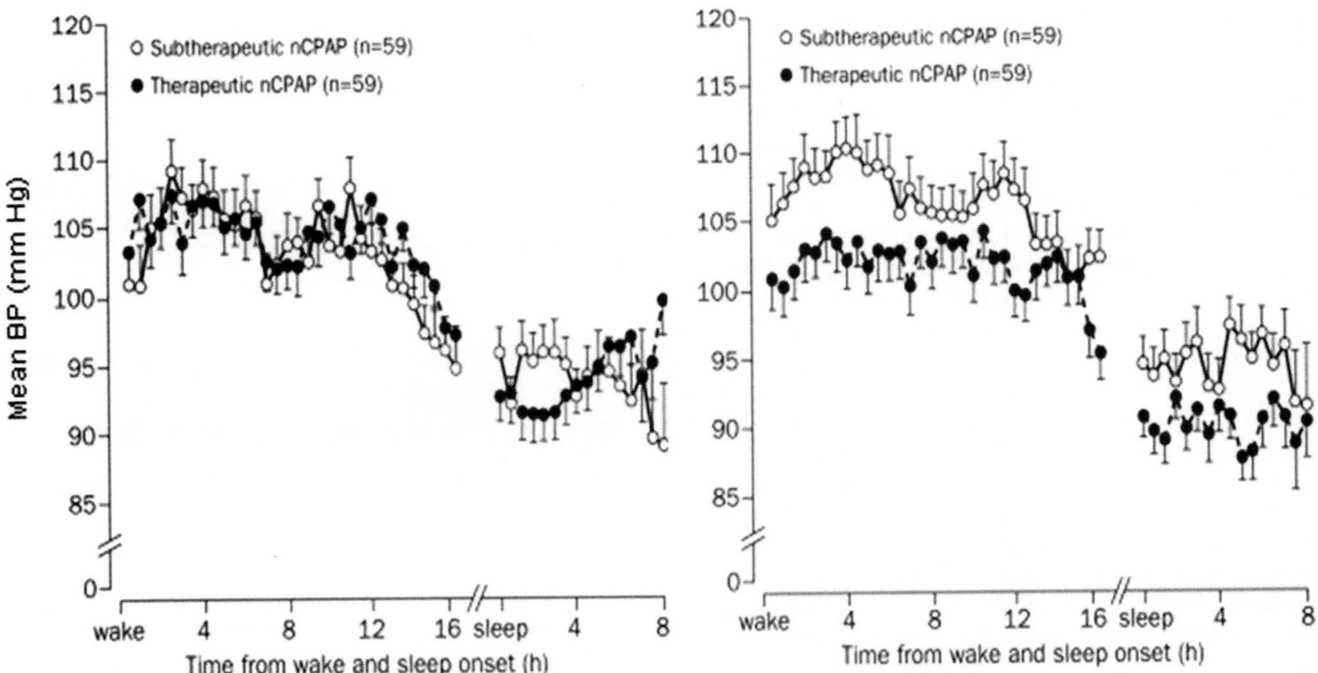


**Figure 43–2** Randomized trial comparing treated (therapeutic versus subtherapeutic CPAP (1 cm $H_2O$ over a 1-month period) and untreated men with sleep apnea. Bars are standard errors for every 30-minute period, synchronized to wake and sleep times. (From Pepperell JC, Ramdassingh-Dow S, Crosthwaite N, et al. Ambulatory blood pressure after therapeutic and subtherapeutic nasal continuous positive airway pressure for obstructive sleep apnoea: a randomised parallel trial. *Lancet*. 2002;359:204–210.)

## TABLE 43–2

### BLOOD PRESSURE CLASSIFICATION AND MANAGEMENT FOR ADULTS AGED 18 YEARS AND OLDER[a]

| | | | | | Initial Drug Therapy Compelling Indications | |
|---|---|---|---|---|---|---|
| **BP Classification** | **SBP, mm Hg** | | **DBP, mm Hg** | **Lifestyle Changes** | **Without** | **With** |
| Normal | <120 | and | <80 | Encourage | | |
| Pre-HYTN | 120–139 | or | 80–89 | Yes | No | Yes[b] |
| Stage 1 HYTN | 140–159 | or | 90–99 | Yes | Yes[c] | Yes[d] |
| Stage 2 HYTN | >160 | or | >100 | Yes | Yes[e] | Yes[f] |

BP, blood pressure; SBP, systolic blood pressure; DBP, diastolic blood pressure; HYTN, hypertension.
[a]Treatment determined by highest BP category.
[b]Treat patients with chronic kidney disease or diabetes to BP goal of <130/80 mm Hg.
[c]Thiazide-type diuretic for most; may consider angiotensin-converting enzyme (ACE) inhibitor, angiotensin-II receptor blocker (ARB), beta-blocker, calcium channel blocker (CCB), or combination.
[d]Other antihypertensive drugs (diuretic, ACE inhibitor, ARB, beta-blocker, CCB) as needed.
[e]Two-drug combination for most (usually thiazide-type diuretic and ACE inhibitor or ARB or beta-blocker or CCB). Initiation of combined therapy should be used cautiously in those at risk for orthostatic hypotension.
[f]Other antihypertensive drugs (diuretic, ACE inhibitor, ARB, beta-blocker, CCB) as needed.
*Source:* From Chobanian AV, Bakris GL, Black HR, et al. The Seventh Report of the Joint National Committee on Prevention, Detection, Evaluation, and Treatment of High Blood Pressure: The JNC 7 Report. *JAMA.* 2003;289:2560–2571.

to 89 mm Hg, prehypertension represents a major public health problem. Vigorous attempts at lifestyle modifications should be undertaken for individuals categorized as prehypertensive. Patients with systolic BPs between 120 and 140 mm Hg are not entirely free from a potential CV event; these prehypertensive individuals have a higher risk for developing hypertension than those with systolic BPs <120 mm Hg. Figure 43–3 shows the importance of matching the initial drug selection with the stage of hypertension and the presence or absence of compelling indications (heart failure, diabetes mellitus type 1 or 2, proteinuria, renal disease, isolated hypertension, myocardial infarction, etc.). The presence of compelling indications not only emphasizes renewed attention to drug selection, but also denotes a need to achieve a more significant decrease in BP (<130/80 mm Hg) in the setting of diabetes, chronic kidney disease (CKD) with proteinuria, congestive heart failure (CHF), and in minority populations.

Findings from recent clinical trials (Table 43–3) point out specific caveats for therapeutic selection in high-risk patients for CVD (33), for those with diabetic renal disease (34,35), and in high-risk ethnic groups (e.g., African Americans) (36). For patients with essential hypertension who are at high risk for CVD, the use of diuretic therapy resulted in outcomes at least equivalent to the use of ACE inhibitors or calcium channel blockers (CCBs) in the ALLHAT study (37). Dihydropyridine calcium blockers should not be used as monotherapy in patients with proteinuric renal disease, whether associated with diabetes mellitus or hypertension. Recent clinical trials with metoprolol and newer vasodilating beta-blockers (carvedilol and bucindolol) have shown benefit in CHF patients when added to standard therapy, including ACE inhibitors (38,39). For patients with type 1 diabetes, ACE inhibitor therapy is the cornerstone of treatment. ACE inhibitors and ARBs have demonstrated favorable results in both diabetic and nondiabetic renal disease. The greatest benefit for slowing progression of type 2 diabetes with renal disease can be seen with angiotensin-II receptor blockers (ARBs), based on findings from the RENAAL and IDNT studies (40,41).

Because patients with chronic kidney disease (serum creatinine ≥1.4 mg/dL or estimated glomerular filtration rate [eGFR] <60 mL/min) are more likely to die from CVD than from ESRD, hypertension should be aggressively controlled (42). Despite this, awareness of kidney disease is low, especially with respect to other chronic diseases. Decreased CKD awareness is most prevalent in first-degree Spanish speakers, male gender, non-Hispanic blacks, and in patients with hypertension (43). The risk for CV and renal disease events starts at systolic BP levels as low as 115 mm Hg (44). ACE inhibitors or angiotensin II receptor blockers (ARBs) should be used in CKD patients whenever possible. An increase in baseline serum creatinine up to 35% on these agents is acceptable unless clinically resistant hyperkalemia develops. Hypertensive patients with eGFR <30 mL/min/1.73 $m^2$ will require increasing doses of loop diuretic in combination with other agents to optimize volume, a critical determinant of elevated BP.

The development of microalbuminuria is associated with abnormal vascular reactivity, salt sensitivity, increased presence of TOD and loss of nocturnal dipping in BP (45). An elevated urine albumin-to-creatinine ratio heralds the need for aggressive BP control.

Effective BP control can be achieved in the majority of patients with hypertension, but more than two (2.7 to 3.8) medications may be needed to reach target BP levels (46).

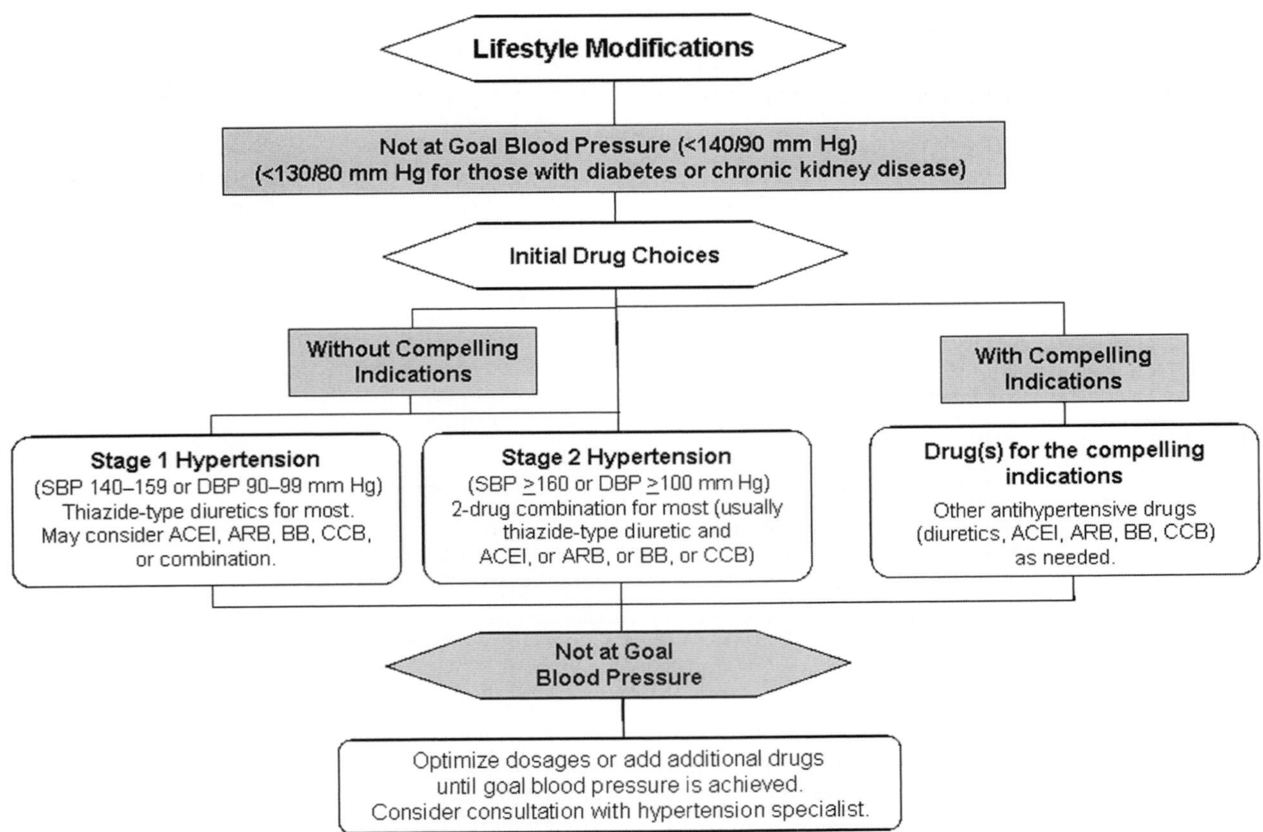


**Figure 43–3** Algorithm for treatment of hypertension, based on randomized controlled trials. SBP, systolic blood pressure; DPB, diastolic blood pressure; ACE, angiotensin-converting enzyme; ARB, angiotensin-II receptor blocker; CCB, calcium channel blocker; HYTN, hypertension. (Adapted from Pepperell JC, Ramdassingh-Dow S, Crosthwaite N, et al. Ambulatory blood pressure after therapeutic and subtherapeutic nasal continuous positive airway pressure for obstructive sleep apnoea: a randomised parallel trial. *Lancet.* 2002;359:204–210; and Chobanian AV, Bakris GL, Black HR, et al. The Seventh Report of the Joint National Committee on Prevention, Detection, Evaluation, and Treatment of High Blood Pressure: The JNC 7 Report. *JAMA.* 2003;289:2560–2571.)

When BP is >20/10 mm Hg above target, consideration should be given to initiating therapy with two drugs. Extensive clinical experience with available antihypertensive agents suggests that any single drug preparation will control only 30% to 65% of patients treated, whereas the addition of a second or third drug to the regimen can improve control rates into the range of 90% to 95%. Patients should return for follow-up monthly until the BP goal is achieved. Serum potassium and creatinine should be monitored at least twice per year (47).

Among older persons, systolic BP is a better predictor of events (coronary heart disease, CVD, heart failure, stroke, end-stage renal disease, and all-cause mortality) than diastolic BP. The initial treatment goal in older patients should be the same as in younger individuals, namely, to achieve a BP below 140/90 mm Hg. However, the concept of a J curve for mortality with exaggerated BP lowering may be of greatest importance in the elderly. Findings from both the SHEP trial (48) and the Rotterdam Study (49) suggest that there may be an increased CV risk in the lowest strata of BP and that reducing systolic BP to <130 mm Hg or diastolic BP to <65 mm Hg may not represent optimal strategy in the elderly.

Electrocardiographic or echocardiographic evidence of left ventricular hypertrophy (LVH) is associated with increased risk of coronary disease, ventricular arrhythmias, and sudden death (50,51), and requires optimal target BP. Most of the antihypertensive drugs used for initial hypertension therapy induce regression of LVH. In the LIFE trial, ARBs were superior to beta-blocker therapy in reducing CV endpoints in hypertensive patients with ECKG evidence of LVH.

Because the risk of heart disease and stroke increases with age among women, increasing attention has been focused on the nearly 30 million American women over age 50 years. In women 50 to 64 years of age, 47% have high BP—this figure increases to 58% in women 65 to 74 years of age, and to 75% for those 75 years and older. African American women have a death rate from hypertension that is approximately 4.5 times higher than the rate for white

**TABLE 43–3**
**SUMMARY OF CARDIOVASCULAR AND KIDNEY OUTCOME TRIALS (2001–2004)**

| Study | Population | Special Note(s) | Effect on Clinical Practice |
|---|---|---|---|
| ALLHAT | North American subjects >55 y | Alpha-blocker terminated due to excess risk for hospitalized CHF | Hypertensive patients respond as well or better to diuretics compared to other agents ACE inhibitors, CCB |
| RENAAL | Type 2 diabetics, 31–70 y with nephropathy | Controlling BP may require 3–4 antihypertensive agents | Greater reduction in proteinuria for losartan vs. placebo |
| IDNT | Type 2 diabetics, hypertensive, proteinuria | | Lower risk of SCr doubling with irbesartan vs. amlodipine or placebo |
| AASK | African Americans, 18–70 y, hypertensive with renal disease | Amlodipine arm terminated due to excess risk of ESRD/death vs. ramipril | Patients with proteinuria should not receive DHP CCB as monotherapy. Lower-than-usual BP control did not slow progression of renal disease. ACE inhibitors more effective at slowing progression compared to CCB or $\beta$-blocker |

y, year(s); CHF, congestive heart failure; ACE, angiotensin-converting enzyme; CCB, calcium channel blocker; SCr, serum creatinine; ESRD, end-stage renal disease; DHP CCB, dihydropyridine calcium channel blocker; BP, blood pressure.
Trial names: ALLHAT, Antihypertensive and Lipid-Lowering Treatment to Prevent Heart Attack Trial; RENAAL, Reduction of Endpoints in NIDDM with the Angiotensin II Antagonist Losartan; IDNT, Irbesartan Diabetic Nephropathy Trial; AASK, African American Study of Kidney Disease and Hypertension.

women, which makes hypertension the probable cause of up to 20% of all deaths in hypertensive African American women. There is no evidence that women respond any differently than men to the risk-reduction effect of antihypertensive drugs (52), and the JNC VII guidelines should be applied equally to women.

## SECONDARY HYPERTENSION

For hypertensive patients who are resistant to treatment with two or more agents, a number of clinical clues can suggest the possible presence of secondary hypertension. Table 43–4 divides the causes of secondary hypertension into four broad categories. Secondary hypertensive disorders can be effectively treated or cured, leading to partial or complete normalization of resistant hypertension in most patients.

### Primary Aldosteronism

Primary aldosteronism is the most common cause of hypertension due to an endocrinopathy. The most common cause of primary aldosteronism is an aldosterone-producing adenoma (70% to 80%). However, glucocorticoid-remediable aldosteronism (GRA), adrenal hyperplasia, and adrenal carcinoma are other considerations. Although the clinical manifestations of primary aldosteronism are not distinctive, the best clues to the presence of primary aldosteronism include hypertension with spontaneous hypokalemia (<3.5 mEq/L), hypertension with provoked hypokalemia (<3.0 mEq/L during diuretic therapy), and hypertension with difficulty in maintaining normokalemia despite potassium supplementation.

Primary aldosteronism should be considered in any patient with both refractory hypertension and hypokalemia with inappropriate kaliuresis (urine potassium >30 mEq/L per 24 hours). One should be especially suspicious of primary aldosteronism if potassium is <3.5 mEq/L despite potassium supplementation, ACE inhibitor or ARB

**TABLE 43–4**
**CLUES TO SECONDARY HYPERTENSION**

Renal
- Renal artery stenosis
- Renal parenchymal obstruction
- Polycystic kidney disease

Endocrine
- Cushing syndrome
- Adrenogenital syndrome
- Pheochromocytoma
- Adrenal and adrenal-like
- Acromegaly
- Hypercalcemia
- Liddle syndrome
- Gordon syndrome

Coarctation of the aorta

Other
- Pre-eclampsia
- Acute intermittent porphyria
- Thyroid (hyper-, hypo-)
- Drugs

**TABLE 43–5**
**BIOCHEMICAL CLASSIFICATION OF PATIENTS WITH HYPERTENSION, HYPOKALEMIA, AND RENAL POTASSIUM WASTING**

| High Renin States | Low Renin States |
|---|---|
| Renovascular disease | Conn syndrome[a] (primary aldosteronism) |
| Malignant hypertension | Bilateral adrenal hyperplasia |
| | Renin-secreting tumors |
| | Glucocorticoid-remediable aldosteronism (GRA)[b] |
| | Mineralocorticoid excess syndrome |
| | Licorice ingestion |
| | Liddle syndrome[c] |

[a]Aldosterone-secreting adrenal adenoma.
[b]Children, early-onset severe hypertension, history of early hemorrhagic stroke, adrenocorticotropic hormone (ACTH) regulates aldosterone secretion, and renin–angiotensin system is suppressed. Suppression of ACTH with glucocorticoids decreases aldosterone and cures the hypertension. Diagnose by high 18-hydroxycortisol/18-oxycortisol.
[c]Hypertension, decreased potassium, alkalosis, decreased aldosterone, sodium channel mutation.

therapy, and/or a potassium-sparing diuretic. In addition, patients may develop muscle spasms, periodic paralysis, or metabolic alkalosis. The clinician needs to remember that not all patients with primary aldosteronism have hypokalemia; 7% to 38% of patients with primary aldosteronism may have normal serum potassium (53). Even 10% to 12% patients with positive tumors may not have hypokalemia during short-term salt loading. Individuals with hypertension and renal potassium wasting can be differentiated into high-renin and low-renin states (Table 43–5). Usually the plasma renin concentration is <1 ng/mL/h in mineralocorticoid excess, and fails to rise above 2 ng/mL/h after salt depletion and upright posture.

The best screening test for primary aldosteronism is the ratio between plasma aldosterone (PA) and plasma renin activity (PRA) (54). Patients with hypokalemia and resistant hypertension should undergo measurement of both PRA and aldosterone concentration. Both specific medications (55) and variability of PA levels may affect the accuracy of the ratio. All diuretics should be discontinued 1 to 2 weeks prior to laboratory workup of hypokalemia. If the patient has uncontrolled hypertension, a CCB or a nonatenolol beta-blocker may be used. Although doxazosin and irbesartan have the least impact on the ratio, atenolol may lead to an increased rate of false-positive aldosterone/renin ratios. Spironolactone and ACE inhibitors also affect this ratio adversely. Physicians may be confused by values measured as PRA versus the new assay of direct renin measurement. The direct renin measurement divided by 8 is roughly equivalent to the PRA. An elevated PA/PRA ratio alone does not establish a diagnosis of primary aldosteronism. The diagnostic suspicion should be confirmed by demonstrating inappropriate aldosterone secretion.

Table 43–6 lists the laboratory evaluation for patients with hypertension, hypokalemia, and kaliuresis. A high

**TABLE 43–6**
**HYPERTENSION; HYPOKALEMIA ($K_S$ <3.5 mEq/L) WITH KALIURESIS ($UK_V$ >30 mEq/24h)**

| Laboratory workup: |
|---|
| Serum electrolytes |
| Serum creatinine, urea |
| Plasma aldosterone, cortisol, PRA |
| 24-h urinary Na, K, Cr, aldosterone and free cortisol during high-salt diet ($U_{Na}V$ >250 mg/kg/d) |
| High salt diet |

$K_S$, serum potassium concentration; $UK_V$, urinary potassium per 24 hrs; PRA, plasma renin activity; Na, sodium; K, potassium; Cr, creatinine; UNaV, urinary sodium per volume of urine.

renin value does not exclude primary aldosteronism. The most important test in diagnosing primary aldosteronism is a nonsuppressed 24-hour urinary aldosterone excretion rate during a salt load. A rate >14 $\mu$g/24 h following 3 days of salt loading (24 mL/kg of physiologic saline over 4 hours for 3 days, or a home oral salt load) distinguishes most cases of primary aldosteronism from essential hypertension. Those specific situations that warrant salt loading (>250 mEq/day) include individuals with hypertension and normal PA, with a PRA ≤1.0, those with high PA and normal–high PRA, and those with spontaneous hypokalemia who have normal PA and normal PRA. Individuals who warrant salt loading can be placed on a high-salt diet (1 level teaspoon of salt each day for 5 days). The urinary aldosterone excretion rate should be determined on days 4 and 5, along with urinary creatinine, potassium and sodium measurements. If the sodium concentration is <250 mEq in 24 hours, mild increases in urinary aldosterone excretion rate may represent inadequate suppression.

Combining urinary aldosterone levels with urinary free cortisol results can distinguish nonaldosterone mineralocorticoid excess from aldosterone mineralocorticoid excess (Table 43–7). Patients with Liddle syndrome usually present with hypertension, hypokalemia, and metabolic alkalosis at an early age. Liddle syndrome is an autosomal dominant disorder associated with low/normal urinary excretion of aldosterone, increased kaliuresis occurring with increased collecting tubular sodium reabsorption via amiloride-sensitive channels, and normal urinary free cortisol measurements. The increased sodium reabsorption in collecting tubules results in increased potassium secretion and hypokalemia. Amiloride has been used to close the sodium channels and correct the defect clinically. Liddle syndrome can be differentiated from congenital adrenal hyperplasia and 11-$\beta$-hydroxysteroid dehydrogenase deficiency (11-$\beta$-OHSD) by analyzing urinary aldosterone and urinary free cortisol values in addition to the clinical presentation.

The mineralocorticoid receptors (MRs) in the distal nephron have equal affinity for both aldosterone and cortisol, but are normally protected from cortisol by the

**TABLE 43–7**

**COMBINING URINARY ALDOSTERONE LEVELS WITH URINARY FREE CORTISOL RESULTS CAN DISTINGUISH NON-ALDOSTERONE MINERALOCORTICOID EXCESS FROM ALDOSTERONE MINERALOCORTICOID EXCESS**

| | | Urinary Free Cortisol | | |
|---|---|---|---|---|
| | | **Low** | **Normal** | **High** |
| Urinary aldosterone | Low-normal | Congenital adrenal hyperplasia | Liddle syndrome<br>Exogenous mineralocorticoids | 11-β-OHSD<br>Cushing syndrome<br>GRA |
| | High | — | Primary aldosterone<br>GRA | Adrenal cancer<br>Primary aldosteronism with Cushing syndrome |

OHSD, hydroxysteroid dehydrogenate deficiency; GRA, glucocorticoid remedial aldosteronism.

presence of 11-β-dehydrogenase, which inactivates the conversion of cortisol to cortisone. The 11-18 hemiacetal structure of aldosterone protects it from the action of 11-β-dehydrogenase so that aldosterone gains specific access to the receptors. When this mechanism (normal 11-β-hydrogenase and aldosterone) is defective, either because of congenital 11-β-OHSD or enzyme inhibition (licorice or carbenoxalone), then intrarenal levels of cortisol increase and inappropriately activate the MRs, resulting in antinatiuresis and kaliuresis associated with hypertension and hypokalemia. Plasma cortisol concentrations in 11-β-OHSD are usually not elevated. The laboratory abnormalities and symptoms are reversed by spironolactone or dexamethasone, but are exacerbated by physiologic doses of cortisone.

Licorice-induced hypermineralocorticoidism has both low PA and low PRA levels. The glycyrrhetinic acid inhibits the enzyme 11-β-dehydroxyase steroid dehydrogenase, allowing cortisol to act as the major endogenous mineralocorticoid avidly binding to the MRs and inducing inappropriate kaliuresis. It is interesting to note that essential hypertension patients are more sensitive to the inhibition of 11-β-hydroxysteroid dehydrogenase by licorice than normotensive subjects, and this inhibition causes more clinical symptoms in women than in men (56). Glycyrrhetinic acid-containing compounds include anti–peptic ulcer medication, carbenoxalone sodium, antituberculosis medication, *p*-aminosalicylic acid, the French alcoholic beverage Boisson de coco, chewing tobacco (57), and some Oriental herbal preparations. Diagnosis depends on the elicitation of a thorough history and laboratory evidence of hypokalemia. In general, regular daily intake of 100 mg of glycyrrhizic acid produces adverse effects in sensitive individuals, whereas consumption of 400 mg/day produces adverse effects in most subjects (58).

Glucocorticoid-remedial aldosteronism (GRA) is an inherited autosomal dominant disorder that mimics a primary aldostoneronism. Aldosterone-like GRA should be suspected in any patient with a primary aldosteronelike presentation who presents with a positive family history and primary aldosteronism, early age (under 21 years) of hypertension onset, or severe hypertension with early death of affected members from a cerebrovascular accident. GRA is usually associated with bilateral adrenal hyperplasia. Patients with GRA have ACTH-sensitive aldosterone production occurring in the zona fasciculata rather than in the zona glomerulosa, which is the normal site of production. The isoenzyme in the zona glomerulosa catalyzes conversion of deoxycorticosterone to corticosterone and of 18-hydroxycorticosterone to aldosterone. The hybrid gene in GRA results from a genetic mutation. This defect allows for an ectopic expression of aldosterone synthesis activity in the ACTH-regulated zona fasciculata. The plasma potassium concentration is normal in more than one half of patients with GRA, in contrast to the pattern seen most commonly with primary aldosteronism. Genetic testing using molecular biologic techniques can detect a chimeric gene responsible for GRA. Standard laboratory testing includes an dexamethasone suppression test and measures of 18-hydroxycortisol and 18-oxycortisol. Both 18-hydroxycortisol and 18-oxycortisol are usually increased. Administration of dexamethasone in doses of 2 mg in 24 hours (0.5 mg every 6 hours) usually results in remission of hypertension and hypokalemia within 7 to 10 days. The suppression of ACTH with exogenous glucocorticoid should correct the metabolic defect and control hypertension in GRA. The use of spironolactone and/or amiloride may be supplemental treatment in addition to exogenous glucocorticoid therapy.

An adrenal computed tomography (CT) scan is helpful in differentiating among adrenal adenoma, adrenal hyperplasia, and adrenal carcinoma. The overall sensitivity of localizing aldosterone-producing tumors by high-resolution CT scanning exceeds 90%. Adrenal carcinomas are typically large (>5 cm) in comparison to a hypodense unilateral macroadenoma (>1 cm). Normally, abnormalities in both glands represent adrenal hyperplasia. Hounsfield units >10 usually indicate adrenal carcinoma, whereas

Hounsfield units <10 most likely suggest an adrenal adenoma. The difference in density results from a vascular tumor versus a lipid-rich adenoma.

Adrenal vein sampling after administration of ACTH may be useful when no adrenal abnormality exists on CT scan or magnetic resonance imaging (MRI) or when there is an asymmetric abnormality in both glands. The sampling of the adrenal vein is technically difficult and should be restricted to experienced centers. It is important to assess both aldosterone and cortisol values at the time of sampling from the right and left adrenal glands and high and low inferior vena cavas. To be certain the samples are from the adrenal veins, cortisol should also be measured in the same samples. Serum cortisol concentrations should be roughly the same in both adrenal veins and approximately 10-fold higher than in the peripheral vein. The aldosterone concentrations should be two times higher from the adrenal vein versus periphery. An aldosterone ratio >10:1 in the presence of a symmetric ACTH-induced cortisol response is diagnostic of an aldosterone-producing adenoma.

Medical therapy with eplerenone (selective aldosterone-receptor antagonist) or spironolactone can be used in patients with bilateral adrenal adenomas, adenomas that cannot be excised surgically (poor surgical risk), in individuals with adrenal hyperplasia, and in those with significant responses to aldosterone-receptor antagonists who do not desire surgery. Surgical removal of an aldosterone-producing adenoma renders normotension and restoration of normal potassium homeostasis in most patients. Adrenal adenomas may be removed laparoscopically. Patients may require drug treatment for 3 to 6 months prior to surgery. Selective hypoaldosteronism usually occurs after aldosterone-producing adenoma removal.

## Cushing Syndrome

Clinical clues for Cushing syndrome include a history of recent change in facial appearance and considerable weight gain, together with complaints of weakness, muscle wasting, peripheral bruising, impotence, and, in women, amenorrhea and hirsutism (59). Typical physical features include truncal obesity, moon face, plethora, and purplish skin stria.

Screening and laboratory studies may indicate glucose intolerance or frank diabetes mellitus, and occasionally neutrophilia with relative lymphocytopenia. Pathologic fractures of a rib are common. A dexamethasone suppression test may be helpful. For diagnosis and localization, a 24-hour urinary free cortisol test, CT, and radioimmunoassay of plasma adrenocorticotropic hormone may be helpful.

The standard of care for most cases of Cushing syndrome is surgical resection of a pituitary gland or an ectopic source of adrenocorticotropic hormone or removal of a cortisol-producing adrenal cortical tumor. Transsphenoidal pituitary adenomectomy or radiation therapy to the pituitary bed may be considered in selected cases.

## Pheochromocytoma

Pheochromocytoma can present in many ways, reflecting variation in the hormone it releases, the pattern of release, and differences in each individual's catecholamine sensitivities. Eighty percent of patients with pheochromocytoma present with headache, 57% with sweating, 48% with paroxysmal hypertension, 39% with persistent hypertension, 64% with palpitations; 13% of patients may be normotensive, and 8% may be completely asymptomatic. In approximately 10% of patients, tumors are discovered incidentally during CT/MRI of the abdomen for unrelated symptoms. Those individuals who warrant a workup for pheochromocytoma include patients with: (a) episodic symptoms of headache, tachycardia, diaphoresis; (b) family history of pheochromocytoma or multiple endocrine neoplasia (MEN) syndrome; (c) unexplained paroxysms of tachy/brady arrhythmias; and/or (d) hypertension during intubation, induction of anesthesia, prolonged or unexplained hypotension after surgery, or adverse CV responses to ingestion or inhalation of certain drugs including: anesthetic agents, glucagon, ACTH, thyrotropin-releasing hormone, antidopaminergic agents, miloxane, phenothiazine, guanethidine, and tricyclic antibiotics.

Currently available tests can establish the diagnosis of pheochromocytoma in >90% of cases. Figure 43–4 illustrates the approach to using plasma catecholamines and urinary metanephrines in the evaluation of patients suspected of having pheochromocytoma (60). Fractionated plasma free metanephrines are the best test for familial (hereditary) pheochromocytoma, whereas 24-hour urinary metanephrines and catecholamines provide adequate sensitivity with low false-positive rates for sporadic pheochromocytoma. The combination of resting plasma catecholamines (NE plus E) at least 2,000 pg/mL and urinary metanephrines (NMN plus MN) at least 1.8 mg in 24 hours has a diagnostic accuracy of approximately 98% in both sporadic and hereditary pheochromocytoma. A number of medications interfere with the biochemical

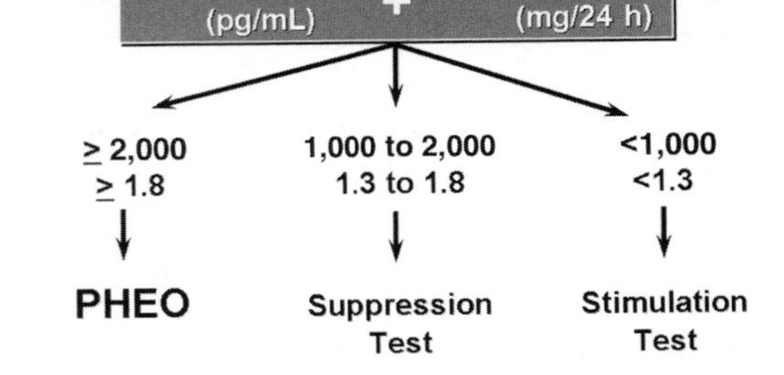


**Figure 43–4** Pheochromocytoma suspected. (Adapted from Bravo EL. Pheochromocytoma. *Cardiol Rev.* 2002;10:44–50.)

diagnosis of pheochromocytoma. Methylglucamine results in a decrease in metanephrines, whereas sotalol increases metanephrine concentration. ARBs, ACE inhibitors, and bromocriptine decrease catecholamine values, whereas $\alpha_1$-blockers, beta-blockers, and labetalol increase catecholamine values. Methyldopa and monamine oxidase inhibitors decrease vanillylmandelic acid (VMA) values, whereas nalidixic acid and anileridine increase VMA values. Phenothiazine, methyldopa, and tricyclic antibiotics have varying effects on these tests. When blood specimens are drawn under standardized conditions, a total plasma catecholamine level ≥2,000 pg/mL is diagnostic of pheochromocytoma, whereas a value of <500 pg/mL excludes pheochromocytoma.

For localization, CT scanning and MRI are equally sensitive (98% versus 100%), whereas $^{131}$I-metaiodobenzylguanadine iothalamate (MIBG) has excellent specificity (100%) but low sensitivity (78%). Pheochromocytomas are typically hyperdense compared to the liver on $T_2$-weighted images, whereas benign tumors are isodense. If no tumor is detected (by either CT or MRI) in a highly suspicious setting, then MIBG scintigraphy should be used.

A provocative test is employed when the clinical findings are highly suggestive of pheochromocytoma but the BP is normal or slightly increased and plasma catecholamines are between 500 and 1,000 pg/mL. The glucagon test has a high specificity (100%) but low sensitivity (81%). Drugs that inhibit central sympathetic outflow (e.g., clonidine, bromocryptine, haloperidol, methyldopa) may decrease plasma catecholamines in normal and hypertensive subjects, but have little effect on the excessive catecholamine secretion by pheochromocytoma. A clonidine suppression test is used for a patient whose plasma catecholamine level is between 1,000 and 2,000 pg/mL, with or without hypertension. A normal clonidine suppression test requires at least a 50% fall of plasma catecholamines from baseline to <500 pg/mL.

Such clinical situations as acute clonidine withdrawal, acute alcohol withdrawal, monotherapy with a pure arterial vasodilator (hydralazine or minoxidil), cocaine abuse, severe CHF, acute myocardial ischemia/infarction, and acute cerebrovascular accident can increase both plasma catecholamines and urine catecholamine metabolites.

Pheochromocytomas may develop in about 50% of patients with multiple endocrine neoplasia (MEN) type 2a and type 2b, in 25% of patients with Von Hippel Lindau (VHL) type 2, and in 5% with Von Recklinghausen disease (neurofibromatosis). However, in patients with Von Recklinghausen disease and hypertension, a pheochromocytoma has been identified in more than one third of patients.

CCBs (nifedipine, verapamil, or diltiazem) are used with or without selective $\alpha_1$-receptor blockers (prazosin, terazosin, doxazosin) in the preoperative management of pheochromocytoma patients. The CCBs relax arterial smooth muscle and decrease peripheral vascular resistance by inhibiting norepinenephrine-mediated release of intracellular calcium and/or calcium transmembrane influx. These agents do not usually produce the overshoot hypotension seen with nonselective $\alpha$-adrenergic blockade. Selective $\alpha_1$-blockers do not enhance norepinenephrine release and usually are not associated with reflex tachycardia. Therefore, CCBs or selective $\alpha_1$-receptor blockers are effective and safe, without the adverse effects associated with the relatively nonspecific complete and prolonged $\alpha_1$-blockade with phenoxybenzamine (61). Phenoxybenzamine, traditionally used to counteract the sudden release of massive quantities of catecholamines during surgical intervention, is associated with dramatic hypertension with tumor manipulation and therefore is used less today than previously.

Current medications and surgical techniques have significantly decreased the risk of surgical intervention in pheochromocytoma. Laparoscopic surgery can be used successfully for tumor removal in the majority of cases. Patients undergoing laparoscopy have less severe intraoperative hypotension, minimal blood loss, shorter duration of hospitalization, and earlier resumption of normal activities.

Several prognostic factors have been suggested for characterizing patients with malignant pheochromocytoma. These characteristics include large tumor size, local tumor extension at the time of surgery, and a DNA ploidy pattern with diploid DNA being benign and DNA anuloploidy tetraploidy having a more progressive nature (62).

## Renal Parenchymal Disease

CKD defined by either a reduction in glomerular filtration rate (GFR) <60 mL/min/1.73 m$^2$ (corresponding male creatinine >1.5 mg/dL or female >1.3 mg/dL) or the presence of albuminuria >300 mg/d or 200 mg of albumin per gram of creatinine has been associated with an increased risk for hypertension.

The HOPE study data demonstrated a continuous relationship between serum creatinine levels and CV outcomes in hypertensive and normotensive patients. An additive risk exists with increased serum creatinine and microalbuminuria (63).

Hypertension is one of the main contributing factors to progressive renal injury, and lowering BP to <130/80 mm Hg is recommended. Patients with renal parenchymal disease usually present with renal insufficiency, proteinuria, or hematuria (64,65). Renal parenchymal disease is a common secondary cause of hypertension, although not often reversible. The clinical clues are easily detected with a carefully performed urinalysis and screening tests of renal function (serum creatinine and eGFR). Verifying proteinuria with sulfosalicylic acid is important because it detects protein light chains present in dysproteinemic states. Urinary protein should be quantitated with a urine protein-to-creatinine ratio to establish the level of the proteinuria. Additional screening studies may include renal ultrasonography. For diagnosis, assessment of the iothalamate GFR and renal biopsy may be helpful.

Baseline systolic BP is a stronger predictor than diastolic BP of renal outcome in patients with type 2 diabetes mellitus and diabetic nephropathy. Patients with the highest baseline pulse pressure have the highest risk for nephropathy progression and experience the greatest risk reduction with systolic BP lowered to $<$140 mm Hg (40). The underlying etiology of the renal disease (focal segmental glomerulosclerosis, chronic interstitial nephritis, amyloidosis, etc.), determines the immediate and long-term management of renal parenchymal disease. Aggressive treatment and control of BP can slow the progression of renal function loss, especially with ACE inhibitors or ARBs as specific additions to the regimen (66). With advanced renal failure (GFR $<$30 mL/min/1.73 $m^2$, corresponding to a serum creatinine of 2.5 to 3.0 mg/dL), the use of loop diuretics is usually warranted to optimize fluid volume, which is critical for BP control. There is a significant opportunity to improve the treatment of hypertension in proteinuric CKD by the increased use of ACE inhibitors and ARBs (67). In diabetics, tight control of blood sugar can also slow the loss of renal function. For patients who do progress to end-stage renal disease, renal replacement therapies, including hemodialysis or peritoneal dialysis, are available, together with renal transplantation for selected patients.

## Renovascular Disease

Renal artery stenosis that results in renovascular hypertension occurs in 1% to 5% of all patients with hypertension (68). The most common causes of renovascular disease are either fibromuscular dysplasia or atherosclerosis.

Atherosclerotic renal artery disease accounts for 90% of all renovascular lesions, usually occurring at the ostium or within the proximal 2 cm of the renal artery (69). Patients with atherosclerotic renal artery stenosis may present with hypertension, renal failure secondary to ischemia, and/or recurrent episodes of CHF, and "flash pulmonary edema."

Fibromuscular dysplasia (FMD) is found predominantly in young women (70). Radiographically it is characterized by a "string of beads" appearance, with the beading extending beyond the normal caliber of the artery, located in the middle to distal portion of the artery. Less common forms of fibrous renal artery stenosis include perimedial fibroplasia, medial hyperplasia, intimal fibroplasia, and adventitial hyperplasia.

Clinical clues for renovascular hypertension include abrupt onset of hypertension, age $<$30 years or $>$55 years, accelerated/malignant hypertension (grade 3 or 4 retinopathy), hypertension refractory to a triple-drug regimen, hypertension and diffuse vascular disease (carotid, coronary, peripheral vascular), systolic/diastolic epigastric bruit, hypertension and unexplained renal insufficiency, renal insufficiency induced by ACE inhibitor therapy, severe

**TABLE 43–8**
**SPECIFICITY AND SENSITIVITY OF SCREENING TESTS FOR RENOVASCULAR HYPERTENSION**

| Test | Sensitivity (%) | Specificity (%) |
|---|---|---|
| Magnetic resonance angiography (MRA) | 100 | 96 |
| Duplex Doppler ultrasonography | 69–96 | 86–90 |
| Spiral computerized tomography angiography | 98 | 94 |
| IVP | ~75 | ~85 |
| Captopril renogram | 70–93 | 95 |
| Captopril-stimulated PRA | 75 | 89 |

IVP, intravenous pyelogram; PRA, plasma renin activity.

hypertension, and recurrent "flash pulmonary edema" (64,71,72).

A number of specialized diagnostic tests have been used to screen patients suspected of having renovascular disease. Duplex Doppler ultrasonography, spiral computed tomography (CT) angiography, and magnetic resonance angiography (MRA) are replacing traditional screening tests (i.e., intravenous pyelogram (IVP), plasma renin activity, captopril renogram). Renal arteriography remains the "gold standard" for diagnosing renal artery stenosis. Renovascular disease can be effectively diagnosed with an acceptable specificity and sensitivity utilizing most forms of newer diagnosis tests (Table 43–8).

Uncontrolled BP and progressive compromise in renal function are the primary indicators for intervention. For younger patients with fibromuscular dysplasia (medial fibroplasia, intimal fibroplasia, periarterial hyperplasia), percutaneous transluminal renal angioplasty is the mainstay of therapy, with surgical revascularization considered a secondary indication. Successful angioplasty results in reduction of both the disease and hypertension (70).

The primary goal of therapy for patients with hemodynamically significant renal artery disease (RAD) is control of hypertension and preservation of kidney function. The four current therapeutic options available to treat patients with RAD include (a) medical management, (b) surgical revascularization, (c) percutaneous transluminal renal angioplasty (PTRA), and (d) stents. The optimal method for treating patients with RAD remains a debatable issue, as there are no randomized controlled trials (RCTs) addressing the risks and benefits of medical versus surgical versus PTRA versus stents. In brief, three RCTs of medical versus PTRA (no stents) demonstrated a slight benefit in BP control with less medication (2.5 versus 3.0), but kidney function was unaffected in patients randomized to PTRA. A recent RCT of medical versus surgical revascularization did not demonstrate any different in composite "stop points," including uncontrolled hypertension,

50% decrease in GFR, CV event, or mortality. Nonetheless, selected patients may derive benefit in BP control and/or kidney function following interventions.

## Hypertension in Women

In the United States, CVD has accounted for more deaths in women than in men every year since 1984 (73). Hypertension is a strong determinant of CVD in women, although CVD is delayed approximately 10 years compared to men (74). Although essential hypertension accounts for the majority of women with hypertension, the primary causes of hypertension that occur only in women are eclampsia in pregnancy and hypertension associated with oral contraceptives.

A point that is frequently forgotten in hypertension diagnosis and treatment is that women have lower brachial systolic BP, diastolic BP, and mean BP than men. Also, they exhibit lower brachial pulse pressure below age 40 years and a higher pulse pressure over age 55 years (75).

Gueyffier et al. compared the effects of antihypertensive drug treatment in 20,802 women and 19,975 men from a meta-analysis of seven previous therapeutic trials (52). The odds ratios for benefit in any category of CV event did not differ between men and women. Because many women with hypertension require more than one medication for optimal BP control, a number of reports have examined the relationship between baseline use of ACE inhibitors, beta-blockers, CCB, or diuretics, or a combination of these, and the incidence of CHD, stroke, and CVD mortality. The Women's Health Initiative Observational Study (WHI-OS) (76) examined differences in CV mortality among postmenopausal women with hypertension but no history of CVD who were treated with different classes of antihypertensive agents, single agent or combination therapy. Among women with hypertension but no history of CVD, a two-drug class regimen of CCB plus diuretics was associated with a higher risk of CVD mortality versus beta-blocker with diuretics. Risks were similar for ACE inhibitors plus diuretics and beta-blockers plus diuretics. Monotherapy with diuretics was equal or superior to other monotherapy in preventing CVD complications of high BP. Further work examining the importance of antihypertensive drug treatment is essential to clarifying the link between treatment strategies and risk in the postmenopausal woman.

Hypertension disorders occur in 6% to 8% of all pregnancies, are the second leading cause of maternal death, and contribute to significant neonatal morbidity and mortality (77). The U.S. National High Blood Pressure Education Program (NHBPEP) recommends the use of four categories in defining pregnancy-related hypertension: "chronic hypertension, pre-eclampsia/eclampsia, pre-eclampsia superimposed upon hypertension and gestational (transient/chronic) hypertension." Chronic hypertension (>140/90 mm Hg) is defined as hypertension that was either present before conception or detected before the 20th week of gestation and did not resolve in the early postpartum period. Diagnosis of pre-eclampsia after the 20th week of gestation denotes the presence of hypertension.

Medication selection in pregnancy is critical to avoiding embryotoxic complications. Methyldopa, hydralazine, and labetalol have been used most often in controlling BP in pregnancy. ACE inhibitors are contraindicated in pregnancy. Angiotensin-II antagonists are believed to raise similar concerns. Beta-adrenergic blocking agents, especially atenolol, may be associated with retardation of fetal growth. CCB may adversely affect uterine placental blood flow. Diuretics have been used for treating hypertension prepregnancy or before midpregnancy. Thiazide diuretics are preferable to loop diuretics. Short-term studies have not found adverse effects from either methyldopa or hydralazine administered during lactation.

Oral contraceptives induce hypertension in approximately 5% of women using high-dose pills containing at least 50 $\mu$g of estrogen and 1 to 4 mg of progestin (78). Systolic BP and diastolic BP are significantly higher in patients who use oral contraceptives for more than 8 years (79). BP should return to pretreatment levels within 3 months of discontinuation of oral contraceptives if the hypertension is attributable to the oral contraceptive. All levels of progestational potency and low levels of estrogen potency have been associated with a significantly increased risk of hypertension.

## Thyroid and Parathyroid Disorders

Thyroid dysfunction together with renovascular hypertension represent the most common forms of reversible secondary hypertension observed in hypertensive individuals >60 years of age (80,81). Thyrotoxic patients have hyperdynamic hypertension and high cardiac output seen predominantly as an elevated systolic BP, whereas elevation in diastolic BP is uncommon. Overall, the prevalence of hypertension in hyperthyroidism varies from 20% to 26%. On the other hand, hypothyroid patients have a high prevalence of elevated diastolic BP, and this can be a valuable clue in the elderly, in whom primary diastolic hypertension is rare. Hypertension in hypothyroid disease is associated with decreased cardiac index, low stroke volume, and increased systemic vascular resistance. Beta-adrenergic receptors are reported to be decreased, while $\alpha$-adrenergic responses are increased.

Most patients with primary hyperparathyroidism are asymptomatic; clinical diagnosis should be strongly suspected in the presence of hypercalcemia. The side effects of hypercalcemia, such as polyuria, polydipsia, renal calculi, peptic ulcer disease, and hypertension, may offer diagnostic clues. Multiple endocrine neoplasia (MEN) syndromes are the exception to the above, and the finding of a thyroid nodule, thyroid mass, or cervical lymphadenopathy should suggest the possibility of a medullary thyroid carcinoma.

Additional screening studies may include assessment of thyroid-stimulating hormone level, serum thyroid hormone level, and serum calcitonin level for thyroid disease. For hyperparathyroidism, serum calcium, serum phosphorus, and serum parathyroid hormone level should be assessed.

For diagnosis, decreased thyroid-stimulating hormone and increased free thyroxine index should be assessed in the hyperthyroid patient; increased thyroid-stimulating hormone, decreased free thyroxine index, presence of medullary thyroid carcinoma, and increased calcitonin in the hypothyroid patient; and hypercalcemia, hypophosphatemia, and increased parathyroid hormone level in the hyperparathyroid patient.

### Coarctation of the Aorta

Although coarctation of the aorta may cause left ventricular failure in early life, adults with coarctation are often asymptomatic (82,83). As a result, the medical history may be of little help in suggesting the presence of coarctation unless the diagnosis is suspected in association with other congenital malformations, such as bicuspid aortic valve, patent ductus arteriosus or ventricular septal defect, and mitral valve abnormalities. The most common location for a coarctation is distal to the left subclavian artery, but it may occasionally involve the origin of the left subclavian artery and may be missed if BPs are not checked in both upper extremities and at least one lower extremity. Absent or reduced pulses in the legs, together with hypertension in the upper extremities and low BP in the lower extremities, are obviously valuable clues to diagnosis. Systolic BPs are elevated disproportionately to the diastolic BP, resulting in wide pulse pressure and bounding pulses proximal to the coarctation. A thrill may be observed in the suprasternal notch, together with palpable pulsations or auscultated bruits over the intercostal arteries.

Additional screening studies may include an abnormal chest x-ray with a "three sign" (proximal aorta, coarctated segment with poststenotic dilation, and indentation of the aortic knob). For diagnosis and localization, two-dimensional echocardiography, aortography, and MRI may be helpful. Management should consist of surgical repair or angioplasty.

## HYPERTENSIVE EMERGENCIES AND URGENCIES

A number of different terms, including "accelerated hypertension," "hypertensive crisis," "malignant hypertension," "hypertension emergencies," and "hypertensive urgencies," generally denote severe hypertension. Conditions associated with systolic BP $>200$ mm Hg and diastolic BP $>110$ mm Hg are associated with TOD (papilledema, CHF, central nervous system dysfunction, etc.). These emergencies require immediate BP reduction, not necessarily to normal, to prevent or limit ongoing TOD.

The primary pathophysiologic abnormalities in patients presenting with hypertensive urgencies stem from defective autoregulation mechanisms of certain vascular beds that lead to arteritis and ischemia. Whereas normal arteries maintain blood flow over a broad range of mean arterial pressures from 60 to 150 mm Hg, excessive abrupt increases in BP above this autoregulation range result in TOD, especially within the brain and kidney. In these settings, the disruption of the blood–brain barrier, diffuse cerebral edema, and subsequent fibrinoid necrosis of medium arteries, small arteries, and arterioles can occur. The abruptness of the BP increase may be more critical than the actual level of BP rise. Because the risk–benefit ratio of immediate therapy for some forms of hypertensive emergencies has not been clearly established, an individual approach should be invoked to guide therapy (clinical setting, absolute level of BP increase, potential for worsening target organ perfusion). The target BP is usually lower for encephalopathy than for an acute stroke in evolution. Hypertensive emergencies are those occasional situations that require immediate BP reduction (not necessarily to normal) to prevent or limit TOD. Examples include hypertensive encephalopathy, intracranial hemorrhage, acute pulmonary edema, or a dissecting aortic aneurysm (84). Hypertensive urgencies are those situations in which reduction of BP over several hours to 24 hours is desirable. Examples include patients with upper levels of stage II hypertension and those with progressive target organ complications but not acute deterioration in target organ disease. Elevated BP alone, in the absence of symptoms or new or progressive TOD, rarely requires emergency therapy. A number of effective agents are available for the management of hypertensive emergencies and urgencies (Table 43–9).

Hypertensive emergencies during pregnancy warrant careful drug selection and hemodynamic monitoring to avoid any increase in fetal risk. Hydralazine, methyldopa, and magnesium sulfate are traditional therapeutic agents in pregnancy; however, labetalol has been used more recently. Bolus injections may achieve therapeutic BP-lowering goals sooner than continuous infusion. Consideration of timely delivery of the infant will often help with BP control.

Most hypertensive urgencies represent patients who are noncompliant with therapy or who are inadequately treated patients with essential hypertension. In most cases, immediate resumption of medication with appropriate outpatient follow-up represents appropriate therapy.

The use of fast-acting nifedipine in hypertensive urgencies has been discouraged by the U.S. Food and Drug Administration. A number of reported serious adverse effects and the inability to control the rate or degree of decline in BP make this agent unacceptable (85,86). The routine use of sublingual or oral nifedipine in patients with chronic hypertension, when BPs increase beyond a predetermined level, is also considered unacceptable.

**TABLE 43–9**
**DRUGS FOR THE MANAGEMENT OF HYPERTENSIVE EMERGENCIES AND URGENCIES**

| Agent | Dose | Onset/Duration of Action (After Discontinuation) | Precautions |
|---|---|---|---|
| | | **Parenteral vasodilators** | |
| Sodium nitroprusside | 0.25–10.0 μg/kg/min as IV infusion,[a] maximal dose for 10 min only | Immediate/2–3 min after infusion | Nausea, vomiting, muscle twitching; with prolonged use may cause thiocyanate intoxication, methemoglobinemia acidosis, cyanide poisoning; bags, bottles, and delivery sets must be light resistant |
| Fenoldopam mesylate | 0.1–0.3 mg/kg/min as IV infusion | <5 min/30 min | Headache, tachycardia, flushing, local phlebitis |
| Glyceryl trinitrate | 5–100 μg as IV infusion[a] | 2–5 min/5–10 min | Headache, tachycardia, vomiting, flushing, methemoglobinemia; requires special delivery system due to drug binding to polyvinyl chloride tubing |
| Nicardipine | 5–15 mg/h IV infusion | 1–5 min/15–30 min, but may exceed 12 h after prolonged infusion | Tachycardia, nausea, vomiting, headache, increased intracranial pressure; hypotension may be protracted after prolonged infusions |
| Verapamil | 5–10 mg IV; can follow with infusion of 3–25 mg/h | 1–5 min/30–60 min | First-, second-, third-degree heart block, concomitant digitalis or beta-blockers, bradycardia |
| Diazoxide | 50–150 mg as IV bolus, repeated, or 15–30 mg/min by IV infusion | 2–5 min/3–12 h | Hypotension, tachycardia, aggravation of angina pectoris, nausea and vomiting, hyperglycemia with repeated injections |
| Hydralazine | 10–20 mg as IV bolus or 10–40 mg IM, repeat every 4–6 h | 10 min IV/>1 h IV; 20–30 min IM/4–6 h IM | Tachycardia, headache, vomiting, aggravation of angina pectoris |
| Enalaprilat | 0.625–1.250 mg every 6 h IV | 15–60 min/12–24 h | Renal failure in patients with bilateral renal artery stenosis, hypotension |
| | | **Parenteral Adrenergic Inhibitors** | |
| Labetalol | 20–80 mg as IV bolus every 10 min; 2 mg/min as IV infusion | 5–10 min/2–6 h | Bronchoconstriction, heart block, orthostatic hypotension |
| Esmolol | 500-mg/kg bolus injection IV or 25–100 mg/kg/min by infusion; may rebolus after 5 min or increase infusion rate to 300 mg/kg/min | 1–5 min/15–30 min | >First-degree heart block, congestive heart failure, asthma |
| Methyldopa | 250–500 mg as IV infusion every 6 h | 30–60 min/4–6 h | Drowsiness |
| Phentolamine | 5–15 mg as IV bolus | 1–2 min/10–30 min | Tachycardia, orthostatic hypotension |
| | | **Oral Agents** | |
| Captopril | 25 mg PO, repeat as needed SL, 25 mg | 15–30 min/6–8 h SL 15–30 min/2–6 h | Hypotension, renal failure in bilateral renal artery stenosis |
| Clonidine | 0.1–0.2 mg PO, repeat hourly as required to total dose of 0.6 mg | 30–60 min/8–16 h | Hypotension, drowsiness, dry mouth |
| Labetalol | 200–400 mg PO, repeat every 2–3 h | 30 min to 2 h/2–12 h | Bronchoconstriction, heart block, orthostatic hypotension |
| Prazosin | 1–2 mg PO, repeat hourly as needed | 1–2 h/8–12 h | Syncope (first dose), palpitations, tachycardia, orthostatic hypotension |

[a]Requires special delivery system.
*Source:* From Vidt DG. Treatment of hypertensive urgencies and emergencies. In: Izzo JL Jr, Black HR, eds. *Hypertension Primer: The Essentials of High Blood Pressure*. Dallas, TX: Council on High Blood Pressure Research, American Heart Association; 2003.

For patients who present with a hypertensive emergency, parenteral therapy may be initiated in the Emergency Department under supervision. Most patients with true hypertensive emergencies should be admitted to an Intensive Care Unit (ICU) for continuous monitoring. The initial goal for BP reduction is not to immediately reduce the BP to normal, but rather to achieve a controlled, progressive decrease in BP to a safer level and to minimize the risk of hypoperfusion in the cerebral, coronary, and renal vascular circulation.

## CONCLUSION

Hypertension is a major public health problem worldwide, affecting over 50 million individuals in the United States alone. Hypertension may result from a number of different pathophysiologic factors that lead to both microvascular and, in time, macrovascular damage. Discovering genetic, environmental, and demographic factors that truly affect both the development and the maintenance of BP should offer hope for future medication development. The classification of patients into a prehypertensive BP category has re-emphasized the need for earlier recognition of patients who may have or develop blood pressure elevations that warrant intervention. A significant percentage of hypertensive patients warrant two or three medications to achieve a 90% control rate. Physicians should not sacrifice BP control in their desire to limit the number of medications used in treating hypertension. In the case of resistant hypertension, a series of clinical clues suggests the presence of secondary hypertension, and in specific situations, a comprehensive workup is necessary. Since the early 1980s, coronary vascular disease has accounted for more deaths among women than among men, so renewed emphasis on the importance of diagnosing and effectively treating hypertension in the female population is paramount. Although the availability of medications and increased public awareness of hypertension have decreased the total number of hypertensive emergencies, the importance of appropriate medication selection and achieving blood pressure–lowering rates is critical to the success of avoiding end-organ damage in this setting. Even though hypertension requires simple diagnostic maneuvers and basic clinical skills, it remains a significant medical problem, with the potential for limiting long-term patient survival.

## REFERENCES


1. Oparil S, Zaman MA, Calhoun DA. Pathogenesis of hypertension. *Ann Intern Med.* 2003;139:761–776.
2. Johnson RJ, Herrera-Acosta J, Schreiner GF, et al. Subtle acquired renal injury as a mechanism of salt-sensitive hypertension. *N Engl J Med.* 2002;346:913–923.
3. Sealey JE, Blumenfeld JD, Bell GM, et al. On the renal basis for essential hypertension: nephron heterogeneity with discordant renin secretion and sodium excretion causing a hypertensive vasoconstriction-volume relationship. *J Hypertens.* 1988;6:763–777.
4. Mazzali M, Hughes J, Kim YG, et al. Elevated uric acid increases blood pressure in the rat by a novel crystal-independent mechanism. *Hypertension.* 2001;38:1101–1106.
5. Cicila GT. Strategy for uncovering complex determinants of hypertension using animal models. *Curr Hypertens Rep.* 2000;2:217–226.
6. Hunt SC, Hopkins PN, Lalouel JM. Hypertension. In: King RA, Roubenoff R, Motulsky AG, eds. *The Genetic Basis of Common Diseases* (2nd ed). New York: Oxford; 2002;127–154.
7. Wilk JB, Djousse L, Arnett DK, et al. Genome-wide linkage analyses for age at diagnosis of hypertension and early-onset hypertension in the HyperGEN study. *Am J Hypertens.* 2004;17:839–844.
8. Cusi D, Barlassina C, Azzani T, et al. Polymorphisms of alpha-adducin and salt sensitivity in patients with essential hypertension. *Lancet.* 1997;349:1353–1357.
9. Hunt SC, Geleijnse JM, Wu LL, et al. Enhanced blood pressure response to mild sodium reduction in subjects with the 235T variant of the angiotensinogen gene. *Am J Hypertens.* 1999;12:460–466.
10. Turner ST, Schwartz GL, Chapman AB, et al. C825T polymorphism of the G protein beta(3)-subunit and antihypertensive response to a thiazide diuretic. *Hypertension.* 2001;37:739–743.
11. Lifton RP. Molecular genetics of human blood pressure variation. *Science.* 1996;272:676–680.
12. Luft FC. Present status of genetic mechanisms in hypertension. *Med Clin North Am.* 2004;88:1–18,vii.
13. Black HR. The paradigm has shifted, to systolic blood pressure [editorial; comment]. *Hypertension.* 1999;34:386–387.
14. Swales JD. Systolic vs. diastolic blood pressure: paradigm shift or cycle? *J Hum Hypertens.* 2000;14:477–479.
15. Beevers DG. Epidemiological, pathophysiological and clinical significance of systolic, diastolic and pulse pressure. *J Hum Hypertens.* 2004;18:531–533.
16. Franklin SS, Khan SA, Wong ND, et al. Is pulse pressure useful in predicting risk for coronary heart disease? The Framingham Heart Study. *Circulation.* 1999;100:354–360.
17. Turner ST, Bielak LF, Narayana AK, et al. Ambulatory blood pressure and coronary artery calcification in middle-aged and younger adults. *Am J Hypertens.* 2002;15:518–524.
18. Staessen JA, Gasowski J, Wang JG, et al. Risks of untreated and treated isolated systolic hypertension in the elderly: meta-analysis of outcome trials. *Lancet.* 2000;355:865–872.
19. Vaccarino V, Berkman LF, Krumholz HM. Long-term outcome of myocardial infarction in women and men: a population perspective. *Am J Epidemiol.* 2000;152:965–973.
20. Mitchell GF, Moye LA, Braunwald E, et al. Sphygmomanometrically determined pulse pressure is a powerful independent predictor of recurrent events after myocardial infarction in patients with impaired left ventricular function. SAVE investigators. Survival and Ventricular Enlargement. *Circulation.* 1997;96:4254–4260.
21. Franklin SS, Larson MG, Khan SA, et al. Does the relation of blood pressure to coronary heart disease risk change with aging? The Framingham Heart Study. *Circulation.* 2001;103:1245–1249.
22. Clement DL, De Buyzere ML, De Bacquer DA, et al. Prognostic value of ambulatory blood-pressure recordings in patients with treated hypertension. *N Engl J Med.* 2003;348:2407–2415.
23. Kaplan NM, Izzo JL. Refractory hypertension. In: Izzo JL, Black HR, eds. *Hypertension Primer.* Dallas TX: American Heart Association; 2003.
24. Yakovlevitch M, Black HR. Resistant hypertension in a tertiary care clinic. *Arch Intern Med.* 1991;151:1786–1792.
25. Taler SJ, Textor SC, Augustine JE. Resistant hypertension: comparing hemodynamic management to specialist care. *Hypertension.* 2002;39:982–988.
26. Nieto FJ, Young TB, Lind BK, et al. Association of sleep-disordered breathing, sleep apnea, and hypertension in a large community-based study. Sleep Heart Health Study. *JAMA.* 2000;283:1829–1836.
27. Pepperell JC, Ramdassingh-Dow S, Crosthwaite N, et al. Ambulatory blood pressure after therapeutic and subtherapeutic nasal continuous positive airway pressure for obstructive sleep apnoea: a randomised parallel trial. *Lancet.* 2002;359:204–210.

28. Hajjar I, Kotchen TA. Trends in prevalence, awareness, treatment, and control of hypertension in the United States, 1988–2000. *JAMA*. 2003;290:199–206.
29. Abbott KC, Bakris GL. What have we learned from the current trials? *Med Clin North Am*. 2004;88:189–207.
30. Chobanian AV, Bakris GL, Black HR, et al. The Seventh Report of the Joint National Committee on Prevention, Detection, Evaluation, and Treatment of High Blood Pressure: The JNC 7 Report. *JAMA*. 2003;289:2560–2571.
31. Chobanian AV, Bakris GL, Black HR, et al. Seventh report of the Joint National Committee on Prevention, Detection, Evaluation, and Treatment of High Blood Pressure. *Hypertension*. 2003;42: 1206–1252.
32. Joint National Committee. The sixth report of the committee on the Prevention, Detection, Evaluation and Treatment of High Blood Pressure (JNC-VI). *Arch Intern Med*. 1997;157:2413–2446.
33. Major outcomes in high-risk hypertensive patients randomized to angiotensin-converting enzyme inhibitor or calcium channel blocker vs diuretic: The Antihypertensive and Lipid-Lowering Treatment to Prevent Heart Attack Trial (ALLHAT) *JAMA*. 2002;288:2981–2997.
34. Brenner BM, Cooper ME, de Zeeuw D, et al. Effects of losartan on renal and cardiovascular outcomes in patients with type 2 diabetes and nephropathy. *N Engl J Med*. 2001;345:861–869.
35. Parving HH, Lehnert H, Brochner-Mortensen J, et al. The effect of irbesartan on the development of diabetic nephropathy in patients with type 2 diabetes. *N Engl J Med*. 2001;345:870–878.
36. Wright JT Jr, Bakris G, Greene T, et al. Effect of blood pressure lowering and antihypertensive drug class on progression of hypertensive kidney disease: results from the AASK trial. *JAMA*. 2002;288:2421–2431.
37. Psaty BM, Lumley T, Furberg CD, et al. Health outcomes associated with various antihypertensive therapies used as first-line agents: a network meta-analysis. *JAMA*. 2003;289:2534–2544.
38. Hjalmarson A, Waagstein F. The role of beta-blockers in the treatment of cardiomyopathy and ischaemic heart failure. [Review]. *Drugs*. 1994;47(suppl 4):31–39; discussion 39.
39. Eichhorn EJ. The paradox of beta-adrenergic blockade for the management of congestive heart failure. *Am J Med*. 1992;92:527–538.
40. Bakris GL, Weir MR, Shanifar S, et al. Effects of blood pressure level on progression of diabetic nephropathy: results from the RENAAL study. *Arch Intern Med*. 2003;163:1555–1565.
41. Hornig B, Landmesser U, Kohler C, et al. Comparative effect of ace inhibition and angiotensin II type 1 receptor antagonism on bioavailability of nitric oxide in patients with coronary artery disease: role of superoxide dismutase. *Circulation*. 2001;103:799–805.
42. Thomas MC, Cooper ME, Shahinfar S, et al. Dialysis delayed is death prevented: a clinical perspective on the RENAAL study. *Kidney Int*. 2003;63:1577–1579.
43. Nickolas TL, Frisch GD, Opotowsky AR, et al. Awareness of kidney disease in the US population: findings from the National Health and Nutrition Examination Survey (NHANES) 1999 to 2000. *Am J Kidney Dis*. 2004;44:185–197.
44. Lewington S, Clarke R, Qizilbash N, et al. Age-specific relevance of usual blood pressure to vascular mortality: a meta-analysis of individual data for one million adults in 61 prospective studies. *Lancet*. 2002;360:1903–1913.
45. Clausen P, Jensen JS, Jensen G, et al. Elevated urinary albumin excretion is associated with impaired arterial dilatory capacity in clinically healthy subjects. *Circulation*. 2001;103:1869–1874.
46. Bakris GL. Maximizing cardiorenal benefit in the management of hypertension: achieving blood pressure goals. *J Clin Hypertens (Greenwich)*. 1999;1:141–147.
47. Bakris GL, Weir MR, on behalf of the Study of Hypertension and Efficacy of Lotrel in Diabetes (SHIELD) Investigators. Achieving goal blood pressure in patients with type 2 diabetes: conventional versus fixed-dose combination approaches. *J Clin Hypertens (Greenwich)*. 2003;5:202–209.
48. Forette F, Lechowski L, Rigaud AS, et al. Does the benefit of antihypertensive treatment outweigh the risk in very elderly hypertensive patients? *J Hypertens*. 2000;18:S9–S12.
49. Voko Z, Bots ML, Hofman A, et al. J-shaped relation between blood pressure and stroke in treated hypertensives. *Hypertension*. 1999;34:1181–1185.
50. Koren MJ, Devereux RB, Casale PN, et al. Relation of left ventricular mass and geometry to morbidity and mortality in uncomplicated essential hypertension. *Ann Intern Med*. 1991;114:345–352.
51. Liao Y, Cooper RS, McGee DL, et al. The relative effects of left ventricular hypertrophy, coronary artery disease, and ventricular dysfunction on survival among black adults. *JAMA*. 1995;273:1592–1597.
52. Gueyffier F, Boutitie F, Boissel JP, et al. Effect of antihypertensive drug treatment on cardiovascular outcomes in women and men. A meta-analysis of individual patient data from randomized, controlled trials. The INDANA investigators. *Ann Intern Med*. 1997;126:761–767.
53. Biglieri EG, Irony I, Kater CE. Identification and implications of new types of mineralocorticoid hypertension. *J Steroid Biochem*. 1989;32:199–204.
54. Montori VM, Young WF Jr. Use of plasma aldosterone concentration-to-plasma renin activity ratio as a screening test for primary aldosteronism. A systematic review of the literature. *Endocrinol Metab Clin North Am*. 2002;31:619–632, xi.
55. Mulatero P, Rabbia F, Milan A, et al. Drug effects on aldosterone/plasma renin activity ratio in primary aldosteronism. *Hypertension*. 2002;40:897–902.
56. Sigurjonsdottir HA, Manhem K, Axelson M, et al. Subjects with essential hypertension are more sensitive to the inhibition of 11 beta-HSD by liquorice. *J Hum Hypertens*. 2003;17:125–131.
57. Blachley JD, Knochel JP. Tobacco chewer's hypokalemia: licorice revisited. *N Engl J Med*. 1980;302:784–785.
58. Stormer FC, Reistad R, Alexander J. Glycyrrhizic acid in liquorice—evaluation of health hazard. *Food Chem Toxicol*. 1993;31:303–312.
59. Kaye TB, Crapo L. The Cushing syndrome: an update on diagnostic tests. *Ann Intern Med*. 1990;112:434–444.
60. Bravo EL. Pheochromocytoma. *Cardiol Rev*. 2002;10:44–50.
61. Brauckhoff M, Gimm O, Dralle H. Preoperative and surgical therapy in sporadic and familial pheochromocytoma. *Front Horm Res*. 2004;31:121–144.
62. Nativ O, Grant CS, Sheps SG, et al. The clinical significance of nuclear DNA ploidy pattern in 184 patients with pheochromocytoma. *Cancer*. 1992;69:2683–2687.
63. Mann JF, Gerstein HC, Pogue J, et al. Renal insufficiency as a predictor of cardiovascular outcomes and the impact of ramipril: the HOPE randomized trial. *Ann Intern Med*. 2001;134:629–636.
64. National High Blood Pressure Education Program (NHBPEP) Working Group. 1995 Update of the Working Group Reports on Chronic Renal Failure and Renovascular Hypertension. *Arch Intern Med*. 1996;156:1938–1947.
65. Moore MA, Porush JG. Hypertension and renal insufficiency: recognition and management. *Am Fam Phys*. 1992;45:1248–1256.
66. Bakris GL, Williams M, Dworkin L, et al. Preserving renal function in adults with hypertension and diabetes: a consensus approach. National Kidney Foundation Hypertension and Diabetes Executive Committees Working Group. *Am J Kidney Dis*. 2000;36:646–661.
67. Giverhaug T, Falck A, Eriksen BO. Effectiveness of antihypertensive treatment in chronic renal failure: to what extent and with which drugs do patients treated by nephrologists achieve the recommended blood pressure? *J Hum Hypertens*. 2004;18:649–654.
68. Olin JW. Renal artery disease: diagnosis and management. *Mt Sinai J Med*. 2004;71:73–85.
69. Olin JW. Atherosclerotic renal artery disease. *Cardiol Clin*. 2002; 20:547–562, vi.
70. Slovut DP, Olin JW. Fibromuscular dysplasia. *N Engl J Med*. 2004; 350:1862–1871.
71. Mann SJ, Pickering TG. Detection of renovascular hypertension. State of the art: 1992. *Ann Intern Med*. 1992;117:845–853.
72. Conlon PJ, O'Riordan E, Kalra PA. New insights into the epidemiologic and clinical manifestations of atherosclerotic renovascular disease. *Am J Kidney Dis*. 2000;35:573–587.

73. Safar ME, Smulyan H. Hypertension in women. *Am J Hypertens.* 2004;17:82–87.
74. Lerner DJ, Kannel WB. Patterns of coronary heart disease morbidity and mortality in the sexes: a 26-year follow-up of the Framingham population. *Am Heart J.* 1986;111:383–390.
75. Smulyan H, Asmar RG, Rudnicki A, et al. Comparative effects of aging in men and women on the properties of the arterial tree. *J Am Coll Cardiol.* 2001;37:1374–1380.
76. Wassertheil-Smoller S, Psaty B, Greenland P, et al. Association between cardiovascular outcomes and antihypertensive drug treatment in older women. *JAMA.* 2004;292:2849–2859.
77. Peters RM, Flack JM. Hypertensive disorders of pregnancy. *J Obstet Gynecol Neonatal Nurs.* 2004;33:209–220.
78. Chasan-Taber L, Willett WC, Manson JE, et al. Prospective study of oral contraceptives and hypertension among women in the United States. *Circulation.* 1996;94:483–489.
79. Lubianca JN, Faccin CS, Fuchs FD. Oral contraceptives: a risk factor for uncontrolled blood pressure among hypertensive women. *Contraception.* 2003;67:19–24.
80. Richards AM, Espiner EA, Nicholls MG, et al. Hormone, calcium and blood pressure relationships in primary hyperparathyroidism [published erratum appears in *J Hypertens.* 1988 Nov;6(11):ii]. *J Hypertens.* 1988;6:747–752.
81. Streeten DH, Anderson GH Jr, Howland T, et al. Effects of thyroid function on blood pressure. Recognition of hypothyroid hypertension. *Hypertension.* 1988;11:78–83.
82. Serfas D, Borow KM. Coarctation of the aorta: anatomy, pathophysiology, and natural history. *J Cardiovasc Med.* 1983;8:575–581.
83. Rocchini AP. Coarctation of the aorta. In: Izzo JL Jr, Black HR, eds. *Hypertension Primer.* Dallas, TX: American Heart Association; 1999.
84. Vidt DG. Management of hypertensive urgencies and emergencies. In: Izzo JL Jr, Black HR, eds. *Hypertension Primer: The Essentials of High Blood Pressure.* Dallas, TX: American Heart Association; 1999.
85. Furberg CD, Psaty BM, Meyer JV. Nifedipine. Dose-related increase in mortality in patients with coronary heart disease. *Circulation.* 1995;92:1326–1331.
86. Grossman E, Messerli FH, Grodzicki T, et al. Should a moratorium be placed on sublingual nifedipine capsules given for hypertensive emergencies and pseudoemergencies? *JAMA.* 1996;276:1328–1331.
87. Vidt DG. Treatment of hypertensive urgencies and emergencies. In: Izzo JL Jr, Black HR, eds. *Hypertension Primer: The Essentials of High Blood Pressure.* Dallas, TX: Council on High Blood Pressure Research, American Heart Association; 2003.
88. Dahlof B, Devereux RB, Kjeldsen SE, et al. Cardiovascular morbidity and mortality in the Losartan Intervention for Endpoint reduction in hypertension study (LIFE): a randomised trial against atenolol. *Lancet* 2002;359:995–1003.
89. Major cardiovascular events in hypertensive patients randomized to doxazosin vs. chlorthalidone: the Antihypertensive and Lipid-Lowering Treatment to Prevent Heart Attack Trial (ALLHAT). ALLHAT Collaborative Research Group. *JAMA.* 200;283:1967–1975.
90. Gerstein HC, Mann JF, Yi Q, et al. Albuminuria and risk of cardiovascular events, death, and heart failure in diabetic and nondiabetic individuals. *JAMA.* 2001;386;421–426.
91. Effects of ramipril on cardiovascular and microvascular outcomes in people with diabetes mellitus: results of the HOPE study and MICRO-HOPE substudy. HOPE Study Investigators. *Lancet* 2000;355:253–259.
92. Nakajima F, Shibahara N, Arai M, et al. Intracranial aneurysms and autosomal dominant polycystic kidney disease: followup study by magnetic resonance angiography. *J Urol.* 2000: 164:311.3. PMID: 10893572.
93. Huston J 3rd, Torres VE, Wiebers DO, Schievink WI. Follow-up of intracranial aneurysms in autosomal dominant polycystic kidney disease by magnetic resonance angiography. *J Am Soc Nephrol.* 1996;7:2135–2142. PMID: 8915973.
94. Butler WE, Barker GF 2nd, Crowell RM. Patients with polycystic kidney disease would benefit from routine magnetic resonance angiographic screening for intracerebral aneurysms: a decision analysis. *Neurosurgery.* 1996;38:506–515. PMID: 8837803.
95. Walker BR, Edwards CR. Licorice-induced hypertension and syndromes of apparent mineralocorticoid excess. *Endocrinol Metab Clin N Am.* 1994;23:359–377. PMID: 8070427.

## QUESTIONS

1. A 55-year-old white man is referred for evaluation of hypertension (BP 185/95 mm Hg), discovered during a blood pressure screening at his workplace. The patient states that he is well and has not seen a physician in many years. He describes himself as "a fitness freak," as he is an active jogger, abstains from alcohol, and limits his salt and fat intake. He denies any knowledge of hypertension, cardiovascular disease, renal disease, or diabetes mellitus. He takes no medications regularly. Family history is significant in that his father was known to be hypertensive and died of a stroke. His older brother is being treated for hypertension.

On examination, the patient appears well, with a blood pressure of 178/96 mm Hg while seated and standing. Body weight is 71 kg (157 lb), and height is 178 cm (70 in). Optic fundus examination is significant for grade II hypertensive retinopathy. The remainder of the examination is normal.

Complete blood count, electrolyte panel, blood urea nitrogen level, creatinine concentration, thyroid-stimulating hormone level, and results of urinalysis are normal. Electrocardiography demonstrates normal sinus rhythm with left ventricular hypertrophy.

To reduce the patient's cardiovascular morbidity and mortality, which therapy would you prescribe?

a. Hydralazine
b. Atenolol
c. Losartan
d. Doxazosin

Answer is c: The educational objective of this question is to recognize the superiority of therapy with an angiotensin-receptor blocker over a traditional beta-blocker for cardiovascular morbidity and mortality in treating patients with primary hypertension and electrocardiographic evidence of left ventricular hypertrophy.

Most previous antihypertensive trials that demonstrated reductions in cardiovascular morbidity and mortality were based on a "stepped care" approach using diuretics and beta-blockers. The recent Losartan Intervention for Endpoint Reduction in Hypertension Study compared the angiotensin-receptor blocker losartan with the beta-blocker atenolol in patients with primary hypertension who had evidence of left ventricular hypertrophy. Despite similar reductions in blood pressure between the groups, losartan recipients had fewer primary cardiovascular events (death, myocardial infarction, or cerebrovascular accident), experienced a lower rate of new-onset diabetes mellitus, and tolerated the medication with fewer side effects (88).

**2.** A 51-year-old white man transfers to your practice after a change of insurance status. His medical history is positive for primary hypertension without target organ damage. He has no history of renal or prostatic disease. Laboratory values obtained from his former primary care physician show normal results for blood urea nitrogen, serum creatinine, electrolytes, urinalysis, prostate-specific antigen, and electrocardiography. He takes the $\alpha$-blocker doxazosin, 2 mg at bedtime.

On examination, blood pressure is 152/93 mm Hg seated and standing. Body weight is 84 kg (185 lb). The remainder of the examination is normal.

What is the appropriate course of action regarding the patient's antihypertensive therapy?

a. Advise a low-sodium diet.
b. Discontinue doxazosin therapy and consider an alternative agent.
c. Advise high dietary intake of calcium and potassium.
d. Increase the doxazosin to 4 mg a day.

Answer is b: The objective of this question is to recognize that withdrawal of monotherapy with an $\alpha$-blocker is recommended to treat hypertension. The Antihypertensive and Lipid-Lowering Treatment to Prevent Heart Attack Trial documented an increased risk of cardiovascular events (especially congestive heart failure) with use of $\alpha$-blockers. This adverse finding was published before completion of the full trial. The authors recommended that clinicians discontinue use of $\alpha$-blocker monotherapy for hypertension and consider alternative therapy. Use of $\alpha$-blocker therapy in combination with other antihypertensive agents and as therapy for symptomatic benign prostatic hyperplasia were not precluded (89).

**3.** Which of the following statements about microalbuminuria is true?

a. To be of clinical value, microalbuminuria must be measured in a timed 12- to 24-hour sample.
b. Microalbuminuria is a cardiovascular risk factor that is independent of traditional Framingham risk factors.
c. Microalbuminuria is present when the "spot" urine albumin-to-creatinine ratio is >500 mg/g.
d. Microalbuminuria is a predictor of cardiovascular risk only in patients with diabetes.

Answer is b: The educational objective is to identify microalbuminuria as a cardiovascular risk factor and appreciate its measurement in clinical practice.

Further analysis of data from the Heart Outcomes Prevention Evaluation (HOPE) trial demonstrated that microalbuminuria was an independent predictor of cardiovascular events in both diabetic and nondiabetic persons at risk for such events.

Clinical measurement of microalbuminuria is an important tool for assessment of chronic kidney disease and estimation of cardiovascular risk. Recent guidelines from the National Kidney Foundation suggest that timed urine collections are not required and that a "spot" urine sample to calculate the albumin-to-creatinine ratio is preferred. The albumin-to-creatinine ratio varies by gender because of differences in muscle mass. The established criteria for albumin-to-creatinine ratios for normal, microalbuminuria, and overt clinical proteinuria are as follows: in men, a normal albumin-to-creatinine ratio is <17 mg/g, whereas in women, <25 mg/g is normal. In microalbuminuria, the ratio is 17 to 250 mg/g in men and 25 to 355 mg/g in women; in clinical proteinuria, the ratio is >250 mg/g in men, whereas in women, it is >255 mg/g (90,91).

**4.** A 37-year-old woman calls Monday morning seeking help with "the worst headache ever" Friday night and Saturday. The headache was associated with severe lethargy and intermittent confusion. She recovered and has felt well for the past 24 hours. She states that she does not have fever or neurologic or cardiovascular symptoms. Her medical history is significant for hypertension, and recurrent urinary tract infections related to her known autosomal dominant polycystic kidney disease. She is concerned because her father died of a stroke during dialysis. Her serum creatinine concentration is 2.6 mg/dL. Blood pressure at home currently is 146/92 mm Hg.

What do you recommend for this patient?

a. Arrange urgent magnetic resonance angiography of her head.
b. Order computed tomography of her head without contrast.
c. Arrange a consultation with the neurology/headache clinic.
d. Make an office appointment for her to see you

Answer is a: The educational objective is to recognize the presentation and diagnosis of berry aneurysm in a patient with autosomal dominant polycystic kidney disease.

The patient's neurologic symptoms 48 hours earlier probably represent a "sentinel bleed" from a berry aneurysm. The likelihood of central nervous system bleeding after such an event is high and warrants urgent evaluation. Magnetic resonance angiography with gadolinium provides acceptable imaging of the carotids, circle of Willis, and central nervous system vasculature to identify or exclude berry aneurysm, which might require intervention. Overall, aneurysm is found in approximately 10% of all patients with autosomal dominant polycystic kidney disease and in about 24% of patients with polycystic kidney disease who have a positive family history of aneurysm. Routine screening with magnetic resonance angiography is often recommended for patients with this family history and autosomal dominant polycystic kidney disease. All patients with autosomal dominant polycystic kidney disease who have central nervous system symptoms should undergo magnetic resonance angiography evaluation to exclude a life-threatening condition (92–94).

**5.** A 52-year-old rodeo rider is referred by his primary care physician for hypertension and hypokalemia over the past 6 months. Blood pressure and routine chemistries were normal last year at the time of a company physical. He has no history of cardiovascular disease, stroke, or renal disease. Family history is negative for hypertension. He uses alcohol socially and does not smoke, but chews tobacco. He takes no medications regularly.

On examination the patient weights 77 kg (168 lb). Blood pressure is 184/102 mm Hg seated and standing. Except for trace pedal edema, the remainder of examination is normal.

The primary care physician provides the following laboratory values:

Blood urea nitrogen: 21 mg/dL
Serum creatinine: 0.9 mg/dL
Serum sodium: 141 mEq/L
Serum potassium: 3.1 mEq/DL
Serum chloride: 100 mEq/L
Serum bicarbonate: 28 mEq/L

A 24-hour urine test during salt loading reveals the following values:

Creatinine: 1.1 g
Sodium: 252 mEq
Potassium: 128 mEq

The daily aldosterone excretion rate is 6 mg (normal, 5 to 10 mg), plasma renin activity is 1 $\mu$g/L/h, and plasma aldosterone level is 9 ng/dL.

Which diagnostic test would you order next?

a. Adrenocorticotropin hormone stimulation test
b. Magnetic resonance angiography with gadolinium
c. Serum cortisol and urinary free cortisol measurement
d. Computed tomography of the adrenal glands

Answer is c: The educational objective of this question is to recognize corticoid excess in a patient with hypertension and hypokalemia.

This patient presents with hypertension, metabolic alkalosis with hypokalemia, and a low normal plasma and urinary aldosterone suggestive of corticoid excess due to tobacco chewing. Chewing tobacco is adulterated with licorice-containing glycyrrhizic acid. Licorice and its derivatives cause hypertension by inhibiting inactivation of cortisol by 11-$\beta$-dehydrogenase. This results in increased activation of corticosteroid receptors by cortisol, an effect that is most obvious for renal mineralocorticoid receptors, resulting in sodium retention and kaliuresis. Modest increases in the serum cortisol level and urinary level of free cortisol are diagnostic of the licorice-containing products. The biochemical data do not support the diagnosis of primary hyperaldosteronism. The low plasma renin activity and clinical presentation do not suggest renal artery stenosis (95).

# 44 Selected Topics in Pulmonary/Critical Care Medicine for an Intensive Review of Cardiology

***James K. Stoller***

The selection of topics for this chapter has been driven by two goals: (a) to present issues at the interface between pulmonary/critical care medicine and cardiology, and (b) to present topics that include information considered both "testable" for the certifying and recertifying examinations in cardiology and relevant to clinical practice. To enhance its Board relevance, the material is presented in a case-based format. In this context, cases are presented with multiple-choice answers concerning the interpretation of hemodynamics, issues in weaning from mechanical ventilation, and diagnostic considerations regarding pulmonary embolism, including the alveolar–arterial oxygen gradient. Because questions with clean, quantitative answers lend themselves to Board examinations, several of the questions posed in this chapter require simple calculations in order to best prepare the reader.

Although this selection of material has been undertaken carefully and with attention to Board relevance, there is no pretense that every pulmonary/critical care issue relevant to cardiologists is included. Indeed, other topics that may warrant review include the management of primary pulmonary hypertension, assessment of a patient's candidacy for cardiac surgery, and the interpretation of cardiopulmonary exercise testing, especially regarding the diagnosis of a ventilatory limitation to exercise.

## INTERPRETING HEMODYNAMIC PROFILES

As presented below, the first series of questions asks the reader to match one of the four hemodynamic profiles (Table 44–1) with one of the four patient profiles (Table 44–2). Each patient profile can be the correct answer once, more than once, or not at all.

### Problem 1

Which patient profile (Table 44–2) best matches hemodynamic profile 1?

In the first case, the hemodynamic profile indicates a mean arterial blood pressure of 85 mm Hg, a mean pulmonary artery pressure of 60 mm Hg, a central venous

**TABLE 44–1**
**MATCH THE HEMODYNAMIC PROFILE**

| | Mean BP | Mean PA | CVP | PAOP | CO |
|---|---|---|---|---|---|
| 1. | 85 | 60 | 15 | 10 | 5 |
| 2. | 80 | 15 | 5 | 7 | 8 |
| 3. | 90 | 50 | 10 | 20 | 2.5 |
| 4. | 70 | 20 | 10 | 8 | 5 |

BP, blood pressure; PA, pulmonary artery pressure; CVP, central venous pressure; PAOP, pulmonary artery occlusion pressure; CO, cardiac output.

pressure of 15 mm Hg, a pulmonary artery occlusion pressure (PAOP) of 10 mm Hg, and a cardiac output of 5 L/min. The best answer is number 4, a 35-year-old woman with dysphagia and sclerodactyly. Specifically, the hemodynamic profile asks the reader to recognize pulmonary hypertension as a potential complication of progressive systemic sclerosis or scleroderma, particularly in patients with the so-called CREST variant. The CREST variant is characterized by calcinosis, Raynaud syndrome, esophageal dysmotility, sclerodactyly, and telangiectasia. Pulmonary complications of scleroderma include interstitial lung disease, which occurs in 70% of patients, and pulmonary hypertension, the prevalence of which ranges from 10% to 80% in various series. The frequency of pulmonary hypertension is perhaps slightly higher in patients with the CREST variant. Also, pulmonary hypertension may occur in the absence of interstitial lung disease. This case also invites the reader to consider the differential diagnosis of pulmonary hypertension. Table 44–3 presents the recent World Health Organization (WHO) classification of pulmonary hypertension.

This specific diagnosis of idiopathic pulmonary artery hypertension, which is defined by a mean pulmonary artery pressure 25 mm Hg at rest or >30 mm Hg with exercise, requires exclusion of other causes of pulmonary hypertension (see Table 44–3). Clinical features of idiopathic pulmonary artery hypertension include a frequency of 1 to 2 cases per million, a slight female predominance (1.7:1), and usually sporadic causation, but with recognition that 6% to 10% of patients with idiopathic pulmonary artery hypertension have a familial, autosomal dominant condition with variable penetrance. Available studies suggest the presence of a PPH 1 gene on chromosome 2, which may be responsible for at least some familial cases.

**TABLE 44–2**
**PATIENT PROFILES**

1. 45-year-old nonsmoker with asthma
2. 50-year-old cirrhotic male with orthodeoxia
3. 75-year-old man with a history of multiple myocardial infarctions (MIs)
4. 35-year-old woman with dysphagia and sclerodactyly

**TABLE 44–3**
**WHO CLASSIFICATION OF PULMONARY HYPERTENSION (PH)**

1. Pulmonary artery hypertension
   - 1.1. Sporadic
     - Familial
   - 1.2. Related to
     - Collagen-vascular disease (e.g., systemic lupus erythematosus, progressive systemic sclerosis)
     - Congenital systemic-to-pulmonary shunt
     - Portal hypertension
     - HIV infection
     - Drugs/toxins (e.g., anorexigens)
     - Persistent pulmonary hypertension of the newborn
     - Other
2. Pulmonary venous hypertension
   - 2.1. Left-sided atrial or ventricular heart disease
   - 2.2. Left-sided valvular disease
   - 2.3. Extrinsic compression of central fibrosing mediastinitis
   - 2.4. Pulmonary veno-occlusive disease
   - 2.5. Other
3. PH associated with disorders of the respiratory system and/or hypoxemia
   - 3.1. Chronic obstructive pulmonary disease
   - 3.2. Interstitial lung disease
   - 3.3. Sleep-disordered breathing
   - 3.4. Alveolar hypoventilation disorders
   - 3.5. Chronic exposure to high altitude
   - 3.6. Neonatal lung disease
   - 3.7. Alveolar-capillary dysplasia
   - 3.8. Other
4. Pulmonary hypertension caused by chronic thrombotic and/or embolic disease
   - 4.1. Thromboembolic obstruction of proximal pulmonary arteries
   - 4.1. Obstruction of distal pulmonary arteries
     - Pulmonary embolism (thrombus, tumor, ova, etc.)
     - *In situ* thrombosis
     - Sickle-cell disease
5. Pulmonary hypertension due to disorders directly affecting the pulmonary vasculature
   - 5.1. Inflammatory
     - Schistosomiasis
     - Sarcoidosis
     - Other
   - 5.2. Pulmonary capillary hemangiomatosis

Optimal interpretation of the hemodynamic profiles in Table 44–1 requires facility with calculation of the pulmonary vascular and systemic vascular resistances. Therefore, the reader is next asked to calculate the pulmonary vascular resistance in hemodynamic profile 1 (see Table 44–1).

## Problem 2

What is the pulmonary vascular resistance?

a. 60 dyne-s-cm$^{-5}$
b. 45 dyne-s-cm$^{-5}$
c. 10 Wood units

**TABLE 44–4**
**CALCULATING THE PULMONARY VASCULAR RESISTANCE**

Resistance = pressure/flow
PVR (in dyne-s-$cm^{-5}$) = 80 (mean PA − PAOP)/CO
Normal values of PVR:
  0.25–1.5 Wood units
  20–120 dyne-s-$cm^{-5}$
To convert Wood units to dyne-s-$cm^{-5}$, multiply by 80

PVR, pulmonary vascular resistance; PA, pulmonary artery pressure; PAOP, pulmonary artery occlusion pressure; CO, cardiac output.

d. 850 dyne-s-$cm^{-5}$
e. 8 Wood units

Of the choices provided, the correct answer is c, or 10 Wood units.

Tables 44–4 and 44–5 review the formulas for calculating pulmonary vascular resistance and the specific calculations in this patient. Notably, the conversion from Wood units to dyne-s-$cm^{-5}$ is achieved by multiplying the Wood units by 80.

Similarly, calculation of the systemic vascular resistance requires knowledge of the appropriate formula.

## Problem 3

What is the systemic vascular resistance?

a. 1020 dyne-s-$cm^{-5}$
b. 840 dyne-s-$cm^{-5}$
c. 650 dyne-s-$cm^{-5}$
d. 1,120 dyne-s-$cm^{-5}$
e. None of the above

Of the choices given, the correct answer is d: 1,120 dyne-s-$cm^{-5}$.

Again, Tables 44–6 and 44–7 present the appropriate formulas and the specific calculation in this case.

## Problem 4

The reader is asked to identify the patient profile (see Table 44–2) that best matches the following hemodynamic profile: mean arterial blood pressure 80 mm Hg, mean pulmonary artery pressure 15 mm Hg, central venous pressure (CVP) 5 mm Hg, pulmonary artery occlusion pressure 7 mm Hg, and cardiac output 8 L/min.

The correct answer is 2, a 50-year-old cirrhotic male with orthodeoxia.

This case invites the reader to consider the hepatopulmonary syndrome, which is characterized by low pulmonary vascular resistance related to the development of intrapulmonary dilatations, or channels that decompress the pulmonary circulation and allow a mechanism of hypoxemia called perfusion-diffusion impairment. In intrapulmonary vascular dilatations, red cells pass through dilated pulmonary vessels, avoiding complete oxygenation because of the large vessel caliber. The hepatopulmonary syndrome consists of the triad of liver disease, increased alveolar–arterial oxygen gradient, and the presence of intrapulmonary vascular dilatations, the diameter of which may extend up to 500 $\mu$m. The prevalence of the hepatopulmonary syndrome in patients with chronic liver disease who are deemed transplant candidates has been estimated to be up to 45%. Other important clinical clues may be the presence of clubbing and the unusual symptom of platypnea, which is the development of dyspnea on assuming the upright posture. This may be accompanied by orthodeoxia, which is desaturation by 10% or 10 mm Hg on assuming upright posture. The cardiologist's role in diagnosing the hepatopulmonary syndrome is critical, as the entity is sensitively detected by a bubble echocardiogram in which there is evidence of right-to-left intrapulmonary shunt, with the delayed appearance of bubbles in the left-sided chambers by at least 3 to 6 systoles after injection of agitated saline.

**TABLE 44–5**
**PULMONARY VASCULAR RESISTANCE OF THIS PATIENT**

PVR (in Wood units) = (mean PA − PAOP)/CO
PVR = (60 mm Hg − 10 mm Hg)/5 L/min
PVR = (60 − 10)/5
PVR = 10 Wood units or 800 dyne-s-$cm^{-5}$

PVR, pulmonary vascular resistance; PA, pulmonary artery pressure; PAOP, pulmonary artery occlusion pressure; CO, cardiac output.

**TABLE 44–6**
**CALCULATING THE SYSTEMIC VASCULAR RESISTANCE**

Resistance = pressure/flow
SVR (in dyne-s-$cm^{-5}$) = 80 (mean BP − CVP)/CO
Normal value of SVR = 770–1,500 dyne-s-$cm^{-5}$

SVR, systemic vascular resistance; BP, blood pressure; CVP, central venous pressure; CO, cardiac output.

**TABLE 44–7**
**SYSTEMIC VASCULAR RESISTANCE OF THIS PATIENT**

SVR (in dyne-s-$cm^{-5}$) = 80 (mean BP − CVP)/CO
SVR = 80 (85 − 15)/5
SVR = 1,120 dyne-s-$cm^{-5}$

SVR, systemic vascular resistance; BP, blood pressure; CVP, central venous pressure; CO, cardiac output.

### Problem 5

Which patient profile best matches hemodynamic profile 3?

The third hemodynamic profile (see Table 44–1) features a mean arterial pressure of 90 mm Hg, a mean pulmonary artery pressure of 50 mm Hg, a CVP of 10 mm Hg, a PAOP of 20 mm Hg, and a cardiac output of 2.5 L/min. Of the choices in Table 44–2, the best choice is 3, a 75-year-old man with a history of multiple myocardial infarctions. This case highlights the hemodynamic profile of left ventricular failure with secondary pulmonary hypertension. The systemic hypertension is presumably a substrate for ischemic heart disease, and the elevated pulmonary artery occlusion pressure of 20 mm Hg bespeaks left ventricular dysfunction, along with an impaired cardiac output of 2.5 L/min.

### Problem 6

Which patient profile best matches hemodynamic profile 4?

The last hemodynamic profile features a mean arterial blood pressure of 70 mm Hg, a mean pulmonary artery pressure of 20 mm Hg, a CVP of 10 mm Hg, a PAOP of 8 mm Hg, and a cardiac output of 5 L/min. The best choice for this normal hemodynamic profile in Table 44–2 is choice 1, a 45-year-old nonsmoker with asthma. In the absence of other relevant disease, asthma is not expected to cause hemodynamic abnormality.

## WEANING FROM MECHANICAL VENTILATION

### Problem 7

In this problem, concerning weaning from mechanical ventilation, the reader is asked to consider the scenario of a 72-year-old man who developed respiratory failure after a community-acquired pneumonia for which he was intubated. Now, despite his being afebrile and with only scant secretions after 3 days of mechanical ventilation, efforts to liberate him from mechanical ventilation have been unsuccessful. Attempts to wean have been accompanied by marked tachypnea and anxiety, though he shows no abdominal paradox and his $PaO_2$ is 75 mm Hg on 40% oxygen. He denies chest pain. His rapid shallow breathing index (the respiratory rate [breaths per minute] divided by the tidal volume [in liters] measured with the patient breathing spontaneously over 1 minute) at the time of his weaning failure is 75. Electrolytes, including serum phosphate, are normal. His past medical history is notable only for hypertension and hypercholesterolemia. You are asked to consider the likeliest causes of this patient's failure to wean, which might include the following choices:

a. Uncontrolled pneumonia
b. Oversedation
c. Ventilatory muscle dysfunction
d. All of the above
e. None of the above

The correct answer is e (None of the above), recognizing that the clinical message is to suspect myocardial ischemia as a cause of weaning failure.

In evaluating the difficult-to-wean patient, many etiologies must be considered, including metabolic derangement (e.g., hypokalemia, hypophosphatemia), persistent neuromuscular weakness, oversedation, ongoing infection, and so on. Beyond the "conventional" causes of weaning failure, myocardial ischemia should also be considered, as studied by Chatila et al. and by Srivastava et al. In the first of these series, 93 patients (mean age 66.5 years, with a known history of coronary artery disease in 53%) were weaned from mechanical ventilation, with successful liberation achieved in 60% in the first trial. The prevalence of ischemia during weaning by ST-segment analysis was 6% (6 of 93 patients); five of these six patients were known to have prior coronary artery disease. Among these six patients with ischemia detected during weaning, four (66%) failed to wean on the initial trial, but all were successfully weaned later, after escalation of their antianginal regimen.

In a follow-up study from the same institution, Srivastava et al. reported an observational study of 83 patients being weaned from mechanical ventilation. In this more recent series, 9.6% (8/83) experienced ischemia during weaning, but only two of the eight experienced chest pain. The likelihood of weaning success was lower on the initial effort in ischemic patients (risk ratio 2.1 [95% confidence interval 1.4–3.1]), leading to the conclusions that:

1. Ischemia during weaning is fairly common and often unaccompanied by chest pain,
2. Ischemia was associated with a higher rate of weaning failure on initial weaning attempts.
3. Attention to treating unsuspected ischemia can enhance the likelihood of successful liberation from mechanical ventilation.

On the basis of these findings, cardiac ischemia should be included in the clinician's "review of systems" in assessing the difficult-to-wean patient. The current patient demonstrates none of the "conventional" causes of weaning failure. Indeed, his rapid shallow breathing index $<105$ favors weaning success at a time when he is unable to wean, suggesting a limiting step other than neuromuscular function. In the context of this patient's risk factors for coronary artery disease, including hypercholesterolemia and hypertension, myocardial ischemia should be considered.

## DIAGNOSIS OF PULMONARY THROMBOEMBOLISM

### Problem 8

This problem involves a 34-year-old never-smoking male who presents with pleuritic pain 5 days after a tibial fracture

**TABLE 44–8**

**THE CLUMSY SKIER: WHAT IS THE BEST CONCLUSION?**

a. His normal alveolar-arterial oxygen gradient ($AaDO_2$) rules out pulmonary embolism (PE).
b. A workup for PE is needed. If an acute PE is found, anticoagulate for 3 to 6 months and stop.
c. A workup for PE is needed. If an acute PE is found, suspect prior PE.
d. He must have chronic obstructive pulmonary disease (COPD).
e. None of the above.

sustained while skiing. He lives an otherwise sedentary life and has not previously seen a doctor. His physical examination is normal except for tachypnea and a leg cast. A room-air arterial blood gas shows a $PaO_2$ of 80 mm Hg, $PaCO_2$ of 36 mm Hg, and a pH of 7.38. An echocardiogram shows normal left ventricular systolic function, mild right ventricular dilatation, and an estimated right ventricular systolic pressure of 78 mm Hg. The question for this problem is: What is the best conclusion regarding diagnosis and management? Table 44–8 presents the options.

The best answer is c: A workup for pulmonary embolism is needed. If an acute pulmonary embolism is found, suspect prior pulmonary embolism.

The "take-home" points regarding pulmonary embolism in this patient are as follows:

1. In a previously normal individual, the right ventricle cannot sustain an acute rise in mean PA pressure to exceed 40 mm Hg.
2. As such, finding a mean pulmonary artery pressure >40 mm Hg (as is likely the case here, where the right ventricular systolic pressure is 78 mm Hg) in this patient with an acute pulmonary embolism should prompt consideration of prior pulmonary embolism.
3. Finally, a normal alveolar–arterial oxygen gradient ($AaDO_2$) does not rule out pulmonary embolism.

Pulmonary embolism poses a significant diagnostic challenge, especially given the acute mortality rate and the higher risk of mortality in undiagnosed individuals. An important and frequently misunderstood point is that, as in the current patient, individuals with pulmonary embolism may present with apparently normal values of $PaO_2$. For example, in a series by Rodger et al., an abnormal alveolar–arterial oxygen gradient was found in only 84% of patients with angiographically proven pulmonary emboli. The diagnostic features associated with the greatest sensitivity for the diagnosis of pulmonary embolism were a $PaO_2 < 80$ mm Hg, D-dimer positivity, <u>or</u> respiratory rate exceeding 20. Ninety-seven percent of patients with angiographically proven pulmonary embolism had one of these three criteria present.

**TABLE 44–9**

**CALCULATING THE ALVEOLAR–ARTERIAL OXYGEN GRADIENT ($AaDO_2$)**

$AaDO_2$ (mm Hg) = $PAO_2 - PaO_2$
$PAO_2 = (FIO_2)(760 - 47 \text{ mm Hg}) - PaCO_2/RQ$, where RQ ~0.8
On room air, $PAO_2 = (0.21)(713) - (1.25)\ PaCO_2$
$AaDO_2 = 149 - [(1.25)(PaCO_2) + (PaO_2)]$
$AaDO_2 = 149 - [(1.25)(36) + 80] = 24$
Normal $AaDO_2 = (\text{age}/4) + 4 = 15$ mm Hg here

$AaDO_2$, alveolar-arterial oxygen gradient; RQ, respiratory quotient; $PAO_2$, alveolar oxygen tension; $PaO_2$, arterial oxygen tension; $PaCO_2$, arterial carbon dioxide tension.

Calculation of the alveolar–arterial oxygen gradient is an important concept in approaching patients with pulmonary embolism. Table 44–9 presents the relevant equation.

In the current patient, the alveolar–arterial oxygen gradient ($AaDO_2$) is 24 mm Hg. Documentation of the $AaDO_2$ must be made with knowledge of the patient's age, as normal values increase with age. Specifically, the normal mean alveolar–arterial oxygen gradient can be approximated by the expression (age/4) + 4. In this patient, the mean value was 15 mm Hg, so his observed alveolar–arterial oxygen gradient is elevated and consistent with pulmonary embolism. In the PIOPED study, the frequency of a room-air $PaO_2$ exceeding 80 mm Hg was 27% in patients with a pulmonary infarction and 11% in patients with dyspnea, thus confirming that a reasonably normal value of $PaO_2$ does not exclude pulmonary embolism.

The critical finding in the current patient is the right ventricular systolic pressure of 78 mm Hg, which is distinctly elevated. The observation that previously normal patients with acute pulmonary embolism cannot sustain a new pulmonary artery pressure exceeding 40 mm Hg comes from studies by McIntyre and Sasahara. In a series of 20 previously normal patients with angiographically proven pulmonary emboli, none of the patients demonstrated a mean pulmonary artery pressure >40 mm Hg. This led to the conclusion that "it appears that the upper limit of pulmonary artery pressure which the normal right ventricle can maintain acutely is approximately 40 mm Hg. As a corollary, it may be stated that a mean pulmonary artery pressure level over 40 mm Hg after pulmonary embolism should suggest either chronic recurrent embolization or prior non-embolic causes of pulmonary hypertension." In the patient presented, no prior co-morbidity is described, so prior pulmonary embolism should be suspected.

Finally, additional diagnostic issues pertaining to pulmonary embolism include features of the electrocardiogram and plain chest radiograph. In a series by Stein and Henry, electrocardiographic features of 155 patients with angiographically proven pulmonary embolism were evaluated. As shown in Table 44–10, a normal electrocardiogram may be seen more frequently (46%) in patients with pulmonary infarction than with dyspnea (10%).

**TABLE 44–10**
**ELECTROCARDIOGRAPHIC FEATURES OF PATIENTS WITH PULMONARY EMBOLISM**

| Feature | Infarction ($N = 119$) | Dyspnea ($N = 31$) | Collapse ($N = 5$) |
|---|---|---|---|
| Normal ECG | 46% | 10% | 20% |
| ST-seg/T-wave | 40% | 57% | 60% |
| Left axis | 13% | 14% | 0% |
| LVH | 9% | 0% | 0% |
| Inc RBBB | 4% | 10% | 0% |
| Acute MI pattern | 2% | 5% | 20% |
| Low voltage | 3% | 5% | 20% |
| P pulmonale | 1% | 5% | 20% |
| Right axis | 1% | 0% | 0% |
| RVH | 1% | 1% | 0% |

Inc RBBB, incomplete right bundle branch block; LVH, left ventricular hypertrophy; RVH; right ventricular hypertrophy.
$p < 0.01$ infarction vs. dyspnea.
*Source:* From Stein PD, Henry J. Clinical characteristics of patients with acute pulmonary embolism stratified according to their presenting syndromes. *Chest.* 1997;112:974–979.

**TABLE 44–11**
**PLAIN CHEST RADIOGRAPHIC FINDINGS IN PATIENTS WITH PULMONARY EMBOLISM**

| Feature | Infarction ($N = 119$) | Dyspnea ($N = 31$) | Collapse ($N = 5$) |
|---|---|---|---|
| Normal film | 14% | 26% | 40% |
| Atelectasis | 75% | 52% | 20% |
| Pleural effusion | 56% | 26% | 0% |
| Pleural-based opacity | 36% | 23% | 0% |
| Elevated diaphragm | 26% | 19% | 20% |
| Decreased vascularity | 20% | 26% | 0% |
| Prominent central pulmonary artery | 14% | 16% | 0% |
| Cardiomegaly | 8% | 16% | 40% |
| Westermark sign | 6% | 6% | 0% |

*Source:* From Stein PD, Henry J. Clinical characteristics of patients with acute pulmonary embolism stratified according to their presenting syndromes. *Chest.* 1997;112:974–979.

Other observed ECG changes include ST-segment/T-wave changes in 40% to 60% of individuals, left-axis deviation in 13% to 14%, and incomplete right bundle branch block pattern in 4% to 10% of individuals. No individual in this series was described with the S1, Q3, T3 pattern, which is said to be specific albeit not sensitive for pulmonary embolism.

Regarding characteristics of the chest x-ray, Table 44–11 presents the findings from this same series.

Notably, normal chest x-rays may be seen in between 14% and 40% of individuals, depending on the clinical presentation as either being infarction, dyspnea, or cardiopulmonary collapse. Atelectasis is the commonest finding, seen in 20% to 75% of individuals, with pleural effusions observed in 26% to 56%. Pleural-based opacities (e.g., Hampton hump) were observed in 23% to 36% of individuals. The remaining abnormalities are seen in lower frequency, as reviewed in Table 44–11.

## BIBLIOGRAPHY

**Chatila W, Ani S, Guanglione D, et al.** Cardiac ischemia during weaning from mechanical ventilation. *Chest.* 1996;109:1577–1583.

**Farber HW, Loscalzo J.** Pulmonary arterial hypertension. *N Engl J Med.* 2004;351:1655–1665.

**Lange PA, Stoller JK.** The hepatopulmonary syndrome. *Ann Intern Med.* 1995;122:521–529.

**McIntyre KM, Sasahara AA.** Determinants of right ventricular function and hemodynamics after pulmonary embolism. *Chest.* 1974;65:534–543.

**McIntyre KM, Sasahara AA.** The hemodynamic response to pulmonary embolism in patients without prior cardiopulmonary disease. *Am J Cardial.* 1971;28:288–294.

**Rodger MA, Cabrier M, Jones GM, et al.** Diagnostic value of arterial blood gas measurement in suspected pulmonary embolism. *Am J Respir Crit Care Med.* 2000;162:2105–2108.

**Srivastava S, Chatila W, Amaoteng-Adjepong Y, et al.** Myocardial ischemia and weaning failure in patients with coronary artery disease: an update. *Crit Care Med.* 1999;27:2109–2112.

**Stein P, Henry J.** Clinical characteristics of patients with acute pulmonary embolism stratified according to their presenting syndromes. *Chest.* 1997;112:974–979.

# Cardiac Electrophysiology

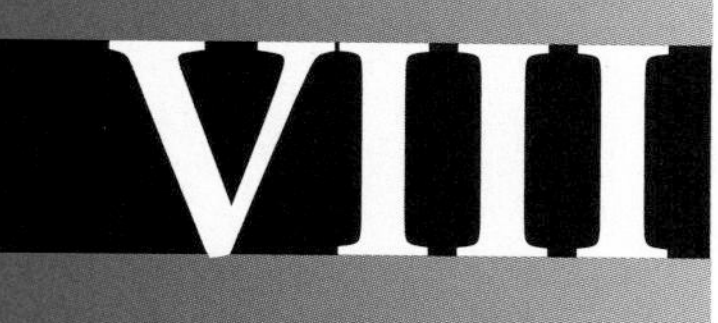

# Twelve-Lead Electrocardiography

45

***Gregory G. Bashian*** ***Curtis M. Rimmerman***

The electrocardiogram (ECG) is an essential diagnostic test. In many ways it is an ideal diagnostic modality because it is noninvasive, is readily performed without discomfort or potential patient injury, is inexpensive, and its results are immediately available. Most important, it provides a diagnostic window of cardiovascular surveillance for a multitude of cardiac pathophysiologic problems, including valvular, myocardial, pericardial, and ischemic heart disease. The electrocardiogram's diagnostic utility is critically dependent on its accurate interpretation. This chapter addresses the diagnostic possibilities encountered in routine electrocardiogram interpretation, including a broad collection of clinical examples. A clinical history, detailed interpretation, and diagnostic summary are included for each tracing. A detailed review of this chapter will provide comprehensive preparation for the Cardiovascular Medicine Subspecialty Board Examination.

## BOARD PREPARATION

To receive a passing score on the Cardiovascular Medicine Subspeciality Board Examination, the examinee must also receive a passing score on the electrocardiogram subsection. To best prepare for the electrocardiogram section, familiarization with the scoring sheet is essential. The scoring sheet is sent to each examinee before the test date, with diagnoses grouped systematically for easy reference. In preparation, understanding and being able to recognize each diagnosis is a "foolproof" preemptive approach.

## A RECOMMENDED APPROACH TO ELECTROCARDIOGRAM INTERPRETATION

To ensure accurate and consistent ECG interpretation, a systematic approach is required. Electrocardiogram interpretation is not an exercise in pattern recognition. To the contrary, employing a methodical strategy based on a thorough knowledge of the cardiac conduction sequence, cardiac anatomy, cardiac physiology, and cardiac pathophysiology can be applied to all electrocardiograms, regardless of the findings.

One systematic approach to each electrocardiogram is to ascertain the following in this recommended order:

1. Assess the standardization and identify the recorded leads accurately.
2. Determine the atrial and ventricular rates and rhythms.
3. Determine the P-wave and QRS-complex axes.
4. Measure all cardiac intervals.
5. Determine if cardiac chamber enlargement or hypertrophy is present.
6. Assess the P-wave, QRS-complex, and T-wave morphologies.
7. Draw conclusions and correlate clinically.

Cardiac pathology is manifest differently on the surface ECG, depending on which lead is interrogated. Each lead provides an "electrical window of opportunity," and by this virtue, offers a unique electrical perspective. The experienced electrocardiographer amalgamates these different windows into a mental three-dimensional electrical assessment, drawing accurate conclusions pertaining to conduction system and structural heart disease. For example, precordial lead $V_1$ predominantly overlies the right ventricle, explaining why right ventricular cardiac electrical events are best observed in this lead. Likewise, precordial lead $V_6$ overlies the left ventricle. This lead optimally represents left ventricular cardiac electrical events.

## 1. Assess the Standardization and Identify the Recorded Leads Accurately

Standard ECG graph paper consists of 1-mm × 1-mm boxes divided by narrow lines, which are separated by bold lines into larger, 5-mm × 5-mm boxes. At standard speed (25 mm/s), each small box in the horizontal axis represents 0.040 second (40 milliseconds) of time and each large box represents 0.200 second (200 milliseconds). At standard calibration (1 mV/10 mm), each vertical small box represents 0.1 mV and each vertical large box represents 0.5 mV. One must be very careful to inspect the standardization square wave (1 mV in amplitude) at the left of each ECG to determine the calibration of the ECG. ECGs with particularly high or low voltages are often recorded at half-standard or twice standard, respectively. In these cases, the 1-mV square wave possesses an amplitude of either 5 or 20 mm. This distinction is important because it will affect the interpretation of all other voltage criteria. All further references to amplitude in this chapter will be under the assumption of the default or preset standardization (1 mV/10 mm).

## 2. Determine the Atrial and Ventricular Rates and Rhythms

The first step in determining the rate and rhythm is to identify atrial activity. If P waves are present, it is important to measure the P-wave to P-wave interval (P–P interval). This determines the rate of atrial depolarization. To estimate quickly either an atrial or ventricular rate on a standard 12-lead ECG, one can count the number of 5-mm boxes in an interval, and divide 300 by that number. For example, if there are four boxes between P waves, the rate is 300 divided by 4, or 75 complexes per minute.

Once the atrial activity and rate are identified, the P-wave frontal plane axis should be ascertained. A normal P-wave axis (i.e., −0 to 75 degrees) typically reflects a sinus node P-wave origin. A simple way of determining a normal P-wave axis is to confirm a positive P-wave vector in leads I, II, III, and aVF. An abnormal P-wave axis supports an ectopic or non–sinus node P-wave origin.

Several possible atrial and junctional rhythms are listed below. They are grouped by cardiac rhythm origin and subsequently subcategorized by atrial rate. Distinguishing features are italicized for emphasis.

### *Rhythms of Sinus Nodal and Atrial Origin*

#### 1. Normal Sinus Rhythm (NSR)

A normal sinus rhythm (NSR) is defined as a *regular* atrial depolarization rate between *60 and 100 per minute* of *sinus node origin*, as demonstrated by a positive P-wave vector in leads I, II, III, and aVF.

#### 2. Sinus Bradycardia

Sinus bradycardia is characterized by a *regular* atrial depolarization rate *less than 60 per minute* of *sinus node origin*, as demonstrated by a positive P-wave vector in leads I, II, III, and aVF. (This is similar to NSR, except the rate is slower.)

#### 3. Sinus Tachycardia

Sinus tachycardia is characterized by a *regular* atrial depolarization rate *≥100 per minute* of *sinus node origin*, as demonstrated by a positive P-wave vector in leads I, II, III, and aVF. (This is similar to NSR, except the rate is faster.)

#### 4. Sinus Arrhythmia

Sinus arrhythmia is characterized by an *irregular* atrial depolarization rate between *60 and 100 per minute* of *sinus node origin*, as demonstrated by a positive P-wave vector in leads I, II, III, and aVF. (This is similar to NSR, except there is *irregularity in the P–P interval >160 milliseconds*.)

#### 5. Sinus Arrest or Pause

Sinus arrest or pause is characterized by a pause of >2.0 seconds without identifiable atrial activity. This may be caused by frank sinus arrest, or may be simply a sinus pause secondary to:

- Nonconducted premature atrial contraction (PAC), in which case a P wave can be seen deforming the preceding T wave.
- Sinoatrial block (SA block), which, like atrioventricular (AV) nodal block, has several forms.

First-degree SA block involves a fixed delay between the depolarizing SA node and the depolarization exiting the node and propagating as a P wave. Because the delay is fixed, this delay cannot be detected on the surface ECG.

Second-degree SA block has two varieties. In Type I (Wenckebach) SA block, there is a progressive delay between SA nodal depolarization and exit of the impulse to the atrium. This is manifest as a progressive shortening of the P–P interval until there is a pause, reflecting an SA node impulse that was blocked from exiting the node. In Type II SA block, there is a constant P–P interval with intermittent pauses. These pauses also represent an SA node impulse that was blocked from exiting the node. However, in this case the duration of the pause is a multiple of the basic P–P interval.

Third-degree SA block demonstrates no P-wave activity, as no impulses exit the sinus node. On the surface ECG, this is indistinguishable from sinus arrest, in which there is no sinus node activity.

#### 6. Sinus Node Re-entrant Rhythm

Sinus node re-entrant rhythm is characterized by a *re-entrant circuit involving the sinus node* and perisinus nodal tissues. Given the sinus origin, the *P-wave morphology and axis are normal and indistinguishable from a normal sinus P wave*. The rate is regular at a rate of *60 to 100 per minute*. (This is very similar to NSR, except characterized by abrupt onset and termination.)

### 7. Sinus Node Re-entrant Tachycardia

Sinus node re-entrant tachycardia is characterized by a *re-entrant circuit involving the sinus node* and perisinus nodal tissues. Given the sinus origin, the *P-wave morphology and axis are normal and indistinguishable from a normal sinus P wave*. The rate is regular at a rate of $\geq$*100 per minute*. (This is very similar to sinus tachycardia, except characterized by abrupt onset and termination.)

### 8. Ectopic Atrial Rhythm

Ectopic atrial rhythm is characterized by a *regular* atrial depolarization at a rate of *60 to 100 per minute* from a *single nonsinus origin,* as reflected by an abnormal P-wave axis. The PR interval may be shortened, particularly in the presence of a low ectopic atrial origin, closer to the atrioventricular node with a reduced intra-atrial conduction time. In the presence of slowed atrial conduction, the PR interval may be normal or even prolonged.

### 9. Ectopic Atrial Bradycardia

Ectopic atrial bradycardia is characterized by a *regular* atrial depolarization at a rate of $\leq$*60 per minute* from a *single nonsinus origin,* as reflected by an abnormal P-wave axis. (This is similar to an ectopic atrial rhythm, except slower.)

### 10. Atrial Tachycardia

Atrial tachycardia is characterized by a *regular,* automatic tachycardia from a *single, ectopic atrial focus* typically with an atrial rate of *180 to 240 per minute*. The ventricular rate may be regular or irregular, depending on the atrioventricular conduction ratio. The P-wave axis is abnormal, given the ectopic atrial focus. (This is similar to an ectopic atrial rhythm, except faster.)

### 11. Wandering Atrial Pacemaker

A wandering atrial pacemaker (WAP) has a rate of *60 to 100 per minute* from multiple ectopic atrial foci, as evidenced by at least *three different P-wave morphologies* on the 12-lead ECG, possessing *variable P–P, PR, and R–R intervals*. Be careful not to confuse this dysrhythmia with atrial fibrillation. Unlike atrial fibrillation, discrete P waves are identifiable.

### 12. Multifocal Atrial Tachycardia

Multifocal atrial tachycardia (MAT) is characterized by a rate of >*100 per minute* with a P wave preceding each QRS complex from multiple atrial ectopic foci, as evidenced by at least *three different P-wave morphologies* on the 12-lead ECG possessing *variable P–P, PR, and R–R intervals*. The ventricular response is irregularly irregular, given the unpredictable timing of the atrial depolarization and variable atrioventricular conduction. Nonconducted atrial complexes during the ventricular absolute refractory period are also often present. Be careful not to confuse this dysrhythmia with atrial fibrillation. Unlike atrial fibrillation, discrete P waves are identifiable. (This is similar to wandering atrial pacemaker, but the atrial rate is faster.)

### 13. Atrial Fibrillation

Atrial fibrillation (AF) is characterized by a *rapid, irregular, and disorganized atrial depolarization* rate of 400 to 600 per minute *devoid of identifiable discrete P waves, instead characterized by fibrillatory waves*.

In the absence of fixed atrioventricular block, the ventricular response to atrial fibrillation is *irregularly irregular*. Be careful not to confuse this dysrhythmia with wandering atrial pacemaker or multifocal atrial tachycardia. The key is the lack of identifiable P waves.

### 14. Atrial Flutter

Atrial flutter (AFL) is characterized by a *rapid, regular atrial depolarization* rate of *250 to 350 per minute*, representing an intra-atrial re-entrant circuit. The atrial waves are termed "flutter waves" and often demonstrate a *"sawtoothed"* appearance, best seen in leads $V_1$, II, III, and aVF.

Although the atrial rate is regular, the *ventricular response rate may be either regular or irregular,* depending on the presence of fixed versus variable atrioventricular conduction. Common atrioventricular conduction ratios are 2:1 and 4:1.

## *Rhythms of Atrioventricular Nodal and Junctional Origin*

### 1. Atrioventricular Nodal Re-entrant Tachycardia

Atrioventricular nodal re-entrant tachycardia (AVNRT) is a micro–re-entrant dysrhythmia that depends on the presence of *two separate atrioventricular nodal pathways*. Slowed conduction is present in one pathway and unidirectional conduction block is present in the second pathway. *This is a regular rhythm* with a typical *ventricular rate of 140 to 200* per minute, with abrupt onset and termination. Its onset is *often initiated by premature atrial complexes (PACs)*. Atrial activity typically consists *of inverted or retrograde P waves occurring either before, during, or after the QRS* complex, *best identified in lead* $V_1$. The QRS complex may be conducted normally or aberrantly.

### 2. Atrioventricular Re-entrant Tachycardia

Atrioventricular re-entrant tachycardia (AVRT) is a *macro–re-entrant circuit that consists of an atrioventricular nodal pathway and an accessory pathway*. This dysrhythmia may conduct antegrade down the atrioventricular nodal pathway with retrograde conduction through the accessory pathway (orthodromic AVRT), or antegrade down the accessory pathway with retrograde conduction up the atrioventricular nodal pathway (antidromic AVRT). As opposed to AVNRT, the *P wave is always present after the QRS* complex. With antidromic AVRT, the QRS complex, by definition, is aberrantly conducted (wide).

### 3. Junctional Premature Complexes

Junctional premature complexes are *premature* QRS complexes of AV nodal origin that may have resultant *retrograde*

*P waves* (a negative P-wave vector in leads II, III, and aVF) occurring immediately *before (with a short PR interval), during, or after the QRS* complex.

#### 4. AV Junctional Bradycardia

AV junctional bradycardia is characterized by QRS complexes of AV nodal origin that occur at a regular rate of <*60 per minute*. These represent a *subsidiary pacemaker* and may have resultant *retrograde P waves* (negative P-wave vector in leads II, III, and aVF) that occur immediately *before (with a short PR interval), during, or after the QRS* complex.

#### 5. Accelerated AV Junctional Rhythm

Accelerated AV junctional rhythm is characterized by QRS complexes of AV nodal origin that occur at a regular rate of *60 to 100 per minute*. These represent a *subsidiary pacemaker* and may have resultant *retrograde P waves* (negative P-wave vector in leads II, III, and aVF) that occur immediately *before (with a short PR interval), during, or after the QRS* complex. (This dysrhythmia is similar to AV junctional bradycardia, except faster.)

#### 6. AV Junctional Tachycardia

AV junctional tachycardia is characterized by QRS complexes of AV nodal origin that occur at a regular rate of *typically 100 to 200 per minute*. This dysrhythmia emanates from the AV junction and serves as a dominant cardiac pacemaker sith an inappropriately rapid rate. *Retrograde P waves* may be identified (negative P-wave vector in leads II, III, and aVF) that occur immediately *before (with a short PR interval), during, or after the QRS* complex. (This dysrhythmia is similar to AV junctional rhythm, except faster.)

### *Rhythms of Ventricular Origin*

#### 1. Idioventricular Rhythm

Idioventricular rhythm is a regular escape rhythm of ventricular origin that possesses a typically *widened QRS* complex (>100 milliseconds) at a rate *of less than 60* per minute. This is often seen in cases of high-degree AV block, in which the ventricle serves as a subsidiary pacemaker.

#### 2. Ventricular Parasystole

Ventricular parasystole is an independent, automatic ventricular rhythm that emanates from a single ventricular focus characterized by a *widened QRS* complex with regular discharge and ventricular depolarization. Because the rhythm is independent and not suppressible, ventricular parasystole is characterized by *varying coupling intervals and unchanged interectopic R–R intervals*. Fusion complexes can be observed when the parasystolic focus discharges simultaneously with native ventricular depolarization. When the ventricle is absolutely refractory, the parasystolic focus is not recorded on the surface electrocardiogram, but its discharge remains unabated.

#### 3. Accelerated Idioventricular Rhythm

Accelerated idioventricular rhythm (AIVR) is a regular rhythm of ventricular origin that typically has a *widened QRS* complex at a *rate of 60 to 100 per minute*. It is often seen in cases of high-degree AV block, in which the ventricle serves as a subsidiary pacemaker plus in cases of coronary artery reperfusion. (AIVR is similar to idioventricular rhythm, except faster.)

#### 4. Ventricular Tachycardia

Ventricular tachycardia (VT) is a sustained cardiac rhythm of ventricular origin that occurs at a typical rate of 140 to 240 per minute. In differentiating this from supraventricular tachycardia with aberrant conduction, the following features suggest VT:

- AV dissociation
- Fusion or capture complexes
- Wide QRS (≥140 milliseconds if right bundle branch block [RBBB] morphology; ≥160 milliseconds if left bundle branch block [LBBB] morphology)
- Left-axis QRS complex deviation
- Concordance of the precordial-lead QRS complexes
- QRS morphologies similar to those of PVCs on the current or previous ECG
- Tachyarrhythmia initiated by a PVC
- If RBBB morphology, possessing a RSr′ pattern (as opposed to an rSR′ pattern)

#### 5. Polymorphic Ventricular Tachycardia

Polymorphic ventricular tachycardia is a paroxysmal form of VT with a *nonconstant R–R interval*, a ventricular rate of 200 to 300 per minute, QRS complexes of alternating polarity, and a changing QRS amplitude that often resembles a sine-wave pattern (*torsades de pointes*). It is often associated with a *prolonged QT* interval at arrhythmia initiation.

#### 6. Ventricular Fibrillation

Ventricular fibrillation (VF) is a terminal cardiac rhythm with chaotic ventricular activity that lacks organized ventricular depolarization.

## 3. Determine the P-Wave and QRS-Complex Axes

A normal P-wave axis varies from 0 to 75 degrees, but is usually between 45 and 60 degrees. P waves with a normal axis are upright in leads I, II, III, and aVF and inverted in lead aVR. An abnormal P-wave axis should prompt the interpreter to consider non–sinus nodal rhythms, dextrocardia, or limb lead reversal, among other causes.

To ascertain the frontal-plane axis of the QRS complex, the QRS-complex vector is assessed in each of the limb leads. A recommended approach is to search for the limb lead in which the QRS complex is isoelectric (i.e., the area of positivity under the R wave is equal to the area of negativity above the Q and S waves). The QRS-complex frontal-plane axis will be perpendicular to the isoelectric lead, thus narrowing down the axis to one of two possibilities (90 degrees clockwise or 90 degrees counterclockwise of the isoelectric lead's axis). Next, one examines a limb lead whose vector is close to one of the two possible axes. Based on whether the QRS is grossly positive or negative in that lead, one can deduce which of the two possible axes is correct.

An alternative approach is as follows:

1. Assess the QRS complex vector in leads I and aVF. If both are positive, the QRS complex is between 0 and +90 degrees, and is therefore normal.
2. If the QRS-complex vector is positive in lead I and negative in aVF, assess the QRS-complex vector in lead II. If it is positive in lead II, the QRS-complex axis is between −30 degrees and 0 degrees, and is leftward but still not pathologically deviated. If the QRS complex is negative in lead II, then the QRS-complex axis is between −90 degrees and −30 degrees, and therefore abnormal left-axis QRS-complex deviation is present.
3. If the QRS-complex vector is negative in lead I and positive in lead aVF, abnormal right-axis QRS-complex deviation is present.
4. If the QRS-complex vector is negative in both leads I and aVF, the QRS-complex axis is profoundly deviated to between −90 degrees and −180 degrees.

## 4. Measure All Cardiac Intervals

### PR Interval

A normal PR interval is between 120 and 200 milliseconds. This represents the interval between P-wave onset and QRS-complex onset. The PR interval represents intra-atrial and AV nodal conduction time. A short PR interval (<120 milliseconds) is suggestive of facile intra-atrial or AV conduction, and may represent ventricular pre-excitation. A prolonged PR interval (>200 milliseconds) reflects delayed intra-atrial or AV conduction. In the setting of a varying PR interval, conduction block or AV dissociation may be present.

### R–R Interval

The R–R interval is inversely proportional to the rate of ventricular depolarization. If AV conduction is normal, the ventricular rate should equal the atrial rate.

### Atrioventricular Block

#### First-Degree AV Block

First-degree AV block occurs when the *PR interval is prolonged (>200 milliseconds)*, and *each P wave is followed by a QRS* complex. Typically the PR interval is constant.

#### Second-Degree AV Block, Mobitz Type I (Wenckebach)

Second-degree AV block, Mobitz Type I (Wenckebach) is characterized by *progressive prolongation of the PR interval, terminating with a P wave followed by a nonconducted QRS* complex. Normal antegrade conduction resumes with a repetitive progressive prolongation of the PR interval with each cardiac depolarization, resuming the cycle. This results in a "grouped beating" pattern. In its most common form, the R–R interval shortens from beat to beat (not including the interval in which a P wave is not conducted). This typically represents conduction block within the atrioventricular node, *superior to the bundle of His.*

#### Second-Degree AV Block, Mobitz Type II

Second-degree AV block, Mobitz Type II is characterized by regular P waves followed by intermittent nonconducted QRS complexes in the absence of atrial premature complexes. The resulting R–R interval spanning the nonconducted complex is exactly double the conducted R–R intervals. This typically represents AV conduction block *below the bundle of His, and has a high propensity to progress* to more advanced forms of AV block.

Note that when there is AV block with a ratio of 2:1, one cannot definitively distinguish between Mobitz Type I and Type II. Longer rhythm strips, maneuvers, and intracardiac recordings may be necessary. A widened QRS complex supports Mobitz Type II but lacks certainty.

#### Third-Degree AV Block (Complete Heart Block)

Third-degree AV block (complete heart block) is characterized by *independent atrial and ventricular activity with an atrial rate that is faster than the ventricular rate.* PR intervals vary with dissociation of the P waves from the QRS complexes. Typically the ventricular rhythm is either a junctional (narrow complex) or ventricular (wide complex) rhythm. (Note this should be distinguished from AV dissociation, which is also characterized by independent atrial and ventricular activity, but the ventricular rate is faster than the atrial rate.)

### QRS Complex Interval

The QRS complex interval is best measured in the limb leads from the onset of the R wave (or Q wave if present) to the offset of the S wave. A normal QRS duration is <100 milliseconds.

If the QRS duration is between 100 and <120 milliseconds, the morphology should be further inspected for features of one or more of the following.

1. *Incomplete right bundle branch block:* QRS complex duration 100 to 120 milliseconds, with a right bundle branch block morphology with an R′ wave duration of ≥30 milliseconds (rsR′ in $V_1$; terminal S-wave slowing in leads I, aVL, and $V_6$).
2. *Left anterior fascicular block (LAFB):*
   - QRS duration <120 milliseconds
   - Significant left-axis deviation (−45 degrees to −90 degrees)

- Positive QRS-complex vector in lead I, negative QRS-complex vectors in the inferior leads (II, III, aVF)
- Absence of other causes of left-axis deviation, such as an inferior myocardial infarction or ostium primum atrial septal defect

3. *Left posterior fascicular block (LPFB):* Early activation along the anterior fascicles produces a small r wave in leads I and aVL, and small q waves inferiorly. Mid and late forces in the direction of the posterior fascicles produce tall R waves inferiorly, deep S waves in I and aVL, and QRS-complex right-axis deviation.
   - QRS duration <120 milliseconds
   - Right axis (>120 degrees)
   - Absence of other clinical causes of right-axis QRS-complex deviation, such as pulmonary hypertension or right ventricular hypertrophy
   - rS QRS-complex pattern in leads I and aVL
   - qR QRS-complex pattern in the inferior leads

If the QRS complex duration is >120 milliseconds, the morphology should be further inspected for features of the following.

1. *Right bundle branch block (RBBB):* The early depolarization vectors in RBBB are similar to normal depolarization reflecting left ventricular electrical events, producing early septal q waves in leads I, aVL, $V_5$, and $V_6$, plus an early RS pattern in leads $V_1$ and $V_2$. Given the right bundle branch conduction block, an unopposed QRS-complex vector representing delayed and slowed right ventricular depolarization is identified. These unopposed delayed left-to right-depolarization forces produce the characteristic broad second R′ wave in leads $V_1$ and $V_2$, plus the deep broad S waves in leads I, aVL, $V_5$, and $V_6$.
   - QRS duration ≥120 milliseconds
   - rsr′, rsR′, or rSR′ in lead $V_1$ ± lead $V_2$
   - Broad (>40 milliseconds) S wave in leads I and $V_6$
   - T-wave inversion and down-sloping ST depression often seen in leads $V_1$ and $V_2$
2. *Left bundle branch block (LBBB)*: LBBB represents an altered left ventricular depolarization sequence. The right ventricle is depolarized in a timely manner via the right bundle branch. The left ventricle is depolarized after right ventricular depolarization via slowed right-to-left interventricular septal conduction. Because left ventricular depolarization initially transpires via the terminal branches of the left-sided conduction system, left ventricular depolarization occurs via an altered sequence with a prolonged QRS-complex duration.
   - QRS-complex duration ≥120 milliseconds
   - Broad and notched and/or slurred R wave in leads aVL, $V_5$, and $V_6$
   - Absent septal Q waves in leads I, avl, $V_5$, and $V_6$
3. *Intraventricular conduction delay:*
   - QRS complex duration >100 milliseconds
   - Indeterminate morphology not satisfying the criteria for either RBBB or LBBB

### *QT Interval*

The QT interval demonstrates heart-rate interdependence. The QT interval is directly proportional to the R–R interval. The QT interval shortens as heart rate increases. To account for this variability with heart rate, the corrected QT interval ($QT_c$) is calculated, in which the QT interval is divided by the square root of the R–R interval. Normative tables for heart rate and gender are available. A normal $QT_c$ is typically <440 milliseconds. A less cumbersome approximation involves measuring the QT interval directly (typically in lead II). If this is >50% of the R–R interval, this supports QT-interval prolongation. In this circumstance, calculating a $QT_c$ interval is appropriate.

Differential diagnosis of a prolonged QT interval includes the following:

- Congenital (idiopathic, Jervell–Lange–Nielsen syndrome, Romano–Ward syndrome)
- Medications (psychotropics, antiarrhythmics, antimicrobials, etc.)
- Metabolic disorders (hypocalcemia, hypokalemia, hypothyroidism, hypomagnesemia, etc.)
- The morphology of QT interval prolongation in hypocalcemia deserves special mention. Typically, hypocalcemia produces prolongation and straightening of the QT interval as a result of prolongation of the ST segment, without frank widening of the T wave.
- Neurogenic, such as an intracranial hemorrhage
- Ischemia

## 5. Determine If Cardiac Chamber Enlargement or Hypertrophy Is Present

If a patient is in sinus rhythm, the atria can be evaluated by analyzing the P-wave morphology in leads II, $V_1$, and $V_2$. Given the superior right atrial location of the sinus node, right atrial depolarization precedes left atrial depolarization. Therefore, right atrial depolarization is best represented in the first half of the surface electrocardiogram P wave. In lead II, if a bimodal P wave is present, the first peak represents right atrial depolarization and the second peak represents left atrial depolarization. In leads $V_1$ and $V_2$, the P wave is typically biphasic. The early portion is upright, representing right atrial depolarization toward lead $V_1$ and $V_2$, with the negative latter half representing left atrial depolarization, away from these leads.

### *Right Atrial Abnormality*

Delayed activation of the right atrium due to hypertrophy, dilation, or intrinsically slowed conduction can result in the summation of right and left atrial depolarization. This typically produces a tall peaked P wave (≥2.5 to 3 mm) in lead II.

### *Left Atrial Abnormality*

Delayed activation of the left atrium due to hypertrophy, dilation, or intrinsically slowed conduction can result in a broadening (>110 milliseconds) and notching of the P wave in lead II, or a deeper inverted phase of the P wave in leads $V_1$ and $V_2$:

- Negative terminal phase of P wave in lead $V_1$ or $V_2$ ≥40 milliseconds in duration and ≥1 mm in amplitude, *or*
- Biphasic P wave in lead II with peak-to-peak interval of ≥40 milliseconds (This is not very sensitive, but is quite specific.)

### *Right Ventricular Hypertrophy*

In right ventricular hypertrophy (RVH), there is a dominance of the right ventricular forces, which produce prominent R waves in the right precordial leads and deeper S waves in the left precordial leads. RVH is suggested by one or more of the following:

- Right-axis QRS-complex deviation (>+90 degrees)
- R:S ratio in lead $V_1$ >1
- R wave in $V_1$ ≥7 mm
- R:S ratio in $V_6$ <1
- ST–T-wave "strain" pattern in right precordial leads supported by asymmetric T-wave inversion
- Right atrial abnormality *in the absence of:*
  - Posterior-wall myocardial infarction
  - Wolff–Parkinson–White syndrome
  - Counterclockwise rotation
  - Dextrocardia
  - Right bundle branch block

### *Left Ventricular Hypertrophy*

Several criteria have been described and validated for the diagnosis of left ventricular hypertrophy (LVH) by electrocardiography.

1. Sokolow and Lyon: Amplitude of the S wave in lead $V_1$ + amplitude of the R wave in $V_5$ or $V_6$ (whichever is the tallest) ≥35 mm
2. Cornell: Amplitude of the R wave in aVL + amplitude of the S wave in $V_3$ >28 mm for men, or >20 mm for women
3. Romhilt–Estes: This is a scoring system in which a total score of 4 indicates "likely LVH," and a score of ≥5 indicates "definite LVH."
   - Voltage criteria = 3 points:
     Amplitude of limb lead R wave or S wave ≥20 mm *or*
     Amplitude of S wave in $V_1$ or $V_2$ ≥30 mm *or*
     Amplitude of R wave in $V_5$ or $V_6$ ≥30 mm
     ST–T-wave changes typical of strain (in which the ST segment and T-wave vector is shifted in a direction opposite to that of the QRS complex vector) = 3 points (only 1 point if patient is taking digitalis)
   - Left atrial abnormality = 3 points:
     Terminal portion of P wave in $V_1$ ≥40 milliseconds in duration and ≥1 mm in amplitude
   - Left-axis deviation = 2 points:
     Axis ≥ −30 degrees
   - QRS duration = 1 point:
     Duration ≥90 milliseconds
   - Intrinsicoid deflection = 1 point:
     Duration of interval from the beginning of the QRS complex to the peak of the R wave in $V_5$ or $V_6$ ≥50 milliseconds

### *Combined or Biventricular Hypertrophy*

Combined ventricular hypertrophy is suggested by any of the following:

- ECG meets criteria for isolated RVH and LVH. This is the most reliable criterion.
- Precordial leads demonstrate LVH by voltage, but there is right-axis deviation (>+90 degrees) in the frontal plane.
- Precordial leads demonstrate LVH, with limb leads demonstrating right atrial abnormality.

## 6. Assess the P-Wave, QRS-Complex, and T-Wave Morphologies

Once the cardiac rate, rhythm, axes, intervals, and chambers have been assessed, one should proceed with the identification of various morphologies that suggest pathologic states. There have been virtually innumerable descriptions of various morphologic criteria for a broad spectrum of pathologic states, but here we discuss those that are most common and/or most important.

### *ECG Abnormalities and Corresponding Differential Diagnoses*

#### Incorrect Lead Placement or Lead Fracture

Incorrect lead placement or lead fracture is most commonly identified in the limb leads, with a negative P-wave vector in leads I and aVL and normal precordial R-wave progression.

#### Low Voltage

Low voltage in limb leads is defined as a QRS-complex amplitude of <5 mm in each of the standard limb leads (I, II, and III). Low voltage of all leads is defined as low voltage in the limb leads plus a QRS-complex amplitude of <10 mm in each of the precordial leads.

Low voltage on the ECG may be of primary myocardial origin or secondary to high-impedance tissue conduction. Differential diagnosis possibilities include:

- Cardiomyopathy (infiltrative or restrictive)
- Pericardial effusion
- Pleural effusion
- Anasarca
- Obesity
- Myxedema
- Chronic obstructive pulmonary disease

### Q Waves

Q waves represent an initial negative QRS-complex vector. Pathologic Q waves are present if they are ≥1 mm (0.1 mV) in depth and ≥40 milliseconds in duration.

Q waves are most commonly associated with a myocardial infarction. To diagnose a myocardial infarction, q waves must be identified in two contiguous leads:

- Inferior leads—II, III, and aVF
- Anteroseptal leads—$V_2$ and $V_3$
- Anterior leads—$V_2$, $V_3$, and $V_4$
- Lateral leads—$V_5$ and $V_6$
- High lateral leads—I and aVL
- Posterior leads $V_1$ and $V_2$ (R-wave amplitude > S-wave amplitude)

Contiguous regions on an electrocardiogram include the following:

- Inferior, posterior, and lateral
- Anteroseptal, anterior, and lateral
- Lateral and high lateral

Other etiologies of Q waves include:

- "Septal" Q waves (small Q waves as a result of the septal left-to-right depolarization vector)—leads I, aVL, $V_5$, and $V_6$
- Hypertrophic cardiomyopathy—any lead
- Left anterior fascicular block—leads I and aVL
- Wolfe–Parkinson–White syndrome—any lead

### ST-Segment Elevation

ST-segment elevation refers to elevation of the segment between the terminal aspect of the QRS complex and the T-wave onset. This elevation is relative to the isoelectric comparative TP segment located between the end of the T wave and the start of the P wave.

Causes of ST-segment elevation include the following.

- *Acute myocardial injury:* convex upward ST-segment elevation in at least two contiguous ECG leads
- *Coronary spasm (Prinzmetal angina):* similar morphology to acute myocardial injury, with the distinction that the ST-segment elevation is typically transient
- *Pericarditis:* diffuse concave upward ST-segment elevation not confined to contiguous ECG leads
- *Left ventricular aneurysm:* most often seen in the right precordial leads, with convex upward ST-segment elevation overlying an infarct zone, with ST-segment elevation persisting for months to years after the initial myocardial infarction
- *Left bundle branch block:* typically discordant from the QRS-complex vector
- *Early repolarization:* manifest as J-point elevation with normal ST segments, best seen in the lateral precordial leads
- *Brugada syndrome:* ST-segment elevation in the right precordial leads with a pattern of right ventricular conduction delay
- *Hypothermia:* Osborne waves

### ST-Segment Depression

The most common causes of ST-segment depression are the following.

- *Myocardial ischemia or non–ST-segment-elevation myocardial infarction (NSTEMI):* Horizontal or down-sloping ST-segment depression demonstrates the greatest specificity for myocardial ischemia. Positive cardiac biomarkers distinguish ischemia versus infarction.
- *Ventricular hypertrophy:* Down-sloping asymmetric ST-segment depression and T-wave inversion is often present in both left and right ventricular hypertrophy.

### Peaked T Waves

The most common causes of peaked, positive T waves are the following.

- Hyperkalemia
- Hyperacute phase of myocardial infarction
- Acute transient ischemia (Prinzmetal Angina)

### U Waves

U waves are seen immediately following the T wave. They are best observed in leads $V_2$, $V_3$, and $V_4$ and are typically up to one quarter the amplitude of the T wave. Prominent U waves are ≥1.5 mm (≥0.15 mV) in amplitude.

Prominent U waves are commonly observed in the presence of:

- Hypokalemia
- Bradyarrhythmias
- Drugs

## *Pathologic States and Corresponding ECG Abnormalities*

### Myocardial Injury and Infarction

- *Acute myocardial infarction:* Q waves and ST-segment elevation. Reciprocal ST segment depression is often observed, but is not necessary.
- *Recent myocardial infarction:* Q waves with ischemic T-wave changes, often inverted; the ST segments are typically no longer elevated.
- *Age-indeterminate myocardial infarction:* persistent Q waves devoid of ST-segment elevation or ischemic T-wave changes.
- *Acute myocardial injury:* regional ST-segment elevation without Q waves.

### Acute Pericarditis

Acute pericarditis is characterized by diffuse ST-segment elevation and/or PR-segment depression. Lead aVR classically demonstrates PR-segment elevation and is highly specific.

- Diffuse ST-segment elevation.
- Diffuse PR-segment depression with PR-segment elevation in lead aVR.
- T-wave inversions typically do not appear until ST segment elevations have resolved.

### Pericardial Effusion

The ECG manifestations of pericardial effusions are a result of the increased impedance of the electrical signal through the pericardial fluid collection coupled with translational cardiac motion within the pericardium. These include:

- Electrical alternans
- Low-voltage QRS complexes

### Digitalis Effect

- Most commonly manifests as ST-segment and T-wave changes
- Concave depression/sagging of the ST segment (usually without frank J-point depression) seen best in leads $V_5$ and $V_6$
- PR-interval prolongation
- T-wave flattening with QT-interval shortening

### Digitalis Toxicity

Digitalis toxicity exerts its effects via a combination of an increase in myocardial automaticity plus suppression of sinus nodal and AV nodal pacemaker function. This manifests as a combination of conduction defects and arrhythmias including but not limited to:

- Atrial tachycardia
- Accelerated junctional rhythm
- First-, second-, or third-degree AV block
- Bidirectional ventricular tachycardia (VT with alternating right and left bundle branch block morphology)
- Ventricular fibrillation

### Hyperkalemia

- Tall, peaked, narrow-based T waves
- PR-interval prolongation
- Advanced conduction block
- Atrial standstill or arrest
- Widening of the QRS complex, which can progress to a "sine wave" pattern
- Ventricular tachycardia or fibrillation

### Hypokalemia

- Prominent U waves, especially in leads $V_2$, $V_3$, and $V_4$
- ST-segment depression
- Decreased T-wave amplitude
- Increase in P-wave amplitude and duration

### Hypercalcemia

- Shortened $QT_c$, predominantly via decreased ST-segment duration

### Hypocalcemia

- Prolonged $QT_c$, predominantly via increased ST-segment duration and straightening without a significant increase in the T-wave duration

### Sick Sinus Syndrome

Sick sinus syndrome is characterized by combinations of the following:

- Marked sinus bradycardia
- Sinus arrest
- Prolonged recovery time of the sinus node following PACs or atrial tachyarrhythmias
- Alternating bradycardia and tachycardia

### Acute Cor Pulmonale

The following suggest acute cor pulmonale:

- Sinus tachycardia
- Anterior precordial T-wave inversion (leads $V_1$–$V_3$)
- Right atrial abnormality
- Right-axis QRS-complex deviation
- An S1, Q3, T3 QRS complex limb lead pattern
- RBBB (may be transient)

### Atrial Septal Defect (ASD), Secundum

The following ECG findings are suggestive of a secundum ASD:

- Right-axis QRS-complex deviation
- Incomplete RBBB
- RVH
- Right atrial abnormality
- PR-interval prolongation

### Atrial Septal Defect (ASD), Primum

The following ECG findings are suggestive of a primum ASD:

- Left-axis QRS-complex deviation
- PR-interval prolongation
- Incomplete RBBB

### Dextrocardia

The following ECG findings suggest dextrocardia:

- Precordial R-wave regression (R-wave amplitude decreases from $V_1$ to $V_6$)
- Negative P-wave vector in leads I and aVL

Wolff–Parkinson–White (WPW) syndrome is suggested by the following ECG findings:

- Shortened PR interval (<120 milliseconds)
- Delta wave representing ventricular pre-excitation (slurring of the initial portion of the QRS complex)
- QRS complex may be wide, representing altered ventricular depolarization

### Hypertrophic Cardiomyopathy

The following ECG criteria are suggestive of hypertrophic cardiomyopathy:

- High-voltage QRS complex
- Deep Q waves not ascribable to a specific coronary artery territory
- ST–T-wave changes including deep T-wave inversions

### Hypothermia

The following ECG criteria are suggestive of hypothermia:

- Osborne waves (elevated J point that is proportional to the degree of hypothermia)
- Bradycardia
- PR-interval, QRS-complex interval, and QT-interval prolongation

### Myxedema

The following ECG criteria are suggestive of myxedema:

- Sinus bradycardia
- PR-interval prolongation
- Low-voltage QRS complexes

## BIBLIOGRAPHY

**Rimmerman CM, Jain AK**, Lippincott Williams & Wilkins. Interactive electrocardiography. In. Philadelphia: Lippincott Williams & Wilkins; 2001.

**Surawicz B, Knilans TK, Chou T-C.** *Chou's Electrocardiography in Clinical Practice: Adult and Pediatric.* 5th ed. Philadelphia: WB Saunders; 2001.

**Topol EJ, Califf RM.** *Textbook of Cardiovascular Medicine.* 2nd ed. Philadelphia: Lippincott Williams & Wilkins; 2002.

# ELECTROCARDIOGRAM CASE HISTORIES

## ELECTROCARDIOGRAM #1

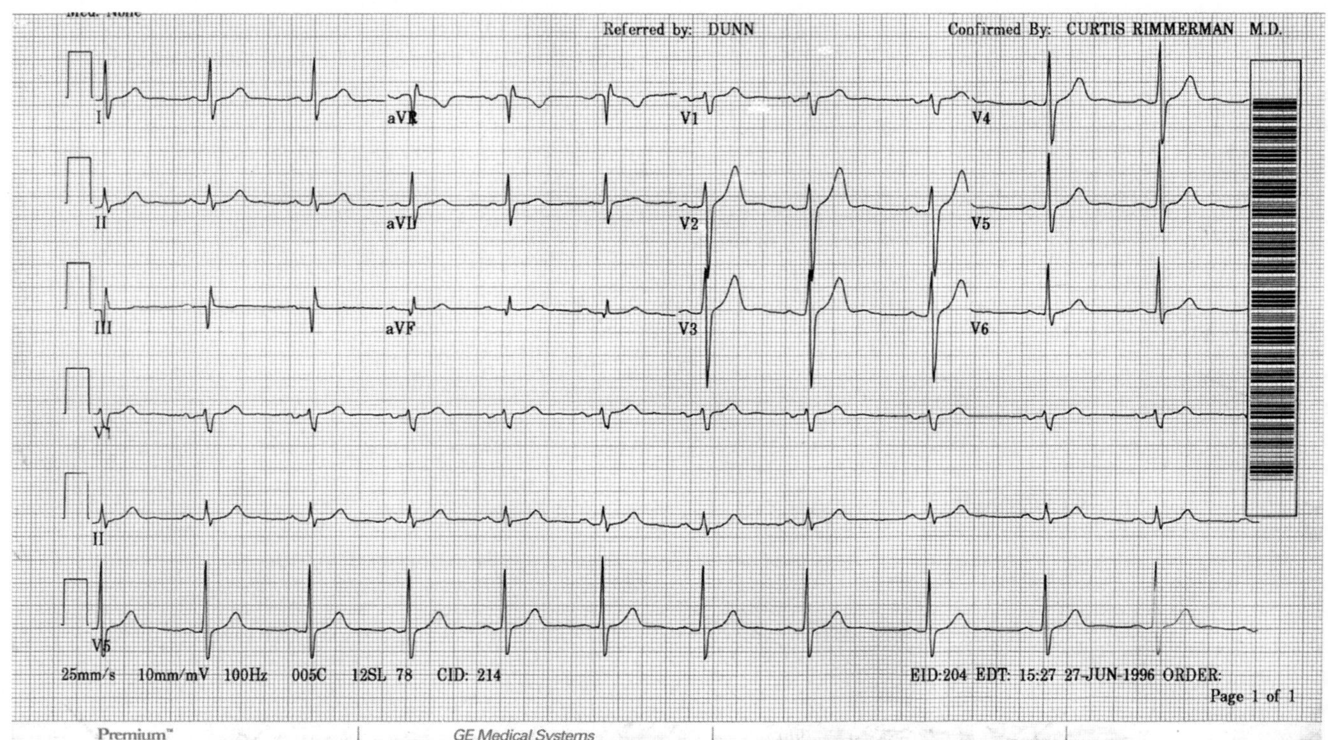


### Clinical History

A 52-year-old man presents for a routine physical examination in the Preventive Medicine Department. His past medical history includes elevated triglycerides and a low HDL cholesterol value. He is otherwise in good health.

### Electrocardiogram Interpretation

The cardiac rhythm is normal sinus rhythm with evidence of sinus arrhythmia best seen in the lead $V_1$ rhythm strip. No pathologic Q waves are present, the ST segments are normal, and all cardiac intervals are normal. This represents a normal electrocardiogram and an example of sinus arrhythmia.

### Commentary

Sinus arrhythmia is a common and normal finding as depicted on this electrocardiogram. The sinus rate increases with inspiration and decreases with expiration.

### Keyword Diagnoses

Normal sinus rhythm
Sinus arrhythmia
Normal electrocardiogram

## ELECTROCARDIOGRAM #2

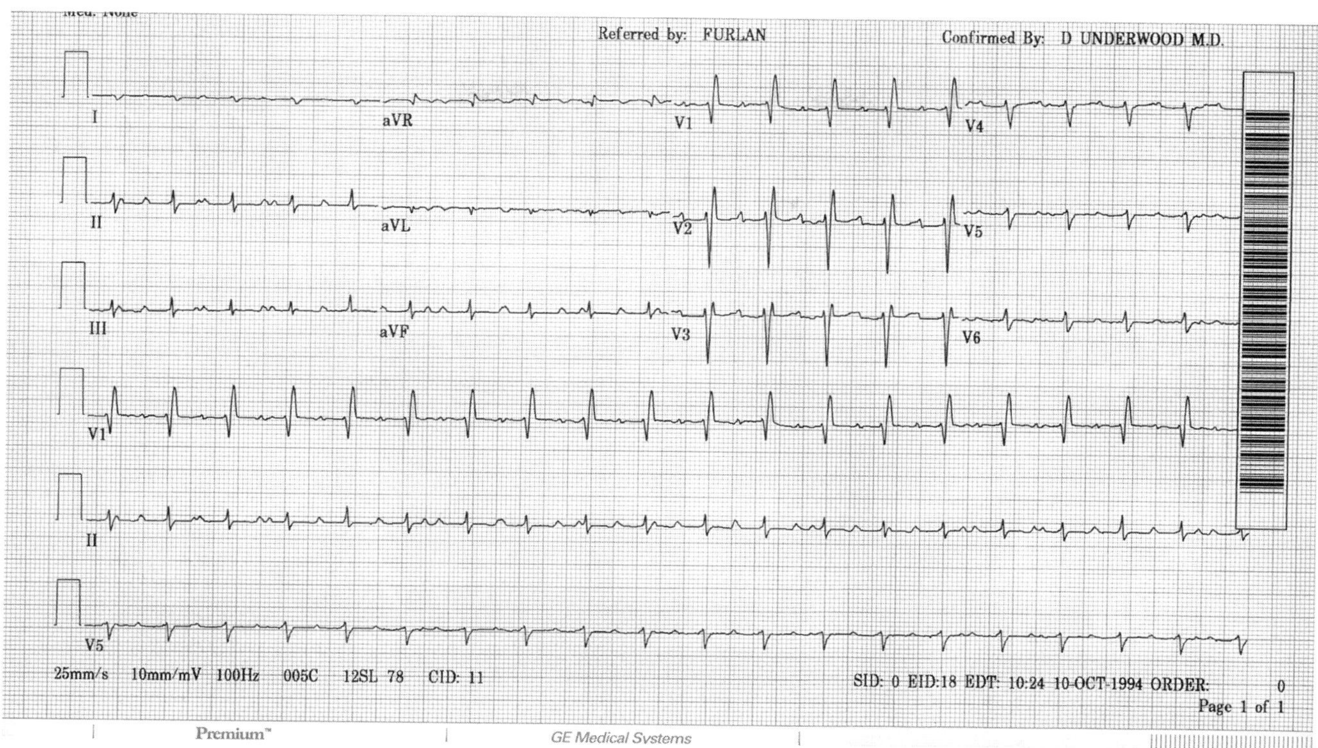


### Clinical History

The patient is a 56-year-old man who underwent a cardiac transplant procedure 6 weeks prior to this electrocardiogram, secondary to an idiopathic nonischemic dilated cardiomyopathy and recurrent ventricular tachycardia. His medications at the time of this electrocardiogram included digoxin, furosemide, lisinopril, potassium, and aspirin.

### Electrocardiogram Interpretation

The cardiac rhythm is sinus tachycardia, in that the P waves demonstrate a normal axis with a constant P–P interval preceding each QRS complex at a regular rate > 100 per minute. A second set of P waves is noted as a constant P–P interval at a slightly longer P–P interval compared to the conducted P waves. This represents the native atrium in this cardiac transplant patient, which is still depolarizing via the native sinus node. The donor P wave that immediately precedes each QRS complex demonstrates first-degree atrioventricular block. Diffuse nonspecific ST–T changes are present. QRS-complex frontal-plane right-axis deviation is present in that the QRS-complex vector is negative in lead I and positive in leads II, III, and aVF. Low-voltage QRS complexes are seen in the limb leads, in that each complex is less than 5 mm in amplitude. A rsR′ QRS-complex morphology is present in lead $V_1$ with an overall normal QRS-complex duration supporting incomplete right bundle branch block.

### Commentary

The presence of dual functioning atria in a recent cardiac transplant patient is a common finding. The native atria gradually extinguish themselves and the donor atria become the dominant atrial pacemaker. The presence of incomplete right bundle branch block in a post–cardiac transplant patient is also a common finding.

### Keyword Diagnoses

Sinus tachycardia
First-degree atrioventricular block
Right-axis deviation
Incomplete right bundle branch block
Nonspecific ST–T changes
Low-voltage QRS
Cardiac transplant

## ELECTROCARDIOGRAM #3

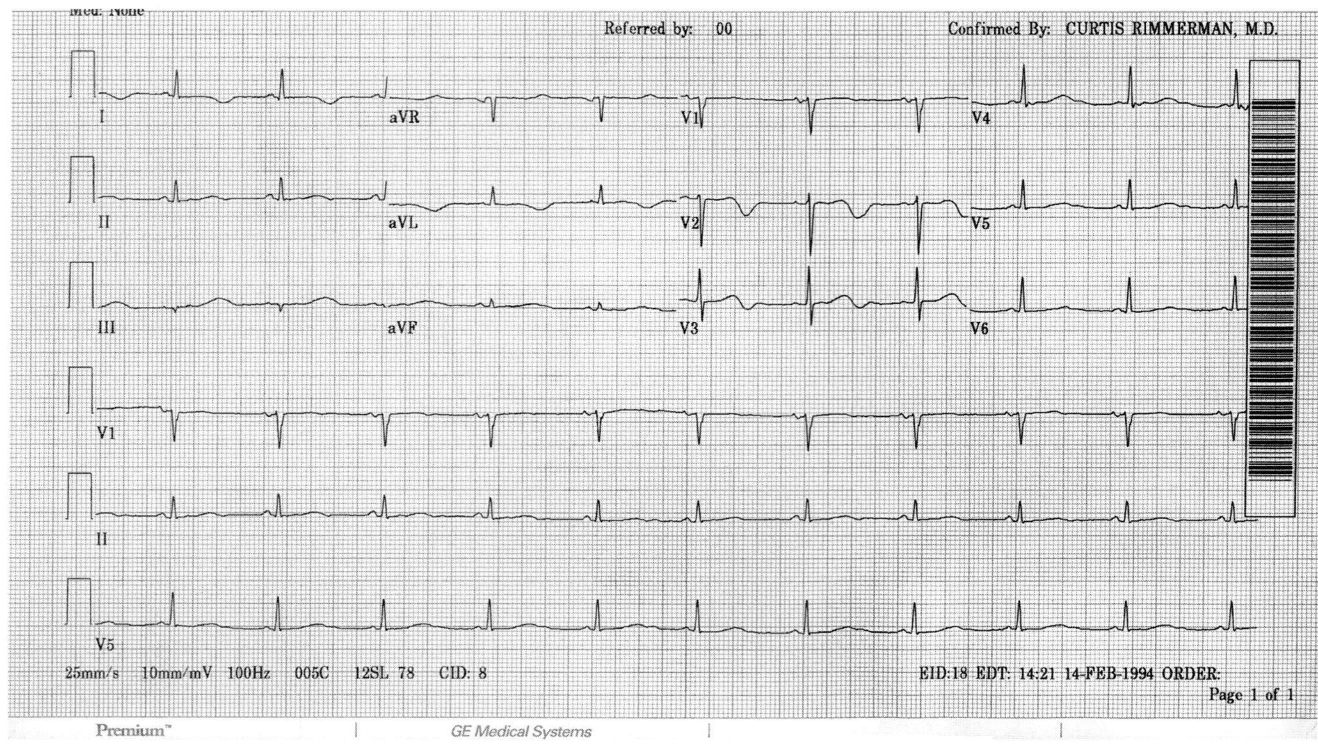


### Clinical History

The patient is a 41-year-old man with myelodysplastic syndrome and insulin-requiring diabetes mellitus, who has been admitted for bone marrow transplantation. His serum potassium at the time of this electrocardiogram was 3.4 mEq/L.

### Electrocardiogram Interpretation

This electrocardiogram emphasizes the necessary methodical approach to interpretation. The ECG demonstrates normal sinus rhythm. In assessing the intervals, it is most notable for a prolonged QT interval.

### Commentary

This electrocardiogram demonstrates the common findings seen in hypokalemia. There is a prolongation of the QT interval, prominent U waves, and T wave flattening.

### Keyword Diagnoses

Normal sinus rhythm
Prolonged QT interval
Nonspecific ST–T changes
U waves
Hypokalemia

## ELECTROCARDIOGRAM #4

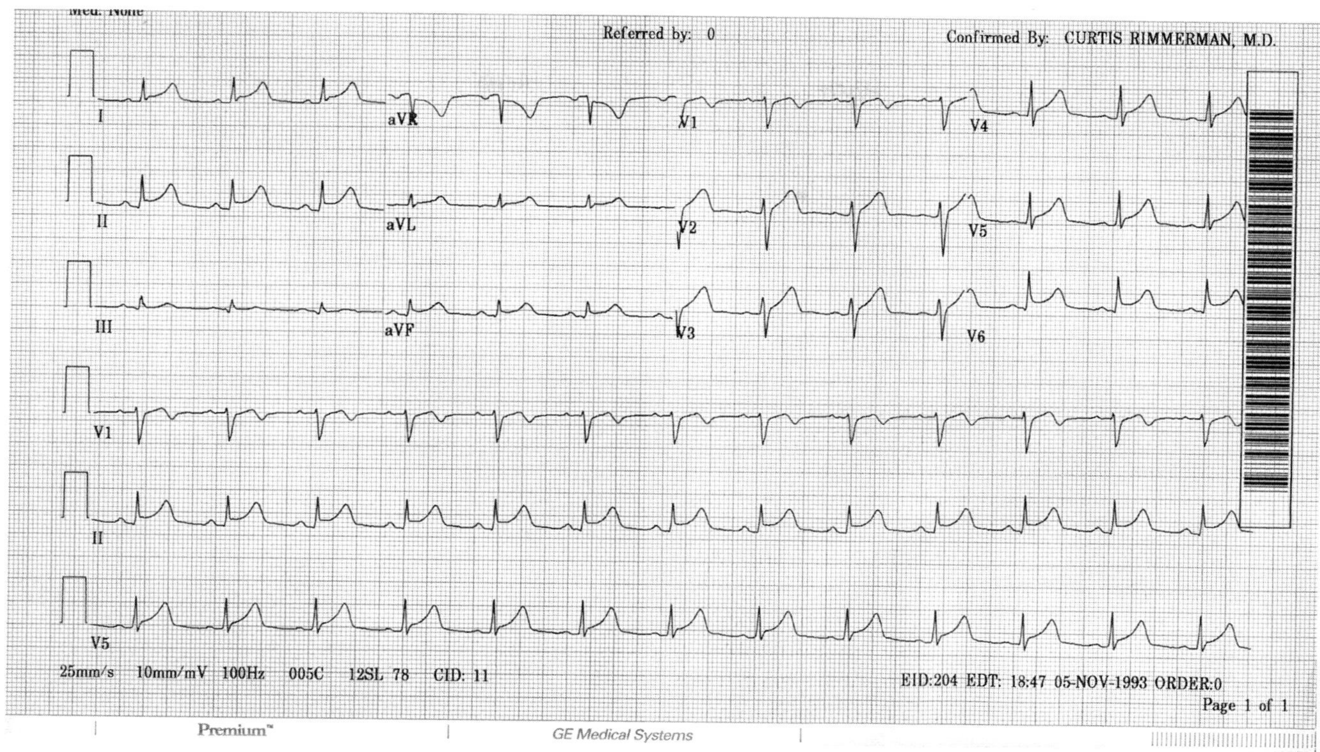


### Clinical History

A 39-year-old woman, an unrestrained passenger in a motor vehicle accident, suffered an aortic transection distal to the left subclavian artery. This electrocardiogram was taken postoperatively, shortly after thoracic aorta repair.

### Electrocardiogram Interpretation

The heart rate and cardiac rhythm are both normal. This represents normal sinus rhythm. This electrocardiogram is most notable for diffuse ST-segment elevation not confined to a particular coronary artery territory, which is most consistent with acute pericarditis. Lead aVR is helpful because there is elevation of the atrial repolarization segment. This segment is termed the PR segment and is located between the terminal aspect of the P wave and QRS-complex onset.

### Commentary

When the PR segment is elevated in lead aVR, this serves as a specific sign for pericarditis. This may be the only electrocardiogram finding supporting pericarditis and remains an important marker to identify.

### Keyword Diagnoses

Normal sinus rhythm
Pericarditis

## ELECTROCARDIOGRAM #5

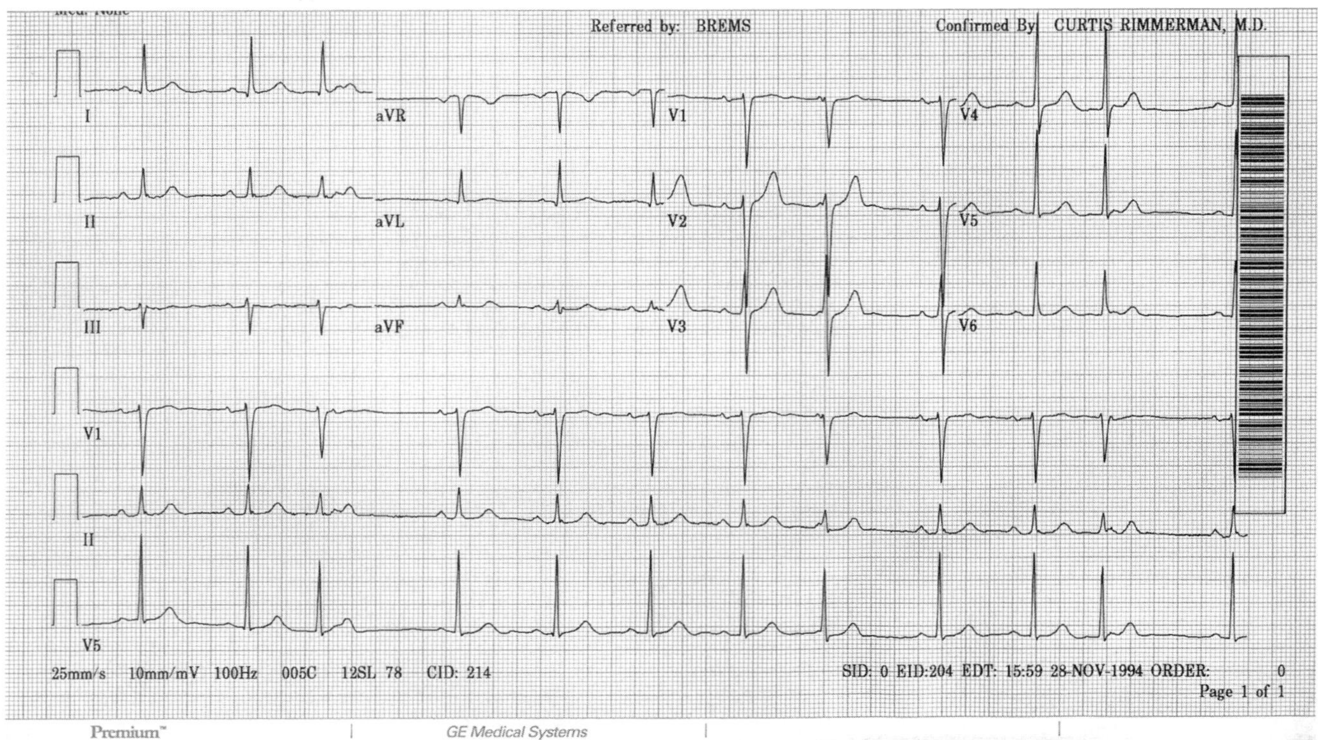


### Clinical History

A 62-year-old man is undergoing preoperative anesthesia clearance prior to planned rotator cuff repair. His past medical history is notable for hypertension but no known cardiac disease. His medications include verapamil.

### Electrocardiogram Interpretation

Normal sinus rhythm is present. The third, eighth, and 11th QRS complexes are premature junctional complexes. A P wave does not precede the third and 11th QRS complexes and demonstrates a similar QRS-complex morphology to the native QRS complex. This is otherwise a normal electrocardiogram.

### Commentary

Premature junctional complexes are an otherwise normal finding. Frequently, retrograde P waves are seen in the presence of premature junctional complexes. An example of retrograde P waves is seen within the ST segment following the third and 11th QRS complexes.

### Keyword Diagnoses

- Normal sinus rhythm
- Premature junctional complex
- Normal electrocardiogram
- Retrograde P waves

## ELECTROCARDIOGRAM #6

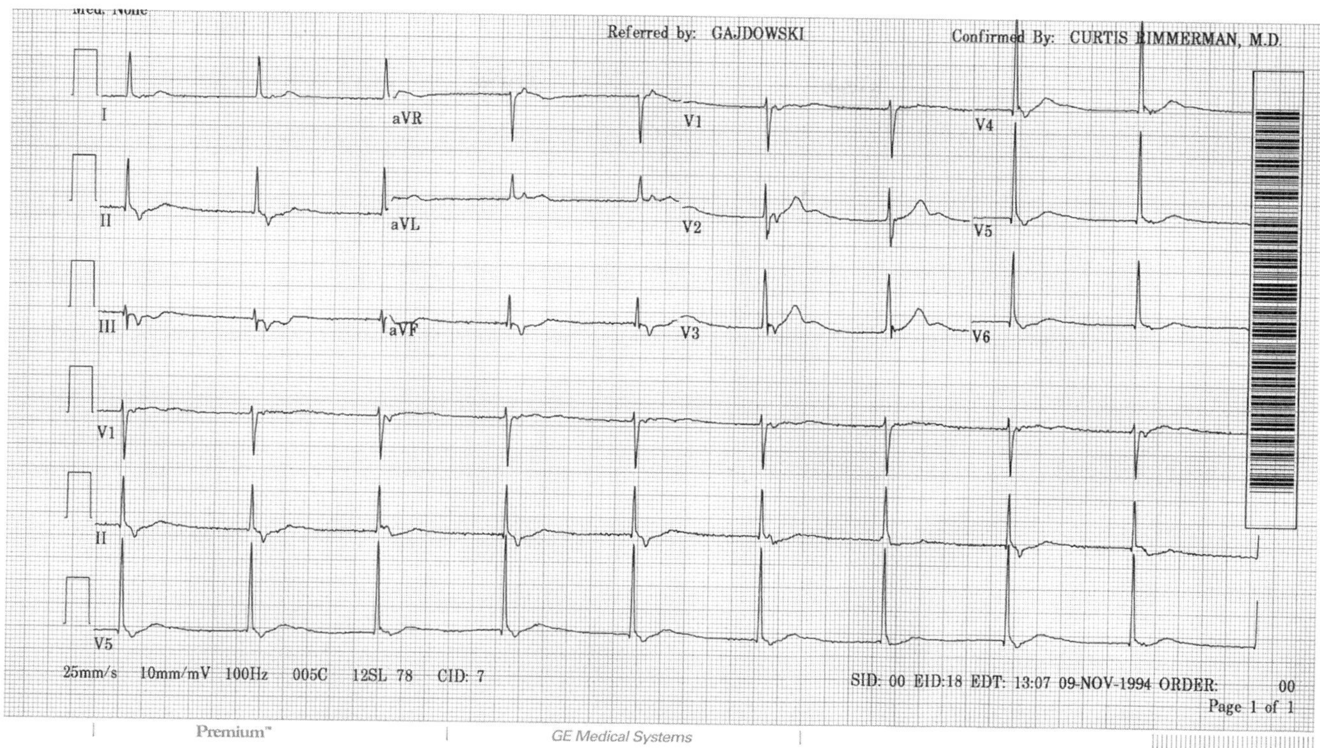


### Clinical History

A 59-year-old man with coronary artery disease status post-remote percutaneous transluminal coronary angioplasty of the right coronary artery re-presents with chest discomfort. A myocardial infarction was excluded by cardiac enzymes and a subsequent stress test was normal. The patient was thought to be suffering from noncardiac musculoskeletal chest discomfort.

### Electrocardiogram Interpretation

The cardiac rhythm demonstrates a regular bradycardia with retrograde P waves after each QRS complex. The P waves possess a negative vector in the inferior leads, as the atrial wave of depolarization is traveling superiorly, opposite the normal direction of conduction. The QRS complex is of normal duration. This represents a junctional bradycardia. The causes of this could be many, including sinus node disease, medication administration, increased vagal tone, atrial conduction system disease, myocardial ischemia, or valvular heart disease. Prominent positive U waves are present in leads $V_2$–$V_4$.

### Commentary

In this case the R–R interval is constant with absent atrial activity prior to each QRS complex. Depending on the relative retrograde–versus–antegrade conduction rates, a retrograde P wave may occur before, within, or after the QRS complex. In this example, antegrade conduction from the atrioventricular junction to the ventricle is faster than retrograde conduction from the atrioventricular junction to the atrium and therefore explains the P wave occupying the proximal ST segment after the QRS complex.

### Keyword Diagnoses

Junctional bradycardia
Retrograde P waves
U waves

## ELECTROCARDIOGRAM #7

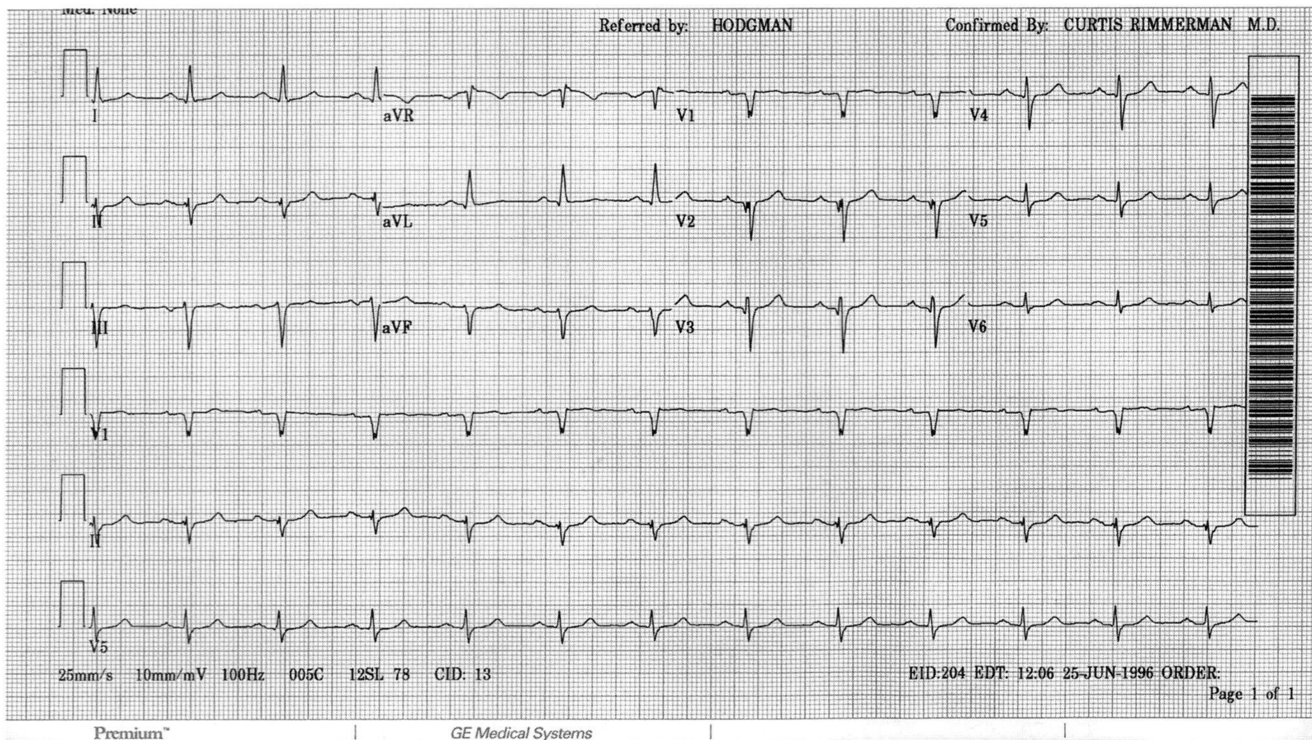


### Clinical History

A 62-year-old man with severe three-vessel coronary artery disease has been referred for coronary artery bypass graft surgery. A recent cardiac catheterization demonstrated normal left ventricular systolic function without evidence of a prior myocardial infarction. Mediations at the time of this electrocardiogram included atenolol, gemfibrozil, and folic acid.

### Electrocardiogram Interpretation

The cardiac rhythm is normal sinus rhythm with a positive QRS-complex vector in lead I and negative QRS-complex vectors in leads II, III, and aVF, consistent with left anterior hemiblock. Q waves are present in leads $V_2$–$V_3$, suggesting an anteroseptal myocardial infarction of indeterminate age. This is a difficult diagnosis in the setting of left anterior hemiblock, as the QRS-complex vector is now displaced inferiorly and posteriorly away from leads $V_2$–$V_3$. This in fact may represent a Q wave based on axis deviation instead of a true myocardial infarction.

### Commentary

Placing leads $V_2$ and $V_3$ one interspace lower and repeating the electrocardiogram may be helpful, as the new presence of an R wave would negate the possibility of a prior anteroseptal myocardial infarction. In this setting an echocardiogram may be helpful to evaluate anteroseptal and septal wall motion. Thus the correct interpretation of this electrocardiogram is normal sinus rhythm with left anterior hemiblock, but cannot exclude a septal myocardial infarction of indeterminate age.

### Keyword Diagnoses

Normal sinus rhythm
Left anterior hemiblock

## ELECTROCARDIOGRAM #8

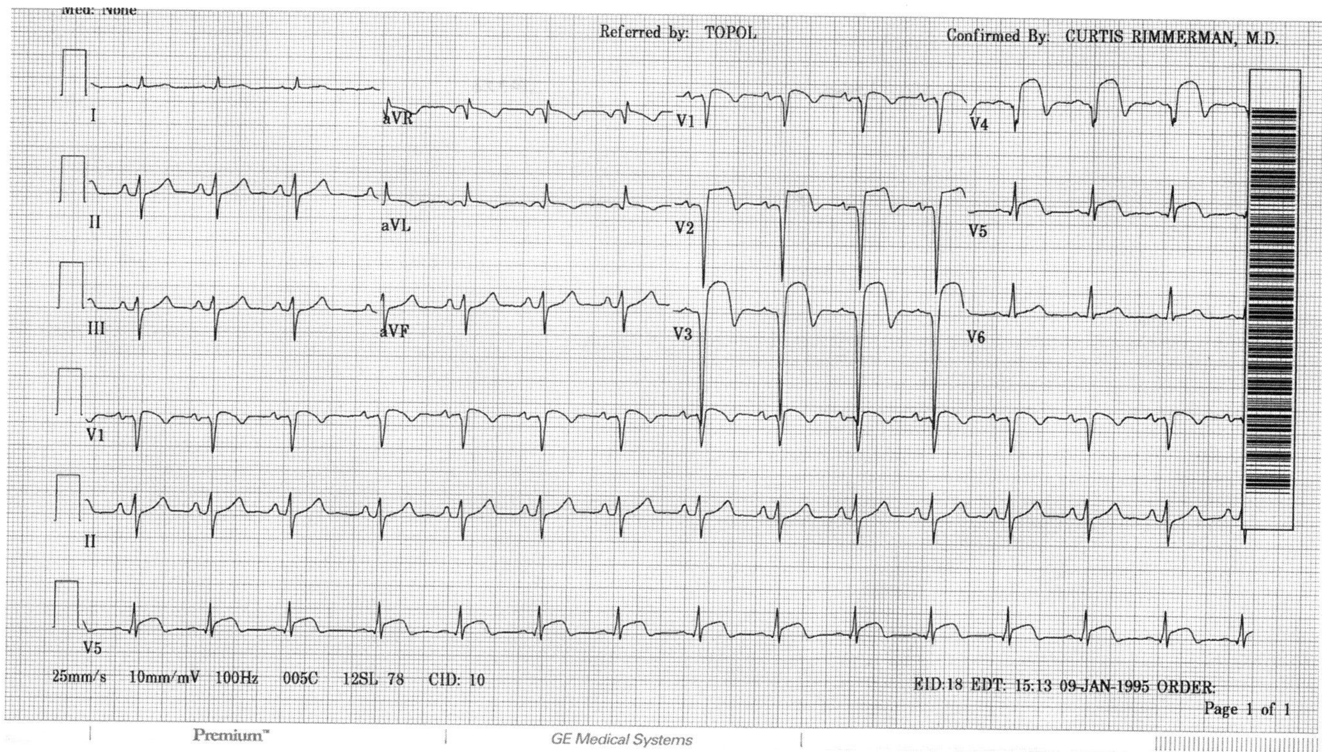


### Clinical History

A 46-year-old man who had a myocardial infarction 2 years before this electrocardiogram presented to the emergency room with a 6-hour history of acute severe substernal chest discomfort. The patient underwent emergency cardiac catheterization and percutaneous transluminal coronary angioplasty of a severe proximal left anterior descending coronary artery stenosis.

### Electrocardiogram Interpretation

The cardiac rhythm is regular, with a normal P-wave axis denoting normal sinus rhythm. A leftward QRS-complex frontal-plane axis is present in the setting of a normal QRS-complex duration, fulfilling the criteria for left anterior hemiblock. Most striking on this electrocardiogram is the maximal 7-mm ST-segment elevation noted in leads $V_2$–$V_5$, I, and aVL with Q-wave formation indicating an extensive acute anterolateral myocardial infarction. There is an ongoing acute myocardial injury pattern with terminal T-wave inversion representing an evolving acute infarction.

### Commentary

This electrocardiogram is an example of an evolving extensive acute anterolateral myocardial infarction. There is concomitant injury and infarction occurring, as prominent Q waves are present with ST-segment elevation. Presumably the left anterior descending obstruction is proximal to the first septal perforator branch, as ST-segment elevation is present in lead $V_1$.

### Keyword Diagnoses

Normal sinus rhythm
Left anterior hemiblock
Anterolateral myocardial infarction, acute
Acute myocardial injury

## ELECTROCARDIOGRAM #9

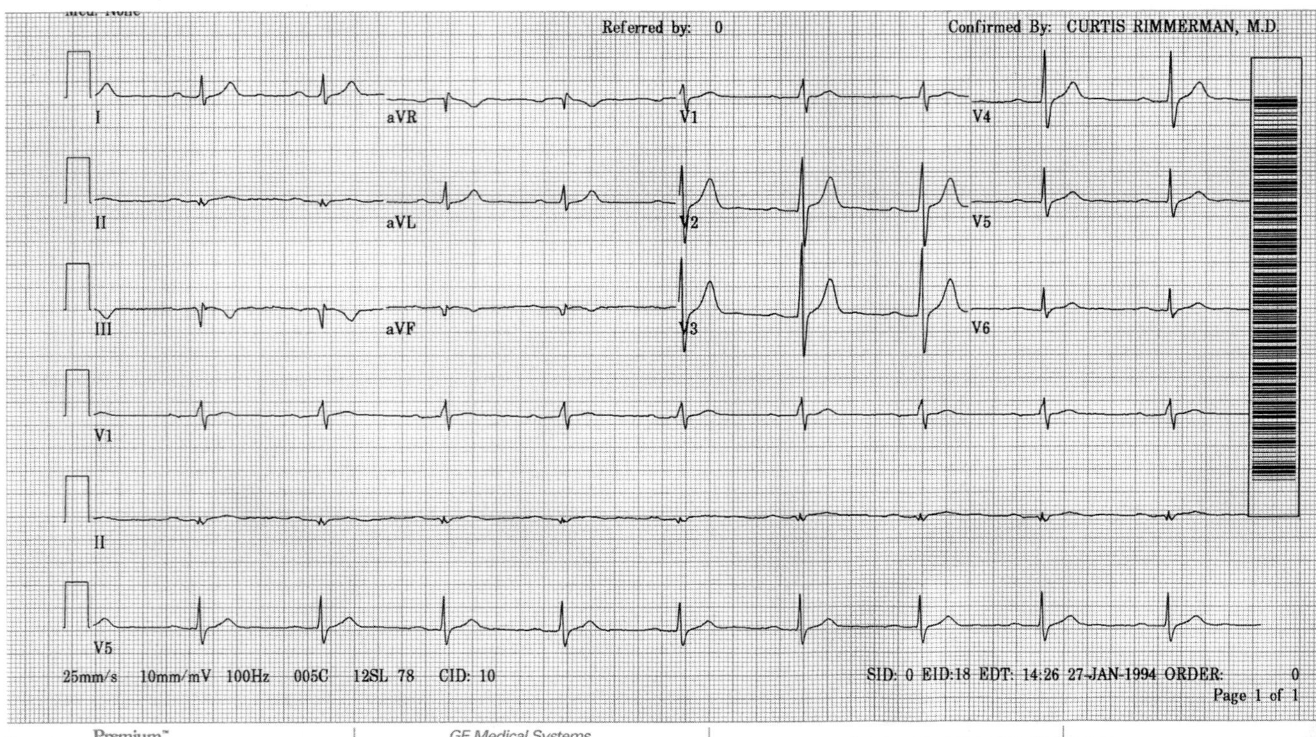


### Clinical History

A 47-year-old man presented to an outside medical facility with an electrocardiogram consistent with an acute inferior myocardial infarction. He received urgent thrombolytic therapy and was accepted in hospital transfer for cardiac catheterization. Co-morbid conditions included long-term tobacco use and hypercholesterolemia. A cardiac catheterization demonstrated severe right coronary artery disease, which was treated with percutaneous coronary intervention.

### Electrocardiogram Interpretation

Important findings on this electrocardiogram include sinus bradycardia with a prolonged PR interval, supporting first-degree atrioventricular block. Pathologic Q waves are present in leads III and aVF, with coved nonelevated ST segments and terminally negative T waves. This supports an inferior myocardial infarction, possibly recent. A tall R wave is noted in leads $V_1$ and $V_2$, and in the setting of an inferior myocardial infarction raises the high likelihood of a concomitant posterior myocardial infarction. This electrocardiogram is best characterized as sinus bradycardia, first-degree atrioventricular block, and a recent inferoposterior myocardial infarction.

### Commentary

In the presence of an inferoposterior myocardial infarction it is important to assess the lateral leads for Q-wave formation. On this electrocardiogram the lateral leads are normal. Given the patient's history of a right coronary artery myocardial infarction, by inference it is likely that leads $V_5$–$V_6$ are represented electrocardiographically by a left circumflex coronary artery.

### Keyword Diagnoses

Sinus bradycardia
First-degree atrioventricular block
Inferoposterior myocardial infarction, recent

## ELECTROCARDIOGRAM #10

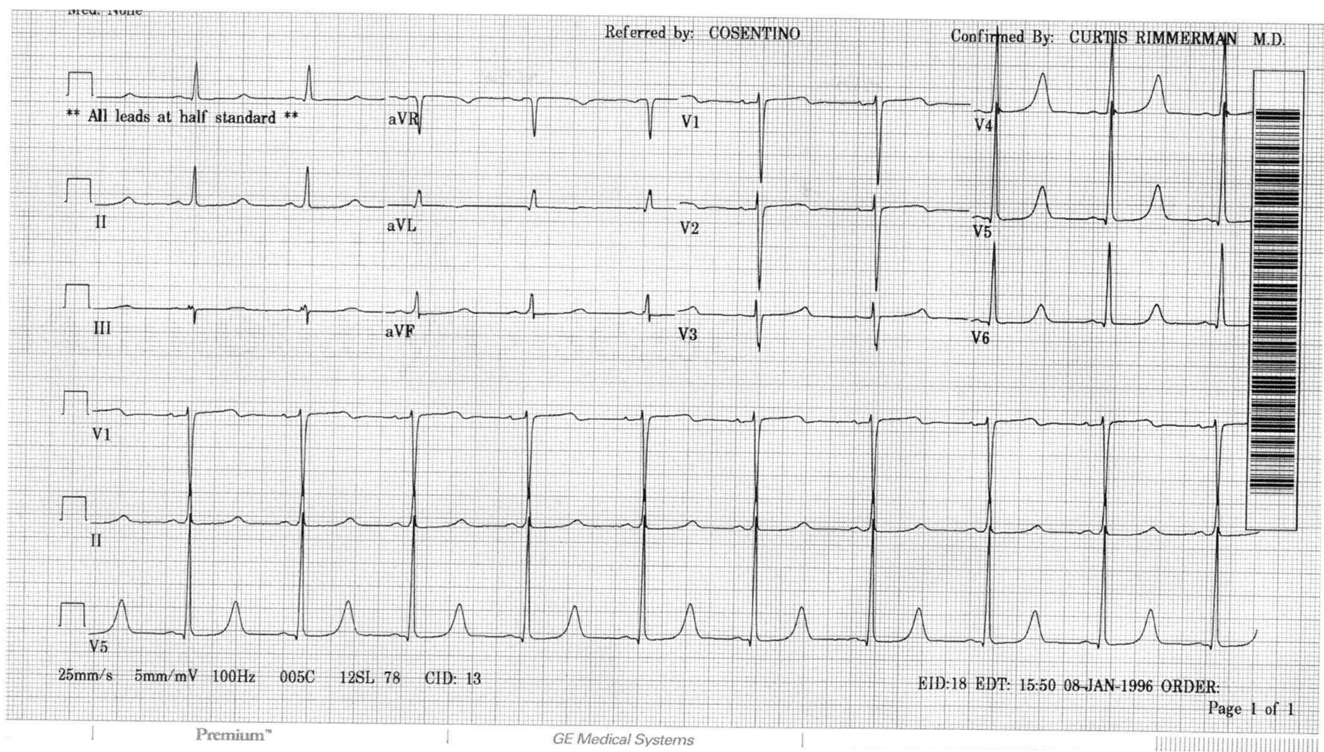


### Clinical History

A 47-year-old woman with dialysis-requiring renal failure secondary to long-standing hypertension has presented to the hospital with recent-onset shortness of breath. At the time of this electrocardiogram her serum calcium level was 7.2 mg/dL and her serum potassium level was 6.4 mEq/L.

### Electrocardiogram Interpretation

This electrocardiogram was obtained at half standardization. Therefore each complex is one half the voltage of a standard electrocardiogram. The atrial rate is 60 per minute, regular and of normal axis. This represents normal sinus rhythm. The QRS complexes are normal. A prolonged QT interval is present, and the ST segment is straightened as seen in patients with hypocalcemia. Peaked T waves, particularly notable in leads $V_4$–$V_6$, are narrow based and symmetric, denoting hyperkalemia.

### Commentary

This combination of findings is commonly seen in a chronic renal failure patient and reflects both hypocalcemia and hyperkalemia. The electrocardiogram may serve as the initial clinical clue to the presence of these electrolyte abnormalities. The patient also demonstrates increased QRS-complex voltage consistent with left ventricular hypertrophy. This is not diagnosed from this electrocardiogram, given the absence of secondary ST–T changes. Diagnosing left ventricular hypertrophy solely on the basis of increased QRS-complex voltage suffers from reduced specificity.

### Keyword Diagnoses

Half standardization
Normal sinus rhythm
Prolonged QT interval
Peaked T waves
Hypocalcemia
Hyperkalemia

## ELECTROCARDIOGRAM #11

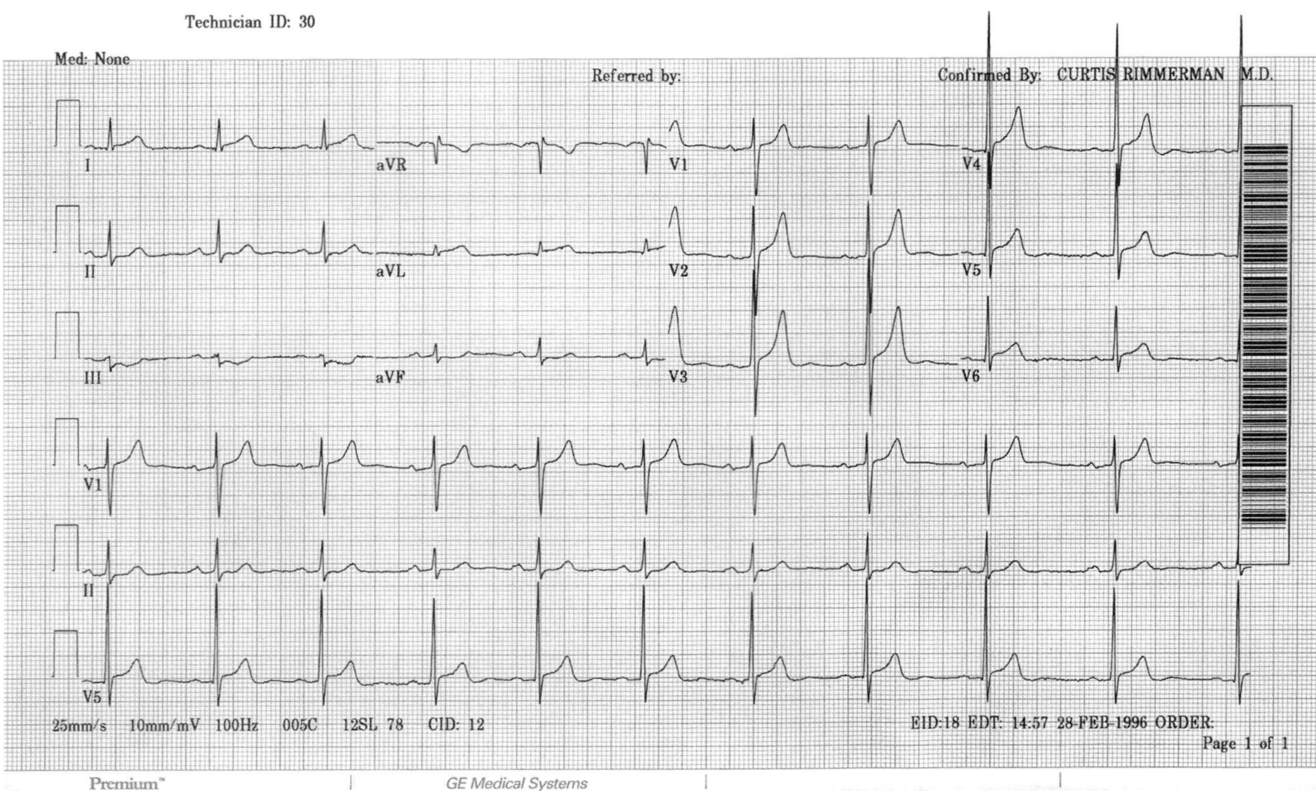


### Clinical History

A 58-year-old man presented to the hospital with an acute chest pain syndrome. He underwent a diagnostic cardiac catheterization that demonstrated an acute occlusion of the left circumflex coronary artery.

### Electrocardiogram Interpretation

Normal sinus rhythm with sinus arrhythmia at a rate slightly greater than 60 per minute is present. ST-segment depression is seen in lead III and less so in lead aVF. In this case, a search for an electrocardiogram explanation is important. ST-segment elevation is seen in leads I and aVL. This represents high lateral acute myocardial injury as seen in an early left circumflex territory acute high lateral myocardial infarction. The initial clue on this tracing is the pronounced reciprocal ST-segment depression best seen in lead III.

### Commentary

Acute myocardial injury patterns can be subtle on an electrocardiogram. Oftentimes reciprocal changes are the first clue, as demonstrated here in lead III. The left circumflex coronary artery territory tends to be the most electrocardiographically silent. A careful search for subtle ST-segment elevation often localizes the abnormality to the high lateral leads.

### Keyword Diagnoses

Normal sinus rhythm
Sinus arrhythmia
High lateral myocardial infarction acute
Acute myocardial injury

## ELECTROCARDIOGRAM #12

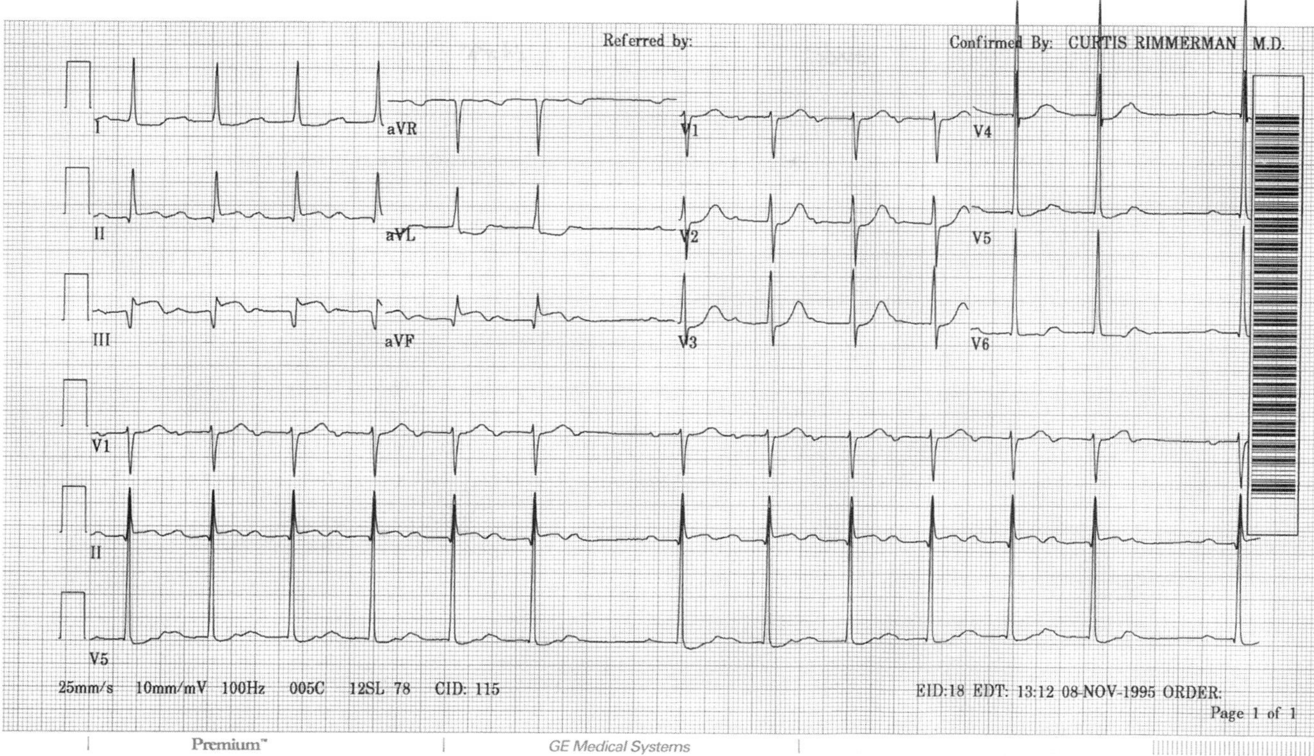


### Clinical History

A 74-year-old man presented to the hospital with sudden-onset anterior chest discomfort and the accompanying electrocardiogram was obtained. An urgent cardiac catheterization was followed by a percutaneous transluminal coronary angioplasty to the right coronary artery, as acute thrombus was present. Medications at the time of this electrocardiogram included intravenous heparin, intravenous nitroglycerin, aspirin, and metoprolol.

### Electrocardiogram Interpretation

Normal sinus rhythm is present. Progressive PR-interval prolongation ensues, with an eventual nonconducted QRS complex. This represents a 7:6 second-degree Mobitz Type I (Wenckebach) atrioventricular block cycle. A 1.5-mm ST-segment elevation with Q waves is seen in the inferior leads, consistent with an acute inferior myocardial infarction. This explains the Wenckebach atrioventricular block, secondary to atrioventricular nodal ischemia during a period of acute myocardial injury. Lead $V_1$ does not demonstrate evidence of ST-segment elevation that would suggest concomitant right ventricular myocardial injury. Reciprocal ST-segment depression is present in leads I and aVL.

### Commentary

Second-degree Mobitz Type I Wenckebach atrioventricular block occurring in the setting of acute myocardial injury does not require temporary pacemaker placement. Close observation of the patient's cardiac rhythm is warranted, as this patient subgroup can progress to more advanced forms of heart block.

### Keyword Diagnoses

Normal sinus rhythm
Second-degree Mobitz Type I Wenckebach atrioventricular block
Inferior myocardial infarction, acute
Acute myocardial injury

## ELECTROCARDIOGRAM #13

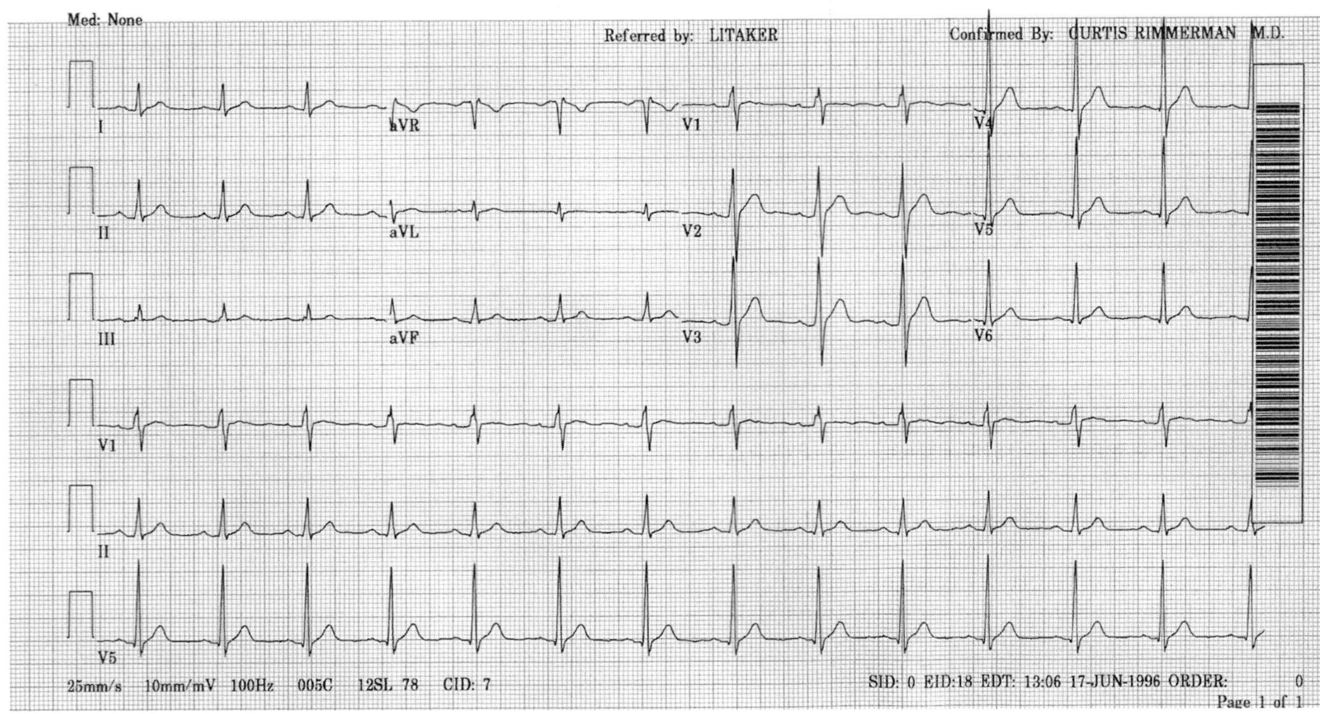


### Clinical History

The patient is a 50-year-old man with recently diagnosed multiple myeloma and a serum calcium level of 13.1 mg/dL.

### Electrocardiogram Interpretation

This electrocardiogram demonstrates normal sinus rhythm. The QRS complexes are normal in both duration and morphology. The only identifiable abnormality is a short QT interval with a truncated ST segment. This is abnormal and represents an electrocardiogram marker of hypercalcemia.

### Commentary

This electrocardiogram emphasizes the need to carefully assess the electrocardiogram intervals on each tracing. The routine electrocardiogram may be the only clinical marker of underlying serum electrolyte disturbances. It is important to identify these abnormalities, as prompt clinical treatment is frequently warranted.

### Keyword Diagnoses

Normal sinus rhythm
Short QT interval
Hypercalcemia

## ELECTROCARDIOGRAM #14

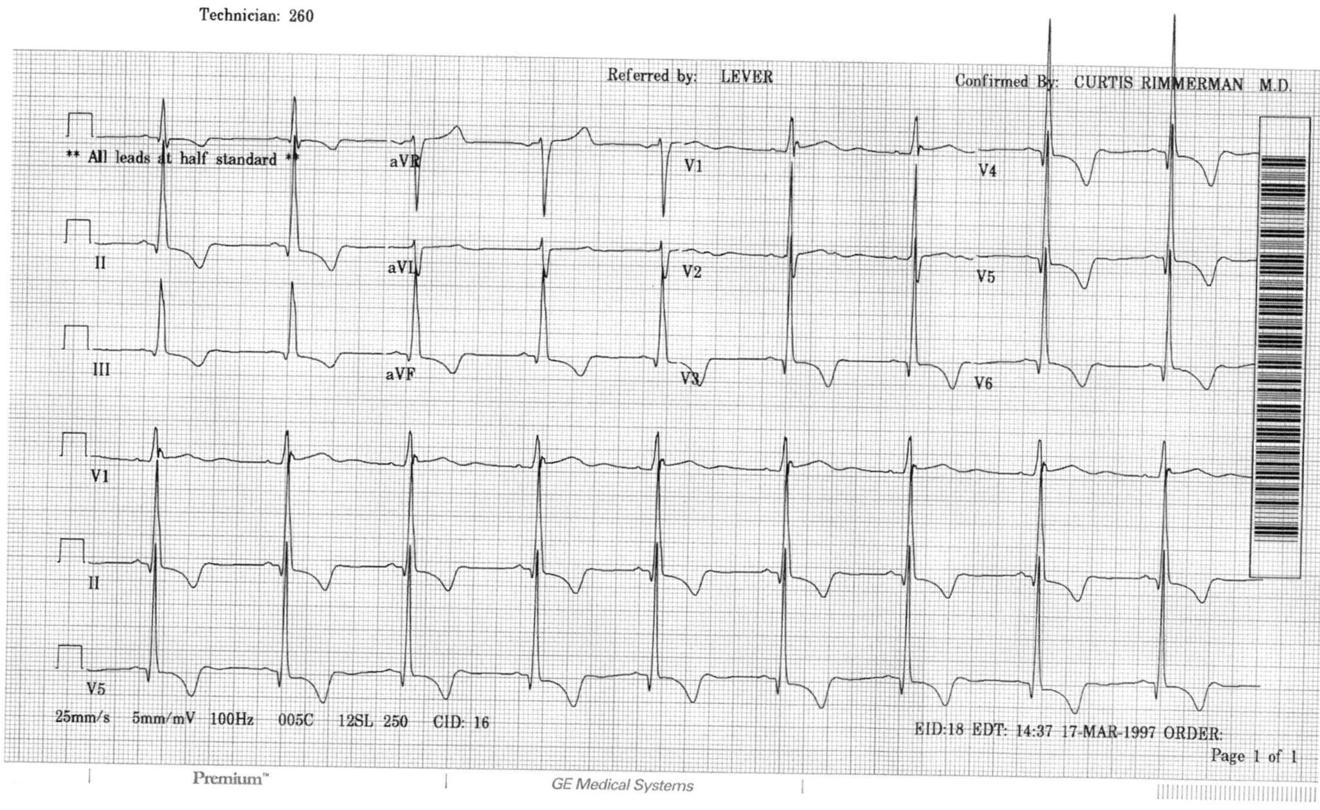


## Clinical History

A 74-year-old man with hypertrophic cardiomyopathy is being seen in follow-up in the Psychiatry Department for chronic depression. His cardiac medications include verapamil and atenolol.

## Electrocardiogram Interpretation

The atrial rhythm is regular, at a rate less than 60 per minute with a normal P-wave axis. This satisfies the electrocardiogram criteria for sinus bradycardia. This electrocardiogram is obtained at half standardization. Despite this, prominent QRS-complex voltage is seen in the precordial leads and inferiorly. A tall R wave is present in leads $V_1$–$V_2$. This suggests the presence of both left ventricular hypertrophy with secondary ST–T changes and right ventricular hypertrophy. This is an example of biventricular hypertrophy with secondary ST–T changes. Prominent Q waves are seen in this patient with hypertrophic cardiomyopathy reflecting septal depolarization.

## Commentary

In this diagnostic setting, prominent septal Q waves are frequently present as seen on this electrocardiogram. It is important to distinguish Q waves secondary to septal depolarization from the possibility of an underlying age-indeterminate myocardial infarction. Oftentimes this is not possible and requires further adjunctive testing.

## Keyword Diagnoses

Half standardization
Sinus bradycardia
Biventricular hypertrophy with secondary ST–T changes
Hypertrophic cardiomyopathy

## ELECTROCARDIOGRAM #15

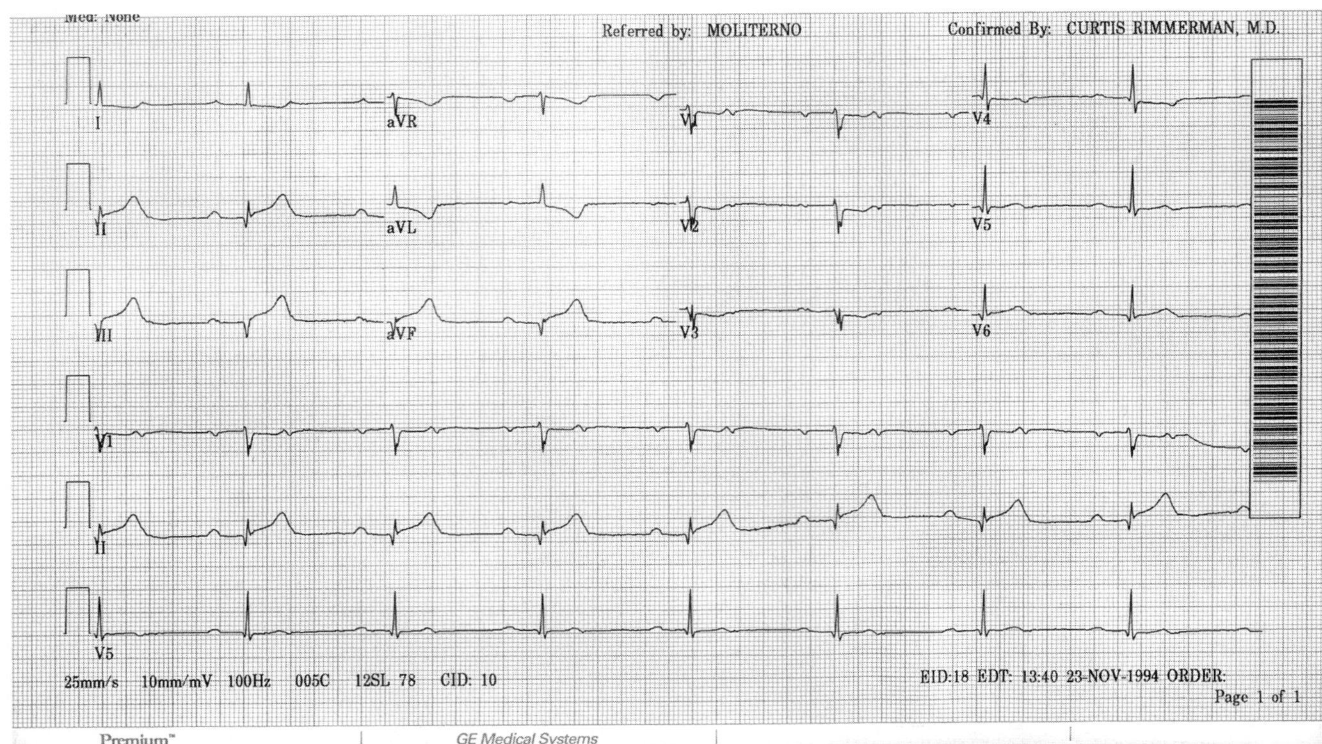


### Clinical History

A 64-year-old man presented to an outside Emergency Room with an acute-onset chest discomfort syndrome and was accepted in urgent hospital transfer for cardiac catheterization. The patient received immediate thrombolytic therapy. A cardiac catheterization demonstrated a 100% distal occlusion of a saphenous vein graft to the right coronary artery, which was successfully angioplastied.

### Electrocardiogram Interpretation

On this tracing the atrial rhythm is best assessed in the lead $V_1$ rhythm strip. Regular P waves occur at a rate of approximately 100 per minute, with a P wave preceding each QRS complex and a P wave following each QRS complex within the terminal aspect of the T wave. This represents normal sinus rhythm with 2:1 atrioventricular block. Inferior Q waves are present with J-point elevation, ST-segment elevation, and ST-segment straightening consistent with an acute inferior myocardial infarction and acute myocardial injury. Reciprocal ST-segment depression is seen in leads I, aVL, and $V_2$–$V_4$. This conduction abnormality is a result of ischemia of the atrioventricular node due to the acute right coronary artery myocardial infarction. Small Q waves approximately 30 milliseconds in duration are present in leads $V_4$–$V_6$. Associated ST–T changes are present. This suggests the possibility of an age-indeterminate anterolateral myocardial infarction. Clinical correlation with the patient's history is necessary.

### Commentary

It is not clear whether this cardiac rhythm is second-degree Mobitz Type I Wenckebach atrioventricular block or second-degree Mobitz Type II atrioventricular block. A longer recording with rhythm strip analysis would be helpful to evaluate for periods of Wenckebach atrioventricular block with varying conduction ratios. In the setting of 2:1 atrioventricular block and acute myocardial injury, temporary pacemaker placement is indicated, as this patient subgroup can proceed to complete heart block and hemodynamic deterioration.

### Keyword Diagnoses

Normal sinus rhythm
2:1 Atrioventricular block
Inferior myocardial infarction, acute
Acute myocardial injury

## ELECTROCARDIOGRAM #16

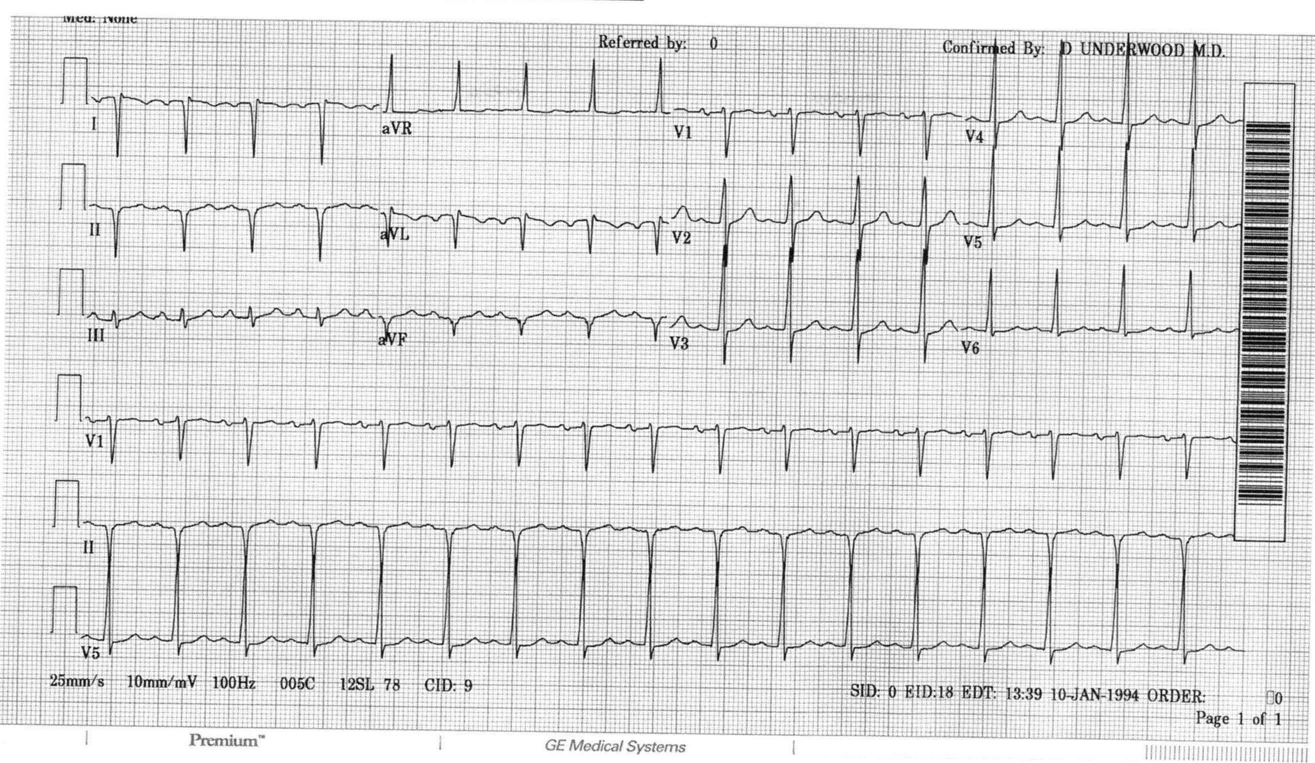


## Clinical History

A 44-year-old man with severe peripheral vascular disease has been admitted for lower-extremity revascularization surgery. He has known coronary artery disease and is status post–myocardial infarction in the remote past, location unknown. His medications included insulin, carbamazepine, amitriptyline, and warfarin.

## Electrocardiogram Interpretation

This electrocardiogram demonstrates a regular atrial rhythm supporting sinus tachycardia at a rate slightly > 100 per minute. The P-wave vector is negative in both leads I and aVL. When the P wave demonstrates a dominant negativity in both leads I and aVL the differential diagnosis includes misplaced limb leads and dextrocardia. Normal R-wave progression is seen in leads $V_2$–$V_6$, which does not support a diagnosis of dextrocardia. Therefore this is an example of misplaced limb leads. The right arm and left arm leads have been reversed. Lead I is inverted. Leads AVR and AVL are reversed, as are leads II and III. Lead AVF is relatively unaffected. Despite this technical error, a dominant Q wave is seen in both leads II and aVF (representing leads III and aVF), possibly suggesting an age-indeterminate inferior myocardial infarction. This does not represent a high lateral myocardial infarction despite the presence of Q waves in leads I and aVL, as these are secondary to the misplaced limb leads.

## Commentary

It is appropriate to repeat this tracing, checking limb lead placement more carefully, to document this patient's electrocardiogram with normally placed leads.

## Keyword Diagnoses

Sinus tachycardia
Misplaced limb leads

## ELECTROCARDIOGRAM #17

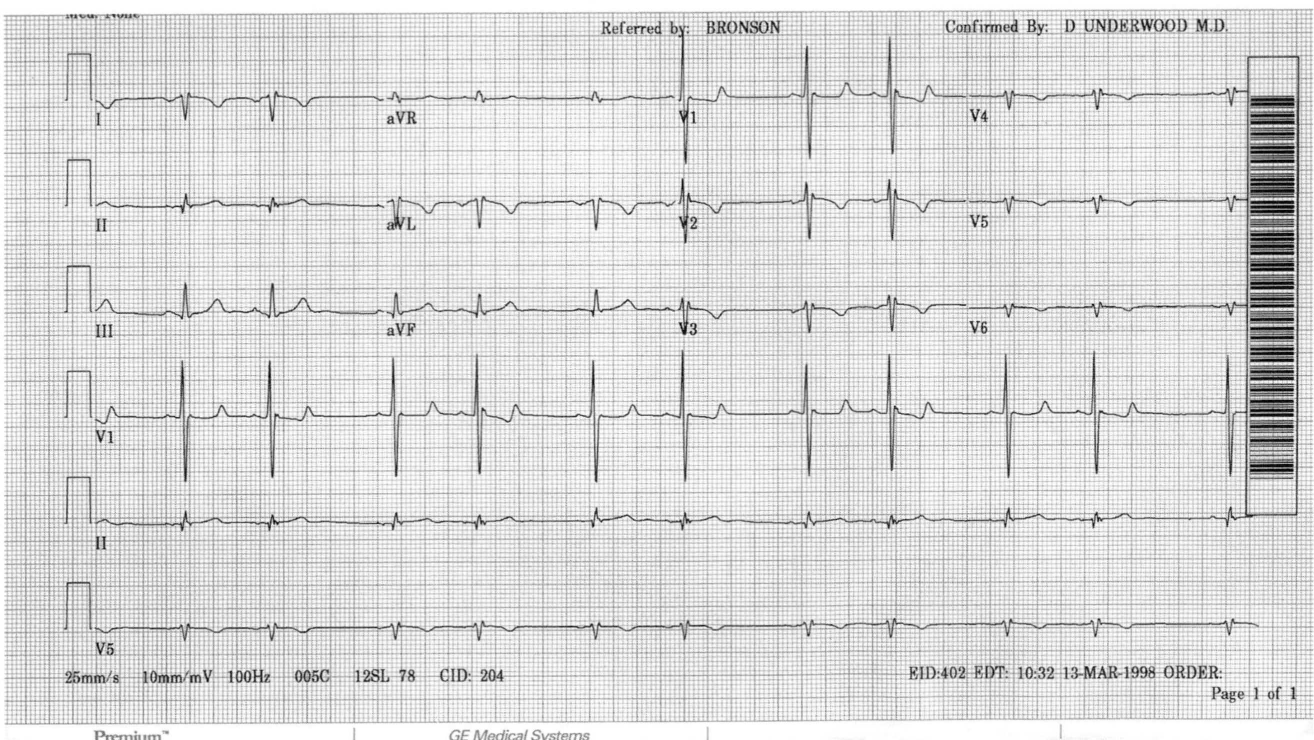


### Clinical History

A 22-year-old woman presents for evaluation of dysplastic nevi. She has known dextrocardia but is on no current medications.

### Electrocardiogram Interpretation

This tracing demonstrates an abnormal P-wave axis with a negative P-wave vector in leads I and aVL. The differential diagnoses for this finding are misplaced limb leads versus dextrocardia. A prominent R wave is seen in lead $V_1$, with R-wave regression as one proceeds from leads $V_2$–$V_6$. A premature atrial complex is present.

### Commentary

Recognizing the presence of dextrocardia is important, because normal electrocardiograms can be interpreted as significantly abnormal. Upon first glance the frontal-plane QRS-complex axis appears deviated extremely rightward, possibly even suggesting a high lateral myocardial infarction. The important diagnostic clue present on this electrocardiogram is the negative P-wave vector in leads I and aVL. This finding, together with R-wave regression seen in leads $V_2$–$V_6$, confirms the presence of dextrocardia.

### Keyword Diagnoses

Normal sinus rhythm
Premature atrial complex
Dextrocardia

## ELECTROCARDIOGRAM #18

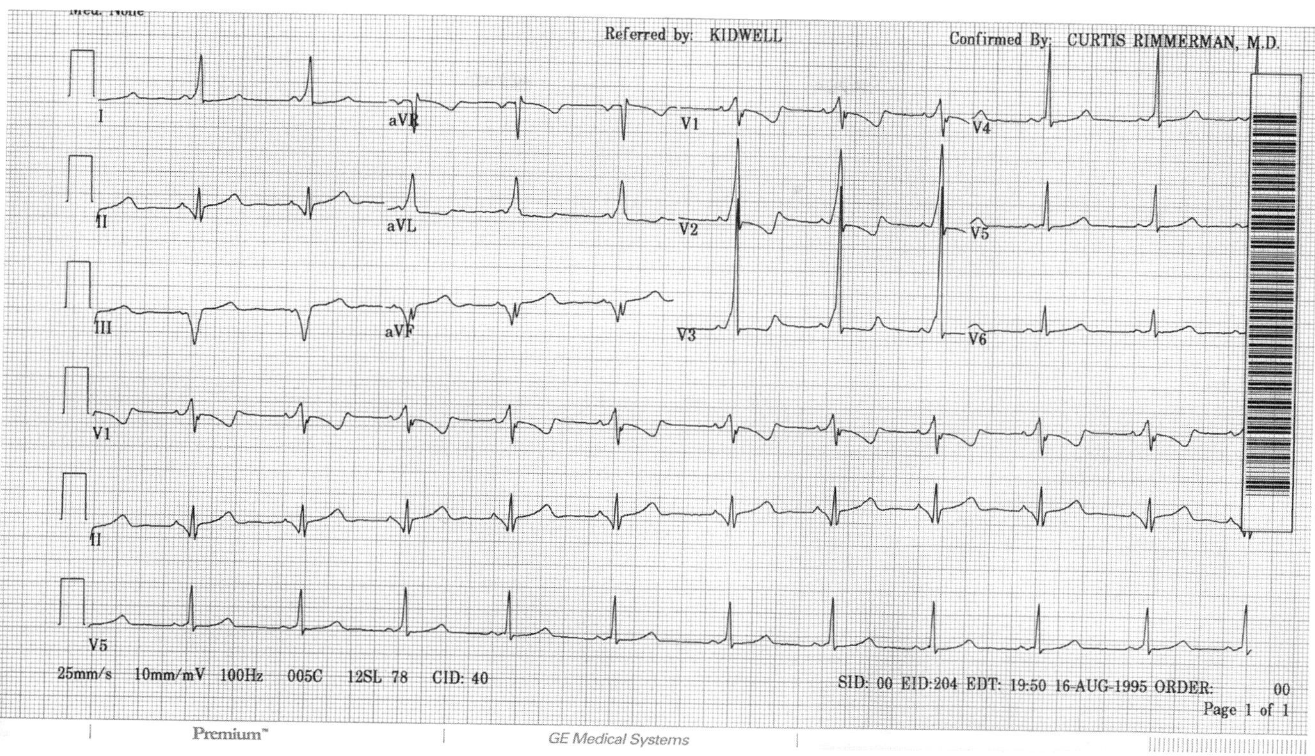


### Clinical History

A 37-year-old woman with Wolff–Parkinson–White syndrome returned for a repeat evaluation in the setting of medication-induced fatigue and persistent palpitations. Her medications include propranolol. The patient subsequently underwent successful radiofrequency ablation of a right ventricular posteroseptal accessory pathway.

### Electrocardiogram Interpretation

Normal sinus rhythm is present. The PR interval is short, with a slurred upstroke to the QRS complex best seen in leads $V_1$–$V_3$, I, and aVL, all supporting ventricular preexcitation and Wolff–Parkinson–White syndrome. Inferior Q waves are present, denoting accessory pathway conduction and a pseudo-infarction pattern. This is not indicative of an inferior myocardial infarction.

### Commentary

Wolff–Parkinson–White syndrome is a common cause of a pseudo-infarction pattern. When the accessory pathway vector is directed opposite an electrocardiogram lead, this generates a negative deflection. The inferior Q waves on this electrocardiogram have a slurred downstroke with a shortened PR interval representing a delta wave.

### Keyword Diagnoses

Normal sinus rhythm
Wolff–Parkinson–White syndrome
Pseudo-infarction pattern

## ELECTROCARDIOGRAM #19

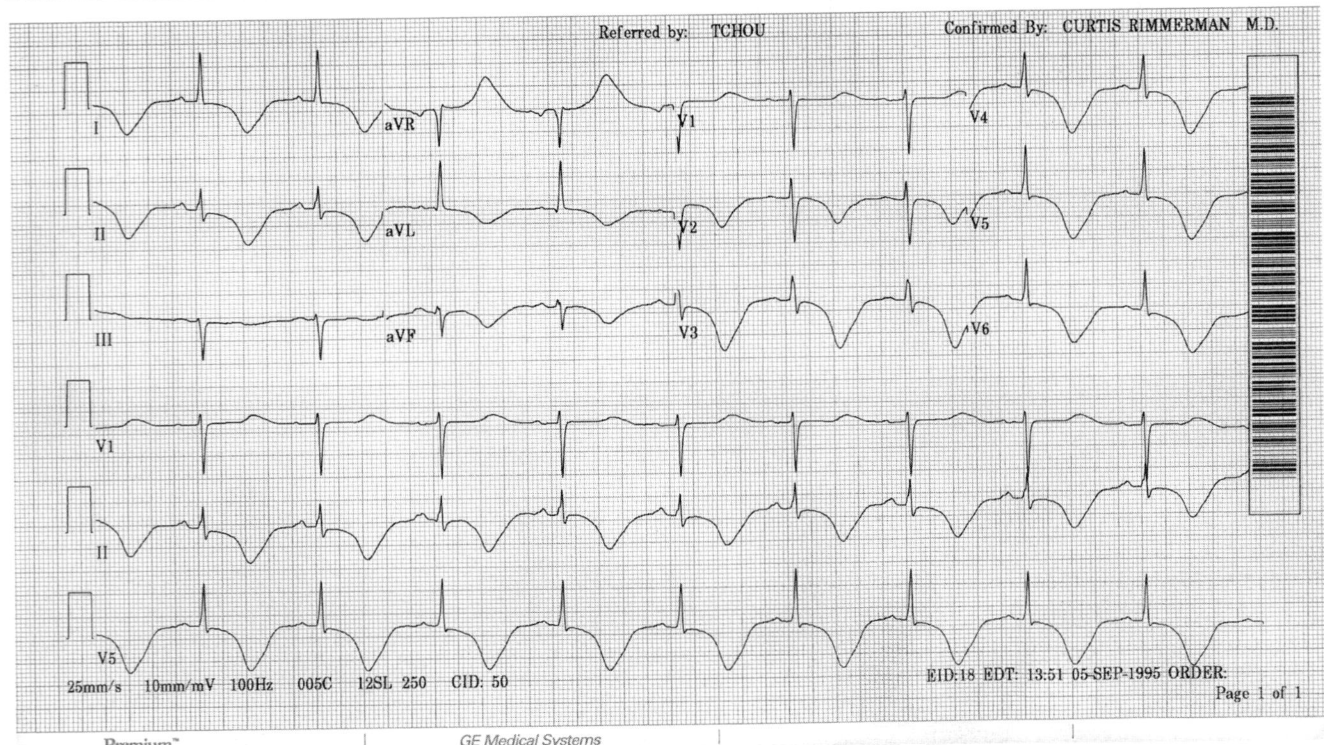


### Clinical History

A 59-year-old woman presented with a chest-discomfort syndrome and the above electrocardiogram. She subsequently underwent cardiac catheterization that demonstrated normal coronary arteries and global mild left ventricular systolic dysfunction. Neurology was consulted about the possibility of a subarachnoid hemorrhage, and this was excluded. Her past medical history includes hypertension.

### Electrocardiogram Interpretation

The atrial rate is regular and slightly less than 60 per minute. The P-wave axis and morphology appear normal, supporting sinus bradycardia. Nonspecific ST–T changes in the form of diffuse T-wave inversion and a prolonged QT interval are present. This is seen in both profound myocardial ischemia and also central nervous system events such as a subarachnoid hemorrhage. Clinical correlation is important. If in fact this represents a myocardial origin, these electrocardiogram findings are most often found in severe subendocardial ischemia or infarction. This is also known as "eggshell" infarct, as a large portion of the subendocardium is infarcted, conferring a worse prognosis on this patient group.

### Commentary

The findings on this electrocardiogram are most consistent with diffuse subendocardial myocardial ischemia or infarction versus a central nervous system event. Both possibilities were excluded in this patient. Given the mild global left ventricular systolic dysfunction, these findings may represent myocarditis or an early form of a cardiomyopathy in which the electrocardiogram demonstrates more pronounced findings. Serial cardiac imaging studies such as echocardiography would be important to evaluate for occult progression of her left ventricular systolic dysfunction.

### Keyword Diagnoses

Sinus bradycardia
Nonspecific ST–T changes
Prolonged QT interval
Ischemia
Central nervous system event

## ELECTROCARDIOGRAM #20

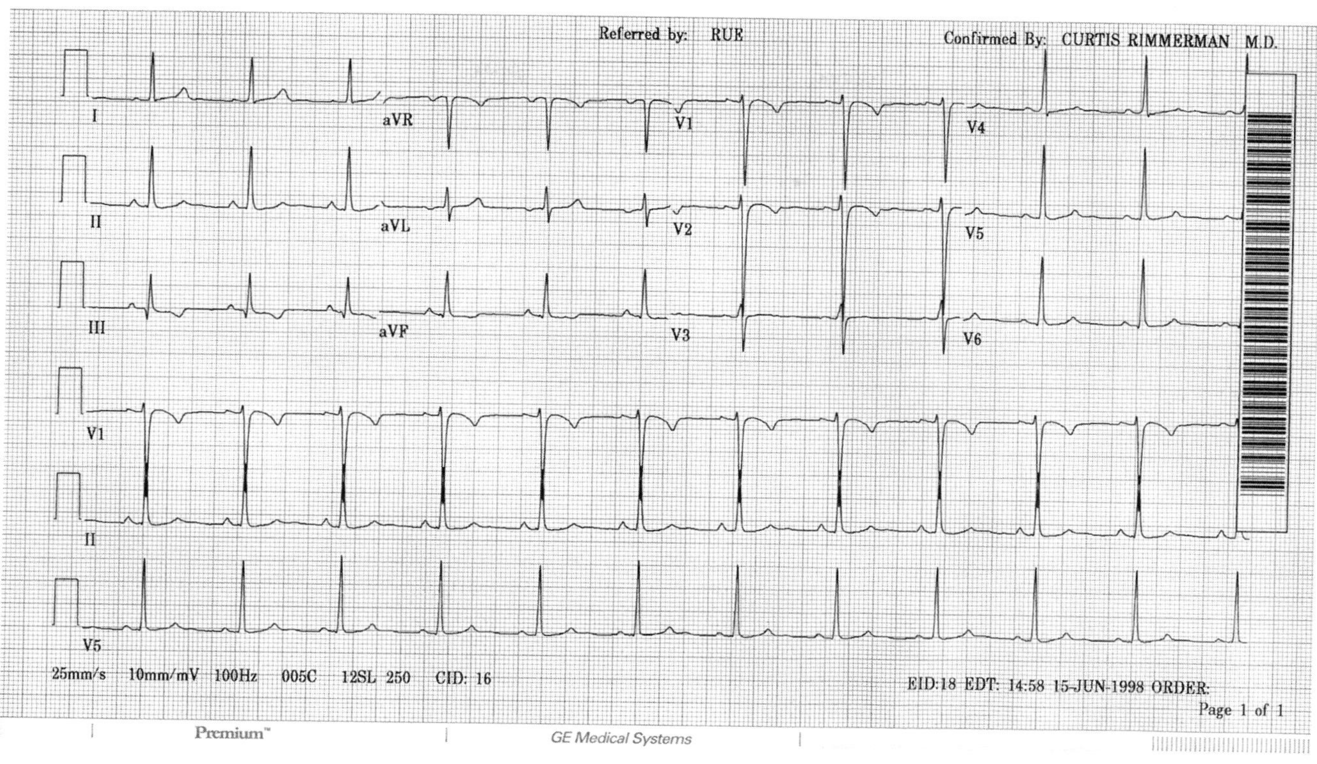


### Clinical History

A 22-year-old woman has been admitted to the hospital for evaluation and treatment of schizophrenia. She is on no current medications.

### Electrocardiogram Interpretation

This is a normal electrocardiogram. The cardiac rhythm is normal sinus rhythm, as the P wave axis in leads I, II, and III is normal and the atrial rate is approximately 70 per minute. T-wave inversion is present in leads $V_1$–$V_2$. In a young patient this is a normal finding and demonstrates a persistent juvenile T-wave pattern.

### Commentary

It is important to recognize normal variants when interpreting electrocardiograms. The persistent juvenile T-wave pattern is a normal variant and should not be confused with underlying cardiac pathology such as myocardial ischemia or a cardiomyopathy.

### Keyword Diagnoses

Normal sinus rhythm
Juvenile T-wave pattern
Normal electrocardiogram

## ELECTROCARDIOGRAM #21

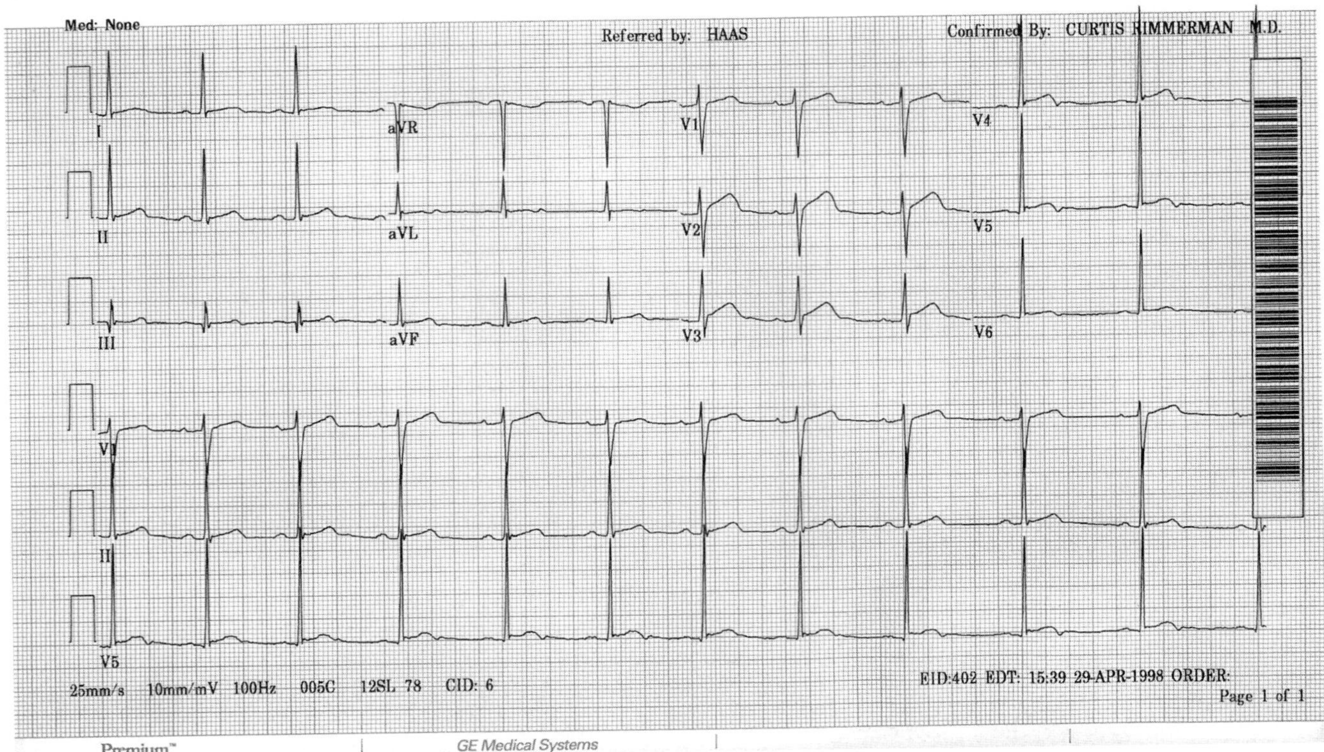


### Clinical History

A 30-old African American man is being evaluated in the presurgical department prior to inguinal hernia repair. He has no known prior cardiac history. An echocardiogram was normal, without evidence of structural heart disease.

### Electrocardiogram Interpretation

Regular P waves with a normal axis at a slightly varying rate of approximately 60 to 75 per minute indicate normal sinus rhythm and sinus arrhythmia. Nonspecific ST–T changes are present throughout the electrocardiogram. J-point elevation and ST-segment elevation are seen in leads $V_2$–$V_6$, I, II, and aVF. This indicates the possibility of an acute myocardial injury pattern but does not support an individual coronary artery territory. The atrial repolarization segment in lead aVR is normal, without evidence to support pericarditis. This represents early repolarization.

### Commentary

The ST–T changes on this electrocardiogram are not normal. However, in younger African American patients, nonspecific ST–T changes with this morphology can represent a normal variant. This was confirmed by the normal resting echocardiogram.

### Keyword Diagnoses

Normal sinus rhythm
Sinus arrhythmia
Normal electrocardiogram
Early repolarization

## ELECTROCARDIOGRAM #22

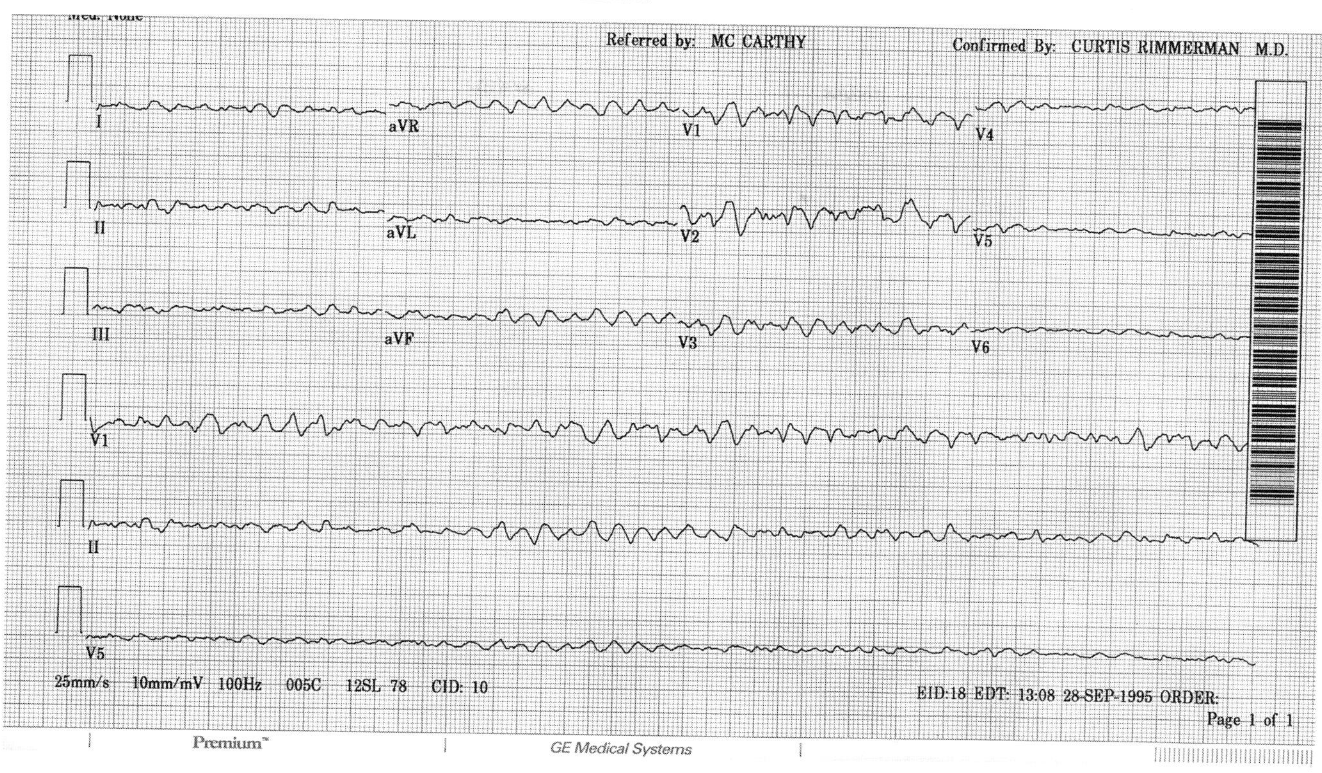


### Clinical History

A 65-year-old man with advanced coronary artery disease and resulting severe left ventricular systolic dysfunction is awaiting cardiac transplantation. This electrocardiogram was obtained while the patient was fully conscious and dependent on a left ventricular assist device. The patient underwent successful cardiac transplantation surgery.

### Electrocardiogram Interpretation

The electrocardiogram baseline is chaotic, without discernible organized atrial or ventricular activity. This represents ventricular fibrillation and is a terminal heart rhythm.

### Commentary

This is a rare opportunity to obtain a recording of ventricular fibrillation on a 12-lead electrocardiogram. There is a complete absence of organized cardiac electrical activity.

### Keyword Diagnose

Ventricular fibrillation

## ELECTROCARDIOGRAM #23

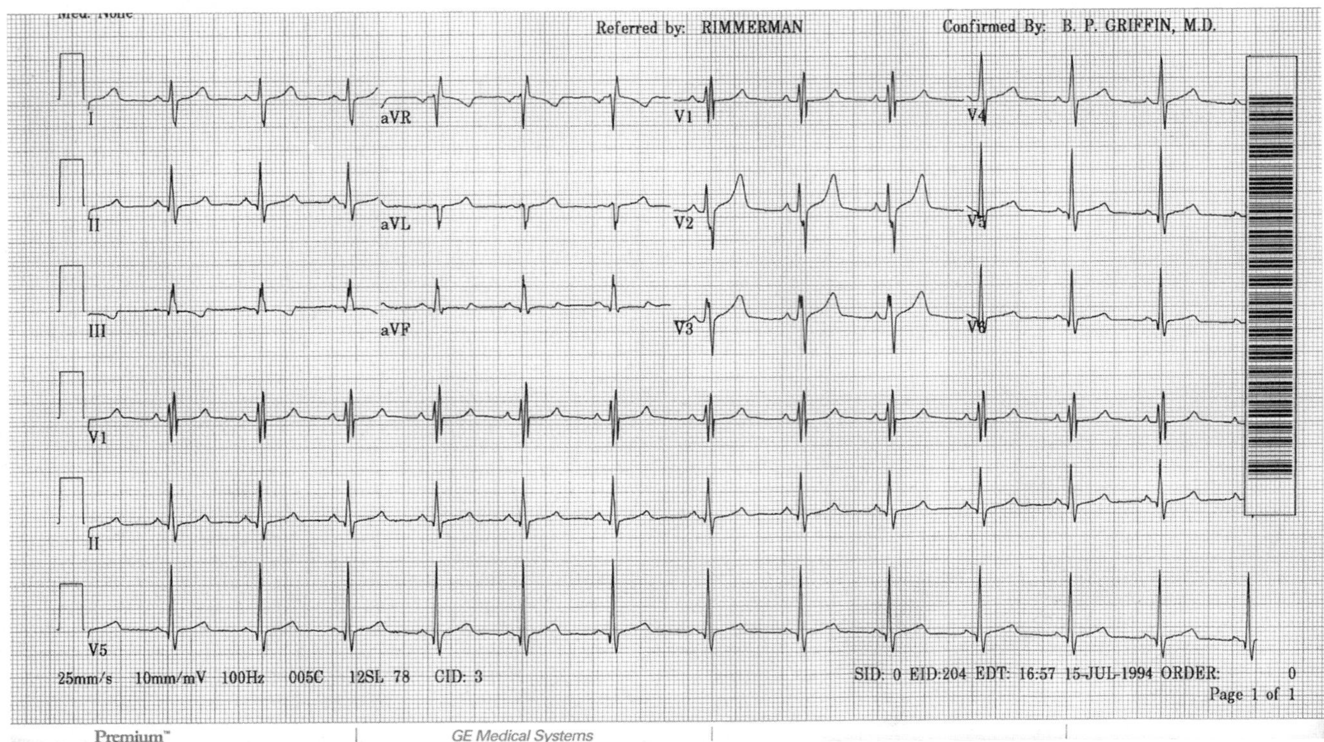


### Clinical History

A 19-year-old man was seen preoperatively, prior to intended ostium secundum atrial septal defect repair. A recent echocardiogram demonstrated a moderate-sized ostium secundum atrial septal defect with left-to-right shunt flow, a dilated right ventricle with normal right ventricular systolic function, and moderate pulmonary hypertension.

### Electrocardiogram Interpretation

The cardiac rhythm is normal sinus rhythm, as a P wave of normal axis precedes each QRS complex. The QRS-complex frontal-plane axis demonstrates right-axis deviation, as the QRS-complex vector is negative in lead I and positive in leads II, III, and aVF. An rsR′ QRS complex morphology is noted in lead $V_1$. This represents an unusual pattern for right ventricular conduction delay, and in the setting of QRS-complex right-axis deviation raises the possibility of an atrial septal defect.

### Commentary

The right ventricular conduction delay as seen in lead $V_1$ is characteristic of an atrial septal defect. Unlike an ostium primum atrial septal defect, in which the QRS-complex frontal-plane axis is deviated leftward, in the setting of an ostium secundum atrial septal defect the QRS-complex vector is normal or deviated rightward. In this circumstance, given the left-to-right interatrial shunt, the rightward deviation of the QRS-complex vector is secondary to the volume overload of the right ventricle.

### Keyword Diagnoses

Normal sinus rhythm
Right-axis deviation
Ostium secundum atrial septal defect

## ELECTROCARDIOGRAM #24

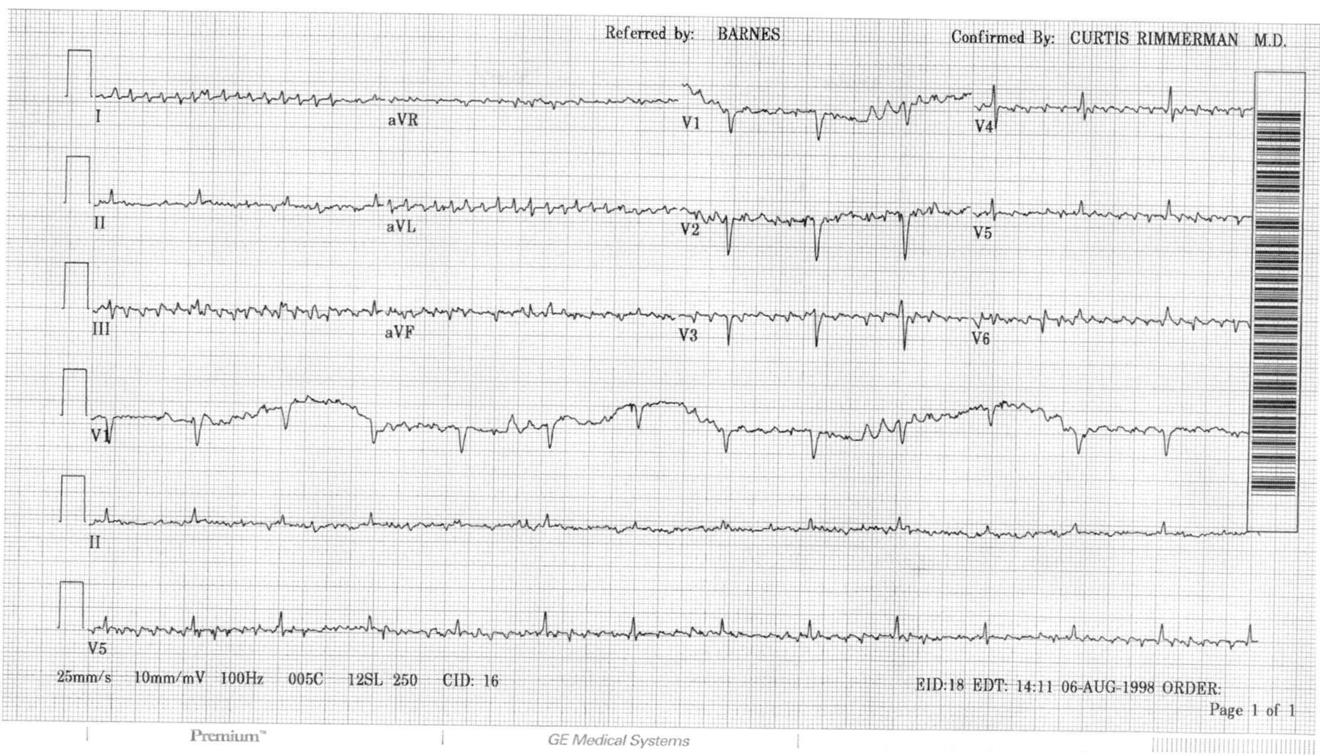


### Clinical History

A 62-year-old woman with fevers and chills of 2 days' duration was admitted with suspected sepsis. Co-morbid conditions include rheumatoid arthritis and chronic obstructive pulmonary disease.

### Electrocardiogram Interpretation

A prominent baseline artifact consistent with electrical interference is present. This significantly compromises the electrocardiogram interpretation. Despite this technical difficulty, QRS complexes occur at regular intervals. Low-voltage QRS complexes are present in the limb leads, as no complex is greater than 5 mm in amplitude. Given the baseline artifact, no identifiable atrial activity is present. The constant QRS-complex cycle length suggests normal sinus rhythm. ST–T-segment and T-wave flattening is suspected, consistent with nonspecific ST–T changes.

### Commentary

The prominent baseline artifact merits a repeat examination, as this artifact interferes significantly with electrocardiogram interpretation.

### Keyword Diagnoses

Baseline artifact
Normal sinus rhythm
Low-voltage QRS—limb leads
Nonspecific ST–T changes

## ELECTROCARDIOGRAM #25

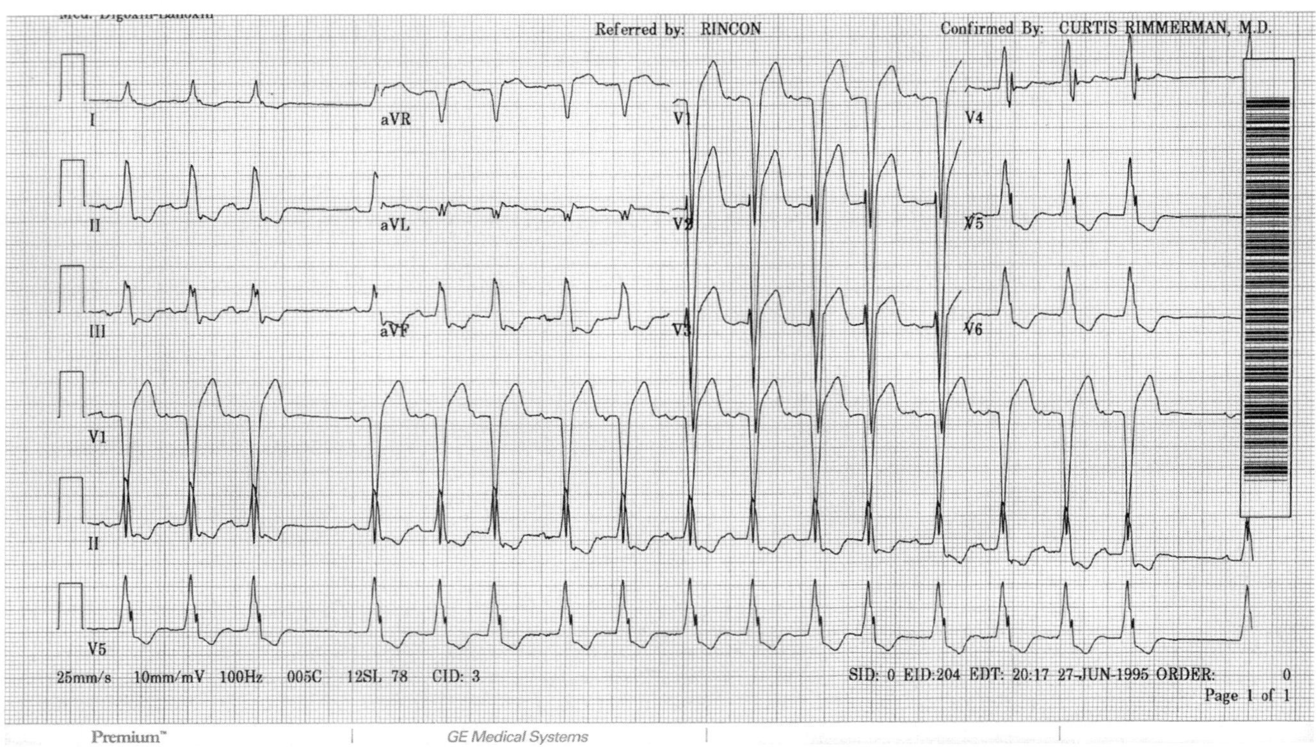


### Clinical History

A 76-year-old man with two prior coronary artery bypass graft surgeries and moderate left ventricular systolic dysfunction has returned for outpatient cardiology follow-up. The patient is being seen preoperatively prior to a planned carotid endarterectomy. His co-morbid conditions include severe chronic obstructive pulmonary disease, paroxysmal atrial fibrillation, and chronic renal insufficiency. His medications included prednisone, digoxin, enalapril, furosemide, and warfarin.

### Electrocardiogram Interpretation

A P wave precedes each QRS complex at a rate greater than 100 per minute, supporting sinus tachycardia. The sixth, eighth, and 12th P waves are premature, reflecting premature atrial complexes. The QRS complex is widened, with a complete left bundle branch block morphology. An apparent pause occurs between the third and fourth QRS complexes. No P wave is identified, but the P–P interval is twice that of the intrinsic P–P interval. The sinus node discharges on time, but the depolarization wave is blocked from exiting the sinus node and depolarizing the atrium. This is known as sinus exit block. No identifiable atrial activity in the form of a P wave is seen. The next P wave occurs when expected, as the sinus node discharges without exit block transpiring.

### Commentary

To diagnose the presence of sinus exit block, the R–R interval encompassing the sinus exit block should be twice the baseline R–R interval. This electrocardiogram also demonstrates significant conduction system disease, given the presence of complete left bundle branch block. This is most likely secondary to the patient's advanced ischemic heart disease.

### Keyword Diagnoses

Sinus tachycardia
Premature atrial complex
Sinus exit block
Complete left bundle branch block

## ELECTROCARDIOGRAM #26

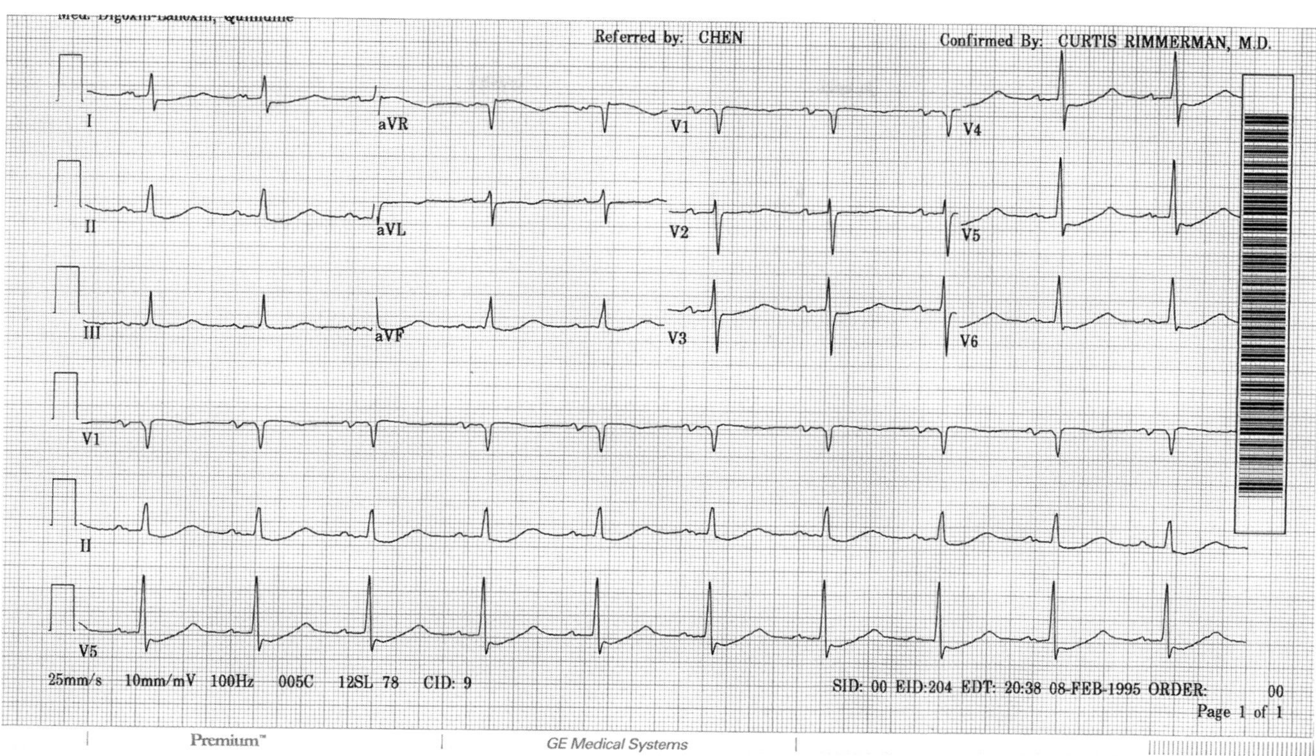


### Clinical History

A 72-year-old man with advanced peripheral vascular disease has been admitted to the hospital for a semielective below-the-knee amputation. His past medical history includes chronic obstructive pulmonary disease, a remote myocardial infarction, and prior pacemaker placement. His medications include quinidine and digoxin.

### Electrocardiogram Interpretation

The cardiac rhythm is normal sinus rhythm, as the P waves occur at regular intervals with a normal axis slightly greater than 60 per minute. The PR interval is prolonged to 220 milliseconds, representing first-degree atrioventricular block. Left atrial abnormality is seen, as the P-wave morphology is terminally negative in lead $V_1$ and bifid in lead II. Diffuse nonspecific ST–T changes are present. Most important, each lead demonstrates a prominent prolonged QT interval. Both the QT-interval prolongation and ST-segment scooping are secondary to the concomitant quinidine effect and digitalis effect.

### Commentary

QT interval prolongation in the setting of quinidine administration may represent quinidine toxicity and near-future proarrhythmia. Comparison with prior electrocardiograms is important to confirm whether this is a new or pre-existing finding.

### Keyword Diagnoses

Normal sinus rhythm
First-degree atrioventricular block
Left atrial abnormality
Prolonged QT interval
Nonspecific ST–T changes
Digitalis effect
Quinidine effect

## ELECTROCARDIOGRAM #27

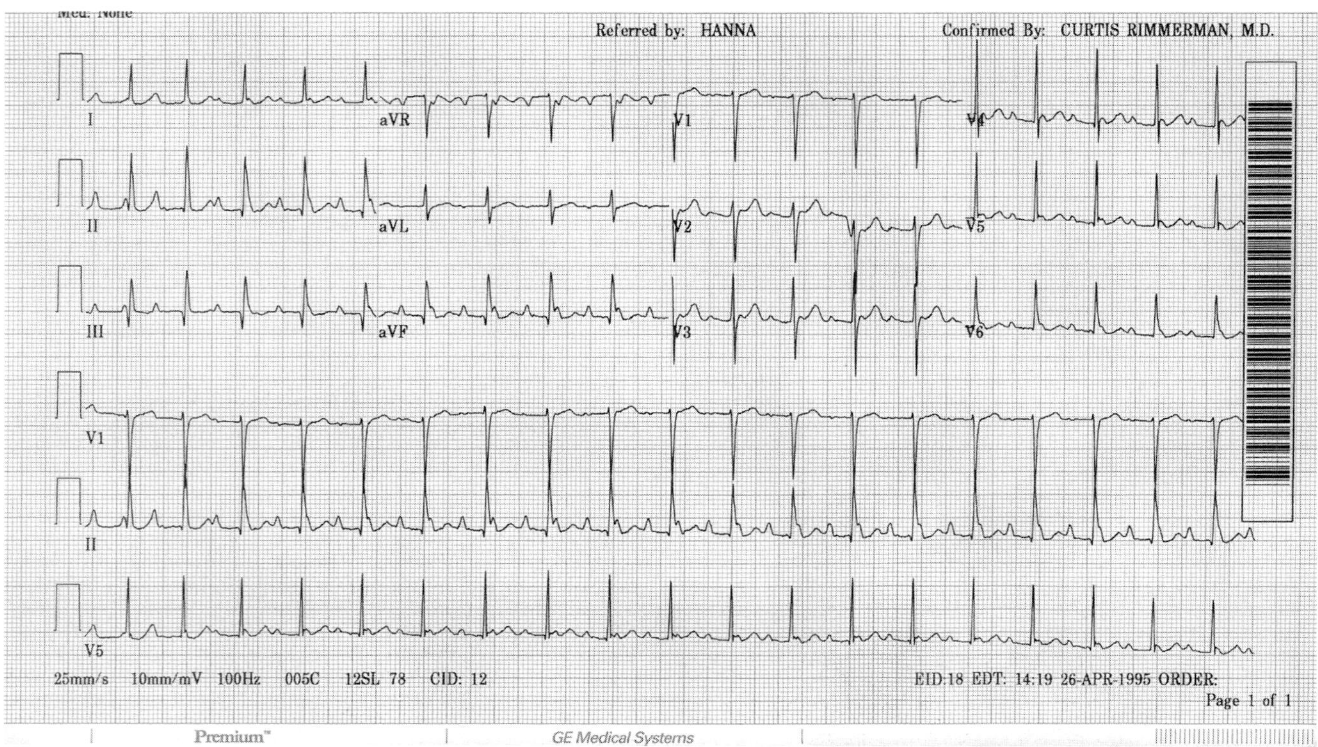


### Clinical History

A 77-year-old woman status post an acute left middle cerebral artery occlusion and urokinase administration is now experiencing recurrent atrial arrhythmias. Medications at the time of this electrocardiogram included diltiazem, topical nitroglycerin, and isosorbide mononitrate. An echocardiogram performed during this hospitalization demonstrated moderate left atrial enlargement and normal left ventricular systolic function without evidence of a prior myocardial infarction.

### Electrocardiogram Interpretation

This electrocardiogram demonstrates two P waves for each QRS complex, best seen in lead aVF. The second P wave occurs on the downslope of the S wave at the beginning of the ST segment. This represents ectopic atrial tachycardia with 2:1 atrioventricular conduction. There are small narrow inferior Q waves that are not of diagnostic significance.

### Commentary

When interpreting electrocardiograms that show arrhythmias, it is important to survey each lead, which may yield a subtle and different clue. For this tracing, regular atrial activity is seen best in the inferior leads. Other leads such as lead $V_1$ demonstrate nearly isoelectric atrial activity and suggest a junctional tachycardia. When a tachycardia is present, it is important to ascertain the shortest P–P interval and compare it to the R–R interval. Without this approach, 2:1 atrioventricular conduction may be overlooked.

### Keyword Diagnoses

Ectopic atrial tachycardia
2:1 Atrioventricular conduction

## ELECTROCARDIOGRAM #28

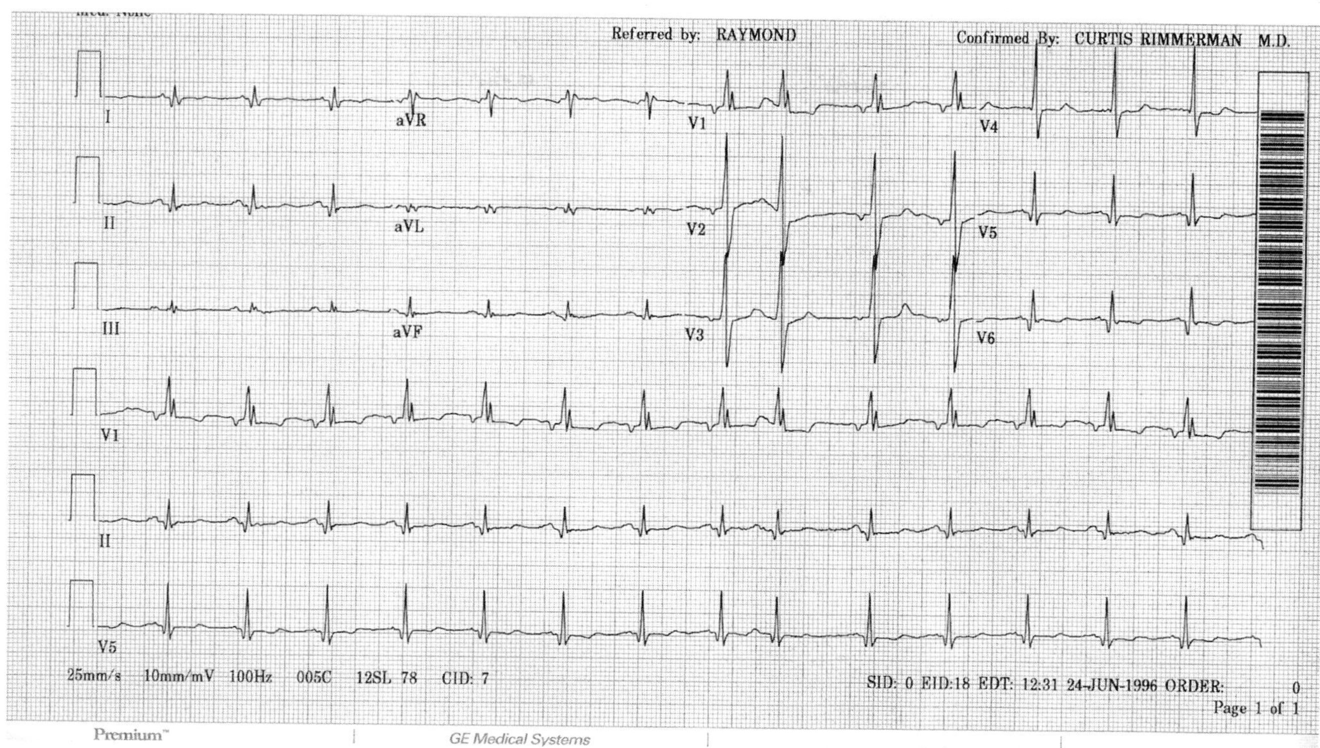


### Clinical History

A 66-year-old man status post recent coronary artery bypass graft surgery, paroxysmal atrial fibrillation, and a cerebrovascular accident has returned for a follow-up evaluation after his bypass surgery. Other co-morbidities include hypertension, non–insulin-requiring diabetes mellitus, and hyperlipidemia.

### Electrocardiogram Interpretation

Normal sinus rhythm is present. The ninth P wave is premature, reflecting a premature atrial complex with a similar QRS-complex morphology. The QRS-complex duration is prolonged but less than 120 milliseconds. Lead $V_1$ demonstrates an Rsr′ QRS-complex pattern indicating an incomplete right bundle branch block. Q waves of diagnostic duration are present in the inferior, lateral, and high lateral leads, indicating an inferolateral myocardial infarction of indeterminate age. R waves are prominent in leads $V_1$–$V_2$, suggesting an age-indeterminate posterior myocardial infarction. This is likely one event and is best characterized collectively as an age-indeterminate inferoposterolateral myocardial infarction. Left atrial abnormality is seen in lead $V_1$, as the terminal P-wave vector is negative.

### Commentary

The most important findings on this electrocardiogram are the diagnostically wide Q waves present in leads I, aVL, and $V_5$–$V_6$, consistent with an age-indeterminate lateral myocardial infarction. In the presence of a lateral myocardial infarction, it is important to identify other potential areas of infarction. Typically, lateral infarctions may extend both posteriorly and inferiorly. The inferior Q waves are of diminutive depth and of only 30 milliseconds duration. In the setting of prominent R waves in leads $V_1$–$V_2$ and prominent lateral Q waves, these findings together suggest an associated inferoposterior myocardial infarction.

### Keyword Diagnoses

- Normal sinus rhythm
- Premature atrial complex
- Left atrial abnormality
- Incomplete right bundle branch block
- Inferoposterolateral myocardial infarction, age-indeterminate

## ELECTROCARDIOGRAM #29

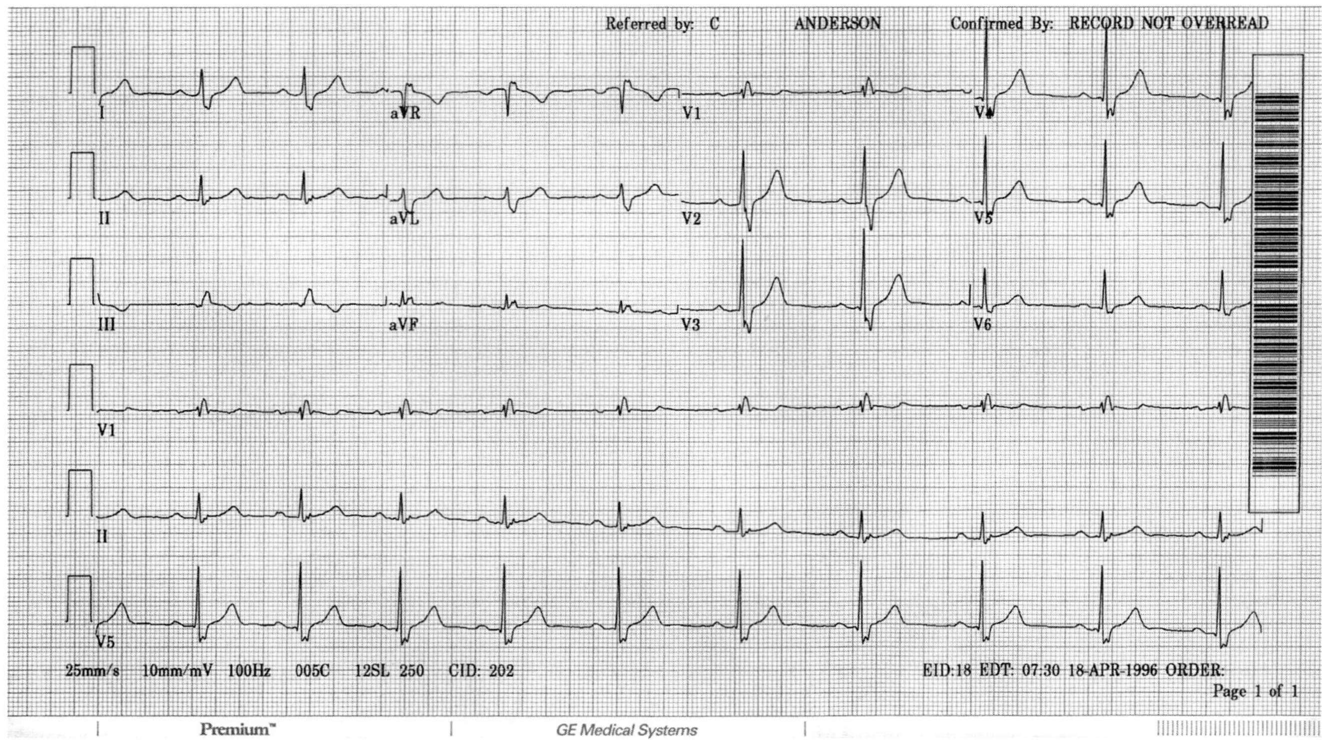


### Clinical History

A 40-year-old man with a history of "an enlarged heart" since a young age is seeking a cardiac evaluation. A prior echocardiogram demonstrated evidence of Ebstein anomaly.

### Electrocardiogram Interpretation

The cardiac rhythm is normal sinus rhythm. This PR interval is borderline prolonged. Right ventricular conduction delay is evidenced by complete right bundle branch block. This is best seen in lead $V_1$, with an rsr′ QRS complex, and also in leads I, aVL, and $V_6$, with a widened QRS complex and terminal S wave indicative of right ventricular conduction delay. Leads $V_2$–$V_3$ demonstrate primary T-wave changes, as depolarization and repolarization demonstrate similar polarity.

### Commentary

Ebstein anomaly is characterized by apical right ventricular displacement of the tricuspid valve septal and/or posterior leaflets, resulting in "atrialization" of the right ventricle. Frequently, these patients suffer from tricuspid insufficiency, right ventricular systolic dysfunction, and resulting slowed right ventricular conduction as evidenced by complete right bundle branch block and 1° AV block. These patients also frequently have one or more accessory pathways.

### Keyword Diagnoses

Normal sinus rhythm
Complete right bundle branch block
Primary T-wave changes
Ebstein anomaly

## ELECTROCARDIOGRAM #30

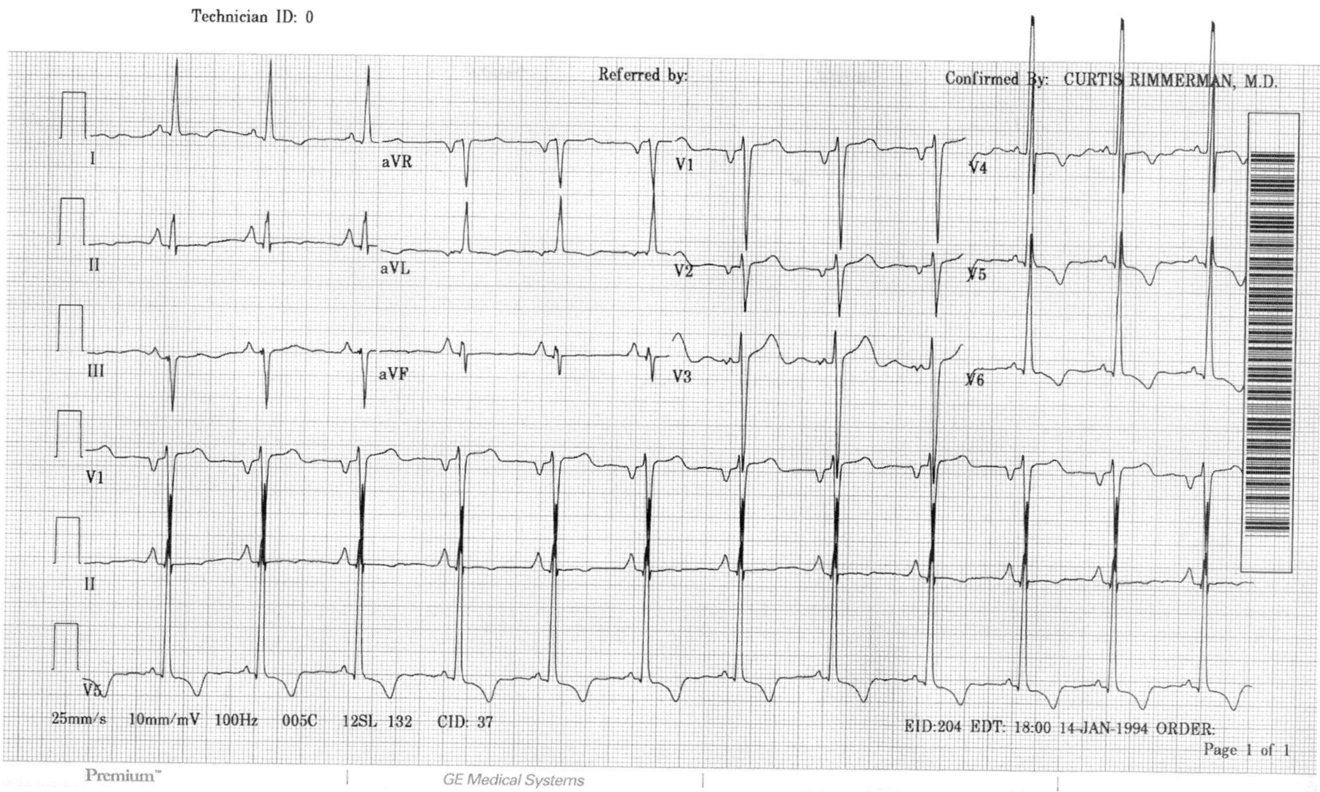


### Clinical History

A 63-year-old man with an approximately 25-year history of hypertension presents to the hypertension clinic for further evaluation. He has noticed recent dyspnea upon exertion. Medications at the time of this tracing included lisinopril.

### Electrocardiogram Interpretation

Normal sinus rhythm is present, as each QRS complex is preceded by a P wave of normal axis. The P-wave morphology is abnormal, with a terminal negativity in lead $V_1$ consistent with left atrial abnormality. In lead II, the P-wave amplitude is >3 mm, consistent with right atrial abnormality. Prominent precordial QRS-complex voltage is present, with asymmetric ST–T changes indicative of left ventricular hypertrophy with secondary ST–T changes. Negative U waves are seen in the lateral precordial leads, supporting the presence of left ventricular hypertrophy.

### Commentary

This electrocardiogram satisfies many criteria for left ventricular hypertrophy. In addition to the prominent QRS-complex voltage and asymmetric T-wave inversion indicative of a strain pattern, a slightly prolonged QRS complex and prominent left atrial abnormality are also present. Negative U waves are readily seen. The differential diagnosis of negative U waves includes coronary artery disease and left ventricular hypertrophy. With the associated electrocardiogram findings, the negative U waves are secondary to left ventricular hypertrophy.

### Keyword Diagnoses

- Normal sinus rhythm
- Left atrial abnormality
- Right atrial abnormality
- Left ventricular hypertrophy with secondary ST–T changes
- Negative U waves

## ELECTROCARDIOGRAM #31

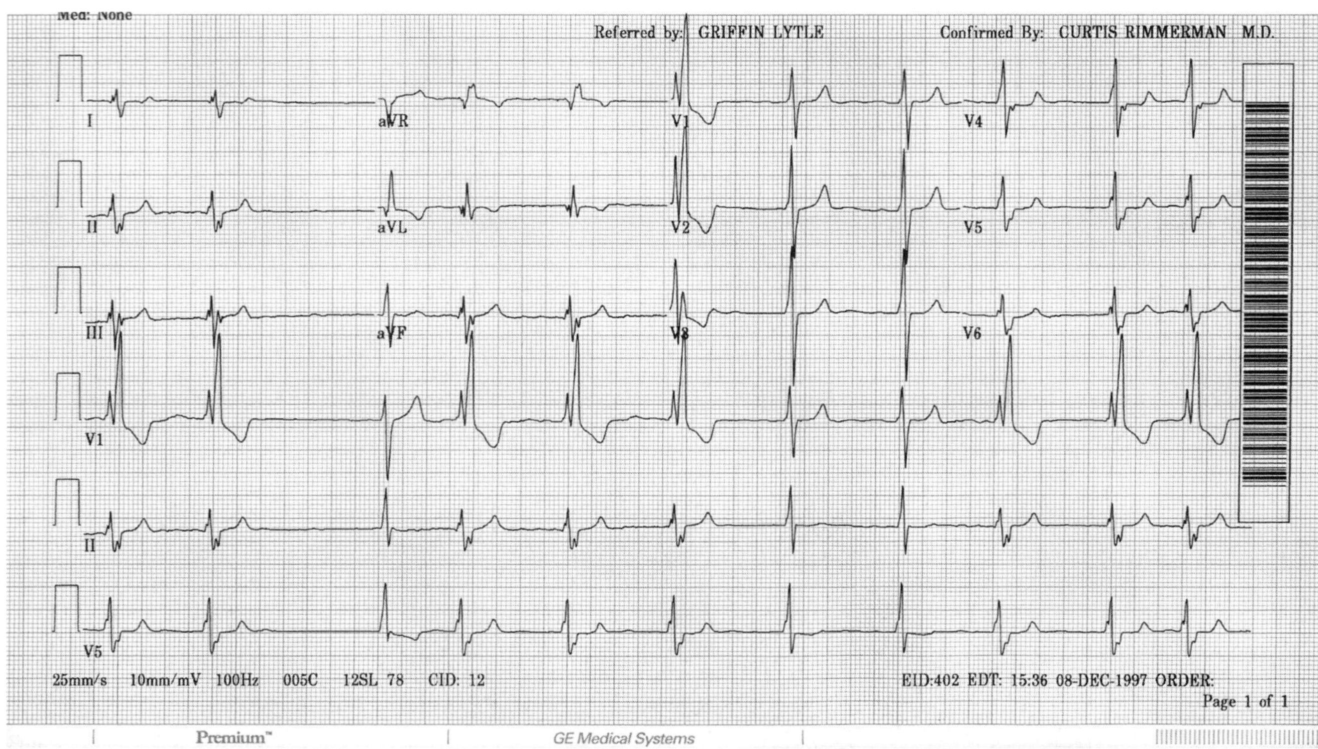


### Clinical History

A 47-year-old man with a history of aortic stenosis status post prior aortic valve replacement re-presents with perivalvular moderately severe aortic insufficiency and congestive heart failure. Co-morbid conditions include insulin-requiring diabetes mellitus and a recently repaired rectal fistula. His medications included insulin, potassium, metolazone, metoprolol, captopril, and digoxin.

### Electrocardiogram Interpretation

The electrocardiogram baseline demonstrates an absence of organized atrial activity. The ventricular response is irregularly irregular, representing atrial fibrillation. An intermittent complete right bundle branch block pattern is seen at shorter R–R intervals. Note that the initiation of the complete right bundle branch block occurs at a shorter R–R interval than does sustaining the complete right bundle branch block. This is a typical finding in acceleration-dependent complete right bundle branch block. With QRS-cycle length slowing, the complete right bundle branch block transiently disappears. There is no evidence of a prior myocardial infarction. High lateral nonspecific ST–T changes are present.

### Commentary

Acceleration-dependent complete right bundle branch block is a common electrocardiogram finding. The right bundle branch has a longer refractory period than the left bundle branch and therefore rate-dependent right bundle branch conduction delay is a more common entity. This may precede permanent complete right bundle branch block.

### Keyword Diagnoses

- Atrial fibrillation
- Acceleration-dependent complete right bundle branch block
- Nonspecific ST–T changes

## ELECTROCARDIOGRAM #32

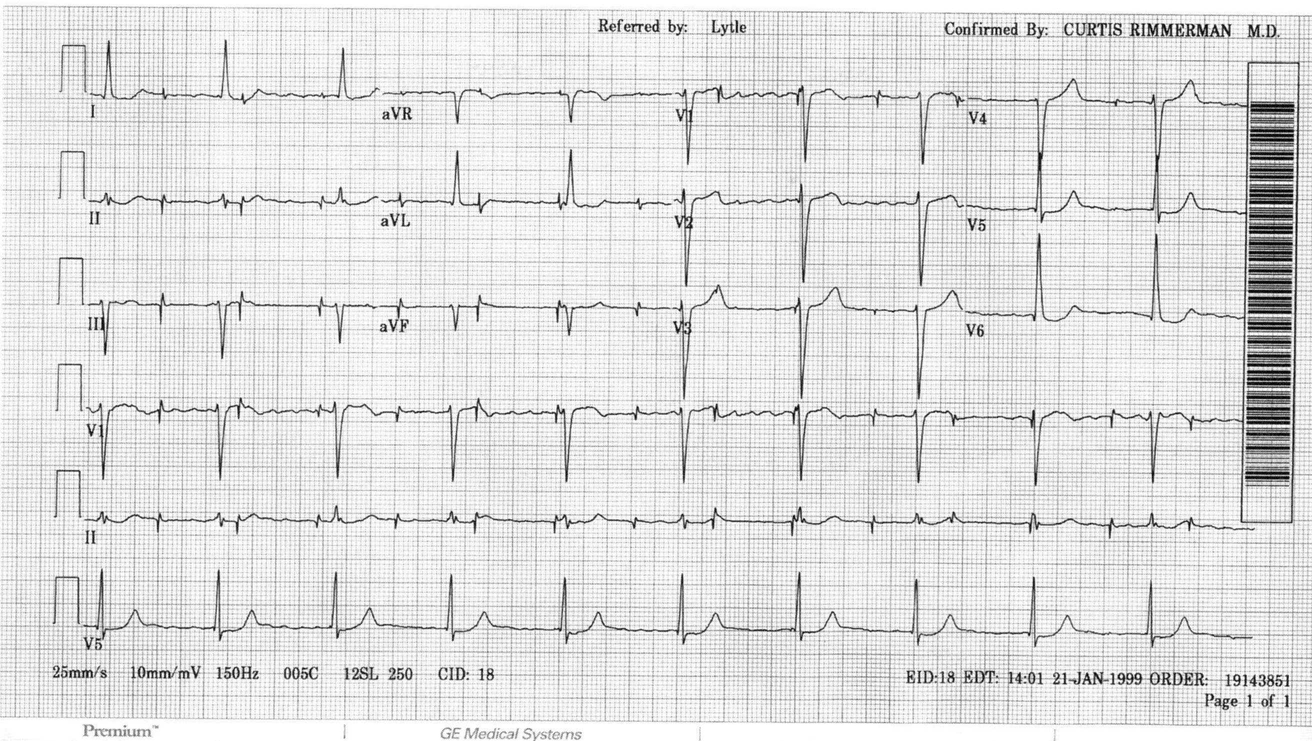


### Clinical History

A 72-year-old woman with advanced atrioventricular block necessitating prior permanent pacemaker placement returns for pacemaker follow-up. Co-morbid conditions include coronary artery disease, hypertension, and hyperlipidemia. Medications at the time of this electrocardiogram included metoprolol, aspirin, digoxin, and simvastatin.

### Electrocardiogram Interpretation

The electrocardiogram baseline is devoid of discrete atrial activity. This represents atrial fibrillation. The QRS complexes occur at regular R–R intervals at a ventricular rate slightly greater than 60 per minute. This is an unexpected finding in the presence of atrial fibrillation. This represents an accelerated junctional rhythm and atrioventricular dissociation. Presumed ventricular pacemaker deflections occur at regular intervals throughout the electrocardiogram with no relationship to the QRS complexes. This represents both pacemaker sensing failure and pacemaker capture failure. Lateral and high lateral nonspecific ST–T changes are demonstrated. The scooping of the ST segments support the presence of digitalis effect.

### Commentary

This electrocardiogram demonstrates abnormal pacemaker function, necessitating further evaluation. This may represent pacemaker lead dislodgement. In the presence of atrial fibrillation, it is important to evaluate the electrocardiogram for a second independent cardiac rhythm. The important clue on this tracing is the constant R–R interval. Atrioventricular dissociation and an accelerated junctional rhythm both support the possible presence of digitalis toxicity, warranting further clinical investigation.

### Keyword Diagnoses

Atrial fibrillation
Accelerated junctional rhythm
Atrioventricular dissociation
Ventricular pacemaker
Pacemaker sensing failure
Pacemaker capture failure
Nonspecific ST–T changes
Digitalis effect

## ELECTROCARDIOGRAM #33

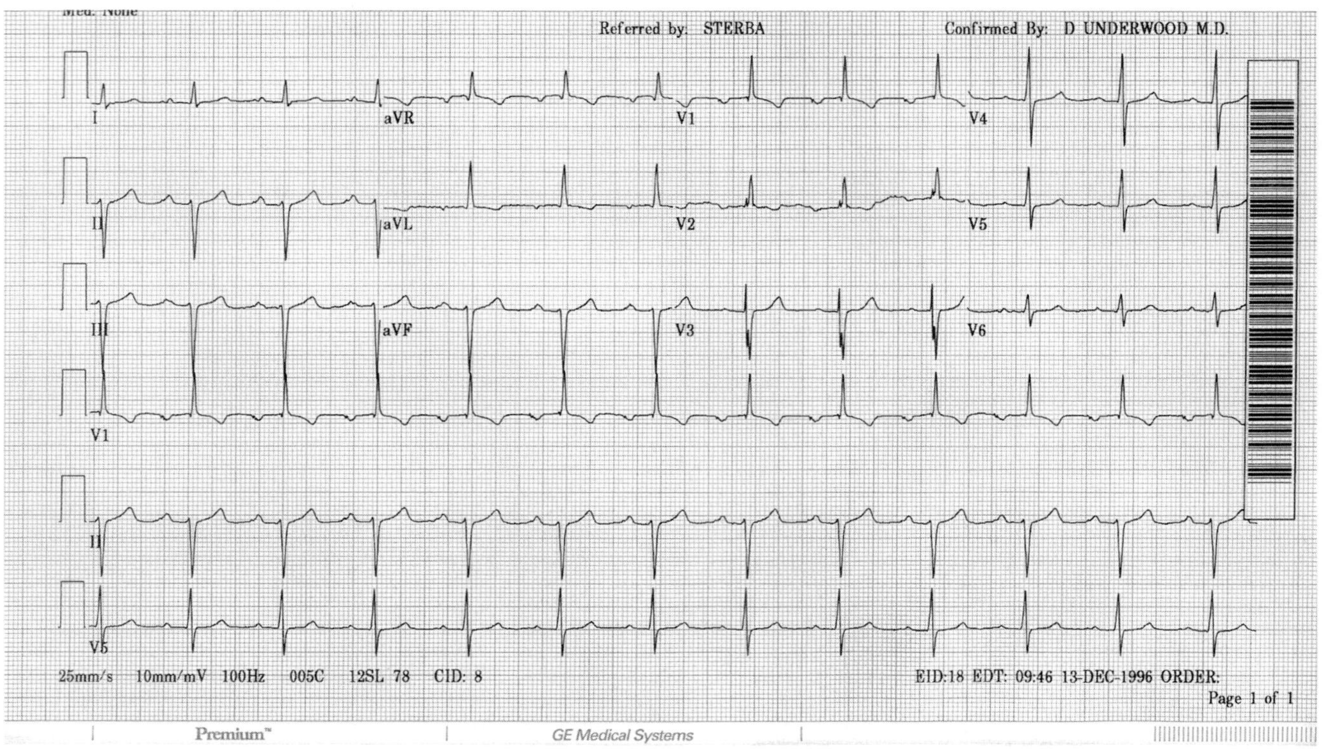


### Clinical History

A 34-year-old woman with a history of an atrioventricular canal and ostium primum atrial septal defect status post surgical repair is readmitted for a cardiac evaluation. She is experiencing paroxysmal atria dysrhythmias and is on no current medications.

### Electrocardiogram Interpretation

This patient is known to have ostium primum atrial septal defect. This electrocardiogram demonstrates a group of findings consistent with this diagnosis. The atrial rhythm is normal sinus rhythm. The PR interval is prolonged at 240 milliseconds, representing first-degree atrioventricular block. The P wave is terminally negative in lead $V_1$ and broadened in lead II, suggesting left atrial abnormality. The QRS-complex axis is deviated leftward, satisfying the criteria for left-axis deviation, as the QRS-complex frontal-plane vector is positive in lead I and deeply negative in leads II, III, and aVF. A rsR′ QRS complex is seen in lead $V_1$ with a normal QRS-complex duration, supporting incomplete right bundle branch block.

### Commentary

A narrow rsR′ QRS complex morphology in the presence of left-axis deviation and left atrial abnormality are a group of findings consistent with the diagnosis of an ostium primum atrial septal defect.

### Keyword Diagnoses

Normal sinus rhythm
First-degree atrioventricular block
Incomplete right bundle branch block
Left atrial abnormality
Left-axis deviation
Ostium primum atrial septal defect

## ELECTROCARDIOGRAM #34

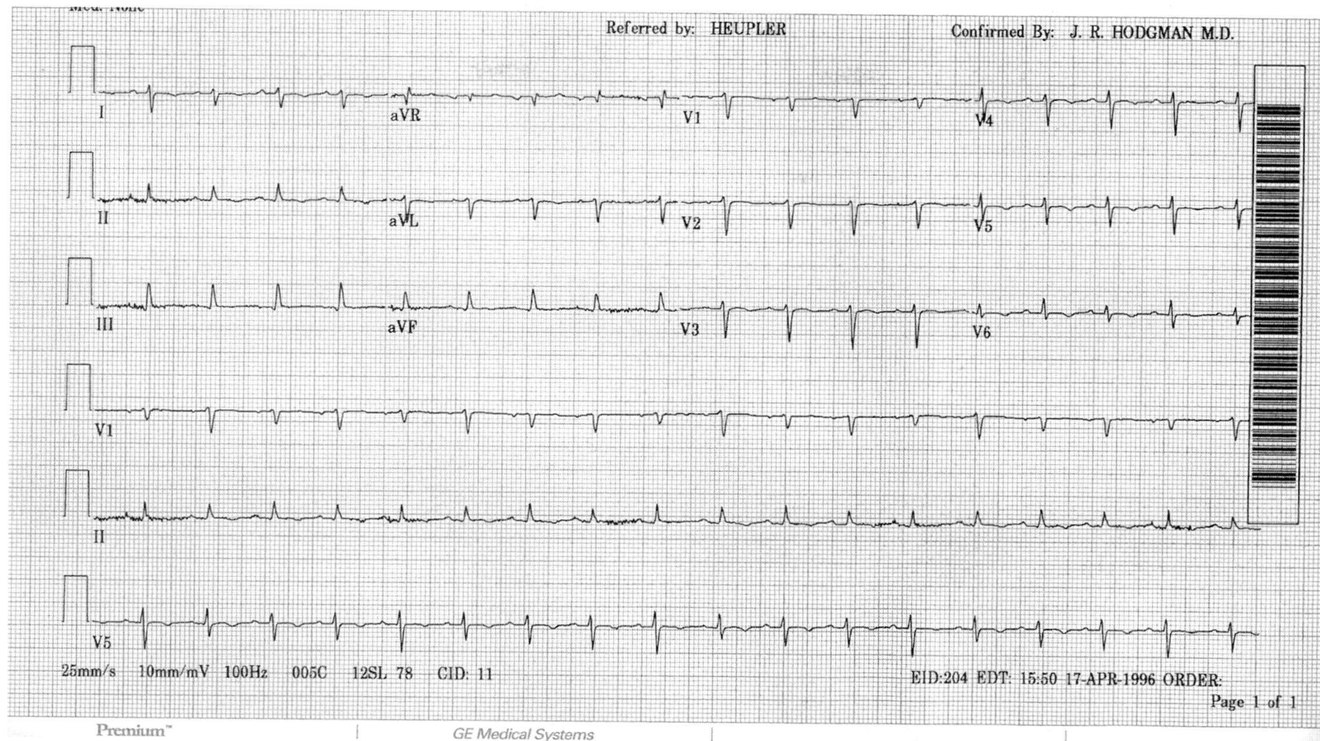


### Clinical History

A 38-year-old man presented with severe dyspnea of 1 week's duration. An echocardiogram demonstrated a large pericardial effusion with evidence supporting cardiac tamponade. The patient underwent urgent surgical pericardial drainage.

### Electrocardiogram Interpretation

The cardiac rhythm is sinus tachycardia, as the P waves are of normal axis and precede each QRS complex at an atrial rate slightly greater than 100 per minute. The frontal-plane QRS-complex axis demonstrates right-axis deviation, as the QRS-complex vector is negative in lead I and positive in leads II, III, and aVF. There are diffuse low-voltage QRS complexes. Nonspecific ST–T changes are also seen. Alternation of the QRS-complex voltage, best seen in rhythm strip lead $V_1$, is apparent. This alternation occurs with every other QRS complex and is termed electrical alternans. Electrical alternans is an electrocardiogram marker of a large pericardial effusion.

### Commentary

The electrocardiogram findings of diffuse low-voltage QRS complexes and electrical alternans suggests the presence of a significant pericardial effusion and cardiac tamponade. The electrical alternans is secondary to the beat- to beat-variability of cardiac position. This is sometimes referred to as a "swinging heart."

### Keyword Diagnoses

Sinus tachycardia
Right-axis deviation
Nonspecific ST–T changes
Low-voltage QRS
Electrical alternans
Pericardial effusion
Cardiac tamponade

## ELECTROCARDIOGRAM #35

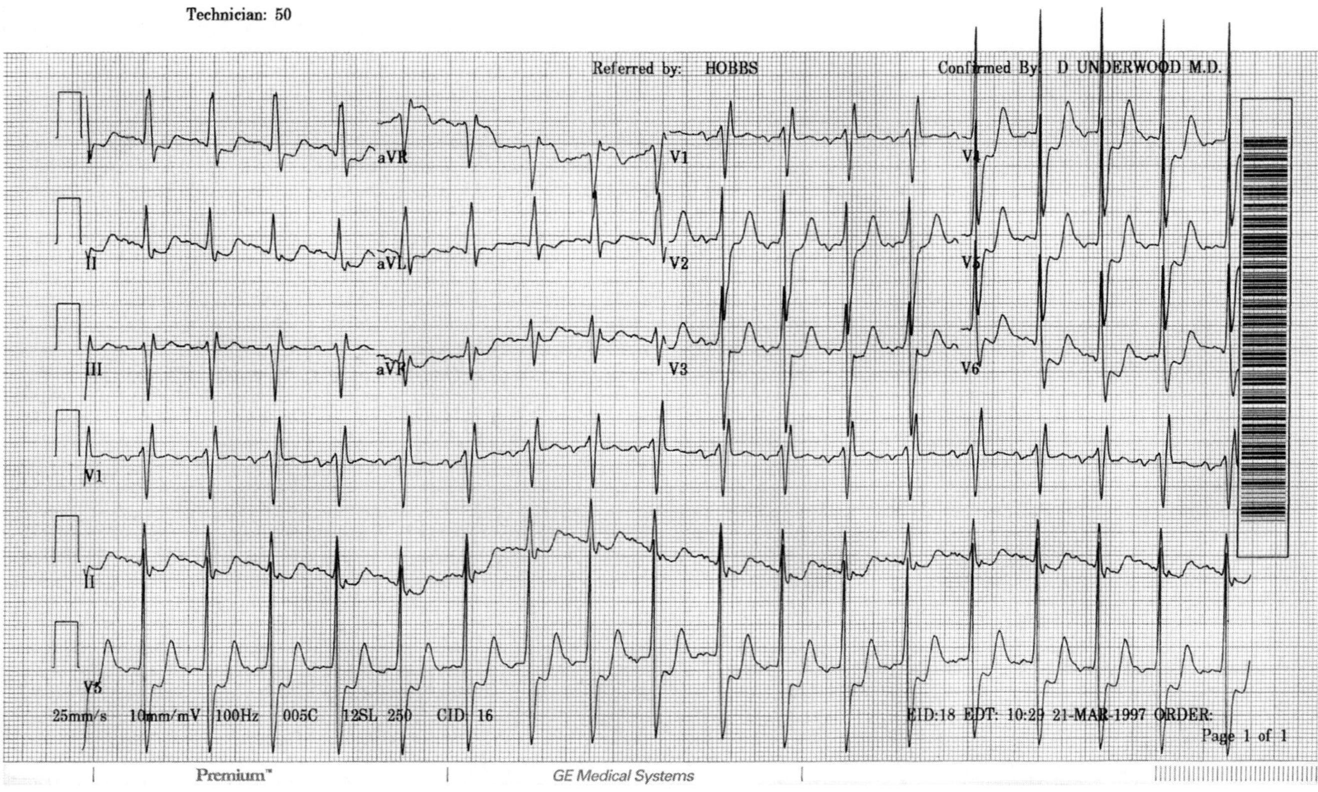


### Clinical History

A 69-year-old woman with a history of severe subaortic stenosis presented to the hospital with a several-day history of dyspnea consistent with congestive heart failure. A cardiac catheterization demonstrated a 100-mm Hg pressure gradient between the left ventricular outflow tract and the left ventricle. Her medications at the time of this electrocardiogram included diltiazem, furosemide, and doxazosin.

### Electrocardiogram Interpretation

A P wave of normal axis precedes each QRS complex at a regular rate of approximately 110 per minute, reflecting sinus tachycardia. An rSR′ QRS complex is present in lead $V_1$ with a QRS-complex duration of 140 milliseconds, consistent with complete right bundle branch block. The P wave in lead $V_1$ demonstrates a terminal negativity and is bifid in lead II, supporting left atrial abnormality. Down-sloping 3- to 4-mm ST-segment depression is present in leads $V_4$–$V_6$, I, and II, consistent with myocardial ischemia and possibly a non–ST-segment-elevation myocardial infarction.

### Commentary

Most often, myocardial ischemia is a bedside diagnosis and requires clinical correlation. In this case the down-sloping ST-segment depression in the setting of a congestive heart failure exacerbation and subaortic stenosis most likely does represent myocardial ischemia. To confirm this suspicion, a follow-up tracing should be obtained after treatment, to demonstrate interval improvement and ST–T-change resolution.

### Keyword Diagnoses

- Sinus tachycardia
- Complete right bundle branch block
- Left atrial abnormality
- Myocardial ischemia

## ELECTROCARDIOGRAM #36

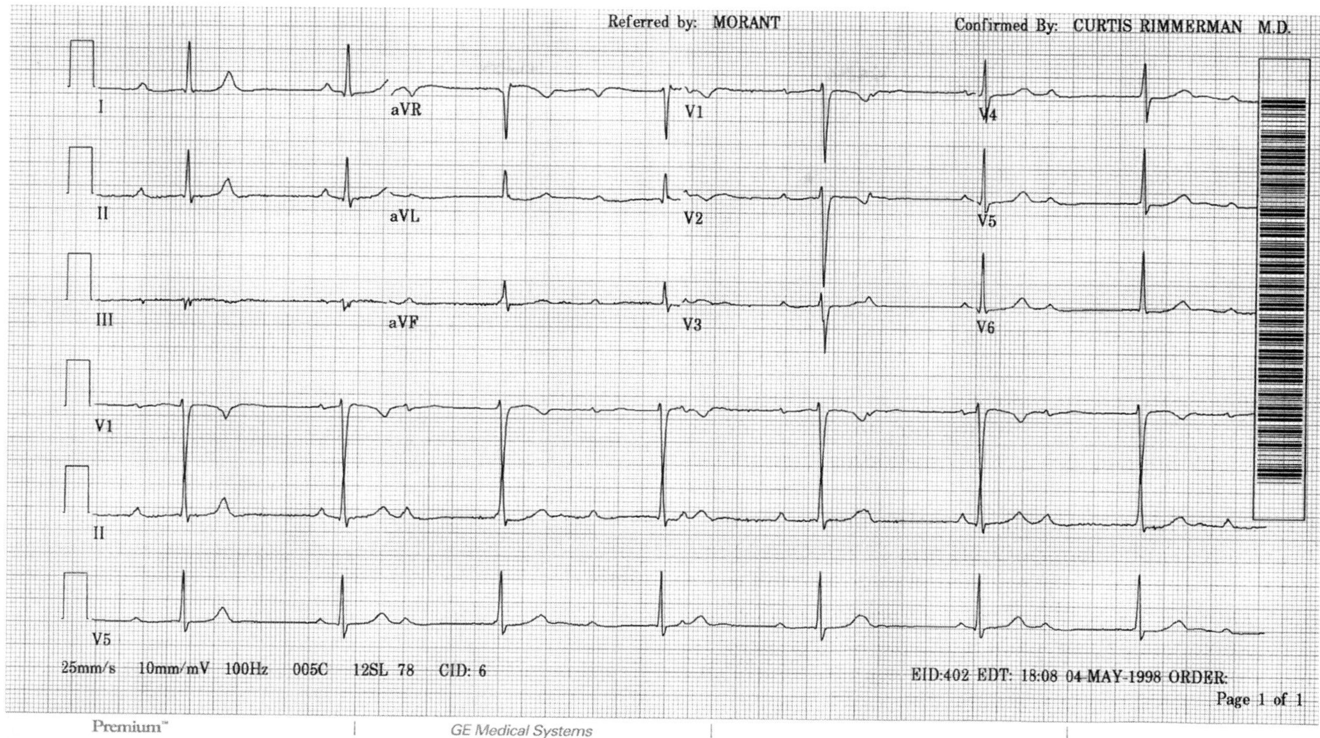


### Clinical History

A 29-year-old woman who was 37 weeks pregnant was admitted to the hospital for close observation of pregnancy-induced hypertension. She has known complete heart block without cardiovascular symptoms requiring no specific treatment or evaluation other than periodic Holter monitoring.

### Electrocardiogram Interpretation

On this tracing the cardiac rhythm is best discerned in rhythm strip lead $V_1$. P waves occur at regular intervals at an atrial rate of approximately 85 per minute. The P-wave axis as ascertained in leads I, II, and aVF is upright and normal. This suggests normal sinus rhythm. The PR interval varies and suggests a lack of association between the P waves and the QRS complexes. The QRS complexes are of normal duration and occur regularly at a rate of approximately 45 per minute. These findings collectively support normal sinus rhythm, junctional bradycardia, and complete heart block.

### Commentary

The electrocardiogram criteria for complete heart block include two independent cardiac rhythms, lack of atrioventricular association, and a noncompeting ventricular rhythm that is slower than the atrial rhythm.

### Keyword Diagnoses

Normal sinus rhythm
Junctional bradycardia
Complete heart block

## ELECTROCARDIOGRAM #37

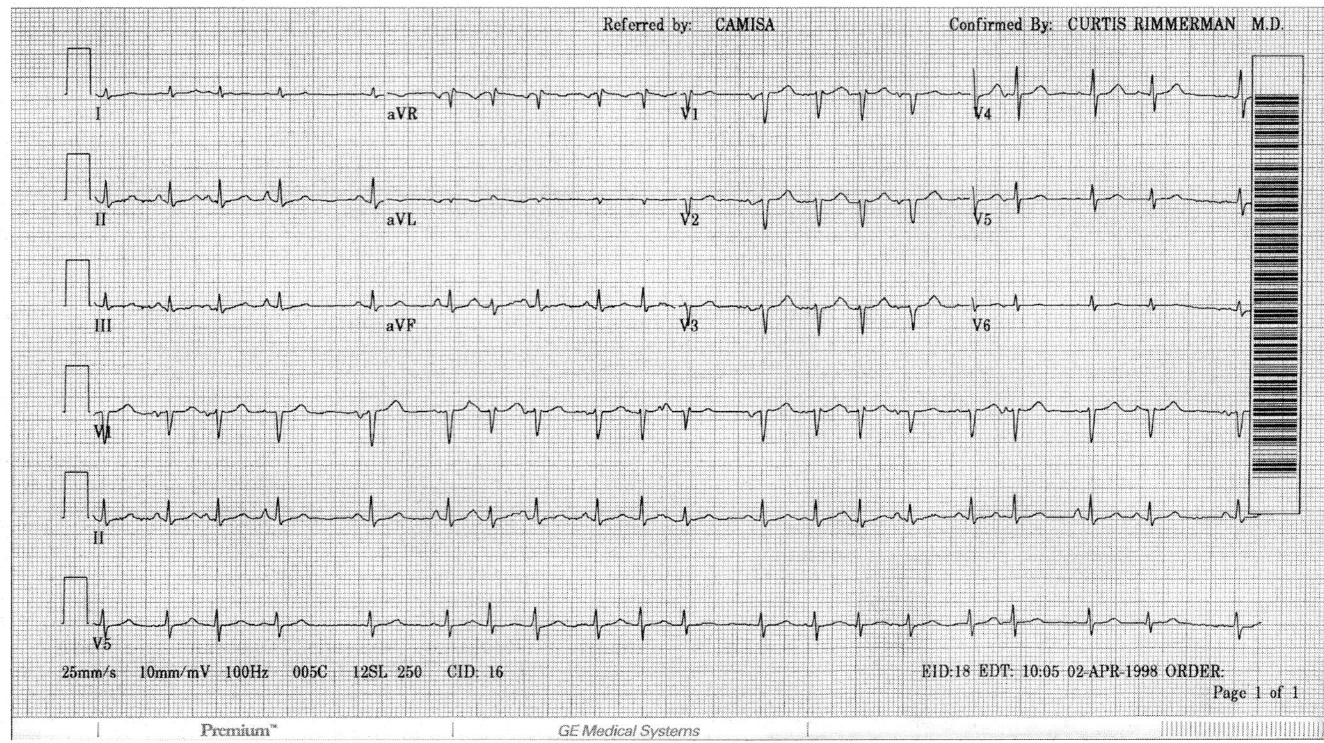


### Clinical History

A 72-year-old man was admitted to the hospital for further evaluation of an erythematous and bullous eruptive rash. His past medical history includes hypertension and chronic obstructive pulmonary disease, for which he takes prednisone and numerous inhalers.

### Electrocardiogram Interpretation

The ventricular rate is rapid, irregular, and >100 per minute, representing a tachycardia. Each QRS complex is preceded by a P wave of differing morphology and PR-interval duration. This represents multifocal atrial tachycardia. Nonspecific ST–T changes are present in the lateral leads.

### Commentary

Multifocal atrial tachycardia is a common dysrhythmia in patients with advanced chronic obstructive pulmonary disease. This dysrhythmia commonly demonstrates resistance to pharmacologic therapy and is best addressed by treating the underlying condition, in this case the chronic obstructive pulmonary disease.

### Keyword Diagnoses

Multifocal atrial tachycardia
Nonspecific ST–T changes

## ELECTROCARDIOGRAM #38

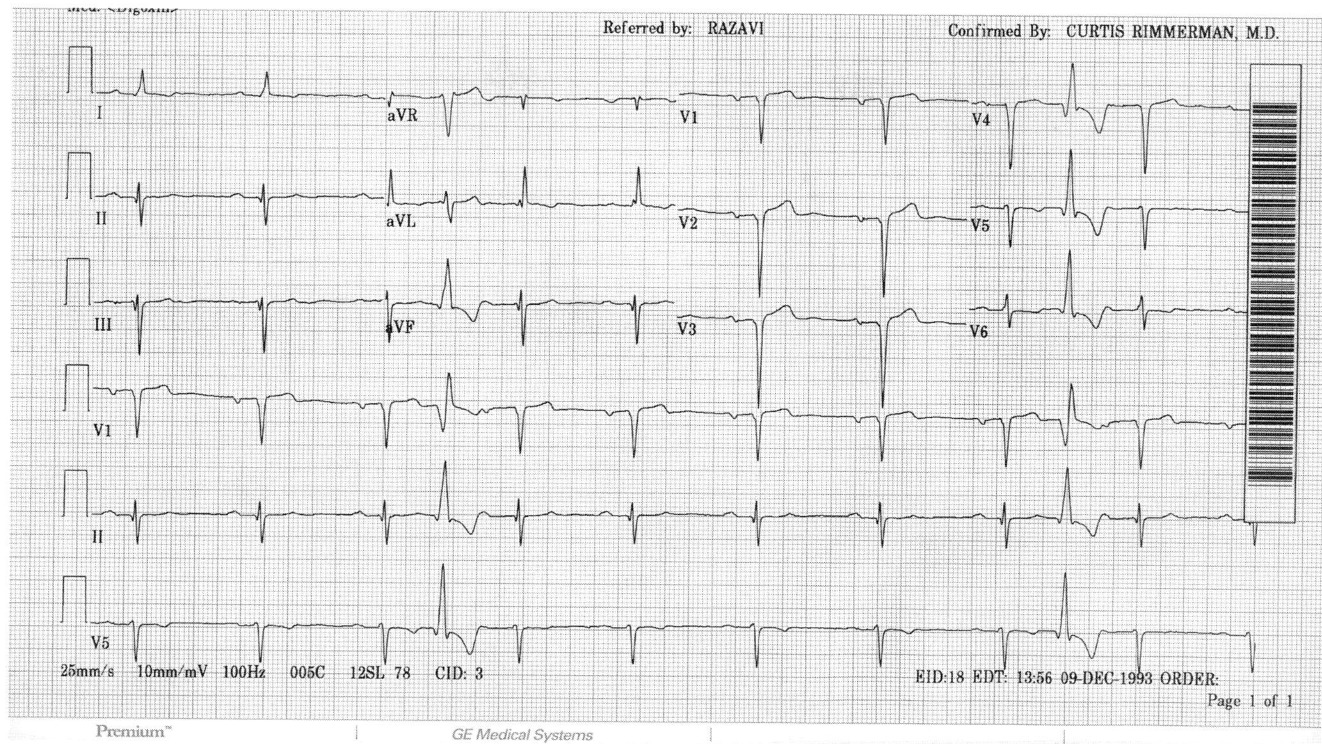


### Clinical History

A 53-year-old man with diffuse coronary artery disease status post inferior and anterior myocardial infarctions 15 years prior to this electrocardiogram returns for routine cardiology follow-up. Subsequent to the myocardial infarctions the patient underwent ventricular aneurysmectomy. He continued with symptoms of stable angina pectoris in the setting of mild mitral insufficiency and moderate left ventricular systolic dysfunction. His medications include digoxin, furosemide, and captopril.

### Electrocardiogram Interpretation

On this tracing, with many findings, a systematic approach is necessary. Sinus bradycardia is present. The PR interval is prolonged, indicating first-degree atrioventricular block. The QRS-complex axis is deviated leftward secondary to diagnostic Q-wave formation in leads II, III, and aVF, supporting an age-indeterminate inferior myocardial infarction. Additional Q waves are noted in leads $V_2$–$V_4$, representing an age-indeterminate anterior myocardial infarction. Premature complexes differing from the native QRS-complex morphology are seen without a preceding P wave. These are premature ventricular complexes. The PR interval immediately following each premature ventricular complex is prolonged and reflects retrograde concealed conduction of the premature ventricular complex into the conduction system slowing antegrade conduction to the ventricle. Unlike most premature ventricular complexes, there is no compensatory pause and therefore these are classified as interpolated premature ventricular complexes.

### Commentary

Frequently, electrocardiograms demonstrate a myocardial infarction in two separate myocardial territories, as demonstrated on this tracing. The premature ventricular complexes are of complete right bundle branch block morphology and therefore are left ventricular in origin. They demonstrate prominent inferior and anterolateral Q waves, supporting the presence of both prior myocardial infarctions.

### Keyword Diagnoses

Sinus bradycardia
First-degree atrioventricular block
Inferior myocardial infarction, age indeterminate
Anterior myocardial infarction, age indeterminate
Interpolated premature ventricular complex
Concealed conduction

## ELECTROCARDIOGRAM #39

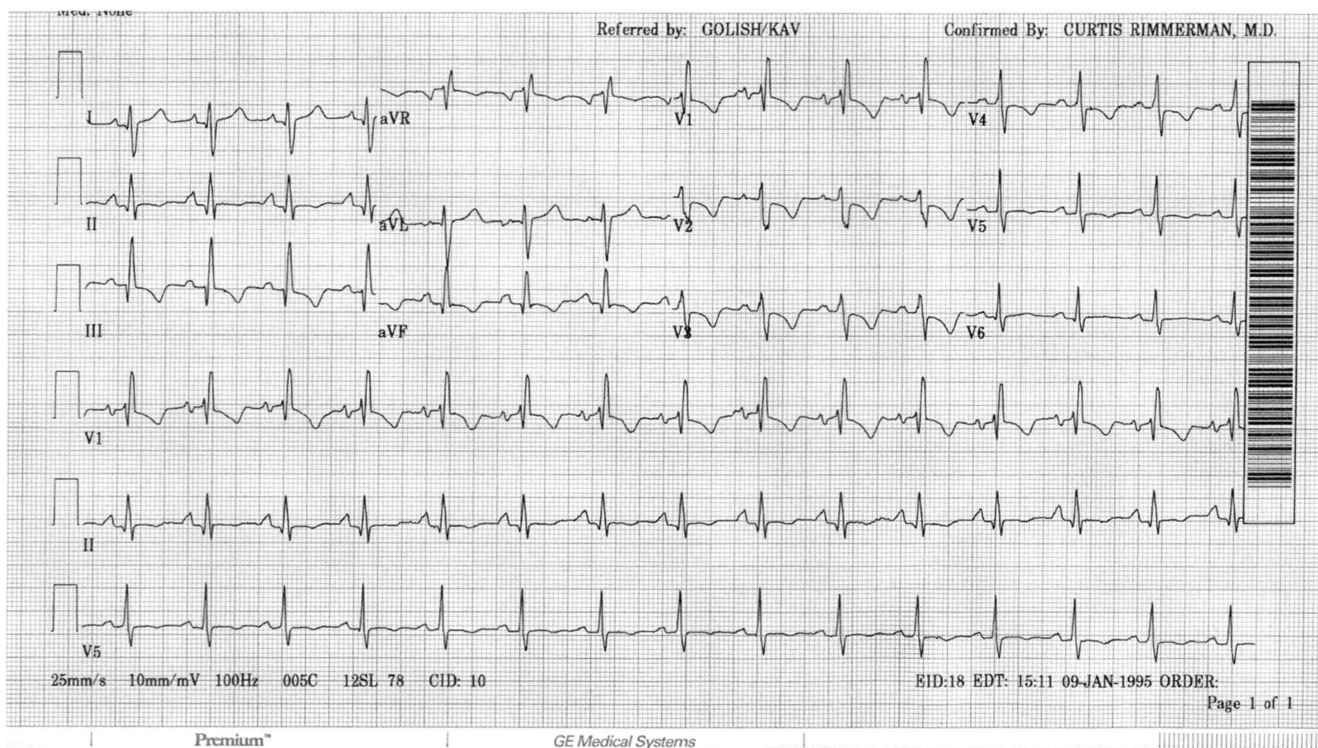


### Clinical History

A 57-year-old woman with a history of adenocarcinoma of the rectum and a pulmonary embolism presented to the hospital urgently, secondary to severe shortness of breath and respiratory failure. Pulmonary angiography demonstrated evidence of both acute and subacute pulmonary emboli and severe pulmonary hypertension. The patient expired shortly after this electrocardiogram.

### Electrocardiogram Interpretation

Normal sinus rhythm is present. Frontal-plane QRS-complex right-axis deviation is noted, given the positive QRS-complex vector in leads II, III, and aVF and a negative QRS-complex vector in lead I. Incomplete right bundle branch block is best seen in lead $V_1$ with an rsR′ QRS-complex pattern. Also notable in lead $V_1$ is a terminally negative P-wave vector suggesting left atrial abnormality. In lead II the P wave is peaked and 3 mm in amplitude, supporting right atrial abnormality. Nonspecific ST–T changes are noted throughout the tracing. Given the incomplete right bundle branch block, right atrial abnormality, and right-axis deviation, right ventricular hypertrophy with secondary ST–T changes merits consideration.

### Commentary

This electrocardiogram is consistent with an acute pulmonary embolism. It demonstrates a dominant S wave in lead I and a Q wave with T-wave inversion in lead III. This is the so-called S1, Q3, T3 QRS-complex pattern described in the setting of an acute pulmonary embolism.

### Keyword Diagnoses

- Normal sinus rhythm
- Right-axis deviation
- Incomplete right bundle branch block
- Left atrial abnormality
- Right atrial abnormality
- Nonspecific ST–T changes
- Pulmonary embolism

## ELECTROCARDIOGRAM #40

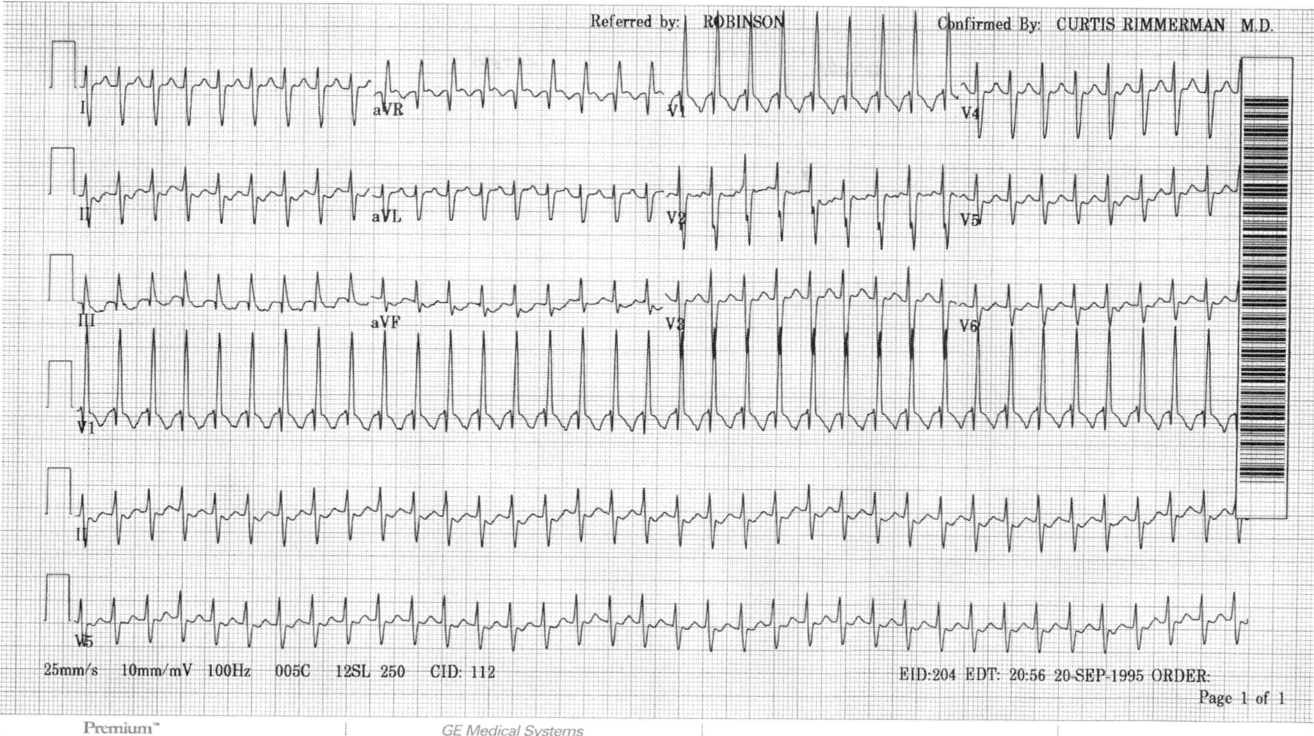


### Clinical History

A 41-year-old man with a history of intravenous substance use, endocarditis, and prior mitral and tricuspid valve replacement re-presents with symptoms and signs of congestive heart failure. He has also noted recent-onset palpitations.

### Electrocardiogram Interpretation

This electrocardiogram demonstrates a regular narrow QRS-complex tachycardia. P waves are possibly seen within the nadir of the ST segment in lead III. Determination of the exact cardiac rhythm is difficult and would require further testing in the form of an electrophysiology study. Therefore, this is best categorized as a supraventricular tachycardia. The QRS-complex frontal-plane axis demonstrates right-axis deviation, as the QRS-complex vector is negative in lead I, isoelectric in lead II, and positive in leads III and aVF. A prominent rsR′ QRS complex of normal duration is seen in lead $V_1$. In the presence of QRS-complex frontal-plane right-axis deviation, this represents right ventricular hypertrophy. Diffuse nonspecific ST–T changes are also present.

### Commentary

This patient was known to have advanced tricuspid valvular heart disease, prosthetic valve mitral stenosis, pulmonary hypertension, and right ventricular hypertrophy. The atrial arrhythmias may be secondary to the cardiac valvular abnormality.

### Keyword Diagnoses

Supraventricular tachycardia
Right-axis deviation
Right ventricular hypertrophy
Nonspecific ST–T changes

## ELECTROCARDIOGRAM #41

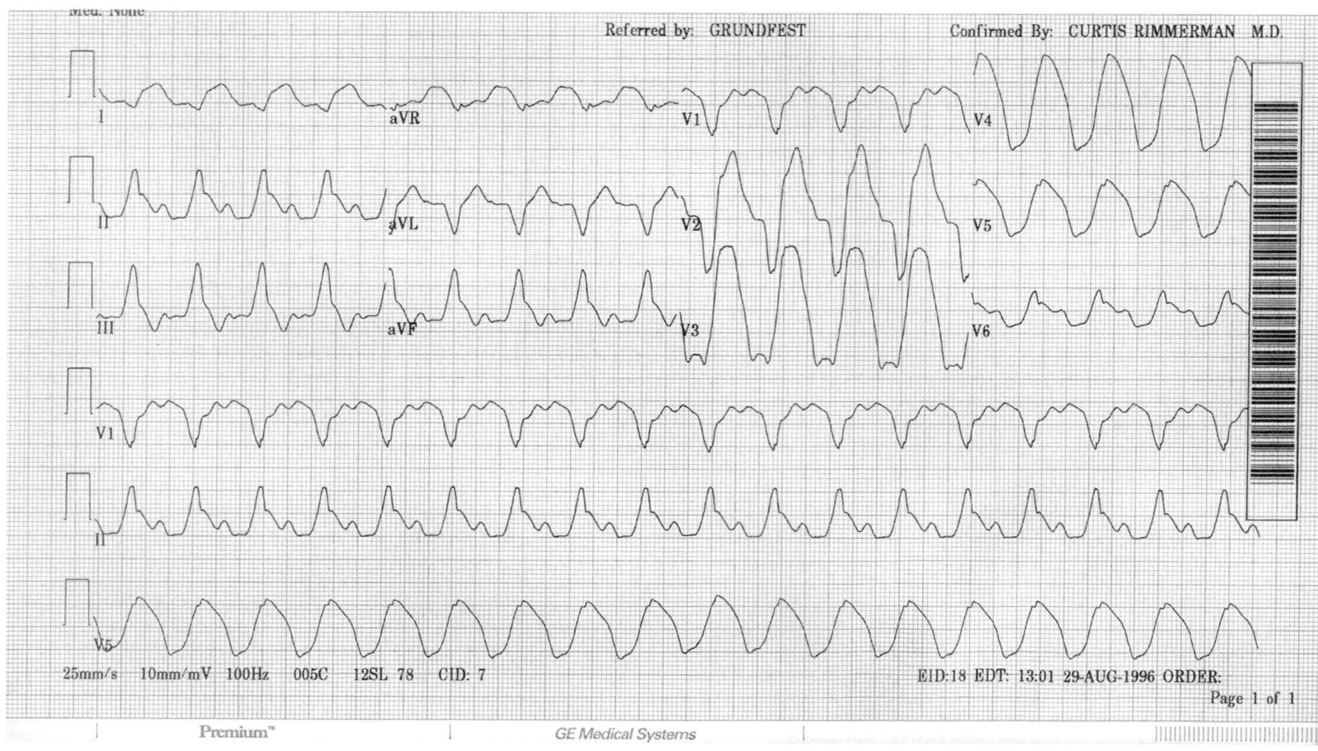


### Clinical History

A 67-year-old woman with dialysis-requiring renal failure is recently postoperative after an exploratory laparotomy for an ischemic bowel. This patient became septic, hypotensive, and hyperkalemic. This electrocardiogram represents her terminal heart rhythm prior to expiring.

### Electrocardiogram Interpretation

Sinus tachycardia is present. The PR interval is prolonged, representing first degree atrioventricular block. The QRS complex is markedly prolonged, demonstrated by a nonspecific intraventricular conduction delay.

### Commentary

In extreme forms of hyperkalemia, ventricular arrhythmias are common, as is profound widening and prolongation of all electrocardiogram intervals. The ST-segment elevation in leads $V_2$–$V_3$ has been termed a dialyzable current of injury.

### Keyword Diagnoses

Sinus tachycardia
First-degree atrioventricular block
Nonspecific intraventricular conduction delay
Hyperkalemia

## ELECTROCARDIOGRAM #42

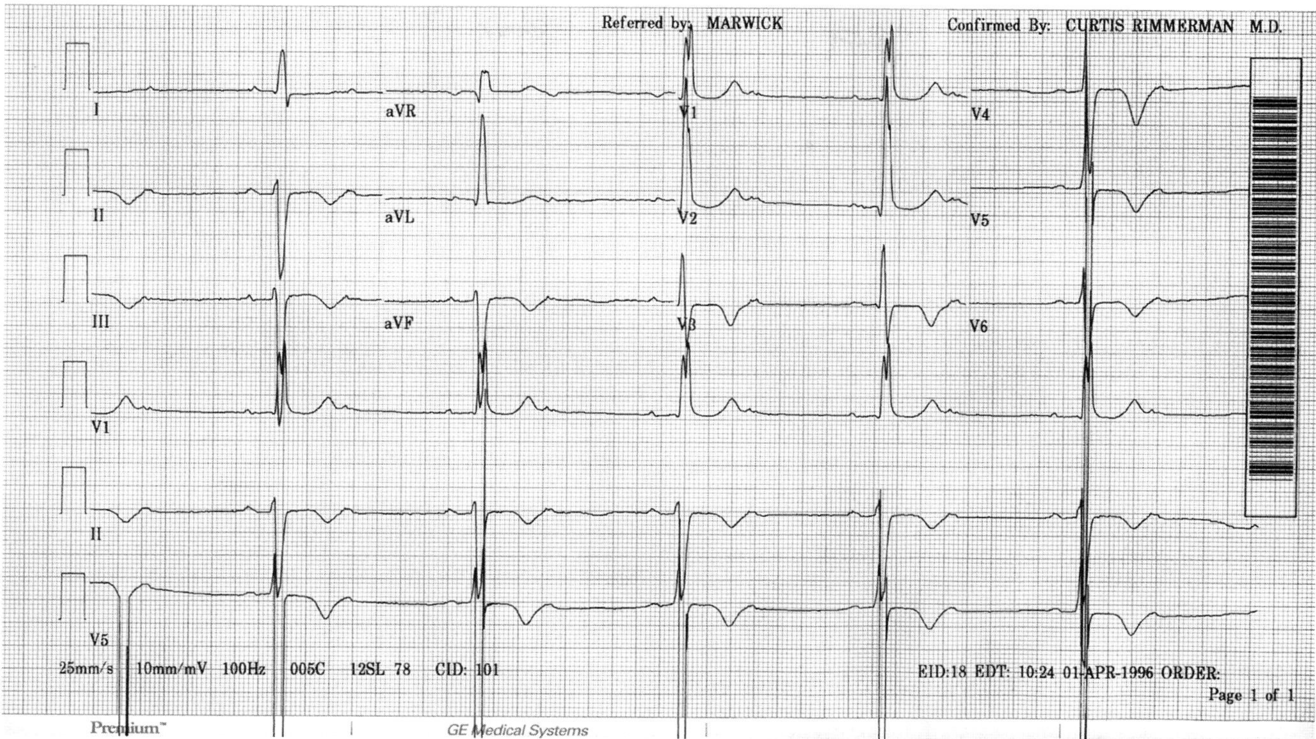


### Clinical History

A 94-year-old woman was admitted to the hospital with acute-onset diarrhea and dehydration. She was noted to have lower-extremity swelling, and venous Doppler studies demonstrated an acute deep venous thrombosis. A subsequent ventilation perfusion scan was interpreted as high probability for an acute pulmonary embolism.

### Electrocardiogram Interpretation

In the lead $V_1$ rhythm strip, a P wave is seen preceding each QRS complex. A P wave is also noted immediately following each T wave. This demonstrates a regular P–P interval at an atrial rate of approximately 70 per minute, denoting normal sinus rhythm. The QRS complex is broadened, with an RSR′ QRS-complex pattern in lead $V_1$, suggesting complete right bundle branch block. The T wave is upright in lead $V_1$, supporting primary T-wave changes. The QRS-complex frontal-plane axis is deviated leftward, with a positive QRS-complex vector in lead I and negative QRS-complex vectors in leads II, III, and aVF, consistent with left anterior hemiblock. Given the bifascicular block, the 2:1 atrioventricular block most likely represents second-degree Mobitz Type II atrioventricular block. Diffuse nonspecific ST–T wave changes are seen. Sinus arrhythmia is also documented. The P–P interval encompassing the QRS complexes is shorter than the P–P interval between the QRS complexes. This is more precisely termed ventriculophasic sinus arrhythmia. This has no known clinical significance.

### Commentary

Given the bifascicular block and 2:1 atrioventricular block, this patient has advanced conduction system disease. It is not known if these findings were new in the setting of her suspected acute pulmonary embolism.

### Keyword Diagnoses

- Normal sinus rhythm
- 2:1 Atrioventricular block
- Complete right bundle branch block
- Left anterior hemiblock
- Nonspecific ST–T changes
- Sinus arrhythmia

## ELECTROCARDIOGRAM #43

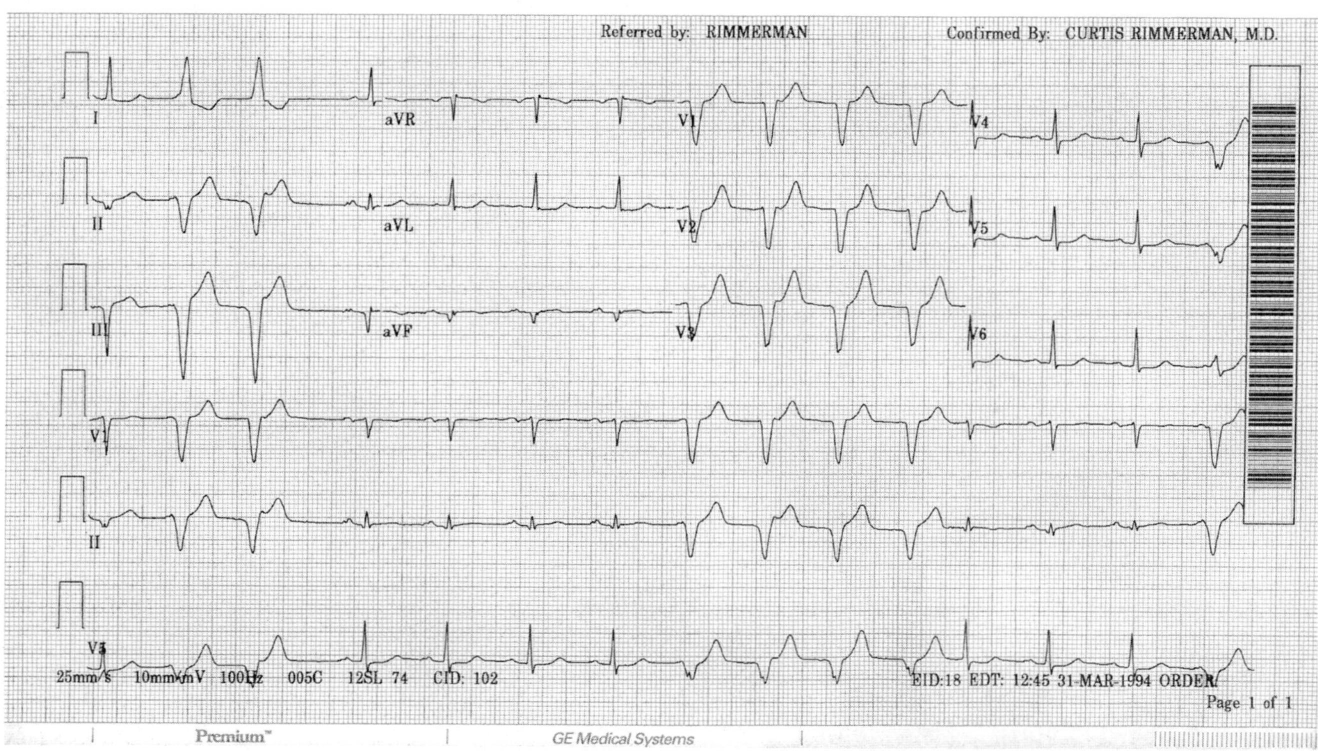


### Clinical History

A 61-year-old man was seen in cardiology outpatient follow-up after an acute inferior myocardial infarction 3 years prior to this electrocardiogram. This was followed by urgent right coronary artery percutaneous transluminal coronary angioplasty. He feels well, with infrequent episodes of angina pectoris. His medications include metoprolol, aspirin, nicotinic acid, simvastatin, and vitamins.

### Electrocardiogram Interpretation

The atrial rhythm is most easily identified in the lead $V_1$ rhythm strip and lead aVF. In these leads, P waves are seen to precede each QRS complex at a rate of approximately 85 per minute, representing normal sinus rhythm. The second, third, eighth, ninth, 10th, and 11th QRS complexes are wide, with a complete left bundle branch configuration. This represents an accelerated idioventricular rhythm. The native QRS complex is abnormal, with a wide Q wave present in leads III and aVF indicating an age-indeterminate inferior myocardial infarction. The first QRS complex is intermediate between the native QRS complex and the accelerated idioventricular rhythm complex and represents a ventricular fusion complex. P-wave activity is seen during the accelerated idioventricular rhythm as a downward deflection within the proximal ST segment of the third QRS complex noted best in leads II, III, and $V_1$. This supports simultaneous atrial activity and atrioventricular dissociation.

### Commentary

This patient also had a history of syncope following his myocardial infarction. An electrophysiology study demonstrated readily inducible sustained monomorphic ventricular tachycardia, and he underwent subsequent defibrillator placement.

### Keyword Diagnoses

Normal sinus rhythm
Accelerated idioventricular rhythm
Fusion complex
Inferior myocardial infarction, age indeterminate
Atrioventricular dissociation

## ELECTROCARDIOGRAM #44

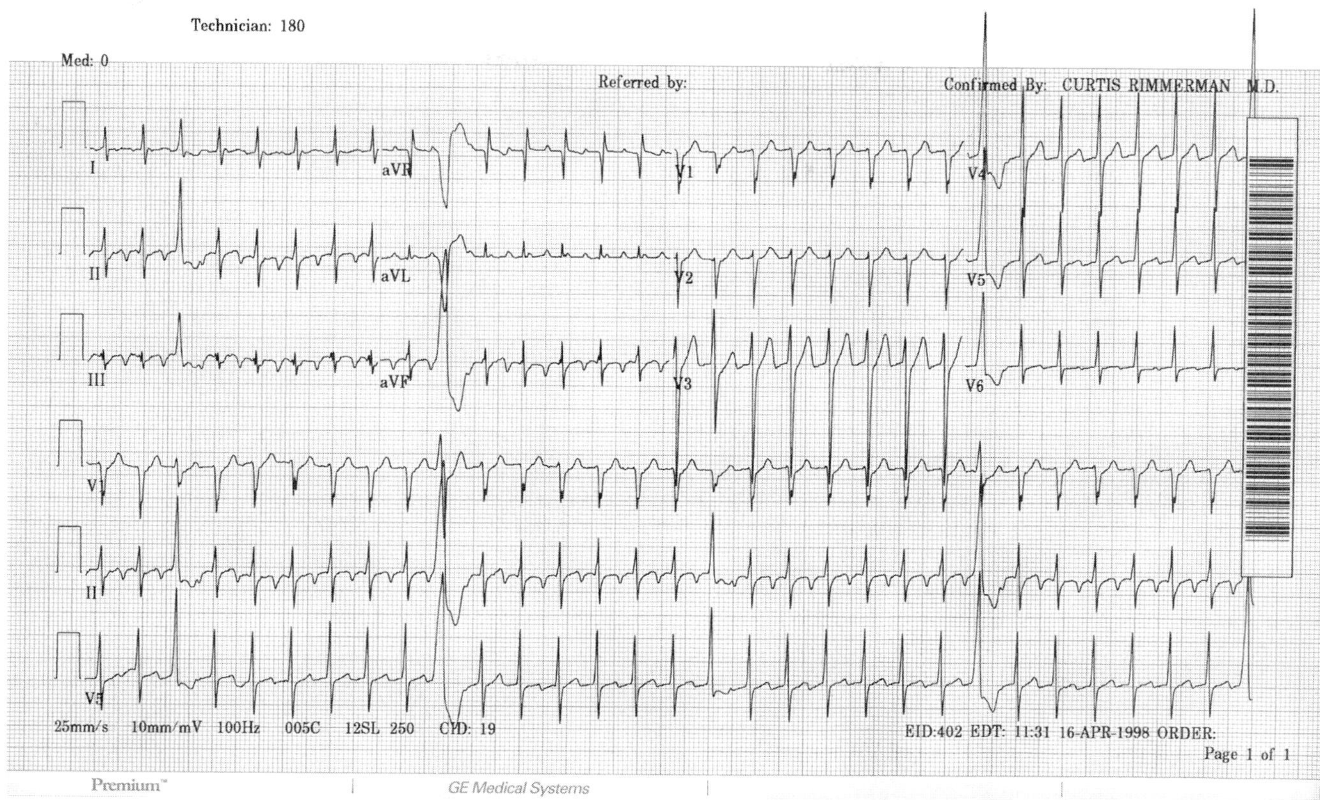


### Clinical History

A 72-year-old man with recently diagnosed myasthenia gravis was admitted for rehabilitation. His past medical history includes diabetes mellitus, chronic obstructive pulmonary disease, recurrent atrial fibrillation, and coronary artery disease.

### Electrocardiogram Interpretation

On this electrocardiogram the atrial rhythm is best discerned in lead aVL. This demonstrates a P wave preceding and immediately following a diminutive QRS complex. This represents atrial flutter with 2:1 atrioventricular conduction. Another possibility is a rapid ectopic atrial tachycardia. Diffuse nonspecific ST–T changes are present, as are frequent premature ventricular complexes. The frequent premature ventricular complexes occur at a constant interectopic interval with a differing coupling interval to the immediately preceding QRS complex. There is evidence of ventricular fusion complexes between the native QRS complex and a premature ventricular complex. These features together confirm the presence of ventricular parasystole.

### Commentary

This is an unusual tracing, as the atrial rhythm is best discerned in lead aVL. This underscores the importance of a systematic evaluation of each electrocardiogram lead, particularly in the setting of an atrial dysrhythmia. The P wave immediately following the QRS complex is best seen in lead aVL and allows for the accurate diagnosis of this atrial dysrhythmia. When frequent premature ventricular complexes are present, it is also important to evaluate for the presence of ventricular parasystole. Ventricular parasystole is an independent automatic dysrhythmia that discharges at a constant rate from the same ventricular focus.

### Keyword Diagnoses

Atrial flutter
2:1 Atrioventricular conduction
Premature ventricular complex
Nonspecific ST–T changes
Ventricular parasystole
Fusion complex

## ELECTROCARDIOGRAM #45

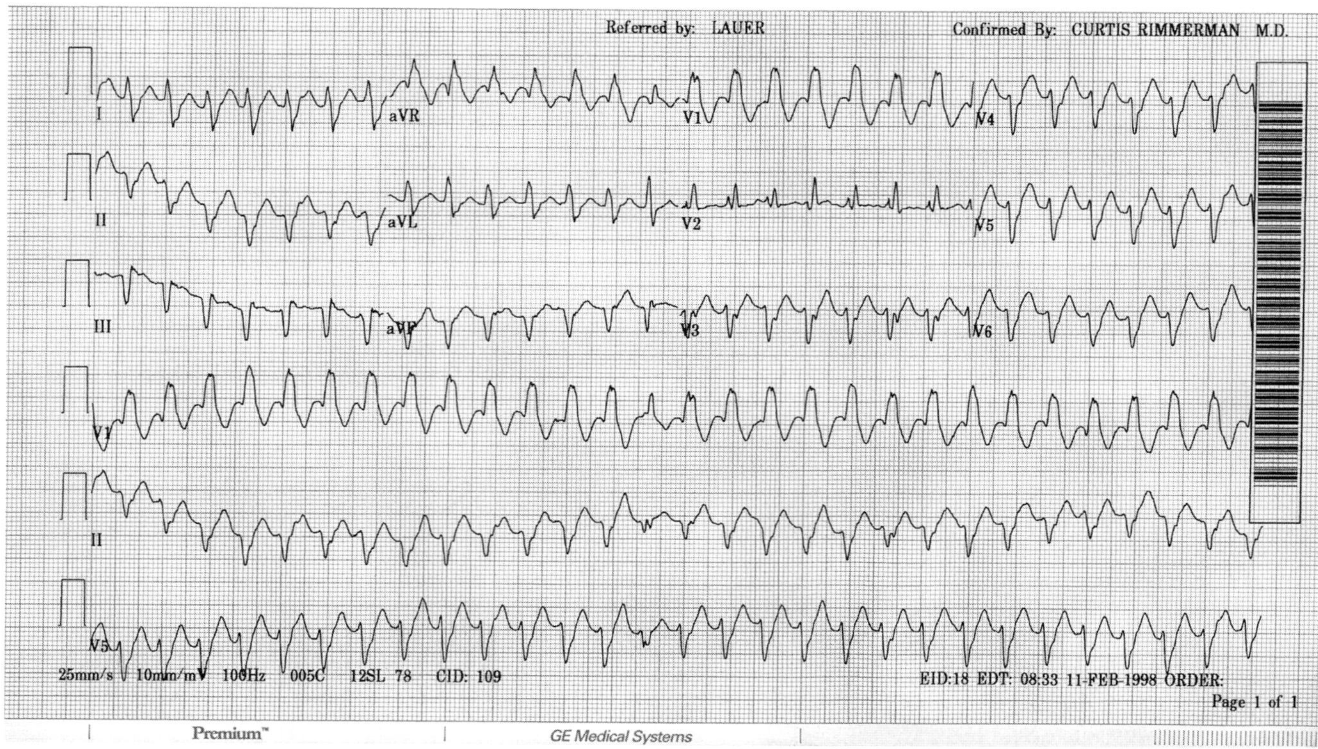


### Clinical History

A 49-year-old man with recurrent idiopathic left ventricular tachycardia was referred for radiofrequency ablation. A recent echocardiogram demonstrated normal left ventricular systolic function without evidence of a prior myocardial infarction. His medications include verapamil, sotalol, simvastatin, and aspirin.

### Electrocardiogram Interpretation

This electrocardiogram demonstrates a regular wide QRS complex tachycardia at a rate of approximately 175 per minute. This tachycardia demonstrates a complete right bundle branch block morphology with a qR QRS complex pattern in lead $V_1$ and terminal S-wave slowing in leads $V_1$ and $V_6$. The QRS-complex frontal-plane axis is deviated far leftward, is prolonged, and has a qR QRS-complex pattern in lead $V_1$, suggestive of ventricular tachycardia. In the center of the tracing, best seen in leads $V_1$ and aVF, a more narrow QRS complex occurs. This is a sinus capture complex and lends greater support to the diagnosis of ventricular tachycardia. In lead aVF, within the sinus capture QRS complex, a prominent Q wave is seen with ST-segment elevation, suggestive of an acute inferior myocardial infarction. Periodic P waves are seen throughout the tracing, suggesting an independent atrial rhythm and atrioventricular dissociation. The precise atrial rhythm diagnosis is not discernible on this tracing. Wandering baseline artifact is also seen.

### Commentary

This electrocardiogram contains important features supporting the presence of ventricular tachycardia. When assessing a wide complex tachycardia, each of these features should be specifically sought. They include atrioventricular dissociation in the presence of an independent atrial rhythm and sinus capture complexes. Not seen on this electrocardiogram but often present in the setting of ventricular tachycardia are ventricular fusion complexes. The apparent Q wave occurring in lead aVF remains unexplained, given the patient's normal heart function and normal regional wall motion on echocardiography.

### Keyword Diagnoses

Ventricular tachycardia
Sinus capture complex
Atrioventricular dissociation
Inferior myocardial infarction acute
Baseline artifact

## ELECTROCARDIOGRAM #46

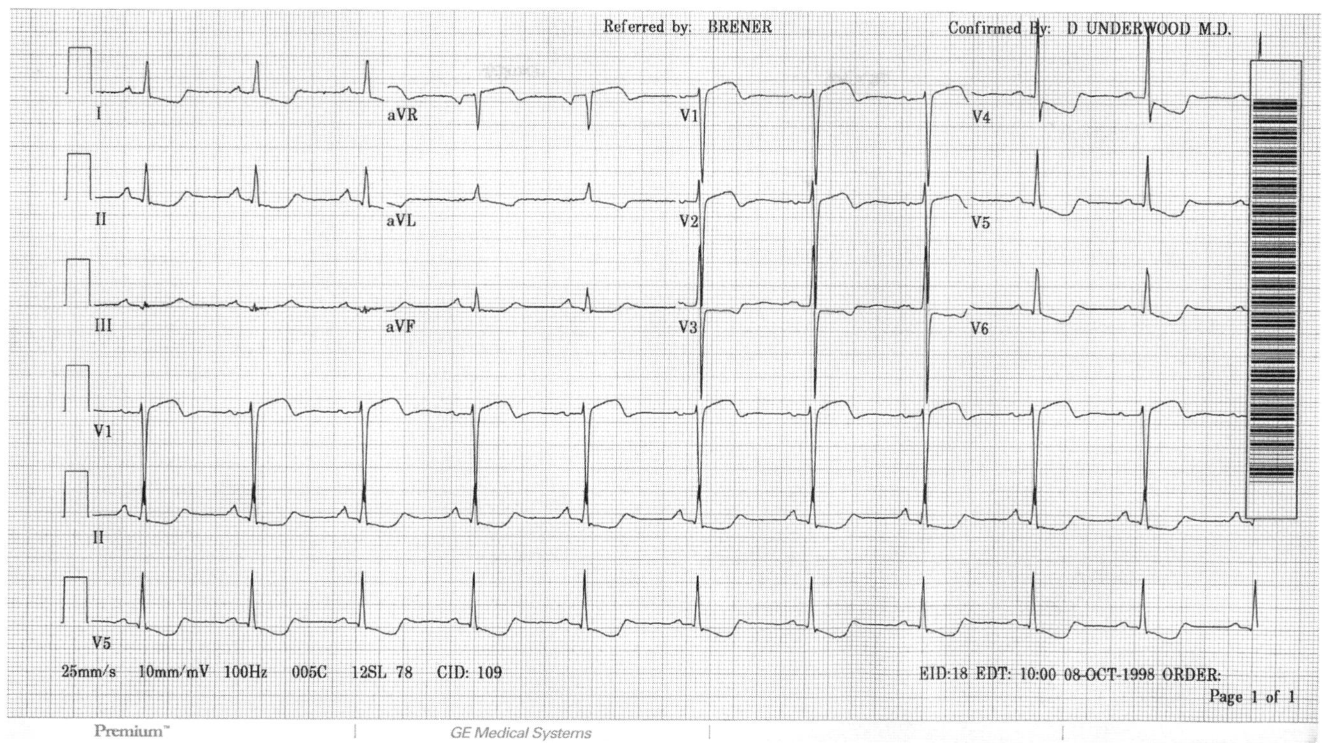


### Clinical History

A 48-year-old woman presented with severe hypertrophic cardiomyopathy and pronounced symptoms of exertional dyspnea and pre-syncope immediately status post–percutaneous alcohol ablation of her first septal perforator branch of the left anterior descending coronary artery. The patient was resting comfortably in the intensive care unit.

### Electrocardiogram Interpretation

The cardiac rhythm is normal sinus rhythm, as the P-wave vector is upright in leads I, II, III, and aVF. The atrial rate is regular and slightly >60 per minute. Approximately 2 mm of ST-segment elevation is seen in lead $V_1$, and 1 mm of ST-segment elevation is present in lead $V_2$. Reciprocal ST-segment depression is seen inferiorly and laterally. This represents an acute septal myocardial infarction and acute myocardial injury.

### Commentary

The ST-segment elevation in leads $V_1$–$V_2$ reflects the proximal septal iatrogenic myocardial infarction created by the alcohol injection. This is a pure proximal septal myocardial injury pattern reflected electrocardiographically. The purpose of this procedure is to infarct the proximal interventricular septum and therefore reduce the degree of left ventricular outflow tract obstruction, avoiding otherwise necessary cardiac surgery.

### Keyword Diagnoses

Normal sinus rhythm
Septal myocardial infarction acute
Acute myocardial injury

## ELECTROCARDIOGRAM #47

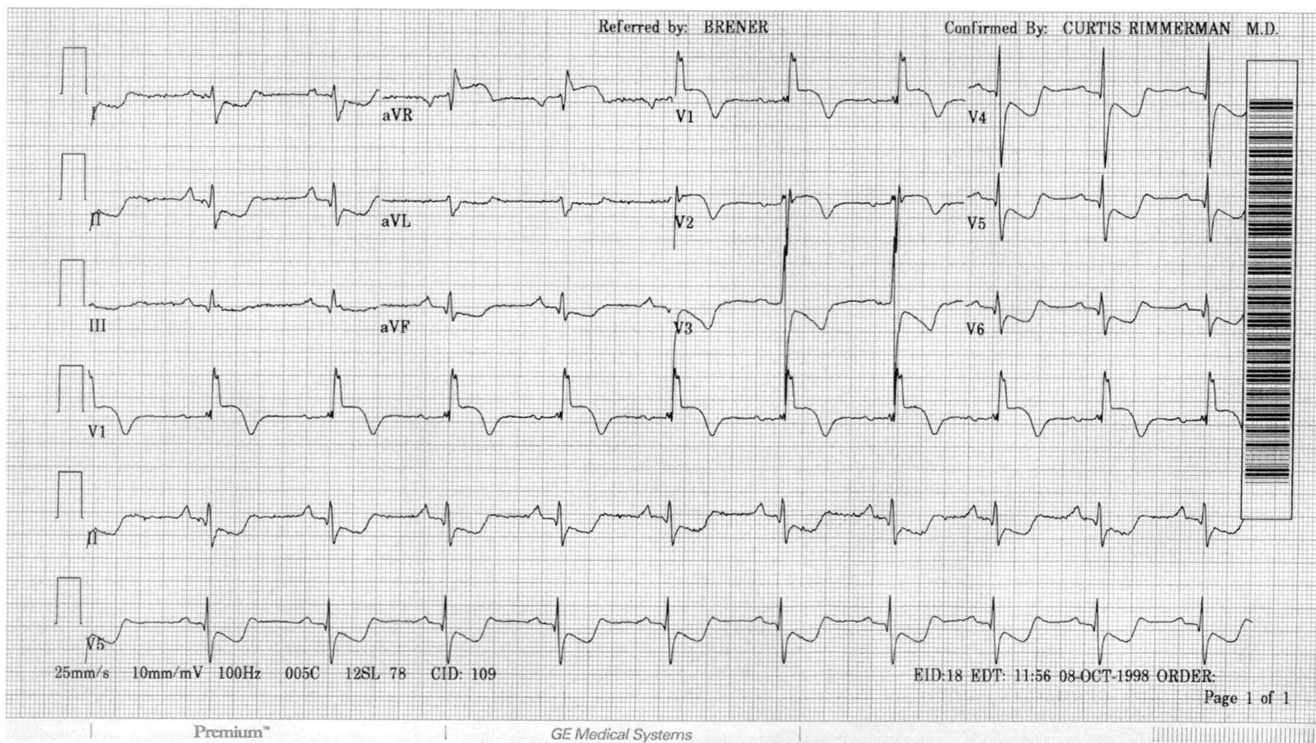


### Clinical History

A 48-year-old woman presented with severe hypertrophic cardiomyopathy and pronounced symptoms of exertional dyspnea and pre-syncope immediately status post-percutaneous alcohol ablation of her first septal perforator branch of the left anterior descending coronary artery. The patient was resting comfortably in the intensive care unit.

### Electrocardiogram Interpretation

The cardiac rhythm is sinus bradycardia with a normal P wave axis slightly <60 minute. An RsR′ QRS complex is seen in lead $V_1$ with terminal S-wave slowing in leads I, aVL, and $V_5$–$V_6$, consistent with complete right bundle branch block. The QRS-complex frontal-plane axis is deviated far rightward, as the QRS-complex vector is negative in lead I and positive in leads III and aVF. Prominent ST-segment elevation of at least 2 mm is seen in leads $V_1$–$V_2$, consistent with an acute septal myocardial infarction and an acute myocardial injury pattern. Diffuse reciprocal ST-segment depression is present.

### Commentary

This electrocardiogram was obtained several hours after electrocardiogram #46 and reflects the same patient. This demonstrates similar findings as tracing #46, with the exception of a newly developed complete right bundle branch block and extreme QRS-complex frontal-plane right-axis deviation. The finding of new extreme right-axis QRS-complex deviation reflects left posterior hemiblock. This is an example of bifascicular block. Inferior Q waves are more prominent on this tracing compared to tracing #46 and reflect the left posterior hemiblock and not the interval development of an inferior myocardial infarction.

### Keyword Diagnoses

Sinus bradycardia
Septal myocardial infarction acute
Complete right bundle branch block
Left posterior hemiblock
Acute myocardial injury

## ELECTROCARDIOGRAM #48

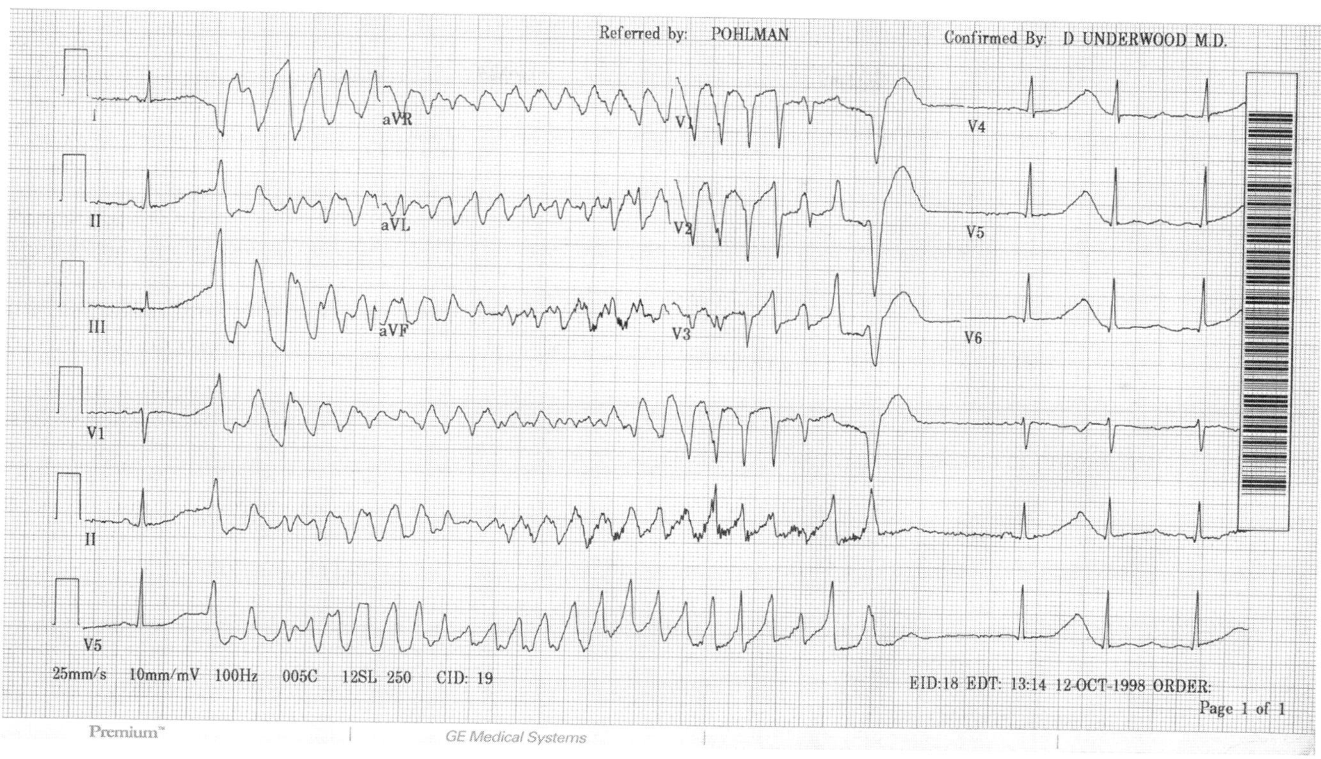


### Clinical History

A 51-year-old woman with metastatic breast carcinoma is undergoing bone marrow transplantation. Her serum potassium level at the time of this electrocardiogram was 2.9 mEq/L.

### Electrocardiogram Interpretation

The extreme left-hand portion of this electrocardiogram demonstrates upright P waves in leads I, II, and III, suggesting normal sinus rhythm. A prolonged QT interval is present, with nonspecific ST–T changes. The first QRS complex is reflective of normal sinus rhythm and a native QRS complex. This is followed by a premature ventricular complex, and a disorganized wide QRS-complex tachycardia ensues. The wide QRS-complex tachycardia has a changing or rotating axis consistent with torsades de pointes. A fine baseline artifact is present.

### Commentary

Torsades de pointes is a potentially fatal ventricular arrhythmia, in this instance triggered by extreme hypokalemia. It is also seen in the presence of antiarrhythmic therapy initiation. It is characterized as a wide QRS-complex ventricular tachycardia with a varying QRS-complex axis as depicted on this electrocardiogram. Prompt correction of any underlying metabolic disturbance and withdrawal of potentially contributing medications is essential.

### Keyword Diagnoses

Normal sinus rhythm
Prolonged QT interval
Torsades de pointes
Baseline artifact
Nonspecific ST–T changes
Hypokalemia

## ELECTROCARDIOGRAM #49

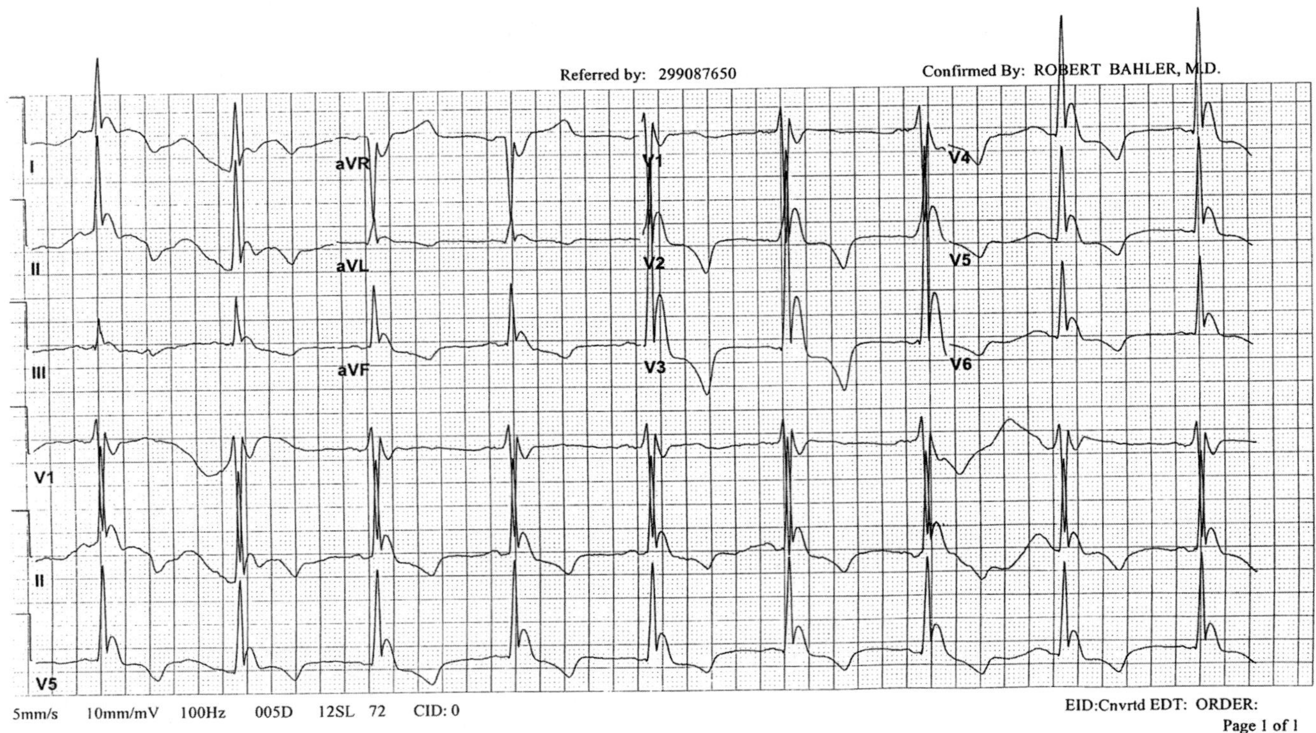


### Clinical History

A 42-year-old man was found unconscious under a bridge and brought to the Emergency Department by ambulance.

### Electrocardiogram Interpretation

Sinus bradycardia is present, as the atrial rate is regular at approximately 50 beats per minute. Baseline artifact, especially in leads I and II, is noted. The QRS complex is significantly widened, with a terminal QRS-complex delay, evident in all leads. Diffuse nonspecific ST–T changes denoting abnormal repolarization are also seen. This is an example of profound hypothermia and Osborne waves. The Osborne or "J" waves represent the terminal QRS-complex conduction delay.

### Commentary

Hypothermia is a medical emergency. This electrocardiogram is a classic example. The etiology of the Osborne wave is not completely clear but is related to slow cardiac conduction. Atrial arrhythmias and PR-interval prolongation are often identified. Osborne waves are named for the person who first identified them and their relationship to hypothermia.

### Keyword Diagnoses

Sinus bradycardia
Baseline artifact
Osborne wave
Hypothermia

46

# Sudden Cardiac Death and Ventricular Tachycardia

**Oussama Wazni** **J. David Burkhardt**

## DEFINITION OF SUDDEN CARDIAC DEATH

Sudden cardiac death (SCD) describes the unexpected natural death from a cardiac cause within a short time period, generally 1 hour from the onset of symptoms, in a person without any prior condition that appears fatal.

## EPIDEMIOLOGY OF SUDDEN CARDIAC DEATH

The incidence of SCD is estimated to be 300,000 to 400,000 per year in the United States. The mortality rate is very high, with only 2% to 15% of patients reaching the hospital alive. Fifty percent of these hospitalized patients die before discharge. There is a high recurrence rate of 35% to 50%. Most sudden cardiac death is associated with a ventricular arrhythmia.

SCD is the first presentation of cardiac disease in 25% of patients. The incidence increases with age at an absolute incidence of 0.1% to 0.2% per year. Men are more commonly affected (3:1). SCD in patients <35 years of age is associated with hypertrophic cardiomyopathy. In patients >35 years old, SCD is most commonly associated with coronary artery disease. The most common arrhythmia is ventricular tachycardia (62%), followed by bradycardia (7%), torsades de pointes (13%), and primary ventricular fibrillation (8%). Only a minority (20% in ideal circumstances) survive to discharge. Determinants of survival are rapid response and bystander cardiopulmonary resuscitation.

## RISK FACTORS AND PATHOPHYSIOLOGY

Risk factors include the following:

- Prior cardiac arrest: high recurrence rate, up to 35% to 50% at 2 years
- Syncope in the presence of coexisting cardiac diseases
- Reduced left ventricular (LV) function and congestive heart failure
- Ventricular premature potentials and nonsustained ventricular tachycardia post–myocardial infarction
- Myocardial ischemia and/or documented scar
- Conduction system disease

The pathophysiology is determined by trigger factors and an underlying substrate conducive to arrhythmia. The mechanism of SCD can be related to any of the following pathophysiologic mechanisms:

- Re-entry around scarred myocardium
- Re-entry using a diseased His–Purkinje system
- Ischemia, electrolyte imbalance, ion channel abnormalities, surges in neurosympathetic tone, antiarrhythmic drugs
- Rapid and irregular ventricular activation: atrial fibrillation in Wolff–Parkinson–White (WPW)

- Bradycardia and asystole-induced arrest are rare except in end-stage congestive heart failure (CHF)

## SUDDEN CARDIAC DEATH IN THE PRESENCE OF CARDIAC DISEASE

Coronary artery disease is present in 80% of those with SCD. Many (75%) have a history of prior myocardial infarction. Sudden death can be the first clinical manifestation in up to 25% of patients with coronary artery disease.

Many (65% of patients) have three-vessel coronary disease (>75% stenosis).Total occlusion of coronaries is rare.

Risk factors include depressed left ventricular systolic function and frequent ventricular premature depolarizations. The Cast study demonstrated that suppression of ventricular premature depolarizations with Class IC medications resulted in higher mortality. The CASS (Coronary Artery Surgery Study) showed improved survival in the group undergoing surgical revascularization compared to the "medical therapy" group.

## SUDDEN CARDIAC DEATH AND HEART FAILURE

In the United States, the heart failure population is expanding, with the population estimated at 4,780,000 and an annual incidence of 400,000 to 465,000 new cases per year. Heart failure total mortality is 25% at 2.5 years, with SCD accounting for 25% to 50% of these cases. Mortality due to SCD is much higher in New York Heart Association (NYHA) Classes II and III than in Class IV patients, who have excess mortality due to pump failure.

### Dilated Cardiomyopathy

Fifty percent of deaths in this patient subgroup are arrhythmic. Ejection fraction is predictive of sudden death, due to either circulatory failure or fatal arrhythmia. Ectopy does not appear to be as predictive of SCD as it is in patients with coronary artery disease. Up to 80% of patients may have nonsustained ventricular tachycardia on Holter monitoring. Electrophysiologic study is of limited use and is less predictive. Primary prevention has recently been evaluated in the SCD HEFT trial. This trial showed a clear mortality benefit for those patients receiving an implantable cardiac defibrillator.

### Hypertrophic Cardiomyopathy

Hypertrophic cardiomyopathy (HCM) is an autosomal dominant disease with incomplete penetrance associated with ever increasingly discovered genetic mutations. The overall incidence of SCD is 2% to 4% in adults and up to 6% in children. It is the most common cause of SCD in young athletes. At present, there are no reliable predictors of SCD, but certain high-risk groups can be identified:

- Young age at disease onset
- Family history of HCM and or sudden cardiac death
- Syncope
- Severe left ventricular hypertrophy
- Abnormal blood pressure drop with exercise
- Nonsustained ventricular tachycardia; rapid and polymorphic is more predictive than monomorphic ventricular tachycardia

EP testing may be useful for risk stratification.

### Arrhythmogenic Right Ventricular Dysplasia

Progressive fibrofatty right ventricular tissue replacement is the pathologic hallmark of this disease. There is a strongly familial pattern; its prevalence may be up to 20% of SCD in young patients (U.S. 3%).

Magnetic resonance imaging (MRI) is the most useful imaging modality to make the diagnosis. Characteristic epsilon waves may be present on the electrocardiogram, as shown in Figure 46–1.

### Long-QT Syndrome

Long-QT syndrome represents a genetic abnormality that affects repolarization. There are several different mutations involving mostly sodium and potassium ionic channels (Table 46–1).

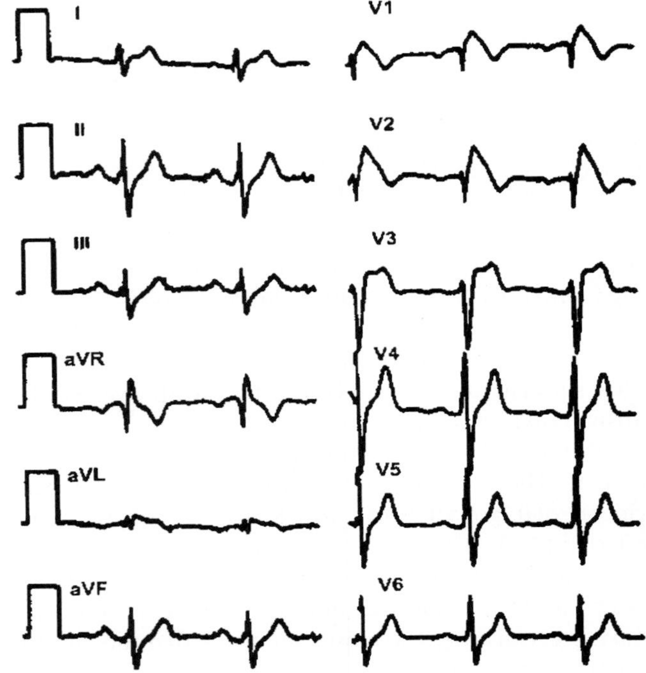


**Figure 46–1** ECG reading in arrhythmogenic right ventricular dysplasia.

**TABLE 46–1**
**FAMILIAL LONG-QT SYNDROMES**

| Syndrome | Chromosome | Channel |
|---|---|---|
| LQT1 | 11p15.5 | $I_{Ks}$ (KVLQT1) |
| LQT2 | 7q35–36 | $I_{Kr}$ (HERG) |
| LQT3 | 3p21–24 | $I_{Na}$ (SCN5A) |
| LQT4 | 4q25–27 | ? |
| LQT5 | 21q22.1–22.2 | minK of $I_{Ks}$ (KCNE) |

Risks associated with Long-QT syndrome are deafness (Jervel and Lange-Nielsen syndrome), female sex, syncope, and documented arrhythmias. Patients usually present with syncope, especially with activity and less commonly at rest. Treatment includes beta-blockers, permanent pacemakers, and implantable cardioverter-defibrillator (ICD) implantation.

The 5-year sudden-death risk in patients on beta-blocker therapy (Long QT Registry) is <1% in asymptomatic patients, 3% in the syncope group, and 13% in the SCD group.

A prolonged QT interval can also be acquired and secondary to a wide range of causes:

- Electrolyte derangements
  - Acute hypokalemia
  - Chronic hypocalcemia
  - Chronic hypokalemia
  - Chronic hypomagnesemia
- Medical conditions
  - Arrhythmias (complete heart block, sick sinus syndrome, bradycardia)
  - Cardiac (myocarditis, tumors)
  - Endocrine: hyperparathyroidism, hypothyroidism, pheochromocytoma
  - Neurologic (cerebrovascular accident, encephalitis, head trauma, subarachnoid hemorrhage)
  - Nutritional (alcoholism, anorexia nervosa, liquid-protein diet, starvation)
- Drugs
  - Antiarrhythmics: Class 1A, Class 3 (sotalol)
  - Dofetilide: torsades de pointes with high initial dosing and approximately 4% overall before renal adjustment
  - Tricyclic antidepressants (amitriptyline, desipramine)
  - Antifungals (itraconazole, ketoconazole)
  - Antihistamines (astemizole, terfenadine)
  - Antimicrobials (bactrim, E-mycin, pentamidine)
  - Neuroleptics (phenothiazines, thioridazine)
  - Organophosphate insecticides
  - Promotility agents (cisapride)
  - Oral hypoglycemics (Glibenclamide)

## Brugada Syndrome

A sodium channel defect (SCN5A) causes Brugada syndrome. It is found most frequently in Southeast Asia, affecting mostly men (4:1). The mode of inheritance is autosomal dominant. On the ECG, ST elevation is present in the right precordial leads (Fig. 46–2). The ST segment may normalize and may change with drugs (ajmaline), which may uncover the characteristic ST elevation of Brugada syndrome. Patients with Brugada syndrome are at increased risk of SCD.

## WPW Syndrome

Wolff–Parkinson–White (WPW) syndrome is caused by accessory atrioventricular connections. There is a 0.1% incidence of SCD per year, with risk related to the conduction properties of the bypass tract. SCD is related to atrial fibrillation that is antegradely conducted over a rapidly

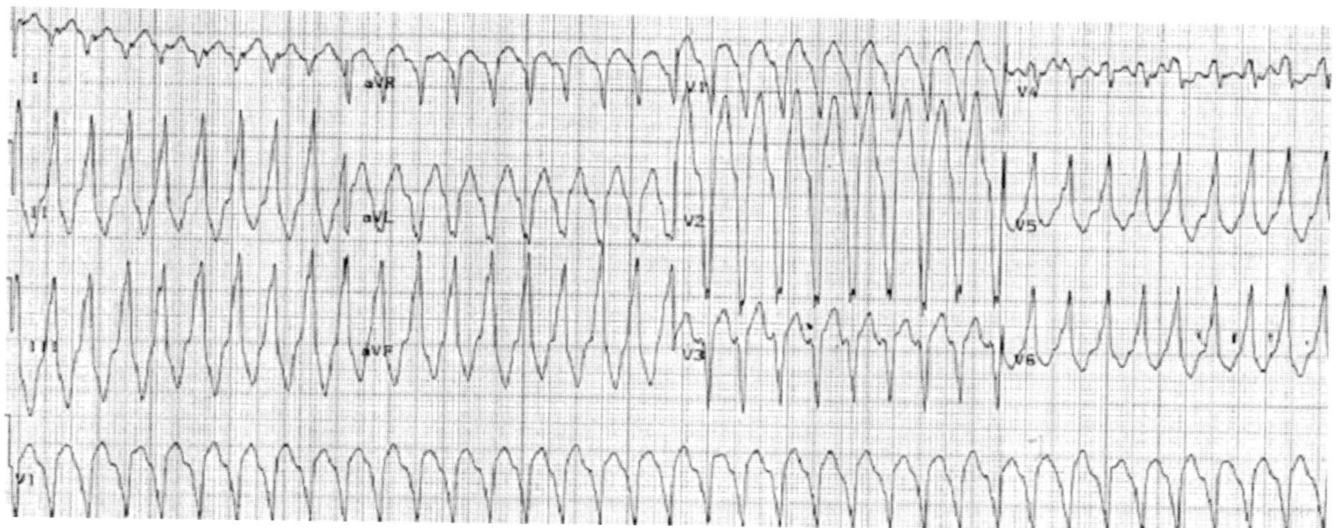


**Figure 46–2** ECG reading in Brugada syndrome.

conducting bypass tract. For symptomatic patients, WPW is curable with ablation with >95% effectiveness. Asymptomatic patients do not require ablation.

### Miscellaneous Causes

There are many other causes of SCD that are not due primarily to electrophysiologic derangements. These include:

- Commotio cordis
- Congenital heart disease
- Right-to-left intracardiac shunts
- Congenital coronary anomalies
- Corrected congenital heart disease
- Sarcoidosis of the heart: ventricular tachycardia from sarcoid lesions, conduction system disease
- Chagas disease: multifocal myocarditis, CHF
- Muscular dystrophies: myocardial scarring, conduction system disease
- Valvular heart disease: ventricular tachycardia and ventricular fibrillation, hypotension, ischemia
- Acute myocarditis
- Severe aortic valve stenosis

## EVALUATION AND MANAGEMENT

### Survivors of Sudden Cardiac Death

A complete history and physical examination focusing on risk factors, medications, drugs, and family history (in the young) should be obtained. A complete cardiac evaluation including ECG, Holter (QT, Brugada), ischemia workup, echocardiography (ejection fraction, valvular abnormalities, right ventricular enlargement), MRI or CT scan and a left heart catheterization with testing for coronary artery spasm and biopsy may be warranted, based on the clinical scenario.

Performing an electrophysiologic (EP) study in those patients with reversible causes for risk stratification is of questionable utility.

In the majority of cases, an ICD is indicated in survivors without identifiable reversible causes.

Workup of patients at risk for sudden cardiac death should be as outlined below, depending on the clinical scenario:

- Echocardiography is currently the most useful initial test.
- EP study is useful in patients with an ejection fraction 35% or greater.
- Drug testing may uncover Brugada/long-QT syndrome
- Signal-averaged ECG may identify possible substrate for re-entry.
  Most useful in ischemics with normal QRS
  Good negative predictive value
  Low positive predictive value
  Limited usefulness
- Event/Holter monitoring.
- Genetic testing is time consuming, expensive, and not widely available. It is not considered routine standard of care.

## VENTRICULAR TACHYCARDIA

### Coronary Artery Disease

Patients with ventricular tachycardia (VT) frequently have a low ejection fraction (EF). Up to two thirds of patients with clinically detected VT post–myocardial infarction have a left ventricularl aneurysm. The mechanism of VT in the majority of cases is myocardial re-entry. In patients with an EF <35%, an ICD is indicated, according to MADIT I and MADIT II. Current ICD therapy can terminate up to 80% of all spontaneous VT with antitachycardia pacing (ATP). However, up to one third of patients will still require antiarrhythmic medications to suppress VT and to minimize shocks and ATP. Catheter ablation of re-entrant circuits is reserved for patients with VT that is refractory to medications and requiring multiple ICD shocks. Patients with nonsustained ventricular tachycardia (NSVT) and EF >45% require treatment with beta-blockers, cholesterol-lowering agents, and angiotensin-converting enzyme inhibitors. Patients with EF <45% and >35% and NSVT require an electrophysiologic study. If this reveals monomorphic VT, then an ICD is indicated.

### Dilated Cardiomyopathy

More than a quarter of patients with dilated cardiomyopathy (DCM) have NSVT on Holter monitoring during a 24-hour period. Currently, an ICD is indicated for primary prevention in patients with DCM and a left ventricularl EF ≤35%. Electrophysiologic study is not helpful in patients with DCM, so it is not pursued in patients with DCM and EF >35%. However, as in patients with ischemic heart disease, if there is a history of hemodynamically significant VT, then an ICD is indicated.

An important factor to consider when assessing VT in DCM is bundle branch re-entry VT. This is a ventricular tachycardia with left bundle branch bundle morphology. This is readily diagnosed in the EP lab. Electrophysiologic testing reveals an abnormal His bundle conduction with long HV intervals. Most frequently, the right bundle is used as the antegrade limb and the left bundle as the retrograde limb. Treatment is ablation of the right bundle.

### Ventricular Tachycardia and the Structurally Normal Heart

#### *Idiopathic Left Ventricular VT with RBBB Morphology*

This is a paroxysmal and sustained VT that occurs predominantly in men. It is a fascicular VT and is the most common left-sided VT. This type of VT is characterized by the following triad: (a) easily induced by atrial pacing, (b) RBBB morphology, and (c) absence of structural heart disease.

This type of VT is highly sensitive to verapamil. The earliest left ventricular activation sites are at the cardiac apex and the mid-interventricular septum. Ventricular activation at the earliest site is usually preceded by high-frequency potentials termed the Purkinje potentials. Ablation at these sites is highly successful in terminating this arrhythmia.

### *Outflow-Tract Ventricular Tachycardia*

Outflow-tract tachycardia may be induced with programmed stimulation. Ithas a characteristic electropharmacologic response. This tachycardia is adenosine sensitive and terminates with beta-blockers, calcium channel blockers, and the Valsalva maneuver. Two clinically distinct features are recognized: exercise-induced ventricular tachycardia and ventricular tachycardia at rest. Most of this ventricular tachycardia is of right ventricular outflow-tract origin, suggested by a left bundle branch block morphology. A left ventricular outflow origin is suggested by right bundle branch block QRS-complex morphology associated with early precordial transition. It originates below the aortic valve in the posterior region of the left ventricular outflow tract. Other foci may be the anterior mitral valve annulus and the superior basal septum. Another potential origin is the aortic valve cusps, most frequently at the left cusp of the aortic valve. Mapping and ablation of the sites of origin is highly successful in abolishing this type of ventricular tachycardia (Fig. 46–3).

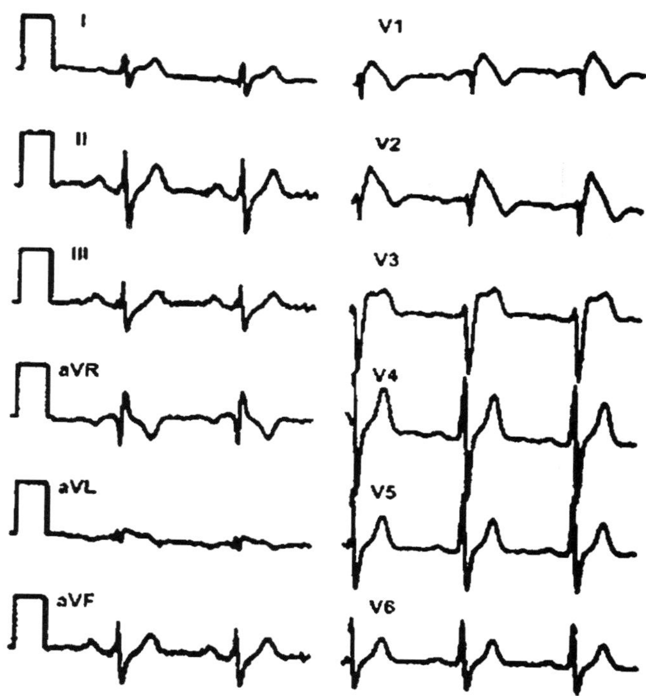


**Figure 46–3** ECG reading in RVOT VT.

### *Short-QT Syndrome*

The short-QT syndrome is a new entity. The corrected QT intervals are <300 milliseconds. There is a high incidence of ventricular tachycardia and fibrillation. Gain-of-function mutations (i.e., a mutation resulting in a new protein, overexpression of a protein, or inappropriate expression of a protein with resultant added or increased function of the mutant protein) in the gene for outward potassium currents have been shown to be responsible for this congenital syndrome. HERG (or KCNH2) and KCQN1 gene mutations have been identified in some families. Management consists of implantation of an ICD and possibly quinidine, which can prolong the QT interval and prevent VT.

## BIBLIOGRAPHY

**Faramarz, Samie H, Jalife J.** Mechanisms underlying ventricular tachycardia and its transition to ventricular fibrillation in the structurally normal heart. *Cardiovasc Res.* 2001;50:242–250.

**Nogami A.** Idiopathic left ventricular tachycardia: assessment and treatment. *Cardiac Electrophysiol Rev.* 2002;6:448–457.

**Wever EFD, Robles de Medina EO.** Sudden death in patients without structural heart disease. *J Am Coll Cardiol.* 2004;43(7).

## QUESTIONS

**1.** Which of the following will most likely respond to verapamil?

a. RVOT ventricular tachycardia
b. Idiopathic left ventricular tachycardia
c. Bundle branch re-entry tachycardia
d. ARVD ventricular tachycardia

Answer is b: Idiopathic left VT with RBBB morphology. This is a paroxysmal and sustained VT that occurs predominantly in en. It is a verapamil-sensitive fascicular VT and is the most common left VT. This type of VT is characterized by the following triad: (a) easily induced by atrial pacing, (b) RBBB morphology, and (c) absence of structural heart disease.

**2.** Which of the following ventricular tachycardias is most amenable to ablation?

a. Ischemic cardiomyopathy VT
b. ARVD VT
c. Brugada syndrome VT
d. Exercise-induced VT

Answer is d: Exercise-induced ventricular tachycardia. This is an outflow-tract tachycardia. Mapping and ablation of the origin site is highly successful in abolishing this type of ventricular tachycardia.

3. Sudden cardiac death in patients >35 years old is most commonly associated with:

a. Hypertrophic cardiomyopathy
b. Coronary artery disease
c. Long-QT syndrome
d. Long QT secondary to various medications

Answer is b: Coronary artery disease. In patients >35 years old, the most common cause of VT is scar related to previous myocardial infarctions.

4. Bundle branch re-entry ventricular tachycardia is most commonly associated with:

a. Enhanced automaticity in the right bundle
b. Enhanced automaticity in the left bundle
c. Supranormal conduction in the His bundle
d. Abnormally slow conduction in the His bundle

Answer is d: Abnormally slow conduction in the His bundle sets up the conditions of re-entry required to sustain this kind of tachycardia.

5. The following ECG is consistent with:

I
II
III
aVR
aVL
aVF
V1
V2
V3
V4
V5
V6

a. Acute anteroseptal myocardial infarction
b. Abnormal SCN5A channel
c. Abnormal KCQN1 channel
d. Old anteroseptal myocardial infarction with an aneurysm

Answer is b: Abnormal SCN5A channel, which causes the Brugada syndrome.

# 47

# Electrophysiologic Testing, Including His Bundle and Other Intracardiac Electrograms

***Mina K. Chung***

This chapter summarizes the components of a comprehensive electrophysiology study. However, the components of a diagnostic electrophysiology study are usually selected based on the indications for the study. Readers who are aiming primarily to prepare for a Board certification exam should direct their attention to components listed in the Summary to this chapter and to the Questions.

## INDICATIONS FOR ELECTROPHYSIOLOGIC TESTING

Indications for performance of an electrophysiology (EP) study have evolved somewhat in recent years, with the indications for implantable cardioverter-defibrillators (ICDs) expanding to defined populations without the need for a "positive" EP study. Thus, the use of EP studies for risk stratification of patients at possible high risk for sudden cardiac death has become more limited. Based on recent multicenter trials, reviewed in Chapter 52, ICDs have become indicated for primary prevention of sudden cardiac death in: (a) patients with coronary artery disease, prior myocardial infarction, left ventricular ejection fraction (LVEF) $\leq$35%, >3 months from revascularization and >1 month from an acute myocardial infarction; and (b) patients with nonischemic cardiomyopathy, LVEF $\leq$35% (with requirements for time from diagnosis for medicare coverage). These patients do not require EP studies to qualify for ICD implantation. However, based on the MUSTT trial (1), patients with LVEF $\leq$40% with coronary artery disease (CAD) after myocardial infarction, and who have nonsustained ventricular tachycardia, benefit from an ICD if, at EP study, sustained ventricular tachycardia (or ventricular fibrillation if reproducibly induced by double extrastimuli) is induced. Thus, EP studies can be indicated for risk stratification of patients who do not yet have indications for an ICD. These patients include patients with CAD, prior myocardial infarction, LVEF $\leq$40%, and nonsustained ventricular tachycardia. Clinical guidelines regarding the use of EP studies in the risk stratification of patients prior to device implantation may be inferred from the ACC/AHA/NASPE 2002 guidelines for device implantation (2).

An EP study is also helpful in the diagnosis of patients presenting with syncope of undetermined etiology and in the diagnosis of wide complex tachycardia. EP studies may also be used to assess for bradyarrhythmias, including sinus node or AV conduction system disease, particularly in patients with possible infra-Hisian conduction system disease.

The most common application for EP studies, however, is for the diagnosis and mapping of tachyarrhythmias as part of a catheter mapping and ablation procedure. The diagnosis of supraventricular tachycardia type and localization of ablatable supraventricular and ventricular substrates are integral parts of ablation procedures [see ACC/AHA/ESC guidelines for management of patients with supraventricular arrhythmias (3)].

Clinical competency guidelines are reported in the ACC/AHA clinical competence statement on invasive electrophysiology studies, catheter ablation, and cardioversion (4).

## THE BASICS OF ELECTROPHYSIOLOGY STUDIES

During an EP study, multipolar catheters are positioned, typically in the right ventricular apex and/or right ventricular outflow tract, the His bundle, the coronary sinus, and/or the right atrium (Fig. 47–1). Programmed electrical stimulation is performed by pacing from bipolar electrodes at various rates and by introduction of premature extrastimuli. Typical baseline recordings include the surface electrocardiograms, particularly leads I, aVF, $V_1$, and $V_6$, as well as intracardiac electrograms from the high right atrium (HRA), His bundle (His, or HBE), right ventricular apex (RVA), and coronary sinus (CS). The electrodes are by convention numbered consecutively, with the most distal electrode being number 1.

### Intracardiac Electrograms

When approaching the interpretation of intracardiac electrograms, it is useful to understand the differences between the surface electrocardiogram and intracardiac electrograms. The surface electrocardiogram (ECG) is recorded on the body surface and reflects the summation of electrical activity. The intracardiac electrogram (EGM) is recorded *within* the heart and is usually filtered differently from surface ECGs to remove high-frequency noise and low-frequency interference (e.g., from respiration). The intracardiac EGM reflects local electrical activity in the heart closest in proximity to the recording electrodes. The display or paper speed is generally faster than the conventional 25-mm/s surface 12-lead ECG speed. Time markers are generally present at the top or bottom of electrogram tracings.

When interpreting intracardiac EGMs, the reader should orient him/herself to the tracings, using the labels, which are usually displayed on along the left margin. Atrial and ventricular activity can be identified by correlation with the surface ECG recordings. Electrograms from atrial or ventricular catheters show local atrial or ventricular depolarization, respectively. Electrograms recorded at either the mitral or tricuspid annulus show *both* atrial and ventricular depolarization. Thus, electrograms from the CS show both atrial and ventricular EGMs. In the CS, the atrial EGMs

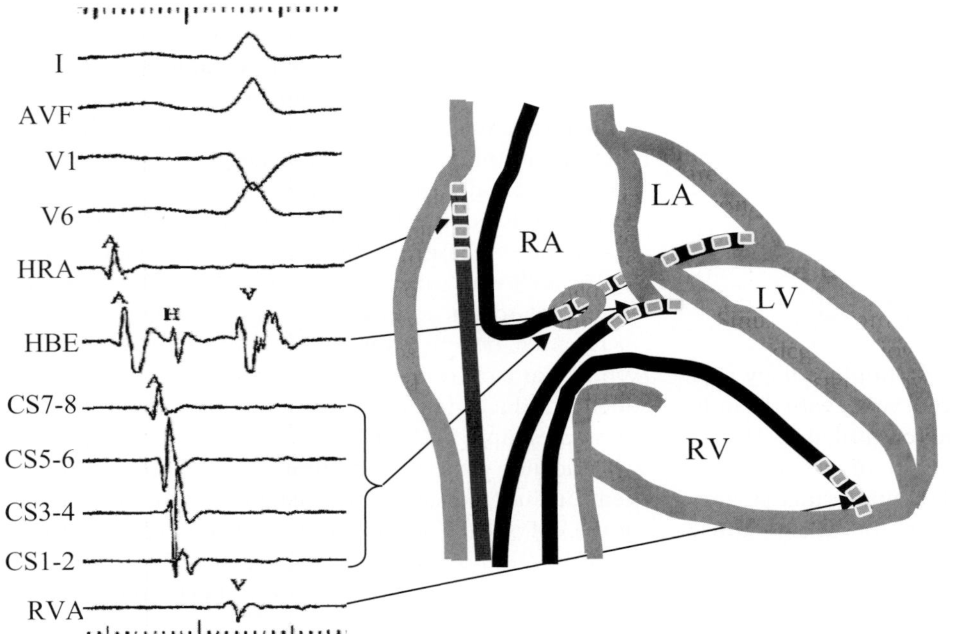


**Figure 47–1** Typical catheter positions and recordings during electrophysiology studies. RA, right atrium; LA, left atrium; LV, left ventricle, RV, right ventricle.

are typically large in amplitude and the ventricular EGMs smaller, unless the catheter is advanced into a ventricular branch. His bundle EGMs are recorded at the tricuspid annulus and typically display atrial, His, and ventricular EGMs, with the size of the atrial or ventricular component dependent on whether the recording electrodes are situated more proximally in the atrium or distally in the ventricle.

## Cycle Lengths versus Rates

During an EP study, intervals are more commonly measured than rates. The "cycle length" of pacing drives or rhythms are measured. The conversion between cycle length and rates is

$$\text{Cycle length (ms)} = 60{,}000/\text{rate (beats/min)}$$

Conversely,

$$\text{Rate (beats/min)} = 60{,}000/\text{cycle length (ms)}$$

Thus, a rate of 60 beats/min corresponds to a cycle length of 1,000 milliseconds, 100 beats/min corresponds to 600 milliseconds, 120 beats/min corresponds to 500 milliseconds, 150 beats/min to 400 milliseconds, and 200 beats/min to 300 milliseconds.

## Baseline Intervals

Typical baseline intervals reported in EP studies include the sinus cycle length (SCL), defined as the interval between sinus atrial electrograms (A–A interval or P–P interval), the surface PR, QRS, and QT intervals. The AH and HV intervals are the most commonly measured intervals (Fig. 47–2). The *AH interval* is measured on the His bundle catheter (HBE) as the time interval from the first major deflection at its baseline crossing to the onset of the His bundle electrogram. The AH interval estimates conduction time across the AV node. The AH interval is highly variable and dependent on vagal tone, medications, and preceding atrial rates, but typically ranges from 50 to 130 milliseconds. The *HV interval* is also measured on the His bundle catheter. The HV interval is the interval from the onset of the His deflection to the *earliest* onset of ventricular activation on any surface lead or intracardiac electrogram. The normal HV interval ranges from 35 to 55 milliseconds. Other baseline intervals are less commonly measured unless they are markedly abnormal. These include the PA interval, defined as the earliest onset of surface P wave to the earliest intracardiac atrial EGM (normal, 20 to 60 milliseconds). The His width from the beginning to end of the His deflection generally ranges from 10 to 25 milliseconds. The RB–V interval measures the interval from the onset of the right bundle potential to the earliest ventricular activation on any surface lead or intracardiac EGM.

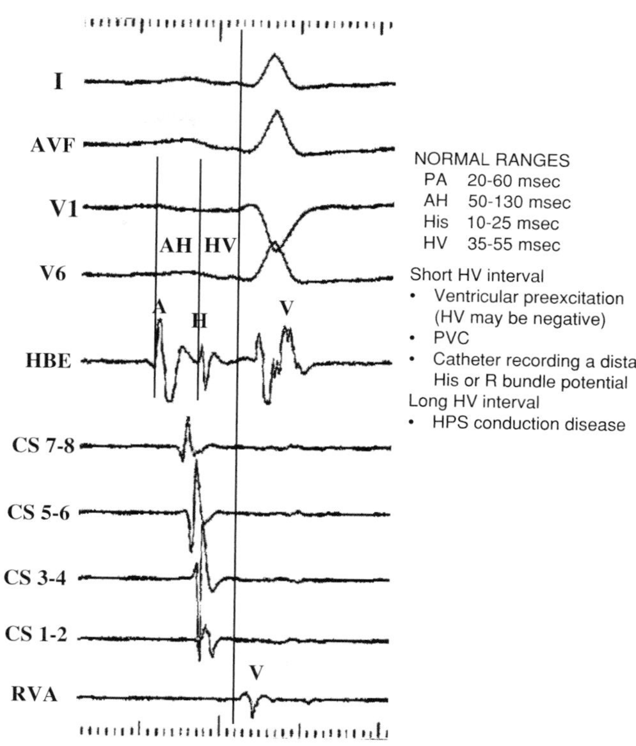


**Figure 47–2** AH and HV intervals.

## Normal Activation Sequences

### *Anterograde Atrial and Ventricular Activation Sequence*

Normal atrial activation during sinus rhythm is from the high right atrium to low RA and then concentrically from proximally to distally along the coronary sinus. Normal ventricular activation is from the RV apex and concentrically from proximal to distal along the coronary sinus (Fig. 47–3, left panel).

### *Retrograde Atrial Activation Sequence*

The sequence of atrial activation during ventricular pacing is from the septum proximally to distally along the CS and from low right atrium in the midline to high RA (Fig. 47–3, right panel).

## Programmed Electrical Stimulation

During an EP study, pacing at various cycle lengths (or rates) or various intracardiac sites is performed. The length of this pacing train and extrastimuli can be programmed and is called programmed electrical stimulation (PES). Common paced cycle lengths are at 600 milliseconds (100 beats/min), 500 milliseconds (120 beats/min), and 400 milliseconds (150 beats/min). The stimuli during the fixed drive train are termed S1. Premature extrastimuli may be introduced in intrinsic rhythm or after a fixed paced drive train (Fig. 47–4). The first extrastimulus is termed S2. The second extrastimulus, when introducing double

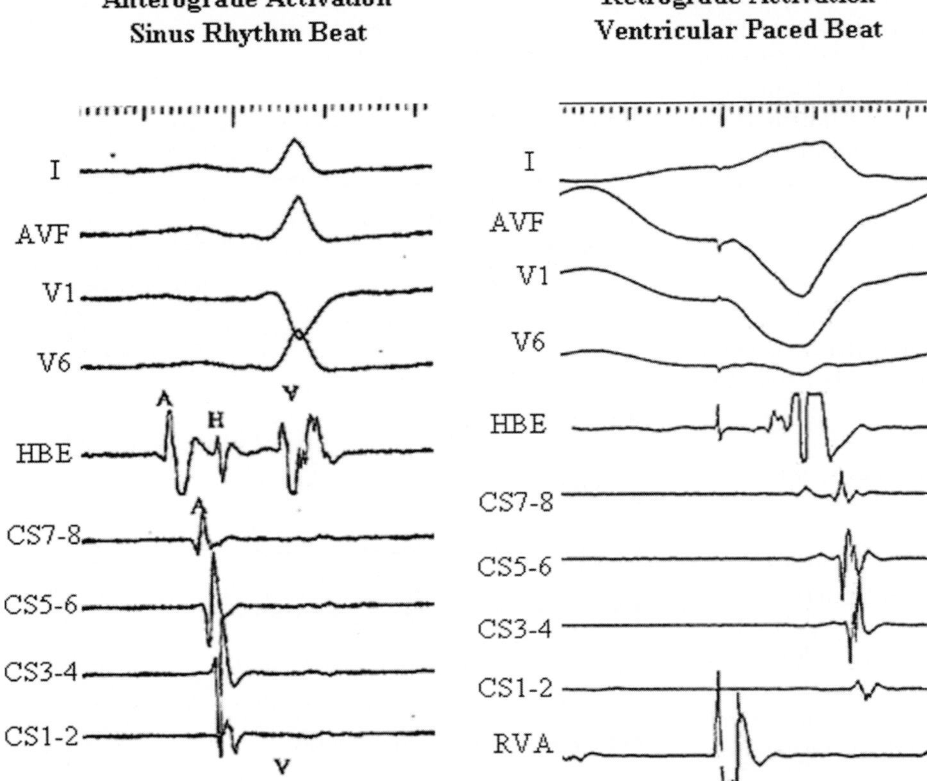


Figure 47–3 Normal activation patterns: anterograde and retrograde activation.

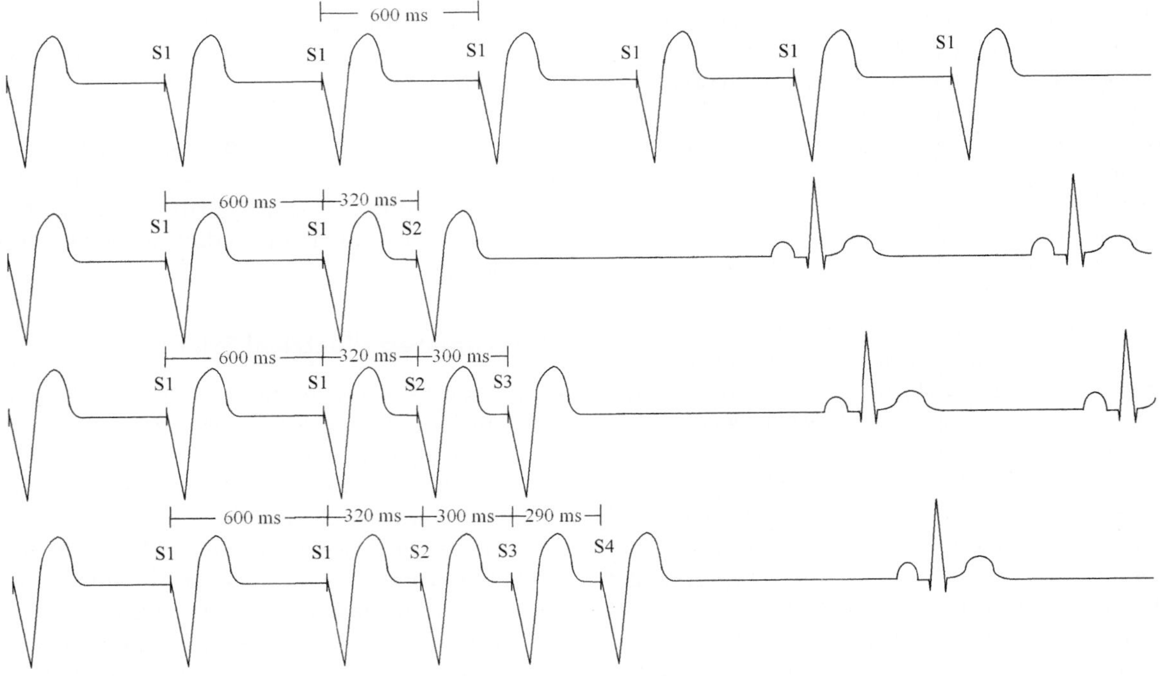


Figure 47–4 Programmed ventricular stimulation.

extrastimuli, is termed S3. The third extrastimulus, when introducing triple extrastimuli, is termed S4, and so on. The common terminology of the paced stimuli, their subsequent intracardiac electrograms, and their intervals are summarized in the following.

### *Pacing Drive Trains and Extrastimuli*

S1 = drive train pacing stimulus
- Continuous overdrive burst, or
- During programmed extrastimuli, typically eight pacing stimuli at a fixed paced cycle length (PCL)

PCL = paced cycle length (e.g., PCL 600 milliseconds = S1S1 interval, pacing rate 100 beats/min)
S2 = first extrastimulus (S1–S2 = coupling interval between S1 and S2)
S3 = second extrastimulus (S2–S3 = coupling interval between S2 and S3)
S4 = third extrastimulus (S3–S4 = coupling interval between S3 and S4)
A1 = atrial electrogram associated with S1 drive or spontaneous atrial rhythm
A2 = atrial electrogram associated with S2 or first spontaneous atrial electrogram after A1
A3 = atrial electrogram associated with S3 or second spontaneous atrial electrogram after A1
H1 = His bundle electrogram associated with S1 drive or spontaneous rhythm
H2 = His bundle electrogram associated with S2 or after second spontaneous depolarization
V1 = ventricular electrogram associated with S1 drive or spontaneous ventricular rhythm
V2 = ventricular electrogram associated with S2 or first spontaneous ventricular electrogram after V1
V3 = ventricular electrogram associated with S3 or second spontaneous ventricular electrogram after V1

### *Refractory Periods*

The *effective refractory period* (ERP) is defined as the longest interval after onset of depolarization that fails to propagate. The ERP is usually determined during programmed electrical stimulation with the delivery of single extrastimuli after paced drive trains. With each successive drive train, the coupling interval is progressively shortened, until the extrastimulus fails to capture the stimulated tissue. This coupling interval identifies the ERP (Fig. 47–5). This interval represents the longest coupling interval that fails to capture the conduction system or myocardium distal to the stimulus (e.g., in the ventricle, S1–S2 interval that produces a V1 but no V2). The *relative refractory period* (RRP) is the longest S1–S2 interval that results in conduction delay distal to the stimulus—for example, when the output interval (V1–V2) is longer than the S1–S2 interval (e.g., when "latency" of ventricular activation is observed). The *functional refractory period* (FRP) is the minimum interval between two consecutively conducted impulses—that is, the shortest output possible (e.g., the shortest V1–V2 interval). A summary and the normal ranges of ERPs are as follows:

- *Effective refractory period* (ERP)—longest interval (e.g., S1–S2 interval) that fails to propagate:

  S1–S2 = V1–no V2 (input measurement)

- *Relative refractory period* (RRP)—longest S1–S2 interval that results in conduction delay:

  S1–S2 ≠ V1–V2 (input ≠ output)

- *Functional refractory period* (FRP)—minimum interval between two consecutively conducted impulses:

  Shortest V1–V2 (shortest output possible)

### *Normal Effective Refractory Periods*

Atrial ERP: 170 to 300 milliseconds
AVN ERP: 230 to 430 milliseconds
His ERP: 330 to 450 milliseconds
Ventricular ERP: 170 to 290 milliseconds

## BRADYARRHYTHMIA EVALUATION BY EPS

Electrophysiologic study to assess bradyarrhythmias is not indicated if symptomatic bradycardia has already been documented or if the patient already has a clear indication for a permanent pacemaker. However, EP study may be helpful for (a) patients with sinus node or AV conduction disease and symptoms but for whom noninvasive monitoring has failed to document correlation of the bradyarrhythmia with symptoms; (b) patients in whom symptoms might also be due to another arrhythmia (e.g., atrial, supraventricular, ventricular tachycardia); or (c) patients with a permanent pacemaker who continue to have symptoms.

## SINUS NODE FUNCTION

### Sinus Cycle Length

The *sinus cycle length* (SCL) is defined as the A–A interval during sinus rhythm. Assessment of sinus node function may include assessment of the sinus node recovery time (SNRT) and/or the sinoatrial conduction time (SACT).

### *Sinus Node Recovery Time*

Atrial overdrive pacing is performed at a rate faster than the sinus rate for ~30 seconds, usually at multiple paced cycle lengths (e.g., PCL 700, 600, 500, 400 milliseconds). The SNRT is the interval from the last paced atrial electrogram to the return sinus atrial electrogram (Fig. 47–6). SNRT

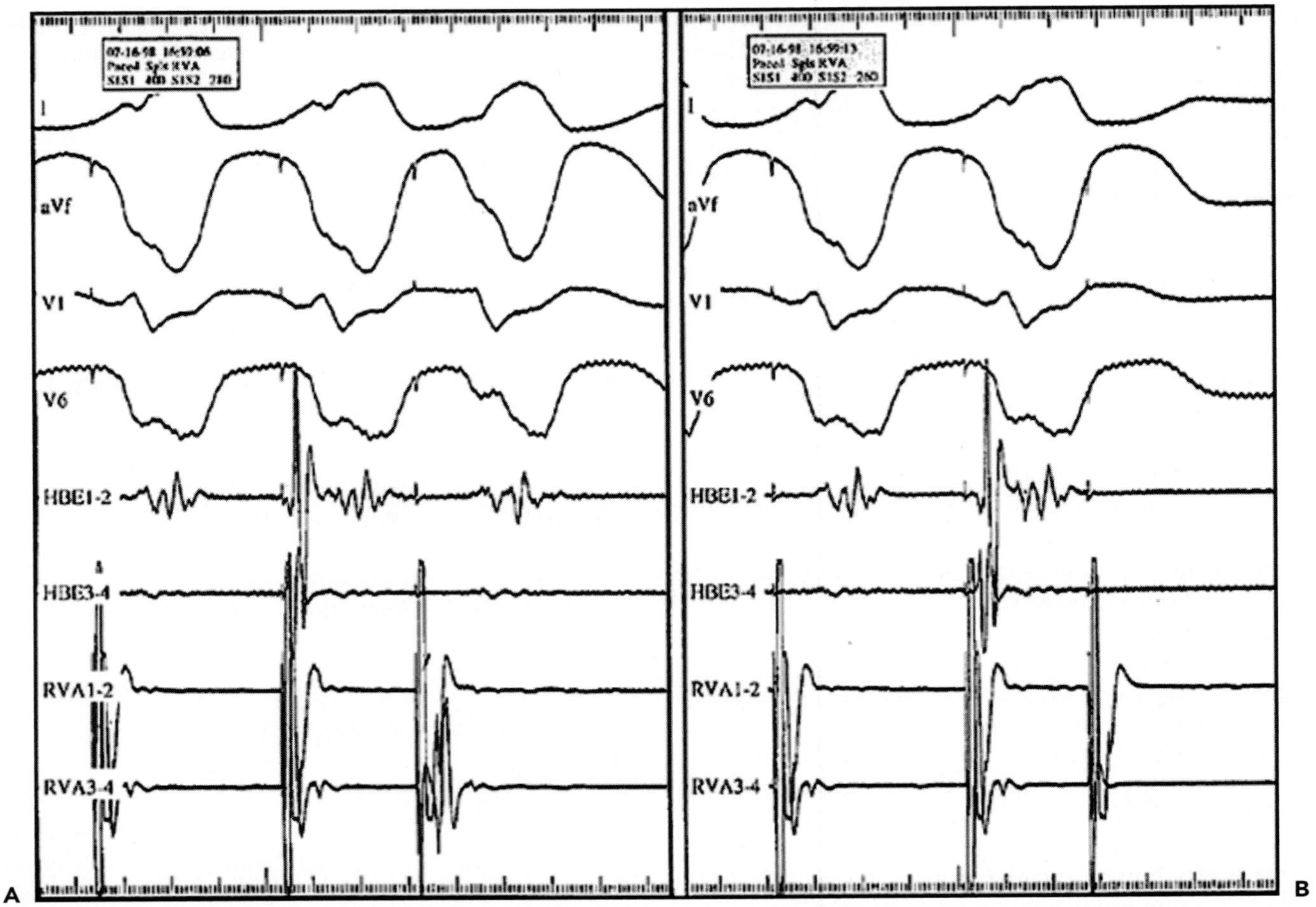

**Figure 47–5** Ventricular effective refractory period (VERP). **A:** PCL 400 milliseconds, CI 280 milliseconds. **B:** PCL 400 milliseconds, CI 260 milliseconds (VERP).

usually lengthens as PCL shortens until retrograde sinus node entrance block occurs, at which point the sinus node is no longer being overdriven as quickly. Then, as PCL shortens further, SNRT typically shortens. Maximal SNRT is the longest SNRT measured after pacing at different PCLs and is reported with the PCL that produces the longest SNRT.

### Corrected Sinus Node Recovery Time

The corrected sinus node recovery time (CSNRT) is the difference between the maximal SNRT and the sinus cycle length (SCL). Normal CSNRT is $<550$ milliseconds. The CSNRT corrects for the variation of SNRT with baseline sinus cycle length.

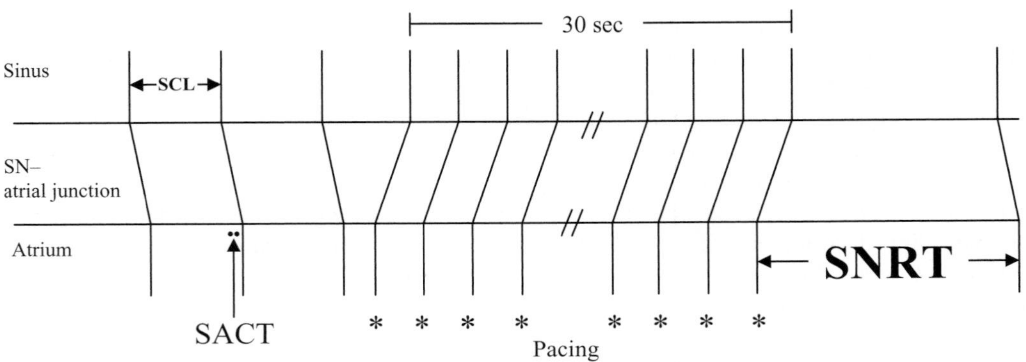


**Figure 47–6** Determination of sinus node recovery time (SNRT).

### Total Sinus Node Recovery Time

After overdrive atrial pacing, the time from the last paced atrial electrogram until the sinus cycle length returns to prepaced rate represents the total sinus node recovery time. Normal is <5 seconds.

### Secondary Pauses

The presence of secondary pauses should be noted after testing for sinus node recovery time. A secondary pause represents an interval longer than the initial sinus node recovery time interval that occurs after the initial sinus recovery beat after overdrive atrial pacing.

## *Sinoatrial Conduction Time*

The SACT is a measure of conduction time from sinus activation to local atrial activation in the region surrounding the sinus node. SACT can be estimated by pacing and recording close to the sinus node and measuring the time to the first spontaneous atrial beat after a single premature beat or slow overdrive train of atrial pacing. (Normal is 50 to 125 milliseconds.)

### Indirect SACT—Narula Method (Fig. 47–7)

From a catheter placed in the high right atrium in the region of the sinus node, a drive train (commonly eight beats) of atrial overdrive pacing is delivered at a PCL ~50 ms (50 to 150 milliseconds) faster than the sinus rate. This rate is assumed to be fast enough that the last beat will capture the sinus node but slow enough to avoid significant prolongation of sinus node recovery time. The interval from the last paced stimulus to the first return sinus activation recorded by the atrial electrogram on the pacing catheter is measured. The estimated SACT = (escape interval − SCL)/2. This assumes that the conduction times into and out of the sinus node are equal.

### Indirect SACT—Strauss Method (Fig. 47–8)

During sinus rhythm (A1), single premature atrial beats (A2) are delivered, starting with a long coupling interval and decrementing by 10 milliseconds. The atrial electrogram of the sinus return beat (A3) is recorded. The sinus return intervals after the premature beats (A2–A3) are plotted against A1–A2 intervals (Fig. 47–8E). Four zones can be described:

*Zone of collision or nonreset (Zone 1, Fig. 47–8A):* Very late-coupled premature atrial beats (A2) collide with the preceding sinus node outgoing activation (A1) and do not penetrate into the sinus node. Thus, the sinus node is unaffected and the next sinus activation (A3) occurs on time (i.e., the sinus node timing is not reset). In this A1–A2 zone of collision, as A1–A2 coupling interval shortens, A2–A3 prolongs by the same amount. Thus, (A1–A2) + (A2–A3) = 2 × (A1–A1).

*Zone of reset (Zone 2, Fig. 47–8B):* In this zone, the premature atrial extrastimuli (A2) penetrate the sinus node and reset the timing of the sinus node, resulting in an advancement in the time of the next sinus activation (A3). During this zone, A2–A3 interval stays relatively constant, representing a plateau in the plot of A1–A2 versus A2–A3. This A2–A3 interval consists of the escape interval of the sinus node and the two-way SACT (A2–A3 = A1–A1 + two-way SACT). The two-way SACT is estimated as the difference between the plateau A2–A3 and the sinus cycle length (A1–A1). Thus, two-way SACT = A2–A3 − A1–A1.

*Zone of interpolation (Zone 3, Fig. 47–8C):* As the premature atrial extrastimulus (A2) coupling interval (A1–A2) shortens further, entrance block may occur in the tissue surrounding the sinus node. In this zone, the premature atrial impulse may not penetrate the sinus node. The escape or return sinus interval (A2–A3) shortens, because A2 does not reset the node. The A1–A3 interval may be the same as the A1–A1 interval (sinus cycle length). In other words, A1–A2 + A2–S3 = A1–A1. However, if A2 conducts to the perinodal tissue, causing the return or escape sinus beat to conduct more slowly on its way out of the sinus node, then A2–A3 may be slightly prolonged, so the sum of A1–A2 + A2–S3 may be slightly longer than A1–A1 during some parts of this zone.

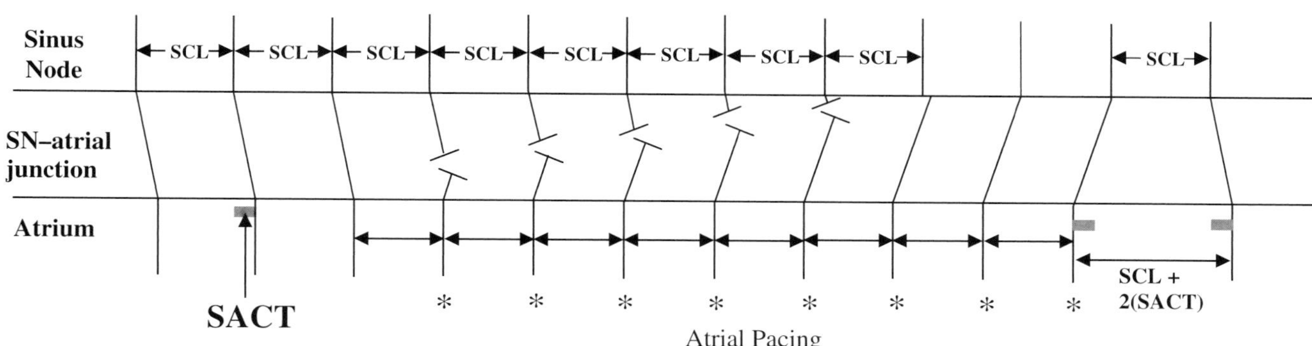


**Figure 47–7** Estimation of sinoatrial conduction time (SACT), Narula method.

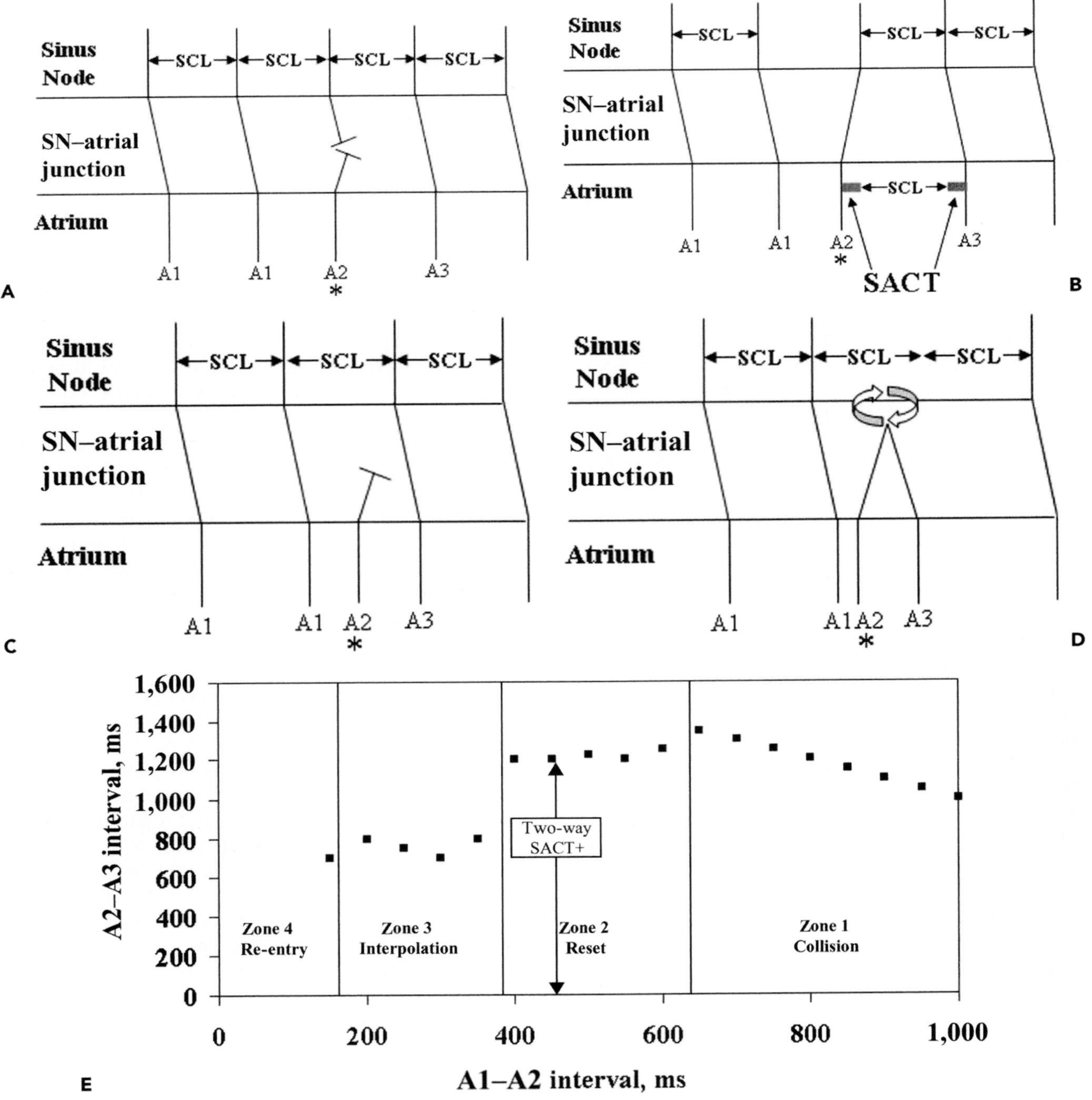


**Figure 47–8** Estimation of sinoatrial conduction time (SACT), Strauss method. **A:** Zone 1, zone of collision. **B:** Zone 2, zone of reset. **C:** Zone 3, zone of interpolation. **D:** Zone 4, zone of re-entry. **E:** A1–A2 versus A2–A3.

*Zone of re-entry (Zone 4, Fig. 47–8D):* In some patients, a re-entrant beat is induced by a short-coupled atrial extrastimulus. In this zone, A1–A3 is shorter than the sinus cycle length A1–A1.

The SACT by Strauss method may be estimated in a shorter protocol by introducing atrial premature beats (A2) at ~40% to 60% of the sinus cycle length and measuring A2–A3 at several A1–A2 coupling intervals. If the A2–A3 intervals are relatively constant (variation <50 milliseconds), then it is assumed that these have been delivered during the plateau phase (Zone 2) and the SACT can be calculated. However, if a stable A2–A3 is not achieved, then the Strauss SACT should not be reported.

### Sinus Node Refractory Period

Sinus node depolarization may be recorded directly, but is technically difficult. Recording may not be successful even with use of high gains and filtering to allow low-frequency signals. Sinus node refractory period (SN ERP) may be estimated indirectly as the A1–A2 interval at which Zone 3 interpolation begins in the Strauss SACT method. At this A1–A2 interval, neither sinus node reset nor activation occurs.

### Intrinsic Heart Rate

The intrinsic sinus rate is inferred as the sinus rate after application of autonomic blockade, using both atropine and propranolol to block vagal and sympathetic inputs, respectively. Intrinsic heart rate (IHR) varies with age and can be estimated by the formula IHR = 118.1 − 0.57(age).

The sensitivity for sinus node dysfunction causing symptoms is ~54% for CSNRT, ~51% for SACT, and ~64% for combined CSNRT + SACT with specificity ~88%. The low sensitivity and specificity of EP study for detection of sinus node dysfunction limits its value in prediction of future events in asymptomatic patients.

### Response to Carotid Sinus Massage

Right and left carotid sinus massage may be performed in patients with syncope of undetermined etiology and no evidence of carotid vascular disease. A sinus pause or AV block >3 seconds with reproduction of clinical symptoms is considered a positive response to carotid sinus massage. A cardioinhibitory response occurs in >70% of patients with a positive response, a vasodepressor response (BP drop <50 mm Hg) in ~15%, and both in others.

## ASSESSMENT OF AV CONDUCTION

The AV node and His–Purkinje system (HPS) function are tested using atrial pacing, atrial extrastimuli, and pharmacologic challenge techniques. The AH interval estimates conduction time through the AV node. The HV interval assesses infra-Hisian conduction and estimates conduction time from the His bundle to the first onset of ventricular activation. Retrograde conduction is tested by ventricular pacing and ventricular extrastimuli.

### Baseline AV Conduction

#### *AH Interval*

The AH interval (Fig. 47–2), an estimation of the conduction time through the AV node, is measured on the His bundle catheter (HBE) from the first major deflection as it crosses baseline to the onset of the His bundle electrogram. Normal range is greatly variable depending on autonomic tone and medications. The input to the AV node is estimated by the atrial electrogram and the output of the AV node by the His deflection on the HBE tracing.

#### *HV Interval*

The HV interval (Fig. 47–2) is measured on the His bundle catheter (HBE) from the onset of the His deflection to the earliest onset of ventricular activation seen on any surface lead or intracardiac electrogram. The normal range for HV intervals is 35 to 55 milliseconds. A *short HV* interval may be seen in ventricular preexcitation syndromes, in which HV may be negative when ventricular activation is pre-excited by anterograde conduction through an accessory pathway that beats out ventricular activation by the AVN to the His–Purkinje system. A short HV may also be measured if a premature ventricular depolarization occurs prior to ventricular activation, and also if the His bundle catheter is placed distally and is recording a distal His or right bundle potential. A *long HV interval* suggests His–Purkinje system conduction disease.

#### *RB–V Interval*

The RB–V interval measures the onset of the right bundle potential to the earliest ventricular activation on any surface lead or intracardiac electrogram.

### Incremental Atrial Pacing

Anterograde AV conduction can be studied during incremental atrial pacing, which refers to atrial pacing at shorter and shorter paced cycle lengths. The presence of decremental AV conduction, typical of AV node conduction, and the pattern of ventricular activation are determined to help distinguish whether anterograde conduction occurs via the AV node or via an accessory pathway.

#### *AH Decrement*

The AH interval normally prolongs as atrial pacing rate increases (as PCL is shortened). This is termed *decremental conduction* and is a property of AV nodal tissue. Failure to decrement AV conduction (AH may decrement but AV interval may stay constant with shortening of the HV interval) suggests the presence of an accessory pathway. Conduction through a typical accessory pathway is usually *nondecremental.*

#### *Pattern of Ventricular Activation*

Conduction through the AV node and His–Purkinje system inscribes a narrow QRS in the absence of aberrancy, or block in a component of the His–Purkinje system. Conduction through a typical accessory pathway usually does not decrement. However, as atrial paced cycle length shortens (at faster paced rates), conduction through the AV node will decrement. In the presence of an accessory pathway, slower conduction through the AV node may allow a larger contribution of ventricular activation to occur via the accessory pathway. This may be manifest as a wider QRS, with greater pre-excitation becoming evident at faster PCLs.

### *PCL of AV Block*

The longest atrial PCL associated with a failure of AV conduction is considered to be the PCL of AV block. This PCL is sometimes termed the *Wenckebach PCL* when conduction block occurs in a second-degree Mobitz Type I AV block pattern, which is the normal response of the AV node to atrial pacing at shorter PCLs. A typical accessory pathway generally blocks in a 2:1 fashion rather than in a Wenckebach pattern.

### *PCL of HV Block*

The PCL of HV block interval is the longest atrial PCL at which block occurs below the His bundle (His deflection without following ventricular activation). This represents an abnormal finding if infra-Hisian block or HV prolongation occurs at atrial PCLs longer than 400 milliseconds.

## AV BLOCK: AV NODE VERSUS INFRA-HISIAN BLOCK

Electrophysiologic studies can be useful in determining the level of AV block. Block in the AV node is usually associated with a narrow QRS. On intracardiac electrograms recorded at the His bundle catheter, an atrial electrogram that blocks with no His deflection indicates block occurred in the AV node (Fig. 47–9, left panel). Infra-Hisian block is usually associated with a wider QRS. At the His bundle catheter, an atrial electrogram and His deflection is inscribed, but with no succeeding ventricular activation. Thus, activation proceeds from the atrium, through the AV node, to the His bundle, with subsequent block occurring below the His bundle (Fig. 47–9, right panel).

AV block occurs when the atrial impulse either is not conducted to the ventricle or is conducted with delay at a time when the AV junction is not refractory. It is classified on the basis of severity into three types.

### First-Degree AV Block

In first-degree AV block, conduction is prolonged (PR interval >200 milliseconds), but all impulses are conducted. The conduction delay may be due to conduction slowing in the AV node, the His–Purkinje system, or both. If the QRS complex is narrow and therefore normal, the AV delay usually occurs in the AV node. This may be determined on baseline His bundle recordings, where AH or HV interval prolongation indicates the level of delayed conduction (Fig. 47–10).

### Second-Degree AV Block

In second-degree AV block, intermittent conduction block occurs. In *Mobitz Type I (Wenckebach)* second-degree AV block, progressive prolongation of the PR interval occurs before the block in conduction. In the usual Wenckebach periodicity (Fig. 47–11), the PR interval gradually increases, but with a decreasing increment, thus leading to a gradual shortening of the RR intervals. The longest PR interval usually precedes the block, and the shortest PR interval usually occurs after the block. The long RR interval of the blocked impulse is usually shorter than twice the basic PP interval. Variants of this pattern are not uncommon. In *Mobitz Type II* second-degree AV block, PR intervals before the block are constant, and there are sudden blocks in P-wave conduction. Advanced or high-degree AV block refers to a block of two or more consecutive impulses. In Mobitz Type I block, the level of the block is almost always at the AV node, particularly with a narrow QRS complex. Rarely, type I Wenckebach periodicity in the His–Purkinje

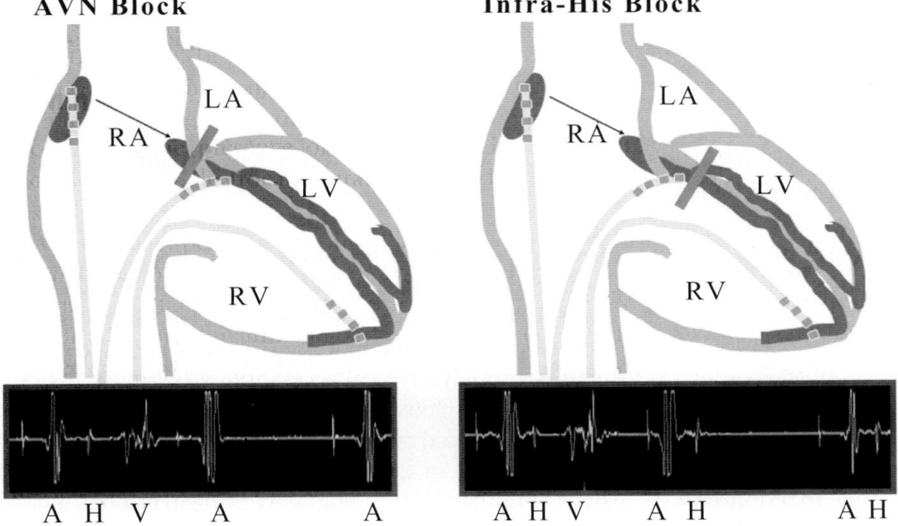


**Figure 47–9** Level of AV block.

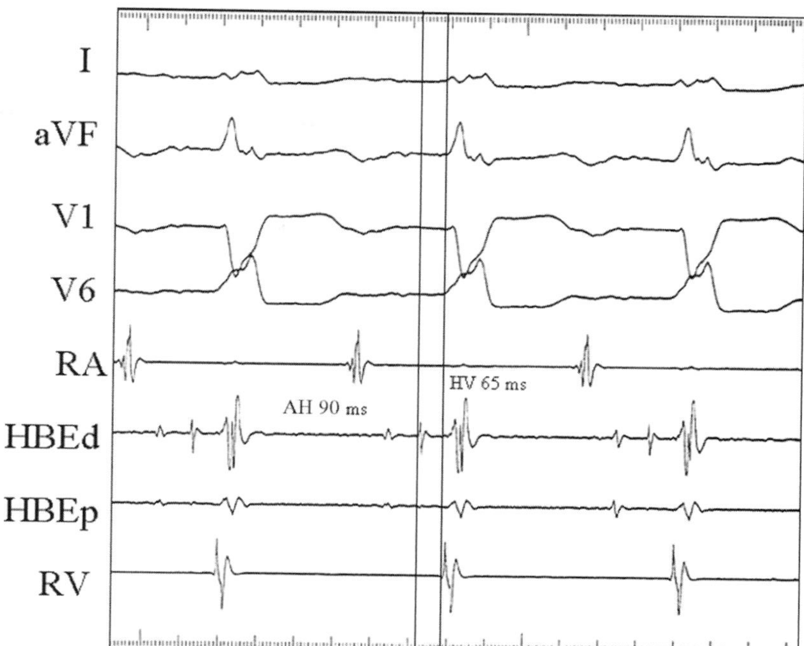


**Figure 47–10** First-degree AV block. In this example, the PR interval is 255 milliseconds. The AH interval is 90 milliseconds and the HV interval is 65 milliseconds. At least part of the prolonged conduction is due to delay in the His–Purkinje system.

system may be seen in patients with a wide QRS or bundle branch block. In contrast, Mobitz Type II block is almost always at the level of the His–Purkinje system and has a higher risk of progressing to complete AV block. In 2:1 AV block, conduction block may occur in either the AV node or the His–Purkinje system. Again, a narrow QRS suggests that the level of block is at the AV node and a wide QRS suggests that the block is infra-Hisian; however, there are exceptions, as can be confirmed by His bundle recordings (Figs. 47–12 and 47–13). It should also be noted that block can occur at both the AV node and infra-Hisian levels.

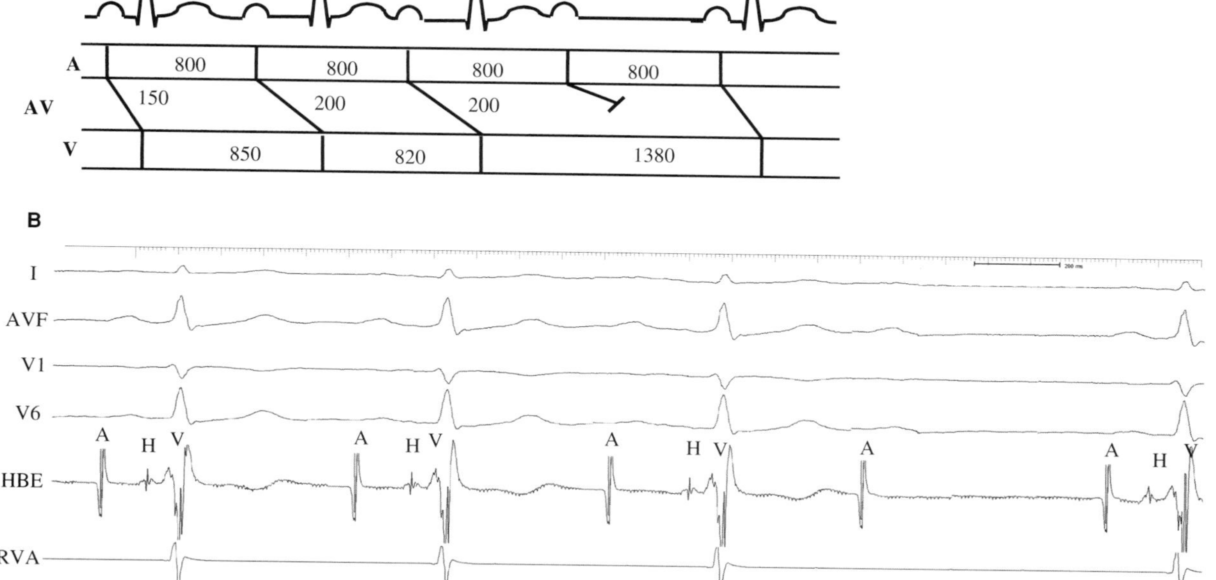


**Figure 47–11** Second-degree AV block, Mobitz Type I (Wenckebach) periodicity. **A:** Ladder diagram of Wenckebach periodicity. The AV interval gradually prolongs prior to the blocked beat. **B:** Intracardiac electrograms of second-degree AV block with Wenckebach block. The AH gradually prolongs prior to the blocked atrial impulse. The block occurs in the AV node.

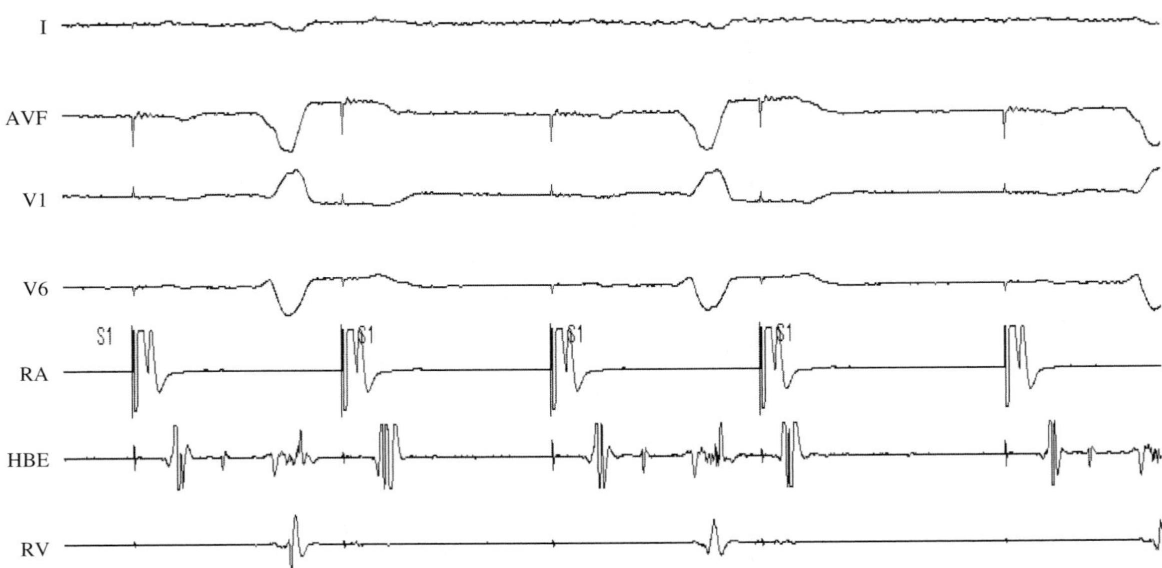


**Figure 47–12** 2:1 AV block in the AV node during atrial pacing.

## Third-Degree AV Block

In third-degree (complete) AV block, no impulses are conducted from the atria to the ventricles. The level of the block can occur at the AV node (usually congenital), His bundle, or in the His–Purkinje system (usually acquired). Escape beats that are junctional (often with narrow QRS) at rates of 40 to 60 beats/min generally occur with congenital complete AV block. Escape beats that are ventricular in origin (with wide QRS) often are slow, ranging from 30 to 40 beats/min. The level of block can again be confirmed by His bundle recordings.

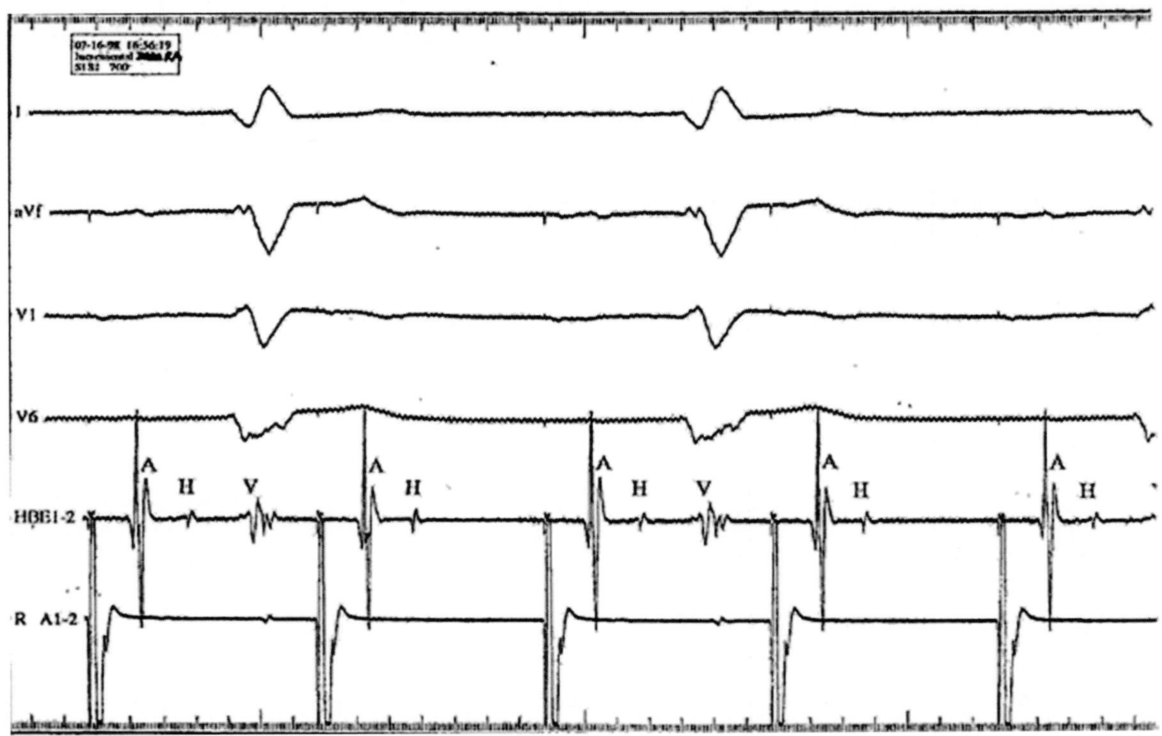


**Figure 47–13** 2:1 AV block due to infra-Hisian block during atrial pacing.

### Atrioventricular Dissociation

It should be noted that AV dissociation, which refers to independent depolarization of the atria and ventricles, is not always due to complete AV block. It may be caused by:

1. Physiologic interference resulting from slowing of the dominant pacemaker (e.g., sinus node) and escape of a subsidiary or latent pacemaker (e.g., junctional or ventricular escape)
2. Physiologic interference resulting from acceleration of a latent pacemaker that usurps control of the ventricle (e.g., accelerated junctional tachycardia or VT)
3. AV block preventing propagation of the atrial impulse from reaching the ventricles, thus allowing a subsidiary pacemaker (e.g., junctional or ventricular escape) to control the ventricles.

Patients with complete AV block have AV dissociation and, generally, a ventricular rate that is slower than the atrial rate. Patients with AV dissociation, however, may have complete AV block or dissociation resulting from physiologic interference, with the latter typically having a ventricular rate that is faster than the atrial rate.

## ASSESSMENT OF AV NODE PHYSIOLOGY

Besides incremental atrial pacing to assess the AV node conduction, including the point at which block occurs (Wenckebach cycle length), AV node physiology can be more carefully dissected and studied using atrial extrastimulus testing.

### Atrial Extrastimulus Testing

AV nodal physiology assessment is generally performed at several atrial PCLs (e.g., PCL 600, 500, 400 milliseconds) with eight-beat trains of atrial overdrive pacing (A1), followed by delivery of a premature atrial extrastimulus (A2). The coupling interval of the extrastimulus (A1–A2) is shortened by 10 to 20 milliseconds with each succeeding drive train.

### Dual AVN Pathway Physiology

AV nodal conduction curves (Fig. 47–14) can be plotted (A1–A2 versus A2–H2 or A1–A2 versus H1–H2). A discontinuous AV nodal conduction curve (AH interval jump of >50 milliseconds after a decrease in A1–A2 coupling interval of 10 milliseconds) suggests the presence of two conduction pathways (typically a fast-conducting AV nodal pathway with a longer refractory period than a slow-conducting AV nodal pathway) (Fig. 47–15). Dual AVN physiology is confirmed by the occurrence of an *AV nodal echo beat*, in which anterograde conduction down the slow AVN pathway is followed by retrograde conduction to the atria via the fast pathway (Fig. 47–15). This typical echo beat occurs with atrial activation occurring within 70 milliseconds of the onset of ventricular activation; on intracardiac electrograms, atrial and ventricular activation occur nearly simultaneously.

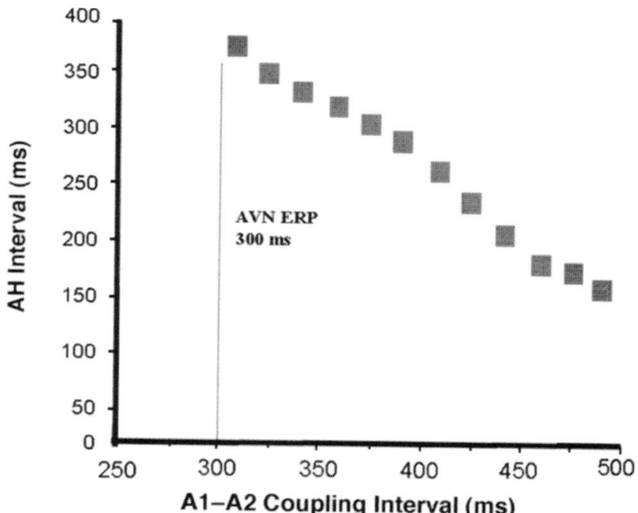


**Figure 47–14** Normal AV node conduction curve.

### AV Nodal Refractory Periods

The *AV nodal effective refractory period* (AVN ERP) is the longest A1–A2 interval that fails to conduct through the AV node (Fig. 47–16). Prolongation may occur with high vagal tone or concomitant medications. Other refractory periods that can be measured include the *AV nodal relative refractory period* (AVN RRP), which represents the longest A1–A2 interval that results in an H1–H2 > A1–A2 during atrial extrastimulus testing. The *AV nodal functional refractory period* (AVN FRP) is the shortest H1–H2 interval (AVN output) observed during extrastimulus testing.

### Incremental Ventricular Pacing

Although it is not a component of EP testing that assesses anterograde AV conduction directly, incremental ventricular pacing (pacing in the ventricle at faster and faster cycle lengths) can help determine whether retrograde conduction occurs via the AV node (Fig. 47–17) or an accessory pathway (Fig. 47–18). Atrial activation occurring with a midline activation pattern that decrements with more rapid pacing rates or a shorter premature extrastimulus coupling interval suggests conduction via the His–Purkinje–AV node system. In this pattern, concentric activation is seen in the coronary sinus leads, with earliest atrial activation occurring at the AV node, septal region, and later activation occurring at more lateral atrial sites (Fig. 47–17). In contrast, retrograde conduction via a left lateral free wall accessory

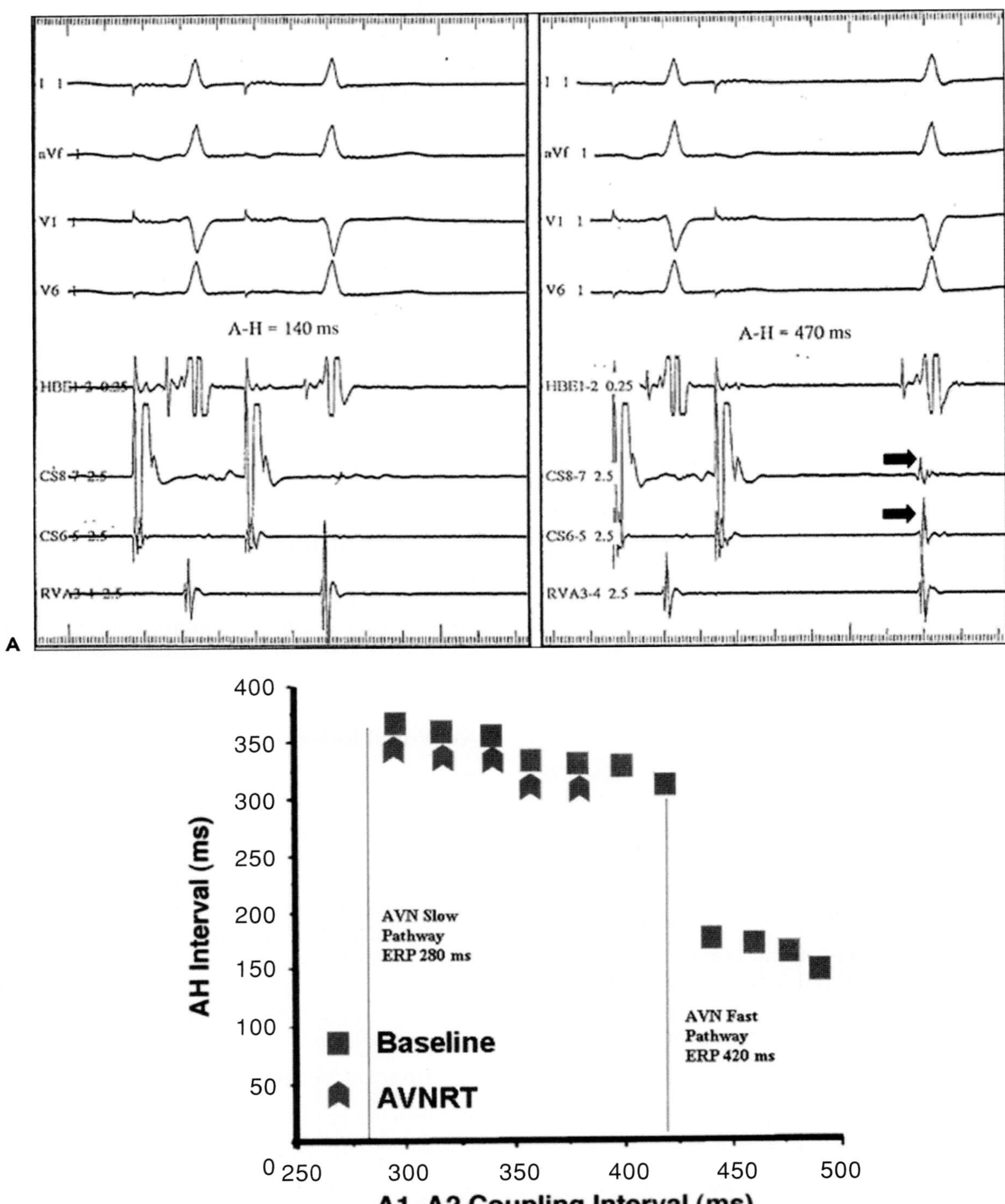


**Figure 47–15** AH jump and AV node echo beat. **A:** Single atrial premature extrastimuli are delivered after eight-beat paced drive cycles. The AH interval is 140 milliseconds with a coupling interval of 290 milliseconds. After a coupling interval of 280 milliseconds, the AH interval "jumps" to 470 milliseconds, indicating the presence of dual AVN pathway physiology. The atrial electrograms evident in the CS leads (arrows) indicate the AVN echo beat with retrograde conduction to the atria. **B:** AV node conduction curve demonstrating an AH jump at the fast pathway effective refractory period (ERP) of 420 milliseconds and induction of echo beats and AVNRT.

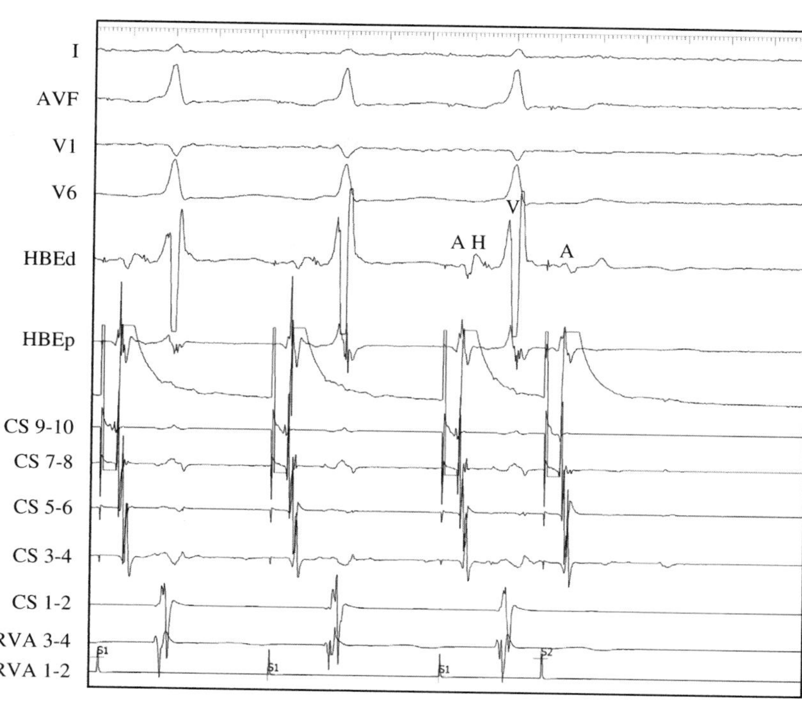


**Figure 47–16** AV node effective refractory period (AVN ERP).

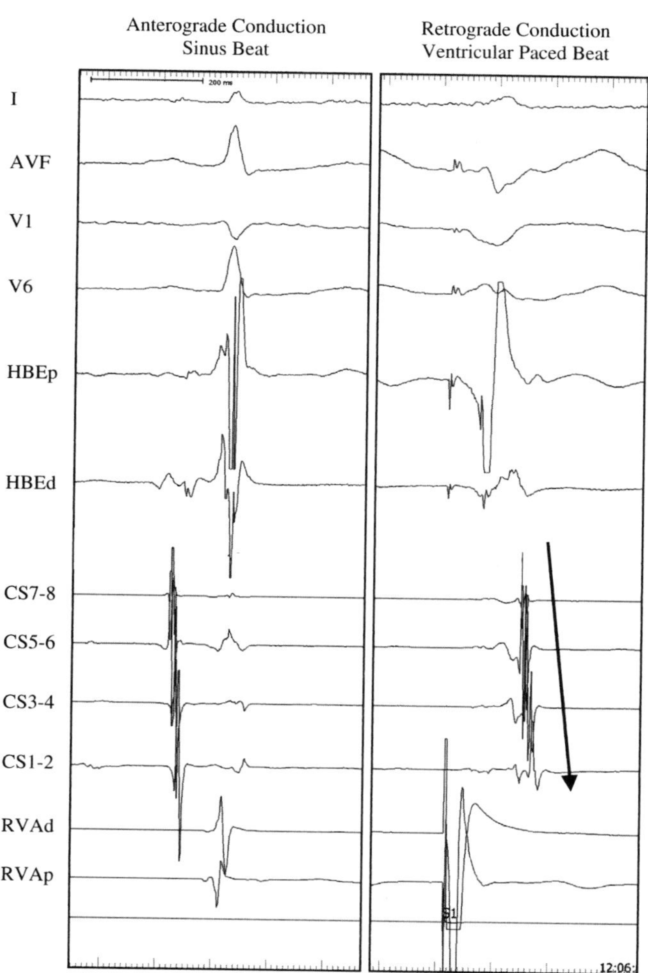


**Figure 47–17** Normal anterograde and retrograde activation.

pathway (Fig. 47–18) will cause an eccentric activation pattern with earliest ventricular activation occurring near the accessory pathway in the lateral coronary sinus leads and earliest retrograde atrial activation in the distal CS.

## PCL of VA Block

The longest ventricular PCL associated with failure of retrograde VA conduction is determined by decremental ventricular pacing. Pacing is performed at shorter and shorter cycle lengths. During retrograde AV nodal conduction, VA intervals gradually increase as pacing cycle length shortens. PCL is shortened until VA block occurs (e.g., retrograde Wenckebach or 2:1 VA block). In the presence of a typical accessory pathway, a constant VA interval is usually observed, and VA block occurs when the accessory pathway refractory period is reached. This usually occurs with a 2:1 VA block pattern, rather than in a retrograde Wenckebach pattern.

## Ventricular Extrastimulus Testing

Analogous to atrial extrastimulus testing, single premature ventricular extrastimuli (V2) are delivered after eight-beat trains of ventricular pacing (V1) at several ventricular PCLs (e.g., PCL 600, 500, 400 milliseconds). The coupling interval of the extrastimulus (V1–V2) is shortened by 10 to 20 milliseconds with each succeeding drive train. In this manner, retrograde VA conduction can be assessed. Decremental retrograde conduction suggests conduction is occurring via the His–Purkinje–AV node system. Retrograde conduction via a typical accessory pathway is generally nondecremental, unless the accessory pathway is an

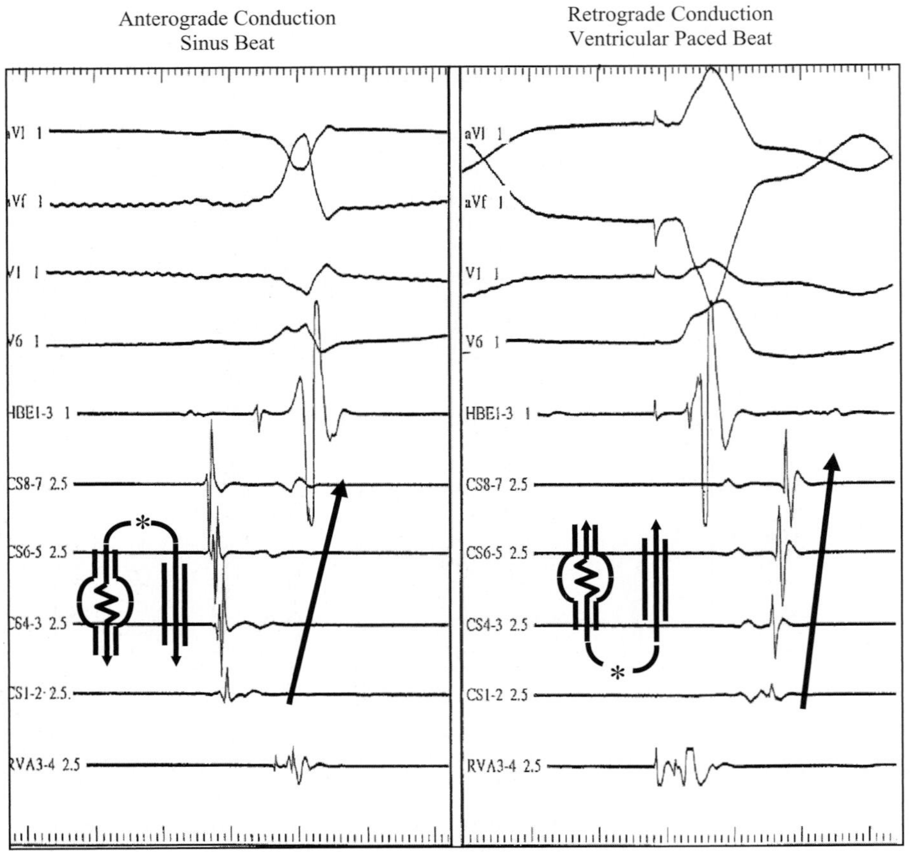


**Figure 47–18** Abnormal anterograde and retrograde activation: left-sided accessory pathway.

atypical, decremental pathway. In addition, retrograde atrial activation patterns are examined to determine if atrial activation occurs with a typical AV nodal midline activation pattern (Fig. 47–17).

## TACHYARRHYTHMIA EVALUATION BY EPS

### Ventricular Tachycardia

Most patients who undergo EP study for assessment of ventricular arrhythmias have coronary artery disease or dilated cardiomyopathy and reduced left ventricular function. EP study may be useful in selected patients for assessment of risk and need for ICD implantation, drug testing, assessment of device/antitachycardia pacing function, or mapping for ablation. EP testing has limited sensitivity and specificity in the prediction of arrhythmic events in nonischemic disease. EP studies have been more useful in risk stratification of patients with CAD after myocardial infarction. Based on data from MUSTT (1) and MADIT (5), survival is improved with ICD implantation in patients with CAD, prior MI, nonsustained VT, and LVEF ≤40%, and inducible sustained VT or reproducibly inducible ventricular fibrillation with double ventricular extrastimuli that is not suppressible with an antiarrhythmic drug (MADIT) (5). These studies provide a rationale for performing EP studies for risk stratification in these patient groups. MADIT II (6) demonstrated the value of prophylactic ICD implantation without EP testing in patients with CAD and LVEF ≤30%. DEFINITE (7) and SCDHeFT (8) studied the value of prophylactic ICD implantation and included patients with nonischemic cardiomyopathy. SCDHeFT demonstrated survival benefits for ICD implantation in ischemic or nonischemic cardiomyopathy patients with heart failure and LVEF ≤35% without the need for EP testing. EP testing is generally not necessary for patients who have criteria that already meet approved ICD indications.

Patients with normal LV function and ventricular tachycardia usually have special types of ventricular arrhythmias that may be studied by EP testing, particularly in conjunction with mapping and ablation.

#### *Ventricular Programmed Stimulation Protocols*

Several stimulation protocols have been useful in stratifying risk for sustained ventricular arrhythmias. Some of the most common are summarized below.

| | |
|---|---|
| Pacing sites | RVA, RVOT |
| Drive cycle lengths | PCL 600 and 400 ms (S1); 8-beat drive trains |
| Number of extrastimuli | 1 to 3 extrastimuli (S2–S4), decrementing extrastimuli by 10 ms starting with last until S2 is refractory |
| Pacing sites | RVA, RVOT |
| Drive cycle lengths | PCL 350, 400, 600 ms (S1); 8-beat drive trains |
| Number of extrastimuli | 4 extrastimuli (S2–S5) beginning at 290, 280, 270, 260 ms, decrementing 10 ms with each drive until S2 is refractory |
| Short–long–short protocol | |
| Pacing sites | RVA, RVOT |
| Drive cycle lengths | PCL 400; 6- or 8-beat drive trains (S1) |
| Number of extrastimuli | S2 at 600 ms; S3 shorter and decrementing until S3 refractory |

### *Ventricular Overdrive Burst Pacing*

#### Ventricular Effective Refractory Period (VERP)

Single ventricular premature extrastimuli are delivered with shortening coupling intervals until the stimulus fails to capture the ventricle (Fig. 47–19). The VERP is the longest ventricular extrastimulus V1–V2 that fails to capture the ventricle during ventricular extrastimulus testing. It is measured from pacing stimulus to pacing stimulus and is recorded at different sites (e.g., RVA, RVOT) and PCLs (e.g., 600, 400 milliseconds).

#### Ventricular Functional Refractory Period (VFRP)

The VFRP is the shortest ventricular coupling interval produced with premature ventricular stimulation. The VFRP is measured from electrogram to electrogram and recorded at different sites (e.g., RVA, RVOT) and PCLs (e.g., 600, 400 milliseconds).

#### Induced Arrhythmias

Definitions of ventricular arrhythmias that can be induced with programmed ventricular stimulation include the following:

- *Repetitive ventricular responses*—one to three PVCs
- *Nonsustained ventricular tachycardia*—three or more ventricular complexes lasting <30 seconds
- *Sustained ventricular tachycardia*—ventricular tachycardia lasting >30 seconds or requiring earlier termination due to hemodynamic compromise
- *Sustained monomorphic VT*—sustained VT of uniform morphology
- *Sustained polymorphic VT*—sustained VT of multiform morphology
- *Pleomorphic VT*—multiple morphologies of monomorphic VT
- *Ventricular flutter*—rapid VT <220 or 240 milliseconds CL with no isoelectric baseline and a sine-wave appearance
- *Ventricular fibrillation*—disorganized chaotic ventricular complexes with loss of organized ventricular contraction

## Morphology

Morphology of ventricular tachycardia can be described by bundle branch block morphology and axis using surface ECG leads I, aVF, and $V_1$:

| | | |
|---|---|---|
| Lead $V_1$ | Positive ⇒ RBBB morphology | Negative ⇒ LBBB morphology |
| Lead I | Positive ⇒ left axis | Negative ⇒ right axis |
| Lead aVF | Positive ⇒ inferior axis | Negative ⇒ superior axis |

### *VA Relationship during Ventricular Tachycardia*

VA dissociation can be readily recognized using intracardiac atrial and ventricular electrograms (Fig. 47–20), helping to confirm the diagnosis of ventricular tachycardia.

## Supraventricular Tachycardia

During EP studies performed for the diagnosis and mapping of supraventricular tachycardia (SVT), multipolar catheters are generally placed in the high right atrium (HRA) or coronary sinus (CS), at the His bundle (HBE), and in the right ventricle (RVA or RVOT). SVT mechanisms include atrial arrhythmias (including ectopic atrial tachycardia, macroreentrant atrial tachycardia, atrial flutter, and atrial fibrillation), AV node re-entrant tachycardia (AVNRT), and atrioventricular reciprocating tachycardia (AVRT) mediated by an accessory pathway.

### *Stimulation Protocols*

Programmed atrial and ventricular stimulation protocols are used in the determination of SVT mechanism and are summarized as follows.

#### Ventricular Pacing

Incremental ventricular pacing at constant rates, but delivered at progressively faster paced cycle lengths, is used for assessment of VA conduction. In particular, the retrograde atrial activation pattern (via AV node versus accessory pathway) is examined to determine the earliest atrial activation site from atrial electrograms recorded on catheters at various atrial sites (Figs. 47–17 and 47–18). The shortest cycle length at which 1:1 VA conduction occurs is recorded and the pattern of VA block at shorter cycle lengths examined. A

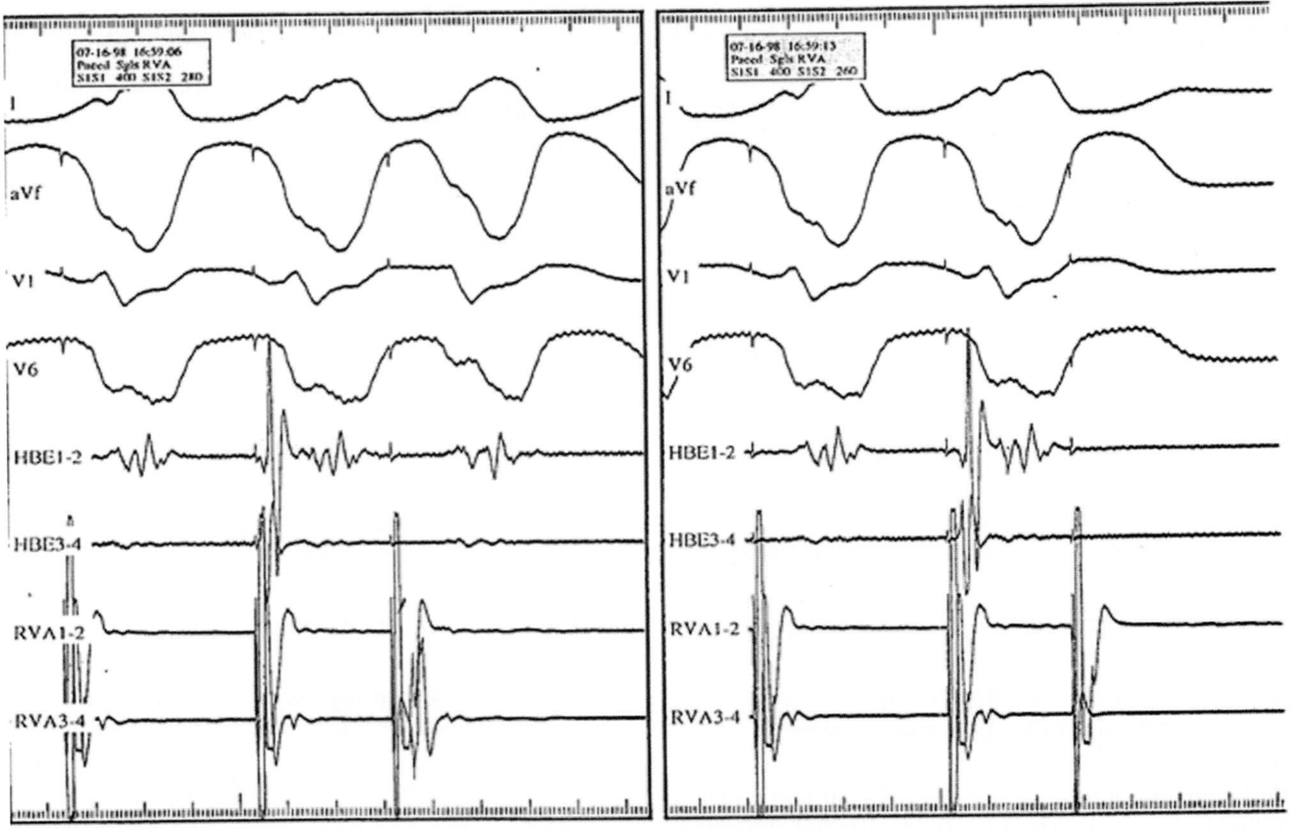


**Figure 47–19** Determination of ventricular effective refractory period (VERP) by ventricular extrastimulus delivery. Single ventricular premature extrastimuli are introduced with shortening coupling intervals until the stimulus fails to capture the ventricle. In this example, at PCL 400 milliseconds, a ventricular premature extrastimulus captures the ventricle at a coupling interval of 280 milliseconds, but fails to capture the ventricle at 260 milliseconds. The VERP is 260 milliseconds at PCL 400 milliseconds.

decremental VA conduction pattern (longer VA times with faster pacing rates) that is concentric (earliest atrial activation in septal leads and later activation in lateral free wall electrodes) suggests that retrograde conduction is occurring via the AV node. Retrograde conduction using an accessory pathway may cause an eccentric atrial activation pattern in the coronary sinus (earliest atrial activation in the posterior or lateral CS in left-sided accessory pathways, Fig. 47–18) or early activation away from the septum in the right atrium. In addition, typical accessory pathways do not display significant decremental conduction, so VA conduction times generally are constant. Exceptions occur for septal accessory pathways in which earliest activation will be at septal leads, and also for decremental accessory pathways in which VA conduction times may be longer at faster pacing rates.

### Programmed Ventricular Stimulation

Single premature ventricular beats are delivered at one or more drive cycle lengths (e.g., 600, 400 milliseconds) to assess retrograde refractory periods, pattern and change in retrograde atrial activation patterns, site of retrograde VA block, and the presence of dual retrograde AV node pathway physiology.

### Atrial Pacing

Assessment of anterograde conduction is performed with atrial pacing and programmed atrial stimulation. Baseline AH and HV intervals are assessed and evidence for decremental AV node conduction sought. Anterograde conduction via the AV node is characterized by increasing AH intervals with faster atrial pacing rates. The shortest paced cycle length at which 1:1 AV conduction occurs and the pattern of anterograde activation and block at paced cycle lengths shorter than this is noted. A Wenckebach AV block pattern and a narrow QRS supports the conclusion that conduction is occurring anterogradely through the AV node. Anterograde ventricular preexcitation by an accessory pathway may become more manifest by atrial pacing, as faster pacing rates will cause decremental, or slower, conduction through

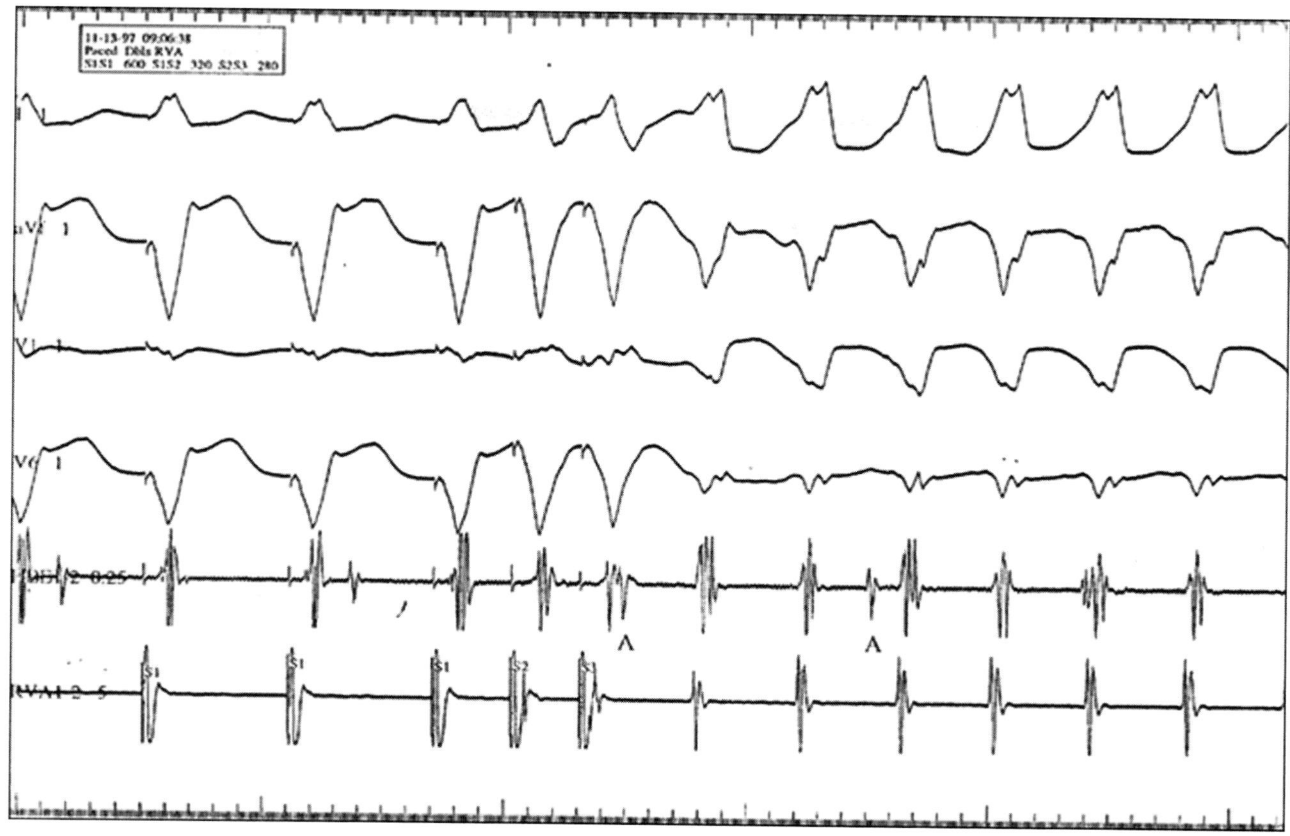

**Figure 47–20** Ventricular stimulation and induction of sustained monomophic ventricular tachycardia (SMVT) with VA dissociation, LB/LSA morphology. VA dissociation is evident during the induction pacing sequence as well as during ventricular tachycardia. A, atrial activation.

the AV node. Thus, at faster atrial pacing rates, the AV node will conduct more slowly, leading to later ventricular activation from the AV node–His–Purkinje system. Because conduction through a typical accessory pathway does not decrement significantly with more rapid pacing rates and ventricular activation, times via the accessory pathway will remain relatively constant, less contribution of ventricular activation will occur via the AV node, and more will occur via the accessory pathway (Fig. 47–21). Another potential important function of burst atrial pacing is the induction of SVT for mapping and ablation.

## Programmed Atrial Stimulation

Delivery of single or double atrial extrastimuli may serve to study AV node physiology, determine the presence of an accessory pathway and its refractory period, and induce SVT. Single premature beats are delivered after fixed drive cycles (e.g., typically after eight-beat 600-, 500-, and/or 400-millisecond PCL atrial drive trains). Normal AV node physiology is characterized by decremental conduction: the faster the stimulation (shorter A1–A2 coupling intervals or faster PCLs), the more slowly the AV node conducts and the longer the AH interval becomes (Fig. 47–22, APD1 and APD2). The following are typical SVT substrates that may be demonstrated:

- *AH jump* (>50 milliseconds over a decrement of 10 in A1–S2) ⇒ dual AVN physiology (Fig. 47–22, APD 2 and APD3)
- *Induction of AV nodal echo beats or AVNRT* by occurrence of block typically in the fast pathway and conduction delay in the slow pathway, allowing recovery for retrograde fast pathway conduction and activation of a retrograde atrial depolarization (Fig. 47–22, APD3, and Fig. 47–23).
- *Induction of orthodromic AVRT* by causing antegrade block in the AP so it is excitable when the impulse returns to conduct retrograde to the atrium.

## Refractory Periods

As in the ventricle, refractory periods of the components of the anterograde conduction system can be determined and are defined as follows:

*Atrial effective refractory period (AERP)* = longest atrial coupling interval (A1–A2) that fails to capture the atrium, measured from pacing stimulus to pacing stimulus

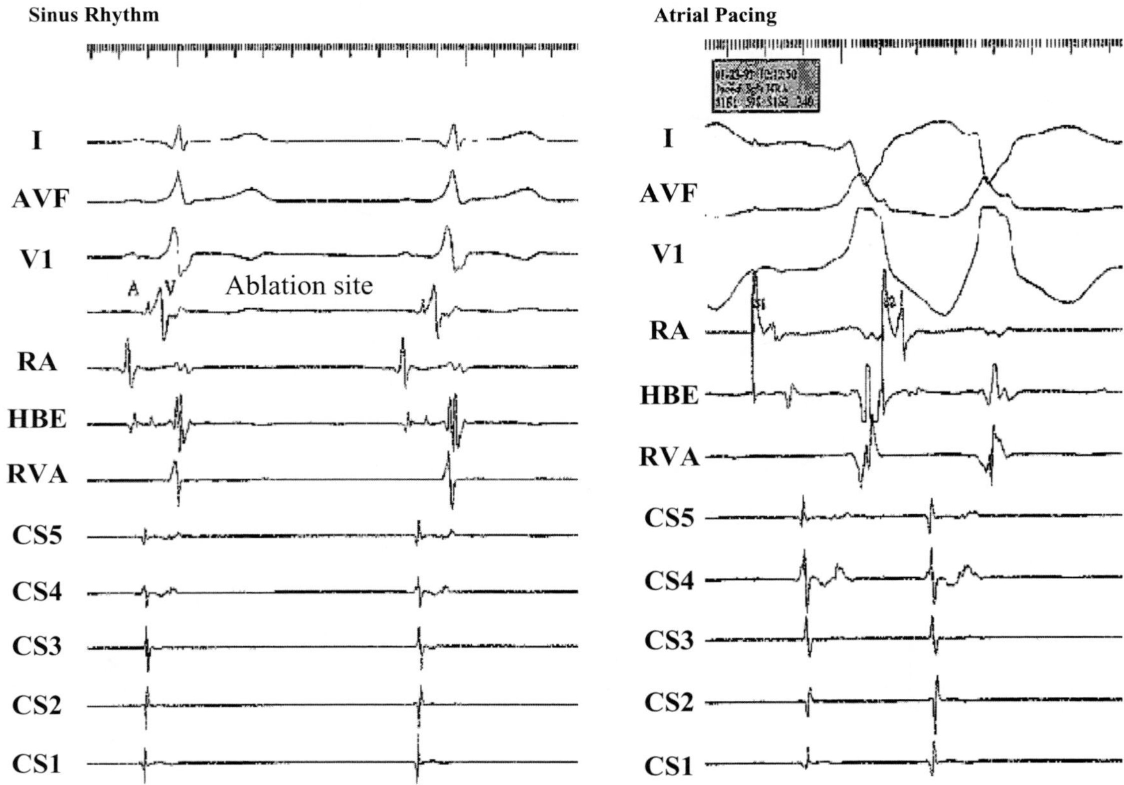


**Figure 47–21** Left free wall accessory pathway. In sinus rhythm **(left panel),** there is fusion of ventricular activation occurring via the atrial node and accessory pathway. During atrial pacing and introduction of premature atrial extrastimuli **(right panel),** pre-excitation becomes more manifest as activation via the AV node decrements and becomes later, leaving a larger component of ventricular activation to occur via the accessory pathway.

*Atrial functional refractory period (AFRP)* = shortest atrial coupling interval during premature atrial stimulation (A1–A2), measured from electrogram to electrogram

*Fast AVN pathway ERP* = longest atrial coupling interval that produces an AH jump to conduction via the slow pathway, measured from electrogram to electrogram during atrial extrastimulus testing

*Slow AVN pathway ERP* = longest atrial coupling interval that produces a block in slow pathway conduction (if only two pathways are present and fast pathway has already blocked, slow AVN pathway ERP = AVN ERP), measured from electrogram to electrogram during atrial extrastimulus testing

*Accessory pathway anterograde ERP* = longest atrial coupling interval that produces a block in accessory pathway conduction, measured from electrogram to electrogram during atrial extrastimulus testing

*Accessory pathway retrograde ERP* = longest ventricular coupling interval that produces a block in retrograde accessory pathway conduction, measured from electrogram to electrogram during ventricular extrastimulus testing.

### Minimum Pre-excited R–R during Atrial Fibrillation

Short R–R intervals suggest a short AP ERP and potentially increased risk.

### Activation Patterns

As discussed above, the pattern of atrial and ventricular activation is examined. The *anterograde ventricular activation sequence* is the sequence of ventricular activation during sinus rhythm, atrial pacing, atrial extrastimuli, or SVT. Eccentric activation of the coronary sinus suggests a left-sided accessory pathway (Fig. 47–18, left panel). The *atrial activation sequence* is the sequence of atrial activation during ventricular pacing, ventricular extrastimuli, or SVT. Eccentric retrograde activation of the coronary sinus suggests a left-sided accessory pathway (Fig. 47–18, right panel; Fig. 47–24).

### Inducible Supraventricular Tachyarrhythmias

Types of SVT that may be induced include the following:

*AV node re-entrant tachycardia (AVNRT):* AVNRT is usually associated with dual AV nodal pathway physiology (discontinuous AVN conduction curves; an AH

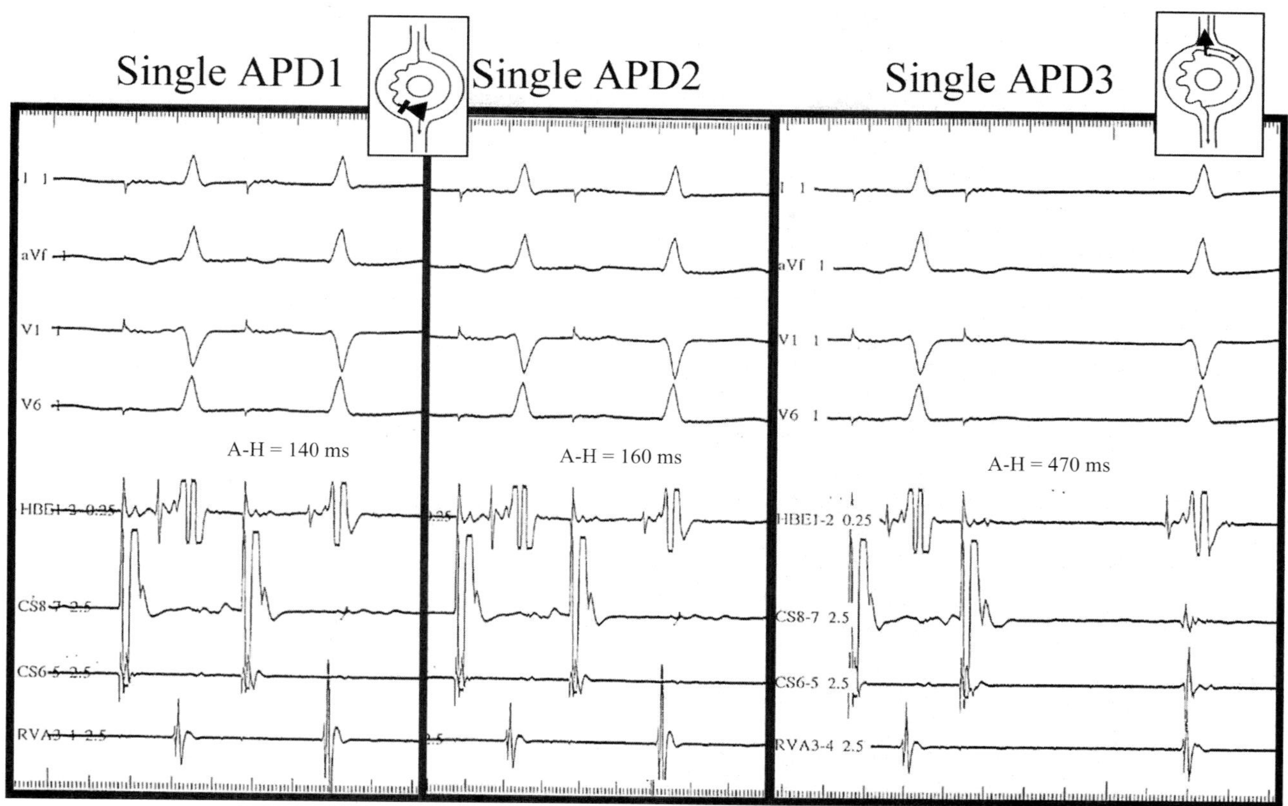


**Figure 47–22** Single atrial extrastimuli. Dual AV node physiology and induction of single typical AV node echo beat. Single APD1 and single APD2: decremental AVN conduction with longer AH interval after shorter A1–A2 coupling interval. Decremental AV node conduction is demonstrated with AH 140 and 160 milliseconds with shortening of APD coupling interval (APD1 to APD2). Single APD3: AH jump (>50-millisecond increase in AH interval for a 10-millisecond decrease in A1–A2 coupling interval) with single typical AV nodal echo (note atrial activation seen in the CS with a short VA interval). APD, atrial premature depolarization.

"jump") (Figs. 47–15, 47–22). In *typical AVNRT*, antegrade conduction occurs via the slow AVN pathway (long AH) and retrograde conduction via the fast AV node pathway with near-simultaneous atrial and ventricular activation (Figs. 47–22, 47–23). In *atypical AVNRT*, antegrade conduction occurs via the fast AVN pathway (with a short PR) and retrograde conduction via the slow AV node pathway (long R–P interval).

*Atrioventricular re-entrant tachycardia (AVRT):* AVRT refers to accessory pathway–mediated re-entrant tachycardia. In AVRT there is 1:1 AV association, as the atria and the ventricles are integral components of the reentrant circuit. In *orthodromic AVRT*, antegrade conduction occurs via the AV node (with a narrow QRS in the absence of bundle branch block/aberration) and retrograde conduction occurs via the accessory pathway (Figs. 47–25 and 47–26). In *antidromic AVRT*, antegrade conduction occurs via the accessory pathway (with wide QRS) and retrograde conduction via the AV node or another accessory pathway.

*Atrial flutter:* In *Type I (typical)* atrial flutter, right atrial activation proceeds in a counterclockwise activation pattern through the posterior isthmus between the inferior vena cava and tricuspid annulus. There may also be clockwise activation utilizing the isthmus. *Type II (atypical)* atrial flutter refers to atrial flutter using non–isthmus-dependent flutter circuits.

*Atrial tachycardia:* Atrial tachycardias may be macro–re-entrant in mechanism, including most incisional or scar-related atrial tachycardias, or due to ectopic (to the sinus node) foci and/or automatic mechanisms.

*Atrial fibrillation:* This most common sustained clinical arrhythmia typically initiates from pulmonary vein ostial or other focal triggering sites or micro–re-entrant circuits. It may sustain with multiple wandering re-entrant circuits.

*Sinus node re-entrant tachycardia:* This tachycardia is characterized by a similar P-wave morphology to sinus rhythm and may be induced and terminated with premature extrastimuli.

*Inappropriate sinus tachycardia (IST):* IST is characterized by inappropriately high resting sinus rate and enhanced sensitivity to adrenergic stimulation.

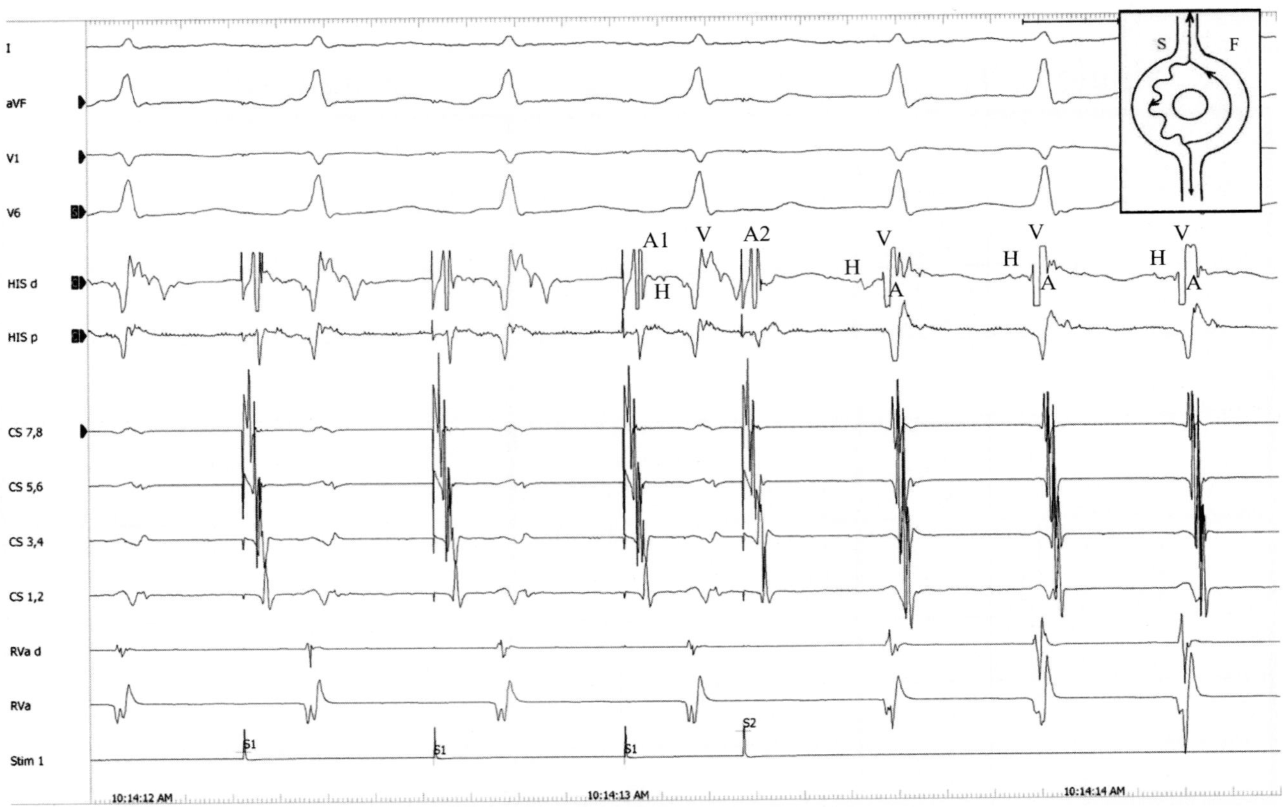


**Figure 47–23** Initiation of AVNRT single APDs CS 400/250 AH jump, initiation of AVNRT.

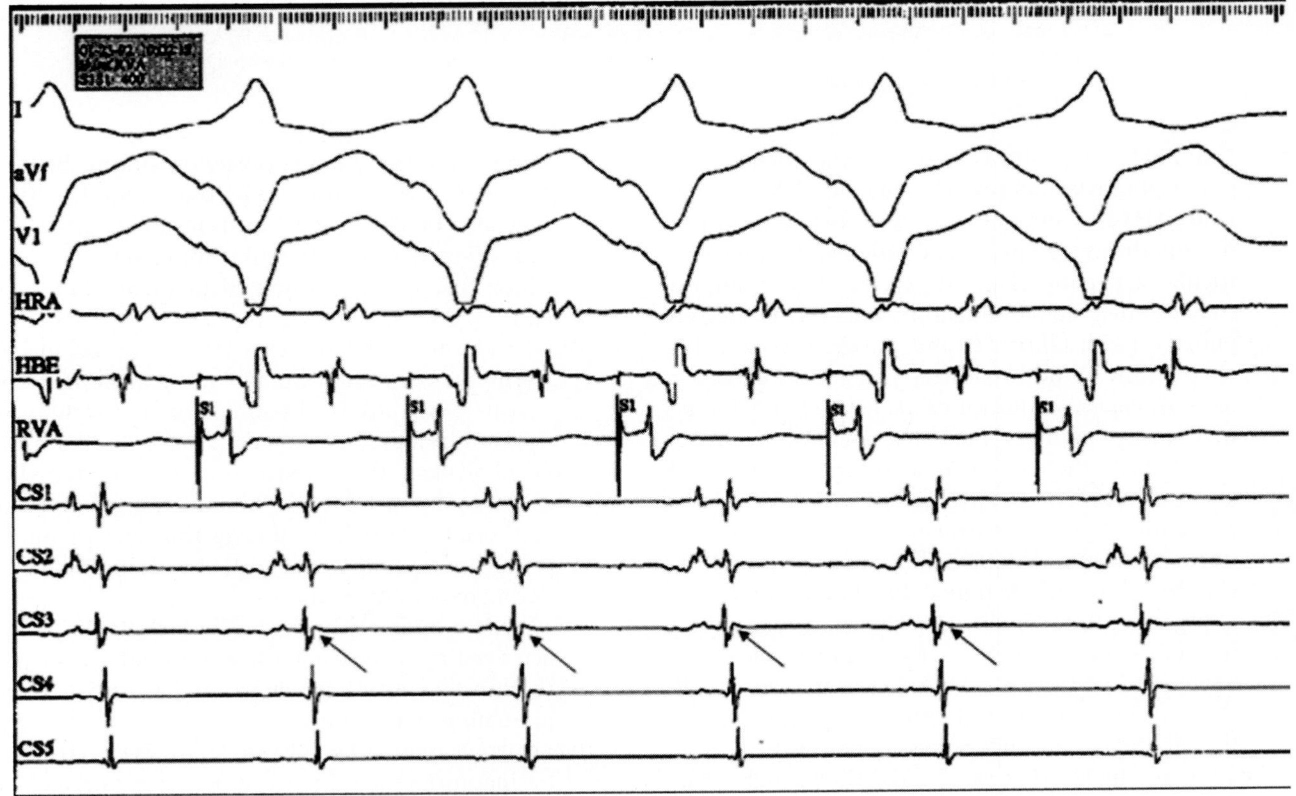


**Figure 47–24** Left-sided accessory pathway. Retrograde atrial activation during ventricular pacing—earliest retrograde atrial activation at CS 3 (*arrows*).

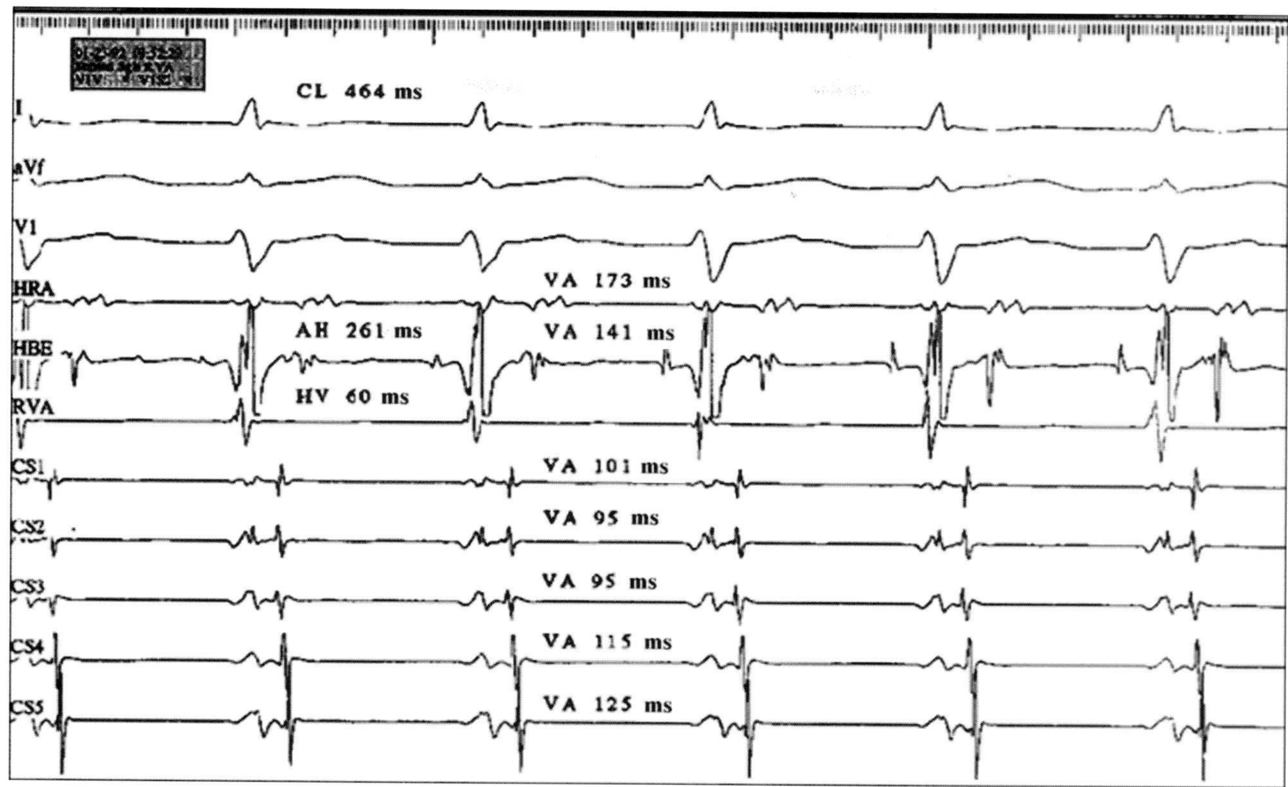


**Figure 47–25** Left-sided accessory pathway mediating orthodromic AVRT—earliest retrograde atrial activation occurs via an accessory pathway at CS 2–3 (VA interval 95 milliseconds).

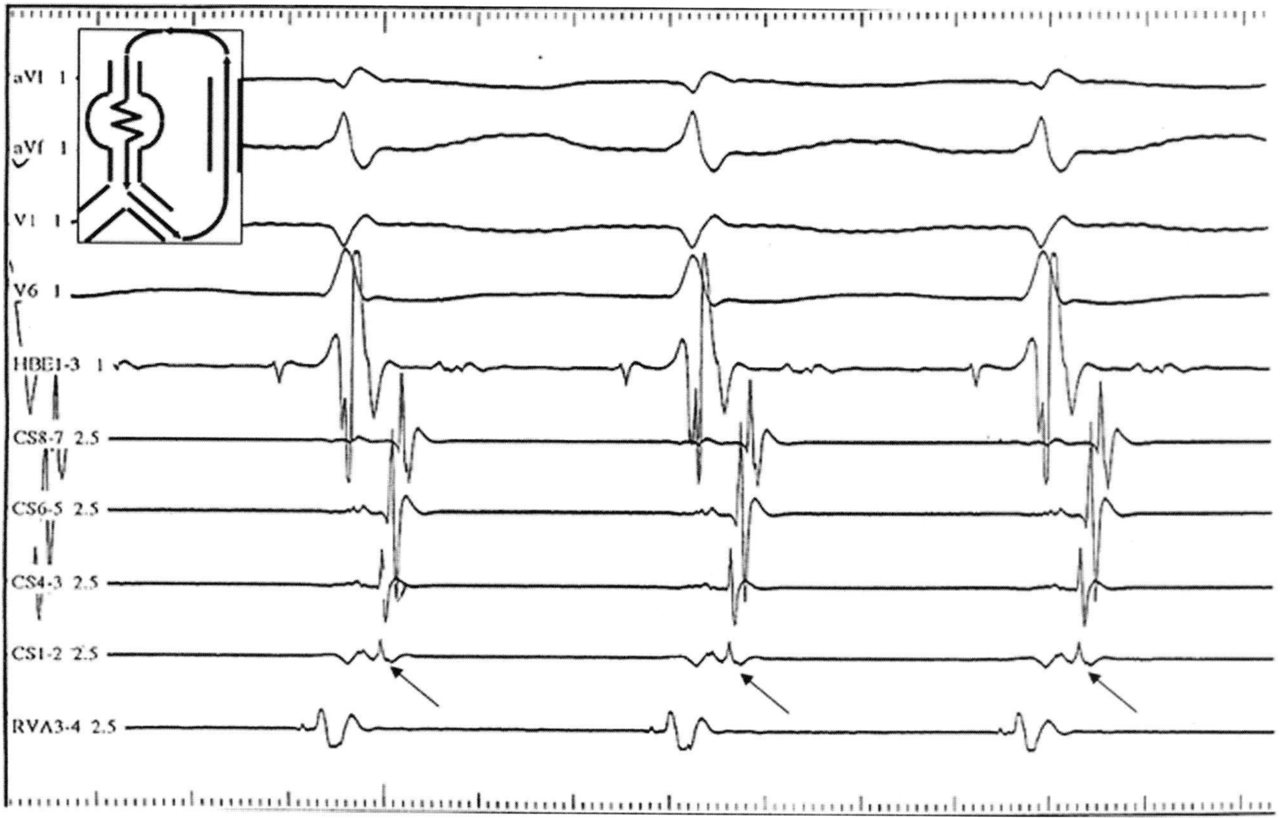


**Figure 47–26** Left free wall accessory pathway mediating orthodromic AVRT—earliest atrial activation occurs in the distal coronary sinus at CS 1–2 (*arrows*).

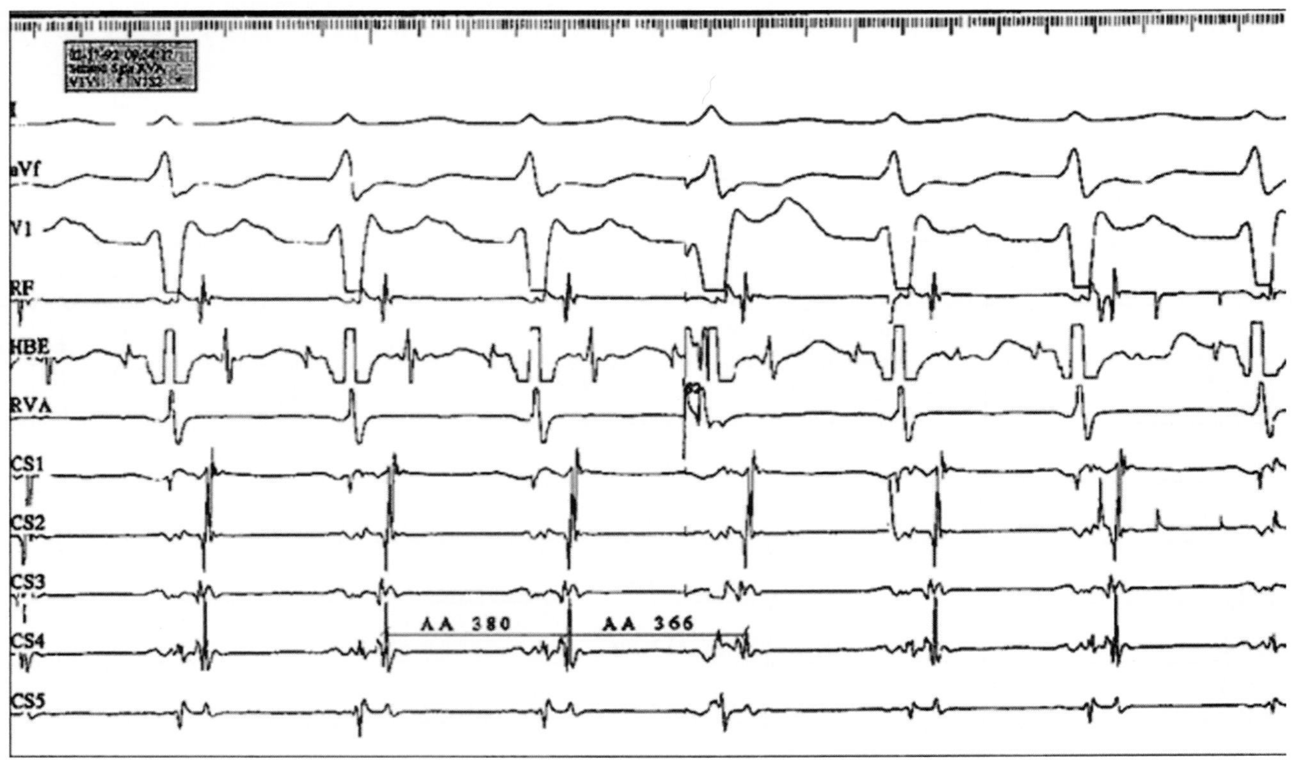


**Figure 47–27** Orthodromic AVRT with single VPD introduced during His refractoriness. The single ventricular extrastimulus delivered during His bundle refractoriness advances retrograde atrial activation, suggesting the presence of a retrogradely conducting accessory pathway, in this case located in the right posteroseptal region.

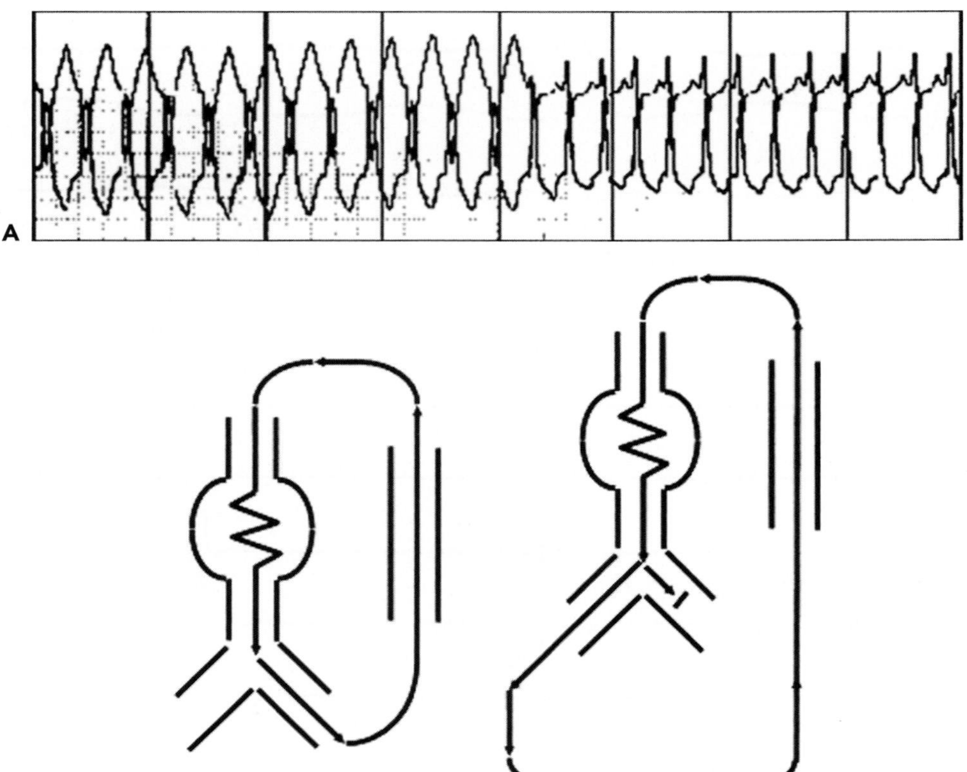


**Figure 47–28** **A:** Conversion of wide complex to narrow complex tachycardia with longer RR interval during wide complex tachycardia. This is diagnostic for AVRT with an accessory pathway ipsilateral to the bundle branch block. **B:** Orthodromic AVRT with ipsilateral BBB. BBB aberration ipsilateral to the accessory pathway results in longer retrograde (VA) activation times as a result of additional time required for transseptal myocardial conduction.

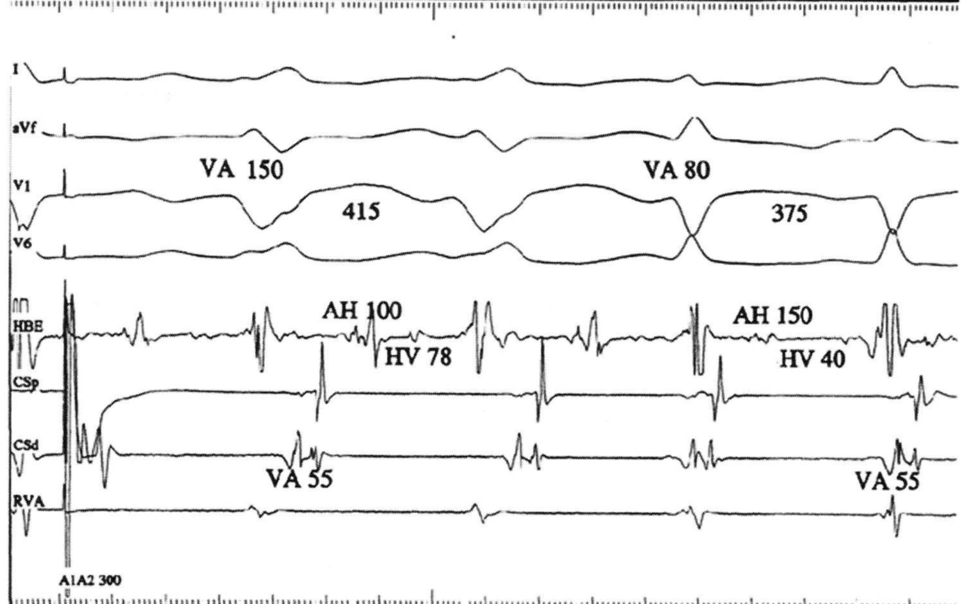


**Figure 47–29** Initiation of orthodromic AVRT with initial LBBB aberration. Retrograde VA activation times are longer during LBBB aberration, indicating participation of a left-sided accessory pathway. Local VA time measured nearest the accessory pathway (CS distal 55 milliseconds) are similar, but earliest V to atrial activation is longer with LBBB aberration.

## Evaluation during Tachycardia

Once a tachycardia is induced, various observations and maneuvers can be performed to help determine the SVT mechanism. These include the following.

- Morphology: Narrow complex, RBBB or LBBB aberrant conduction, or pre-excited
- Atrial activation sequence
- Ventricular activation sequence
- HA or VA interval: Short HA interval (<100 milliseconds) suggests AVNRT, longer HA intervals (>100 milliseconds) suggests orthodromic AVRT mediated by an accessory pathway.

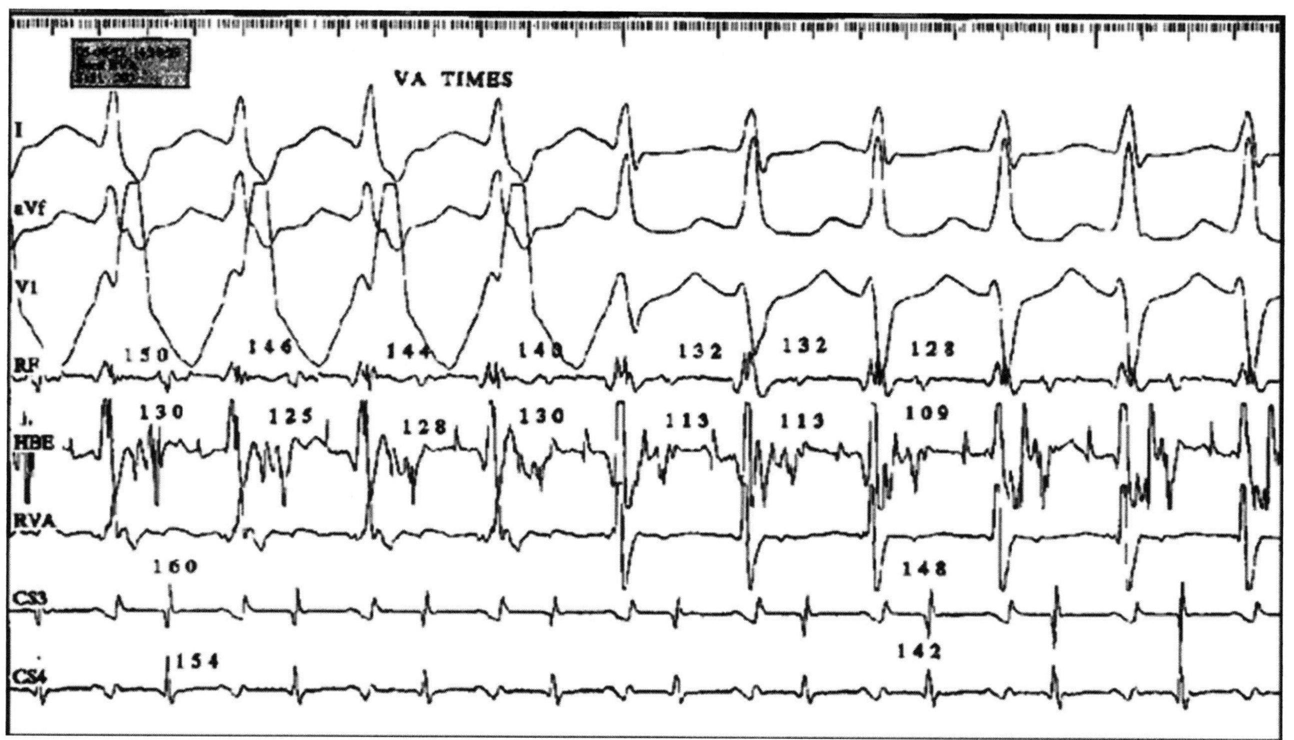


**Figure 47–30** RBBB aberration during AVRT utilizing a right posteroseptal accessory pathway. Retrograde VA activation times are longer during RBBB aberration, confirming the presence of a right-sided accessory pathway.

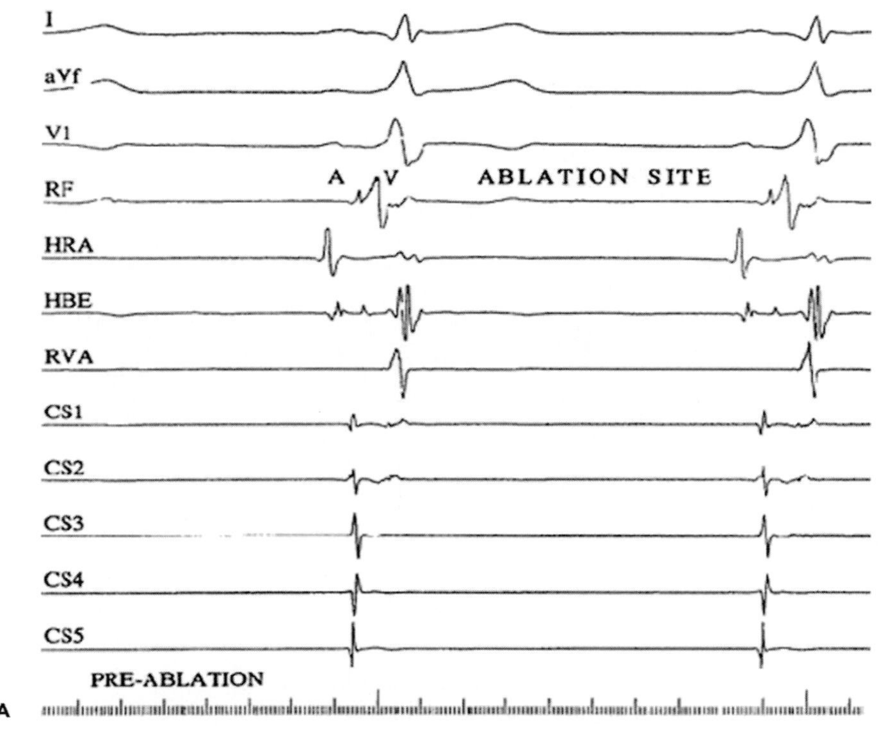


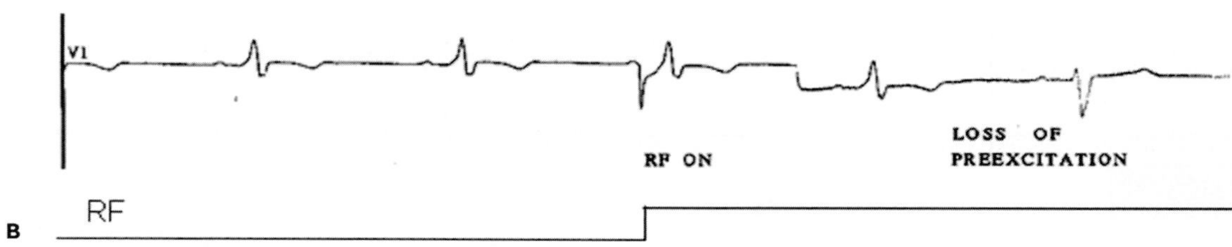


**Figure 47–31** Left-sided accessory pathway. **A:** Successful ablation site. **B:** Radiofrequency ablation.

- Single ventricular premature extrastimuli during SVT (Fig. 47–27): If single ventricular premature extrastimuli delivered during His refractoriness advances retrograde atrial activation, then a retrogradely conducting or concealed accessory pathway is present. However, this only demonstrates the presence of an accessory pathway. It does not prove that the pathway is an integral part of the circuit, as it could be a bystander pathway.
- Bundle branch block aberration in SVT (Figs. 47–28, 47–29, and 47–30): VA interval prolongation during aberration in SVT indicates a retrogradely conducting accessory pathway ipsilateral to the bundle branch block. On a surface ECG recording, this may be manifest by a longer cycle length (slower rate) during the wide complex tachycardia/aberration than during narrow complex conduction (Fig. 47–28). The prolongation of the cycle length occurs as a result of a prolongation of VA conduction times. Bundle branch block aberration ipsilateral to the accessory pathway results in longer retrograde (VA) activation times as a result of the additional time required for transseptal myocardial conduction (Figs. 47–28, 47–29, and 47–30). Demonstration of such a change in VA time with aberration confirms the presence of the accessory pathway ipsilateral to the bundle branch blocked and also indicates that the accessory pathway is a component of the re-entrant circuit.

## Mapping during Ablation

A diagnostic EP study is critical to confirmation and definition of arrhythmia substrate prior to ablation of most supraventricular and ventricular tachycardias. Currently, various mapping techniques based on determination of earliest activation sites include the utilization of electrophysiologic recordings and various electroanatomic, contact catheter, and noncontact mapping systems that can graphically tag and record activation times in three-dimensional space with computer generation of a display of activation or voltage maps. Although ablation of some arrhythmias is based on anatomic location (e.g. slow pathway region for AV node reentrant tachycardia or pulmonary vein antral isolation for atrial fibrillation ablation), successful ablation of other tachycardias often requires determination of the earliest site of activation, which helps to determine the location of the targeted arrhythmia substrate. An example is shown in Figure 47–31, which demonstrates the fusion of atrial and ventricular electrograms on the ablation catheter at the site of an accessory pathway. In this circumstance, ablation using radiofrequency energy resulted in prompt ablation of the pathway, loss of ventricular pre-excitation, and restoration of normal AV conduction.

## SUMMARY

This chapter has summarized the components of a comprehensive diagnostic electrophysiology study. For users of this book preparing for Cardiovascular Board exam review, I suggest focusing on:

- Recognition of the His bundle electrogram and determination of the sites of AV block (AV nodal versus infra-Hisian block)
- Recognition of VA dissociation during wide complex tachycardia using intracardiac electrograms, indicating the rhythm is most likely ventricular tachycardia
- Recognition of the initiation of AV node reentrant tachycardia with demonstration of an "AH jump" and induction of an SVT with near-simultaneous atrial and ventricular activation
- Recognition of a left free wall accessory pathway with abnormal, eccentric early activation via a more distal coronary sinus location (e.g., rather than the normal earliest activation at the septum and later activation in the lateral coronary sinus/left atrial or ventricular free wall)
- Recognition that the ipsilateral bundle branch block during SVT causing a longer cycle length or longer VA time indicates the presence of an accessory pathway

## REFERENCES


1. Buxton AE, Lee KL, Fisher JD, et al. A randomized study of the prevention of sudden death in patients with coronary artery disease. Multicenter Unsustained Tachycardia Trial Investigators. *N Engl J Med.* 1999;341:1882–1890.
2. Gregoratos G, Abrams J, Epstein AE, et al. ACC/AHA/NASPE 2002 guideline update for implantation of cardiac pacemakers and antiarrhythmia devices—summary article: a report of the American College of Cardiology/American Heart Association Task Force on Practice Guidelines (ACC/AHA/NASPE Committee to Update the 1998 Pacemaker Guidelines). *J Am Coll Cardiol.* 2002;40:1703–1719.
3. Blomstrom-Lundqvist C, Scheinman MM, Aliot EM, et al. ACC/AHA/ESC guidelines for the management of patients with supraventricular arrhythmias—executive summary. a report of the American College of Cardiology/American Heart Association Task Force on Practice Guidelines and the European Society of Cardiology Committee for Practice Guidelines (writing committee to develop guidelines for the management of patients with supraventricular arrhythmias) developed in collaboration with NASPE-Heart Rhythm Society. *J Am Coll Cardiol.* 2003;42:1493–1531.
4. Tracy CM, Akhtar M, DiMarco JP, et al. American College of Cardiology/American Heart Association clinical competence statement on invasive electrophysiology studies, catheter ablation, and cardioversion. A report of the American College of Cardiology/American Heart Association/American College of Physicians—American Society of Internal Medicine Task Force on Clinical Competence. *J Am Coll Cardiol.* 2000;36:1725–1736.
5. Moss AJ, Hall WJ, Cannom DS, et al. Improved survival with an implanted defibrillator in patients with coronary disease at high risk for ventricular arrhythmia. Multicenter Automatic Defibrillator Implantation Trial Investigators. *N Engl J Med.* 1996;335:1933–1940.
6. Moss AJ, Zareba W, Hall WJ, et al. Prophylactic implantation of a defibrillator in patients with myocardial infarction and reduced ejection fraction. *N Engl J Med.* 2002;346:877–883.
7. Kadish A, Dyer A, Daubert JP, et al. Prophylactic defibrillator implantation in patients with nonischemic dilated cardiomyopathy. *N Engl J Med.* 2004;350:2151–2158.
8. Bardy GH, Lee KL, Mark DB, et al. Amiodarone or an implantable cardioverter-defibrillator for congestive heart failure. *N Engl J Med.* 2005;352:225–237.


## QUESTIONS

1. Where is the site of the block?

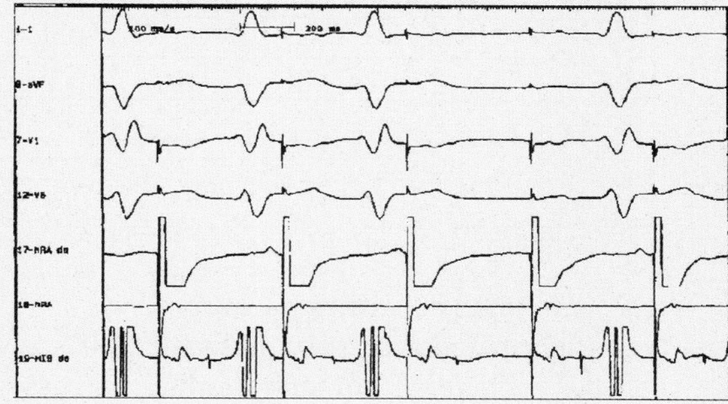

a. AV node
b. Infra-His
c. Intra-His
d. AV node and infra-His

Answer is b: The tracing shows atrial pacing with RBBB and second-degree AV block without prolongation of the PR or AH intervals prior to the blocked beat (third paced beat). On this third paced beat, the His electrode shows an atrial electrogram followed by a His deflection, but no subsequent ventricular electrogram or QRS. Thus, the block occurs below the bundle of His (infra-Hisian block).

**2.** Where is the site of the block?

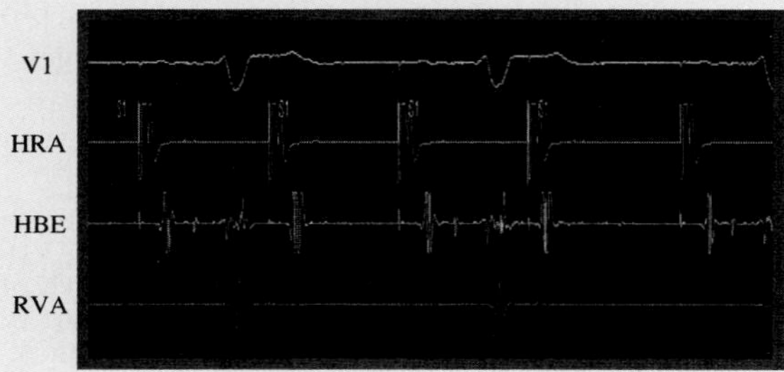


a. AV node
b. Infra-His
c. Intra-His
d. AV node and infra-His

Answer is a: The tracing shows atrial pacing (S1 drive) with 2:1 AV block. Inspection of the His bundle electrogram tracings demonstrate S1 atrial pacing stimuli flowed by atrial electrograms. After the first paced beat, there is a His bundle electrogram followed by a ventricular electrogram and QRS on the surface ECG. After the second paced beat, no His bundle electrogram follows the atrial electrogram. The next paced beats repeat this pattern. The block is at the level of the AV node, because conduction is blocked prior to arrival to the His bundle.

**3.** Where is the site of the block?

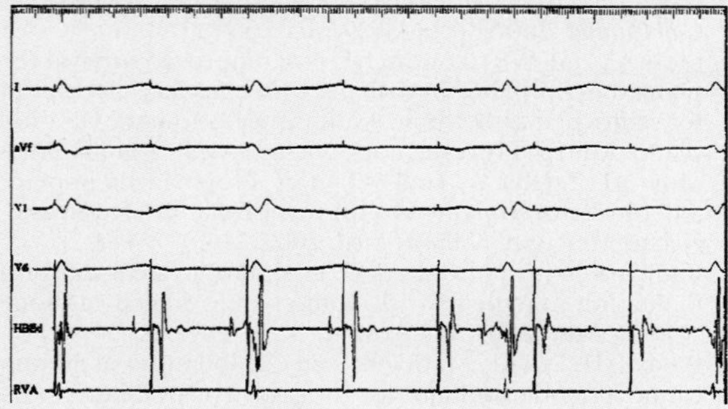


a. AV node
b. Infra-His
c. Intra-His
d. AV node and infra-His

Answer is d: This tracing shows second-degree AV block during atrial pacing. The His bundle electrogram demonstrates the atrial pacing stimuli followed by atrial electrograms. After the first atrial paced beat, there is a long AH interval followed by a His electrogram, but no ventricular electrogram or QRS. This beat blocks below the bundle of His. After the second paced beat there is a slightly longer AH interval followed by a ventricular electrogram on the RVA tracing and a corresponding surface QRS. After the third paced beat, the AH is longer still but there is no conduction after the His electrogram to the ventricles. This beat again shows infra-Hisian block. After the fourth paced beat, there is no His electrogram. This beat blocks in the AV node and the series shows AV node Wenckebach occurring (gradually prolonging AH interval followed by block in the AV node). The fifth paced beat shows conduction after the block with a shorter AH interval followed by conduction to the ventricles. The sixth paced beat shows a small His deflection with slightly longer AH, but infra-Hisian block (no ventricular activation). The seventh paced beat shows a slightly longer AH interval with conduction to the ventricles. Thus, the tracing demonstrates two levels of block, in the AVN (Mobitz I Wenckebach pattern) and infra-Hisian block.

**4.** What is the diagnosis?

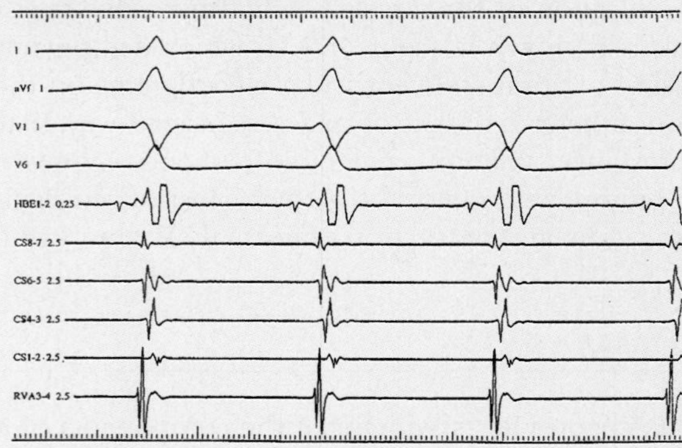


a. Orthodromic AVRT
b. Left-sided accessory pathway
c. Atrial tachycardia
d. AV node re-entrant tachycardia

Answer is d: The tracing shows a narrow QRS-complex tachycardia with a cycle length of 350 milliseconds. The coronary sinus atrial electrograms show a concentric atrial activation pattern (earliest at CS 7–8 at the septum and later at more distal CS electrodes) with near simultaneous activation of the atrium and ventricle. The earliest atrial activation is likely the small deflection at the onset of the QRS on the HBE tracing, which actually slightly precedes the ventricular activation. This pattern is consistent with AV node re-entrant tachycardia.

**5.** What is the diagnosis?

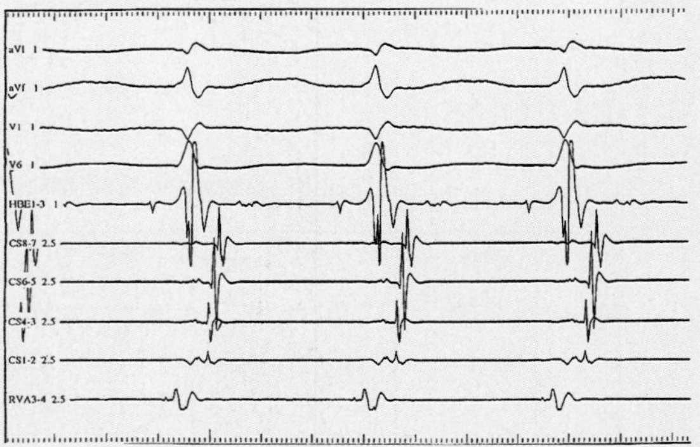


a. Left-sided accessory pathway
b. Right-sided accessory pathway
c. AV node reentrant tachycardia
d. Sinus tachycardia

Answer is a: This tracing shows a narrow complex tachycardia with a cycle length of 370 milliseconds. The anterograde activation occurs via the AV node and His–Purkinje system (AH seen in HBE1–3 with narrow QRS). The earliest atrial activation occurs in the distal CS as CS 1–2. This eccentric activation pattern indicates retrograde activation via a left lateral accessory pathway. The tachycardia is consistent with orthodromic atrioventricular reentrant tachycardia using a retrogradely conducting left-sided accessory pathway.

# Supraventricular Tachycardias

# 48

***Jennifer E. Cummings Robert A. Schweikert***

Supraventricular tachycardias (SVTs) continue to be the most common as well as most diverse type of cardiac arrhythmia. SVTs may occur in all age groups and are associated with a wide range of etiologies, heart rates, frequency, and severity of heart disease. The numerous potential mechanisms and variety of descriptive adjectives for these arrhythmias make establishing a succinct classification system difficult. Approaches to classification of SVT include: (a) clinical behavior (i.e., paroxysmal, persistent, permanent, incessant, sustained, nonsustained, chronic, and repetitive); (b) mechanism (i.e., ectopic, automatic, reentrant, reciprocating, slow/fast, fast/slow, orthodromic, and antidromic); (c) electrocardiographic appearance (i.e., narrow or wide QRS); and finally, (d) location (i.e., sinus, atrial, and atrioventricular [AV] nodal/junctional). The type of classification may provide important information in the diagnosis and treatment of SVTs. Clinicians often have difficulty determining a consistent and inclusive comprehensive management algorithm that may be easily and consistently applied to all forms of SVTs. This chapter briefly reviews not only the most common SVTs but also provides a concise approach to diagnosis that incorporates all four methods of classification.

Symptoms from SVT may range from none to profoundly disabling. SVT generally presents with a variety of symptoms, the most common of which is palpitation. Palpitation may be accompanied by shortness of breath, chest pain, lightheadedness, syncope, and/or near-syncope. The noninvasive cardiac evaluation of palpitation may include ambulatory Holter monitoring, cardiac event recording, transtelephonic monitoring, and, less commonly, an implantable loop recorder. The goals of this noninvasive process are twofold. First, it is necessary to document the arrhythmia for diagnostic evaluation. Second, it is helpful to correlate symptoms with a documented arrhythmia. Although ambulatory Holter monitoring is easy to obtain and thus frequently ordered for patients with suspected SVT, its diagnostic yield is very low. Symptoms and simultaneous electrocardiographic abnormalities are observed in only 2% to 13% of 24-hour ambulatory Holter monitors. In contrast, the patient-activated cardiac event recorder provides a greater yield and is more cost effective than ambulatory Holter monitoring in the correlation of arrhythmia with transient symptoms (1).

The newer implantable loop recorders are placed subcutaneously at a parasternal chest site, similar to a pacemaker. These monitors can record arrhythmias for >1 year. They record both when activated by an external trigger or following automatic programmed parameters within the device. Because implantation of this device is considered invasive, it is reserved for those patients with sudden and dramatic symptom onset associated with tachyarrhythmic episodes or those patients with very rare but debilitating symptoms.

## APPROACHING SUPRAVENTRICULAR TACHYCARDIA: AV NODE DEPENDENT VERSUS ATRIAL AND SINUS NODE DEPENDENT

In terms of evaluating arrhythmias based on site of origin, there are essentially three types of SVT: (a) sinus node dependent (sinus tachycardia, inappropriate sinus tachycardia, and sinus node re-entry); (b) atrial dependent (atrial tachycardia, atrial flutter, and atrial fibrillation); and (c) AV node/junction dependent (AV node re-entry tachycardia [AVNRT] and AV reciprocating tachycardia [AVRT]). The first step in classifying supraventricular tachycardias is to differentiate the sinus and atrial tachycardias from AV node/junctional tachycardias (2,3). This difference is easiest to see if the tachycardia is observed during changes in AV node conduction. AV node conduction can be altered by a change in vagal tone or with medications such as calcium channel blockers or adenosine. If spontaneous changes in vagal tone do not change AV node conduction, maneuvers may be performed to prolong AV node conduction and refractoriness. Physiologic maneuvers include deep breathing, carotid sinus massage, and the strain phase of the Valsalva maneuver. Carotid sinus massage increases vagal tone and is easily performed at the bedside. In older patients, it is important to exclude the presence of significant carotid artery atherosclerotic disease before performing carotid sinus massage. The "diving reflex" can also be used with pediatric patients. This can be done by placing a plastic bag filled with ice water on the patient's face for 15 to 20 seconds. Though this maneuver may be effective, it is less well tolerated and therefore not frequently used.

If physiologic maneuvers are unsuccessful, drugs may also be used to alter AV node conduction. Edrophonium chloride (Tensilon) was used classically because its potent vagotonic effect creates temporary AV node block; however, it is often poorly tolerated and therefore is no longer commonly used. Verapamil and diltiazem can also be used to create temporary AV node block. These calcium channel–blocking medications have a slow onset and, allowing for a "gentler" diagnosis than sudden AV node block. However, calcium channel blockers have potential for side effects such as hypotension. Adenosine is the most commonly used drug for this purpose because of its extremely short half-life (approximately 9 seconds). Adenosine provides a very transient AV node block. This effect is maximized when it is administered in a rapid intravenous bolus via a central vein.

Observing tachycardia behavior during slowed AV conduction or AV block will help differentiate between sinus/atrial and AV nodal/junctional tachycardias. Perpetuation of the tachycardia, despite AV block occurs primarily with atrial/sinus tachycardias (Fig. 48–1). Termination of the tachycardia as a result of AV block often implicates the AV node as an essential part of the tachycardia circuit (thus an AV node/junctional-dependent tachycardia). There are only rare exceptions to this rule. First, there have been reports of atrial tachycardias that terminate with adenosine administration. However, these atrial tachycardias often slow gradually before terminating, as compared to AV node-dependent arrhythmias, which terminate suddenly. Additionally, if the tachycardia breaks spontaneously, examining the termination can provide insight as to whether the tachycardia is atrial/sinus or AV nodal/junctional. If the tachycardia terminates with a P wave that is not followed by a QRS (Fig. 48–2), it is most consistent with an AV nodal/junctional-dependent tachycardia. This is best explained by understanding that if the rhythm had been an atrial tachycardia, it would have had to terminate at the atrial focus and develop AV block simultaneously, which is very unlikely.

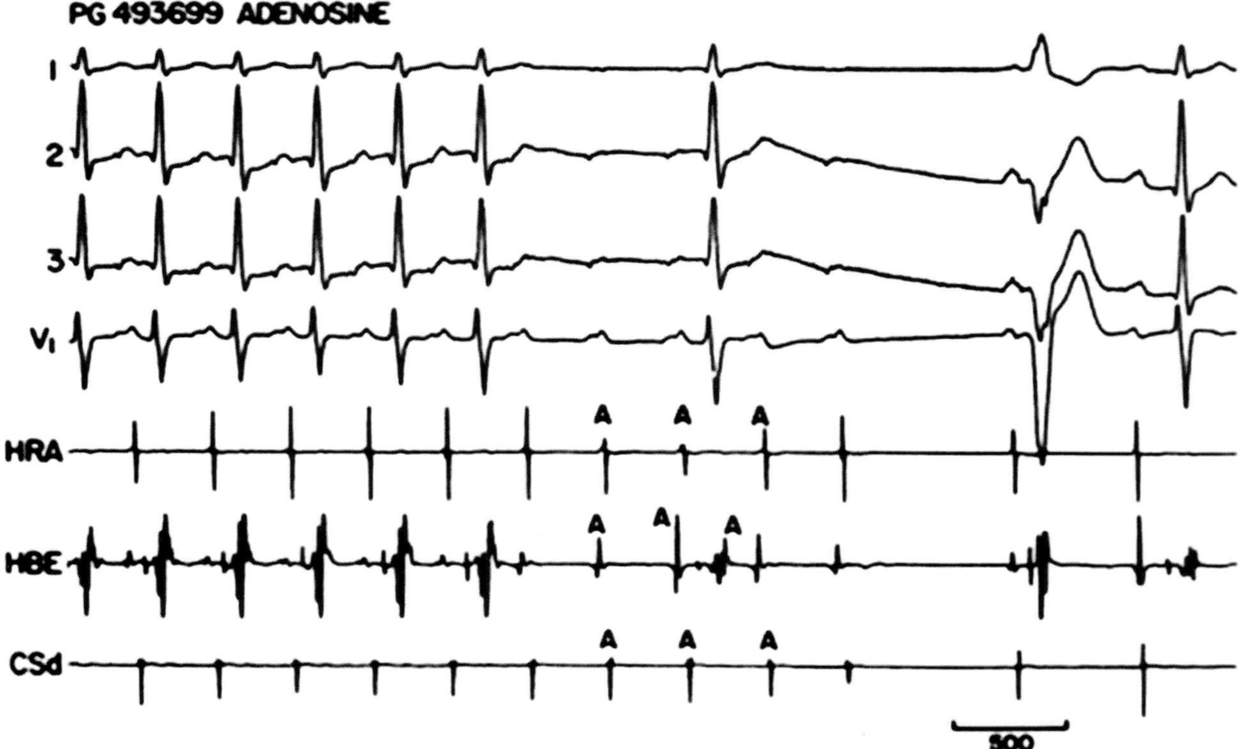


**Figure 48–1** Atrial tachycardia terminating following the administration of adenosine demonstrating continuation of the atrial tachycardia despite block in the AV node. This would imply that the tachycardia is not AV nodal dependant.

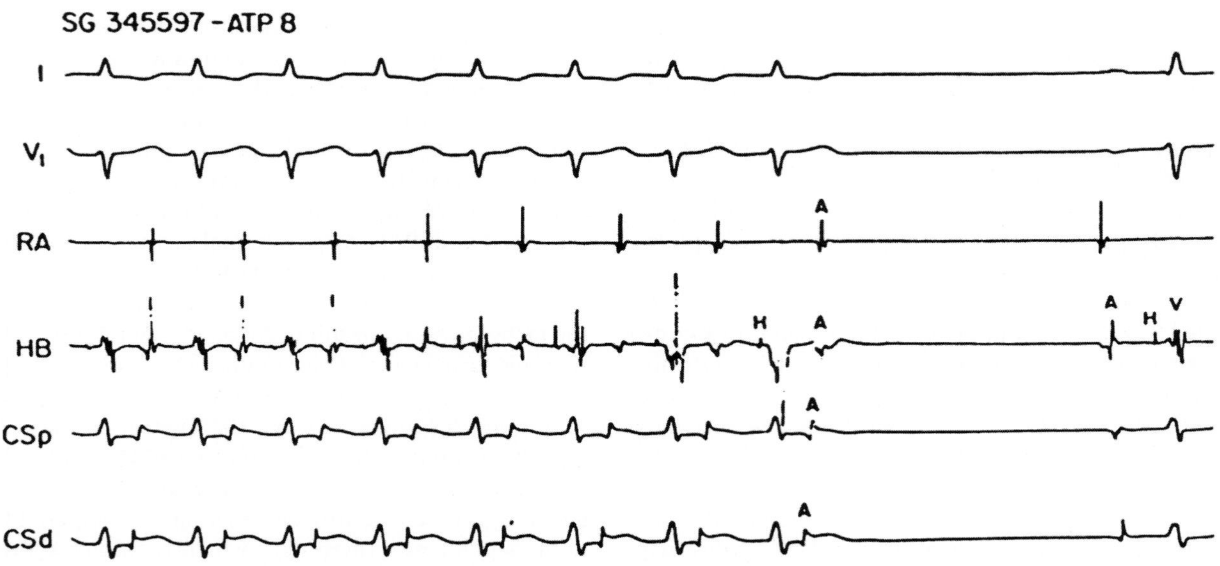


**Figure 48–2** AV nodal/junctional-dependent tachycardia.

Other electrocardiographic findings are helpful in distinguishing sinus/atrial-dependent from AV nodal/junctional-dependent tachycardia. The P-wave axis indicates the origin of atrial depolarization, which may help differentiate sinus/atrial from AV junction tachycardia. A "high to low" activation sequence is manifested by a surface electrocardiogram positive P-wave deflection in leads II, III, and avF. This is most consistent with a sinus or high atrial tachycardia. In contrast, AV junctional tachycardias must activate the atria from the area at the AV ring (often near the AV node), leading to opposite "low to high" activation.

If the tachycardia appears to have a 1:1 P:QRS relationship, examining the relationship of the R wave to the following P wave may provide additional information to differentiate between sinus/atrial versus AV nodal/junctional tachycardias. If the distance from the R to the following P wave is <50% of the R–R distance, the tachycardia is termed "short RP." If the distance from the R to the following P is >50% of the R–R distance, the tachycardia is termed "long RP." A short RP interval is more often seen in AV nodal/junctional-dependent tachycardias (AVNRT and AVRT) and a long RP interval is more often seen in sinus/atrial tachycardias. However, this rule also has exceptions that should be noted. Long RP tachycardias, though typically indicative of sinus/atrial dependence, can be seen in *atypical* (fast–slow) AVNRT (as described later in this chapter) or in an unusual form of AVRT that occurs in an accessory pathway with decremental properties. This is seen in the permanent form of junctional reciprocating tachycardia (PJRT). Also, sinus tachycardia with a long first-degree AV block may present with a short R–P interval.

In <50% of patients, an appreciable P wave may not be clearly distinct from the QRS. This may be because the P wave is hidden within the QRS complex or because the rate and artifact of the tachycardia mask the P wave. In *typical* AV node re-entrant tachycardia the P wave generally occurs simultaneously with the QRS. In this arrhythmia, the P wave is often inscribed in the terminal part of the QRS and results in pseudo-r deflection in V1 or S wave in II, III, and aVF. However, appreciation of this change may require comparison of the QRS during tachycardia with the electrocardiogram (ECG) in normal sinus rhythm.

## AV NODE-DEPENDENT TACHYCARDIAS: AVNRT VERSUS AVRT

Once the above methods have been used to establish whether the rhythm is AV nodal dependent, further evaluation is needed to determine what type of AV nodal/junctional tachycardia is present. Junctional or AV node-dependent tachycardias include: (a) AV node re-entrant tachycardia (AVNRT); and (b) AV reciprocating tachycardia (AVRT) using an accessory pathway.

### AV Nodal Re-entry Tachycardia

#### *Clinical Presentation and Diagnosis*

In patients without ventricular pre-excitation who are in sinus rhythm, typical AVNRT is the most common mechanism of SVT, accounting for >60% of presenting SVTs (4–6).

As shown in Table 48–1, AVNRT is seen in children as well as in the elderly; however, it is most common in the fourth decade. This arrhythmia affects women more often than men, as women represent two thirds of the patients with AVNRT. There is no known association with other structural heart disease. Although palpitation is the primary symptom of this arrhythmia, syncope and

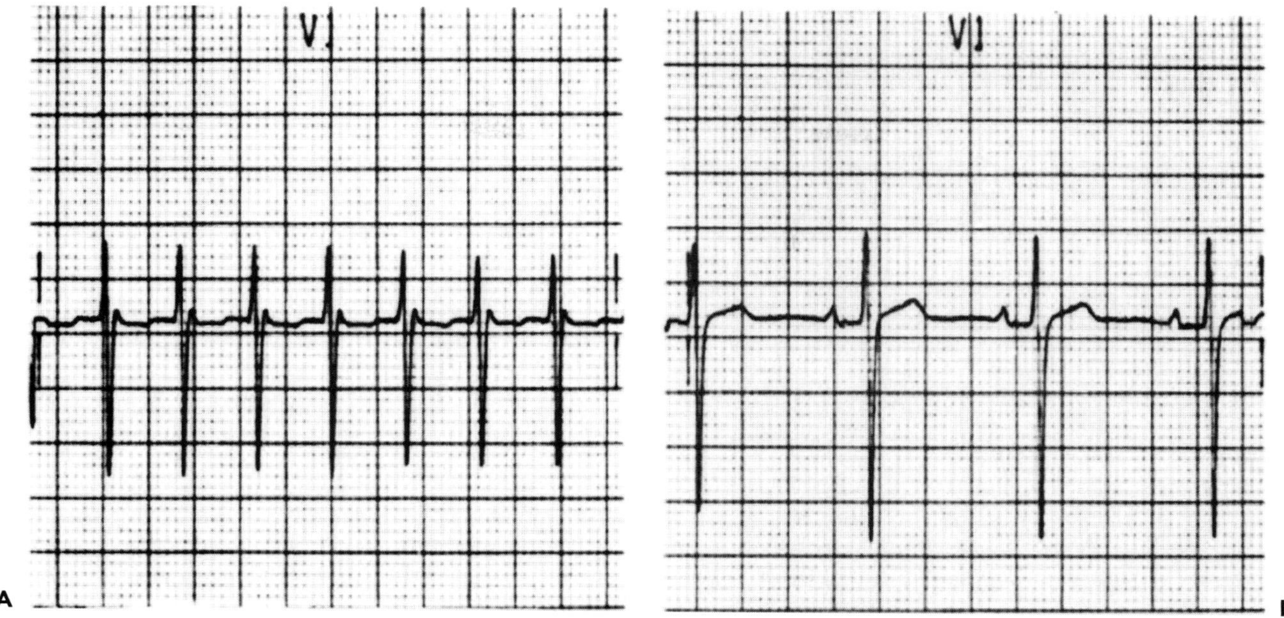


**Figure 48–3** ECG in normal sinus rhythm.

near-syncope have been observed, most notably in elderly patients. Because the right atrium is activated nearly simultaneously with the right ventricle, it is often contracting against a closed tricuspid valve, causing many patients to feel neck fullness. Because this is an AV node-dependent arrhythmia, termination can be achieved with AV nodal blockade, as with Valsalva, carotid sinus massage, or IV adenosine. Termination is characteristically abrupt, often with a retrograde P wave (negative P-wave axis in the inferior leads) without a subsequent QRS. Because a portion or all of the re-entry circuit is within the AV node, the atrial and ventricular activation are nearly simultaneous, thus this is a very "short RP" tachycardia. In fact, the retrograde P wave is frequently hidden in the QRS complex.

### Mechanism

The electrophysiologic circuit of AVNRT uses regions of tissue within or adjacent to the AV node that possess different electrophysiologic properties. Patients with AVNRT have what is termed *dual AV node physiology.* This means that within/near the AV node there is a fast conducting pathway with a long refractory period and a slower conducting pathway with a shorter refractory period. In *typical* AVNRT (slow–fast form) there is antegrade conduction (from the atria to the ventricles) over the slower pathway and retrograde (back from the ventricles toward the atrium) conduction over the fast pathway (Fig. 48–4). AVNRT typically initiates with a premature atrial beat that arrives at the AV node when the fast pathway is still refractory (longer refractory

**TABLE 48–1**

**NARROW-QRS TACHYCARDIA: CLINICAL AND ELECTROPHYSIOLOGIC CHARACTERISTICS**

| | Common AVN Re-entry | Orthodromic Tachycardia | Long-RP Tachycardia | Atrial |
|---|---|---|---|---|
| Age (y) | 56 ± 19 | 35 ± 15 | 56 ± 24 | 61.5 ± 6 |
| Range | 19–80 | 19–56 | 22–78 | 56–70 |
| Female gender (%) | 70 | 54 | 50 | 50 |
| Cycle length (ms) | 357.5 ± 56.8 | 321.25 ± 60 | 510 ± 10 | 373.3 ± 37.3 |
| Range | 230–450 | 220–420 | 500–520 | 320–400 |
| P polarity (%) | — | — | 100% | 70% |
| Typical P location (%) | 100 | 42 | 100 | 70 |
| QRS alternation (%) | 8 | 36 | 0 | 0 |

Diagnostic categories listed in the table represent the final diagnosis made at electrophysiology study. P polarity was not identifiable in AV node re-entry and orthodromic tachycardia.

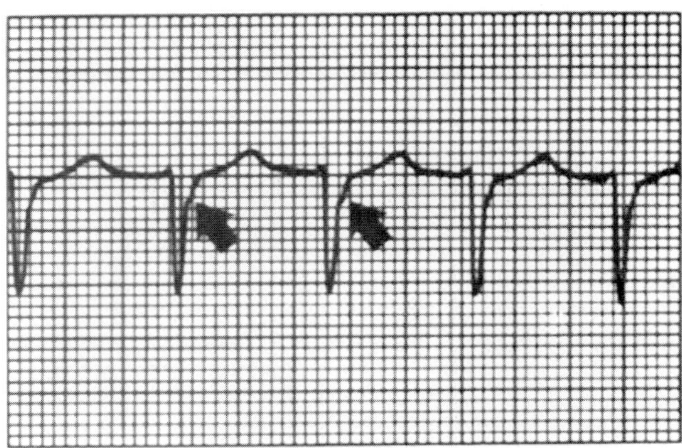

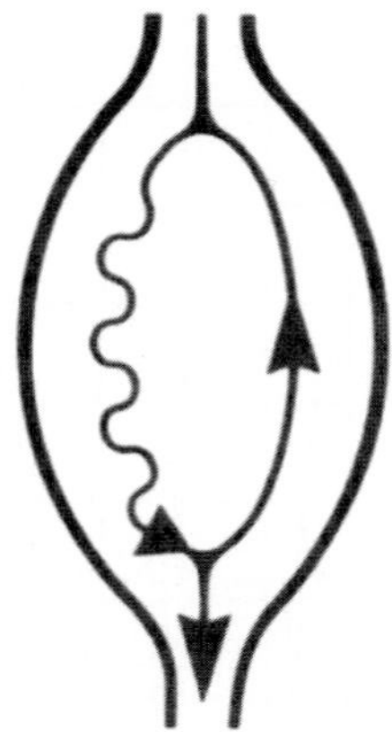

**Figure 48–4** Typical AVNRT.

time), but the slow pathway is able to conduct antegrade. However, because of the slower conduction, by the time the impulse arrives at the ventricular side of the AV node, the fast pathway has recovered and is able to conduct retrograde back up into the atrium. Thus, typical AVNRT is down the slow pathway and up the fast pathway. Because the atria are activated via the fast pathway, the retrograde P wave is very close to (or buried within) the QRS. As mentioned previously, ECG lead V1 may reveal a pseudo-r prime pattern due to deformation of the terminal portion of the QRS complex by the retrograde P wave. This ECG finding is very specific for AVNRT. The concept of a tachycardia using two pathways with different conducting and refractory times is "re-entry." A wide range of both atrial and ventricular arrhythmias are re-entrant circuits. When both pathways are within what is considered the AV node (the fast and the slow pathways), this is termed dual AV node physiology and substrate for AVNRT.

In the unusual variety or "atypical" AVNRT, antegrade conduction occurs over the fast pathway and retrograde conduction over the slow pathway. Though this "atypical" form uses a similar mechanism (dual AV node physiology) at the AV node, it has a long RP (retrograde slow conduction) and a short PR (fast antegrade conduction) interval. This atypical AVNRT is still AV node dependent and thus may terminate with adenosine or during any change in AV node conduction properties.

### *Treatment*

Because both typical and atypical AVNRT are manifestations of dual AV node physiology, they are treated in the same fashion. In the acute setting they usually are responsive to vagal maneuvers and adenosine. If they recur, longer-acting medications that alter AV node conduction (including beta-blockers and calcium antagonists) may be used. Though medications can be successful, catheter ablation is considered the treatment of choice. Catheter ablation of either form of AV node re-entry consists of an anatomic ablation of the slow pathway located at the posterior input to the AV node. This area is most often bordered by the coronary sinus and the tendon of Todaro posteriorly and the tricuspid valve anteriorly. Once identified anatomically, radiofrequency ablation of the slow pathway is performed and subsequent conduction occurs only down the fast pathway.

## AV Reciprocating Tachycardia and Ventricular Pre-excitation (Wolff–Parkinson–White Syndrome)

### *Clinical Presentation and Diagnosis*

Accessory atrioventricular connections or pathways may also participate in AV nodal-dependent re-entrant arrhythmias. The presence of such an accessory pathway may be apparent by surface ECG. Because of the rapid and nondecremental conduction properties of these pathways, they may "pre-excite" the ventricle. This ventricular pre-excitation results in a short PR interval and slurring of the upstroke of the QRS ("delta wave"). This ECG abnormality is termed Wolff–Parkinson–White (WPW) *pattern*. In contrast, the term WPW *syndrome* is reserved for such patients who also have clinical SVT. It is estimated that 1 to 1.5 in 1,000 ECGs show a WPW pattern. Population-based studies have indicated that 50% to 60% of patients with WPW pattern demonstrate symptoms that may include palpitations or more severe symptoms such as syncope (7). Approximately 85% of such symptomatic patients have AV re-entrant tachycardia using the AV node as the antegrade limb and the accessory pathway as the retrograde limb of the circuit (8,9). Approximately 30% to 40% of patients with WPW pattern develop atrial fibrillation.

This type of tachycardia is not only dependent on the AV node but requires the presence of an accessory pathway. This pathway provides an additional connection between the atria and ventricles, other than the AV node. The term "pre-excitation" stems from the fact that the ventricle receives electrical activation from both the AV node–His–Purkinje system and the accessory pathway. Because

**TABLE 48–2**
**DISTRIBUTION OF MOST ACCESSORY PATHWAYS**

| | Left Lateral | Posteroseptal | Right Anterior | Right Lateral |
|---|---|---|---|---|
| Gallagher (1978) | 47% | 27% | 9% | 17% |
| Milstein (1987) | 51% | 32% | 14% | 3% |

conduction antegrade via the accessory pathway is not decremental as with the AV node, the ventricle is pre-excited prior to AV nodal activation. This pre-excitation is represented by the delta wave on the ECG. When there is evidence of ventricular pre-excitation by ECG at baseline, the accessory pathway is described as "manifest." This pre-excitation tends to be more evident at more rapid atrial rates, when AV nodal conduction is slowed, making pre-excitation even more apparent. Occasionally, conduction through the AV node is preferred to that over the accessory pathway. This may be secondary to slow or poor antegrade conduction in the accessory pathway. In these patients there may be minimal or no delta wave on the ECG, as the ventricle is predominantly or completely activated via the AV node. The accessory pathway is still present and may be able to conduct retrograde (and thus be able to cause tachycardia), but it is not evident in sinus rhythm. These accessory pathways are termed "concealed."

It is important to remember that the presence of an accessory pathway does not always indicate that this pathway is a critical part of the presenting SVT. For this reason it is important first to determine the role of the AV node (dependent or independent) in the presenting SVT. Accessory pathways provide only an additional connection between the atria and ventricles. Patients with an accessory pathway and even a history of Wolff–Parkinson–White syndrome may also have other SVTs (i.e., AVNRT) that have no relationship to the accessory pathway.

### *Accessory Pathways*

Accessory pathways may be located along either the mitral or tricuspid annulus. These pathways consist of a bundle of myocardial muscle that bypasses the atrioventricular groove with direct insertion on the ventricular myocardium of the right or left ventricle. On rare occasions, the lower insertion is in proximity or attached to the branches of the right bundle. As shown in Table 48–2, of all accessory pathways, almost half are located on the left side of the heart along the mitral annulus, nearly one third are in the posteroseptal region, and the remainder are at the right anteroseptal region or the right lateral wall of the tricuspid annulus.

Multiple electrocardiographic algorithms have been proposed to diagnose the location of the accessory pathway from surface 12-lead ECGs (Fig. 48–5) (9–14). Unfortunately, no algorithm has proven entirely reliable. A general and easy classification proposed by Rosenbaum and Hecht (15) describes a "type A," with a positive delta wave and QRS in the precordial leads (Fig. 48–6), which is usually associated with a left lateral accessory pathway, and a "type B," with a left bundle-type QRS morphology in the precordial leads, which is usually associated with a right-sided pathway (Fig. 48–7).

### *Mechanism*

AVRT is another form of a re-entrant arrhythmia. In AVRT, one limb of the re-entry circuit is the AV node and the other limb is the accessory pathway. The clinical importance of accessory pathways and pre-excitation reside primarily in their predisposition to tachyarrhythmias. The conduction properties of the accessory pathway (speed of conduction and recovery) determine the likelihood of developing a re-entrant circuit (i.e., AVRT). The direction of the circuit differentiates the two types of AVRT: *orthodromic* AVRT and *antidromic* AVRT. Orthodromic reciprocating tachycardia (ORT) comprises the majority of the reciprocating

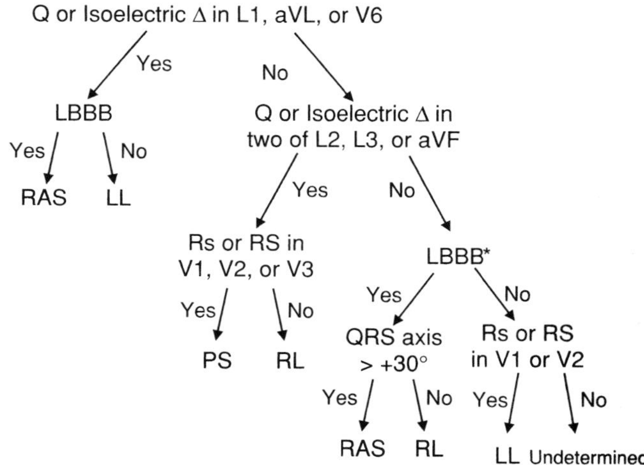


**Figure 48–5** Milstein's algorithm for localization of accessory pathways. LL, left lateral; PS, posteroseptal; RAS, right anteroseptal; RL, right lateral. *LBBB, +QRS LL, rS V1 and V2. (From Milstein S, Sharma AD, Guiraudon GM, et al. An algorithm for the electrocardiographic localization of accessory pathways in the Wolff–Parkinson–White syndrome. *Pacing Clin Electrophysiol.* 1987;10(3 pt 1):555–563.)

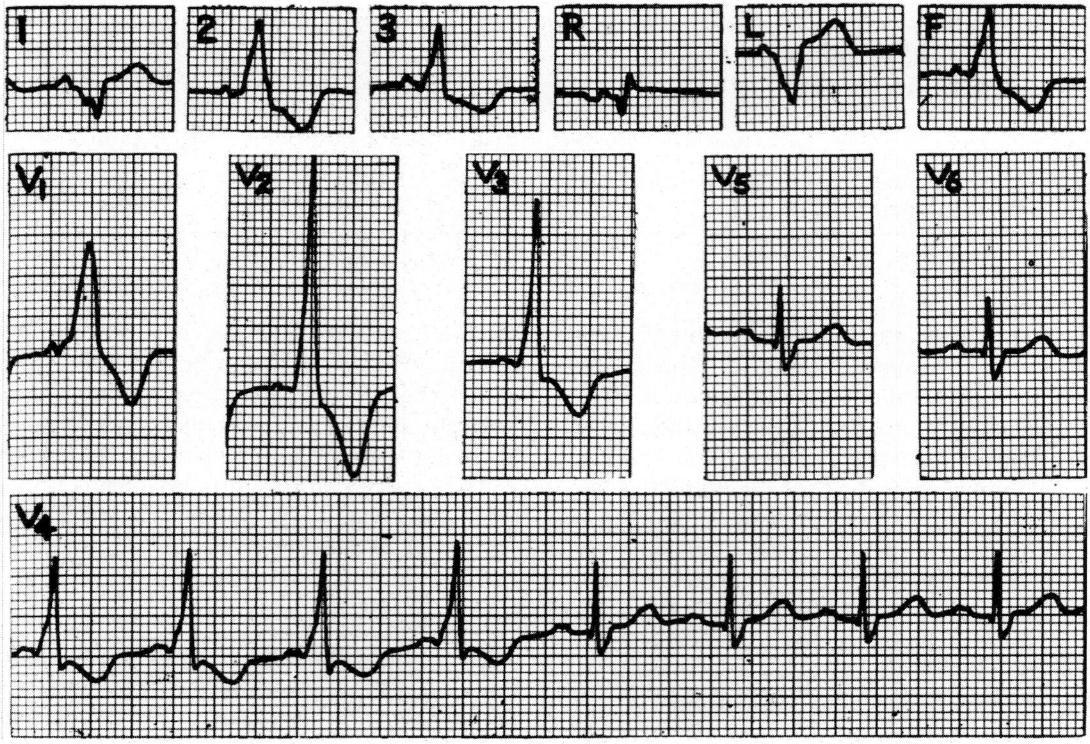


**Figure 48–6** Type A accessory pathway.

tachycardias associated with Wolff–Parkinson–White syndrome. The antegrade limb of this re-entrant circuit is the AV node, whereas the retrograde limb is the accessory pathway. Because the ventricle is activated via the AV node, the QRS complex is narrow. Though it is rare, antidromic reciprocating tachycardia (ART) uses the accessory pathway as the antegrade limb and the AV node as the retrograde limb. Because the ventricle is activated via the accessory pathway, the QRS complex is wide (maximal pre-excitation).

### *Electrophysiologic Characteristics and Diagnostic Maneuvers*

Orthodromic reciprocating tachycardia is typically characterized by a short RP and a long PR interval as the circuit is conducting up the accessory pathway and down the AV node. Because conduction from the atria to the ventricles is via the AV node, the QRS morphology during tachycardia should be similar (in the absence of aberration) to the QRS morphology during normal sinus rhythm.

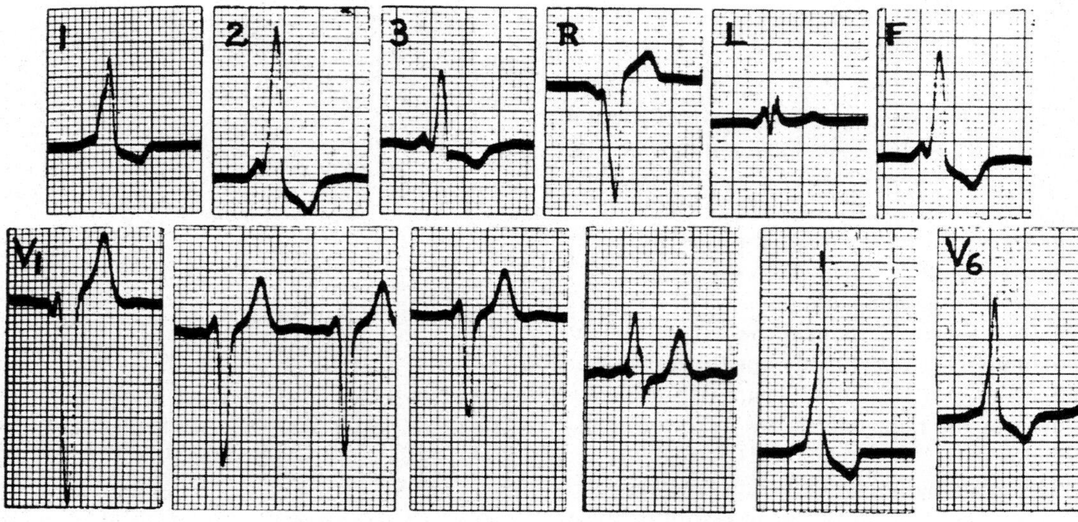


**Figure 48–7** Type B accessory pathway.

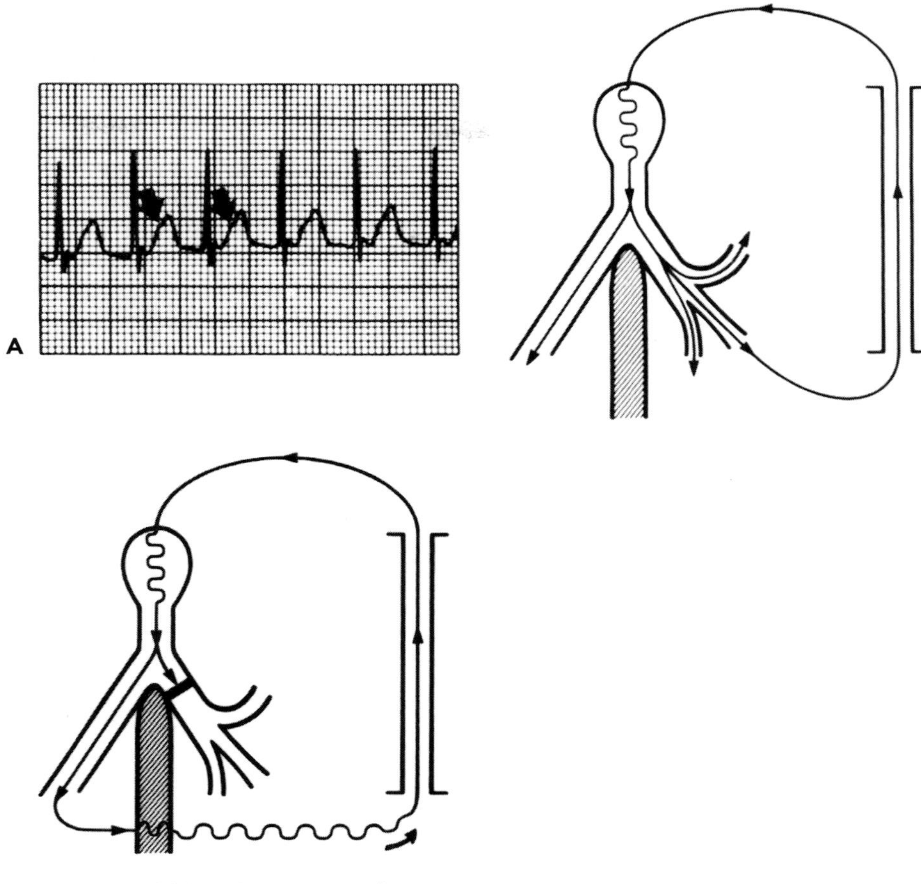


**Figure 48–8** Behavior of the accessory pathway during tachycardia. **A:** Bundle branch block is ipsilateral to a free wall bypass tract. **B:** Bundle branch block is contralateral to a free wall bypass tract.

Though algorithms based on the surface ECG are notoriously inconsistent, behavior of the accessory pathway during tachycardia can provide clinicians with hints as to the location of the pathway. For example, spontaneous or induced functional bundle branch block during ORT can yield a diagnostically useful phenomenon. As demonstrated in Figs. 50–8A,B, if the bundle branch block is ipsilateral to a free wall bypass tract, the retrograde re-entrant impulse is compelled to traverse a greater distance from the His–Purkinje fibers to the ventricular insertion of the bypass tract. As a result, the global VA conduction time during the tachycardia must increase (usually by at least 35 milliseconds). Therefore, the tachycardia cycle length may also increase such that the rate of the tachycardia may become slower. In contrast, if the bundle branch block is contralateral to a free wall bypass tract, there is no change in the distance the retrograde re-entrant impulse has to travel to reach the ventricular insertion of the accessory pathway. Thus there is no effect on the tachycardia cycle length. Therefore, an SVT that slows with the development of bundle branch block should invoke suspicion that the tachycardia is ORT using an accessory pathway located ipsilateral to the site of bundle branch block.

### *Exceptions and Rare Forms of AVRT*

Occasionally, patients present with an incessant ORT in which retrograde conduction up the accessory pathway is decremental. Though it is rare, this type of accessory pathway is associated with a tachycardia called the permanent form of junctional reciprocating tachycardia (PJRT). PJRT typically uses a concealed posteroseptal accessory pathway with a long conduction time and decremental AV node-like properties. These decremental properties prolong the time between the R and P, often making it a "long RP" tachycardia rather than the typical "short RP." Because of the incessant nature of this arrhythmia, it has been associated with tachycardia-induced cardiomyopathy. Tachycardia-induced cardiomyopathy is not related to any one specific SVT, but is associated with any incessant or persistent tachycardia.

Antidromic tachycardia is the least common arrhythmia associated with Wolff–Parkinson–White syndrome, occurring in only 5% to 10% of patients. This tachycardia is characterized by a wide QRS complex that is fully pre-excited with a regular R–R interval. If the diagnosis of WPW is not recognized, this tachycardia may be mistaken for ventricular tachycardia.

Uncommonly, patients may have more than one accessory pathway. In these cases there are multiple potential re-entrant arrhythmia circuits. Of these patients, 33% to 60% will present with antidromic tachycardia. Even less common is a tachycardia involving two accessory pathways as both the antegrade and retrograde limbs of the circuit, without any involvement of the AV node. In these very rare cases, the tachycardia does not terminate with AV node blockade. In patients with more than one pathway, more likely scenarios are one pathway involved in either ORT or ART with the AV node as one limb of the circuit, and the other pathways as "bystanders." The term "bystander" describes accessory atrioventricular pathways that exist, but that are not part of the tachycardia circuit. The typical use of the term "bystander conduction" involves a wide-complex pre-excited SVT that is due to typical AVNRT (antegrade fast AV nodal pathway conduction and retrograde slow AV nodal pathway conduction) with concomitant antegrade conduction through the accessory pathway producing the wide-complex QRS pattern.

Occasionally, the presence of multiple accessory pathways will become apparent only after the dominant pathway has been ablated. The Ebstein anomaly is associated with Wolff–Parkinson–White syndrome in 6% to 26% of patients with this congenital heart defect. In addition, 40% to 55% of patients with WPW and the Ebstein anomaly have multiple accessory pathways (16).

#### Treatment

Treatment of a patient with WPW syndrome (presence of an accessory pathway and AVRT) may involve both drug therapy and catheter ablation. In the acute setting, patients with ORT (conduction down the AV node and thus a narrow QRS complex) can be treated with AV nodal-blocking agents such as adenosine and vagal maneuvers. Chronic treatment may be directed at any essential component of the circuit. Administration of calcium channel antagonists or beta-adrenergic blockers affects the AV node, whereas antiarrhythmic drugs including flecainide, propafenone, quinidine, procainamide, and amiodarone may be chosen to target the accessory pathway. More invasive options such as catheter ablation therapy of the accessory pathway are now playing a more prominent role in management of WPW syndrome. With newer computerized mapping technologies, the acute success rate nears 100%, with a less than 1% risk of significant complications. However, pathway location may play a role in risk during ablative procedures in that some right anteroseptal pathways are very close to the AV node, increasing the possibility of disruption of normal conduction during ablation (possibly requiring pacemaker implantation).

#### Wolff–Parkinson–White Syndrome and Sudden Cardiac Death

In contrast, in patients presenting with pre-excited tachycardia (thus a wide QRS complex), adenosine and AV node-blocking agents are *absolutely* contraindicated. In these rhythms, the ventricles are being activated antegrade via the accessory pathway. Often these rhythms are atrial arrhythmias (atrial tachycardia, atrial fibrillation, and atrial flutter) that are conducting predominantly down the accessory pathway (and partially the AV node). In these scenarios, the "bystander" accessory pathway is conducting the tachycardia to the ventricle. If an AV-blocking agent is administered, conduction may be exclusively through the accessory pathway. Because these pathways typically do not have protective decremental properties as the AV node does, rhythms such as atrial flutter/fibrillation (>300 beats/min) may be conducted to the ventricle in a 1:1 fashion (Fig. 48–9). AV conduction at that rate may degenerate rapidly into ventricular fibrillation and subsequent cardiac arrest. In these patients, procainamide, flecainide, propafenone, or amiodarone should be considered. In case of atrial fibrillation/flutter with rapid response and hemodynamic instability, electrical direct-current cardioversion is the treatment of choice.

As shown in Table 48–3, atrial fibrillation may be a coexisting or presenting arrhythmia in about 20% to 40% of patients with Wolff–Parkinson–White syndrome. Atrial fibrillation in the presence of an accessory pathway with rapid antegrade conduction can result in degeneration to ventricular fibrillation and subsequently result in sudden cardiac death. The risk of sudden death for patients with WPW syndrome is not clear but is definitely not very high. Population-based studies suggest an incidence of 0.15% per year, and sudden death occurs almost exclusively in previously symptomatic patients (7).

This occasional occurrence of ventricular fibrillation as the initial manifestation of Wolff–Parkinson–White syndrome has stimulated interest in the possibility of identifying asymptomatic patients who may be at risk for this complication. These patients possess antegrade conducting accessory pathways (pre-excitation during normal sinus rhythm) and no symptoms of SVT. Screening these patients involves evaluating the conduction properties of the accessory pathway. An easy and noninvasive method is to observe for intermittent ventricular pre-excitation by electrocardiogram, which may involve supervised treadmill stress testing or simply ambulatory Holter monitoring during the patient's daily activities. This intermittent pre-excitation refers to the abrupt loss of the pre-excitation or delta wave from one beat to the next. This phenomenon suggests an accessory pathway that is incapable of extremely rapid antegrade conduction and therefore carries a low risk for sudden cardiac death (17) .

If normalization of the QRS is not observed during Holter monitoring or during exercise, electrophysiologic evaluation must be considered to assess the conduction property of the accessory pathway. The most direct method for such risk stratification is the induction of atrial fibrillation in an electrophysiologic laboratory setting and the determination of the shortest R–R interval. This provides

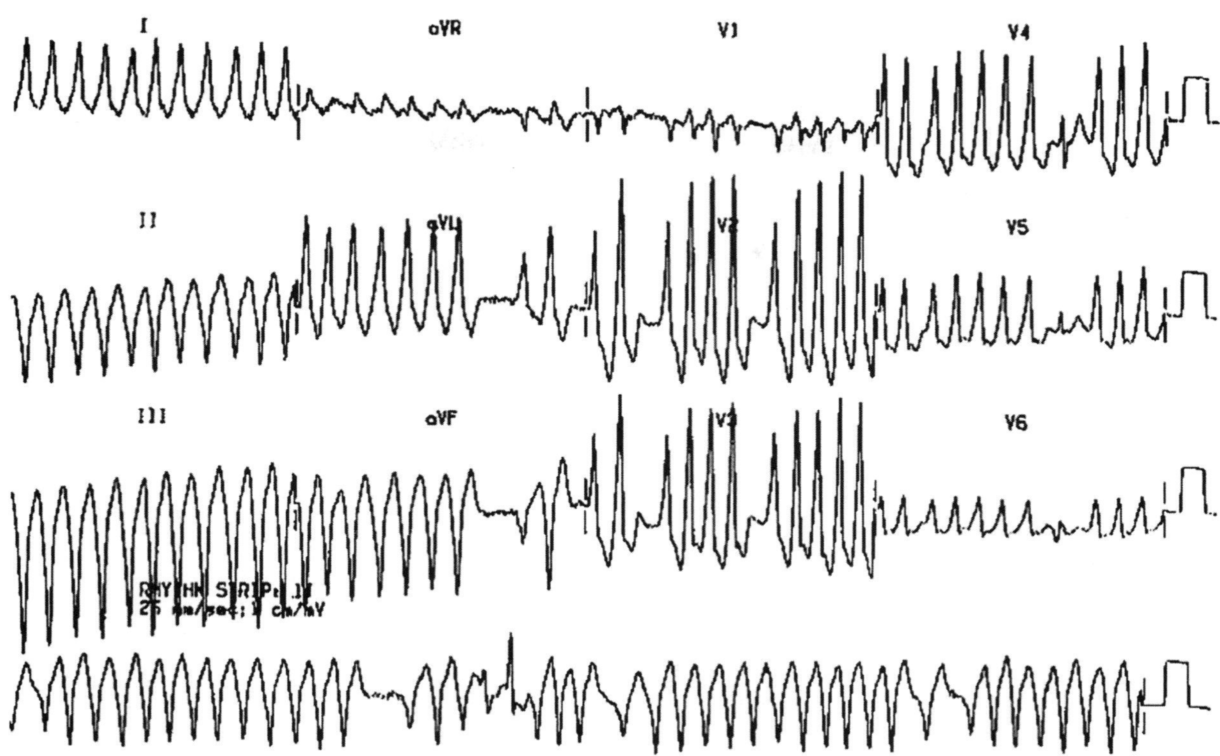


**Figure 48–9** Atrial arrhythmia in Wolff–Parkinson–White syndrome.

information as to the antegrade conduction capabilities of the accessory pathway. Studies have shown that patients with WPW syndrome who experienced and survived an episode of sudden cardiac death had the shortest R–R intervals (18). A shortest R–R interval of <250 milliseconds indicates an accessory pathway that is incapable of dangerously rapid antegrade conduction. However, caution should be exercised about drawing conclusions if the shortest R–R interval is <250 milliseconds, as this does not necessarily confer a high risk of sudden death for a patient with WPW syndrome. The positive predictive value of this finding is only 20%. Therefore, the finding of a shortest R–R interval <250 may mean simply that the patient cannot be told that he or she is excluded from the small subset of patients with WPW syndrome who will ultimately experience sudden cardiac death.

**TABLE 48–3**
**TACHYARRHYTHMIAS IN 161 WPW PATIENTS**

| | |
|---|---|
| RT1 | 89 |
| RT + AF1 | 32 |
| AF | 15 |
| RT + AF + VF | 13 |
| AF + VF | 5 |
| VF | 4 |
| RT + VF | 3 |
| Total WPWs | 161 |

RT, reciprocating tachycardia; AF, atrial fibrillation; VF, ventricular fibrillation.

In addition, because of the very high cure rates achievable with catheter ablation, this approach may be the best treatment option for patients involved in high-performance physical activity or with specific jobs, such as pilots or bus/truck drivers. In symptomatic patients with WPW syndrome, particularly those with frequent SVT, catheter ablation may be considered as the first-line treatment option.

In general, chronic treatment of AV nodal-dependent SVTs includes AV nodal-blocking medications (beta-adrenergic blockers and/or calcium channel antagonists) and catheter ablation. In general, it is recommended that the more invasive strategy of catheter ablation be reserved for those patients in whom medical therapy has failed or is poorly tolerated. However, there is evidence to support the consideration of catheter ablation as a first-line therapy for patients with frequent episodes of SVT, as catheter ablation in these patients is more effective and more cost effective than medical therapy over time.

Radiofrequency catheter ablation of SVT has been shown to be cost effective and to improve quality of life for patients with WPW syndrome who survive cardiac arrest or who experience SVT or atrial fibrillation (19), and for highly symptomatic patients with AV nodal re-entrant tachycardia or AV re-entrant tachycardia using a concealed action potential (20).

## ATRIAL-DEPENDENT ARRHYTHMIAS

There are three predominant types of atrial-dependent arrhythmias: (a) atrial tachycardia, (b) atrial flutter, and (c) atrial fibrillation. This section discusses the first two; the third, atrial fibrillation, is discussed in Chapter 51.

### Atrial Tachycardia

#### *Clinical Presentation and Diagnosis*

Atrial tachycardias require only the atrium for the initiation and maintenance of the arrhythmias. It presents in all age groups and has a wide range of potential mechanisms and clinical presentation. Atrial tachycardia can be completely asymptomatic in some individuals versus recurrent and disabling in others. Short episodes of atrial tachycardia may be seen on ambulatory Holter monitoring in 2% to 6% of normal young subjects and in up to 29% of older subjects. The majority of these episodes are asymptomatic and do not require treatment. However, in about 10% of patients, atrial tachycardia is associated with significant symptoms. As shown in Table 48–1, atrial tachycardia is more prevalent in older patients and is common in patients with underlying heart disease.

#### *Mechanisms*

There are several possible mechanisms for atrial tachycardia. Automatic or focal atrial tachycardia typically originates from a discrete area within the atria. It is suspected to be a cell or group of cells that possesses its own automaticity that independently fires and differs in rate, origin, and behavior from normal sinus rhythm. These ectopic atrial tachycardia foci are typically from either the pulmonary veins or the crista terminalis region. They are often incessant and unresponsive to medical therapy. In fact, the incessant nature of automatic atrial tachycardia may predispose these patients to tachycardia-mediated cardiomyopathy.

Another distinct mechanism is multifocal atrial tachycardia (MAT). MAT is a supraventricular tachycardia characterized by multiple P-wave morphologies (at least three are necessary to establish the diagnosis), a varying PR interval, and an irregular ventricular response. Though the mechanism is not well understood, many feel that it is the result of multiple automatic and/or triggered foci driving the atria at different rates. It is distinct from atrial fibrillation in that there are well-defined P waves. By definition, there are at least three distinct P-wave morphologies and thus at least three different sources of atrial depolarization.

#### *Treatment*

As with most arrhythmias, treatment approaches for atrial tachycardia are twofold: (a) medication and (b) catheter ablation. Medications such as beta-adrenergic blockers and calcium channel antagonists can be used, although most ectopic atrial tachycardias and re-entrant atrial tachycardias are not terminated or prevented by these drugs. These medications can be considered in the acute setting to control the ventricular response by decreasing AV conduction (e.g., creating 2:1 AV block and thus decreasing ventricular response). Unfortunately, they often do little to slow or control the actual atrial focus. Other agents, including Class 1A, 1C, and Class III drugs are more effective in maintaining sinus rhythm or terminating the arrhythmia. Catheter ablative procedures are becoming an alternative treatment strategy for patients in whom medical therapy fails.

MAT is most often observed in chronically ill patients, frequently those with respiratory failure or chronic pulmonary or cardiac disease. It has also been associated with digoxin toxicity, electrolytic imbalance (hypokalemia and hypomagnesemia), acute myocardial infarction, and mitral valve disease. Intravenous verapamil, intravenous potassium, and large doses of magnesium have been used in the acute treatment of this arrhythmia, but with limited success. Low doses of beta-adrenergic antagonists have also been suggested, but may be problematic in the majority of patients with chronic lung disease. Long-term treatment usually involves the use of a calcium channel antagonist, often requiring relatively high doses. However, the most effective therapy for MAT is treatment of the underlying medical condition or abnormality, such as treatment of bronchospasm and hypoxemia and correction of electrolyte disturbances. Cardioversion is generally *ineffective* for this arrhythmia disorder. Targeted catheter ablation is not effective. AV node ablation and permanent pacing may be considered in cases that are refractory to conventional medical therapy.

### Atrial Flutter

#### *Clinical Presentation and Diagnosis*

Atrial flutter is a macro-re-entrant atrial tachycardia. Patients with atrial flutter can be divided into two categories: (a) those with previous ablation or cardiac surgery and (b) those with no previous ablation or cardiac surgery. All atrial flutters typically present with a regular atrial rhythm up to 300 to 350 beats/min conducting to the ventricle at various rates but often a constant multiple of the atrial rate (2:1, 4:1, etc.).

#### *Mechanism*

The mechanism of atrial flutter involves the concept of re-entry (discussed earlier). Similar to the concept of re-entry discussed in AV node-dependent rhythms, this type of re-entry requires two areas of atrial tissue with different conduction and refractory properties. Rather than rotate around the AV groove between the atria and ventricles, atrial flutter circuits rotate around areas of nonconducting

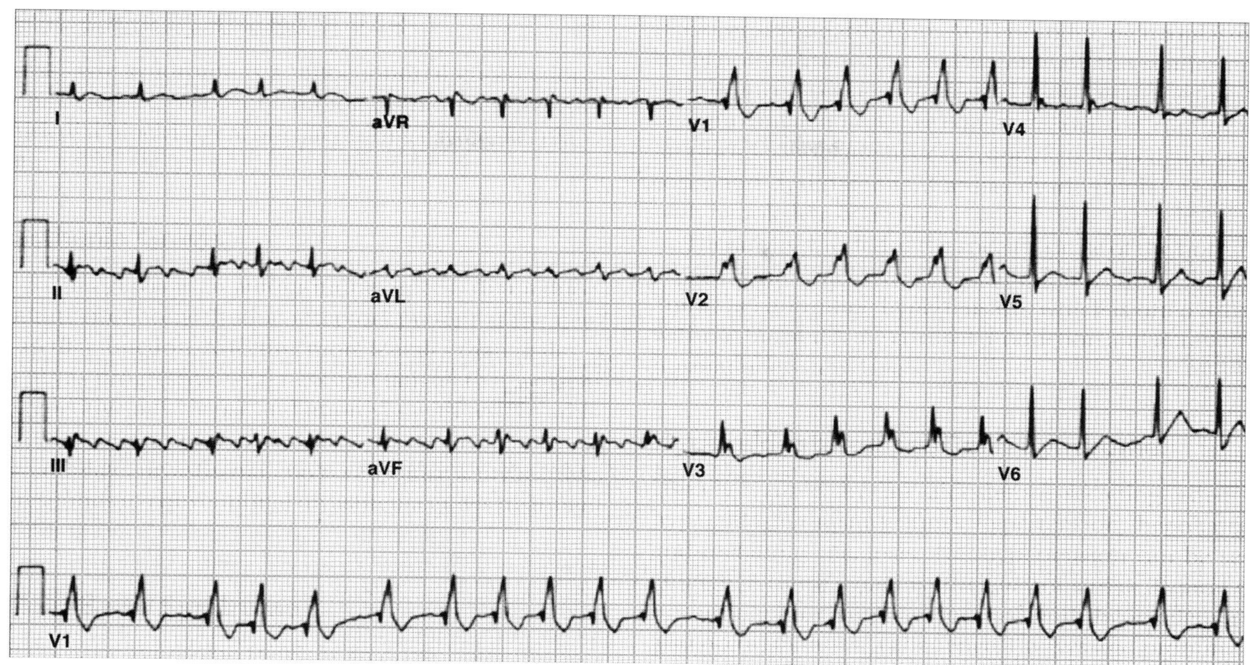


**Figure 48–10** Typical sawtooth pattern of flutter waves.

tissue within the atrium. These rotating circuits then drive the atrial flutter at a cycle length equal to the time it takes for the wavefront to go around the circuit once.

In patients with no history of previous ablation or cardiac surgery, the area of nonconducting tissue is typically anatomic (nonconducting tissue such as the valve rings or great vessels). Typical right atrial flutter most commonly takes a "counterclockwise" rotation as it courses around the crista terminalis, through the isthmus between the tricuspid valve and inferior vena cava, up the septum, and back around to the crista. This gives it the typical sawtooth pattern of flutter waves that are seen in the inferior leads (Fig. 48–10). This circuit may occur in the opposite direction in a "clockwise" direction. Rarely, electrical atrial scarring in the absence of surgery has been documented in patients with atrial flutter. Some have proposed that this scarring may be a result of a myopathic process. Whenever there are areas of nonconducting tissue, atypical flutter circuits may develop. These atypical flutters can develop and rotate around these areas of scar.

In patients with a previous history of ablation or cardiac surgery, the area of nonconducting tissue is usually a site of scar from previous incisions or radiofrequency lesions. Common sites include the right atriotomy scar, the septum, and near areas of previously ablated tissue.

### *Treatment*

Like other atrial-dependent rhythms, atrial flutter is often difficult to manage medically. Beta-adrenergic blockade and calcium channel antagonists are options that can be used in the acute setting to slow conduction via the AV node and thus slow the ventricular response. Antiarrhythmic medications may also be used; however, the use of Class 1C agents (flecanide, propafenone) may slow the cycle length of the flutter, permitting 1:1 atrioventricular conduction. Because of this risk, AV nodal-blocking agents (beta blockers or calcium channel antagonists) should always be given in addition to Class 1C agents. In contrast, Class III drugs may terminate and prevent atrial flutter by prolonging atrial refractoriness. Catheter ablation may be an option for many patients. With use of the newer computerized mapping technology, improved mapping of the macro-re-entrant circuit has increased success rates. During catheter ablation the goal is to interrupt the circuit in such a way that re-entry cannot perpetuate. In typical isthmus-dependent right atrial flutter, a line of block with ablative lesions can be employed between two nonconducting structures (e.g., the tricuspid valve and the inferior vena cava). Once this is in place, the milieu for re-entry ceases to exist.

## SINUS-DEPENDENT ARRHYTHMIAS

Sinus-dependent tachycardias are rare forms of atrial tachycardias that originate at or within the area of the sinus node. These arrhythmias include sinus node re-entrant tachycardia and inappropriate sinus tachycardia. Both need to be differentiated from physiologic sinus tachycardia, which is an increase of heart rate secondary to either cardiac or noncardiac etiology. In the latter form, treatment of the

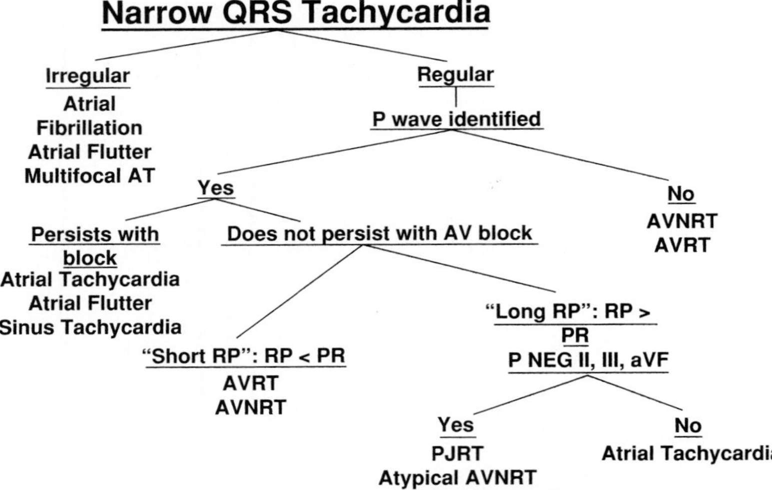


**Figure 48–11** Algorithm for treatment of SVT.

underlying disease may result in resolution of the sinus tachycardia. Occasionally, it is desirable to slow sinus tachycardia for symptomatic relief while the underlying etiology is being addressed. For example, beta-adrenergic blockers may be useful for thyrotoxicosis or for sinus tachycardia associated with acute myocardial infarction in the absence of heart failure. However, both sinus node re-entrant tachycardia and inappropriate sinus tachycardia are arrhythmias that generally behave differently than normal sinus tachycardia. These tachycardias, characterized by a P-wave morphology similar to that observed during normal sinus rhythm, persist without any physiologic cause. Sinus node re-entry is a re-entry mechanism within the sinus node and is usually observed in older patients with concomitant heart disease. In contrast, inappropriate sinus tachycardia in both the chronic and paroxysmal forms is observed mostly in young adult women.

Treatment of these arrhythmias is often very difficult. Like most tachycardias, rate control with medications such as beta-blockers and calcium channel antagonists may be used. Antiarrhythmic drug therapy has not been shown to be highly effective for these tachycardias but may be considered. When medical treatment is ineffective, catheter ablation may be considered. However, particularly for inappropriate sinus tachycardia, success with sinus node modification has been limited and should not be considered primary therapy. These arrhythmias are rare, and evaluation should focus on elucidating a possible physiologic mechanism (i.e., thyroid disease). Inappropriate sinus tachycardia should be differentiated from a specific syndrome called postural orthostatic tachycardia syndrome (POTS), which is characterized by orthostatic hypotension and 40 to 50 beats increase in the heart rate within 10 minutes after assuming a standing position. This is important in that POTS is managed medically, with catheter ablation contraindicated.

## CONCLUSION

Supraventricular tachycardia is a descriptive diagnosis with varying pathologies, mechanisms, and treatments. Many of these underlying mechanisms can be determined from the surface electrocardiogram and via utilization of bedside maneuvers. It is important to implement a systematic approach to SVT, not only to define the underlying mechanism but also to provide rapid, effective, and appropriate treatment (Fig. 48–11).

## REFERENCES

1. Kinlay S, Leitch JW, Neil A, et al. Cardiac event recorders yield more diagnoses and are more cost-effective than 48-hour Holter monitoring in patients with palpitations. A controlled clinical trial. *Ann Intern Med.* 1996;124(1 pt 1):16–20.
2. Blomstrom-Lundqvist C, Scheinman MM, Aliot EM, et al. ACC/AHA/ESC guidelines for the management of patients with supraventricular arrhythmias—executive summary: a report of the American College of Cardiology/American Heart Association Task Force on Practice Guidelines and the European Society of Cardiology Committee for Practice Guidelines (Writing Committee to Develop Guidelines for the Management of Patients with Supraventricular Arrhythmias). *Circulation.* 2003;108(15):1871–1909.
3. Fuster V, Ryden LE, Asinger RW, et al. ACC/AHA/ESC guidelines for the management of patients with atrial fibrillation: executive summary a report of the American College of Cardiology/American Heart Association Task Force on Practice Guidelines and the European Society of Cardiology Committee for Practice Guidelines and Policy Conferences (Committee to Develop Guidelines for the Management of Patients with Atrial Fibrillation) developed in collaboration with the North American Society of Pacing and Electrophysiology. *Circulation.* 2001;104(17):2118–2150.
4. Bar FW, Brugada P, Dassen WR, et al. Differential diagnosis of tachycardia with narrow QRS complex (shorter than 0.12 second). *Am J Cardiol.* 1984;54(6):555–560.
5. Wu D, Denes P, Amat-y-Leon F, et al. Clinical, electrocardiographic and electrophysiologic observations in patients with paroxysmal supraventricular tachycardia. *Am J Cardiol.* 1978;41(6):1045–1051.
6. Josephson ME. Paroxysmal supraventricular tachycardia: an electrophysiologic approach. *Am J Cardiol.* 1978;41(6):1123–1126.

7. Munger TM, Packer DL, Hammill SC, et al. A population study of the natural history of Wolff–Parkinson–White syndrome in Olmsted County, Minnesota, 1953–1989. *Circulation*. 1993;87(3): 866–873.
8. Prystowsky EN. Diagnosis and management of the preexcitation syndromes. *Curr Probl Cardiol*. 1988;13(4):225–310.
9. Gallagher JJ, Pritchett EL, Sealy WC, et al. The preexcitation syndromes. *Prog Cardiovasc Dis*. 1978;20(4):285–327.
10. Milstein S, Sharma AD, Guiraudon GM, et al. An algorithm for the electrocardiographic localization of accessory pathways in the Wolff–Parkinson–White syndrome. *Pacing Clin Electrophysiol*. 1987;10(3 pt 1):555–563.
11. Arruda MS, McClelland JH, Wang X, et al. Development and validation of an ECG algorithm for identifying accessory pathway ablation site in Wolff–Parkinson–White syndrome. *J Cardiovasc Electrophysiol*. 1998;9(1):2–12.
12. Chiang CE, Chen SA, Teo WS, et al. An accurate stepwise electrocardiographic algorithm for localization of accessory pathways in patients with Wolff–Parkinson–White syndrome from a comprehensive analysis of delta waves and R/S ratio during sinus rhythm. *Am J Cardiol*. 1995;76(1):40–46.
13. Fitzpatrick AP, Gonzales RP, Lesh MD, et al. New algorithm for the localization of accessory atrioventricular connections using a baseline electrocardiogram. *J Am Coll Cardiol*. 1994;23(1): 107–116.
14. Xie B, Heald SC, Bashir Y, et al. Localization of accessory pathways from the 12-lead electrocardiogram using a new algorithm. *Am J Cardiol*. 1994;74(2):161–165.
15. Rosenbaum F, Hecht H. The potential variations of the thorax and the esophagus in anomalous atrioventricular excitation (Wolff–Parkinson–White syndrome). *Am Heart J*. 1945(29):281–326.
16. Bardy GH, Packer DL, German LD, et al. Preexcited reciprocating tachycardia in patients with Wolff–Parkinson–White syndrome: incidence and mechanisms. *Circulation*. 1984;70(3):377–391.
17. Klein GJ, Gulamhusein SS. Intermittent preexcitation in the Wolff–Parkinson–White syndrome. *Am J Cardiol*. 1983;52(3):292–296.
18. Klein, GJ, Bashore TM, et al. Ventricular fibrillation in the Wolff–Parkinson–White syndrome. *N Engl J Med*. 1979;301(20):1080–1085.
19. Hogenhuis W, Stevens SK, Wang P, et al. Cost-effectiveness of radiofrequency ablation compared with other strategies in Wolff–Parkinson–White syndrome. *Circulation*. 1993;88(5 pt 2):II437–II446.
20. Cheng CH, Sanders GD, Hlatky MA, et al. Cost-effectiveness of radiofrequency ablation for supraventricular tachycardia. *Ann Intern Med*. 2000;133(11):864–876.

## QUESTIONS

**1.** A 44-year-old patient with no previous cardiovascular history, who presents with a wide-QRS, irregular, and fast tachycardia (on ECG) is best treated with:

a. Lidocaine
b. Procainamide
c. Metoprolol
d. Diltiazem

Answer is b: This patient has atrial fibrillation with pre-excited QRS and should be treated with procainamide. AV node-blocking agents are absolutely contradicted because they will favor conduction over the accessory pathway with increased risk of degeneration into ventricular fibrillation.

**2.** Catheter ablation is an established and well-accepted treatment for each of the following tachycardia *except:*

a. AV node re-entry
b. AV re-entry
c. Permanent junctional tachycardia
d. Sinus tachycardia

Answer is d: Catheter ablation is an established therapy for all the arrhythmias listed except sinus tachycardia.

**3.** Which of the following forms of congenital heart disease is commonly associated with Wolff–Parkinson–White syndrome?

a. Aortic stenosis
b. Ebstein anomaly
c. Pulmonary stenosis
d. Atrial septal defect

Answer is b: Ebstein Anomaly is associated with WPW in 6% of patients with this congenital anomaly.

**4.** Which of the following supraventricular tachycardias is associated with tachycardia-induced cardiomyopathy?

a. Permanent junctional tachycardia
b. Incessant atrial tachycardia
c. Atrial flutter with rapid ventricular response
d. All of the above

Answer is d: All tachycardias of incessant nature can cause tachycardia-induced cardiomyopathy.

**5.** Which test would you consider for an asymptomatic 31-year-old man with intermittent pre-excitation?

a. Holter monitoring
b. Electrophysiologic study
c. Exercise test
d. Catheter ablation
e. None of the above

Answer is e: No further investigation or treatment is indicated for an asymptomatic patient with intermittent pre-excitation.

**6.** Conduction block in the AV node without termination of the tachycardia is compatible with all of the following mechanisms *except:*

a. Atrial tachycardia
b. AV re-entry tachycardia
c. Atrial flutter
d. Sinus tachycardia

Answer is b: The only tachycardia that cannot sustain with conduction block in the AV node is AV re-entry.

**7.** The initial manifestations of Wolff–Parkinson–White syndrome include which of the following?

a. Atrial fibrillation
b. AV re-entry tachycardia
c. Ventricular fibrillation
d. Wide-QRS tachycardia
e. All of the above

Answer is e: All of the above are possible arrhythmias in Wolff–Parkinson–White syndrome.

**8.** Administration of metoprolol is more likely to terminate:

a. Sinus tachycardia
b. Atrial tachycardia
c. Atrial fibrillation
d. AV re-entry tachycardia

Answer is d: Sinus tachycardia will slow down but not terminate. Atrial tachycardia and atrial fibrillation will not be affected by metoprolol.

**9.** Which of the following is the treatment of choice to terminate a narrow-QRS tachycardia?

a. Metoprolol
b. Diltiazem
c. Adenosine
d. Procainamide
e. Cardioversion

Answer is c: Adenosine is the best acute treatment for narrow-QRS tachycardia.

**10.** For a patient with Wolff–Parkinson–White syndrome who presents with a regular wide-QRS tachycardia, all of the following are possible treatment choices *except:*

a. Procainamide
b. Cardioversion
c. Amiodarone
d. Ibutilide
e. Adenosine

Answer is e: Adenosine and AV node-blocking agents are contraindicated in pre-excited arrhythmias.

**11.** Transesophageal recording may help in establishing the diagnosis in which of the following supraventricular tachycardias?

a. Atrial tachycardia
b. AV node re-entrant tachycardia
c. AV re-entrant tachycardia
d. Atrial flutter
e. All of the above

Answer is e: Transesophageal recording can provide information that is helpful in establishing a diagnosis in all of the supraventricular tachycardias listed.

**12.** Change in the tachycardia rate with development of bundle branch block is consistent with:

a. Atrial tachycardia
b. AV node re-entry
c. AV re-entry
d. Sinus tachycardia

Answer is c: AV re-entry due to an accessory bypass tract ipsilateral to the bundle branch block is the only arrhythmia associated with the above behavior.

**13.** The presence of an r prime in V1 during narrow-QRS tachycardia is suggestive of:

a. AV re-entry
b. AV node re-entry
c. Rate-dependent bundle branch block
d. Atrial tachycardia

Answer is a: The correct answer is AV node re-entry.

**14.** The best therapy for multifocal atrial tachycardia is

a. Digoxin
b. Diltiazem
c. Metoprolol
d. Flecainide
e. Treatment of the underlying disorder

Answer is e: No drug therapy will be effective for multifocal atrial tachycardia if the underlying disorder is not corrected.

# Atrial Fibrillation and Flutter

# 49

***Dimpi Patel*** ***Andrea Natale***

Atrial fibrillation is the most common sustained arrhythmia seen in clinical practice. There are estimated to be >2 million patients with atrial fibrillation in the United States. The prevalence and incidence of atrial fibrillation increase with advancing age. The mainstay of therapy includes pharmacologic rate control and antiarrhythmic therapy, cardioversion, and antithromboembolic management. Nonpharmacologic therapies, including ablation, device, and surgical approaches, are also becoming increasingly utilized and potentially curative.

## EPIDEMIOLOGY

### Prevalence

- 0.4% general population
- 0.2% in population 25 to 34 years old
- 2% to 5% in population >60 years old
- 10% in population >80 years old
- 8% to 14% in hospitalized patients

### Incidence

- The incidence of AF increases from less than 0.1% per year (>160,000 new U.S. cases year) in those under 40 years of age to 1.5% per year in females and 2% per year in males over the age of 80 (Kannel et al. 1983).
- 20% to 40% after cardiac surgery

## FACTORS PREDISPOSING TO ATRIAL FIBRILLATION

The most common cardiovascular diseases associated with atrial fibrillation (AF) are hypertension and ischemic heart disease. Other predisposing conditions include:

- Advancing age
- Rheumatic heart disease (especially mitral valve disease)
- Nonrheumatic valvular disease
- Cardiomyopathies
- Congestive heart failure
- Congenital heart disease
- Sick sinus syndrome/degenerative conduction system disease
- Wolff-Parkinson-White syndrome
- Pericarditis
- Pulmonary embolism
- Thyrotoxicosis
- Chronic lung disease
- Neoplastic disease
- Postoperative states
- Diabetes
- Normal hearts affected by high adrenergic states, alcohol, stress, drugs (especially sympathomimetics), excessive caffeine, hypoxia, hypokalemia, hypoglycemia, or systemic infection

## MORBIDITY AND MORTALITY

### Survival

The pressure of atrial fibrillation leads to a 1.5- to 2-fold increase in total and cardiovascular (CV) mortality (Emelia et al. 1998). Factors that may increase mortality include:

- Age
- Mitral stenosis
- Aortic valve disease
- Cardiac artery disease (CAD)
- Hypertension
- Congestive heart failure (CHF)

Patients with myocardial infarction (MI) or CHF have higher mortality if AF is present.

### Stroke/Thromboembolism

Atrial fibrillation predisposes to stroke and thromboembolism.

- 5- to 6-fold increased risk of stroke (17-fold with rheumatic hearts disease (RHD))
- 3% to 5%/year rate of stroke in nonvalvular AF
- Single major cause (50%) of cardiogenic stroke
- 75,000 strokes/year
- Silent cerebral infarction risk
- Risk varies increases with age, concomitant cardiovascular disease, stroke risk factors

### Tachycardia-Induced Cardiomyopathy

Persistent rapid rates can lead to tachycardia-mediated cardiomyopathy and left ventricular (LV) dysfunction. These are, however, reversible with ventricular rate control and regularization. Control can be achieved with medical rate control, atrioventricular (AV) node ablation, or achievement of sinus rhythm.

Atrial cardiomyopathy leads to structural remodeling with an increase in atrial size in patients with AF.

### Symptoms and Hemodynamics

- Rapid ventricular rates
- Irregularity of ventricular rhythm
- Loss of AV synchrony
- Symptoms: limitation in functional capacity, palpitations, fatigue, dyspnea, angina, CHF

## PATHOGENESIS

Current models of the pathogenesis of atrial fibrillation present a competitive interaction between triggers of AF and a substrate that tends to maintain the AF.

- Electrical activation: rapid, multiple waves of depolarization with continuously changing, wandering pathways
- Intracardiac electrograms: irregular, rapid depolarizations, often >300 to 400 beats/min
- Mechanical effects:
  - Loss of coordinated atrial contraction
  - Irregular electrical inputs to the AV node and His–Purkinje system leading to irregular ventricular contraction
- Surface electrocardiogram:
  - No discrete P waves
  - Irregular fibrillatory waves
  - Irregularly irregular ventricular response

### Multiple Wavelet Hypothesis (Moe et al. 1964)

Atrial fibrillation is sustained by the propagation of multiple re-entrant circuits. Electrophysiologic mapping studies in animals and humans have demonstrated the presence of multiple re-entrant wavelets. Continuously changing, wandering pathways are determined by local refractoriness, excitability, and conduction properties of the atrial tissue.

The initiation and perpetuation of AF can depend on increasing atrial size and decreasing re-entrant circuit wavelength, $\lambda$, where $\lambda$ is the distance traveled by the depolarization wavefront during the refractory period. The path length for AF re-entrant circuits, $\alpha$, depends on atrial size. To support re-entry, the path length of the circuit must be $\geq$ the wavelength.

$$\lambda \text{ (wavelength)} = \text{CV (conduction velocity)} \times \text{ERP (effective refractory period)}$$

Structural enlargement of the atria can predispose to persistence of AF by allowing more re-entrant circuits to be sustained in the atria. Small re-entrant circuits from shortened tissue refractoriness may enhance vulnerability to atrial tachyarrhythmias.

### "Atrial Fibrillation Begets Atrial Fibrillation" (Wijffels et al. 1995)

Structural and electrical remodeling leads to increased sustainability of atrial fibrillation. Electrical remodeling leads to shortened atrial ERPs.

According to the Goat model (Allessie et al.), longer periods of atrial burst pacing lead to shortened ERPs, which leads to longer periods of AF sustainability.

Verapamil may abrogate ERP shortening. This effect is not seen with beta-blockers or other antiarrhythmic agents studied and may be due to attenuation of rate-induced calcium overload, because verapamil-induced block of electrical remodeling was overcome by hypercalcemia in an animal model. Reports of verapamil causing an enhancement of AF through shortening of E–F intervals (estimate of ERPs during AF) may be due to sympathetic neurohumoral effects. In an animal model, verapamil did not promote AF when given with beta-blockade.

In structural remodeling, tachycardia-induced cardiomyopathy leads to atrial enlargement, which supports more wavelets.

### Focal Initiating Triggers (From Haissaguerre et al., 1998)

Focal sources that initiate atrial fibrillation have been identified, particularly in patients with lone atrial fibrillation in the absence of structural heart disease. Foci most commonly arise from the ostia of the pulmonary veins and are potential targets for curative ablation.

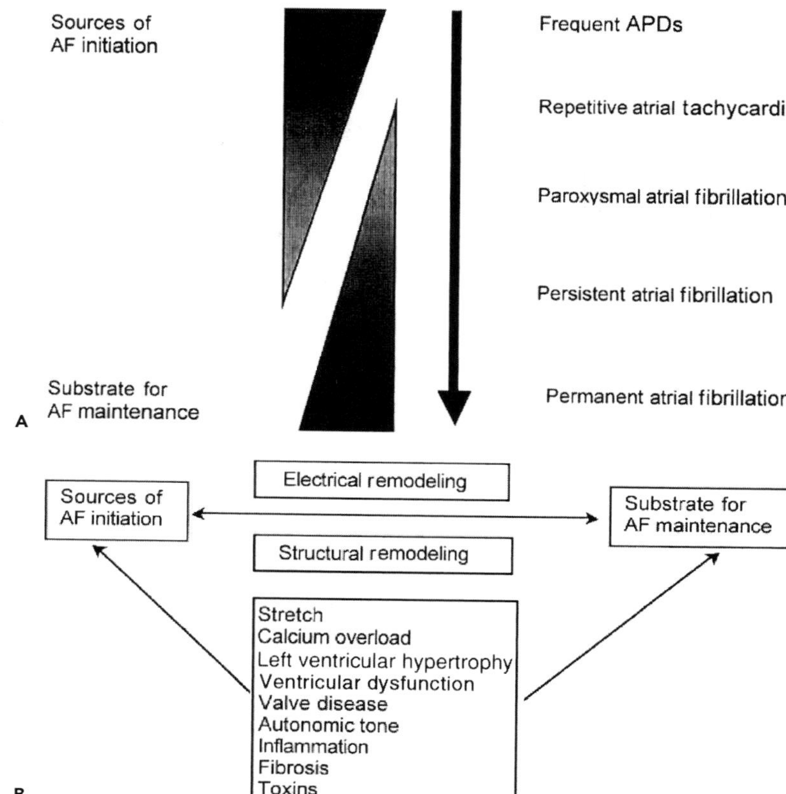


**Figure 49–1** The dual-substrate concept (modified from).

## Dual-Substrate Concept (Modified from Lesh et al. 2000)

Substrates for sources that initiate atrial fibrillation and substrates for maintenance of AF underlie the spectrum and natural history of progression of disease, influenced by structural and electrical remodeling (Fig. 49–1). In some situations, the triggering mechanisms (pulmonary vein tachycardia) may also be the driving mechanism sustaining AF. In such patients, the atria can be thought of as resistant to maintainance of AF and only remain in AF while there is a focal tachycardia driver firing at a rapid rate.

## Atrial Flutter Re-entrant Mechanism

### *Cavotricuspid Isthmus-Dependent (CTI) Atril Flutter*

- CTI dependent flutters refers to circuits which involve the isthmus of tissue in the posterior right atrium between the tricuspid annulus and inferior vena cava (IVC) (Fig. 49–2).
- The circuit can propagate around the isthmus in a clockwise or counterclockwise direction
- Counterclockwise atrial flutter is characterized by dominant negative flutter waves in the inferior leads and positive flutter deflection in lead V1.
- Clockwise atrial flutter is characterized by positive flutter waves in inferior leads and negative flutter waves in lead V1.
- Ablation of the posterior corridor is curative ~90%.

### *Non-Cavotricuspid Isthmus-Dependent (NCTI) Atrial Flutter*

- NCTI dependent flutters do not use cavotricuspid isthmus. NCTI flutters most likely related to atrial scar which creates a conduction block and a central obstacle that allows for reentry.
- NCTI can be found in patients with prior cardiac surgery involving the atrium, such as repair of congenital heart disease, mitral valve surgery or maze procedure.
- NCTI dependent flutters are less common than CTI flutters.

### *Treatment*

- Successful ablation is dependent on identifying a critical portion of the re-entry circuit where it can be interrupted with either one or a line of RF applications.
- Atrial flutter may be difficult to treat medically and may develop with organization of AF re-entrant flutter circuits during treatment with antiarrhythmic therapy.

## ATRIAL FIBRILLATION DEFINITIONS

- Lone: Absence of cardiac or other conditions predisposing to AF
- Acute: <48 hours

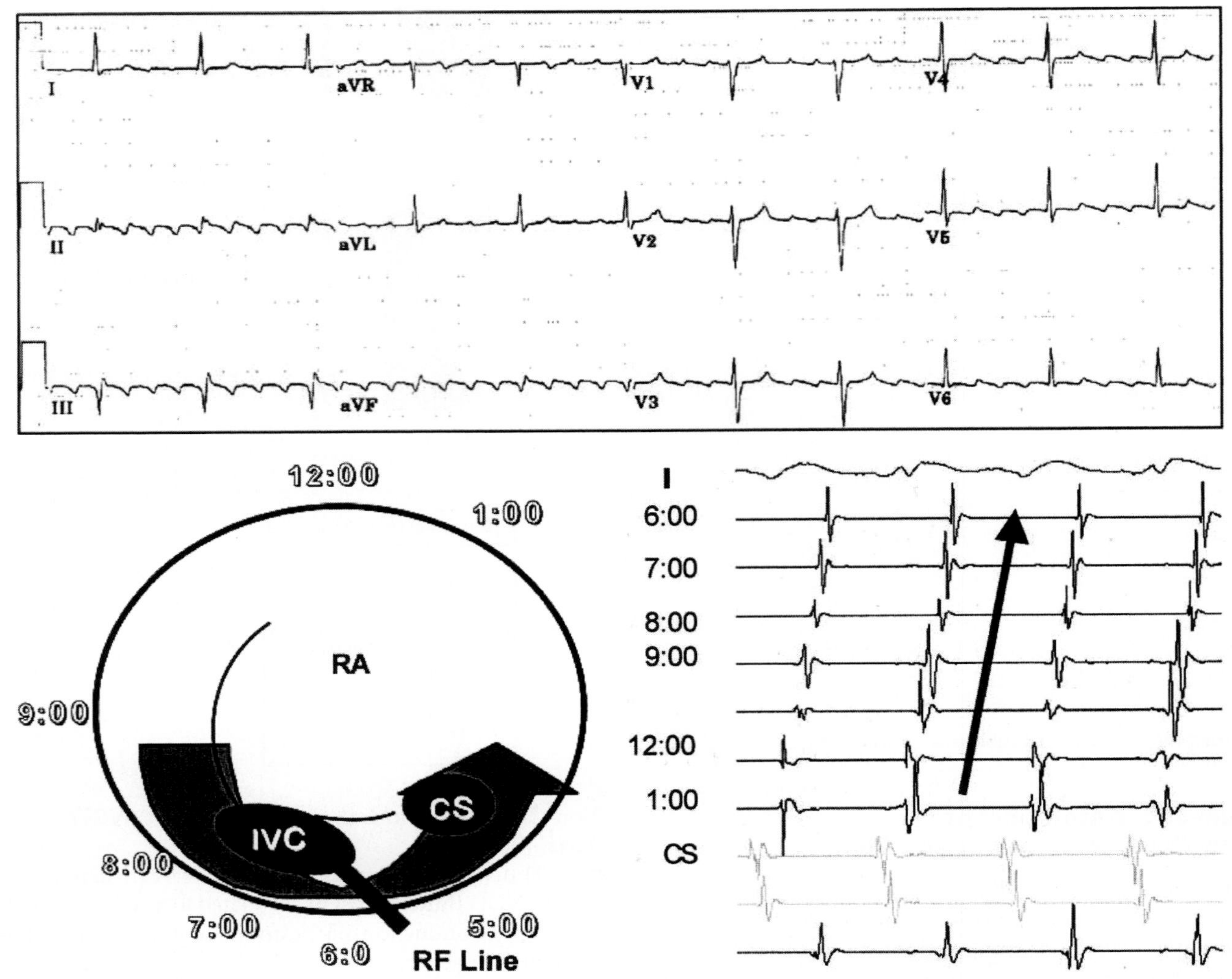


Figure 49–2 Type I counterclockwise right atrial flutter.

- Recurrent: Has two or more paroxysmal or permanent episodes
- Paroxysmal: Self-terminating within 7 days, generally lasting 24 hours
- Persistent: Is not self-terminating within 7 days or is terminated with treatment
- Permanent: Persistent despite cardioversion

## EVALUATION FOR UNDERLYING CONDITIONS

### History

- Precipitating factors and conditions
- Alcohol, caffeine, sympathomimetic, herbal supplements, or other drug use
- Duration and frequency of episodes
- Degree of associated symptoms
- Manner of atrial fibrillation initiation
- Regularity at initiation may suggest tachycardia-induced AF

### Documentation of Atrial Fibrillation and Initiation

- ECGs, rhythm strips
- Transtelephonic (remote) event monitoring
- Evaluation for precipitating bradycardia, PSVT, atrial flutter, atrial ectopy, atrial tachycardia

### Diagnostic Testing

- Lab studies—thyroid function tests, electrolytes
- Echocardiogram—evaluate LV function, valves, atrial size
- Functional stress testing or cardiac catheterization—evaluate for CAD in patients with risk factors and evaluate candidacy for 1C agents

**TABLE 49–1**
**CONSEQUENCES OF ATRIAL FIBRILLATION AND TARGETS OF THERAPY**

| Targets of Therapy | Goals of Therapy |
|---|---|
| Symptoms from palpitations | |
| Irregular heart beats | Maintenance of sinus rhythm |
| Rapid ventricular rates | Control of AV nodal conduction |
| Impaired hemodynamics | |
| Loss of AV synchrony | Maintenance of sinus rhythm |
| Rapid ventricular rates | Control of AV nodal conduction |
| Risk of thromboembolism | Reduction in risk of systemic embolism/stroke |
| Tachycardia-induced cardiomyopathy | |
| Ventricular cardiomyopathy | Control of ventricular rate, AV nodal conduction |
| Atrial cardiomyopathy | Maintenance of sinus rhythm |
| Increase in mortality | Improvement in survival |

## MANAGEMENT OF ATRIAL FIBRILLATION

Consequences of atrial fibrillation and targets of therapy are given in Table 49–1.

### Treatment Strategies

- Ventricular rate control
  - AV nodal blocking drugs
  - AVN modification/ablation and pacing
- Achievement and maintenance of sinus rhythm (SR)
  - Antiarrhythmic drugs
  - Cardioversions
  - Nonpharmacologic therapies
    - Ablation
    - Surgery—Maze procedure
    - Atrial defibrillator
    - Pacing
- Anticoagulation
- Maintenance of SR with antiarrhythmic therapy
  - Potential for more complete relief of symptoms and hemodynamic improvement.
  - Approximately one-half of patients will develop recurrent AF after cardioversion to SR
  - Potential for increased mortality and proarrhythmic potential when antiarrhythmic agents are used.

### Atrial Fibrillation Follow-up Investigation of Rhythm Management (AFFIRM)

The AFFIRM study (Wyse et al. 2002) was a multicenter trial of rate versus rhythm control strategies (Table 49–2). It tested the hypothesis that in patients with AF, total mortality with primary therapy intended to maintain SR is equal to that with primary therapy intended to control heart rate. The study randomized 4,060 patients (>65 years old or with risk factors for stroke), with a primary endpoint of total mortality. No significant difference in total mortality was found among strategies, although there was a strong trend toward better survival in the rate-control arm. The study also showed that continued anticoagulation is important even in the rhythm-control arm, so this may be the best strategy in relatively asymptomatic older patients with good rate control.

**TABLE 49–2**
**RATE CONTROL VERSUS RHYTHM CONTROL**

| | Potential Benefits | Potential Risks |
|---|---|---|
| Maintenance of sinus rhythm | Better control of symptoms<br>Reduced risk from anticoagulation<br>Avoidance of electrical and structural remodeling | Increased risk of adverse effects (including death)<br>Higher cost |
| Control of heart rate alone | Lower risk of adverse effects (including death)<br>Possibly lower cost | Poorer relief of symptoms<br>Increased risk from anticoagulation |

### Control of Ventricular Rate

Rapid ventricular rates can cause symptoms and/or ventricular dysfunction. The goal of treatment, a heart rate of 70 to 100 beats/min at rest, can be achieved pharmacologically with agents that slow AV nodal conduction, such as digoxin, beta-adrenergic blockers, and calcium channel blockers (Table 49–3).

#### *Digoxin*

Digoxin has direct and indirect effects on the AV node, with a primary vagotonic effect. Advantages include that:

- It is inexpensive.
- It can be given intravenously.
- It can be used safely in patients with heart failure.
- It is effective in controlling resting ventricular rates in chronic, persistent AF.

Disadvantages are that:

- Peak onset of heart rate–lowering effect is delayed by 1 to 4 hours.
- The therapeutic window is narrow.
- It is less effective in rate control of paroxysmal AF.
- It is less effective for rapid rates during hyperadrenergic states, when vagal tone is low, e.g., during exercise or in acute and ICU settings, because of increased sympathetic tone.

**TABLE 49–3**
**PHARMACOLOGIC RATE CONTROL FOR ATRIAL ARRHYTHMIAS**

| Agent | Loading Dose | Maintenance Dose | Side Effects Toxicity | Comments |
|---|---|---|---|---|
| Digoxin | 0.25–0.5 mg IV or PP, then 0.25 mg every 4–6 h to 1 mg in first 24 h | 0.125–0.25 mg PO or IV per day | Anorexia, nausea; AV block; ventricular arrhythmias; accumulates in renal failure | Used in CHF; vagotonic effects on the AV node; delayed onset of action; narrow therapeutic window; less effective in postop, paroxysmal AF with high adrenergic states |
| Betal-blockers | | | | |
| Propranolol | 1 mg IV every 2–5 min to 0.1–0.2 mg/kg | 10–80 mg PO t.i.d–q.i.d. | Bronchospasm; CHF; ↓ BP | Effective in heart rate control; rapid onset of action; esmolol is short acting |
| Metoprolol | 5 mg IV every 5 min to 15 mg | 25–100 mg PO b.i.d–t.i.d. | | |
| Esmolol | 500 μg/kg IV over 1 min | 50 μg/kg IV for 4 min; repeat load PRN and ↑ maintenance 20–50 μg/kg/min every 5–10 min | | |
| Calcium channel blockers | | | | |
| Verapamil | 2.5–10 mg IV over 2 min | 5–10 mg IV every 30–60 min or 40–160 mg PO t.i.d or 120–480 mg/d, sustained release | ↓ BP, CHF<br>↑ digoxin lev | Rapid onset, can be used safely in COPD and DM |
| Diltiazem | 0.25 mg/kg over 2 min; repeat PRN every 15 min at 0.35 mg/kg | 5–15 mg/h IV or 30–90 mg PO q.i.d or 120–360 mg sustained release per day | | Often well tolerated with low-LVEF patients |

CHF, congestive heart failure; AF, atrial fibrillation; BP, blood pressure; COPD, chronic obstructive pulmonary disease; DM, diabetes mellitus; LVEF, left ventricular ejection fraction.

Digoxin should be used with caution in elderly patients and in patients with decreased renal function.

### *Beta-Adrenergic Blockers*

Advantages of beta-adrenergic blockers are that they

- Are very effective for heart rate control, even with exercise
- Can be given intravenously
- Have rapid onset of action
- Have long-term benefits in patients with LV dysfunction

Disadvantages of beta-adrenergic blockers are that they

- May provoke bronchospasm
- Are negatively inotropic and may exacerbate CHF
- May reduce exercise tolerance as a result of their negative inotropy and chronotropy

### *Calcium Channels Blockers*

The advantages of calcium channel blockers such as verapamil and diltiazem include:

- Beneficial effects on electrical remodeling
- Verapamil can attenuate the atrial ERP shortening seen with even short-duration AF
- Available intravenously
- Rapid onset of action
- Can be used safely in chronic obstructive pulmonary disease (COPD) and diabetes mellitus

Disadvantages include:

- Negative inotropic effects
- Can cause hypotension
- Long-term safety questioned

### *Class I or III Antiarrhythmic Drugs*

Sotalol, amiodarone, propafenone, and flecainide can contribute to ventricular rate control.

## NONPHARMACOLOGIC RATE CONTROL

### Complete AV Junction Ablation

Radiofrequency catheter ablation is usually technically easy to accomplish.

- Advantages
  - Effectively controls rapid ventricular rates
  - Significant symptomatic relief and improvement in quality of life demonstrated
  - Can reverse tachycardia-mediated cardiomyopathy

**TABLE 49–4**
**PHARMACOLOGIC CONVERSION REGIMENS**

| Drug | Route | Dose | Success Rate |
|---|---|---|---|
| Quinidine | PO | 200–324 mg t.i.d. to 1.5 g/d | 48–86% |
| Procainamide | IV | 1 g over 20–30 min | 48–65% |
| Propafenone | PO | 600 mg | 55–87% |
| | IV | 2 mg/kg over 10 min | 40–90% |
| Flecainide | PO | 300 mg | 90% |
| | IV | 2 mg/kg over 10 min | 65–90% |
| Amiodarone | IV | 1.2 g over 24 h | 45–85% |
| Sotalol | PO | 80–160 mg, then 160–360 mg/d | 52% |
| Dofetilide | PO | 125–500 $\mu$g b.i.d. based on CrCl | 30% |
| Ibutilide | IV | 1 mg over 10 min, repeat in 10 min PRN | 31% |

- Disadvantages
  - Requires a permanent rate-responsive pacemaker
  - Patient is pacemaker dependent
  - Pacing RV alone may significantly worsen ventricular function. Biventricular pacing may be necessary in patients with reduced LV function.

### AV Node Modification

AV node modification may avoid the need for a pacemaker, but it has some disadvantages:

- Significant rate of production of complete AV block
- Higher recurrence rates of return of rapid AV conduction
- Does not improve symptoms due to irregularity of ventricular rates in atrial fibrillation

## RESTORATION OF SINUS RHYTHM

### Electrical Cardioversion

Electrical cardioversion is the most effective method of restoring sinus rhythm. In this technique, shock is synchronized to the R wave. The optimal patch positioning is anterior–posterior (e.g., right parasternal to left paraspinal). For standard monophasic external cardioversion, usual initial energies are 200 J for atrial fibrillation and 50 to 100 J for atrial flutter. Energies can be increased up to 300 J if initial efforts are unsuccessful. Biphasic external conversion, however, requires less energy as a rule.

All electrical cardioversion requires conscious sedation with a short-acting anesthetic such as etomidate or methohexital.

Cardioversion is urgently indicated for patients with clinical instability (e.g., hypotension, ischemia, CHF). It is electively indicated for patients who remain in symptomatic AF after a trial of pharmacologic therapy.

### Pharmacologic Conversion (Table 49–4)

A small randomized controlled study showed no effect of digoxin on conversion rate. However, quinidine, procainamide, flecainide, propafenone, sotalol, amiodarone, dofetilide, and ibutilide showed success rates of 31% to 90%. Procainamide, ibutilide, and amiodarone are available for intravenous administration.

Procainamide is usually administered a dose of 10 to 15 mg/kg IV at ≤50 mg/min, then at 1 to 2 mg/min. It is necessary to monitor blood pressure, as hypotension may require slowing the infusion rate; hemodynamic effects may limit dosing in severe LV dysfunction. It is also necessary to monitor for proarrhythmia—QT prolongation and torsades de pointes. Note that the active metabolite, N-acetyl procainamide (NAPA), may accumulate to toxic levels and cause, renal failure.

Ibutilide is a class III potassium channel blocking agent. In one study it was shown to be more efficacious than procainamide in converting short-term atrial fibrillation/flutter to sinus rhythm. Usual dosing is 1 mg IV over 10 minutes, which can be repeated after another 10 minutes. One should monitor for QT prolongation and torsades de pointes.

Amiodarone is IV form is useful for patients who cannot take oral drugs, though it is more expensive. It may be helpful for hemodynamically unstable patients with recurrent atrial fibrillation despite cardioversion or other antiarrhythmic drugs, for whom rate control is refractory to conventional AV nodal blocking drugs, or who are intolerant of standard antiarrhythmic or rate-controlling drugs as a result of negative inotropy. Rapid oral loading of ibutilide can usually also be achieved in patients with intact gastrointestinal function.

### Maintenance of Sinus Rhythm (Table 49–5)

Maintenance of sinus rhythm often requires an antiarrhythmic agent, particularly in patients with frequent or

**TABLE 49–5**
**DRUGS FOR MAINTENANCE OF SINUS RHYTHM**

| Antiarrhythmic Drug | Dose | % Maintenance SR (6–12 mo) | Side Effects/Comments |
|---|---|---|---|
| Class IA | | | |
| Quinidine | 200–400 mg PO t.i.d.–q.i.d. | 30–79% | ↑ QT, proarrhythmia/TdP, potential ↑ AV node conduction, diarrhea, nausea, ↑ digoxin levels, thrombocytopenia |
| Procainamide | 10–15 mg/kg IV at ≤50 mg/min or 2–6 g/d PO in b.i.d. or q.i.d. sustained release | N/A | ↓ BP, CHF, drug-induced lupus, agranulocytosis; active metabolite NAPA with class III activity accumulates in renal failure |
| Disopyramide | 100–300 mg PO t.i.d. | 44–67% | Anticholinergic effects (e.g., urinary retention, dry eyes/mouth), CHF |
| Class 1C | | | |
| Flecainide | 50–200 mg PO b.i.d. | 34–81% | Proarrhythmia visual disturbance, dizziness, CHF, avoid in CAD or LV dysfunction |
| Propafenone | 150–300 mg t.i.d. | 30–76% | CHF, avoid in CAD/LV dysfunction |
| Class IA/B/C | | | |
| Moricizine | 200–300 mg t.i.d. | N/A | Proarrhythmia, dizziness, GI/nausea, headache, caution in CAD/LV dysfunction |
| Class III | | | |
| Sotalol | 80–240 mg b.i.d. | 37–70% | CHF, bronchospasm, bradycardia, ↑ QT proarrhythmia/TdP |
| Amiodarone | 600–1600 mg/d loading in divided doses, 100–400 mg daily maintenance | 40–79% | Pulmonary toxicity, bradycardia hyper- or hypothryroidism, hepatic toxicity, GI (nausea, constipation), neurologic, dermatologic, and opthalmologic side effects, drug interactions |
| Dofetilide | CrCl (mL/min)<br>>60: 500 μg b.i.d.<br>40–60: 250 μg b.i.d.<br>20–40: 125 μg b.i.d. | 58–71% | Exclude CrCl <20 mL/min, ↑ QT, proarrhythmia/TdP, headache, muscle cramps |

TdP, torsades de pointes; BP, blood pressure; CHF, congestive heart failure; CAD, coronary artery disease; LV, left ventricular.

resistant atrial fibrillation, underlying cardiovascular disease, enlarged atria, or other continuing disease factors that predispose to AF. Antiarrhythmic agents available that can be effective in maintaining sinus rhythm include class IA (quinidine, procainamide, disopyramide), IC (flecainide, propafenone), IA/B/C (moricizine), and III (sotalol, amiodarone, dofetilide) antiarrhythmic drugs. Other new class III antiarrhythmic agents being studied include azimilide, trecetilide, tedisamil, and dronedarone. A substudy of the AFFIRM trial demonstrated that amiodarone is more effective at 1 year for the maintenance of sinus rhythm than sotalol or other class I agents.

## CLASS IA ANTIARRHYTHMIC DRUGS

Class IA antiarrhythmic drugs

- Delay fast sodium channel-mediated conduction with a depression of phase 0
- Prolong repolarization
- Are associated with an incidence of torsade de pointes
- Can enhance AV nodal conduction, potentially increasing ventricular rates during AF
- Usually require concomitant use of AV nodal blocking agents

These drugs are usually not used chronically because of their potential proarrhythmic effects.

### Quinidine

The use of quinidine is limited by proarrhythmia concerns. There is a higher risk in patients on diuretics and those with electrolyte depletion. From a meta-analysis by Coplen et al. 1990, the proportion of patients remaining in SR on quinidine at 1 year was 50% (control, 25%), but total mortality was 2.9% (control, 0.8%). However, only 7 of 12 deaths in the quinidine group died of cardiac causes. Note that in-hospital initiation or systematic QT interval assessment may not have been followed for many of the studies in this analysis.

The SPAF trial 1991 showed increased mortality on antiarrhythmic therapy, which usually consisted of quinidine, with risk seen in patients with a history of congestive heart failure.

Because of the potential for proarrhythmia, including torsades de pointes, in-hospital initiation is recommended, with continuous ECG monitoring and assessment of QT interval.

Quinidine increases serum digoxin levels, so concomitant digoxin dosage usually should be decreased.

Other adverse effects of quinide include gastrointestinal symptoms, particularly diarrhea.

### Procainamide

Procainamide given intravenously, is often a first-line antiarrhythmic agent for AF after cardiac surgery. It's long-term use is usually limited by a high incidence of drug-induced lupus, however, long-term controlled trials are not available.

### Disopyramide

Disopyramide has been shown to be effective for maintenance of SR in ~50% of patients over a follow-up of 6 to 12 months. Its use is limited, however, because of its anticholinergic side effects and, in older males, urinary retention. Disopyramide is also negatively inotropic.

## CLASS IC ANTIARRHYTHMIC DRUGS

The class IC antiarrhythmic drugs markedly slow sodium channel–mediated conduction, with a marked depression of phase 0, but only a slight effect on repolarization.

Flecainide and propafenone have been shown to be equivalent in efficacy in comparative studies. However, proarrhythmia in the form of wide-complex tachycardia due to ventricular tachycardia or slow atrial flutter with 1:1 AV conduction can occur with these agents. They are usually avoided in patients with coronary artery disease or impaired ventricular function.

Patients with underlying heart disease may be at higher risk for proarrhythmia with class IC drugs. The Cardiac Arrhythmia Suppression Trial (CAST) reported increased mortality in patients treated with flecainide and encainide for ventricular arrhythmias after myocardial infarction.

### Flecainide

Flecainide has been shown to be effective in the treatment of atrial fibrillation and is usually well tolerated. Noncardiac effects include visual disturbances, dizziness, and paresthesias.

### Propafenone

Propafenone has weak beta-blocking activity and is effective in the treatment of AF. It is now available in a slow-release form that can be taken twice a day.

### Moricizine

Moricizine has class I/IC properties, but controlled data on its efficacy in AF is sparse.

## CLASS III ANTIARRHYTHMIC DRUGS

Class III antiarrhythmic drugs are potassium channel blockers that prolong repolarization.

### Amiodarone

Amiodarone affects multiple ion channels. Sodium and potassium channel effects include increased refractoriness in the atria, AV node, and ventricles. It also has noncompetitive beta-blocking and calcium channel blocking activity. The drug inhibits phospholipase and antagonizes thyroid hormone but is effective against AF; it has been reported to be superior to sotalol and quinidine, as well as to flecainide, in a meta-analysis.

Amiodarone has a long half-life, requiring weeks to months to achieve steady state. When used long term, however, it has a potential for organ toxicity. It can cause significant bradycardia, but proarrhythmia is uncommon. The risk for pulmonary toxicity appears to be dose related.

Associated with high discontinuation rates.

Other potential side effects include hypothyroidism or hyperthyroidism, liver function test elevation or toxicity, skin changes and photosensitivity, peripheral neuropathy, and, very rarely, optic neuritis. Patients with CHF and prior proarrhythmia/torsade de pointes are at higher risk.

The usual maintenance dose of amiodarone for atrial arrhythmias is <400 mg q.i.d., often 100 to 200 mg q.i.d.

### Sotalol

Sotalol is a nonselective beta-blocker with class III activity that is effective in AF. It has significant beta-blocking activity with potential for bradycardia and negative inotropic effects. Monitoring for QT interval prolongation and torsade de pointes is recommended.

The d-isomer of sotalol (d-sotalol) studied in Survival with Oral D-Sotalol (SWORD) increased mortality in patients after myocardial infarction (MI) (d-sotalol) was withdrawn from development).

### Dofetilide

Dofetilide is a potent inhibitor of $I_{kr}$, the rapid component of the delayed rectifier. In the DIAMOND trials of patients after MI or with CHF, it did not increase mortality. During this study, it was also found to be beneficial in maintaining sinus rhythm.

In-hospital initiation is mandated, and dosage should be adjusted in the presence of renal insufficiency.

## NEW CLASS III ANTIARRHYTHMIC DRUGS UNDER DEVELOPMENT

### Azimilide

Azimilide prolongs action potential duration by blockade of $I_{Ks}$ as well as $I_{Kr}$. It may be less reverse use dependent than other $I_{Kr}$ blockers. Theoretically, at least, it may have a lower risk for proarrhythmia.

Azimilide is being studied in ALIVE, a trial of azimilide use after myocardial infarction.

### Tedisamil

Tedisamil blocks $I_{Kr}$ and $I^{to}$ and may have effects on $I_{KATP}$ openers. It prolongs action potential duration and refractory periods in atrial but not ventricular myocardium.

### Dronedarone

Dronedarone is a deiodinated derivative of amiodarone in late stages of development and clinical testing.

## ANTIARRHYTHMIC DRUG SELECTION

Strategies for the approach to antiarrhythmic drug selection should provide adequate rate control and minimization of thromboembolism risk. The decision to use an antiarrhythmic drug should include consideration of frequency and duration of the AF, symptoms, reversibility of the arrhythmia, and the presence of structural heart disease. In addition, the risk of side effects, including organ toxicity and proarrhythmia, should be weighed against the benefits and efficacy rates of the drugs.

### Antiarrhythmic Drug Considerations

Recurrences can be expected (50% at 6 to 36 months) but are generally not life threatening. Total suppression of symptoms and/or recurrences risks drug toxicity, so safety is important. Reductions and improvements in quality of life are reasonable goals for treatment.

### Approach to Antiarrhythmic Drug Selection

Consider

- Frequency and duration of AF
- Symptoms
- Reversibility
- Structural heart disease
- Risk of side effects
- Proarrhythmia
- Organ toxicity
- Age and activity level
- Assessment of risky versus benefits
- Efficacy

#### *Frequency, Duration, and Symptoms*

##### First Episode

After a first episode, the future pattern of recurrence cannot be predicted. The success rate and rate of recurrence are more favorable on an antiarrhythmic drug, but antiarrhythmic drug therapy may not be necessary after a first occurrence, unless factors such as structural heart disease, large atria, or advanced age suggest a high risk of recurrence.

A first episode can be converted either pharmacologically or electrically. If there is early recurrences of AF after cardioversion, then consider prescribing an antiarrhythmic drug. One may also consider stopping the antiarrhythmic drug after a few weeks or months.

##### Recurring, Paroxysmal Atrial Fibrillation

For recurring, paroxysmal AF, assess the frequency and associated symptoms. If the patient is asymptomatic, consider rate control or antiarrhythmic therapy and warfarin, if indicated. If the patient is symptomatic, consider further rate control or antiarrhythmic drug therapy.

For infrequent episodes in a patient with a normal heart, consider intermittent drug therapy (e.g., 150 to 300 mg flecainide PO or 300 to 600 mg propafenone PO). For frequent symptomatic episodes, consider an antiarrhythmic drug.

##### Chronic, Persistent Atrial Fibrillation

For chronic, persistent AF, assess the duration of the atrial fibrillation, atrial size, symptoms, and anticoagulation status. Based on this assessment, one may want to consider cardioversion. Antiarrhythmic therapy may also be required for successful conversion and maintenance of sinus rhythm at least short term, if not chronically.

#### *Structural Heart Disease*

Patients with coronary artery disease and/or ventricular dysfunction are at higher risk of proarrhythmia. For these patients:

- Avoid class IC drugs (based on CAST).
- Consider dofetilide, for which no harmful outcomes were reported in the DIAMOND MI and CHF trials.
- Consider sotalol for patients with preserved LV function who can tolerate its beta-blocking activity.
- Consider amiodarone, which has a low proarrhythmic profile and can be used as a first- or second-line agent with safety, based on the results of the EMIAT, CAMIAT, CHF-STAT, and GESICA trials.

**TABLE 49–6**
**PROARRHYTHMIA IN STUDIES OF ANTIARRHYTHMIC DRUGS FOR ATRIAL FIBRILLATION**

| Drug | *n* | TdP | VT/SCD | I:IAFL | Brady | Total |
|---|---|---|---|---|---|---|
| Quinidine | 1,043 | 0.6 | 1.2 | 0 | 0 | 1.7 |
| Flecainide | 1,634 | 0 | 0.4 | 0.4 | 0.4 | 1.8 |
| Propafenone | 788 | 0 | 0.2 | 0 | 0 | 0.9 |
| Sotalol | 260 | 1.5 | 0.8 | 0 | 1.1 | 2.3 |
| Amiodarone | 816 | 0 | 0 | 0 | 0 | 0 |

TdP, torsades de pointes; VT, ventricular tachycardia; SCD, sudden cardiac death; I:IAFL.
Adapted from Thibault, Nattel. *J CV EP* 1999;10:472–481.

Patients with left ventricular hypertrophy (LVH) may have a higher risk of torsades de pointes. Class IC drugs may be preferred as first-line therapy in these patients.

### *Other Drug Considerations—Efficacy, Organ Toxicity, and Proarrhythmia*

#### Efficacy

Class IA and class IC drugs have efficacy rates of ~50% in maintaining SR at 6 months. The class III drugs have slightly higher efficacy rates (50% to 70%).

#### Side Effects

Side effects are common with the use of antiarrhythmic agents. The side effect profile and risk for organ toxicity often limits continuation, although not necessarily, initiation of a particular drug.

- Amiodarone has significant potential for organ toxicity. Risk is dose and duration related, and side effects often limit its use, particularly in younger patients.
- Sotalol has negative inotropy, negative chronotropy, and bronchospastic side effects.
- Procainamide has a high frequency of drug-induced lupus, which seriously limits its long-term use. There is also a small risk of agranulocytosis.
- Quinidine has a small risk of agranulocytosis, thrombocytopenia, and/or lupus with procainamide and of thrombocytopenia and lupus with quinidine.

#### Proarrhythmic Risk (Table 49–6)

Patients with normal hearts and non–life threatening AF are at low risk for proarrhythmia. They may be treated with drugs with the lowest risk of proarrhythmia or organ toxicity. For these seasons, class IC drugs are often used as the first line of treatment. Class IA drugs and sotalol (class III) are lower-tier choices.

Patients with CAD or ventricular dysfunction are at higher risk for proarrhythmia from class IC drugs, so one should consider dofetilide, sotalol, or amiodarone for these patients.

Risk factors for proarrhythmia include structural heart disease, LV dysfunction, CHF, prior MI or CAD, LVH, female gender, prior torsades de pointes or CHF (amiodarone), and older age (Fig. 49–3).

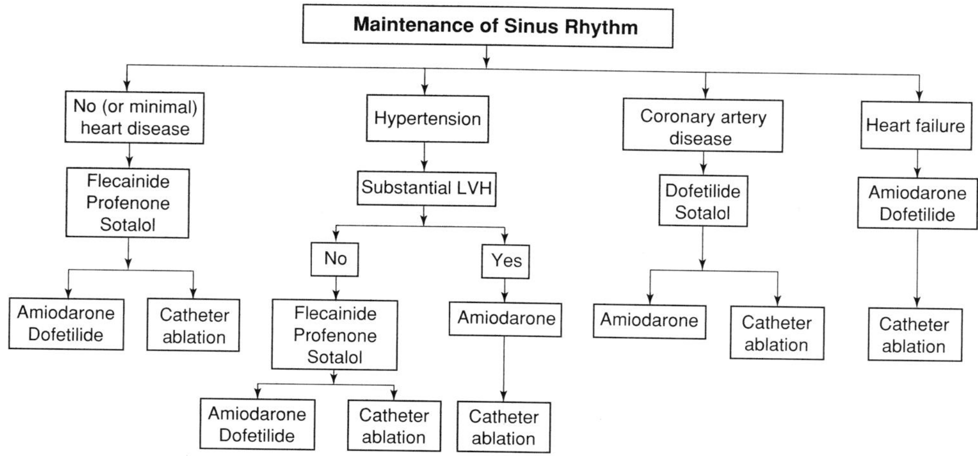


**Figure 49–3** AFASAKI, atrial fibrillation, aspirin, anticoagulation study; SPAFI, stroke prevention in atrial fibrillation; BAATAF, boston area anticoagulation trial; CAFA, canadian atrial fibrillation anticoagulation trial; SPINAF, stroke prevention in non-rheumatic atrial fibrillation study; AFI, atrial fibrillation investigators; EAFT, european atrial fibrillation trial.

## INPATIENT VERSUS OUTPATIENT INITIATION OF ANTIARRHYTHMIC DRUGS

The choice between initiating antiarrhythmic drug therapy on an inpatient or outpatient basis remains controversial, but inpatient initiation is usually recommended for:

- Patients with LV dysfunction
- Patients with persistent AF
- Patients at risk for proarrhythmia (see above risk factors)
- Class IA and III antiarrhythmic agents other than amiodarone: dofetilide (mandated in-hospital initiation), sotalol, quinidine, procainamide, or disopyramide
- CHF patients with a history of torsades de pointes starting amiodarone
- Prior history of proarrhythmia
- Prolonged QT at baseline when initiating class IA and class III drugs
- Propensity to bradycardia
- History of ventricular arrhythmias in a patient with significant LV dysfunction and no ICD

## PROARRHYTHMIA RISK BY STRUCTURAL HEART DISEASE AND ANTIARRHYTHMIC DRUG

- No structural heart disease: class IC, amiodarone < sotalol, class IA
- Structural heart disease: amiodarone < sotalol, class IA < class IC (except LVH)

## ANTIARRHYTHMIC DRUG SELECTION

### Chronic Anticoagulation and Antithrombotic Therapy

Atrial fibrillation is associated with thromboembolic events and stroke; AF is one of the most potent risk factors for stroke in the elderly and is the most common cause of cardiogenic stroke.

The risk of stroke in nonvalvular AF varies with age and the presence of concomitant cardiovascular disease and other risk factors. In general, patients with nonvalvular AF have about a sixfold increased risk of stroke. From the Framingham Heart Study, over 30 years of follow-up, the annual rate of stroke was 4.2% per year, and increased relative risk of stroke was associated with hypertension, CAD, CHF, and AF.

In patients younger than age 60 years and without hypertension or cardiovascular disease, the risk of stroke is low. Meta-analysis (five major primary prevention trials for stroke in atrial fibrillation) indicated that the risk of stroke is ~1% per year for patients under age 65 without risk factors of hypertension, diabetes, or prior stroke or transient ischemic attack. For patients who are older, who have risk factors for stroke or concomitant cardiovascular disease, the risk of stroke is ~3% to 5% per year. Older patients (>75 years old) with risk factors for stroke are at higher risk (8% per year).

Most strokes associated with AF appear to result from cardiac emboli, presumably from thrombi formed in fibrillating atria. The rate of stroke is clustered at the onset of the arrhythmia, with 25% of patients suffering a stroke, whereas another 14% have a stroke within the first year.

Several large clinical trials have identified risk factors for stroke when AF is present:

- Transient ischemic attack (TIA) or previous stroke
- Diabetes
- Hypertension
- Age
- Left ventricular dysfunction
- Increased left atrial size
- Rheumatic mitral valve disease
- Prosthetic valves
- Women >75 years old
- Mitral annular calcification
- Increased wall thickness
- Thyrotoxicosis

### Paroxysmal Atrial Fibrillation

Patients with paroxysmal AF have a stroke rate of 3.7% per year. Events are clustered at the onset of the arrhythmia, the incidence of embolism is 6.8% in the first month, decreasing to 2% per year over the subsequent 5 years.

Patients with paroxysmal AF appear to be at similar risk as patients with chronic, persistent AF and generally are treated similarly with regard to anticoagulation.

Patients with a single AF event, with no other risk factors or structural heart disease and <65 years old have a low stroke event rate of 1% per year.

### Stroke/Thromboembolism Prevention Trials (Tables 49–7, 49–8, and 49–9)

Primary prevention trials include:

- Atrial Fibrillation, Aspirin, Anticoagulation Study (AFASAK)
- Stroke Prevention in Atrial Fibrillation Trial (SPAF)
- Boston Area Anticoagulation Trial (BAATAF)
- Canadian Atrial Fibrillation Anticoagulation Trial (CAFA)
- Stroke Prevention in Non-rheumatic Atrial Fibrillation Study (SPINAF)
- Second phase of the Stroke Prevention in Atrial Fibrillation study (SPAF 2)
- Third phase of the Stroke Prevention in Atrial Fibrillation study (SPAF 3)
- Second phase of the Atrial Fibrillation, Aspirin, Anticoagulation Study (AFASAK 2)

Secondary prevention trials include:

- European Atrial Fibrillation Trial (EAFT)
- Atrial Fibrillation Investigators (AFI)

**TABLE 49–7**
**STROKE/THROMBOEMBOLISM REDUCTION IN ATRIAL FIBRILLATION: WARFARIN VS. CONTROL**

| | Warfarin | Control | RRR% | *p* Value |
|---|---|---|---|---|
| AFASAKI | 2.7 | 6.2 | 56 | < 0.05 |
| SPAFI | 2.3 | 7.4 | 67 | 0.01 |
| BAATAF | 0.4 | 3.0 | 86 | 0.002 |
| CAFA | 3.4 | 4.6 | 26 | 0.25 |
| SPINAF | 0.9 | 4.3 | 79 | 0.001 |
| AFI | 1.4 | 4.5 | 68 | <0.001 |
| EAFT | 8.5 | 16.5 | 47 | 0.001 |

RRR%, relative risk ratio (percent).

The AFI trial reported results pooled from five primary prevention trials, and found a 68% reduction in stroke risk with warfarin and borderline significant reduction in risk with aspirin.

## AMERICAN COLLEGE OF CHEST PHYSICIANS GUIDELINES FOR ANTITHROMBOTIC THERAPY FOR ATRIAL FIBRILLATION

Risk stratification schemes for antithrombotic therapy from the American College of Chest Physicians are given in Table 49–10, and their recommendations are summarized in Table 49–11.

### Summary (Fig. 49–4)

1. Anticoagulation is an important consideration for patients with AF, particularly those in whom atrial fibrillation persists >48 hours or continues to recur after cardioversion.
2. AF is known to increase the risk of stroke.
3. Anticoagulation is recommended if AF persists >48 hours, particularly if cardioversion is anticipated after this time.
4. Anticoagulation with warfarin (target PT/INR 2.5, range 2.0 to 3.0 for AF) should be recommended for all anticoagulation-eligible patients >75 years old, as well as for patients <75 years old who have any of the following risk factors for thromboembolism:
   - Prior TIA, systemic embolus, or stroke
   - Hypertension
   - Poor LV function
   - Rheumatic mitral valve disease
   - Prosthetic heart valves
5. Patients aged 65 to 75 years with no risk factors can be treated with aspirin or warfarin.
6. Aspirin is recommended for patients <65 years old and who have no risk factors.
7. These recommendations apply to paroxysmal as well as chronic, persistent AF.

### Recommendations for Anticoagulation in Patients Undergoing Cardioversion

1. The risk of emboli after cardioversion is 0.6% to 5.6% without and 0.8% to 1% with anticoagulation.
2. The anticoagulation recommendations of the American College of Chest Physicians for electrical cardioversion are
   - For AF >48 hours in duration, anticoagulate with warfarin (target INR 2.5, range 2.0 to 3.0) for 3 weeks before elective cardioversion.

**TABLE 49–8**
**STROKE/THROMBOEMBOLISM REDUCTION IN ATRIAL FIBRILLATION: ASPIRIN VS. CONTROL**

| | Aspirin | Control | RRR% | *p* Value |
|---|---|---|---|---|
| AFASAKI | 5.2 | 6.2 | 16 | NS |
| SPAFI | 3.6 | 6.3 | 42 | 0.02 |
| EAFT | 15.5 | 19.0 | 17 | 0.12 |
| AFI | 6.3 | 8.1 | 21 | 0.05 |
| ESPS2 | 13.8 | 20.7 | 33 | 0.16 |

RRR%, relative risk ratio (percent).
AFASAKI, atrial fibrillation, aspirin, anticoagulation study; SPAFI, stroke prevention in atrial fibrillation; EAFT, european atrial fibrillation trial; AFI, atrial fibrillation investigators; ESPS2, european stroke prevention study 2.

**TABLE 49–9**
**STROKE/THROMBOEMBOLISM REDUCTION IN ATRIAL FIBRILLATION WARFARIN VS. ASPIRIN**

| | Warfarin | Aspirin | RRR% | *p* Value |
|---|---|---|---|---|
| AFASAKI | 2.7 | 6.2 | 48 | <0.05 |
| SPAF2 | | | | |
| ≤75 | 1.3 | 1.9 | 48 | 0.24 |
| >75 | 3.6 | 4.8 | 33 | 0.39 |
| EAFT | NA | NA | 40 | 0.008 |
| AFASAK2 | 3.4 | 2.7 | −21 | NS |

| | Warfarin | Low Dose Warfarin + Aspirin | RRR% | *p* Value |
|---|---|---|---|---|
| SPAF3 | 1.9 | 7.9 | 74 | <0.0001 |
| AFASAK2 | 3.4 | 3.2 | −6 | NS |

RRR%, relative risk ratio (percent).
AFASAKI, atrial fibrillation, aspirin, anticoagulation study; SPAF2, stroke prevention in atrial fibrillation phase 2; EAFT, european atrial fibrillation trial; AFASAK2, atrial fibrillation, aspirin, anticoagulation study phase 2.

- Continue warfarin until SR has been maintained for 4 weeks (allows time for mechanical atrial transport to resume and for possible recurrence of AF).
- In some circumstances, a transesophageal echocardiography (TEE) protocol may be substituted for conventional therapy, but adjusted-dose warfarin should be continued until SR has been maintained at least 4 weeks.

3. Consideration should be given to managing anticoagulation for atrial flutter similar to that for atrial fibrillation.
4. Long-term anticoagulation beyond the 4 weeks after cardioversion should be considered if there also is cardiomyopathy, history of previous embolism, mitral valve disease, or other indications for long-term anticoagulation as listed above.
5. Heparin anticoagulation followed by oral anticoagulation may be indicated for patients requiring emergency cardioversion for hemodynamic instability. For AF of <48 hours duration, the risk of embolism after cardioversion appears to be low, but pericardioversion anticoagulation is recommended. (From Albers et al., 2001.)

## ROLE OF TRANSESOPHAGEAL ECHOCARDIOGRAPHY

The ACUTE trial compared conventional anticoagulation versus a TEE-guided approach before cardioversion. It randomized 1,222 patients to conventional anticoagulation with therapeutic warfarin for 3 weeks prior to cardioversion or to a TEE-guided approach. Recently reported results show no significant difference in thromboembolic complications occurring after cardioversion in the two arms.

## NONPHARMACOLOGIC MANAGEMENT OF ATRIAL FIBRILLATION AND FLUTTER

Electrical cardioversion is the most effective method of conversion to sinus rhythm and is the method of choice for

**TABLE 49–10**
**RISK STRATIFICATION SCHEMES FOR NONRHEUMATIC ATRIAL FIBRILLATION**

| AF Investigators | | SPAF3 | |
|---|---|---|---|
| **Risk Strata** | **Annual Stroke Rate (%)** | **Risk Strata** | **Annual Stroke Rate (%)** |
| <65 y, no other RF | 1.0 | No RF, no hx HTN[a] | 1.1 |
| <65 y, ≥1 other RF | 4.9 | | |
| 65–75 y, ≥1 other RF | 4.3 | No RF, hx HTN[a] | 3.6 |
| >75 y, no other RF | 3.5 | | |
| >75 y, ≥1 other RF | 8.1 | >1 RF[b] | 7.9 |

RF, risk factors; HTN, hypertension; SPAF3, stroke prevention in atrial fibrillation phase 3.

**TABLE 49–11**
**AMERICAN COLLEGE OF CHEST PHYSICIANS GUIDELINES FOR ANTITHROMBOTIC THERAPY FOR ATRIAL FIBRILLATION**

| Risk Factors | No. | Recommendation |
|---|---|---|
| High[a] | 1 | Warfarin |
| Moderate[b] | >1 | Warfarin |
| | 1 | Warfarin or aspirin |
| None | 0 | Aspirin |

hemodynamically compromising AF. It is necessary, however, to evaluate the need for anticoagulation before cardioversion.

For elective direct-current cardioversion:

- Fast for at least 6 to 8 hours.
- Correct electrolyte imbalances.
- Exclude toxic drug levels.
- Generally, hold digoxin the morning of the procedure.

Electrode positioning should assure an appropriate vector for atrial defibrillation:

- Anterior–posterior
- R subclavicular/parasternal–L posterior patch position

Conscious sedation should be produced with a short-acting anesthetic (e.g., etomidate, methohexital, or propofol). Vital signs, ECG, respiratory status, and pulse oximetry must be closely monitored.

In performing the procedure, synchronize to the QRS complex to minimize risk of inducing ventricular fibrillation.

Atrial flutter may require less energy for successful cardioversion (e.g., 50 to 100 J) than atrial fibrillation (usually begin at 200 J). If atrial pacing electrodes are present,

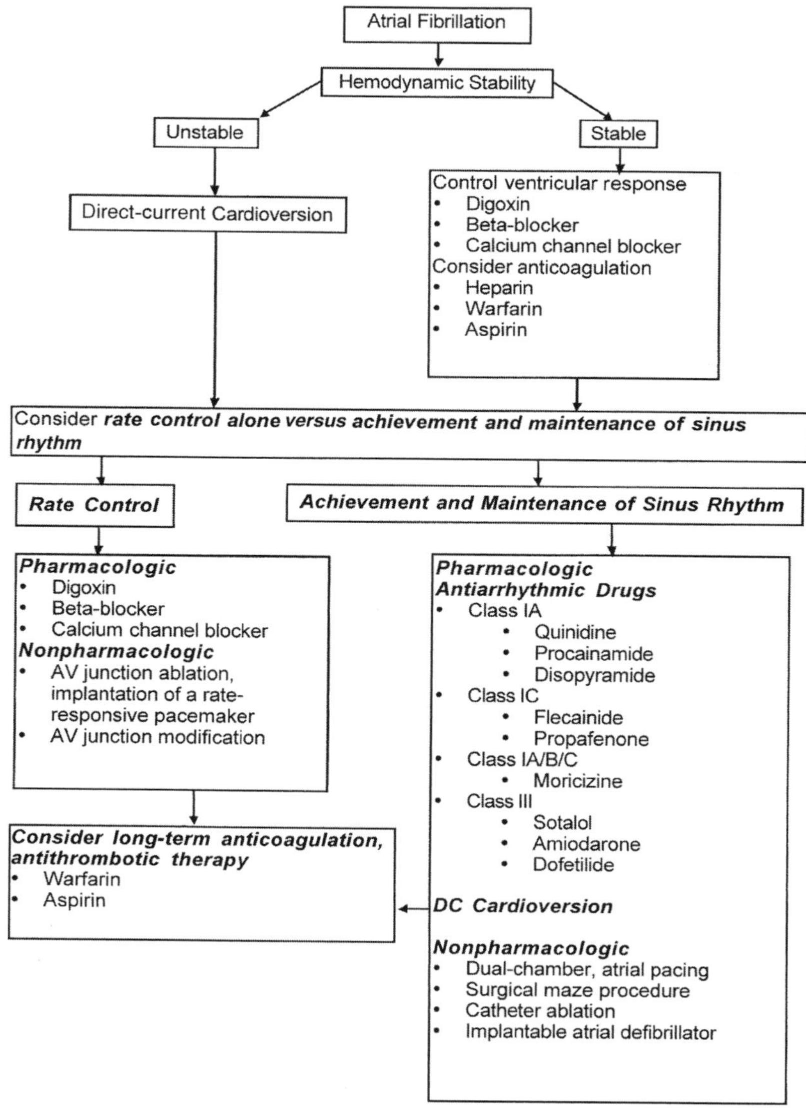


**Figure 49–4** Strategies for management of atrial fibrillation.

atrial overdrive pacing may be attempted to terminate atrial flutter.

Internal cardioversion may be used for atrial fibrillation that is refractory to standard external cardioversion. In this case, high-energy (200 to 360 J) transcatheter direct-current shocks are used. Lower-energies (2 to 10 J) have been successful using catheters placed in the right atrium and coronary sinus.

Biphasic external defibrillators can be used with decreased atrial defibrillation thresholds. At our institution we have achieved sinus rhythm in >99% of patients with this method.

## AV NODE ABLATION OR MODIFICATION

Complete AV nodal (or His bundle) ablation with implantation of a permanent rate-responsive pacemaker was initially achieved with direct-current ablation. Now it is performed primarily using radiofrequency catheter ablation methods. The procedure is successful in up to 100% of patients, and most experience significant symptomatic improvement. Complete ablation is most appropriate and successful for patients whose symptoms are secondary to difficult–to-control rapid ventricular rates.

AF patients who have undergone AV node junctional ablation and have a severely depressed ejection fraction should have a biventricular pacemaker implanted (PAVE study).

Advantages of complete AV node ablation include:

- High rate of procedural success, nearing 100%
- Only a low rate of recurrent rapid ventricular conduction (0% to 14%)
- Improvement in symptoms and quality of life reported in 84% to 100% of patients
- Ventricular dysfunction also shown to improve

When compared to pharmacologic rate control, symptoms improved in both groups, although the improvements were greater in the AV junction ablation and pacing groups.

Disadvantages of complete AV node ablation are

- Dependence on a permanent pacemaker
- Lack of effects on AV dissynchrony
- No reduction in risk of thromboembolism

A possible small risk of late sudden death, primarily reported after direct-current ablation, has been reported, although the deaths may have been related to significant underlying structural heart disease.

In AV nodal modification without complete ablation, transcatheter radiofrequency energy is applied to the region of slow-conducting pathway AV nodal inputs in the right posterior atrial septum. AV nodal tissue in this region, although slower conducting, is believed to have shorter refractory periods than fast-conducting-pathway AV nodal inputs located in the anterior atrial septal region. Since AV nodal conduction during atrial fibrillation may be limited by AV nodal refractoriness, elimination of tissue conducting with short refractoriness may slow conduction to the ventricles by limiting conduction to AV nodal tissue that has longer refractory properties.

Advantages of AV nodal modification include:

- Has been successful in controlling ventricular rates
- May avoid need for permanent pacing

Disadvantages are

- Significant rate of inadvertent complete or high-degree AV block requiring permanent pacemakers in 16% to 36% of patients
- Lower acute success rates, 15% to 81%
- Higher rates of recurrent rapid ventricular conduction in 16% to 68% when compared to complete AV junction ablation

Increased cardiac output has been reported with regularization of ventricular rates, which would be achieved by complete AV junction ablation, but might not be attained after successful modification alone.

## CATHETER ABLATION OF ATRIAL ARRHYTHMIAS

Radiofrequency catheter ablation may be used for the ablation of supraventricular tachycardias (SVTs) that may degenerate to atrial fibrillation, for AV nodal re-entrant tachycardia, and for accessory pathway–mediated atrioventricular re-entry.

Radiofrequency ablation of atrial flutter consists of application of radiofrequency energy along a line from the tricuspid annulus to the inferior vena cava (IVC) and/or from the coronary sinus os to the IVC and can effectively prevent the occurrence of typical, isthmus-dependent atrial flutter in approximately 90% of patients. It has been used successfully in patients with concomitant atrial fibrillation that can be controlled with antiarrhythmic medication but whose recurrences on medication may be in the form of atrial flutter, often occurring at a slow atrial rate that may facilitate 1:1 AV conduction.

Atypical atrial flutter or tachycardias arising from the right or left atria have also been successfully ablated, particularly those associated with atrial scar or incisions, and which can be mapped with newer mapping systems.

## ABLATION OF ATRIAL FIBRILLATION

### Catheter Maze—Right and Left Atrial Linear Ablation

A surgical maze procedure can be used to compartmentalize the right and left atria into corridors that limit the development of re-entry. For the catheter maze, radiofrequency energy is delivered in linear applications to the right and left atria.

Acute success rates of 50% to 80% have been reported, with a recent report of 57% long-term success (Schwarz et al.). However, procedures were long, recurrence rates were high, and repeat procedures were required in one third to two thirds patients.

The procedure is limited by excessively high serious complication rates of 20% to 50% (perforation/tamponade, thromboembolism/CVA, pulmonary vein stenosis). A more limited set of linear ablations in combination with pulmonary vein isolation may be helpful in more resistant patients, where the atrial subtrate may be more receptive to AF because of disease.

### Pulmonary Vein and Other Venous–Atrial Interface Isolation to Suppress the Triggers of AF

These procedures target local initiation sites of atrial fibrillation, because 89% to 95% of AF triggers arise from pulmonary vein ostial regions, possibly associated with the ligament of Marshall as well as the superior vena cava (SVC) and IVC insertions into the right atrium. Multiple pulmonary vein foci have been found in over one half of patients, and radiofrequency ablation is targeted to isolate these sites or to eliminate the tachycardia foci that trigger and possibly maintain AF.

Acute success rates of 87% to 95%, long-term success rates of 60% to 90% have been reported. Current methods, however, require long procedure times, with a high rate of recurrence and need for repeat procedures compared to other forms of radiofrequency ablation. There is also a risk of symptomatic pulmonary vein stenosis from ablation within the pulmonary vein (approximate risk 1% to 2%).

Improvements in techniques for mapping and ablation have improved of the safety and success of this procedure. Circumferential ablation methods using alternative delivery techniques and/or energy sources (e.g., ultrasound energy), laser, and cyroablation are under investigation.

The success of application of these procedures to the spectrum of AF patients remains to be defined. Highest success rates tend to be in paroxysmal lone atrial fibrillation. Success rate may be substantially lower in AF associated with other cardiac disease, especially in patients with marked atrial scarring.

## SURGICAL APPROACHES

Surgical approaches to AF include left atrial isolation, corridor, pulmonary vein isolation, and maze procedures.

### Maze Procedure

The maze procedure divides the atria into "mazelike" corridors and blind alleys that limit the development of re-entry by limiting available pathlength. Part of its success may be due to the pulmonary vein isolation that is part of the operation. In some cases, atrial transport function may be preserved but reduced.

A high degree of curative success (>80% to 90%) has been reported, but the procedure has had limited use and has been reserved primarily for patients with symptomatic refractory AF or performed in conjunction with mitral valve surgery.

Surgical and minisurgical approaches to isolating the PV ostia are being developed that may accomplish the same results as catheter-based approaches.

### Pacemaker Therapy

Permanent pacing may become necessary for sick sinus syndrome, tachy-brady syndromes, bradyarrhythmias occurring as a result of drug therapy, or after AV junction ablation.

Newer programming options may restrict upper tracking limits during atrial arrhythmias, but allow higher rate-responsive, sensor-driven upper rate limits. New "mode-switching" algorithms can change operation from dual-chamber pacing to single-chamber (VVI or VVIR) or DDIR pacing at the onset of atrial arrhythmias. Today's pacemakers also provide atrial overdrive pacing algorithms.

Studies suggest that dual-chamber or atrial pacing that maintains atrioventricular synchrony may reduce the incidence of AF when compared to single-chamber ventricular pacing. These studies have consisted largely of patients with sick sinus syndrome who require permanent pacing.

A prospective randomized trial of atrial versus ventricular pacing in 225 patients with sick sinus syndrome reported the frequency of AF and the thromboembolic event rate to be higher in the ventricular-paced group. However, another randomized study showed no difference in outcome.

Although most studies have been nonrandomized, comparisons of patients with physiologic dual-chamber, atrial synchronous (DDD, DDI, or AAI) pacing versus ventricular paced (VVI) modes suggest a decreased incidence in the development of AF in the physiologically paced groups.

A recent review reported the incidence of AF to be 0 to 23% in AAI and dual-chamber–paced patients, and 14% to 57% in VVI-paced patients.

Atrial fibrillation that occurs via vagally mediated mechanisms has also been successfully controlled by atrial overdrive pacing. Novel pacing approaches include atrial overdrive pacing and dual atrial pacing modalities.

### Implantable Atrial Defibrillator

Initial implantable atrial defibrillators provided automatic or patient-activated low-energy ventricular-synchronous atrial defibrillation. They were shown to be capable of effective, safe atrial defibrillation even without backup ventricular defibrillation.

Current devices provide ventricular as well as atrial defibrillation, as well as higher-output shocks, which may be required particularly if coronary sinus defibrillation leads are not used.

A major limitation of these devices is intolerance to the pain associated with the shock. These devices are practical only if AF occurs infrequently, at least with concurrent medication therapy.

## BIBLIOGRAPHY

### Current Practice Guidelines

**Albers GW, Dalen JE, Laupacis A, et al.** Antithrombotic therapy in atrial fibrillation. *Chest.* 2001;119(suppl):194S–206S.

**Fuster V, Ryden L, Cannom D, et al.** ACC/AHA/ESC 2006 Guidelines for the Management of Patients with Atrial Fibrillation. A Report of the American College of Cardiology/American Heart Association Task Force on Practice Guidelines and the European Society of Cardiology Committee for Practice Guidelines (Writing Committee to Revise the 2001 Guidelines for the Management of Patients with Atrial Fibrillation) Developed in Collaboration with the European Heart Rhythm Association and the Heart Rhythm Society. *Circulation.* 2006;15:114(7).

**Prystowsky EN, Benson D Jr, Woodrow MD, et al.** Management of patients with atrial fibrillation: a statement for healthcare professionals from the Subcommittee on Electrocardiography and Electrophysiology, American Heart Association. *Circulation.* 1996;93:1262–1277.

### Epidemiology

**Emelia J, Benjamin, MD, ScM; Philip A, Wolf, MD; Ralph B. D'Agostino, PhD; Halit Silbershatz, PhD; William B. Kannel, MD; Daniel Levy, MD.** Impact of Atrial Fibrillation on the Risk of Death The Framingham Heart Study. *Circulation* 1998;98:946–952.

**Kannel WB, Abbott RD, Savage DD, McNamara PM.** Coronary heart disease and atrial fibrillation: The Framingham Study. *Am Heart J* 1983;106:389–396.

### Pharmacologic Management

**Coplen SE, Antman EM, Berlin JA, et al.** Efficacy and safety of quinidine therapy for maintenance of sinus rhythm after cardioversion: a meta-analysis of randomized control trials. *Circulation.* 1990;82:2248–2250.

**Farshi R, Kistner D, Sarma JS, et al.** Ventricular rate control in chronic atrial fibrillation during daily activity and programmed exercise: a crossover open-label study of five drug regimens. *J Am Coll Cardiol.* 1999;33:304–310.

**Jung F, DiMarco JP.** Treatment strategies for atrial fibrillation. *Am J Med.* 1998;104:272–286.

**Kassotis J. Costeas C, Blitzer M, Reiffel JA.** Rhythm management in atrial fibrillation—with a primary emphasis on pharmacologic therapy: part 3. *Pacing Clin Electrophysiol.* 1998;21:1133–1145.

**Masoudi FA, Goldschlager N.** The medical management of atrial fibrillation. *Cardiol Clin.* 1997;15:689–719.

**Olgin JE, Viskin S.** Management of intermittent atrial fibrillation: drugs to maintain sinus rhythm. *J Cardiovasc Electrophysiol.* 1999;10:433–441.

**Reiffel JA.** Selecting an antiarrhythmic agent for atrial fibrillation should be a patient-specific, data-driven decision. *Am J Cardiol.* 1998;82:72N–81N.

**Singh BN.** Current antiarrhythmic drugs; an overview of mechanisms of action and potential clinical utility. *J Cardiovasc Electrophysiol.* 1999;10:283–301.

**Torp-Pedersen C, Moller M, Bloch-Thomsen PE, et al.** Dofetilide in patients with congestive heart failure and left ventricular dysfunction. Danish Investigations of Arrhythmia and Mortality on Dofetilide Study Group. *N Engl J Med.* 1999;341:857–865.

**Wyse DG, Waldo AL, DiMarco JP, Domanski MJ, Rosenberg Y, Schron EB, Kellen JC, Greene HL, Mickel MC, Dalquist JE, Corley SD**; Atrial Fibrillation Follow-up Investigation of Rhythm Management (AFFIRM) Investigators. A comparison of rate control and rhythm control in patients with atrial fibrillation. *N Engl J Med* 2002 Dec 5;347(23):1825–1833.

### Pathogenesis

**Daoud EG, Knight BP, Weiss R, et al.** Effect of verapamil and procainamide on atrial fibrillation-induced electrical remodeling in humans. *Circulation.* 1997;96:1542–1550.

**Friedman HS, Rodney E, Sinha B, et al.** Verapamil prolongs atrial fibrillation by evoking an intense sympathetic neurohumoral effect. *J Investig Med.* 1999;47:293–303.

**Goette A, Honeycutt C, Langberg JJ.** Electrical remodeling in atrial fibrillation. Time course and mechanisms. *Circulation.* 1996;94:2968–2974.

**Lesh MD, Guerra P, Roithinger FX, Goseki Y, Diederich C, Nau WH, Maguiro M, Taylor K.** Novel catheter technology for ablative cure of atrial fibrillation. *J Interv Card Electrophysiol.* 2000 Jan;4 Suppl 1:127–139.

**Moe GK, Rheinboldt WC, Abildskov JA.** A computer model of atrial fibrillation. *Am Heart J* 1964;67:200–220.

**Tieleman RG, De Langen C, Van Gelder IC, et al.** Verapamil reduces tachycardia-induced electrical remodeling of the atria. *Circulation.* 1997;95:1945–1953.

**Tieleman RG, Van Gelder IC, Crijns HJ, et al.** Early recurrences of atrial fibrillation after electrial cardioversion: a result of fibrillation-induced electrical remodeling of the atria? *J Am Coll Cardiol.* 1998;31:167–173.

**Yu WC, Chen SA, Lee SH, et al.** Tachycardia-induced change of atrial refractory period in humans: rate dependency and effects of antiarrhythmic drugs. *Circulation.* 1998;97:2331–2337.

**Wijffels MC, Kirchhof CJ, Dorland R, Allessie MA.** Atrial fibrillation begets atrial fibrillation. A study in awake chronically instrumented goats. *Circulation.* 1995 Oct 1;92(7):1954–1968.

### Stroke Incidence and Anticoagulation

**Albers GW, Dalen JE, Laupacis A, et al.** Antithrombotic therapy in atrial fibrillation. *Chest.* 2001;119(suppl):194S–206S.

**Atrial Fibrillation Investigators.** Echocardiographic predictors of stroke in patients with atrial fibrillation: a prospective study of 1066 patients from 3 clinical trials. *Arch Intern Med.* 1998;158:1316–1320.

**Atrial Fibrillation Investigators.** Risk factors for stroke and efficacy of antithrombotic therapy in atrial fibrillation. Analysis of pooled data from five randomized controlled trials. *Arch Intern Med.* 1994;154:1449–1457.

**Connolly SJ, Laupacis A, Gent M, et al.** Canadian Atrial Fibrillation Anticoagulation (CAFA) Study. *J Am Coll Cardiol.* 1991;18:349–355.

**EAFT (European Atrial Fibrillation Trial) Study Group.** Secondary prevention in non-rheumatic atrial fibrillation after transient ischaemic attack or minor stroke. *Lancet.* 1993;342:1255–1262.

**Ezekowitz MD, Bridgers SL, James KE, et al.** Warfarin in the prevention of stroke associated with nonrheumatic atrial fibrillation. Veterans Affairs Stroke Prevention in Nonrheumatic Atrial Fibrillation Investigators. *N Engl J Med.* 1992;327:1406–1412.

**Gullov AL, Koefoed BG, Petersen P, et al.** Fixed minidose warfarin and aspirin alone and in combination vs adjusted-dose warfarin for stroke prevention in atrial fibrillation: Second Copenhagen Atrial Fibrillation, Aspirin, and Anticoagulation Study. *Arch Intern Med.* 1998;158:1513–1521.

**Laupacis A, Albers G, Dalen J. et al.** Antithrombotic therapy in atrial fibrillation. *Chest.* 1998;114:579S–589S.

**Petersen P, Boysen G, Godtfredsen J, et al.** Placebo-controlled, randomised trial of warfarin and aspirin for prevention of thromboembolic complications in chronic atrial fibrillation. The Copenhagen AFASAK study. *Lancet.* 1989;1:175–179.

**Stroke Prevention in Atrial Fibrillation Investigators.** Warfarin versus aspirin for prevention of thromboembolism in atrial fibrillation: Stroke Prevention in Atrial Fibrillation II Study. *Lancet.* 1994;343:687–691.

**The Stroke Prevention in Atrial Fibrillation Investigators.** Predictors of thromboembolism in atrial fibrillation: I. Clinical features of patients at risk. *Ann Intern Med.* 1992;116:1–5.

**The Stroke Prevention in Atrial Fibrillation Investigators.** Predictors of thromboembolism in atrial fibrillation: II. Echocardiographic features of at risk. *Ann Intern Med.* 1992;116:6–12.

**The Stroke Prevention in Atrial Fibrillation Investigators.** Stroke Prevention in Atrial Fibrillation Study. Final results. *Circulation.* 1991;84:527–539.

**Takahashi N, Seki A, Imataka K, Fujii J.** Clinical feature of paroxysmal atrial fibrillation: an observation of 94 patients. *Jpn Heart J.* 1981;22:143–149.

**The Boston Area Anticoagulation Trial for Atrial Fibrillation Investigators.** The effect of low-dose warfarin on the risk of stroke in patients with nonrheumatic atrial fibrillation. *N Engl J Med.* 1990;323:1505–1511.

**The SPAF III Writing Committee for the Stroke Prevention in Atrial Fibrillation Investigators.** Patients with nonvalvular atrial fibrillation at low risk of stroke during treatment with aspirin: Stroke Prevention in Atrial Fibrillation III Study. *JAMA.* 1998;279:1273–1277.

**Wolf PA, Kannel WB, McGee DL, et al.** Duration of atrial fibrillation and imminence of stroke: the Framingham study. *Stroke.* 1983;14:664–667.

**Wolf PA, Abbott RD, Kannel WB.** Atrial fibrillation as an independent risk factor for stroke: the Framingham Study. *Stroke.* 1991;22:983–988.

## Ablation for Atrial Flutter/Fibrillation

1. **Chen SA, Tai CT, Tsai CF, et al.** Radiofrequency catheter ablation of atrial fibrillation initiated by pulmonary vein ectopic beats. *J Cardiovasc Electrophysiol.* 2000;11:218–227.
2. **Feld GK, Fleck RP, Chen PS, et al.** Radiofrequency catheter ablation for the treatment of human type 1 atrial flutter. Identification of a critical zone in the reentrant circuit by endocardial mapping techniques. *Circulation.* 1992;86:1233–1240.
3. **Haissaguerre M, Gencel L, Fischer B, et al.** Successful catheter ablation of atrial fibrillation. *J Cardiovasc Electrophysiol.* 1994:5:1045–1052.
4. **Haissaguerre M, Jais P, Shah DC, et al.** Right and left atrial radiofrequency catheter therapy of paroxysmal atrial fibrillation. *J Cardiovasc Electrophysiol.* 1996;7:1132–1144.
5. **Haissaguerre M, Jais P, Shah DC, et al.** Spontaneous initiation of atrial fibrillation by ectopic beats originating in the pulmonary veins. *N Engl J Med.* 1998;339:659–666.
6. **Marrouche NF, Dresing T, Cole C, et al.** Circular mapping and ablation of the pulmonary vien for treatment of atrial fibrillation: impact of different catheter technologies. *J Am Coll Cardiol.* 2002;40(3):464–474.
7. **Marrouche NF, Schweikert R, Saliba W, et al.** Use of different catheter ablation technologies for treatment of typical atrial flutter: acute results and long-term follow-up. *Pacing Clin Electrophysiol.* 2003;26(3):743–746.

# Wide-Complex Tachycardia: Ventricular Tachycardia versus Supraventricular Tachycardia

50

***Walid Saliba  Anne Kanderian***

Wide-complex tachycardia (WCT) is defined as a tachyarrhythmia with a rate >100 beats/min and a QRS duration greater than 120 milliseconds on a 12-lead electrocardiogram (ECG). Utilizing the ECG, the correct mechanistic diagnosis of a wide-complex tachycardia rhythm is often difficult. Besides being an intellectual exercise, it is very important to establish the correct diagnosis in order to deliver appropriate acute therapy and to plan subsequent long-term patient management. Several criteria and algorithms have been developed to help distinguish among different causes of wide-complex tachycardia. When used individually, none of these criteria reaches 100% specificity; however, when properly applied together and in conjunction with the clinical history and presentation, the algorithms serve as a guide to the correct diagnosis in the majority of the cases.

Wide-complex tachycardia can result from either a ventricular or a supraventricular mechanism. Ventricular tachycardia (VT) originates below the level of the His bundle. Supraventricular tachycardia (SVT) originates in or involves structures above the His bundle. SVT may involve atrial tachycardia, atrial fibrillation, atrial flutter, atrioventricular (AV) node re-entrant tachycardia, or AV re-entrant tachycardia (Fig. 50–1). AV re-entrant tachycardia may be either orthodromic re-entrant tachycardia or antidromic re-entrant tachycardia (Fig. 50–2). Orthodromic re-entrant tachycardia occurs when antegrade ventricular conduction occurs via the AV node and retrograde conduction to the atrium is via the accessory pathway. Antidromic re-entrant tachycardia occurs when ventricular antegrade conduction occurs over the accessory pathway and retrograde conduction occurs via the AV node.

## DIFFERENTIAL DIAGNOSIS

Wide-complex tachycardia can occur by three different mechanisms.

1. Ventricular tachycardia is the most common cause of WCT in the general population, accounting for >80% of all cases. It is even more common in patients with

Atrial Tachycardia

RA LA RV LV

Atrial Fibrillation

RA LA RV LV

Flutter circuit

RA LA RV LV

Atrial Flutter

AVNRT Circuit

RA LA RV LV

AV Node Re-entrant Tachycardia

**Figure 50–1** Supraventricular tachycardia.

structural heart disease, and it may occur in 98% in patients with a prior history of a myocardial infarction. Ventricular tachycardia may be either monomorphic or polymorphic. Monomorphic VT occurs when the QRS morphology is stable and uniform, whereas polymorphic VT occurs when the QRS complexes vary in morphology.

2. The second mechanism of WCT occurs when the tachycardia originates above the ventricle and has abnormal ventricular activation, also known as SVT with aberrancy. It accounts for 15% to 20% of all cases of WCT and includes a variety of disorders.

   a. The first example is SVT with bundle branch block aberration, which may be either a right bundle branch (RBBB) or a left bundle branch (LBBB) morphology (Fig. 50–3). Activation of the ventricle through the His–Purkinje system (His bundle and both bundle branches) results in a narrow QRS complex. Activation of the ventricle unilaterally via one bundle branch results in a wide QRS complex, because activation of the remainder of the ventricular myocardium is dependent on slow myocardial conduction. Aberration occurs when there are abnormalities of intraventricular conduction in response

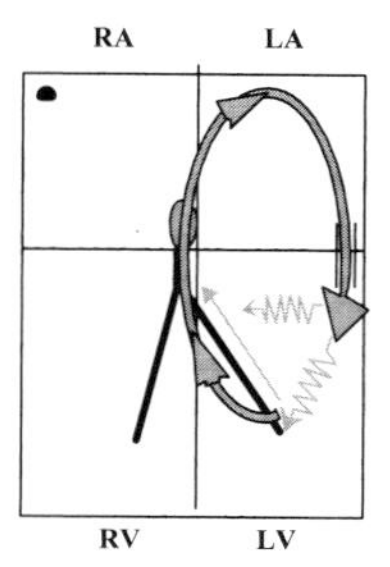


Antidromic Re-entrant Tachycardia

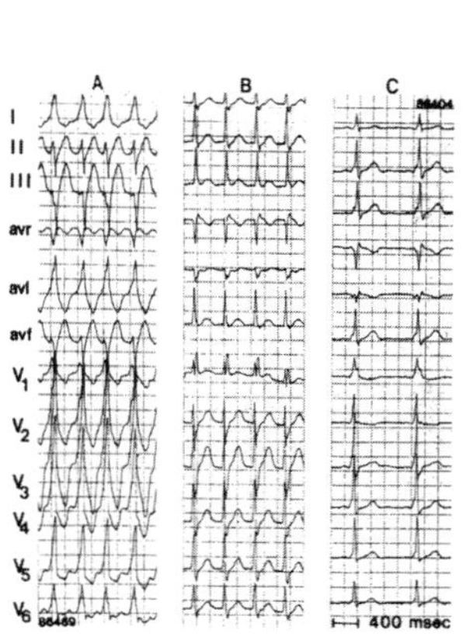


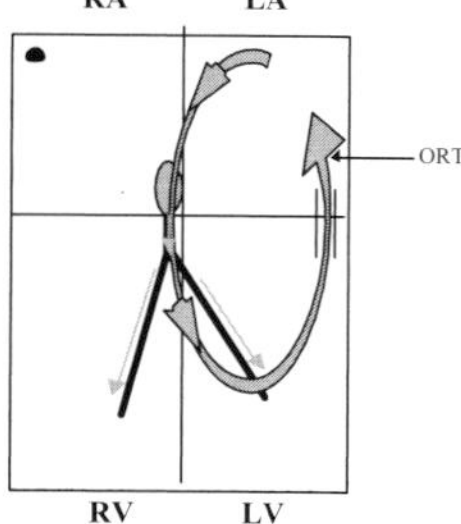


Orthodromic Re-entrant Tachycardia

**Figure 50–2** AV re-entrant tachycardia.

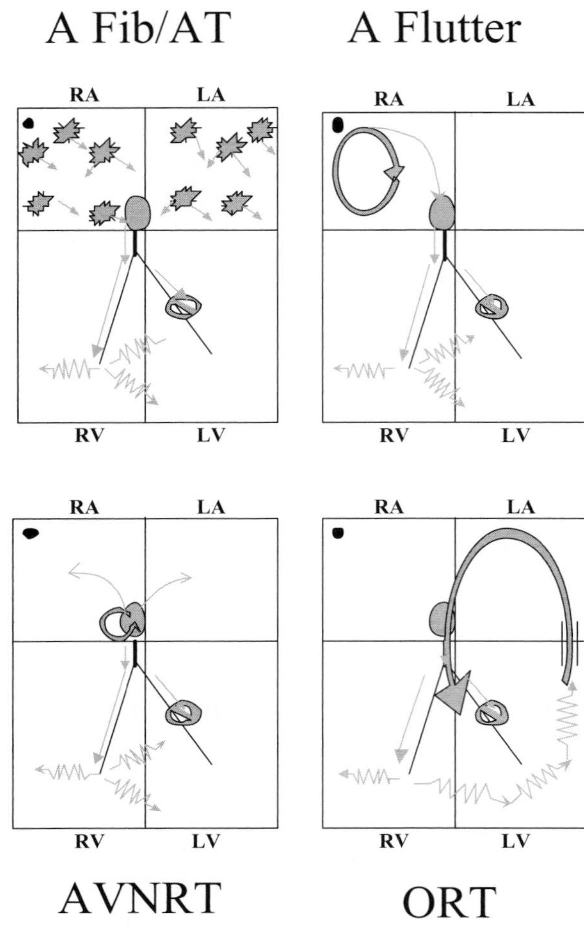


**Figure 50–3** SVT with bundle branch block.

to changing heart rate, and when the conduction over the His–Purkinje conduction system is delayed or blocked in either the right or left bundle branch. RBBB is more common, occurring in 80% of cases. The aberration may be fixed, occurring in normal sinus rhythm at a slow heart rate, or it may be functional and present only during tachycardia.

b. SVT with antegrade conduction via an accessory pathway, such as in Wolff–Parkinson–White syndrome, accounts for 1% to 5% of all WCT. The accessory pathway is an anomalous AV connection that inserts directly into ventricular myocardium at the base of the ventricle along the mitral or tricuspid valve annulus. Ventricular activation is initiated at this insertion point and is termed ventricular pre-excitation. Pre-excitated tachycardia can occur with SVT with antegrade conduction via the accessory pathway. The accessory pathway is not part of the tachycardia circuit and is not essential for its perpetuation. The other form of pre-excited tachycardia can occur with antidromic reciprocating tachycardia, in which the accessory pathway is part of the tachycardia circuit (Fig. 50–4).

c. Another form of WCT is SVT with an intraventricular conduction delay. This can occur in patients with cardiomyopathy, corrected congenital heart disease such as tetralogy of Fallot, or Ebstein anomaly, in which myocardial conduction is further impaired. The conduction abnormality is usually apparent during normal sinus rhythm.

d. Some drugs are capable of producing nonspecific widening of the QRS complex during SVT. These include $Na^+$ channel blockers, especially Class IC agents (flecainide, encainide), less so Class IA antiarrhythmics (quinidine, procainamide, disopyramide), and amiodarone. The most common example is a patient with atrial flutter being treated with flecainide. Flecainide can induce flutter rate slowing to permit 1:1 AV nodal conduction and a secondary increase in the ventricular rate with a wide QRS complex. This is as a result of the slow ventricular conduction in response to the $Na^+$channel blockade. This can be easily and erroneously interpreted as VT.

e. Electrolyte abnormalities such as hyperkalemia can cause widening of the QRS complex and can be mistakenly interpreted as VT. The morphology is typically LBBB.

3. Ventricular paced rhythms can also mimic WCT (Fig. 50–5). Most pacemakers are dual chamber, with a lead in the right atrium and one in the right ventricle. Pacing of the right ventricle causes a LBBB QRS morphology. The surface ECG representation of the pacing stimulus is less apparent with the use of bipolar pacing modes and a resultant decrease in the energy requirement for reliable ventricular pacing. Therefore the pacing spike may be overlooked or even absent from ECG tracings. A wide QRS tachycardia can occur in any SVT with atrial tracking, in which the ventricle is paced in response to atrial sensing. In these cases, it is essential to obtain an adequate history and to analyze a previous ECG to evaluate the baseline morphology of the QRS complex.
4. Pacemaker-mediated tachycardia can also produce a WCT. The pacemaker is itself responsible for the tachycardia when ventricular pacing results in retrograde conduction to the atrium. The pacemaker senses the atrial conduction, resulting in ventricular pacing, which in turn is followed by retrograde conduction to the atrium, resulting in "endless loop tachycardia" (Fig. 50–6).
5. Lastly, artifacts from recording equipment problems (such as fast-sweep speed recording) or from external repetitive motion (such as brushing teeth) can present as "WCT" (Fig. 50–7).

## DIAGNOSIS

### Clinical Presentation

In order to diagnose the etiology of the wide-complex tachycardia, it is important to look at the clinical

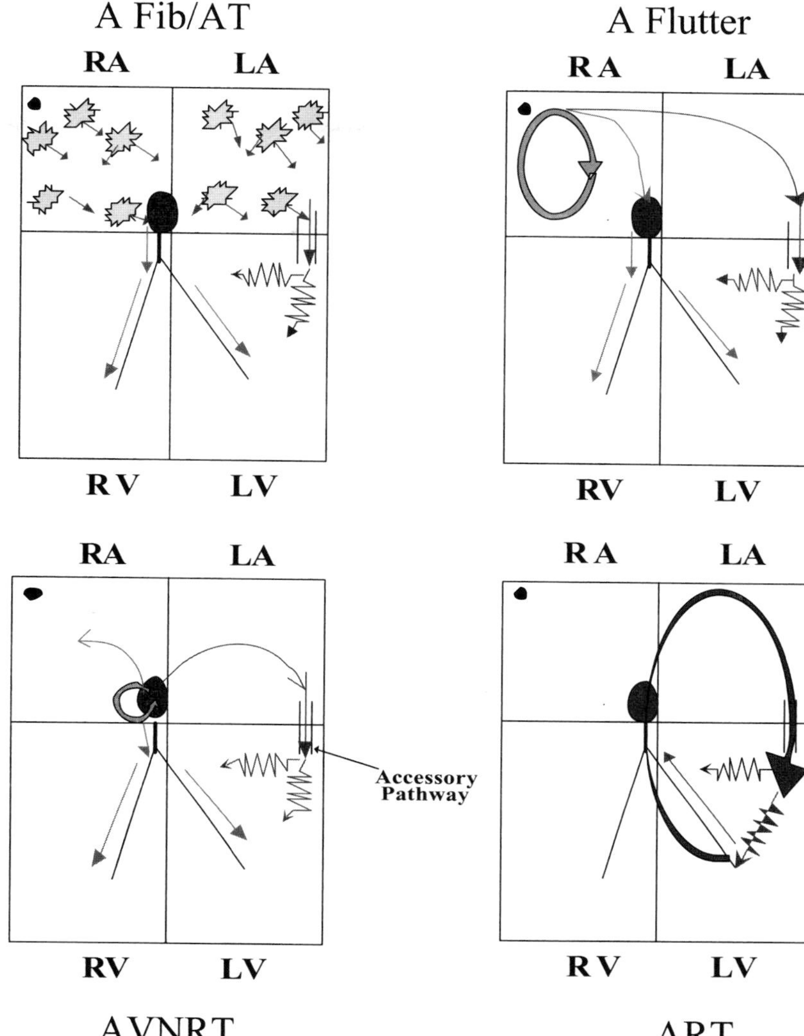


**Figure 50–4** SVT with pre-excitation.

presentation. As mentioned before, obtaining an accurate patient history is crucial in formulating an accurate rhythm diagnosis. A prior history of heart disease, myocardial infarction, or congestive heart failure makes the diagnosis of ventricular tachycardia highly suggestive as the cause of the WCT. Akhtar et al. have reported that the positive predictive value of a WCT representing VT in a patient with a prior history of myocardial infarction as 98%. Tchou reported that of patients who had a prior myocardial infarction and a first episode of tachycardia occurring after the infarction, 28 of 29 patients presented with VT and were diagnosed correctly. The older the patient is, the more likely that the tachycardia is ventricular; however there is a significant overlap with SVT patients. It is also helpful to know if there is any presence of congenital heart disease, or if the patient has a pacemaker or defibrillator. Knowing that the patient has an implantable cardioverter-defibrillator (ICD) raises a concern for pacemaker-associated tachycardia, but more important, the presence of the device suggests that the patient has risk factors for VT. A history of a prior similar episode may also be useful. The first occurrence of the arrhythmia after a myocardial infarction is highly suggestive of VT, whereas SVT may be more likely if there is recurrence of the arrhythmia over several years. The presence of other medical conditions can point to a diagnosis of WCT. For example, in a patient with renal failure, the WCT may be attributable to hyperkalemia. In a patient with known peripheral vascular disease, the WCT may be indicative of VT, because such patients are likely to have underlying coronary artery disease.

Knowing what medications the patient is taking, especially cardiac medications, is vital when evaluating WCT. It is important to identify drugs that prolong the QT interval, such as sotalol, quinidine, and erythromycin, which can all cause torsade de pointes, a form of polymorphic VT. Electrolyte abnormalities caused by certain drugs such as diuretics (hypokalemia and hypomagnesemia) or ACE inhibitors (hyperkalemia) may predispose to VT. Patients

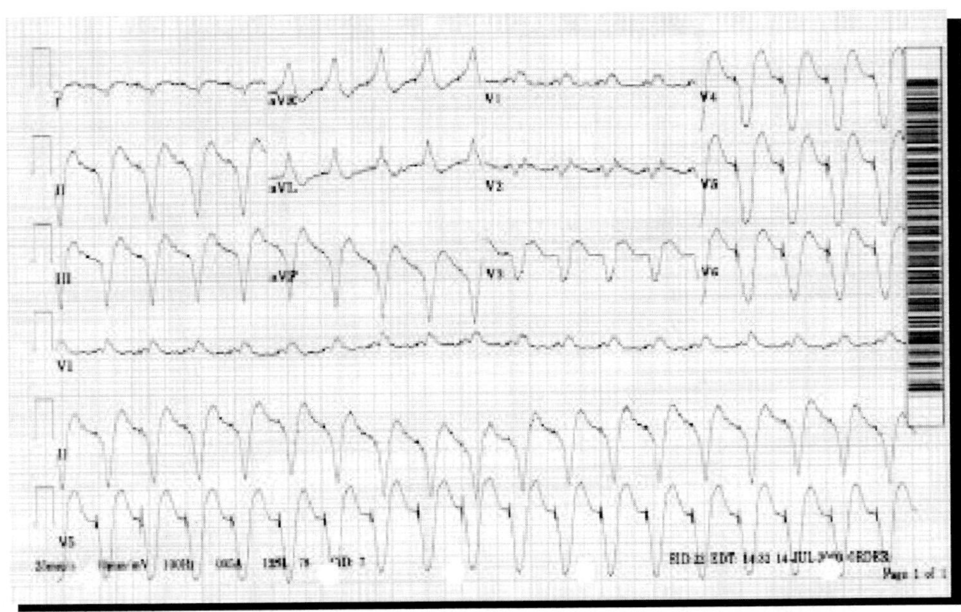

Figure 50–5 Ventricular paced tachycardia.

who are on digoxin are more susceptible to an arrhythmia when hypokalemia is present. The most common arrhythmias are monomorphic VT, bidirectional tachycardia, and junctional tachycardia, and typically occur when the plasma digoxin concentration is >2.0 ng/mL. As stated earlier, Class IC agents can cause rate-related aberrant conduction during SVT. Symptoms such as palpitations, lightheadedness, or chest pain are generally not useful in evaluating the etiology of the WCT.

One of the priorities in evaluating a patient with WCT is determining if the patient is hemodynamically stable or unstable. This requires knowing the patient's blood pressure and heart rate. In a patient who is unstable, emergency cardioversion is required and the mechanism of the arrhythmia may not necessarily be known. VT can be present when the patient is hemodynamically stable and should not be mistaken for SVT, lest the patient be given inappropriate medical therapy (such as adenosine or verapamil) that can lead to hemodynamic compromise with VT. When the patient is hemodynamically stable, a more detailed physical exam can be performed. Inspection of the chest can point to underlying cardiovascular disease when there is a sternal incision, a pacemaker, or defibrillator.

Atrioventricular dissociation occurs in 60% to 75% of patients with VT and is a result of the atria and ventricle depolarizing independently. It almost never occurs in SVT. This finding is usually seen on the surface ECG. However, it is also possible to make this diagnosis on physical exam by assessing the jugular venous pulsation. Cannon A waves are irregular pulsations that are of greater amplitude than the normal jugular venous waves, and occur intermittently when the atrium and ventricle contract simultaneously.

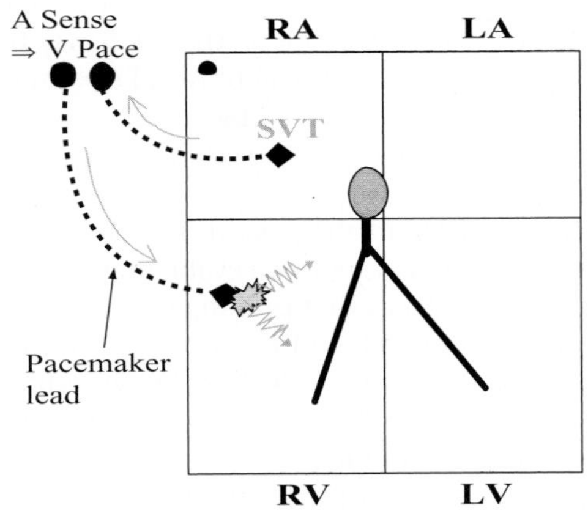


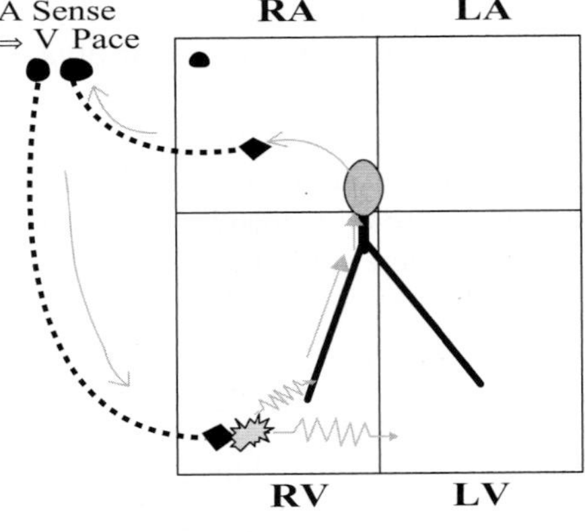


Figure 50–6 Ventricular paced tachycardia. **Left:** Atrial tracking. **Right:** Pacemaker-mediated tachycardia.

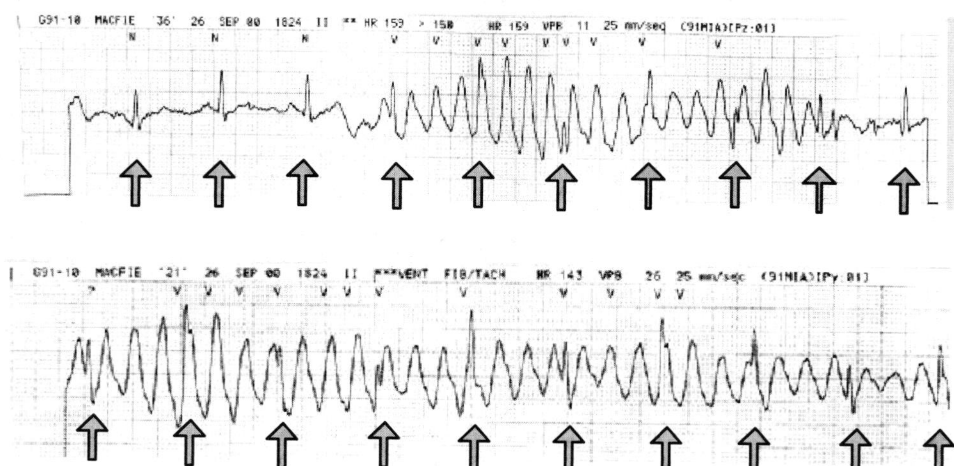

**Figure 50–7** Artifact mimicking WCT.

When the tachycardia rate is slower, there can be variable intensity of the first heart sound. However, evaluating this may not be practical in an acute situation.

Laboratory tests should be performed for patients with WCT to determine potassium and magnesium levels. If the patient is on digoxin, it is also important to obtain the serum digoxin level. If a chest x-ray is available, one can readily identify the presence of a pacemaker, defibrillator, or sternal wires that might point to underlying structural heart disease.

## Provocative Maneuvers

Certain bedside maneuvers can be performed to distinguish VT from SVT. The Valsalva maneuver or carotid sinus massage enhances vagal tone, which depresses sinus nodal and AV nodal activity. These maneuvers will slow the heart rate during sinus tachycardia, but once they are completed, the heart rate will increase again. If the patient is in SVT, these maneuvers may terminate the rhythm. If the patient is in an atrial tachycardia or flutter, the rhythm will persist though the ventricular rate may be slower, thus uncovering the background atrial activity. These maneuvers can also elicit VA conduction block, which can induce AV dissociation during VT.

Certain drugs can be used to diagnose the tachyarrhythmias. For example, adenosine, given in 6- to 12-mg boluses intravenously during WCT, can result in one of the following scenarios:

1. The tachycardia terminates, making it more likely to be supraventricular in etiology, invoking AV node participation. Some atrial tachycardias may also terminate with adenosine.
2. AV block occurs, uncovering the background atrial activity such as atrial tachycardia, flutter, or fibrillation, thus allowing the diagnosis of an atrial tachyarrhythmia.
3. If 1:1 AV association is present and not evident during WCT, adenosine-induced VA block results in AV dissociation, thus making the diagnosis VT (Fig. 50–8).

Adenosine has a short half-life of about 10 seconds. However, this drug has to be used with caution, because it may cause hemodynamic compromise in a patient with VT. Some paroxysmal VT in structurally normal hearts may terminate with adenosine.

Termination of the rhythm with lidocaine suggests VT as the mechanism. Amiodarone and procainamide, however, will not diagnose the rhythm if the WCT is terminated. Beta-blockers may be given as well. They can terminate SVT or uncover AV dissociation during VT in a manner similar to adenosine. It is important that verapamil not be given if the diagnosis is in question, because it can lead to significant hemodynamic compromise in VT and induce ventricular fibrillation and cardiac arrest.

## ECG Criteria

The most reliable way to differentiate VT from SVT is by evaluating the ECG. A 12-lead ECG is more helpful than a rhythm strip. A rhythm strip may be additive as a result of analyzing the beginning and termination of the tachycardia. A previous ECG during a normal rhythm will help to identify the baseline QRS morphology and the presence of

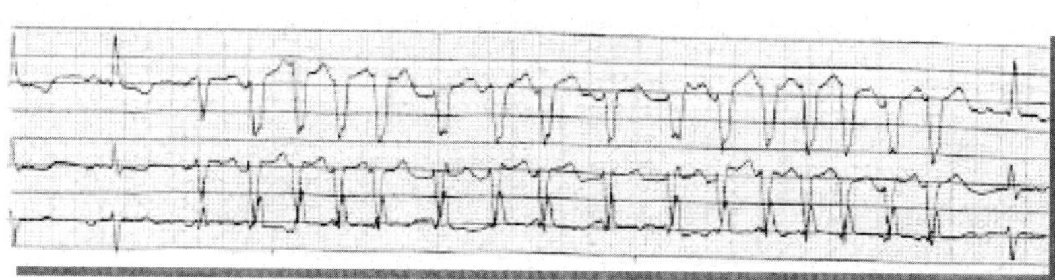

**Figure 50–8** Irregular VT.

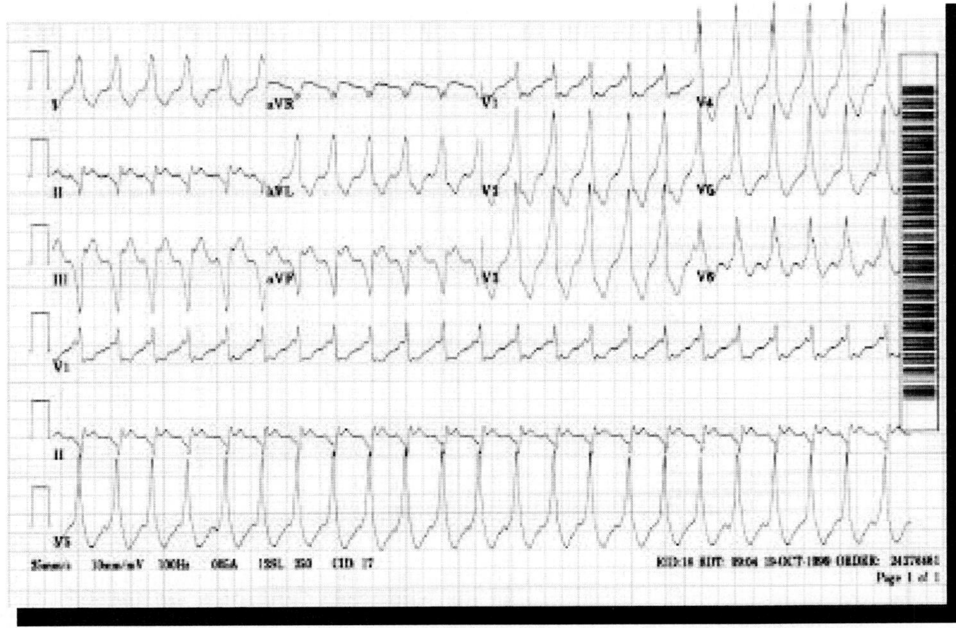

Figure 50–9 VT: QRS concordance.

Q waves that might suggest a prior myocardial infarction. Ventricular preexcitation may be suggested if there is the presence of delta waves.

There are several ECG criteria and different algorithms that may be used to differentiate VT from SVT in WCT.

1. The tachycardia rate has no diagnostic value in determining the mechanism of the WCT.
2. Regularity of the RR intervals is also not a useful criterion, because VT can be irregular in patients on antiarrhythmic medications.
3. QRS-complex duration can be useful in differentiating VT from SVT. The WCT is more suggestive of VT when the QRS duration is >140 milliseconds with a RBBB morphology and >160 milliseconds with a LBBB morphology. A study by Wellens showed that all of 70 patients with WCT due to SVT had QRS-complex durations <140 milliseconds, whereas 66% of patients with WCT due to VT had QRS-complex duration >140 milliseconds. Another study, by Akhtar, showed that 15% of patients with VT had QRS-complex duration <140 milliseconds and that QRS duration >140 milliseconds with RBBB pattern

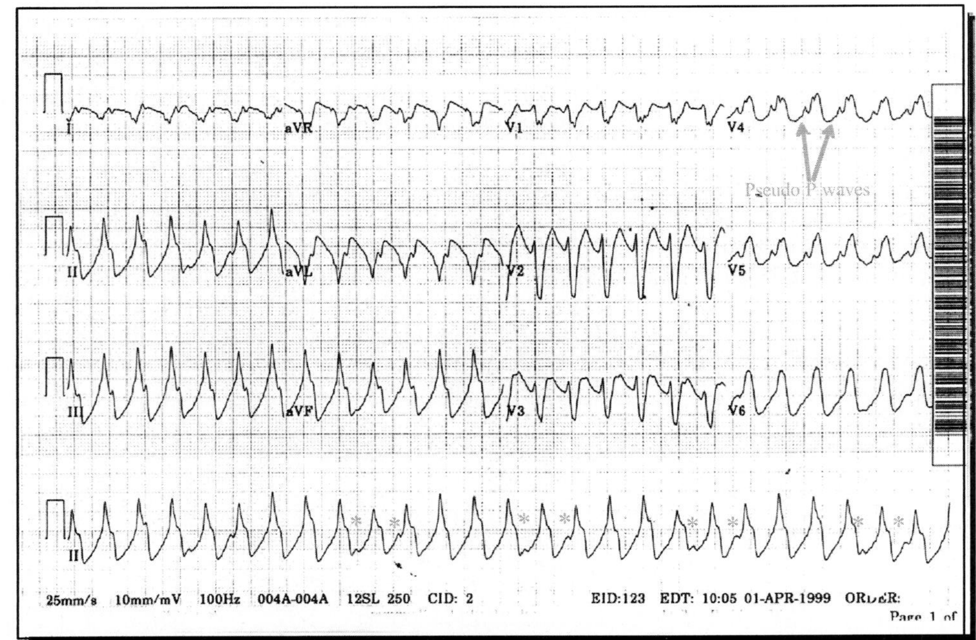


Figure 50–10 VT: AV dissociation.

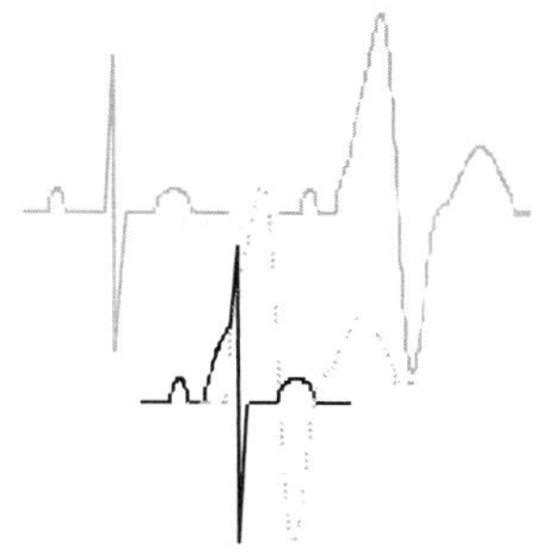


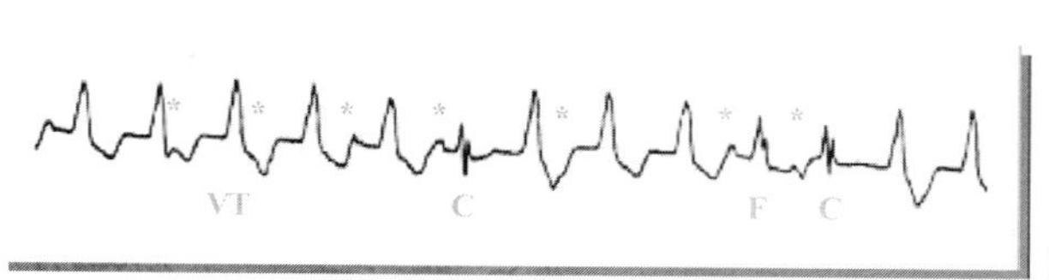


**Figure 50–11** **A:** Fusion complex. **B:** Fusion and capture complexes.

or >160 milliseconds with LBBB pattern correlates with VT. Wide QRS-complex duration can still be seen with pre-excitation, ventricular pacing, use of antiarrhythmic drugs, and marked baseline intraventricular conduction delays. VT in structurally normal hearts may have a relatively narrow QRS complex in a case with idiopathic left ventricular VT.

4. The QRS-complex axis may also be helpful in diagnosing WCT. A right superior QRS-complex axis in the frontal plane is more suggestive of VT. Presence of LBBB and right-axis deviation is also almost always due to VT. Presence of Q waves that are also present in normal sinus rhythm suggests prior myocardial infarction, which makes the diagnosis of VT more likely. Pseudo-Q waves can be seen in SVT, which represents retrograde atrial activation.
5. QRS-complex concordance in the precordial leads is highly predictive of VT, with a specificity as high as 90% or greater. The sensitivity is low because it is only present in <20% of patient with VT. Concordance occurs when all the QRS complexes in the precordial leads (V1 to V6) have the same polarity, either positive or negative (Fig. 50–9). It is important to remember that 1% to 2% of patients with pre-excited tachycardia involving left lateral accessory pathways possess positive QRS-complex concordance.
6. AV dissociation is the most useful criterion to distinguish VT from SVT (Fig. 50–10). It occurs in up to 60% of patients with VT but is apparent on the surface ECG in only 20% to 30% of patients. The specificity is 99%, but again, the sensitivity is only 20%. AV dissociation occurs in <1% of all SVTs. Several methods can be used to maximize atrial recordings, such as using an esophageal lead, utilizing temporary epicardial atrial pacemaker wires post–cardiac surgery, changing arm lead position, and utilizing a pacemaker programmer for atrial and ventricular electrogram display in patients with permanent dual-chamber devices. Thirty percent of VT patients may have 1:1 AV association, and this cannot be differentiated from SVT. Transient AV dissociation can be elicited with carotid sinus massage or IV adenosine, which helps to confirm the diagnosis of VT.
7. The presence of capture and fusion complexes on an ECG during WCT makes the diagnosis of VT more likely. A ventricular fusion complex results from simultaneous activation of the ventricle by two or more impulses originating from the same or different chambers of the heart. An example is the fusion of a ventricular impulse with a sinus or other supraventricular conducted impulse, or another ventricular impulse. The resulting QRS-complex morphology is variable and depends on the relative contribution of each of the sources of ventricular activation. During WCT, a change in the morphology of the QRS complex is indicative of fusion and suggests the diagnosis of VT. A fusion complex is not pathognomonic for VT and can occur when a premature ventricular contraction occurs during SVT with aberrancy. A capture complex is a ventricular QRS complex that results from conduction of a supraventricular impulse to the ventricle and ventricular depolarization before the ventricle is depolarized by the VT circuit. It is usually a narrower complex and is identical to the sinus QRS complex. It indicates that the normal conduction system has temporarily captured and depolarized the ventricle before the next VT complex. Although fusion and capture complex are seen infrequently, when they are present, they strongly indicate the etiology of WCT as VT, with the specificity being 99% and the sensitivity 5% for capture complex (Fig. 50–11A,B).
8. The absence of a precordial RS pattern on a 12-lead ECG is suggestive of VT. This is the first criterion in Brugada's algorithm. Brugada performed an analysis on 554 patients with WCT. Fifteen percent of all cases had an absent RS pattern, and 100% of these cases were due to VT. Though the specificity remains high (100%), the sensitivity is quite low (21%). If an RS pattern is present, a RS duration (as measured from the beginning of the R wave to the nadir of the S wave) of >100 milliseconds suggests VT (Fig. 50–12). This is the second step in Brugada's algorithm. This finding is present in 32% of patients with WCT and has a specificity of 98%. Combining these two criteria can correctly diagnose 47% of all WCT and identify 66% of all VT.

**TABLE 50–1**
**MORPHOLOGY CRITERIA**

| | RBBB | | LBBB | |
|---|---|---|---|---|
| | **VT** | **SVT** | **VT** | **SVT** |
| V1 | Monophasic R<br>R (>30 ms) + any S<br>qR | Triphasic<br>rSR′<br>rSr′<br>rsr′ | rS (Broad r >30 ms)<br>Notching/delay in S<br>QS ≥70 ms<br>RT taller than RS | rS, QS<br>(rapid downstroke) |
| V6 | RS (R < S)<br>QS, Q rs<br>QR<br>Monophasic R | Triphasic<br>Rs<br>RS (R > S)<br>qRs | QR, QS<br>QrS, qR<br>Rr′ | rR′<br>Monophasic R<br>No Q waves |

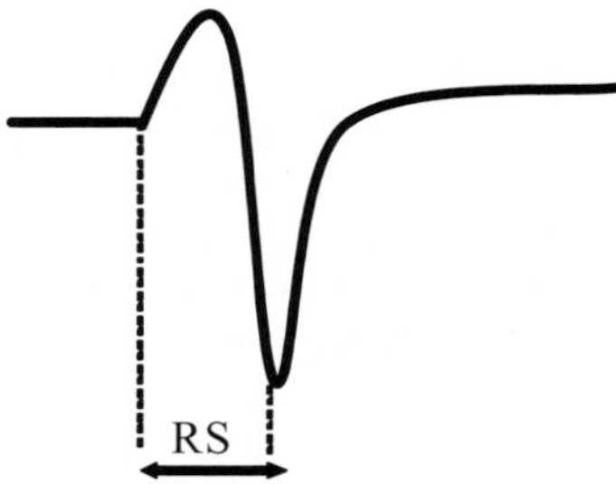


**Figure 50–12** RS.

9. QRS morphology: Different criteria for RBBB and LBBB morphologies can also help distinguish VT from SVT (Table 50–1; Fig. 50–13). This is based predominantly on the QRS-complex analysis in the precordial leads: V1, V2, and V6. If the QRS complex is predominantly positive in V1, a "RBBB-like" pattern is observed and the corresponding morphology criteria are applied. Alternatively, if the QRS complex is predominantly negative in V1, a "LBBB-like" pattern is observed and the corresponding morphology criteria are applied.

## ALGORITHMS

The most commonly used approach for the differential diagnosis of WCT is the aforementioned algorithm by Brugada (Fig. 50–14). This algorithm is comprised of four steps and has a sensitivity of 98.7% and a specificity of 96.5%. The four sequential steps assess for the presence of RS QRS complexes in the precordial leads, the RS interval, AV dissociation, and specific morphology criteria for VT in V1 and V6 (Fig. 50–15).

A second-level algorithm (Brugada's criteria II) helps to distinguish VT from pre-excited SVT. This algorithm has three steps and has a sensitivity of 75% and specificity of 100% (Figs. 50–16 and 50–17).

## SPECIAL CASES

There are other miscellaneous ECG criteria that can help differentiate VT from SVT.

- When the QRS complex during WCT is narrower than in normal sinus rhythm, this is more suggestive of VT.

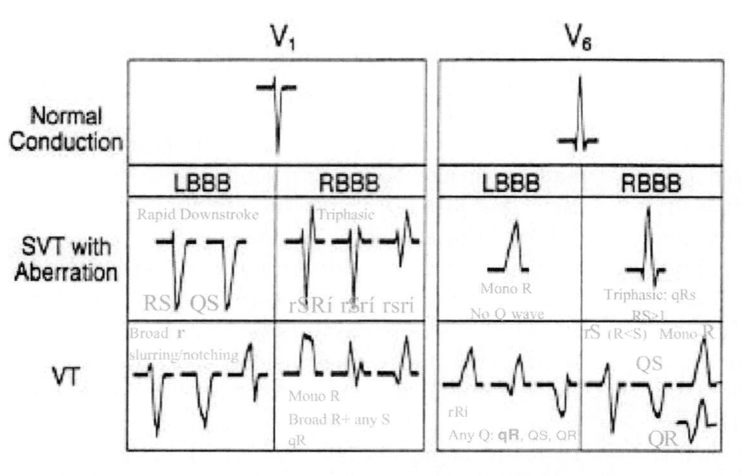


**Figure 50–13** Morphology criteria.

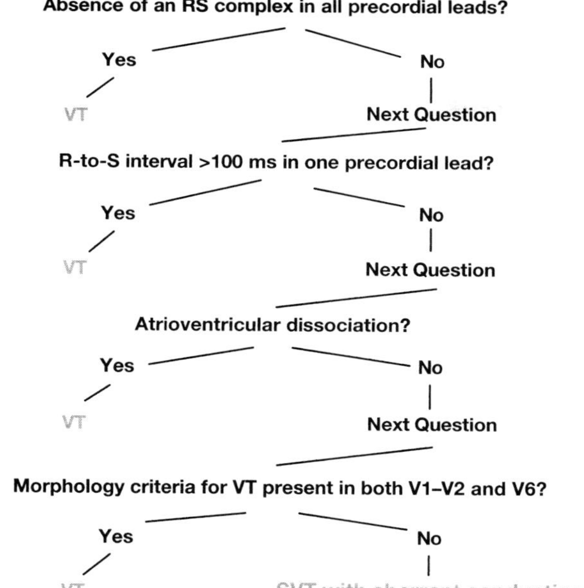


**Figure 50–14** Brugada's criteria I.

- The WCT is more likely to be VT if there is contralateral bundle branch block in normal sinus rhythm rather than during the WCT.
- Although regularity in itself does not help to distinguish SVT from VT, rapid irregular WCT with beat-to-beat QRS-duration variation is suggestive of atrial fibrillation with WPW (Fig. 50–18)
- Misdiagnosis of SVT as VT using morphology criteria can occur when the WCT is a result of pre-excited tachycardia or a paced ventricular rhythm.

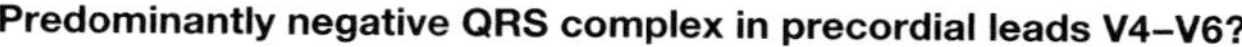

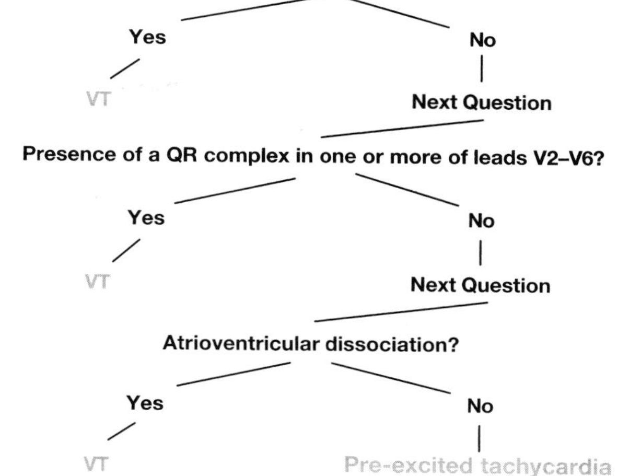


**Figure 50–16** Brugada's criteria II.

- VT can be misdiagnosed as SVT in cases of bundle branch re-entrant VT (BBR-VT). This occurs when ventricular activation begins via the RBBB and produces a LBBB QRS morphology. The conduction spreads transseptally to retrogradely, reentering the LBBB and establishing the re-entry circuit of BBR-VT. Following the morphology criteria for LBBB QRS complexes will lead to an incorrect diagnosis of SVT with LBBB aberrancy. However, if AV dissociation is present, the correct diagnosis of VT will be made.
- A narrow QRS VT can occur with QRS durations <140 milliseconds. This can occur in 12% of VTs. A possible explanation is when the origin of the VT comes from the septum, which causes simultaneous spread of ventricular activation. Such is the case when idiopathic left

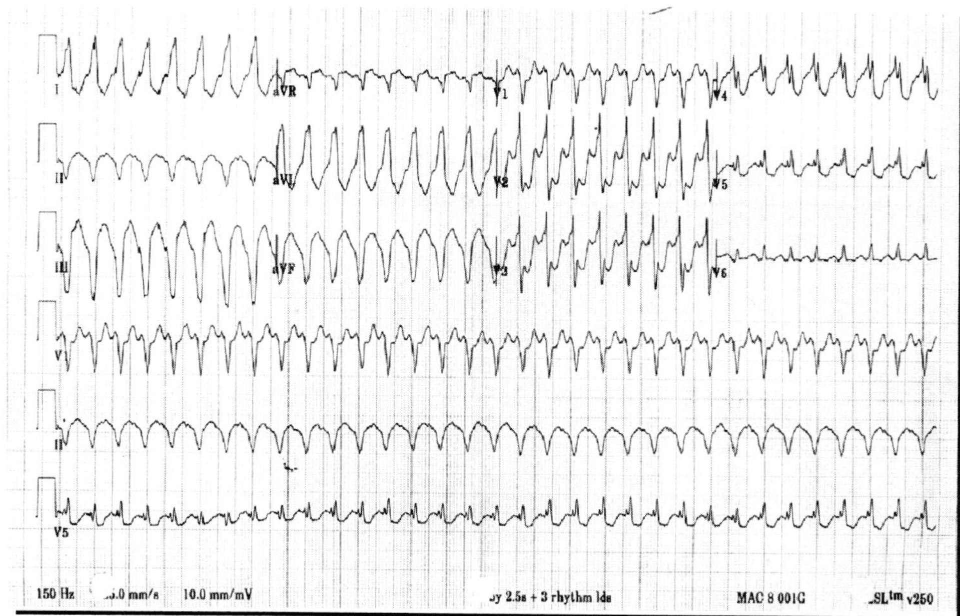


**Figure 50–15** This ECG shows an RS pattern in $V_1$–$V_5$. The RS interval measures 140 msec in $V_4$, which suggests a diagnosis of VT with 98% specificity.

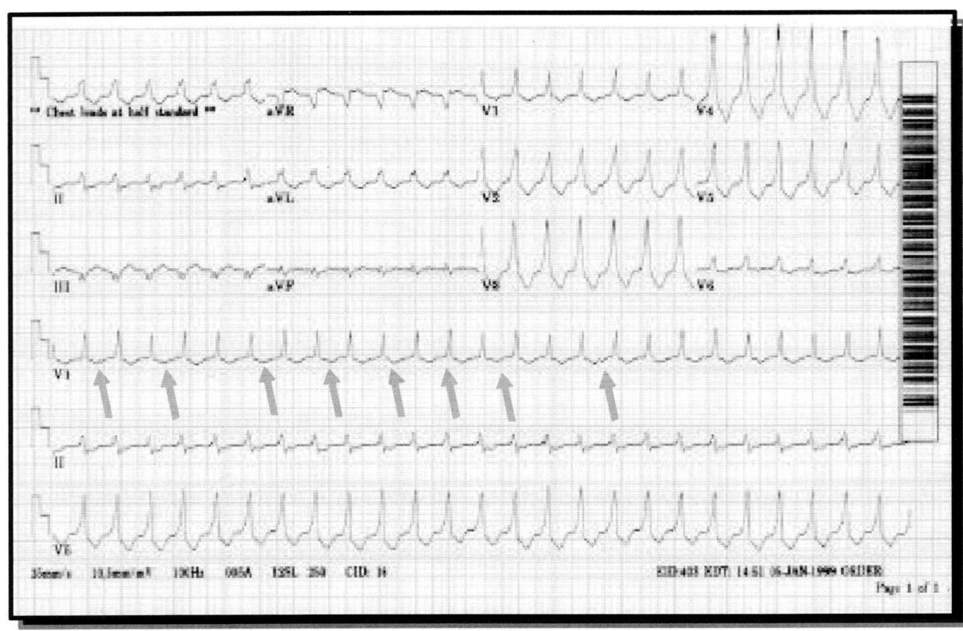

Figure 50–17 ECG: AV dissociation.

ventricular tachycardia (fascicular VT) is present. This type of VT can be terminated with IV verapamil and is therefore misdiagnosed as SVT.

## CONCLUSIONS

Despite multiple diagnostic tools, the determination of WCT etiology can be difficult. Morphology criteria are difficult to remember with certainty. The widespread use of antiarrhythmic medications with secondary intraventricular conduction delay has reduced the accuracy of currently available algorithms. Certain key points that should be committed to memory:

- If the configuration of the WCT is not compatible with aberration, then it is likely to be VT.
- If structural heart disease is present, WCT is most likely VT.
- Certain type of treatments (verapamil, adenosine) can potentially worsen the patient's situation. So if the diagnosis remains in question, treat it as though it is VT.

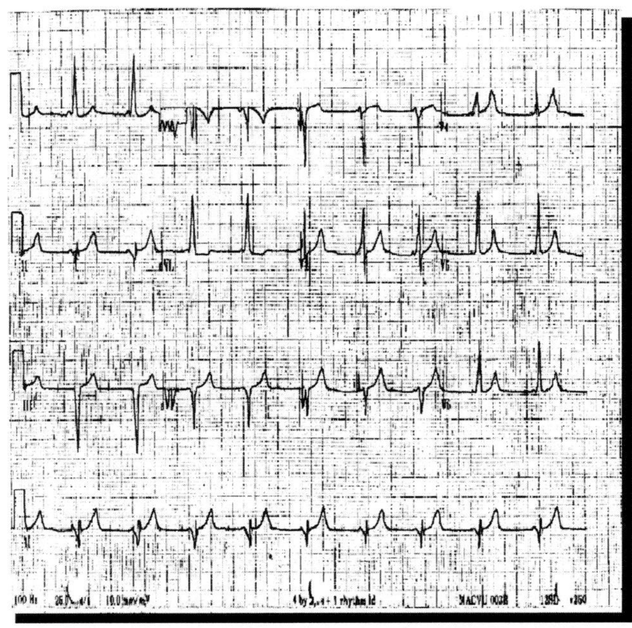

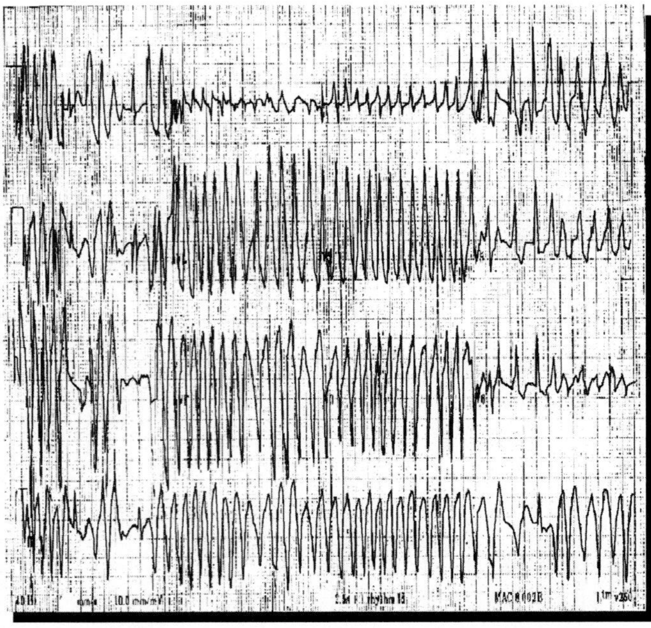

Figure 50–18 Examples of other ECG criteria.

- Using morphology criteria, pre-excited tachycardias and paced ventricular rhythms may be easily mistaken for VT.
- AV dissociation remains the most important and most specific criterion for the diagnosis of VT.
- In some situations, "I don't know" is the correct answer. In these cases, an electrophysiology study may necessary for an accurate arrhythmic diagnosis

## BIBLIOGRAPHY


**Akhtar M, Shenasa M, Jazayeri M, et al.** Wide QRS complex tachycardia: reappraisal of a common clinical problem. *Ann Intern Med.* 1988;109:905–912.

**Baerman JM, Morady F, DiCarlo LA, et al.** Differentiation of ventricular tachycardia from supraventricular tachycardia with aberration: value of the clinical history. *Ann Emerg Med.* 1987;16: 40–43.

**Belhassen B, Rotmensch HH, Laniado S.** Response of recurrent sustained ventricular tachycardia to verapamil. *Br Heart J.* 1981;46: 679–682.

**Brugada P, Brugada J, Mont L, et al.** A new approach to the differential diagnosis of a regular tachycardia with a wide QRS complex. *Circulation.* 1991;83:1649–1659.

**Buxton AE, Marchlinski FE, Doherty JU, et al.** Hazards of intravenous verapamil for sustained ventricular tachycardia. *Am J Cardiol.* 1987;59:1107–1110.

**Coumel P, Leclercq JF, Attuel P, et al.** The QRS morphology in post-myocardial infarction ventricular tachycardia: a study of 100 tracings compared with 70 cases of idiopathic ventricular tachycardia. *Eur Heart J.* 1984;5:792–805.

**Curione M, Fuoco U, Borgia C, et al.** An electrocardiographic criterion to detect AV dissociation in wide QRS tachyarrhythmias. *Clin Cardiol.* 1988;11:250–252.

**Gelband H, Waldo AL, Kaiser GA, et al.** Etiology of right bundle branch block in patients undergoing total repair of tetralogy of Fallot. *Circulation.* 1971;44:1022–1033.

**Kindwall KE, Brown J, Josephson ME.** Electrocardiographic criteria for ventricular tachycardia in wide complex left bundle branch block morphology tachycardias. *Am J Cardiol.* 1988;61:1279–1283.

**Miller JM, Marchlinski FE, Buxton AE, et al.** Relationship between the 12-lead electrocardiogram during ventricular tachycardia and endocardial site of origin in patients with coronary artery disease. *Circulation.* 1988;77:759–766.

**Miller JM.** The many manifestations of ventricular tachycardia. *J Cardiovasc Electrophysiol.* 1992;3:88–107.

**Miller JM.** Ventricular tachycardia: ECG manifestations. In Zipes DP, Jalife J, eds. *Cardiac Electrophysiology: From Cell to Bedside.* 2nd ed. Philadelphia: WB Saunders; 1995:990–1008.

**Morady F, Baerman JM, DiCarlo LA, et al.** A prevalent misconception regarding wide-complex tachycardias. *JAMA.* 1985;254:2790–2792.

**Nathan AW, Hellestrand KJ, Bexton RS, et al.** Proarrhythmic effects of the new antiarrhythmic agent flecainide acetate. *Am Heart J.* 1984;107:222–228.

**Pick A, Langendorf R.** Differentiation of supraventricular and ventricular tachycardias. *Prog Cardiovasc Dis.* 1960;2:391–407.

**Rankin AC, Oldroyd KG, Chong E.** Value and limitations of adenosine in the diagnosis and treatment of narrow and broad complex tachycardias. *Br Heart J.* 1989;62:195–203.

**Reddy GV, Leghari RU.** Standard limb lead QRS concordance during wide QRS tachycardia: a new surface ECG sign of ventricular tachycardia. *Chest.* 1987;92:763–765.

**Steinman RT, Herrera C, Schuger CD, et al.** Wide QRS tachycardia in the conscious adult: ventricular tachycardia is the most frequent cause. *JAMA.* 1989;261:1013–1016.

**Wellens HJJ, Bar FWHM, Lie K.** The value of the electrocardiogram in the differential diagnosis of a tachycardia with a widened QRS complex. *Am J Med.* 1978;64:27–33.

**Wellens HJJ, Brugada P.** Diagnosis of ventricular tachycardia from the 12 lead electrocardiogram. In Barold SS, ed. *12-Lead Electrocardiography.* Cardiology Clinics, vol 5, no 3. Philadelphia: WB Saunders; 1987:511–525.

Wide-Complex Tachycardia: VT versus SVT Worksheet

1. QRS-Complex Duration
   VT: QRS >140 ms for RBBB, QRS >160 ms for LBBB
2. QRS-Complex Axis
   VT: right superior
3. Capture and Fusion Complexes
4. QRS Precordial Concordance
5. WCT: Brugada's Criteria I

   Step 1. Absence of an RS complex in all precordial leads?
   Step 2. R-to-S interval >100 ms in one precordial lead?
   Step 3. AV dissociation?
   Step 4. Morphology criteria for VT present in *both* V1–V2 *and* V6?

RBBB morphology

| | VT | | SVT |
|---|---|---|---|
| V1 | Monophasic R | V1 | Triphasic |
| | R (>30 ms) + any S | | rSR′, rSr′ |
| | qR | | rR′, rsr′ |
| V6 | RS (R < S) | V6 | Triphasic |
| | QS, Qrs | | Rs, RS (R > S) |

LBBB morphology

| | VT | | SVT |
|---|---|---|---|
| V1 | rS: Broad r > 30 ms | V1 | rS, QS (rapid downstroke) |
| | Notching/delay in S | | |
| | QS ≥ 70 ms | | |
| | RT taller than RS | | |
| V6 | QR, QS, QrS, qR | V6 | rR′ |
| | Rr′ | | Monophasic R |
| | | | No Q waves |

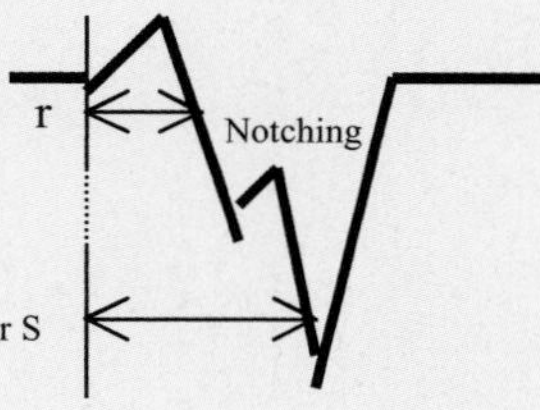


6. WCT: Brugada's Criteria II

   Step1. Predominantly negative QRS complex in precordial leads V4–V6?
   Step2. Presence of a QR complex in one or more of leads V2–V6?
   Step3. Atrioventricular dissociation?

7. Diagnosis: ECG Criteria Miscellaneous Conditions
   1. QRS complex during WCT narrower than during NSR: suggests VT.
   2. Contralateral BBB in NSR and WCT: suggests VT.
   3. Rapid irregular WCT + beat-to-beat QRS-to-QRS interval variation: atrial fibrillation with WPW.

8. Special Cases
   1. Misclassification of SVT for VT: Pre-excited tachycardia, paced ventricular rhythm.
   2. Misclassification of VT for SVT: BBR-VT (without evidence of AV dissociation).
   3. Narrow QRS VT: ILV-VT

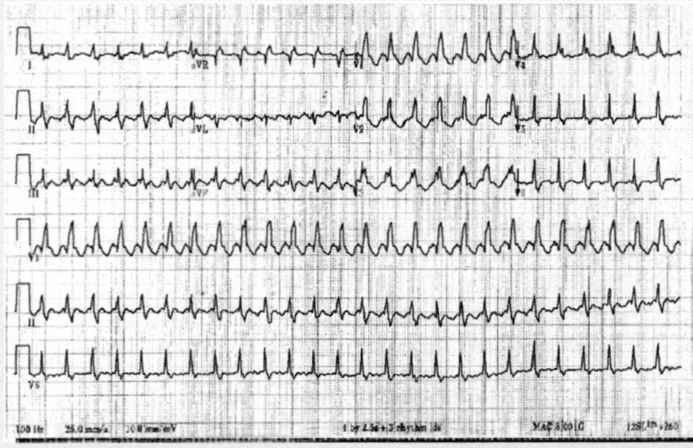

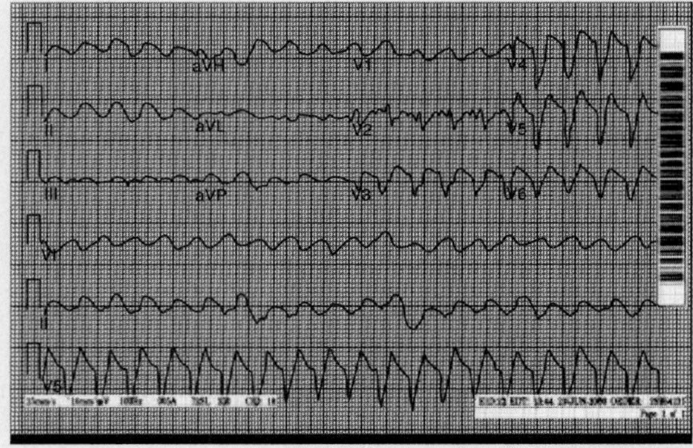

# Pacemakers and Defibrillators

51

*John S. Zakaib*    *Bruce L. Wilkoff*

## CARDIAC PACING

Cardiac pacing is the only definitive therapy for symptomatic bradycardia. Whether iatrogenic, ischemic, or intrinsic conduction system disease is present, cardiac pacing can be a temporary bridge to recovery, a backup safety therapy, or a permanent therapy, depending on the clinical scenario. What follows is a review of major topics in cardiac pacing.

### Indications

Indications for cardiac pacing vary with the clinical scenario. The major determinant of need for permanent pacing is the anticipated duration of the pacing indication. For example, symptomatic bradycardia associated with a toxic ingestion of a nodal blocking drug (e.g., digitalis) can be anticipated to resolve as the drug is cleared. Temporary pacing may be indicated in the short term, but a permanent device should not be needed. Alternatively, a transient neurocardiogenic (cardioinhibitory) bradycardic episode may resolve spontaneously, and temporary pacing should not be needed. However, if episodes recur on medical therapy to the point of causing recurrent syncope, a permanent pacemaker is indicated to protect the patient from subsequent syncopal episodes.

### Temporary Pacing

In the emergency department setting, transcutaneous pacing can be used as a bridge to a more definitive transvenous temporary pacing system in the setting of symptomatic bradycardia of any etiology with hemodynamic compromise.

In the critical care setting, temporary pacing can be a lifesaving bridge to recovery or, further, to a definitive therapy for the underlying cause of bradycardia. The indications can roughly be divided into those related to ischemia, and all other categories.

In the setting of myocardial infarction, up to 25% of patients will have a rhythm disturbance. A smaller subset of these patients develop bradycardia or atrioventricular (AV) nodal conduction block requiring temporary pacing. Some of these patients do eventually require permanent pacing after they have been treated for their acute infarction. In general, the "high-degree" heart blocks such as Mobitz Type II second-degree heart block and third-degree heart block warrant temporary pacing during the throes of anterior (LAD territory) infarcts or inferior (RCA territory) infarcts. Further, new bundle branch block or alternating bundle branch block reflect ischemia within the interventricular septum and warrants temporary pacing as a backup in case of progression to complete heart block. Refractory bradycardia in the setting of an infarct in any territory necessitates temporary pacing.

Absent an acute myocardial infarction, symptomatic bradycardia with or without AV dissociation and third-degree AV block with ventricular escape warrants temporary pacing. Backup pacing indications include temporary ventricular pacing during right heart catheterization in the setting of pre-existing left bundle branch block (LBBB), new bundle branch block or AV block in the setting of endocarditis, and essential pharmacologic therapies that may induce or exacerbate bradycardia.

Temporary pacing systems with temporary epicardial atrial and ventricular wires are routinely used in the setting of open heart surgery. These systems are used to optimize cardiac output coming off cardiopulmonary bypass, and subsequently as a backup system in case AV nodal conduction block occurs postoperatively, especially in the setting of valvular heart surgery.

## Permanent Pacing

The indications for permanent pacing are listed in detail in the American College of Cardiology/American Heart Association ACC/AHA/NASPE 2002 Guideline Update for Implantation of Cardiac Pacemakers and Antiarrhythmia Devices: Summary Article: A Report of the American College of Cardiology/American Heart Association Task Force on Practice Guidelines (ACC/AHA/NASPE Committee to Update the 1998 Pacemaker Guidelines). This document is summarized in Table 51–1.

## Device Features

Single-chamber devices that only pace the ventricle or atrium have fallen by the wayside in favor of more sophisticated atrioventicular pacing devices that have the ability to track the sinus node rate when appropriate and pace the ventricle after a set delay. They also switch modes to ventricular backup pacing when the atrial signal falls outside of set parameters, as in paroxysmal atrial fibrillation and sick sinus syndrome. Further, cardiac resynchronization therapy with biventricular pacing has a role in symptomatic heart failure (New York Heart Association [NYHA] Class III–IV) and evidence of left ventricular dysynchrony (LBBB or echo dyssynchrony parameters). Despite the predominance of dual-chamber pacemakers, there is increasing data suggesting that right ventricular stimulation increases the incidence of heart failure, hospitalization, and death in various patient subsets. However, if the ventricle needs to be stimulated, the vast majority of patients tolerate right ventricular stimulation, as dual-chamber stimulation is preferred over sole ventricular stimulation. Figure 51–1 shows a schematic of pacemaker timing cycles.

### *Rate-Adaptive Pacing*

A variety of methods have been employed to allow for implantable pacemakers to increase their pacing rate in the setting of metabolic demand for increased cardiac output. The most commonly employed methods include motion sensing, acceleration sensing, and minute ventilation sensing. These techniques utilize motion, acceleration, and/or minute ventilation, respectively, as a surrogate for increased metabolic demand for oxygen delivery. In patients with chronotropic incompetence, or the inability to increase cardiac output in response to exercise, rate-adaptive devices can utilize these surrogates to increase pacing rate and therefore increase cardiac output.

There are advantages and disadvantages to each type of sensor system. Motion sensors and accelerometers provide an almost immediate rise in rate and therefore cardiac output when they detect activity. However, they can be "fooled" by stimuli external to the patient that mimics patient activity (i.e., turbulence during flight, etc.). The accelerometer tends to respond more specifically to patient activity than does the motion sensor. The advantage of the minute ventilation sensor is that it responds specifically to the patient's respiratory rate—a parameter that is controlled by the brainstem. Although this parameter perhaps more reliably reflects the degree of patient exertion, it tends to lag behind the initiation of strenuous activity. Dual-sensor systems that utilize data collected from an accelerometer and minute ventilation detection may actually be best suited for effective rate-adaptive pacing.

### *Mode Switching*

Another feature of dual-chamber cardiac pacemakers that allows the devices to respond to changes in the physiology of the patient is mode switching. Mode switching is the ability of the device to revert to a separate, backup pacing mode in the event that the primary pacing mode no longer best serves the patient's pacing need. For example, in a patient with AV nodal block, a dual-chamber device may be programmed to sense or track the patient's intrinsic sinoatrial rate and to pace the ventricle after a set delay within the range of 60 to 120 beats/min. If the atria begin to fibrillate, the sensed atrial rate would exceed the rate parameter and the device would switch modes to a backup ventricular-only mode with a set rate sufficient to prevent hemodynamic compromise. If the patient reverted to sinus rhythm subsequently, the device would recognize the atrial rate back within the set parameter range and switch back to the primary mode, tracking the atrium and pacing the ventricle. Mode switching allows for the maximum responsiveness to the patient's intrinsic rhythm. These devices are most commonly programmed DDDR and revert to VVIR during periods of high atrial rates.

### *Other Programmable Features*

Modern pacemakers now include a myriad of programmable features to better match the patient's physiologic status. They can be programmed to pace at a lower "sleep" rate during typical sleeping hours, with absence of strenuous activity confirmed by the devices metabolic sensing system. Programmable pulse width and output allow the programmer to optimize the impulse specifications to ensure capture while preserving battery power. Diagnostic information and event data including mode-switching data can be stored and retrieved later to assess for the presence and prevalence of atrial arrhythmias and other events. Atrial and ventricular electrograms can be obtained and stored. Device status data can also be retrieved, including battery usage and projected battery life given current settings.

### *Leads*

The pacing leads conduct the electrical pacing impulse to the myocardium, and conduct the intrinsic electrical

**TABLE 51–1**
**INDICATIONS FOR PERMANENT PACEMAKERS**

Class I

- Symptomatic third-degree AV block and advanced second-degree AV block with bradycardia, documented asystole longer than 3 seconds, escape rhythm less than 40 beats/min, status post-AV nodal ablation, or postoperative AV block anticipated to persist
- Neuromuscular disease associated with AV block, such as Erb's dystrophy, myotonic muscular dystrophy, Kearns-Sayre syndrome, peroneal muscular atrophy with or without symptomatic bradycardia
- Any second-degree AV block with symptomatic bradycardia
- Intermittent third-degree AV block, Type II second-degree AV block, or alternating bundle branch block in the setting of chronic bi- or trifascicular block
- Third-degree AV block within or below the His after acute MI
- Persistent and symptomatic second- or third-degree AV block after acute MI
- Symptomatic SND, iatrogenic drug induced, absent any alternative drug therapy
- Symptomatic chronotropic incompetence
- Documented pause-dependent VT
- Recurrent syncope with carotid sinus massage
- Symptomatic bradycardia/chronotropic incompetence after cardiac transplantation

Class IIa

- Asymptomatic third-degree AV block with average awake V rate ≥40 beats/min, especially in the setting of cardiomegaly or LV dysfunction
- Asymptomatic Type II second-degree AV block with narrow QRS complex
- Asymptomatic Type I second-degree AV block at intra- or infra-His level at EPS
- First- or second-degree AV block with symptoms similar to pacemaker syndrome
- Syncope not attributable to AV block when other causes excluded, especially VT, when bi- or trifascicular block is present
- Prolonged HV (>100 ms) at EPS or evidence of pacing-induced infra-His block when bi- or trifascicular block is present
- Spontaneous or drug-induced SND and symptoms of bradycardia, absent a clear association of the two
- Syncope of unexplained origin and SND documented or provoked at EPS
- High-risk congenital long QT
- Recurrent syncope with hypersensitive cardioinhibitory response
- Unexplained syncope with SND or AV nodal dysfunction discovered at EPS
- Symptomatic, recurrent neurocardiogenic syncope with bradycardia
- CRT in refractory NYHA Class III-IV DCM or ICM with QRS >130 ms and LVEF <35%

Class IIb

- Marked first-degree AV block in patients with LV dysfunction and congestive heart failure, when a shorter AV interval may improve hemodynamics
- Neuromuscular diseases with any degree of AV block with or without symptoms
- Neuromuscular diseases with any degree of fascicular block
- Persistent AV block at the AV nodal level after acute MI
- Minimally symptomatic patients with awake heart rate <40 beats/min
- Prevention of symptomatic, drug-refractory atrial fibrillation in coexisting SND
- Neurally mediated syncope with significant bradycardia reproduced by tilt testing
- Medically refractory, symptomatic HOCM with significant outflow obstruction
- Symptomatic, refractory DCM with prolonged PR and documented improvement with pacing
- Symptomatic bradycardia/chronotropic incompetence after transplantation that may resolve

AV, atrioventricular; MI, myocardial infarction; SND, sinus node dysfunction; VT, ventricular tachycardia; LV, left ventricular; EPS, electrophysiology study; CRT, cardiac resynchronization therapy; NYHA, New York Heart Association; HV, Histo ventricular conduction time; DCM, dilated cardiomyopathy; LVEF, left ventricular ejection fraction; HOCM, hypertrophic obstructive cardiomyopathy.

*Source:* After Gregoratos G, Abrams J, Epstein AE, et al. ACC/AHA/NASPE 2002 guideline update for implantation of cardiac pacemakers and antiarrhythmia devices: summary article. A report of the American College of Cardiology/American Heart Association Task Force on Practice Guidelines (ACC/AHA/NASPE Committee to Update the 1998 Pacemaker Guidelines). *Circulation.* 2002;106:2145–2161.

activity of the myocardium to the sense amplifiers within the device. Unipolar leads have a single electrode at their tip, and therefore they direct current from their tip to the can of the device through the patient's tissues, or vice versa. For this reason, problems such as pectoral, intercostal, or diaphragmatic stimulation are more likely to occur, particularly in implants requiring higher outputs to capture the ventricle. Bipolar leads have two electrodes with close proximity at their tip and direct current proximal to distal or distal to proximal over much smaller distances. These leads can achieve capture of the myocardium with lower output energies and thus are more efficient. They are capable of unipolar function as well, but with the same limitations as standard unipolar leads. Of note, bipolar leads are by

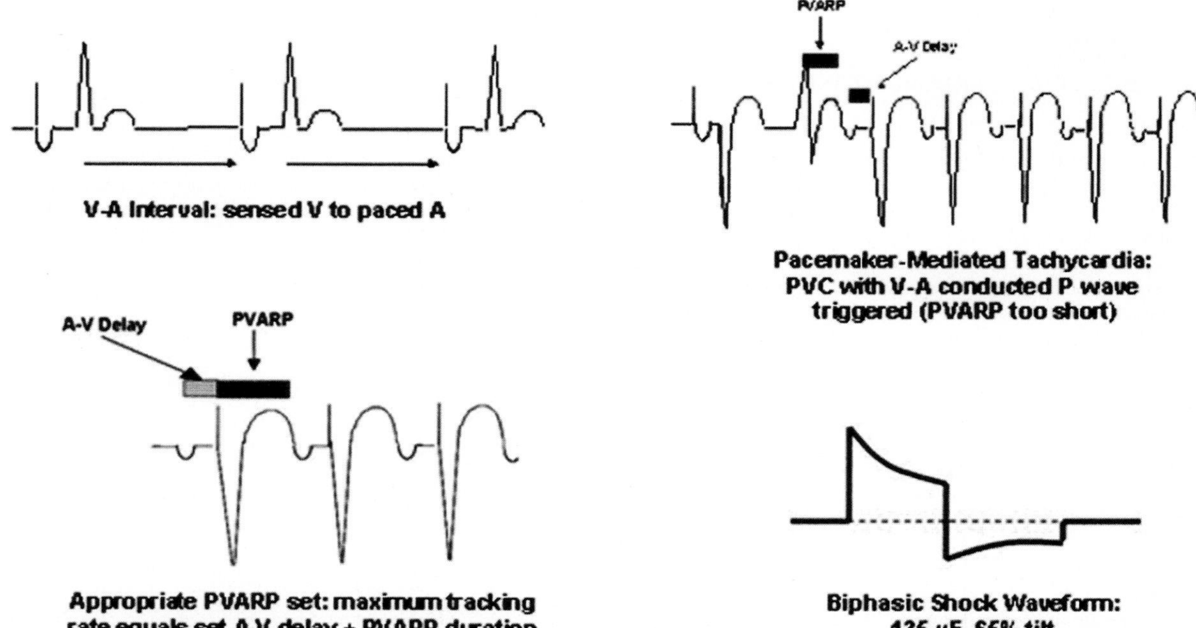


**Figure 51–1** Schematic of important device timing cycles and impulses.

necessity larger and stiffer than unipolar leads, and are more prone to mechanical failures than unipolar leads.

Coronary sinus leads are small, highly flexible unipolar or bipolar leads. They can be directed from the right atrium via the coronary sinus into a branch cardiac vein for the purpose of pacing the left ventricle in synchrony with the right ventricle in patients with ventricular dysfunction and delayed intraventricular conduction, usually manifest as a left bundle branch block.

Epicardial leads can be placed surgically using minimally invasive techniques or during open heart surgery for another indication and subsequently utilized instead of transvenous leads for standard pacing or more commonly for cardiac resynchronization therapy (biventricular pacing). Often two leads are placed at the time of surgery and one of the two is subsequently utilized for biventricular pacing, depending on the thresholds and pacing characteristics of each at the time of device implant.

A variety of fixation techniques are utilized to maintain the contact of the lead tip with the myocardium. Active fixation leads employ a fixed extended or retractable screw or plastic projections (tines) at the lead tip that usually entrap in the trabeculations of the right ventricle or the right atrial appendage. These systems allow for better maintenance of the lead tip at the desired site of implantation during deployment of the fixation tine. Passive fixation systems utilize fixed tines that intercalate into the trabeculae of the ventricle to maintain the position of the lead. As lead implants "mature" over time, pacing thresholds tend first to rise due to inflammation and then improve as healing continues and the inflammation resolves. Most leads have a small amount of steroid impregnated at the lead tip that reduces the size of the fibrotic tissue capsule.

## Basic Concepts of Impulses and Timing

Following is a review of some basic concepts in pacemaker theory that are central to an understanding of the clinical application of pacing technology.

*Stimulation threshold:* The minimum amount of electrical energy that consistently produces a cardiac depolarization. The energy is a combination of voltage and pulse duration. It can be expressed in terms of amplitude (milliamperes or volts), pulse duration (milliseconds), charge (microcoulombs), or energy (microjoules).

*Voltage output:* The amount of voltage being delivered to the heart every time the pacemaker emits a stimulus. It is expressed in volts.

*Pulse width (or pulse duration):* The length in milliseconds the voltage is delivered to the heart.

*Strength–duration curve:* The hyperbolic relationship between the voltage output and the pulse width that defines the stimulation threshold (Figure 51–2).

*Atrial sensing/sensitivity:* A programmed parameter that defines the largest signal that will be ignored by the device and thus determines which signals are detected by the pacemaker or implantable cardioverter/defibrillator (ICD) in the atrial channel. Atrial sensing in the dual-chamber pacing mode, DDD, will inhibit the atrial stimulus which would occur at the end

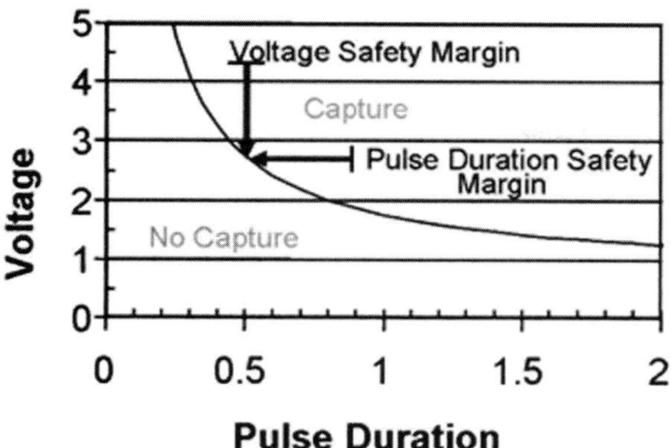


**Figure 51–2** The strength–duration curve.

of the atrial escape interval (V-to-A interval), initiate the AV interval, and trigger the ventricular output at the end of the AV interval.

*Ventricular sensing/sensitivity:* A programmed parameter that defines the smallest signal that will be ignored by the device and thus determines which signals are detected by the pacemaker or ICD in the ventricular channel. Ventricular sensing in the dual-chamber pacing mode, DDD, will inhibit both atrial and ventricular stimuli that were scheduled to be output at the end of the atrial escape interval (atrial) or AV interval (ventricle) and initiate a new atrial escape interval (V-to-A interval).

*Atrial oversensing:* Sensing on the atrial channel that occurs due to signals on the atrial lead either related to signals originating outside the atrium, such as far-field ventricular signals, myopotentials from the pectoralis major muscle or diaphragm, or from noise originating from a dysfunctional lead (insulation or conductor fractures or a loose set screw). Depending on the mode of pacing, atrial oversensing will either inhibit or trigger atrial and/or ventricular stimuli.

*Ventricular oversensing:* Sensing on the ventricular channel that occurs due to signals on the ventricular lead either relating to signals originating outside the ventricle, such as myopotentials from the pectoralis major muscle in a unipolar lead system or from lead dysfunction secondary to insulation or conductor fracture or loose set screws. Sometimes the ventricular channel will oversense the atrial paced output and inhibit the ventricular output. This is called crosstalk inhibition and is usually prevented by a blanking of the ventricular sensing amplifier during the atrial paced outputs.

*Chronotropic competence:* The ability to match cardiac output to the metabolic needs of the body by appropriate modification of the heart rate.

*Minimum rate:* Also called the escape rate, this is the slowest rate at which the pacemaker will allow the heart to beat. The minimum paced rate is calculated by the ventricular paced or sensed event to atrial paced output interval plus the programmed A–V delay measured in milliseconds and converted to rate by dividing that sum into 60,000.

*V–A interval:* Also called the atrial escape interval, this is calculated by subtracting the paced AV interval from the minimum rate interval. It is initiated by a paced or sensed ventricular event and concludes with a paced atrial event or is interrupted by either an atrial or ventricular sensed event.

*A–V delay:* This programmed interval is initiated by an atrial sensed or paced event and is terminated with a ventricular paced stimulus unless interrupted by a ventricular sensed event (either a conducted beat through the AV node or a premature ventricular beat). Often AV delays initiated by sensed atrial events are programmed to be shorter than AV delays initiated by atrial paced events.

*Upper rate limit:* The fastest rate at which the ventricular channel can track intrinsic P waves or, in the case of rate-adaptive pacing on the basis of a sensor, the fastest rate at which the ventricular channel can track the sensor rate algorithm. The atrial tracking or upper rate limit is constrained by dividing 60,000 by the sum of the sensed AV delay and the PVARP.

*PVARP:* This is the Post-Ventricular Atrial Refractory Period. The PVARP is the timeframe during which the atrial channel is refractory after either a paced or sensed (R-wave) ventricular event. Its purpose is to prevent atrial sensing and tracking of any V–A (retrograde) conduction of ventricular events to the atrium that would trigger a pacemaker-mediated tachycardia (see later).

## Programming

Device programming has become more complex as dual-chamber pacing systems have become ubiquitous and biventricular pacing is becoming commonplace. It is important to note that the basic parameters discussed above can usually be derived with caliper measurements of the intervals observed on a 12-lead electrocardiogram (ECG) or rhythm strip. Following is a concise review of programming codes and timing cycles that provide the underpinnings of device programming.

### Codes

A standard coding system has been adopted to delineate the basic settings of the device as follows: The first designation is the chamber paced, the second designation is the chamber sensed, the third designation is the device response to a sensed event, and the final designation reflects the rate-adaptive status of the device. There is a fifth position in the code that is rarely used, but is reserved for indicating the

**TABLE 51–2**
**MODE CODES FOR CARDIAC PACEMAKERS**

| I<br>Chamber Paced | II<br>Chamber Sensed | III<br>Response to Sensed Event | IV<br>Program Rate Response | V<br>Tachycardia Therapy |
|---|---|---|---|---|
| O: none | O: none | O: none | O: none | O: none |
| A: atrium | A: atrium | I: inhibited | S: simple | P: pace |
| V: ventricle | V: ventricle | T: triggered | M: multiple | S: shock |
| D: dual (A + V) | D: dual (A + V) | D: dual (T + I) | C: communicating | D: dual (P + S) |
| S: single | S: single | — | R: rate response | — |

response that the device will provide during a tachycardia. Table 51–2 reviews the mode codes in detail.

As an example, a DDIR pacemaker can pace in both the atrium and the ventricle, and sense activity in both the atrium and the ventricle. Further, it will inhibit upon sensing intrinsic activity, and it has rate-adaptive functionality as well. A VOO device will pace the ventricle asynchronously, without sensing intrinsic activity.

### *Timing Cycles*

When a dual-chamber device paces the atrium, the ventricular channel is blanked for a period of 20 to 40 milliseconds as a safety feature to prevent inhibition of the ventricular channel by far-field (ventricular) sensing of the atrial paced output. The blanking period prevents "crosstalk inhibition," which could cause, in patients with complete lack of AV conduction, a string of atrial paced events and ventricular asystole. After the blanking period, the ventricular channel is open to sensed events, typically for 100 milliseconds. If, during this alert period a sensed event occurs, then the AV interval is abbreviated, usually to 120 milliseconds. This abbreviated AV delay is designed to prevent pacing during the vulnerable period of the ventricle, for instance, when the sensed event is caused by a premature ventricular depolarization. During the remainder of the AV delay (after the blanking and safety alert period), any sensed ventricular event will cause the ventricular output to be inhibited and reinitiate the atrial escape interval. If by the end of the programmed AV interval no event has been sensed, the device will pace the ventricle. After every paced or sensed ventricular event, a postventricular atrial refractory period (PVARP) is initiated. During this period, the atrial channel is refractory to detecting atrial activity. The purpose of the PVARP is to prevent detection of atrial activity produced by retrograde conduction through the AV node. Without making the atrium refractory to retrograde atrial events (V-to-A conducted beats) an endless loop cycle can be set up that continues until the retrograde conduction fails. This endless loop tachycardia is one of several types of pacemaker-mediated tachycardia (see Fig. 51–1 for a schematic of pacemaker timing cycles in comparison to the surface ECG).

### *Diagnostics*

Modern pacing devices are capable of storing tremendous amounts of data and reporting data in a variety of usable formats. Following is a brief review of device diagnostics and their applications.

*Histograms.* Histograms are a statistical report of a parameter describing the relative frequency of an event relative to time, heart rate, or another parameter. Histograms do not correlate symptoms to specific events, and from them one can only *infer* cause and effect (Fig. 51–3).

*Trends.* Trends evaluate the progression of a parameter over time. They are not a statistical representation but instead describe the correlation of an activity over time with symptoms. Trends can document concurrence of patient and rhythm events if interrogated quickly after the event occurs. Trends require *extrapolation* to connect patient and rhythm events. (See Fig. 51–3).

*Event monitoring:* Event monitoring captures an exact record of an event as characterized by electrograms, marker channel, and intervals. These monitored records are not statistical reflections of data but the actual recordings. Therefore, they can capture the relationship of symptoms and objective data. They require neither inference nor extrapolation (see Fig. 51–3).

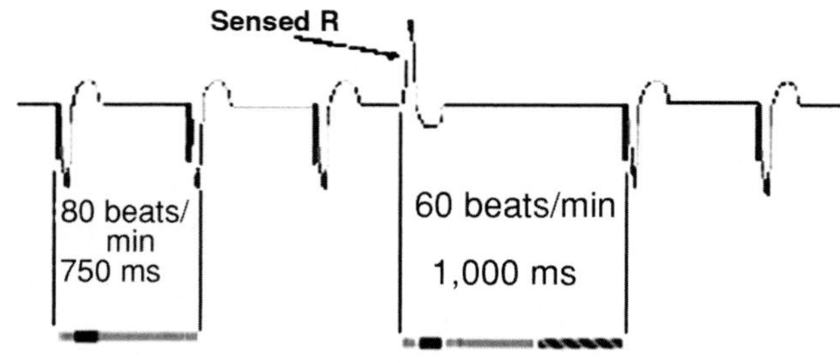


**Figure 51–3** Histogram: ventricular hysteresis.

## Troubleshooting and Complications

Device troubleshooting most often involves interrogation of the device and adjustment of the pacing mode or timing cycles in order to optimize device function. Further, device interrogation using a programmer can reveal diagnostic information about the integrity of the leads, status of the battery, and performance of the device's algorithms, including the behavior of the rate-adaptive sensor function. A review of some specific device troubleshooting issues follows.

### *Endless Loop Tachycardia*

Endless loop tachycardia is a type of pacemaker-mediated tachycardia specific to dual-chamber devices programmed to the VDD or DDD mode. Endless loop tachycardia is triggered by the atrial channel sensing retrograde conduction of a paced ventricular impulse. In response to the sensed event, the ventricle is paced again after the set AV interval, and retrograde conduction to the atrium recurs. As the atrium senses the retrograde V–A signal, the cycle begins again. The phenomenon is terminated by either applying a magnet to the device, thus reverting the device to nominal asynchronous pacing, or by reprogramming the device to lengthen the PVARP so that the atrial channel is refractory during the retrograde (V–A) conduction.

### *Pacemaker Syndrome*

The so-called pacemaker syndrome is a constellation of physical symptoms and signs associated with loss of AV synchrony, most commonly associated with VVI pacing. Affected patients suffer weakness, dizziness, lightheadedness, dyspnea on exertion, and sometimes even orthopnea and dyspnea at rest, independent of their underlying ventricular function. The symptoms result from ventricular pacing, typically with retrograde atrial conduction, which produces atrial contraction against a closed AV valve. The decrease in efficiency associated with loss of atrial kick as well as the increased back pressure within the pulmonary circuit both contribute to the symptomatology. Similar symptoms and physiology can result from atrial pacing with delayed AV conduction. The result is also related to atrial contraction against a closed AV valve. The treatment for pacemaker syndrome is device upgrade to a dual-chamber device. An atrial tracking ventricular pacemaker eliminates the physiologic underpinnings of pacemaker syndrome and typically alleviates the symptoms.

### *Lead Fracture/Failure*

Lead fracture is the term used to describe failures in the integrity of the lead wires, insulation, and/or coil. Fractures often occur at the ingress of the lead into the thorax within the subclavian vein as it passes between the clavicle and the first rib, particularly at the suture sleeve, due to tight ligatures or a sharp angulation of the lead in the pacemaker pocket. Crush injuries and chronic abrasion at this site are common etiologies of lead fracture. Disruption of the insulation causes a reduction of the pacing impedance and is often manifest by intermittent oversensing and either failure to produce a paced output or failure to capture the heart. Disruption of the lead conductor causes an increase in the pacing impedance and can also be manifest by intermittent oversensing and either failure to produce a paced output or to capture the heart. After the ECG, the chest x-ray is often the first diagnostic modality to reveal a lead fracture. Device interrogation typically suggests the diagnosis (abnormally high or low lead impedance, as noted above).

### *Infection/Erosion*

Device infection occurs most commonly from bacterial contamination at the time of device implantation. Most infections do not present within the first month after implantation but are manifest within the first 2 years after implantation. Some infections can be indolent and persist for years before becoming apparent. The most commonly responsible organisms are *Staphylococcus* species, with gram-negative organisms occurring predominantly in diabetic patients or those otherwise immunocompromised. Physical findings associated with device infection may range from normal pocket appearance to mildly erythematosus overlying tissue, to a swollen, boggy pocket and incision line. Occasionally a device will erode through the skin in the setting of a chronic device infection. When the pocket appears normal, the infection is typically unmasked by the presence of fevers and positive blood cultures. The treatment for device pocket infection with or without endocarditis is with antibiotics and device and lead explantation. The replacement device cannot be reimplanted at the time of device and lead extraction but 2 to 7 days later, usually contralaterally. Less commonly, device infection can occur secondary to bacterial endocarditis or other bloodstream infection. Vegetations can sometimes be observed on the leads, most commonly utilizing transesophageal echocardiography.

### *Extraction*

The most compelling reason for lead extraction is pacing system infection, either localized to the pocket or with associated bacteremia or endocarditis. Multiple leads can compromise the venous flow, risking subclavian or SVC occlusion with symptoms, or prevent the addition of leads for upgrade to an ICD or BiV system. Lead extraction can range from simply applying traction to a relatively recently implanted lead, to the use of mechanical, electrosurgical, or excimer laser extraction sheaths to facilitate the removal of fibrosed leads from the endovascular surface. Lead extraction using these devices can be complicated by serious bleeding complications leading to tamponade and even death, and are thus best relegated to experienced operators.

## IMPLANTABLE CARDIOVERTER-DEFIBRILLATORS

Implantable cardioverter-defibrillators (ICDs) initiated a new era in the treatment of ventricular tachyarrhythmias. In contrast to modern devices, the early ICD systems were implanted via thoracotomy with epicardial placement of defibrillating patches and sensing electrodes and abdominal implantation of the device can. The devices themselves had no programmability, no significant diagnostics, and an abbreviated battery life of about 1 year. Patients requiring permanent pacing had to have a separate pacing device implanted. Over time, ICDs have grown geometrically smaller, allowing for prepectoral implantation with transvenous leads, have bradycardia and antitachycardia pacing, and hundreds of programmable parameters, diagnostics, and event storage, all while device longevity has expanded to 5 to 7 years. The devices now have full pacing capabilities and some are CRT capable as well.

### Indications

Indications for implantation of ICDs have expanded greatly over the past decade, based on data collected from the major ICD trials. The Center for Medicare and Medicaid Services (CMS) published updated guidelines on in 2005 for reimbursement for ICD implantation, recognizing the data from the primary and secondary prevention trials of ICDs with and without capacity for cardiac resynchronization. The clinical trials that provide the underpinnings for the currently accepted indications for implantation will be addressed elsewhere, as will the indications for CRT therapy. For the purpose of thorough Board review, the ACC/AHA/NASPE Guideline document referenced in the Bibliography is a critical, high-yield reference but represents recommendations that preceded the publication of the SCD-HeFT, DEFINITE, DINAMIT, COMPANION, and CARE-HF trials. The practical (reimbursed) indications for ICD implantation are listed in Table 51–3. In brief, ICDs are indicated for secondary prevention after a cardiac arrest or in patients with sustained spontaneous or sustained EPS-inducible ventricular arrhythmias. In addition, ICDs are indicated for primary prevention in patients with left ventricular dysfunction (LVEF <36%) with or without coronary artery disease with several limitations and in patients with inherited or familial conditions that increase the risk of sudden cardiac death.

### Devices

The current generation of ICDs includes single-chamber VVI devices, dual-chamber devices with fully programmable pacing capabilities, and CRT devices capable of biventricular pacing and antitachycardia therapies. As technology has progressed, these devices have become smaller, have better longevity, and are more programmable. The diagnostics available allow for extensive troubleshooting and event monitoring.

**TABLE 51–3**
**CENTER FOR MEDICARE AND MEDICAID SERVICES (CMS)–APPROVED (REIMBURSED) INDICATIONS FOR ICD THERAPY**

- Documented VF arrest not due to a reversible cause
- Documented sustained VT, spontaneous or induced by EPS, absent acute MI or reversible cause
- Documented familial or inherited conditions with a high risk of life-threatening VT (e.g., long QT, HCM)
- Coronary artery disease with prior MI, LVEF ≤35%, and inducible VT or VF at EPS
- Documented prior MI and LVEF ≤30%, except NYHA Class IV, shock, MI within 40 days or CABG/PCI within 90 days, or any noncardiac disease associated with <1-y survival
- Ischemic heart disease, prior MI, NYHA Class II–III symptoms, LVEF ≤35%
- DCM >9 mo duration, LVEF ≤35%, NYHA Class II–III symptoms
- DCM >3 mo duration, LVEF ≤35%, NYHA Class II–III symptoms if enrolled in an approved clinical trial or approved national registry

VF, ventricular fibrillation; VT, ventricular tachycardia; EPS, electrophysiology study; MI, myocardial infarction; HCM, hypertrophic cardiomyopathy; LVEF, left ventricular ejection fraction; NYHA, New York Heart Association; CABG, coronary artery bypass grafting; PCI, percutaneous coronary intervention; DCM, dilated cardiomyopathy. Providers must be able to justify the medical necessity of devices other than single-lead devices.

### Lead Systems

Typically, single-chamber ICD systems are implanted using active- or passive-fixation multipolar leads with shocking coils that lie in the right ventricle (RV) apposed to the endocardium as well as the superior vena cava (SVC). With this configuration, the device can deliver energy from the RV (+) coil to the SVC (−) coil or vice versa, or from either coil (+) to the ICD can (−) itself or vice versa. Various investigations have demonstrated that defibrillation thresholds (DFTs) can be reduced using optimal polarity and an "active can" configuration.

ICDs can be attached to epicardial leads or patches implanted during surgery. These leads are typically placed using minimally invasive techniques for patients with high defibrillation thresholds or during open heart surgery performed for other indications. Subcutaneous arrays and even azygous vein leads can be placed. Virtually all ICDs are implanted with transvenous in lieu of surgically placed leads.

Dual-chamber devices possess an atrial lead in addition to the ventricular shocking coil lead. The atrial lead is typically a standard bipolar pacing lead without a shocking coil and plays no role in defibrillation.

### Implantation

The most common site for device implantation is the left prepectoral space. This site gives access to the left subclavian vein for transvenous lead placement. Especially in "active can" configurations, this site of implantation allows for lower DFTs as the path for energy transmission from can to coil or vice versa traverses the LV myocardium. In the case of prior device infection, scarring, subclavian stenosis, or mastectomy on the left side, the right prepectoral space may be used. Lead implantation technique is much like that used for standard pacing lead implantation; however, there is an impetus to implant the lead tip at the RV apex so that the RV shocking coil rests completely within the right ventricle. In dual-chamber ICD implantations, the atrial lead is typically a standard bipolar pacing lead and has no role in cardioversion of ventricular arrhythmias.

## Device Function

### *Detection*

ICDs have a variety of programmed routines designed to aid in the detection and verification of ventricular tachycardia (VT) and ventricular fibrillation (VF), and to minimize the number of inappropriately delivered therapies. The device must be able to sense low-amplitude high-rate signals in VF, while not oversensing far-field atrial activity or ventricular repolarization. Appropriate sensing thresholds must be achieved at the time of implantation, or the device cannot be relied on to appropriately detect and treat malignant ventricular arrhythmias.

Detection algorithms utilize counters, and detection criteria are based on signal counts registered faster than the tachycardia threshold criterion programmed into the device. For example, if an ICD is programmed to detect VT at cycle lengths of less than 400 milliseconds and the device senses consecutive R waves with a cycle length of 390 milliseconds, it begins to count consecutive R waves until it reaches the programmed detection criterion, perhaps 15 beats. If the device detects 15 consecutive R waves with cycle length less than 400 milliseconds, it registers a VT event and administers therapy. VF is a more unstable arrhythmia, with shorter cycle lengths, and smaller and more variable wavelet amplitudes. The device cannot be assured of sensing *consecutive* signals to meet the VF criterion, so the criterion is often programmed to detect VF if *15 of 20* R waves are detected with a cycle length below the VF threshold cycle length.

Single-chamber devices use these cycle length criteria in addition to analyzing the suddenness of arrhythmia onset, the duration and persistence of the arrhythmia, and the morphology of the sensed R waves. Dual-chamber devices have the advantage of being able to compare ventricular sensed activity to atrial sensed activity, so rates and relationship of A to V can be compared in the detection criteria. Further, dual-chamber devices can detect AV dissociation. So the detection algorithms can be more sophisticated and potentially more accurate in the detection of VT requiring therapy and the discrimination of SVT or AF not requiring ICD therapy (Fig. 51–4).

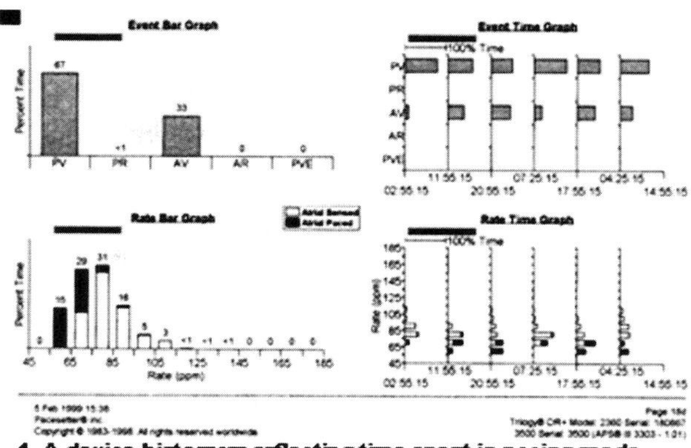

**1. A device histogram reflecting time spent in pacing mode and rate**

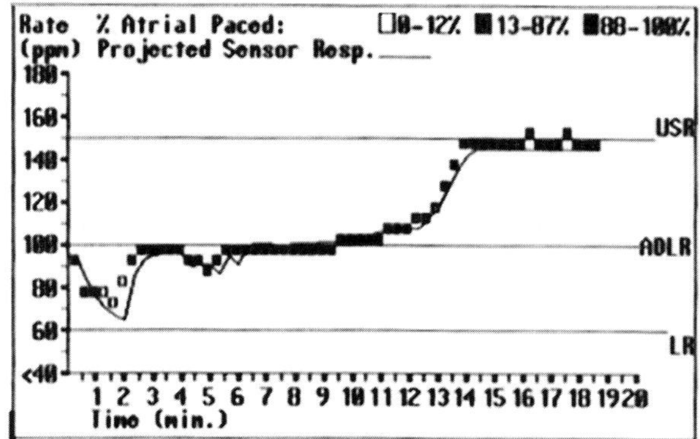

**2. A Trend reflecting atrial pacing rates over a period of time**

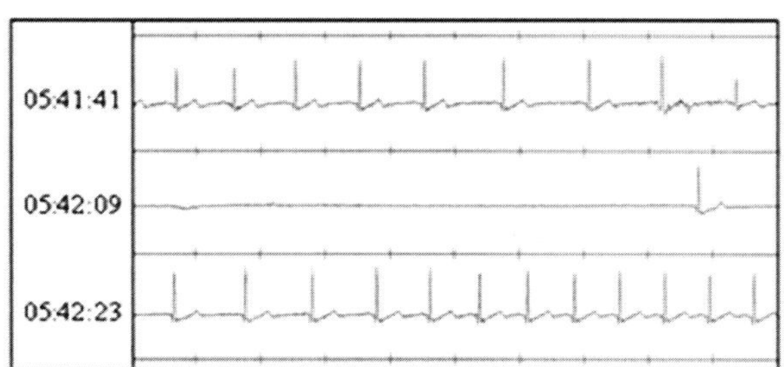

**3. An event recording revealing a long sinus pause**

**Figure 51–4** Device diagnostics: histograms, trends, and event monitoring.

For example, a dual-chamber device set to apply VT therapies at ventricular cycle lengths of 400 milliseconds or less may detect VT as in the previous example while at the same time detecting atrial signals with a cycle length of 200 milliseconds. Recognizing the atrial tachycardia (flutter) and the 2:1 ventricular response, the device monitors but does not "detect and treat" VT. If, in the same example, the device senses atrial signals with a cycle length of 400 milliseconds, it monitors the sinus tachycardia or SVT but does not deliver therapy for VT.

### *Therapies*

The therapy for VF is defibrillation upon detection with consecutive high-energy shocks pending redetection until the arrhythmia is terminated. Upon meeting the detection criteria, the device begins to charge its capacitor to the programmed output for the initial shock. Upon completion of capacitor charging, the device then rechecks for the presence of the arrhythmia and if present, it delivers the shock. After the initial shock, the device monitors for arrhythmia meeting criteria and if present, it charges again, typically to a higher or maximum output. If after charging the arrhythmia persists, the device again delivers therapy. The cycle continues until the arrhythmia is terminated.

Therapies for VT include low-energy synchronized cardioversion as well as antitachycardia pacing (ATP). The advantage of ATP is that it is painless and is not often perceived by the patient. When an ATP device detects VT, it can deliver a programmed burst of pacing impulses at a cycle length just shorter than the detected arrhythmia in an attempt to interrupt the re-entrant ventricular tachycardia circuit. After the burst, the device monitors for persistence of the arrhythmia. If VT persists, further bursts of ATP can be delivered, followed if necessary by low- or high-output cardioversion. ATP bursts can be programmed at a fixed cycle length representing a percentage of the VT cycle length, or at a progressively shorter (accelerating) cycle length for a programmed number of pulses. The number of ATP attempts prior to administration of shocks can be programmed too. Low-output cardioversion shocks are typically synchronized to the intrinsic R wave of the VT. Based on a variety of investigations, ATP is not inferior to low-energy cardioversion in terms of efficacy, and because it is painless, it has become the preferred therapy for "slow VT." In addition, recent data have documented that faster tachyarrhythmias, between 200 and 250 beats/min, can be successfully pace terminated approximately 50% of the time.

### *Waveforms*

The shock waveform for VT and VF is the same: a prolonged (relative to a pacing impulse) biphasic waveform lasting 5 to 20 milliseconds. The waveform is a truncated exponential decay voltage wave with a drop from the initial voltage to the trailing-edge voltage, called the tilt. A typical tilt is a 65% reduction of the voltage at the end of the first phase of the biphasic pulse. Then the capacitor polarity is reversed, producing a leading-edge negative voltage for the second phase equal to the trailing-edge positive voltage of the first phase. The second phase also has a tilt and is truncated after a few milliseconds. Biphasic waveforms with second phases equal to or shorter in duration than the first phase have been associated with significantly lower defibrillation thresholds as compared with monophasic waveforms. Thus, all current production ICDs utilize a biphasic waveform (Fig. 51–5).

### *Polarity*

Modern ICDs have the programmability to add or subtract various electrodes from the circuit (can or SVC electrode) or change the initial (positive or negative) polarity of the leads and the can, as well as the polarity of the waveform. Polarity changes are sometimes undertaken to reduce DFTs in patients with high DFTs.

### *Programming*

Device programming for ICDs involves programming pacing modes as well as detection parameters and therapies for VT and VF. Modern ICDs have full pacing capabilities and, depending on the device and indication for implantation, may be programmed for ventricular backup pacing, dual-chamber tracking and pacing, and even resynchronization pacing. The following review focuses on the antiarrhythmia features of ICDs. Refer to the pacing section of the chapter for more on pacemaker programming.

#### Detection Criteria

Therapies for VT and VF are administered only after detection criteria are met. Therefore, the criteria programming is critical to optimal device function. The concepts of arrhythmia detection have been presented previously. What remains is the actual interface programming between the device and the physician. As a practical matter, the detection criteria sets are typically divided into VT parameters and VF parameters. The VT parameters may further be broken down into "slow" VT and "fast" VT zones, based on the premise that slower VT may be more amenable to painless therapies (ATP) and faster VT may be more prone to acceleration or failure of ATP to convert the rhythm back to the baseline rhythm. Furthermore, "monitor zones" can be established so that rhythms in a given rate zone can be recorded as "events" and retrieved later for analysis. So the task of the device programmer is to match the detection criteria and therapies to the anticipated needs of the patient.

For example, if an 80-year-old patient with prior myocardial infarction and LV dysfunction has a device implanted after a documented VT episode with a VT cycle length of 380 milliseconds, and the patient is now being treated with amiodarone and long-acting beta-blockers, the physician programmer may opt for VVI backup pacing at 40 beats/min, a "slow VT" zone of 400 to 320 milliseconds, and a "fast VT" zone of 319 to 290 milliseconds, with a VF zone of anything less than 290 milliseconds. Therapies may include three attempts at ATP at 81% of the VT cycle length, followed by 20 J, 30 J, maximum output shocks if ATP fails to convert the "slow" VT. The fast VT zone may be programmed for 20 J, 30 J, maximum output for six shocks, and the VF zone may be programmed likewise, 20 J, 30 J, maximum output for six shocks.

Now suppose the patient goes home and comes back to the Emergency Department with "weakness" but has received no shocks as far as he can tell. Telemetry reveals NSR 60 beats/min. Interrogation of the device reveals nominal function and no recorded events. Perhaps the patient is

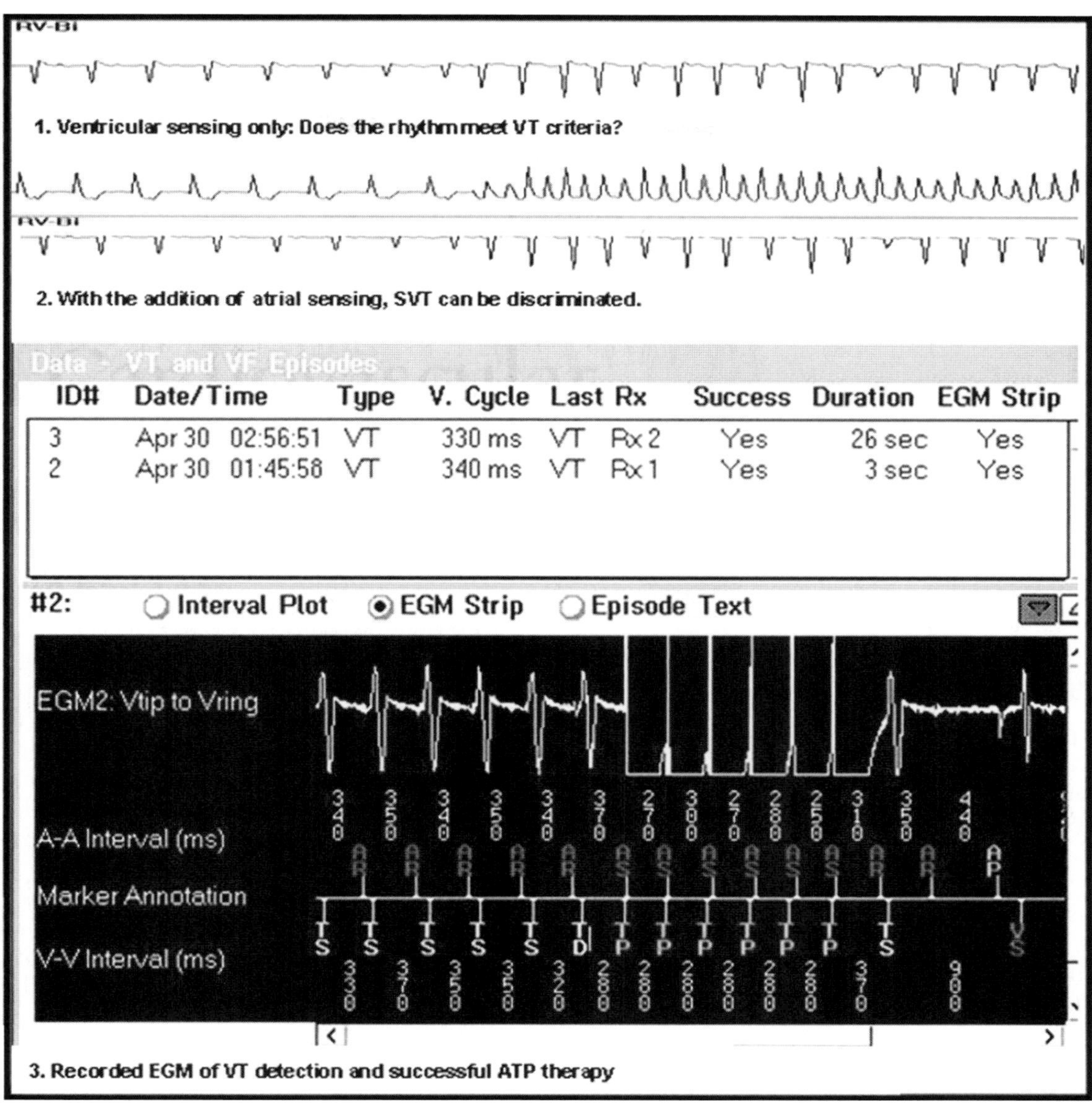


**Figure 51–5** ICD detection: dual-chamber discrimination and event report.

having VT that has now slowed below the detection criteria as a result of the addition of negative chronotropes and antiarrhythmic drugs. Rather than simply change the slow VT zone and risk treating a stable sinus tachycardia, a monitor zone can be applied to record events occurring in the 480- to 401-millisecond zone so that at follow-up, the physician can identify slow VT occurring below the detection zone and adjust the "slow VT zone" parameters accordingly.

Another patient with a similar profile but no history of arrhythmia may have a single-chamber device implanted for primary prevention. In this case, the physician programming the device may simply try to protect the patient from any arrhythmia reasonably anticipated to be inappropriately fast and hemodynamically unstable, and set a single zone below 320 milliseconds with six maximum output shocks.

### Therapies—ATP

Antitachycardia pacing as described previously is typically programmed to be administered in a burst of constant cycle length impulses or as a "ramp" of decreasing cycle length impulses. Typically, the device is programmed to initial ATP at a cycle length of 80% to 85% of the arrhythmia cycle length. To date no benefit has been demonstrated of "ramp" ATP over static cycle length ATP, and both achieve termination of VT in up to 90% of attempts. Typical bursts are 8 to 12 impulses, with reapplication of detection criteria after the burst to redetect persistent arrhythmias. Posttherapy criteria are often less stringent than initial detection criteria so as to shorten time to redetection and retreatment of persistent arrhythmias. The programmer decides the number of attempts at ATP prior to reverting to a cardioversion strategy, but typically several attempts at ATP are made before administering shocks in an initial program. Rates of acceleration of VT are low, in the 1% to 3% range, but are quite variable among patients, among cycle lengths, and among morphologies of tachycardias within a single patient.

Therapies—Cardioversion and Defibrillation

Low-energy synchronized cardioversion may be programmed for detected VT with outputs typically between 5 and 20 J. These synchronized therapies are preferred because they are effective, have shorter charge times, are less likely to cause VF via an R-on-T mechanism, thus preventing some syncopal events. If the ATP or low-energy shocks are unsuccessful or accelerate the rhythm to VF, then the device delivers high-energy synchronized shocks. Devices can be programmed to deliver five or six distinct therapies in sequence, each often more aggressive than the previous therapy. Therapies delivered at or above the DFT have a high probability of converting the rhythm back to baseline, with repeat therapies sometimes necessary to convert successfully.

## Troubleshooting

### *High Defibrillation Thresholds*

Because delivered therapies convert the malignant rhythm as a probability function based on delivered energy in excess of the defibrillation threshold or DFT, it is important to estimate the DFT at the time of device implantation. Initial device therapies are typically programmed with a margin of safety above the estimated DFT to increase the chance of conversion with the first shock delivered. A variety of scenarios can lead to high DFTs, but they can be divided into device-related and patient-related categories.

Device-related causes of high DFTs may include inappropriate lead positioning at implantation or subsequent dislodgement of the lead. Loose header screw or lead failure/fracture may result in high-impedance failure of defibrillation. Inappropriate shocking vector, such as in the case of an active can system implanted in the right prepectoral pocket, may result in unacceptably high DFTs. In this case, a subcutaneous array on the left side or an azygous vein shocking coil could be implanted and the system reprogrammed to shock from RV to azygous or vice versa or from RV to subcutaneous array or vice versa. Waveform morphology, polarity, and tilt may also be reprogrammed if the device nominal setting leads to high DFTs.

Patient-related characteristics that may lead to higher DFTs include the use of drugs that may increase the defibrillation threshold, including Class I agents, nonselective beta-blockers, nondihydropyridine calcium antagonists, and especially amiodarone. Hypoxia and ischemia may both lead to refractory VF and failure of internal and even high-energy external shocks, so it is imperative that these clinical parameters be treated and optimized prior to elective DFT testing. A potential procedural complication, pneumothorax, may affect DFTs in active can configurations when air is interposed between the heart and the device. Recognition of this phenomenon is critical so that the situation is remedied prior to repositioning of leads or addition of extra coils or arrays. Finally, multiple prior attempts at defibrillation may raise DFTs during subsequent attempts within a brief period of time. Retesting hours to days after implantation may reveal lower DFTs than initially observed at implantation.

### *Evaluating Inappropriate Shocks*

The evaluation of an ICD shock begins with an appropriate history and physical examination focusing on the circumstances of the discharge in question and the integrity of the device implantation and the patient's cardiopulmonary status. The history should assess for antecedent anginal and presyncopal symptoms, dyspnea, nausea/vomiting/diarrhea, and other potential causes of electrolyte imbalances as well as external factors such as proximity to sources of electromagnetic interference (EMI). The physical examination should assess for decompensated heart failure, rate and regularity of rhythm, trauma to the device or the anatomic location of the leads (often beneath the clavicle).

Interrogation of the device is paramount, and evaluation of stored events and electrograms should reveal the nature of the episode during which the therapy was administered. If the therapy was appropriate, one should determine whether it was successful and assess potential reasons why subsequent therapies may have been required. If the therapy was inappropriate, a determination should be made as to whether it was in response to a conducted supraventricular arrhythmia, a far-field oversensing of myopotentials or atrial arrhythmias, or noise from lead fracture or failure.

### *Failure to Detect*

The most common cause of failure to detect ventricular arrhythmias is inappropriate programming of tachycardia zones and detection criteria. Very often a device is implanted and antiarrhythmic drug therapy is initiated at the same time. Subsequent symptomatic arrhythmias may occur at rates lower than observed prior to implantation and initiation of drug therapy, as a consequence of drug therapy. The resulting scenario is that of an implanted device blinded to the culprit arrhythmia because of the programmed tachycardia zone. Ventricular arrhythmias can therefore be slowed into a rate range where physiologically normal tachycardia may occur. An example might be an athlete with an ICD implanted for symptomatic Brugada syndrome. The patient could potentially have physiologic sinus tachycardia below the 400- to 380-millisecond range, but could also develop VT with a similar cycle length. Detection algorithms utilizing atrial channel activity would be imperative in discriminating malignant ventricular arrhythmias in this patient.

### *ICD Management during Surgical Procedures and MRI Scanning*

The ICD detection algorithms can be "spoofed" by high-frequency signals such as those delivered during electrocautery use intraoperatively. As a result, inappropriate therapies could be delivered by the device during a surgical procedure. Device detection can be turned off through the use of a device programmer or a magnet applied to the implant site, so long as telemetry monitoring and external defibrillation are available during the procedure.

MRI scanners can be a source of EMI in addition to inactivating device therapies while the patient is inside the scanner. In the past, this fact and the vulnerability of the devices to high-energy field magnets have precluded ICD patients from undergoing MRI scans. Further study is needed in this area to determine the appropriateness of this exclusion.

## SUMMARY OF IMPORTANT ISSUES FOR THE BOARD EXAMINATION

The issues discussed in this chapter are the technical aspects of pacemaker and defibrillator therapy. All of the issues discussed are important for patient care, but for the examination, the indications for pacemaker and defibrillator implantation and the supporting multicenter clinical trials are of primary importance. In addition, pacemaker electrocardiography, which depends on understanding the basic timing cycles and intervals, is likely to be both important to the cardiologist in practice as well as in test material. In a parallel way, evaluation of the appropriateness of defibrillator therapy, ATP and shock therapies, determining the presence or absence of a ventricular or supraventricular arrhythmia, lead dysfunction, and the appropriateness of the programmed parameters, as well as the effectiveness of the therapy, are central to patient care and for the examination. A list of essential facts is provided as bulleted points.

### Essential Facts

- Ohm's law: Voltage = current × resistance ($V = IR$).
- All pacemaker intervals are initiated and terminated by a sensed event (usually silent to the electrocardiogram) or by a pacemaker output (usually apparent on the electrocardiogram).
- Pacemakers make decisions on a beat-to-beat basis, on the basis of the current interval and not as a result of the heart rate. Therefore each beat and each interval must be analyzed separately.
- Conversion of intervals to rate equivalents or back are done as follows:

$$\text{Heart rate (beats/min)} = \frac{60{,}000}{\text{cycle length (ms)}}$$

$$\text{Cycle length (ms)} = \frac{60{,}000}{\text{heart rate (beats/min)}}$$

- Pacemaker magnets close the "reed switch." Closing the "reed switch" will almost always disable sensing for pacemakers and cause the pacemaker to function at a fixed rate regardless of the intrinsic rhythm.
- Pacemaker magnets, when placed over an ICD, will disable detection and therapy of tachyarrhythmias. This is most commonly only temporary, i.e., while the magnet is over the "reed switch." However, in some devices, depending on the programming of the device, it can turn off arrhythmia detection and therapy *until the device is reprogrammed*.

## BIBLIOGRAPHY

**Ellenbogen KA, Kay GN, Wilkoff BL.** *Clinical Cardiac Pacing and Defibrillation.* 2nd ed. Philadelphia: WB Saunders; 2000.

**Ellenbogen KA, Wood MA.** *Cardiac Pacing and ICDs.* 3rd ed. Blackwell Science; 2002.

**Gregoratos G, Abrams J, Epstein AE, et al.** ACC/AHA/NASPE 2002 guideline update for implantation of cardiac pacemakers and antiarrhythmia devices: summary article. A report of the American College of Cardiology/American Heart Association Task Force on Practice Guidelines (ACC/AHA/NASPE Committee to Update the 1998 Pacemaker Guidelines). *Circulation.* 2002;106: 2145–2161.

## QUESTIONS

1. The AV delay is 200 milliseconds and the time from a paced QRS to the next atrial paced event is 800 milliseconds. To what basic or lower rate has the pacemaker been programmed?

   a. 100 beats/min
   b. 90 beats/min
   c. 80 beats/min
   d. 70 beats/min
   e. 60 beats/min

Answer is e: The cycle length consists of the AV interval + VA interval. These two intervals added together and converted to a heart rate yield the lower rate or base rate programmed for this pacemaker patient.

200 ms + 800 ms = 1,000 ms = cycle length

Base heart rate = 60,000/1,000 ms = 60 beats/min

Note that the AV interval can be dynamically shortened (based on the sensor and or the atrial rate) and there can be a shortening of the AV interval if there is a sensed P wave instead of an atrial paced beat. In addition, the rate of the pacemaker can be increased with apparent increases in the base rate if the sensor detects a need to increase the paced rate.

**2.** A 20-year-old college student loses consciousness during math class. She has had an average of two syncopal spells a year for as long as she can remember. She has no warning before her spells, and she has dislocated her thumb and chipped a tooth in the past during similar spells. The patient's indication for a pacemaker is

a. Class I
b. Class II
c. Class III

Answer is b: Despite the controversy about the use of pacemakers for vasovagal (neurocardiogenic) syncope, it is appropriate to implant a pacemaker in this situation. The Vasovagal Syncope Pacemaker (VPS) study demonstrated a marked reduction in syncope in patients with at least six syncopal spells in their lifetime. Clearly, this patient has a history consistent with neurocardiogenic syncope with severe spells. The VPS study required a tilt study with relative bradycardia. There did not need to be asystole.

**3.** The sensed AV interval is 150 milliseconds and the PVARP (postventricular atrial refractory period) is 350 milliseconds. What is the most rapid atrial rate that the pacemaker can track 1:1?

a. 300 beats/min
b. 250 beats/min
c. 200 beats/min
d. 150 beats/min
e. 120 beats/min

Answer is e: The maximal rate at which a DDD pacemaker can track an atrial rhythm is limited by the shortest interval in which the atrium can be detected. By adding together the PV interval (the AV interval initiated by a P wave and terminated with a ventricular pacemaker output) and the PVARP (the time during which the atrium cannot sense another P wave after a ventricular sensed or paced event), the total refractory period can be calculated. That interval converted to a heart rate is the maximal rate at which the pacemaker can participate in producing a paced rhythm. Both the PV delay and the PVARP can vary on the basis of atrial rate and sensor rate, but in this example the intervals are fixed. Thus,

$$\text{AV interval} + \text{PVARP} = 150\text{ ms} + 350\text{ ms} = 500\text{ ms}$$

Converting this to heart rate, we see that the maximal paced rate = 60,000/500 milliseconds = 120 beats/min. To increase the upper tracking rate it would be necessary to shorten the sensed AV interval, the PVARP, or enable rate-adaptive shortening of these intervals.

**4.** A pacemaker-dependent 65-year-old woman says that her activity-sensing pacemaker programmed to the DDDR mode (unipolar) makes her heart race every time she sweeps the floor. Which of the following could remedy the patient's situation?

a. Increase the rate response slope.
b. Program the atrial channel to bipolar paced configuration.
c. Program the ventricular channel to bipolar sensed configuration.
d. Decrease the atrial sensitivity from 1 mV to 3 mV.
e. Decrease the ventricular sensitivity from 1 mV to 4 mV.

Answer is d: This woman is using her upper body, which has the potential to activate her activity sensor and to produce myopotentials from use of the pectoralis major muscle. Increasing the rate response slope will increase the heart rate increase related to her activity. Programming the atrium to bipolar paced configuration would not affect her heart rate but could help if her complaint was secondary to stimulation of the pectoral muscles. Programming the ventricle to bipolar sensed configuration would reduce the likelihood that the ventricular channel would detect myopotentials, because the muscle would no longer be within the antennae being sensed by the ventricle. Sensed events on the ventricular channel would inhibit ventricular output and could be responsible for syncope due to bradycardia. Decreasing the ventricular sensitivity would potentially decrease the likelihood that myopotentials would be sensed, but this would cause inhibition of the ventricular output and a decreased heart rate. Decreasing the atrial sensitivity from 1 mV to 3 mV will likely decrease the probability of sensing myopotentials on the atrial channel. These atrial sensed events would have been tracked to the ventricle and cause the patient to perceive a tachycardia rhythm.

**5.** The VVI pacemaker is programmed to a lower rate of 80 beats/min. There are PVCs and usually the heart rate is paced at 80 beats/min, but intermittently there are intervals between intrinsic R waves of 960 milliseconds. Which of the following could be the explanation for the electrocardiographic findings?

a. Paced bipolar impedance of 300 ohms
b. Hysteresis rate of 60 beats/min
c. Sleep rate of 55 beats/min
d. Paced unipolar impedance of 250 ohms
e. PVC response

Answer is b: The rate of 80 beats/min needs to be converted to an interval. Cycle length = 60,000/80 = 750 milliseconds. The interval of 960 is longer than the 750 (80 beats/min). Longer intervals than the lower rate (base rate) of the pacemaker suggest (a) inhibition, (b) failure of output by the pacemaker (lead or generator related), or (c) an algorithm that explains the particular circumstance. A paced bipolar impedance of 300 ohms is relatively low, but normal. If this represented a marked drop from previous measurements, then it is possible that there is a short within the pacing lead. The hysteresis rate of 60 beats/min translates to a sensed escape interval of 1,000 milliseconds. This could explain the ECG as long as the paced intervals between ventricular events were 750 milliseconds. If the ECG findings occurred only at night, then intervals of 960 milliseconds would be normal, but would not explain the other paced intervals at 750 milliseconds. A unipolar pacing impedance cannot be too low to work. This is low but does not explain the findings. PVC responses can extend the PVARP to avoid initiating a pacemaker-mediated tachycardia, but would not change the escape interval of the pacemaker.

# Syncope

52

***Fredrick J. Jaeger***

This chapter focuses on core material related to the evaluation of patients who present with syncope of unknown origin. It reviews the indications and contraindications for various salient procedures and diagnostic maneuvers to evaluate patients who present with syncope. Highlighted among these are head-up tilt table testing to provoke and confirm neurocardiogenic syncope and electrophysiologic testing to assess atrioventricular (AV) node and sinoatrial (SA) node dysfunction, and inducibility of supraventricular tachycardia (SVT) and ventricular tachycardia (VT), which could be responsible for recurrent syncope. It is critical, in this era of evidence-based medicine and quality outcomes, health maintenance organizations (HMOs), DRGs, and limitations of diagnostic testing availability, that a concise, logical, streamlined approach to the evaluation of patients with syncope be employed. Several useful algorithms can be found in the literature (Fig. 52–1) (1). Recently, it was proposed that emergency departments adopt a streamlined approach to syncope patients that will allow more efficient utilization of resources, identifying high-risk patients and avoiding unnecessary admissions for low-risk patients (2).

Syncope, defined as the transient loss of consciousness with complete reversibility without subsequent focal neurologic deficit, is a frequent clinical conundrum for cardiologists, internists, and electrophysiologists (3,4). The approach to the syncopal patient is comprised of several algorithms, the aggressiveness of which depend on the seriousness of the syncopal spells, and the presence or absence of structural heart disease. Although the most common etiology of all syncope from all causes and in all groups is probably benign vasovagal syncope, a syncopal event in a patient with significant coronary disease, prior myocardial infarction (MI), severe left ventricular (LV) dysfunction, congestive heart failure, or in the context of known complex ventricular arrhythmias may be malignant and a harbinger of subsequent sudden cardiac death.

## EPIDEMIOLOGY OF SYNCOPE

In the early 1980s it was recognized that syncope is a common reason for emergency room visits and admissions (5). Many of these patients were suspected to have either reflex or neurocardiogenic/vasovagal syncope, but testing was limited. Simultaneously, techniques of electrophysiologic testing were being developed, ambulatory monitoring was in its infancy, and tilt table tests were still a research tool. Then, as today, the workup for patients with unexplained syncope was extremely expensive. Even with recent constraints, DRGs, and so on, the evaluation of patients with syncope still has been estimated to be $1 billion annually. Although syncope for the most part was probably suspected to be due to underlying neurocardiogenic syncope, in the 1980s there was no good test or "gold standard" to determine which patients were susceptible or truly vasovagal. When the tilt table was introduced and recognized as a valuable electrophysiologic modality, it entered intense and extensive utilization. The late 1980s and early 1990s represent the probable zenith of its use. Between 1992 and 1994, tilt table procedures escalated from approximately 6,000 per year to 14,000 per year. Recent years have seen a downtrend in the number of tilt table tests being performed, particularly as our clinical acumen has become better at identifying patients who are experiencing vasovagal syncope. Patients with syncope and a normal heart virtually always have underlying vasovagal syncope, even despite a negative tilt table test. Given the constraints of limited reproducibility, specificity, and sensitivity, tilt table tests, although still frequently performed, are reserved for those patients who meet specific criteria of recurrent syncope, for which no ready explanation can be provided.

In general, determination of the underlying etiology for syncope is almost always largely presumptive. Rarely do spontaneous clinical events occur during cardiac or telemetric monitoring. The goal in the evaluation of syncope is

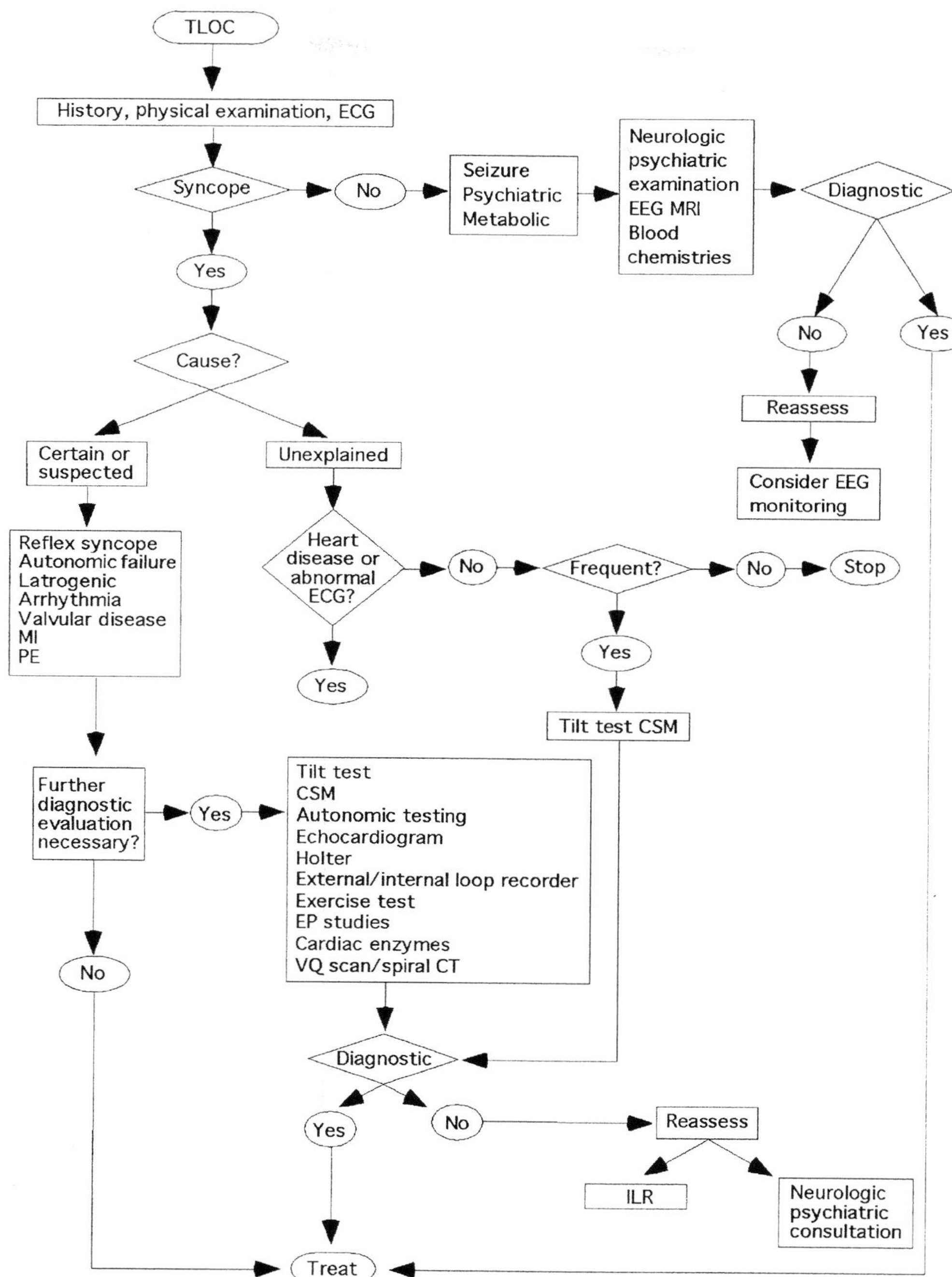


**Figure 52–1** Example of diagnostic algorithm for patients with loss of consciousness. TLOC, transient loss of consciousness; ECG, electrocardiogram; EEG, electroencephalogram; MRI, magnetic resonance imaging; MI, myocardial infarction; PE, pulmonary embolism; CSM, carotid sinus massage; EP studies, electrophysiologic studies; VQ scan, ventilation perfusion scan; CT, computed tomography; ILR, insertable loop recorder. (From: Kaufmann H, Wieling W. Syncope: a clinically guided diagnostic algorithm. *Clin Auton Res.* 2004;14:I/87–I/90.)

therefore not only to determine a likely underlying diagnosis with a relative degree of certainty and alacrity, but also to ensure that no life-threatening issues are responsible. Diagnostic studies such as head-up tilt table tests, electrophysiologic studies (EPS), and so on, are merely tools to examine various components of the autonomic nervous system and the cardiac electrical system, and the results must be interpreted with cautious skepticism. Although it is reassuring to convince oneself of a relatively benign type of syncope, as in vasovagal, it is axiomatic that the patient should always be assumed to have more malignant underlying causes of syncope until proven otherwise. Merely assuming that a positive tilt table test explains syncope in a patient with an ejection fraction (EF) of 25% from known coronary artery disease is clearly clinically inappropriate and fraught with danger. To further confound the differential diagnosis, many patients have syncope that is multifactorial. For example, an elderly patient with tendency toward sinus node dysfunction and carotid sinus hypersensitivity may also be on medications that result in hypovolemia and a tendency toward orthostatic hypotension. All can lead to syncope.

Syncope results from the many potential causes of cerebral hypoperfusion, and textbooks and review articles frequently display long, comprehensive lists of possible etiologies of syncope (Table 52–1) (6). In general, these lists can be synthesized and concentrated into five potential causes: (a) reflex syncope, of which vasovagal is the index hallmark and most common cause; (b) orthostatic hypotension; (c) arrhythmic syncope; (d) mechanical structural disease such as coronary artery obstructive and valvular cardiac disease; and (e) cerebrovascular causes. Using this framework and a precise definition of syncope differentiates it from other causes of loss of consciousness, including transient ischemic attacks (TIAs) and strokes, hypoglycemia and other metabolic causes, seizure disorders, psychogenic syncope, or vertebral basilar insufficiency (drop attacks). Traditionally, etiologies of syncope have also been even more broadly divided into cardiac and noncardiac causes. This simple paradigm has been utilized to predict clinical outcomes and prognosis. Cardiac causes of syncope may lead to increased mortality compared to noncardiac causes, in which the prognosis is normal and survival is assured (7). However, there is certainly considerable overlap between the cardiac and noncardiac causes. For example, it is now understood that aortic stenosis can cause syncope not only from heart block, or fixed cardiac output, but through reflex mechanisms similar to the Bezold–Jarisch reflex (8).

It is often difficult to differentiate an episode of true syncope from other causes of loss of consciousness. These include seizure disorders or epilepsy, metabolic abnormalities, cerebral vascular accidents (CVAs) or TIAs, and factitious syncope/pseudo-seizures or conversion reactions. The prototypical tonic-clonic movements of epilepsy are well known. Aura, urinary incontinence, and tongue biting are also frequently reported during seizures. Prior head trauma and concussion also may suggest seizures as the cause of loss of consciousness. Syncope is frequently accompanied by a few involuntary movements of the head and extremities, which can mimic a seizure disorder. This has been termed "convulsive syncope" and "anoxic seizures" and results from loss of oxygen to the central nervous system (CNS) and brainstem motor centers, and does not reflect an epileptiform phenomenon. These jerking movements are also frequently observed during ventricular fibrillation induced during electrophysiologic testing or during tilt-induced profound vasovagal episodes. Witnesses to clinical episodes of syncope also frequently report similar movements and ascribe them to seizures. Even trained medical personnel may be quick to assume, incorrectly, that seizures are occurring in these situations.

**TABLE 52–1**
**CAUSES OF SYNCOPE**

Neurally mediated (reflex)
Vasovagal syncope (common faint)
- Classical
- Nonclassical

Carotid sinus syncope
Situational syncope
- Acute hemorrhage
- Cough, sneeze
- Gastrointestinal stimulation (swallow, defecation, visceral pain)
- Micturition (postmicturition)
- Postexercise
- Postprandial
- Other (e.g., brass instrument playing, weightlifting)

Glossopharyngeal neuralgia
Orthostatic hypotension
Autonomic failure
- Primary autonomic failure syndromes (e.g., pure autonomic failure, multiple-system atrophy, Parkinson's disease with autonomic failure)
- Secondary autonomic failure syndromes (e.g., diabetic neuropathy, amyloid neuropathy)

Postexercise
Postprandial
Drug (and alcohol)-induced orthostatic syncope
Volume depletion
- Hemorrhage, diarrhea, Addison disease

Cardiac arrhythmias as primary cause
Sinus node dysfunction (including bradycardia/tachycardia syndrome)
Atrioventricular conduction system disease
Paroxysmal supraventricular and ventricular tachycardias
Inherited syndromes (e.g., long-QT syndrome, Brugada syndrome)
Implanted device (pacemaker, implantable cardioverter-defibrillator) malfunction
Drug-induced proarrhythmias
Structural cardiac or cardiopulmonary disease
Cardiac valvular disease
Acute myocardial infarction/ischemia
Obstructive cardiomyopathy
Atrial myxoma
Acute aortic dissection
Pericardial disease/tamponade
Pulmonary embolus/pulmonary hypertension
Cerebrovascular
Vascular steal syndromes

*Source:* From Brignole M, Lavagna I, Paolo A, et al. Guidelines on management (diagnosis and treatment) of syncope—update 2004. *Eurospace.* 2004;6:467–537.

## HISTORY

When a patient presents with syncope of unknown origin, the single most important piece of information is the history. Specific detailed questioning regarding the presence or absence of structural heart disease, valvular heart disease, coronary artery disease, previous myocardial infarctions, prior syncope (9), family history, and so on, can quickly delineate the high-risk patient from those at low risk. Historical factors related to a syncopal event can also help point in a specific direction. Situational syncope during phlebotomy, during prolonged standing, in a dentist's office, in a restaurant, in church, following alcohol ingestion, and so on, are almost universally vasovagal or neurocardiogenic. The presence of prodromal symptoms, such as nausea or diaphoresis, usually also heralds the onset of the vasovagal reflex. Frequently, the patient with vasovagal syncope may have postsyncopal symptoms that can last from hours to a day or so, including weakness, nausea, fatigue, and a tendency to recurrent syncope.

In contrast, a lack of prodrome or presence of previous myocardial infarction or heart failure certainly points to more malignant etiology of syncope, usually mandating hospital admission. Complete and immediate recovery after a syncopal event suggests an arrhythmic etiology, such as VT, SVT, or AV block. Injuries are uncommon with vasovagal syncope, as the patient usually tends to crumble to the ground, rather than fall abruptly. In contrast, severe injuries and automobile accidents are suggestive of a more serious arrhythmic etiology such as extreme tachycardia or bradycardia.

Calkins et al. have retrospectively evaluated the value of the history and the differentiation of patients with recurring syncope (10). Eighty patients with recurrent syncope undergoing a comprehensive evaluation were given comprehensive questionnaires focusing on the features of their syncopal spells. Patients underwent extensive electrophysiologic testing, tilt table testing, and ambulatory recording when appropriate, with the diagnosis confirmed in these 80 patients. The origin of syncope was broadly broken down into two varieties: relatively benign syncope due to vasovagal or neurocardiogenic etiology versus a more serious type of syncope due to underlying AV block or ventricular tachycardia. As expected, symptoms prior to the onset of syncope, such as blurred vision, palpitations, nausea, and generalized warmth or diaphoresis, were more consistent with neurocardiogenic syncope. Similar symptoms after the syncopal event were also more consistent with neurocardiogenic syncope. In contrast, little or no warning prior to the syncopal event was more consistent with AV block or ventricular tachycardia. Patients with AV block or VT tended to be older and of male gender, owing to the predominance of atherosclerotic disease. In addition, patients with more dangerous syncope etiologies generally reported no prior episodes, specifically having less than two episodes of syncope in their lifetime. These features, together with a history, can help determine whether a patient requires admission for further investigation.

## CLINICAL FEATURES OF SYNCOPE

Often, witnesses to the syncopal event can provide other clues as to the possible cause, particularly regarding the duration of syncope. Prolonged episodes of unresponsiveness, such as 7 to 10 minutes or more, are unlikely to be due to vasovagal or arrhythmic etiologies and instead suggest neurologic processes. Sudden loss of consciousness followed by fairly quick resumption of consciousness suggests tachyarrhythmias, such as VT, SVT, or atrial fibrillation with a postconversion pause. Patients who experience vasovagal syncope frequently have several minutes of prodromal symptoms, followed by loss of consciousness. The episode of unconsciousness with vasovagal syncope varies but may last 3 to 4 minutes, particularly if the patient cannot be rendered supine. A patient with vasovagal syncope may arouse slowly, with considerable confusion and postsyncopal vagal symptoms.

## PHYSICAL EXAMINATION

The physical examination of patients with syncope is generally directed toward cardiac auscultation for the presence of valvular disease, carotid bruits, pulses, irregular pulse and rhythm from atrial fibrillation, and so on. For patients with vasovagal syncope, the physical exam and the cardiovascular exam will generally be entirely normal. However, the presence of murmurs, S3 or S4 gallops, and displaced point of maximal intensity (PMI) may point to the presence of LV dysfunction. Similarly bigeminal rhythms, trigeminy, may also suggest the presence of LV dysfunction in a patient with syncope. Findings of congestive heart failure, jugular venous distention, heptojugular reflux, heptosplenomegaly, and bibasilar pulmonary rales also point to the presence of LV dysfunction in a patient with syncope. The finding of atrial fibrillation on physical examination or during electrocardiography (ECG) is very important and suggests tachybrady syndrome or sick sinus syndrome. Gross neurologic evaluation showing evidence of lateralization or focal neurologic deficits is also important, suggesting either cardioembolic phenomena from atrial fibrillation or carotid atherosclerotic disease, both of which can cause episodic loss of consciousness.

Carotid sinus massage can be performed safely at the bedside, but is contraindicated in the presence of carotid bruits, known carotid stenosis, TIAs, and CVAs. During ECG monitoring, sequential bilateral gentle carotid massage can be performed for 5 to 10 seconds, with the patient in a supine, slightly elevated head position. Positive responses consist of cardioinhibitory responses of pauses >3 seconds. Patients with true carotid sinus syndrome frequently show an instantaneous and abrupt response with a prolonged cardioinhibitory response to massage with loss of consciousness (LOC).

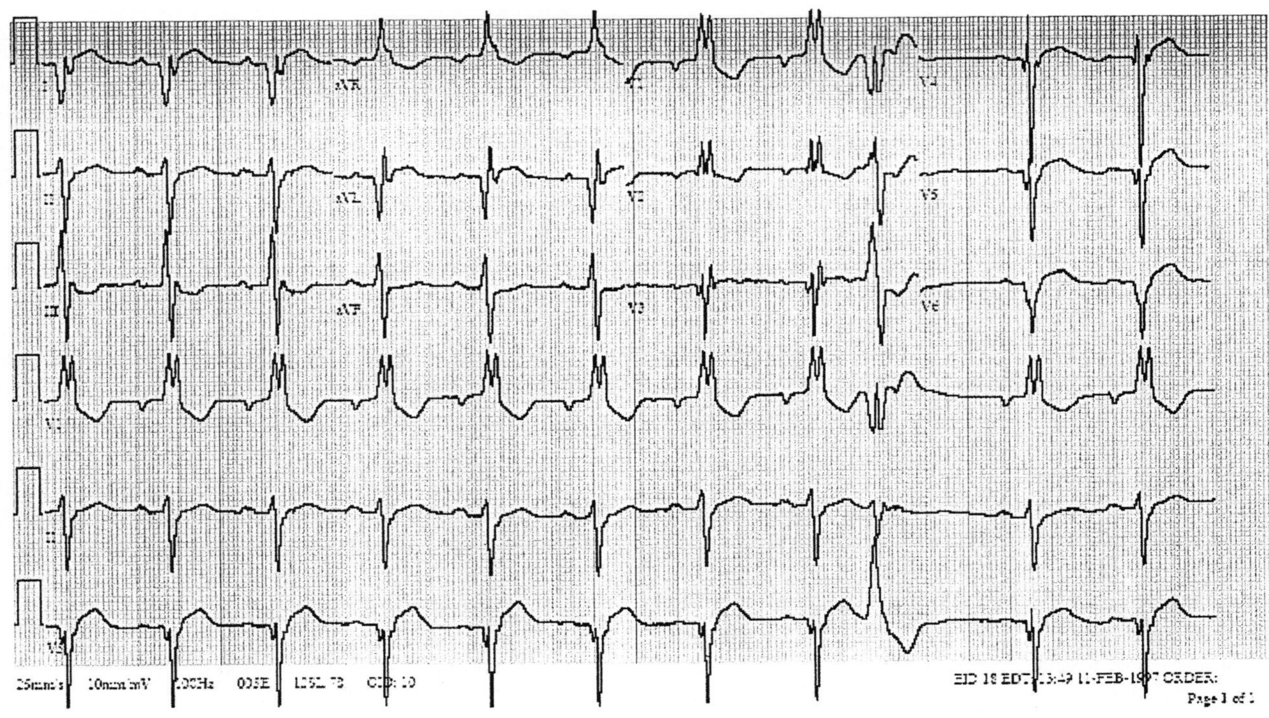

**Figure 52–2** Complete right bundle branch block, left anterior hemiblock, and first-degree AV block, so-called trifasicular block. This finding in patients with syncope suggests intermittent high-degree AV block and may indicate a need for a permanent pacemaker.

Careful observations of postural responses of blood pressure and heart rate are often useful when evaluating patients with syncope. The presence of marked orthostatic hypotension (OH) in patients with syncope is highly suggestive. Orthostatic hypotension is defined as a systolic blood pressure decline of >20 to 30 mm Hg or a diastolic blood pressure decline of >10 mm Hg. These can be elicited either immediately on assuming an upright posture from supine baseline or can occur more gradually at 1 to 3 minutes. Orthostatic hypotension is very common, particularly in the elderly, and may be multifactorial, often resulting from medications (diuretics, vasodilators, etc.) and intrinsic dysfunction of autonomic reflexes that can occur with aging, strokes, diabetes, alcohol use, and atherosclerosis of cardiopulmonary, aortic arch, and carotid sinus baroreceptors. Marked abrupt or instantaneous OH is particularly prominent in multisystem atrophy (MSA, previously called Shy–Dragger syndrome) or in pure or primary autonomic failure (PAF, previously called Bradbury–Eggleston syndrome). Patients with MSA may exhibit features of Parkinsons disease (PD), but PD itself is an important etiology for OH as well, either from intrinsic autonomic failure or from antiparkinson medications (11). Patients with PD often experience unexplained falls, which may result from OH, gait disturbances, or "on–off" phenomena.

## DIAGNOSTIC TESTING FOR SYNCOPE

Laboratory investigation for syncope of undetermined etiology begins with an ECG to identify arrhythmias or previous myocardial infarctions. The presence of Q waves indicative of previous MI, long QT interval, left bundle branch block, ventricular pre-exitation, or left anterior hemiblock are all significant and may suggest the need for further invasive investigation. Syncope in a patient with trifascicular block (Fig. 52–2) is a Class 2A indication for implantation of a permanent pacemaker (12,13). Signal-averaged ECG, although once touted as a major advancement in diagnostic capability for syncope, is now reserved largely for the detection of late potentials, predominantly in patients with transient ventricular ectopy, which may signify underlying arrhythmogenic right ventricular dysplasia (ARVD). Unfortunately, most of these patients have an intrinsic QRS abnormality consistent with a right bundle branch block, which makes the signal-averaged ECG less specific.

### Stress Testing and Echocardiography

When clinically indicated, particularly with physical findings or an ECG suggesting the presence of structural heart disease, initial testing often includes functional studies to assess for an ischemic etiology. Echocardiography is useful to assess for mechanical or structural lesions, such as hypertrophic cardiomyopathy, aortic stenosis, occult LV systolic dysfunction, or in the case of ARVD or RV dysfunction. Routine incorporation of these modalities is costly and unnecessary in the vast majority of syncope cases, particularly when the clinical history, ECG, and physical examination are normal and suggest a benign cause.

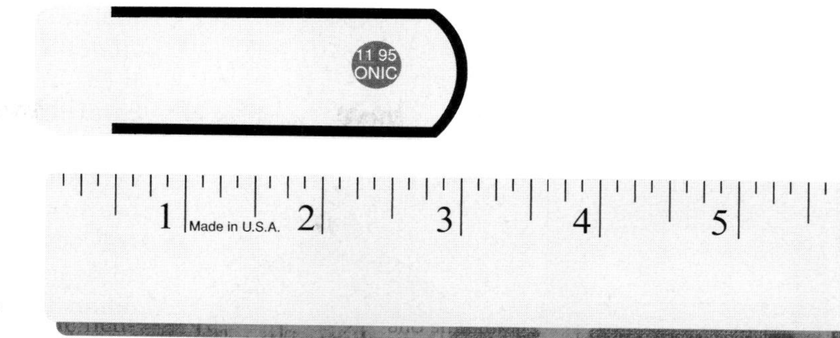


**Figure 52–3** Reveal (Medtronic) implantable loop recorder.

## Ambulatory Electrocardiographic Monitoring

Ambulatory electrocardiographic monitoring as a baseline may be helpful, particularly for those patients with recurrent syncopal episodes, and may disclose paroxysmal atrial fibrillation, SVT, or nonsustained ventricular tachycardia. Routine Holter monitoring in the absence of structural heart disease is frequently unrewarding. Newer systems utilizing event-recording technology, such as the King of Hearts (Instromedix) and others may be more helpful to disclose intermittent episodes of brady- or tachyarrhythmias. Ambulatory blood pressure monitor devices are also available and are frequently utilized for patients suspected of having intermittent orthostasis. However, these devices can be quite clumsy and burdensome, and often do not react quickly enough to record substantive data. Future ambulatory and implantable ECG event recorders currently in development may also allow simultaneous blood pressure recording.

## Reveal

The implantable loop recorder (Fig. 52–3) was designed specifically for patients with infrequent syncopal episodes in which Holter monitoring or 30-day event recordings fail to demonstrate the etiology of their syncope. The ideal patient is one who has recurrent syncope, palpitations, or suspected SVT once or twice a year, escaping conventional monitoring. Current indications are for patients with syncope of undetermined etiology with a structurally normal heart. It should not be implanted in high-risk patients with syncope and severe LV dysfunction. It has also been used in patients with fleeting or suspected SVTs for whom electrophysiologic testing is contemplated. An emerging indication is for patients who have drug-refractory seizures in whom an arrhythmic etiology from either tachy- or bradycardia is suspected.

Several studies have utilized the implantable loop recorder in their diagnostic algorithms to determine the cause of syncope. The RAST (Randomized Assessment of Syncope Trial) evaluated 60 patients randomized through either the conventional diagnostic paradigm of electrophysiologic testing, tilt table test, and extensive recording or accelerated loop recorder implants (14–16). Follow-up was for 1 year. Patients with loop recorder implants had an earlier time to diagnosis. The ISSUE investigators (International Study of Syncope of Undetermined Etiology) examined the use of the loop recorder implant in several important patient subgroups, including those with: (a) syncope and a normal heart who had a negative tilt table test; (b) syncope and a bundle branch block and a negative EPS; and (c) syncope with cardiomyopathy and a negative EPS. The first cohorts of the ISSUE study consisted of 82 patients with syncope and a negative tilt and 29 patients with syncope and a positive tilt (17). Both groups received implantable loop recorders. During follow-up, there was an approximate 34% syncope recurrence rate in both groups despite treatment. Interrogation of the implantable loop recorders showed that the underlying electrocardiographic abnormalities during syncope were consistent with a vasovagal etiology in the vast majority of patients. This suggested that in patients with a normal heart, syncope is still most likely due to underlying vasovagal phenomena, despite a negative tilt test. With this observation, as well as others on tilt test limitations, it has become apparent that the tilt table test may be superfluous in the evaluation of patients with syncope and a normal heart. The ISSUE study further went on to implant lopp recorders in patients who had bundle branch block, syncope, and a negative electrophysiologic test, including a challenge with Ajmaline (18). During follow-up, syncope recurred in >40% of patients, and the most common finding was AV block or asystole, although sinus arrest was also observed. Therefore, this supported the current practice of implanting pacemakers in patients with syncope, normal LV function, and bundle branch block, which is currently a Class IIA indication. Finally, the ISSUE investigators implanted loop recorders in patients with ischemic and dilated cardiomyopathies and syncope following a negative EPS (19). These patients usually now receive a defibrillator. A total of 35 patients were implanted with loop recorders following a negative EPS. During a relatively short follow-up of 6 ± 5 months, there was a 17% recurrence of syncope, predominately due to bradyarrhythmias. No VT was observed, although the follow-up was short. Therefore, it still would be prudent to consider implanting a

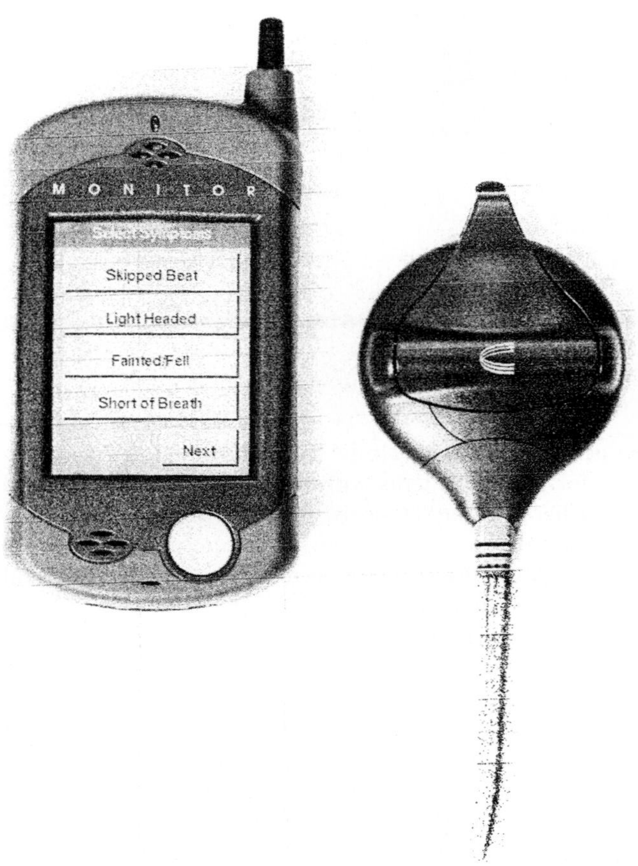


**Figure 52–4** Cardionet ambulatory arrhythmia monitor.

defibrillator in patients with severe LV dysfunction and syncope.

Currently, Medicare requires that in order to receive a loop recorder a patient have recurrent syncope, not presyncope; have at least 2 to 4 weeks of external event recording; have a tilt table test if appropriate; and electrophysiologic testing. Future studies may help support the incorporation of the implantable loop recorder in a more expedited fashion in those patients felt to be at low risk for significant ventricular arrhythmias.

Recently, a new wireless ambulatory monitoring system called the Cardionet has been introduced. The patient wears a wireless two-channel/lead ECG harness that transmits to a PDA (personal digital assistant)-size device that communicates constantly with a central monitoring center via the cellular telephone network (Fig. 52–4). The device utilizes arrhythmia detection algorithms to determine arrhythmia severity and are GPS (Global Positioning System) and altimeter capable. Feedback to the ordering physician can be immediate if certain "panic" arrhythmia criteria are met, as well as routine Internet strip transmission provided on a secure connection. Ideally, it is aimed at the low-risk patient, that is, one without structural heart disease in whom syncope or periodic palpitations are suspected to be benign arrhythmias such as sick sinus syndrome, SVT, or atrial fibrillation. It is also useful for detection of asymptomatic but clinically important arrhythmias such as atrial fibrillation. It has been helpful to detect such rhythms disturbances, particularly in patients who have had cryptogenic strokes.

No further investigations are probably required in a patient with historical absence of structural heart disease who has a normal ECG and a single episode of syncope that is typically vasovagal, However, if there are risk factors for coronary artery disease, such as a male aged >50 years, additional testing frequently includes assessment of LV function with an echocardiogram as well as an exercise test. In the absence of structural heart disease, for a single episode of syncope without malignant features, no other testing is typically required. However, if any of the above significant indicators of structural heart disease are present, then further investigation such as Holter monitoring and possibly EPS are warranted. The finding of nonsustained VT in the presence of LV dysfunction, and an EF <40%, especially in the setting of syncope, is indicative of the need for electrophysiologic testing and defibrillator implantation.

## Electrophysiologic Testing

For patients who present with syncope of undetermined etiology, electrophysiologic testing has been described as the "gold standard" for demonstration of supraventricular and ventricular arrhythmias, AV nodal or His–Purkinje disease, and bradyarrhythmias, all of which can be responsible for syncope. Indications for electrophysiologic testing in patients with syncope are given in Table 52–2 (20). This procedure, introduced clinically in the late 1970s, involves the insertion of several intravascular catheters to record intracardiac atrial electrograms, His potentials, and ventricular electrograms. Atrial and ventricular programmed electrical stimulation may induce sustained monomorphic VT or SVT. Measurement of AV node refractoriness and Wenckebach cycle length may demonstrate significant AV nodal

**TABLE 52–2**
**CLINICAL FEATURES SUGGESTING NEED FOR ELECTROPHYSIOLOGIC TESTING OF PATIENTS WITH SYNCOPE**

Prior myocardial infarction
Left ventricular dysfunction/cardiomyopathy
Wide-QRS complex/left or right bundle branch block
Systemic Illness
  Sarcoid
  Lyme
Prolonged P–R interval
"Complex" ventricular ectopy—nonsupraventricular tachycardia
Supraventricular tachycardia
Family history of sudden cardiac death
Electrocardiogram suggestive of Brugada syndrome
Suspected supraventricular tachycardia
Delta wave/Wolff–Parkinson–White syndrome

**TABLE 52–3**
**ELECTROPHYSIOLOGY STUDY—COMPONENTS**

Sinus node recovery time (SNRTS)
AV node function—effective refractory period, Wenckebach of AV node
His–Purkinje assessment—measurement of HV intervals
  Infra-His block—procainamide challenges
  Intra-His block
Inducibility of supraventricular tachycardia
Inducibility of ventricular tachycardia
Atrial fibrillation, postconversion pauses
Brugada syndrome—pharmacologic challenge with intravenous procainamide

disease that could be responsible for intermittent Mobitz type I, II, or high-degree AV block, particularly in elderly patients. Similarly, a prolonged His–ventricular (HV) interval suggests that syncope may be due to heart block. His–Purkinje conduction can be challenged by administration of IV procainamide with subsequent marked HV prolongation (21). In general, electrophysiologic testing is less helpful in the evaluation of the sinus node (Table 52–3). Occasionally, sinus node recovery times (SNRTS) can demonstrate prolonged pauses indicative of sinus node dysfunction. Attempted induction of sustained monomorphic ventricular tachycardia (SMVT) consists of programmed electrical stimulation of the right ventricle at two sites (RV apex and RV outflow tract), usually with sequential repetitive drive trains of 400 to 600 milliseconds followed by one, two, or three ventricular extra-stimuli. Other protocols attempt to induce SMVT by using more rapid repetitive bursts (300 to 350 milliseconds) in the ventricle. The finding of sustained monomorphic ventricular tachycardia is significant and suggests the need for an implantable cardioverter-defibrillator (ICD).

Almost every tachyarrhythmia is amenable to some form of radiofrequency catheter ablation. AV nodal re-entry, AV re-entry via accessory pathways, and atrial tachycardias are frequently mapped and ablated in a straightforward fashion. In previous decades, EPS was performed much more frequently for syncope evaluation than it is at present. Current clinical practice reserves EPS for a few select cases, such as patients with LV dysfunction, suspected SVTs, conduction abnormalities, and those who may be candidates for radiofrequency ablation. Rarely is EPS performed for syncope in patients with normal hearts and normal ECGs, given the likelihood of a vasovagal cause in this patient subset. Patients who present with syncope in the presence of LV dysfunction, a previous MI, or an EF <35% to 40% qualify for empiric ICDs given the MADIT 2 and SCD-Heft data (22). There are still several clinical situations in which EPS is performed to evaluate syncope patients (see Table 52–2). American College of Cardiology/American Heart Association (ACC/AHA) guidelines are listed in Table 52–4.

**TABLE 52–4**
**GUIDELINES FOR ELECTROPHYSIOLOGIC STUDIES FOR PATIENTS WITH SYNCOPE**

Class I: General agreement
  Patients with suspected structural heart disease and syncope that remains unexplained after appropriate evaluation
Class II: Less certain, but accepted
  Patients with recurrent unexplained syncope without structural heart disease and with a negative head-up tilt test
Class III: Not indicated
  Patients with a known cause of syncope for whom treatment will not be guided by electrophysiologic testing

*Source:* From Zipes DP, DiMarco JP, Gillette PC, et al. Guidelines for clinical intracardiac electrophysiological and catheter ablation procedures: a report of the American College of Cardiology/American Heart Association Task Force on Practice Guidelines (Committee on Clinical Intracardiac Electrophysiologic and Catheter Ablation Procedures), developed in collaboration with the North American Society of Pacing and Electrophysiology. *J Am Coll Cardiol.* 1995;26:555–573.

## SPECIFIC ETIOLOGIES OF SYNCOPE

### Neurally Mediated Syncope

Vasovagal syncope (also called neurocardiogenic syncope, empty heart syndrome, and ventricular syncope) is the most common of the neurally mediated syncopes. All of these syndromes result from disturbances or perturbations of the autonomic nervous system. A partial list of some of the more commonly observed neurally mediated syncopes is given in Table 52–5. Syncope arising from aortic stenosis or hypertrophic obstructive cardiomyopathy is felt to have a

**TABLE 52–5**
**NEURALLY MEDIATED SYNCOPE**

Vasovagal/neurocardiogenic syncope
Carotid sinus syncope
Tussive/cough syncope
Glossopharyngeal neuralgia/deglutition syncope (Elias)
Pallid breath-holding spells (Jaeger)
Aortic stenosis
Hypertrophic obstruction cardiomyopathy
Pacemaker syncope
Syncope secondary to pulmonary hypertension
Micturition syncope
"Mess trick"/fainting lark-self—induced hyperventilation and Valsalva syncope
Diving reflex—reflex bradycardia/vasoconstriction, especially in cold water, causing loss of consciousness
Syncope with atrial fibrillation, supraventricular tachycardia, and ventricular tachycardia—may have neurally mediated component resulting from atrial fibrillation vasodepressor reflexes

significant neurally mediated component and may precipitate the stimulation of C fibers in the posterior left ventricle in a fashion similar to vasovagal syncope (Bezold–Jarisch reflex) (8). In addition, it is suspected that in patients with syncope due to recurrent atrial fibrillation, SVT, or VT, there may also be a neurally mediated component in which atrial vasodepressor reflexes result in significant vasodepression, causing a drop in blood pressure and contributing to the loss of consciousness independent of a low cardiac output.

Symptoms preceding the vasovagal response are typical and can serve as clues to the nature of the syncopal spell. Vagal symptoms such as diaphoresis, nausea, vomiting, and diarrhea are common both before and after the syncopal spell. The patient may be observed to be very pale, and may complain of either being cold or excessively warm. Frequently, patients report presyncopal loss of vision, which may persist for a variable amount of time. This has been described as "graying out." Tinnitus or loss of hearing is frequently described as occurring prior to the syncopal event. Patients can be observed, both spontaneously and during head-up tilt table tests, to be hyperventilating and may complain of shortness of breath, representing an autonomic trigger reflex. The onset of yawning during a head-up tilt table test can often herald the onset of a vasovagal event. Sinus tachycardia associated with the episode may be perceived as palpitations and be confused with SVT, or may mimic a chest discomfort complaint.

During unconsciousness, patients may be observed to experience a generalized myoclonic jerking, the so-called anoxic seizure or convulsive syncope. This may mimic the features of epilepsy to both medical and nonmedical bystanders, and may complicate the differential diagnosis. When patients awaken, there may be a slight confusion, which can also mimic a postictal state. If patients try to ambulate too quickly, they may experience another episode of syncope.

The most common precipitant of vasovagal syncope is from so-called noxious stimuli, such as flight or fight, pain, venipuncture, fear, or anxiety. Other situations in which marked venous pooling or sequestration of blood volume in lower extremities or splanchnics takes place may also precipitate the vasovagal response. These include prolonged rigid standing, as in soldiers at attention; pregnancy, in which the gravid uterus prevents venous return from the inferior vena cava (IVC) compression; or from inadequate venous return, such as in hypovolemia, diuretic treatment, anemia, or acute hemorrhage. Prolonged bed rest, as in patients recovering from illness, can also lead to a propensity for vasovagal syncope. It has been known for several decades that astronauts returning from even brief exposure to microgravity are also predisposed to a vasovagal-type syndrome. The "first-dose phenomenon," such as occurs with certain vasodilators and nitrates, has also been shown to precipitate a vasovagal-type response, as does beta-blocker withdrawal (3).

The clinical scenario of typical vasovagal syncope begins with abrupt vasodepression, followed by a marked cardioinhibitory response. Similar to cardioinhibitory responses observed during carotid sinus hypersensitivity testing, cardioinhibitory responses can also occur during head-up tilt table testing. These include sinus pauses of 3.5 seconds or more, as well as junctional rhythm, marked sinus bradycardia, or also commonly AV block of the first-, second-, or even third-degree variety. Less commonly, vasodepressor syncope occurs in which an isolated drop in blood pressure accompanies the syndrome. Even during pure vasodepressor syncope and hypotension, the heart rate can be observed to be inappropriate for the degree of hypotension. Cardioinhibitory responses that accompany vasovagal syncope have also been called "extrinsic sick sinus syndrome" and are myriad. We have frequently observed prolonged episodes of asystole, incidentally recorded by monitoring. Asystolic events occurring during vasovagal syncope can also be observed during phlebotomy-provoked fainting. Reflex asystolic pauses are occasionally mistaken for intrinsic SA or AV node disease and may promulgate erroneous consideration and referral for a permanent pacemaker. However, reflex-mediated asystolic pauses are benign, with a favorable prognosis, and pacemaker implantation is not usually necessary (23). Other types of bradyarrhythmia can be observed both clinically during vasovagal syncope and during tilt table testing, including junctional bradycardia, marked sinus bradycardia, and first-, second-, or third-degree AV block. A unique form of atrial fibrillation can be initiated by or cause a vasovagal response. This form of atrial fibrillation is felt to be vagal in origin, resulting from marked parasympathetically mediated inhomogeneity of atrial refractoriness, leading to precipitation of atrial fibrillation. The heightened or augmented parasympathetic autonomic status can then trigger concomitant vasovagal fainting (3).

The natural history of recurrent vasovagal syncope is heterogenous, but some clinical observations merit specific mention. Vasovagal episodes tend to cluster. It is not uncommon for patients to have relative quiescence of their episodes of syncope, only to have episodes re-emerge with increasing frequency, particularly around times of major life stressors. Patients with previously recurrent vasovagal syncope may have no further episodes following an initial positive tilt table test. In this respect, demonstration of the underlying etiology provides reassurance to the patient of the relatively benign nature of the syncope and may have a therapeutic affect. The occurrence of frequent spontaneous resolution of vasovagal syncope, even in untreated patients, can make the evaluation of the efficacy of subsequent pharmacologic interventions spurious. Similarly, up to 75% of patients may have a negative tilt table test on subsequent tests performed months or years later, which makes obtaining reproducibility difficult. Natale et al. observed 54 patients with neurocardiogenic syncope who declined

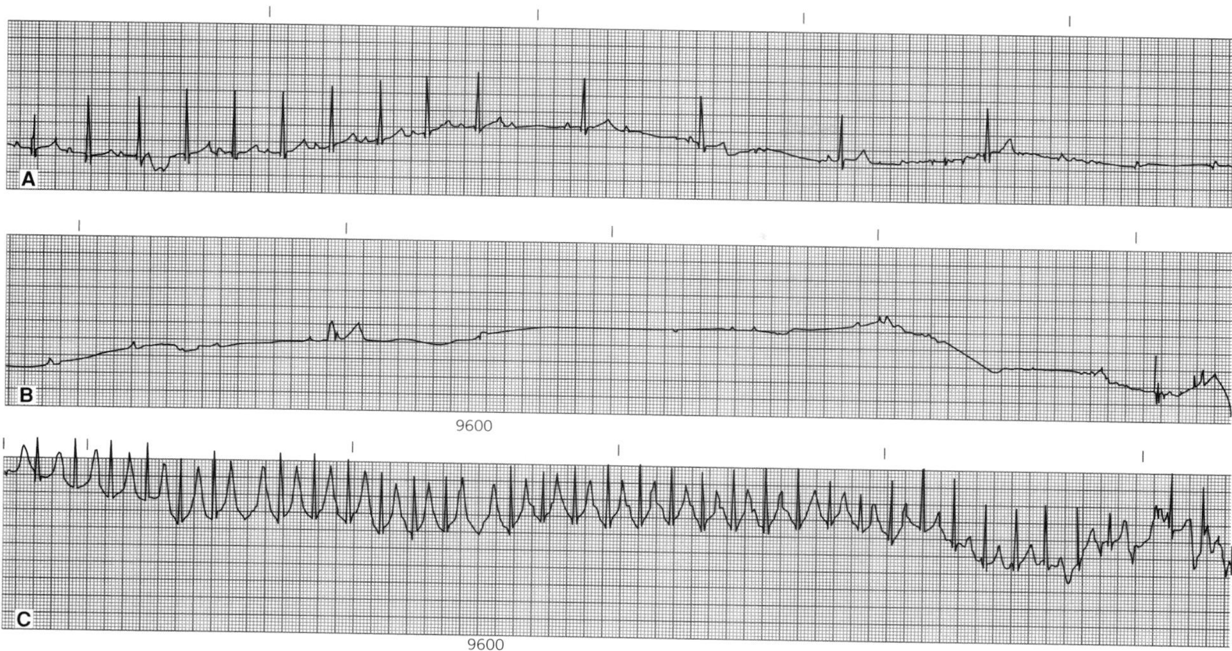


**Figure 52–5** Example of prolonged asystole and cardioinhibitory response during a vasovagal syncope provoked by tilt table testing.

treatment. During follow-up, nearly 70% of the patients had no further episodes (24).

The pathophysiology of vasovagal syncope historically has been attributed to the activation of C fibers in the posterior and inferior wall of the left ventricle during a vigorous contraction of a relatively empty ventricle (Bezold–Jarisch reflex) (8). This initiates a reflex-mediated sympathetic withdrawal, leaving the heightened parasympathetic activation relatively unopposed. Withdrawal of sympathetic activation causes peripheral arterial and arteriolar vasodilation and hypotension, and the parasympathetic predominance causes bradycardia (Fig. 52–5) (25). This concept has been challenged by the observation of a vasovagal-type response in cardiac transplant patients, who presumably would not have intact afferent and efferent innervations capable of propagating the vasovagal reflex (26). Alternative theories for vasovagal pathogenesis have been proposed, including various neurohumoral and neuroendocrine peptides, epinephrine, and the ubiquitous nitric oxide (27). There also appears to be a genetic predisposition to vasovagal susceptibility. Patients with fainting episodes frequently report that their parents or siblings also were fainters. As yet, no specific gene markers have been identified. A recent intriguing but highly conjectural proposal to explain genetic origins of the vasovagal repose was that during the times of humans as hunter-gatherer-warriors, the tendency to faint, especially during battles, may have have afforded a survival benefit by feigning death and avoiding mortal wounds. This has been called the "Paleolithic threat hypothesis" (28).

Vasovagal syncope can be divided into two categories: a relatively benign form in which patients have a recognized precipitating stimulus; and a more malignant variety in which there is no recognized stimulus but the patient may have prolonged asystole and severe injuries, with loss of driving privileges and employment (29). This latter variety is frequently found to have some underlying autonomic abnormalities or blood volume distribution abnormalities, such as hypovolemia or marked venous pooling. In many cases, no abnormalities can be found. Future advances in the understanding and treatment of vasovagal syncope will require a better delineation of the pathophysiology.

### *Head-Up Tilt Testing for Vasovagal Syncope*

The head-up tilt table test was initially devised in the mid-1980s as a research tool for the evaluation of postural reflexes. Subsequently, it was recognized as an important clinical tool to induce and provoke vasovagal syncope in susceptible individuals, thereby establishing a diagnosis. In the 1980s and early 1990s, extensive and divergent tilt table protocols were proposed for vasovagal syncope provocation, including protocols with 90-degree tilt for up to 90 minutes and those using tilt tables with saddle support. Some of these protocols were extremely effective at inducing the vasovagal response but possessed spurious specificity. Recently, several consensus panels have convened to standardize the nomenclature and head-up tilt protocol, which currently consists of at least 30 minutes of 70-degree tilt. Higher degrees of tilt (80 to 90 degrees) or more prolonged tilting durations may decrease specificity. Following an initial drug-free tilt test, intravenous administration of the $\beta$-agonist isoproterenol can increase the yield but may sacrifice specificity (30,31). An ACC expert panel document regarding tilt table testing for assessing syncope has established indications (30), including recurrent syncope that is thought to be vasovagal but has not been clearly demonstrated to be so. In general, the tilt table test is not utilized in patients with structural heart disease until other causes of syncope have been excluded. Tilt table testing may also be appropriate for patients with a single syncope spell, if they are felt to be high risk—that is, the syncope resulted in, for example, injury or an automobile accident, or for a patient with a high-risk occupation. Furthermore, tilt table testing may be helpful for patients who are demonstrated to have intermittent episodes of AV block, sinus bradycardia asystole, and in whom the intrinsic form of sick sinus syndrome could be present. Tilt table testing is probably not indicated for a patient with structural heart disease, a patient with a single episode of syncope with typical classic clinical features, or in whom other causes of syncope have been demonstrated. There are several specific indications for tilt table testing, including the differentiation of convulsive syncope or anoxic seizures from true epilepsy; in evaluating a patient with unexplained falls, faints, or injuries; to assess the impact of autonomic dysfunction or neuropathies; or to determine the presence of orthostatic hypotension. Although it has been speculated that tilt table testing may be helpful in assessing effects of therapy affect, it is not highly predictive.

In addition to these indications, our center frequently utilizes tilt table testing to assess for the presence of overt or covert orthostatic hypotension and to gauge response to therapy. Frequently, the orthostatic response is relatively latent and can only be observed after a prolonged period of upright posture. These nonvasovagal drops in blood pressure are often caused by medication, venous pooling, or autonomic insufficiency.

Proposed tilt table testing protocols include adjunctive pharmacologic challenges with edrophonium, adenosine (32), clomipramine, or sublingual nitroglycerin (The Italian Protocol) (6,33) to accelerate onset of vasovagal syncope.

### *Vasovagal Syncope—Pharmacologic Therapy*

The initial treatment for vasovagal syncope consists of reassurance, recognition and avoidance of precipitating factors, expansion of salt and fluid intake, and avoidance of sympathomimetics (cold remedies, caffeine, tobacco), dehydration, and alcohol. Patients can be instructed to recognize the premonitory symptoms of vasovagal faint plus a few techniques to avoid syncope, such as immediately assuming a supine position with elevated and moving legs to decrease venous return. During their prodromal phase, fainters are frequently incorrectly admonished by onlookers to "put their head between their legs" or "go outside to get some fresh air." Such actions universally result in syncope and are to be discouraged. Although it has not been rigorously tested, repetitive coughing has been observed to abort the faint, and recently a variety of leg crossing and arm movements have also been proposed (34). When episodes are recurrent and recalcitrant to these simple maneuvers, pharmacologic treatment is often required. Initial empiric therapy usually consists of beta-blockers, serotonin reuptake inhibitors, $\alpha$-agonists (Midodrine, ProAmatine) (35), anticholinergics, or volume expanders such as Florinef (Table 52–6) (36,37). Despite extensive observational reports on the efficacy of many medications for the prevention of vasovagal syncope, there are few randomized studies challenging their use (34). Emerging treatment modalities include tilt table training, in which the patient is taught a technique to perform several times daily that simulates the effects of tilt table testing. This approach has shown significant promise in initial reports and is thought to work by allowing postural reflexes to accommodate to the recurrent postural changes, thereby decreasing venous pooling and attenuating and downregulating certain cardiopulmonary baroreceptors, thus increasing the individual's resistance to vasovagal syncope (38). As mentioned, this simple exercise may be more effective than medications for vasovagal prophylaxis, but its use is limited by the substantial time commitment and required compliance.

**TABLE 52–6**
**VASOVAGAL SYNCOPE: PHARMACOLOGIC THERAPY**

Hydrofluorocortisone—mineralocorticoid
Beta-blockers
Disopyramide
Serotonin reuptake inhibitors—sertraline, fluoxetine, paroxetine
Anticholingerics—levsin, transdermal scopolamine
Theophylline—adenosine receptor blockade
Amphetamines
$\alpha$-Agonists—phenylephrine, pseudoephedrine, midodrine
Calcium channel blockers
Epogen, DDAVP—(Grubb)

### *Beta-Blockers for Vasovagal Syncope*

Beta-blockers have long been the mainstay of initial pharmacologic therapy for patients with recurrent vasovagal syncope. Only recently has beta-blockade been subjected to the rigors of clinical trials. In fact, several trials have not shown any significant improvement in nature of syncope or frequency of syncope in patients treated with beta-blockers compared to placebo (34). Nevertheless, beta-blockers are frequently prescribed, particularly when the patient has sinus tachycardia or postural orthostatic tachycardia syndrome (POTS) preceding the vasovagal response as observed on a tilt table test. The mechanism of action is linked to the drugs' negative inotropic and chronotropic properties, which decrease LV contraction, avoid mechanoreceptor C-fiber activation, and inhibit the precipitation of

Bezold–Jarisch reflex. They may also help to partially offset reflex-mediated vasodepression by leaving ambient $\alpha$-receptor–mediated vasoconstriction unopposed. It has also been suggested that beta-blockers may have a CNS effect, working by central serotonin-blocking activity. There has been increased concern about the utilization of beta-blockers in that they may transform relatively benign vasovagal episodes into more malignant occurrences by suppressing intrinsic escape cardiac pacemaker activity and inhibiting automaticity.

### *Treatment of Vasovagal Syncope*

Based on the results of a few additional diagnostic tests performed at our facility, we are also able to further guide pharmacologic therapy. We frequently perform blood volume determination using a radioiodine technique, thereby assessing the autonomic reflexes and the degree of venous pooling. If patients are found to have significant hypovolemia from the blood volume determination, then therapy starts with a high-salt diet and Florinef. If the hemodynamic reflexes reveal a hyperkinetic circulation, as seen in POTS, then beta-blockade is the preferred initial therapy. If there is failure of vasoconstriction during upright posture, then vasoconstricting $\alpha$-agonist medications (midodrine) are initial therapy. Marked venous pooling is frequently found, especially in sedentary patients, and support stocking therapy as well as physical exercise and reconditioning of leg muscles are prescribed. Finally, young patients are frequently "hypervagal," and power spectrum analysis can show a predominance of the vagal component, suggesting some benefit with anticholinergic therapy. Often, severe cases have been found to have multiple abnormalities and to require multiple drug therapy.

### *Pacemakers for Vasovagal Syncope*

For patients with recurrent episodes of syncope that are refractory to pharmacologic therapy, for those who have high-risk occupations, or for those who experience prolonged asystole on head-up tilt table tests, the implantation of a permanent pacemaker with rate-drop algorithms has been a long-time but controversial option (39). Evidence for the efficacy of pacing for vasovagal syncope came from large retrospective studies in small, nonrandomized cohorts. In the early to mid-1990s, several studies were proposed to examine this potential therapeutic modality. It was recognized that although cardioinhibitory components of the vasovagal response were frequently observed, they occurred later in the response, only after very profound hypotension had occurred. Therefore, pacing only when the heart rate was low was superfluous and probably already too late to abort or prevent the faint. Several proposed pacemaker designs were evaluated in the hopes that earlier detection would help ameliorate the fainting process. One was designed to tachypace at high rates (>90 to 100 beats/min) when it detected a rapidly falling heart rate. It was hoped that rapid pacing would bolster or preserve cardiac output and maintain consciousness. The multicenter VPS trial randomized patients with vasovagal syncope to a permanent pacemaker with rate-drop technology or to conventional (i.e., pharmacologic) therapy (40). The results demonstrated a dramatic reduction in syncopal recurrences in the pacemaker group. For a brief time after the publication of this trial, pacemakers became a more prevalent component of vasovagal syncope therapy. However, the VPS2 trial, in which patients were randomized to backup pacing only versus pacemakers with rate drop actively programmed, failed to show any benefit from the rate-drop capability and again relegated pacemaker implantation for vasovagal syncope to a relatively last resort in highly selected patients (3,40,41).

Therefore, given the high rate of spontaneous resolution in the long term, patients can be reassured as to the general eventual favorable prognosis with vasovagal syncope. Pharmacologic therapy is therefore provided as a temporary or short-term solution. Despite the considerable efforts of aggressive pharmacologic therapy and pacemakers, up to 20% to 30% of patients continue to experience recurrent syncope due to vasovagal phenomena.

## Postural Orthostatic Tachycardia Syndrome (POTS)

Postural orthostatic tachycardia syndrome is an emerging but poorly understood syndrome. Patients present with the perception of exaggerated heart rate responses to tilt and exercise, with palpitations, light-headedness, and syncope. This syndrome is different from the inappropriate sinus tachycardia syndrome (14), which may result from intrinsic sinus node hypersensitivity or ectopic atrial tachyarrhythmias. In addition to heart rate responses, patients may have multisystem complaints, including chronic fatigue-type syndrome (42), fibromyalgia, cognitive dysfunctions, sleep disorders, gastrointestinal and gastrourinary abnormalities suggesting a form, albeit mild, of autonomic dysfunction. This syndrome may overlap such historical syndromes as mitral valve prolapse syndrome, the hyper-$\beta$-adrenergic circulatory state, hyperkinetic heart syndrome, soldier's heart, DeCosta syndrome, and neurocirculatory asthenia. They do have a vasovagal susceptibility, particularly on tilt table testing, although syncope frequently occurs during extreme sinus tachycardia without demonstrable cardioinhibitory responses. Therefore these patients appear to experience a more unusual form of vasodepressor syncope, particularly on a tilt table test. Several distinct varieties of POTS due to various underlying etiologies exist, and there are probably heterogeneous cases due to multiple causes, such as mild autonomic dysfunction, hypovolemia, excessive venous pooling, catecholamine hypersensitivity, norepinephrine transporter deficiency, and many other causes (11). Treatment can be very difficult and challenging, relying on volume expanders and beta-blockers or calcium channel blockers, selective serotonin reuptake inhibitors (SSRIs), and a host of relatively investigational and off-label medications (11).

## Carotid Sinus Syndrome

Although it is not as common as recurrent vasovagal syncope, carotid sinus syndrome accounts for a significant proportion of syncopal events, particularly in elderly patients. Carotid sinus syndrome results when an overactive or hypersensitive carotid reflex precipitates sudden bradycardia, pauses, or asystole, frequently with a vasodepressor reflex. Episodes may be precipitated by maneuvers that activate the carotid sinus reflex. Often gentle or mild pressure can elicit this exquisitely sensitive reflex. Activities such as tying a necktie, a tight collar, head turning, and forced exhalation as in playing an instrument may precipitate the reflex. Carotid sinus hypersensitivity is common, considering the definition of a 3-second or longer pause with carotid sinus massage. This reflex is particularly common in patients with coronary artery disease and may reflect the extent of coronary atherosclerosis. Carotid sinus syndrome is defined by clinically recurring episodes of syncope confirmed secondary to carotid sinus hypersensitivity. It has been suggested that alterations in the carotid baroreceptors are responsible for the syndrome and reflex. Recent work has focused on alterations in the mechanoreceptors and proprioceptive receptors in the surrounding denervated sternocleidomastoid muscles (43). Treatment for the majority of cases of carotid sinus syndrome, particularly when accompanied by the typical cardioinhibitory responses, is comprised of a DDD permanent pacemaker. The accompanying vasodepressor reflex frequently requires the addition of a high-salt diets and volume expander plus the elimination of potential offending medications such as diuretics.

## Neurally Mediated Syncope Syndromes

Less common examples of neurally mediated syncope involve various situations with diverse autonomic nervous system inputs. Tussive or cough syncope can be seen in chronic obstructive pulmonary disease (COPD) patients and may occur during violent paroxysms of coughing. This may result from decreased cardiac output from markedly increased intrathoracic pressure or a Valsalva-type precipitation of bradycardia or heart block. There may also be marked turbulence of cerebral vascular blood flow and intracranial pressure during these severe cough episodes. Deglutition syncope, glossopharyngeal neuralgia (44), micturition, and defecation syncope are also reflex syncope episodes that presumably initiate a bradycardic and vasodepressor response. Pacemaker syndrome, which was more frequently observed during the previous decades of VVI pacing, results from atrial vasodepressor reflexes precipitated during retrograde conduction from ventricular pacing with subsequent atrial activation on a closed AV valve, causing canon A waves. These vigorous atrial systoles cause transient hypotension, which may result in syncope. As mentioned previously, aortic stenosis and hypertrophic cardiomyopathy may cause syncope through a fixed cardiac output but may also precipitate the Bezold–Jarisch reflex in a manner similar to a vasovagal cause. Pallid breath-holding spells are unique episodes of syncope, which occur in very young children following a minor injury or startle, after which they hold their breath, becoming pale and faint (45,46). This is probably an infant or pediatric form of vasovagal syncope.

## Orthostatic Hypotension in the Elderly

The elderly can be particularly susceptible to marked fluctuations in systemic blood pressure. They are frequently sedentary, leading to attenuation of their postural reflexes. They may demonstrate supine systolic hypertension and hypotension when upright. Patients may frequently experience marked drops in blood pressure, particularly postprandially, with blood volume sequestration in the splanchnics and abdomen.

## Arrhythmias as a Cause of Syncope

Virtually any tachy- or bradyarrhythmia can cause symptomatic light-headedness, hypotension, and syncope. This is particularly true in the setting of significant LV dysfunction. Sustained monomorphic or polymorphic ventricular tachycardia in the presence of severe LV dysfunction is an ominous cause of syncope and can quickly progress to lethal ventricular fibrillation. Ventricular tachycardia in a normal heart is an unusual cause of syncope, although it is now understood that syncope can result from normal heart VT as well as SVT via the recruitment of vasodepressor-type reflexes akin to vasovagal responses. Sick sinus syndrome, paroxysmal atrial fibrillation with significant postconversion causes, as well as Mobitz type II and complete heart block are also important causes of syncope. Electrophysiologic testing (see section on electrophysiologic testing) and ambulatory monitors are important tools to obtain symptom–syncope correlation. Based on the results of the Madit II, SCD Heft, and Definite trials, patients with depressed LV function from any cause, that is, EF <35%, should receive implantable cardioverter-defibrillators for primary prevention. A patient presenting with syncope who meets these criteria should be presumed to have had ventricular tachycardia as the cause and should receive an ICD in an expedited fashion.

## Long-QT Syndrome (LQTS)

The long-QT syndrome is a genetically transmitted disorder of cardiac ion channels, which results in intermittent or persistent prolongation of the QT interval, predisposing to a specific type of ventricular tachyarrhythmia called

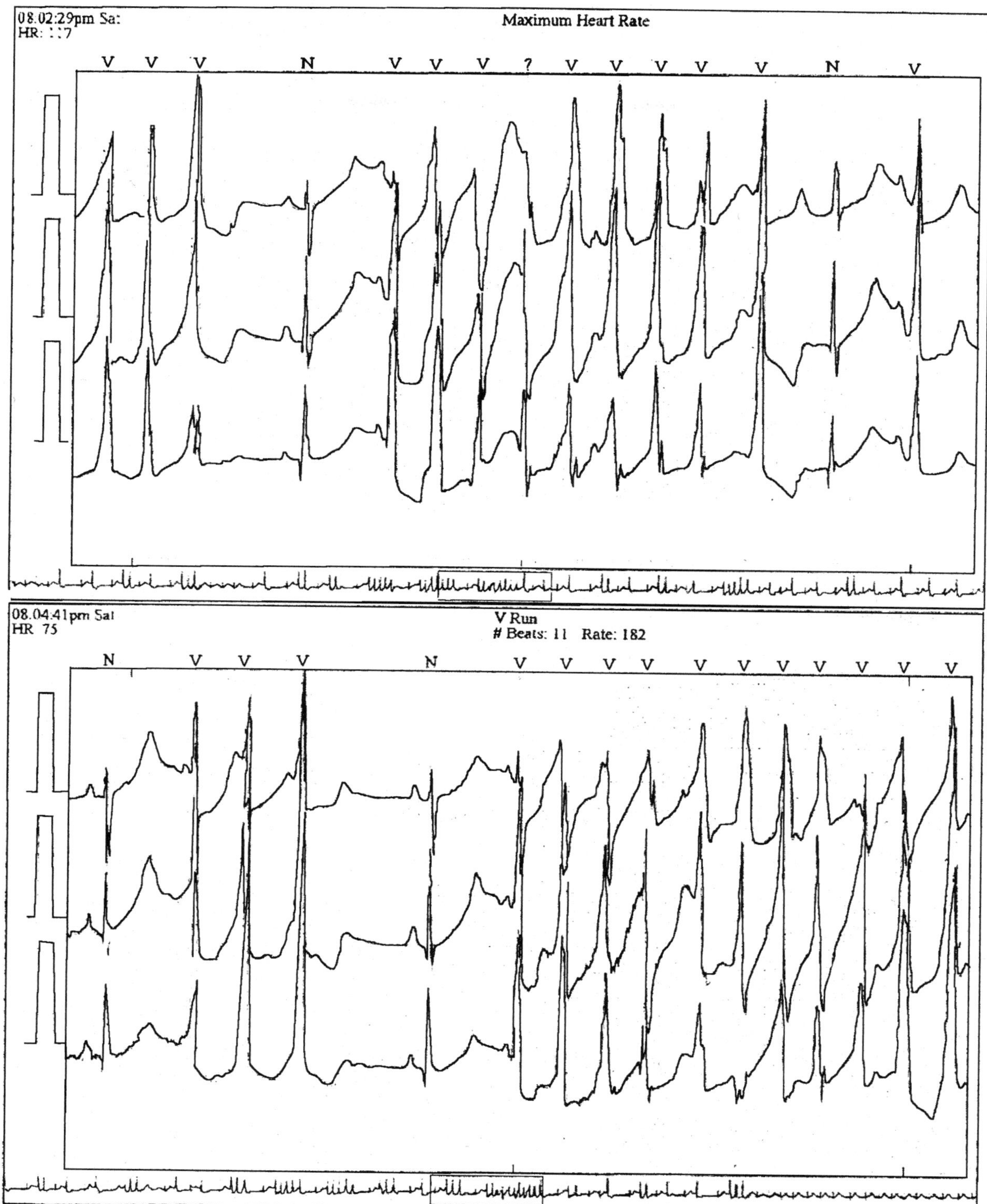


**Figure 52–6** Long-QT syndrome and polymorphic VT in a young patient presenting with syncope.

torsades de pointes (Fig. 52–6) (47). Many distinct subtypes have been described and can be associated with congenital deafness (Jervell–Lange–Nielsen) or with normal hearing (Romano–Ward). Ventricular tachyarrhythmias may be precipitated by bradycardia or catecholamine surges. These ventricular arrhythmias may provoke a syncopal event, and can be associated with sudden cardiac death. Family members of confirmed cases should be carefully evaluated for this disorder. Treatment may consist of beta-blockade, pacemakers, or ICDs. Careful examination of the

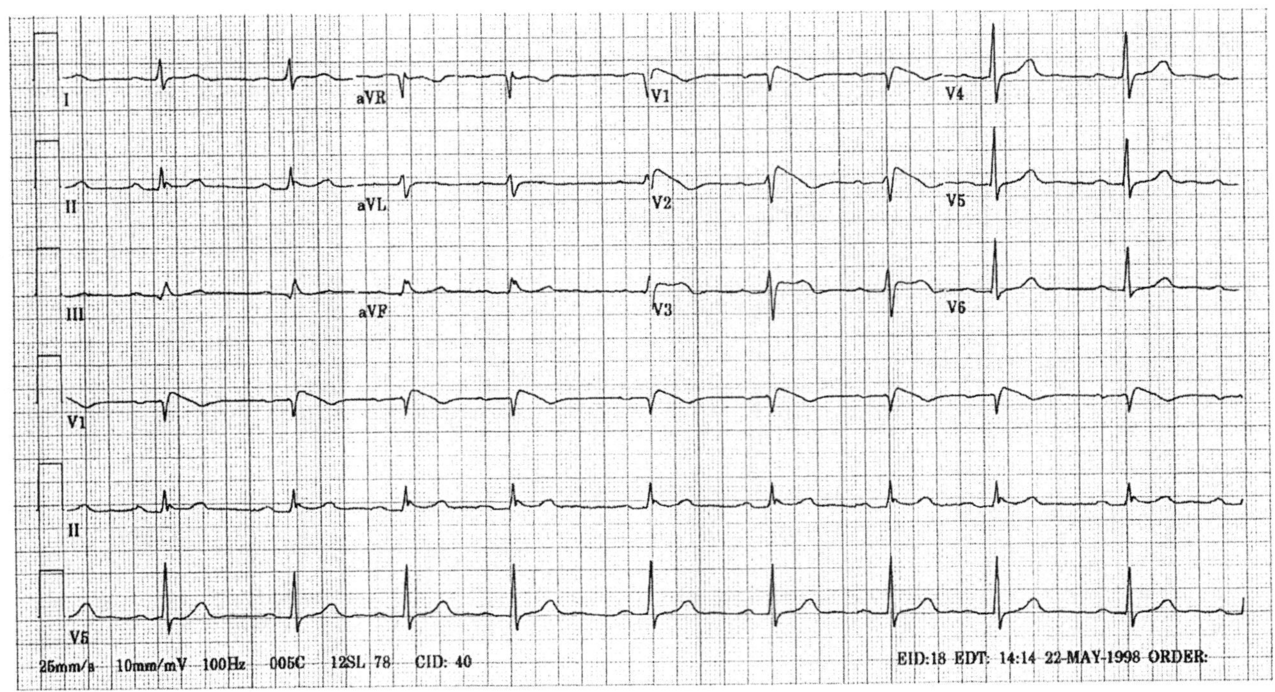


**Figure 52–7** ECG findings of right bundle branch block and precordial ST-segment elevation suggestive of Brugada syndrome.

ECG is paramount in all patients, particularly in young patients with a family history of syncope. Normal QT intervals have been described for males and females. Many drugs have been described that prolong the QT interval and may unmask covert patients (6).

## Syncope and Dilated Cardiomyopathy

Much attention has been focused on the specific clinical scenario of syncope in a patient with a dilated, nonischemic cardiomyopathy. Syncope in patients with dilated cardiomyopathy (DCM) has long been understood to be a poor prognostic sign and portends high mortality, perhaps 50% at 1 year. Electrophysiology testing has poor sensitivity in this group for the provocation of SMVT. Several studies have proposed empiric defibrillators for these patients, and it is now a Class II indication. The recent adoption of SCD-Heft and Definite study guidelines for the implantation of ICDs in DCM patients with an EF <35% has rendered previous arguments for empiric ICDs moot.

## Brugada Syndrome and Arrhythmogenic Right Ventricular Dysplasia

Brugada syndrome is a recently described arrhythmic disorder in which patients are susceptible to ventricular fibrillation and sudden death (48). Patients may present as survivors of sudden cardiac death but may also have symptoms related to transient VT such as palpitations and syncope. Their hearts are structurally normal. The ECG characteristically demonstrates ST-segment elevation and right bundle branch block in the precordial leads (Fig. 52–7). This disorder is most likely due to a genetic abnormality of cardiac ion channels (channelopathy). Brugada syndrome is endemic in Asia, where it is a recognized cause of sudden death and has been observed to occur in families. Sudden death occurs frequently at night, during sleep. Patients with suspicious but nondiagnostic ECGs can be further evaluated in the electrophysiologic laboratory with sodium channel blockade medications such as intravenous procainamide or ajmaline, which may precipitate the characteristic ECG pattern. Flecainide, usually prescribed for atrial arrhythmia, has also been observed to provoke this ECG pattern in otherwise unsuspected patients. Patients diagnosed with Brugada syndrome should receive a defibrillator if they are symptomatic or if there is a family history of sudden cardiac death.

Arrhythmogenic right ventricular dysplasia (ARVD) results from a genetic abnormality of right ventricular myocardium, replaced and infiltrated with fat and fibrous tissue (49). Patients may experience frequent PVCs and ventricular tachycardia, resulting in syncope. Characteristic findings on a CT or MRI are fatty infiltration of the right ventricular myocardium. ECG may show complete or incomplete right bundle branch block, a juvenile T-wave pattern, or an epsilon wave. Major and minor criteria have been proposed to establish the diagnosis (49). Patients with symptomatic ARVD should receive a defibrillator and frequently require antiarrhythmic medications (sotalol, amiodarone) to decrease the frequency of ICD shocks.

## DRIVING AND SYNCOPE

Syncope while driving can have life-threatening consequences for operators, passengers, and other motorists. Patients with syncope are frequently instructed to refrain from driving until a definitive diagnosis is established and successful treatment assured. An expert consensus panel has summarized their suggestions based on specific syncope etiologies and the expected recurrence rates after appropriate therapy is implemented (50). In patients with vasovagal syncope, it is recommended that no driving be done for 3 months following what appears to be successful therapy. Patients with syncope due to VT who receive an ICD should refrain from private driving for an appropriate probationary period; approximarely 6 or 7 months, as loss of consciousness (LOC) can occur very quickly during ventricular tachycardia before the ICD can detect, charge, shock, and terminate. Commercial driving is probably best avoided by patients with ICDs.

## CONCLUSIONS

The evaluation of the patient with syncope requires a thoughtful and logical approach to avoid the pitfalls of unnecessary testing. Syncope in the presence of significant structural heart disease suggests a need for expedited hospitalized evaluation, and if significant LV dysfunction is found, frequently preceding to a defibrillator. Neurocardiogenic or vasovagal syncope, although extremely common, remains a therapeutic challenge. Improved treatment modalities and pharmacologic interventions will require a better understanding of the epidemiology and pathophysiology. The role of tilt table testing in the evaluation of patients with syncope is evolving, and it is hoped that a uniformity of tilt table methodology and testing indications will soon be promulgated and adopted. The role of permanent pacemakers for vasovagal syncope remains uncertain. Improved monitoring technologies for syncope will enhance diagnostic capabilities. Implantable devices that monitor heart rate and blood pressure will greatly enhance the ability to diagnose patients accurately.

## REFERENCES


1. Kaufmann H, Wieling W. Syncope: a clinically guided diagnostic algorithm. *Clin Auton Res.* 2004;14:I/87–I/90.
2. Shen WK, Decker WW, Smars PA, et al. Syncope Evaluation in the Emergency Department Study (SEEDS). A multidisciplinary approach to syncope management. *Circulation.* 2004;110:3636–3645.
3. Sheldon R, Jaeger FJ. Neurally mediated syncope. The role of pacing. In: Ellenbogen KA, Kay GN, Wilkoff BL, eds. *Clinical Cardiac Pacing and Defibrillation.* 2nd ed. Philadelphia: WB Saunders; 2000:455–478.
4. Benditt DG, Van Dijk G, Sutton R, et al. Syncope. *Curr Probl Cardiol.* 2004;29:145–229.
5. Kapoor WN. Syncope. *N Engl J Med.* 2000;343:1856–1862.
6. Brignole M, Lavagna I, Paolo A, et al. Guidelines on management (diagnosis and treatment) of syncope—update 2004. *Eurospace.* 2004;6:467–537.
7. Klein GJ, Gersh BJ, Yee R. Electrophysiological testing. The final court of appeal for diagnosis of syncope. *Circulation.* 1995;92: 1332–1335.
8. Mark AL. The Bezold-Jarisch reflex revisited: clinical implications of inhibitory reflexes originating in the heart. *J Am Coll Cardiol.* 1983;1:90–102.
9. Sheldon R, Rose S, Flanagan P, et al. Risk factors for syncope recurrence after a positive tilt-table test in patients with syncope. *Circulation.* 1996;93:973–981.
10. Calkins H, Shyr Y, Frumin H, et al. The value of the clinical history in the differentiation of syncope due to ventricular tachycardia, atrioventricular block, and neurocardiogenic syncope. *Am J Med.* 1995;98:365–373.
11. Grubb, BP. Neurocardiogenic syncope and related disorders of orthostatic intolerance. *Circulation.* 2005;111:2997–3006.
12. Gregoratos G, Cheitlin MD, Conill A, et al. ACC/AHA guidelines for implantation of cardiac pacemakers and antiarrhythmia devices. *J Am Coll Cardiol.* 1998;31:1175–1209.
13. Gregoratos G, Abrams J, Epstein AE, et al. ACC/AHA/NASPE 2002 guideline update for implantation of cardiac pacemakers and antiarrhythmia devices; summary article: a report of the American College of Cardiology/American Heart Association Task Force on Practice Guidelines (ACC/AHA/NASPE Committee to Update the 1998 Pacemaker Guidelines). *Circulation.* 2002;106:2145–2161.
14. Krahn AD, Yee, R, Klein G, et al. Inappropriate sinus tachycardia: evaluation and therapy. *J Cardiovasc Electrophysiol.* 1995;6:1124–1128.
15. Krahn AD, Klein GJ, Norris C, et al. The etiology of syncope in patients with negative tilt table and electrophysiological testing. *Circulation.* 1995;92:1819–1824.
16. Krahn AD, Klein GJ, Yee R, et al. Randomized Assessment of Syncope Trial. Conventional diagnostic testing versus a prolonged monitoring strategy. *Circulation.* 2001;104:46–51.
17. Moya A, Brignole M, Menozzi C, et al. International Study on Syncope of Uncertain Etiology (ISSUE) Investigators. Mechanism of syncope in patients with isolated syncope and in patients with tilt-positive syncope. *Circulation.* 2001;104:1261–1267.
18. Brignole M, Menozzi C, Moya A, et al. International Study on Syncope of Uncertain Etiology (ISSUE) Investigators. Mechanism of syncope in patients with bundle branch block and negative electrophysiological test. *Circulation.* 2001;104:2045–2050.
19. Menozzi C, Brignole M, Garcia-Civera R, et al. Mechanism of syncope in patients with heart disease and negative electrophysiologic test. *Circulation.* 2002;105:2741–2745.
20. Zipes DP, DiMarco JP, Gillette PC, et al. Guidelines for clinical intracardiac electrophysiological and catheter ablation procedures: a report of the American College of Cardiology/American Heart Association Task Force on Practice Guidelines (Committee on Clinical Intracardiac Electrophysiologic and Catheter Ablation Procedures), developed in collaboration with the North American Society of Pacing and Electrophysiology. *J Am Coll Cardiol.* 1995;26:555–573.
21. Tracy CM, Akhtar M, DiMarco JP, et al. American College of Cardiology/American Heart Association clinical competence statement on invasive electrophysiology studies, catheter ablation, and cardioversion. *J Am Coll Cardiol.* 2000;36:1725–1736.
22. Bardy GM, Lee KL, Mark DB, et al. Amiodarone or an implantable cardioverter-defibrillator for congestive heart failure. *N Engl J Med.* 2005;352:225–237.
23. Natale A, Beheiry S, Wase A, et al. Occurrence of clinical asystole in patients without evidence of structural heart disease. Response to tilt table test and follow-up. *Circulation.* 1999;100:1–245.
24. Natale A, Masood A, Mohammad J, et al. Provocation of hypotension during head-up tilt testing in subjects with no history of syncope or presyncope. *Circulation.* 1995;92:54–58.
25. Kosinski D, Grubb B, Temesy-Armos P. Pathophysiological aspects of neurocardiogenic syncope: current concepts and new perspectives. *PACE.* 1995;18:716–724.
26. Fitzpatrick AP, Banner N, Cheng A, et al. Vasovagal reactions may occur after orthotopic heart transplantation. *J Am Coll Cardiol.* 1993;21:1132–1137.

27. Mosqueda-Garcia R, Furlan R, Tank J, et al. The elusive pathophysiology of neurally mediated syncope. *Circulation*. 2000;102:2898–2906.
28. Bracha HS, Bracha AS, Williams AE, et al. The human fear-circuitry and fear-induced fainting in healthy individuals. The paleolithic-threat hypothesis. *Clin Auton Res*. 2005;15:238–241.
29. Maloney JD, Jaeger FJ, Fouad-Tarazi FM, et al. Malignant vasovagal syncope; prolonged asystole provoked by head-up tilt. *Cleve Clin J Med*. 1988;55:542–548.
30. Benditt DG, Ferguson DW, Grubb B, et al. ACC Expert Consensus Document. tilt table testing for assessing syncope. *J Am Coll Cardiol*. 1996;28:263–275.
31. Kapoor WN, Brant N. Evaluation of syncope by upright tilt testing with isoproterenol. A nonspecific test. *Ann Intern Med*. 1992;116:358–363.
32. Flammang D, Church T, Waynberger M, et al. Can adenosine 5'-triphosphate be used to select treatment in severe vasovagal syndrome? *Circulation*. 1997;96:1201–1208.
33. Kurbaan AS, Franzen A, Bowker TJ, et al. Usefulness of tilt test-induced patterns of heart rate and blood pressure using a two-state protocol with glyceryl trinitrate provocation in patients with syncope of unknown origin. *Am J Cardiol*. 1999;84:665–670.
34. Brignole M. Randomized clinical trials of neurally mediated syncope. *J Cardiovasc Electrophysiol*. 2003;14:64–69.
35. Perez-Lugones A, Schweikert R, Pavia S, et al. Usefulness of midodrine in patients with severely symptomatic neurocardiogenic syncope: a randomized control study. *J Cardiovasc Electrophysiol*. 2001;12:935–938.
36. Atiga WL, Rowe P, Calkins H. Management of vasovagal syncope. *J Cardiovasc Electrophysiol*. 1999;10:874–886.
37. Natale A, Jasbir S, Anwer D, et al. Efficacy of different treatment strategies for neurocardiogenic syncope. *PACE*. 1999;18:655–662.
38. Di Girolamo E, Di Iorio C, Leonzio L, et al. Usefulness of tilt training program for the prevention of refractory neurocardiogenic syncope in adolescents. *Circulation*. 1999;100:1798–1801.
39. Sutton R, Brignole M, Menozzi C, et al. Dual-chamber pacing in the treatment of neurally mediated tilt-positive cardioinhibitory syncope. pacemaker versus no therapy: a multicenter randomized study. *Circulation*. 2000;102:294–299.
40. Connolly SJ, Sheldon R, Roberts RS, et al. The North American Vasovagal Pacemaker Study (VPS). A randomized trial of permanent cardiac pacing for the prevention of vasovagal syncope. *J Am Coll Cardiol*. 1999;33:16–20.
41. Connolly SJ, Sheldon R, Thorpe KE, et al. Pacemaker therapy for prevention of syncope in patients with recurrent severe vasovagal syncope. *JAMA*. 2003;289:2224–2229.
42. Holaigah I, Rowe P, Kan J, et al. The relationship between neurally medicated hypotension and the chronic fatigue syndrome. *JAMA*. 1995;274:961–967.
43. Blanc J, L'Heveder G, Mansourati J, et al. Assessment of a newly recognized association: carotid sinus hypersensitivity and denervation of sternocleidomastoid muscles. *Circulation*. 1997;95:2548–2551.
44. Elias J, Kuniyoshi R, Valadao W, et al. Glossopharyngeal neuralgia associated with cardiac syncope. *Arq Bras Cardiol*. 2002;78:510–519.
45. Jaeger FJ, Schneider L, Maloney JD, et al. Vasovagal syncope: diagnostic role of head-up tilt test in patients with positive ocular compression test. *PACE*. 1990;13:1416–1423.
46. Wieling W, Ganzeboom KS, Saul JP. Reflex syncope in children and adolescents. *Heart*. 2004;90:1094–1100.
47. Camm AJ, Janse MJ, Roden DM, et al. Congenital and acquired long QT syndrome. *Eur Heart J*. 2000;21:1232–1237.
48. Wilde, AAM, Antzelevitch C, Borggrefe M, et al. Proposed diagnostic criteria for the Brugada syndrome. *Circulation*. 2002;106:2514–2519.
49. Corrado D, Basso C, Nava A, et al. Arrhythmogenic right ventricular cardiomyopathy: current diagnostic and management strategies. *Cardiol Rev*. 2001;9:259–265.
50. Epstein AE, Miles WM, Benditt DG, et al. Personal and public safety issues related to arrhythmias that may affect consciousness: implications for regulation and physician recommendations. A medical/scientific statement from the American Heart Association and the North American Society of Pacing and Electrophysiology. *Circulation*. 1996;94:1147–1166.

## QUESTIONS

**1.** An 83-year-old man comes to see you in your office complaining of three episodes of abrupt loss of consciousness in the last year. His PMH is negative. His internist recently performed a stress echo test and Holter monitoring that were normal. His ECG reveals "trifascicular block." What is the next step?

a. Perform EPS, and if negative, implant a Reveal device.
b. Perform EPS, and if negative, implant an ICD.
c. Consider EPS for VT, and if negative, recommend a pacemaker.
d. Schedule a tilt test.

Answer is c: The presence of trifasicular or bifasicular block on the ECG suggests that the underlying etiology of syncope may be intermittent heart block, Mobitz type II, third-degree heart block, so-called Stokes-Adams block. Given a normal stress echo test and normal LV function, electrophysiologic testing will likely be negative for ventricular tachycardia. Based on current ACC/AHA guidelines, when no other cause for syncope is found, implantation is indicated for syncope that has not been demonstrated to be due to AV block.

**2.** A 57-year-old man with dilated cardiomyopathy presents to the emergency department with a facial laceration. He reports that he was urinating during the night and suddenly lost consciousness, falling and sustaining the injury. He felt fine before and after the event. He has an EF of 25% secondary to probable viral myocarditis. His ECG reveals IVCD and occasional multifocal PVCs. What is the next step?

a. Discharge from the emergency department with a 48-hour Holter monitor.
b. Admit, perform EPS, and if negative, implant a Reveal device.
c. Schedule an outpatient tilt test.
d. Admit, perform EPS, and if negative, offer an ICD.

Answer is d: Syncope in a patient with dilated cardiomyopathy is a very poor prognostic sign. Electrophysiologic testing has a low negative predictive value and therefore cannot be wholly relied on to screen patients who need a defibrillator. Implantation of a defibrillator remains a Class 2B indication in the presence of "advanced structural heart disease" denoting severe ischemic or nonischemic cardiomyopathy. In addition, based on the ejection fraction alone, the patient qualifiesy for ICD implantation according to the recent Definite and SCD-Heft data.

3. A 21-year-old female college student presents to her local emergency department because she fainted twice earlier that day. She reports that the first episode occurred while she was in the shower. It was preceded by nausea with diaphoresis, followed by sudden loss of consciousness. After she awoke on the floor, she felt very nauseated, diaphoretic, and vomited. She tried to stand but fainted again. She is otherwise healthy but has had the "flu" for 3 days. You are asked to consult. Her PMH, ECG, physical exam, and lab are normal. She had previously fainted once, while donating blood at a blood drive. What tests should you order?
   a. Tilt test
   b. Holter monitoring
   c. Stress echo test
   d. None of the above

Answer is d: Patients who present with a typical vasovagal episode with a classic prodrome and sequalae, who are otherwise healthy, probably require no other diagnostic testing or therapy, as the most unlikely etiology is vasovagal syncope. Tilt table testing is indicated only if the syncope becomes recurrent, or after single episodes of syncope with atypical features or for a high-risk patient.

4. Treatment for vasovagal syncope usually involves avoiding offending stimuli, dehydration, and prolonged standing; improving or decreasing venous pooling; and high-salt and high-fluid diet. For recurrent episodes, pharmacologic therapy is often employed. Initial pharmacologic therapy consists of all of the following *except:*
   a. Beta-blockers
   b. Disopyramide
   c. Serotonin reuptake inhibitors
   d. Florinef

Answer is b: Disopyramide (Norpace) is a Type 1A sodium channel antiarrhythmic medication. It was proposed to be effective for vasovagal syncope based on its negative inotropic and anticholinergic effects. However, in a very well designed study, using disopyramide loading and repeat tilt table tests, no efficacy was found. In addition, there is genuine concern for proarrhythmia in using the antiarrhythmic agents for treatment of a relatively benign disorder. Therefore, disopyramide may have a role for some patients, but it should not be used as initial therapy.

5. Carotid sinus syndrome is probably the second most common cause of neurally mediated syncope. It results from hypersensitivity of the carotid reflex and causes marked bradycardia and, frequently, concominent hypotension. All of the following are true regarding the features and treatment of carotid hypersensitivity *except:*
   a. The finding of carotid sinus hypersensitivity is extremely specific for the presence of carotid sinus hypersensitivity and syndrome, and mandates pacemaker implantation.
   b. Pacemaker implantation has been shown to significantly reduce the number of syncopal spells.
   c. Patients with recurrent unexplained falls or injuries should be considered to have a neurally mediated syncopal etiology such as carotid sinus hypersensitivity and be tested either with carotid sinus massage testing or tilt table testing.
   d. Carotid sinus hypersensitivity syndrome may result from abnormal proprioception and barrel receptor responses, in the carotid artery and the surrounding sternocleido mastoid.

Answer is a: Although the finding of carotid sinus hypersensitivity in a patient with recurrent syncope is highly suggestive, without the presence of the clinical syndrome the finding is relatively nonspecific. Carotid sinus hypersensitivity has been shown to be prevalent in patients with coronary disease and other forms of atherosclerotic disease as well. The *sine qua non* for carotid sinus syndrome is demonstration of carotid sinus hypersensitivity during carotid sinus massage, and a clinical scenario consistent with syncope resulting from direct stimulation of the carotid sinus baro and vagal reflex.

# Miscellaneous/ Pericarditis

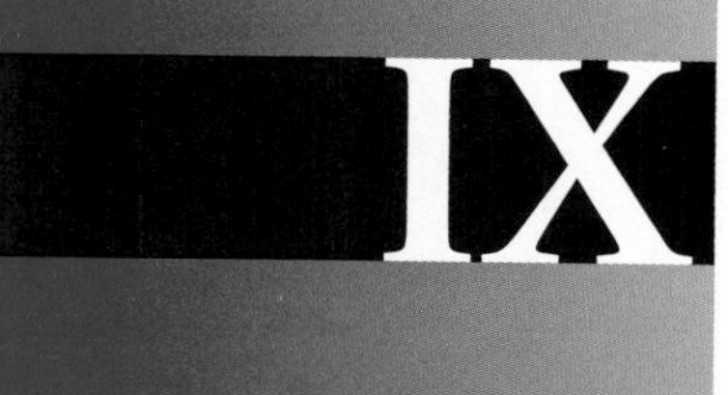

# Pericardial Diseases

# 53

***Oussama Wazni*** ***Allan L. Klein***

The pericardium envelops the cardiac chambers. It is made up of visceral and parietal layers that are separated by straw-colored pericardial fluid. The pericardium can be affected by acute and chronic conditions. These can cause a variety of clinical syndromes, including acute pericarditis, tamponade, recurrent pericarditis, and constrictive pericarditis.

## ACUTE PERICARDITIS

### Clinical Presentation and Workup

Inflammation of the layers of the pericardium, from any of myriad causes, yields a common clinical syndrome termed *acute pericarditis*. The causes of acute pericarditis are listed in Table 53–1. Chest pain from acute pericarditis can radiate to the neck and shoulders. Classically the pain is better with sitting up and leaning forward and worsens with lying supine. It can also be worse with deep inspiration and coughing.

Physical examination usually reveals a pericardial rub that is best heard at the left lower sternal border in end-expiration with the subject leaning forward. It is classically a rasping or creaking sound with a triple cadence, but may be biphasic or monophasic.

Electrocardiographic examination classically shows diffuse concave ST-segment elevation and PR depression. A helpful finding is PR elevation in lead aVR. The electrocardiogram (ECG) changes evolve through four stages. The first stage is diffuse ST elevation, which is followed by resolution of the ST elevation and flattening of the T waves. Stage three reveals inversion of the T waves, and by stage four the T waves are back to normal (Fig. 53–1).

Chest radiography is performed to rule out other mediastinal abnormalities, especially aortic dissection. An enlarged cardiac silhouette in the setting of acute pericarditis could represent the presence of pericardial effusion.

Echocardiography is not required to establish the diagnosis; however, the presence of pericardial fluid on echocardiography helps to confirm the diagnosis. In patients with hemodynamic compromise indicating tamponade, the presence of pericardial fluid mandates pericardiocentesis.

Pericardiocentesis is indicated in patients with tamponade and in those with suspected malignancy or purulent infection. Pericardial fluid should be sent for cytologic examination and analyzed for triglycerides (chylous pericarditis), red cell and white cell counts and pH, and amylase and lipase. If tuberculous pericarditis is suspected, then antituberculous therapy should be initiated promptly and pericardial fluid sent for acid fast bacteria (AFB) cultures. Pericardial biopsy and polymerase chain reaction for AFB may helpful in the diagnosis of tubercuous pericarditis.

### Treatment

The treatment of acute pericarditis depends on the etiology. Nonsteroidal therapy (such as ibuprofen) is used to treat idiopathic viral and postpericardiotomy syndrome. If symptoms do not improve, a different nonsteroidal anti-inflammatory drug (NSAID) should be tried or colchicine should be added. Steroids should be used as a last resort if there is no improvement after colchicine is added.

Steroids should not be used in patients with post–myocardial infarction pericarditis, because steroids interfere with scar formation and may pose a higher risk for rupture. NSAIDS, such as indomethacin, interfere with blood flow and should not be used in the setting of myocardial infarction (MI). Dressler syndrome (fever, malaise, pleuritis, and pericarditis) that occurs several weeks after an MI can be treated with aspirin or NSAIDs and, for resistant cases, with steroids. Dressler syndrome is not associated with worse prognosis.

Malignant pericardial effusions are usually managed by pericardiocentesis or pericardiostomy (pericardial window).

**TABLE 53–1**
**CAUSES OF ACUTE PERICARDITIS**

Malignant tumor
Idiopathic pericarditis
Uremia
Bacteria infection
Anticoagulant therapy
Dissecting aortic aneurysm
Diagnostic procedures
Connective tissue disease
Postpericardiotomy syndrome
Trauma
Tuberculosis
Other:
- Radiation
- Drugs that induce lupuslike syndrome
- Chylopericardium
- Post–myocardial infarction syndrome (Dressler)
- Fungal infections
- Acquired immunodeficiency syndrome–related pericarditis

*Source:* From Fowler NO. Pericardial disease. *Heart Dis Stroke.* 1992;1:85–94, with permission.

### Prognosis and Complications

Several factors have been recognized to indicate poor prognosis. These are fever above 38°C, subacute onset, large pericardial effusion, immunosuppression, trauma, and use of anticoagulants. Complications include recurrent pericarditis in 20% to 30% of patients, tamponade in 15%, and constrictive pericarditis.

## PERICARDIAL EFFUSION AND CARDIAC TAMPONADE

Pericardial effusion can be exudative or transudative and can be caused by a vast list of conditions. Slowly expanding effusions are usually asymptomatic. Patients may have nonspecific symptoms such as fullness and dull ache. The physical exam is usually nonrevealing except in large effusions, which are associated with muffled cardiac sounds and dullness to percussion, bronchial breath sounds, and egophony at the lower edge of the left scapula (Ewart sign). The ECG may show low voltage and, in large effusion, electrical alternans. Diagnostic pericardiocentesis should be performed in patients with large effusions and in cases without a clear etiology. Tests as summarized above should be performed depending on the clinical presentation. The treatment and management depends on the underlying cause as outlined in the previous section.

Cardiac tamponade is a clinical diagnosis, which is a result of increased central venous pressure and poor cardiac output due to compromised diastolic filling. Clinically, patients have tachycardia, hypotension, quiet precordium, and raised jugular pressure with a prominent X descent (rapid ventricular filling during systole) and absent Y descent (absent diastolic filling). Pulsus paradoxus (a decrease >10 mm Hg in systolic blood pressure during inspiration) is an ominous sign of impending hemodynamic compromise. The ECG may show low voltage and, in large effusion, electrical alternans. Tamponade is a life-threatening emergency, and pericardiocentesis should be performed immediately. Echocardiography is the test of

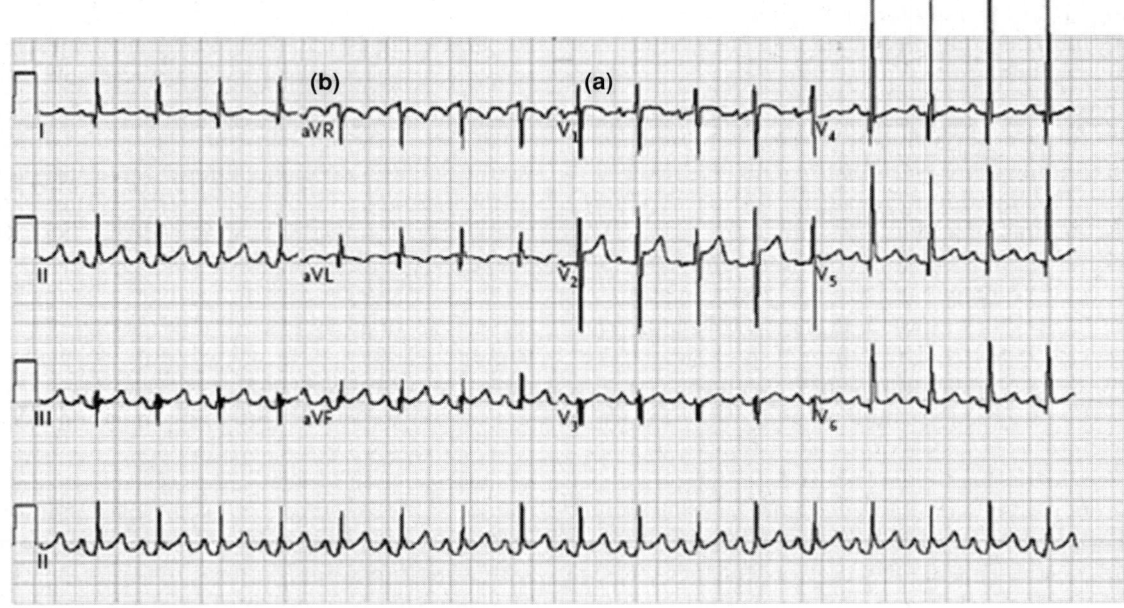


**Figure 53–1** Electrocardiogram of acute pericarditis, demonstrating ST-segment elevation **(a)** and PR-segment depression **(b)**.

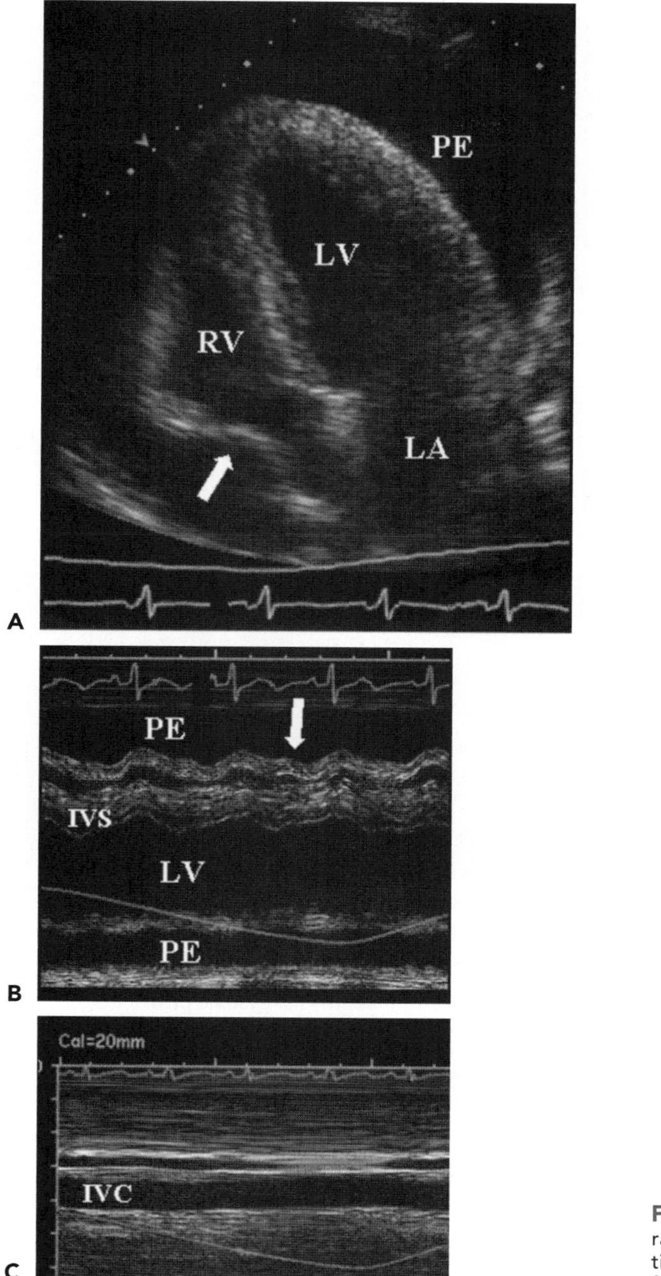


**Figure 53–2** Echocardiographic images of a large pericardial effusion with features of tamponade. **A:** Apical four-chamber view of the left ventricle (LV), left atrium (LA), and right ventricle (RV), demonstrating a large pericardial effusion (PE) with diastolic right atrial collapse (*arrow*). **B:** M-mode image with the cursor placed through the right ventricle, interventricular septum (IVS), and LV in the parasternal long axis. The view demonstrates a circumferential pericardial effusion (PE) with diastolic collapse of the right ventricle free wall (*arrow*) during expiration. **C:** M-mode image from the subcostal window in the same patient, demonstrating inferior vena cava (IVC) plethora without inspiratory collapse. (From Troughton RW, Asher CR, Klein AL. Pericarditis. *Lancet.* 2004;363:717–727.)

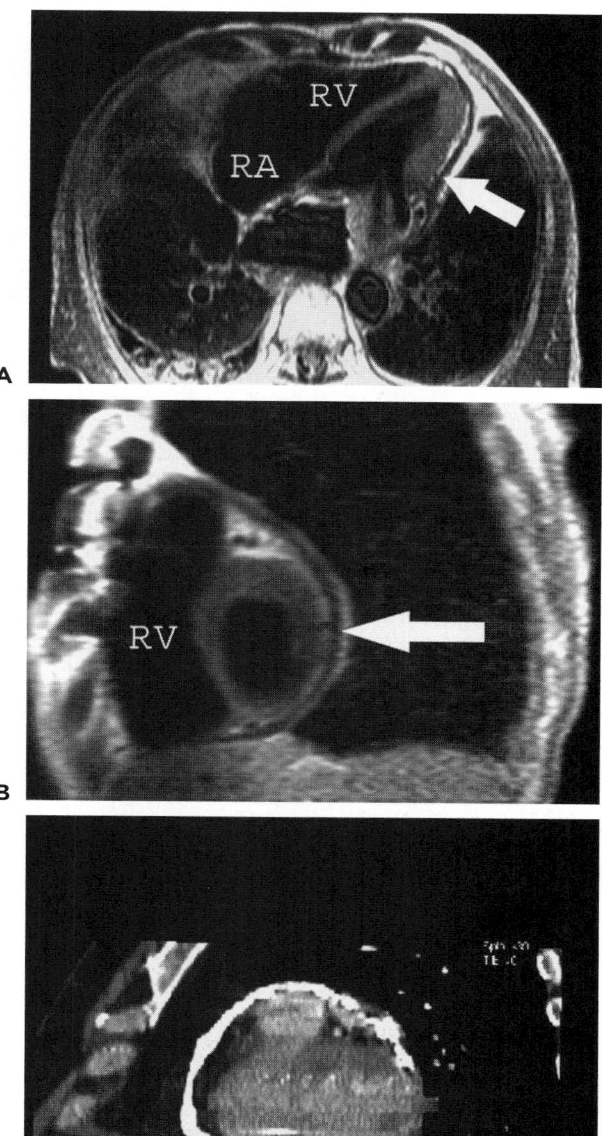


**Figure 53–3** Magnetic resonance (MRI) and computed tomography (CT) images demonstrating features of constrictive pericarditis (CP). **A:** MRI "dark blood" image (spin-echo; axial projection) from a patient with CP, demonstrating pericardial thickening and/or calcification along the posterolateral wall represented by curvilinear signal void (*arrow*) separated by the bright signal of the epicardial and pericardial fat. There is associated conical/tubular compression deformity of the left ventricle. **B:** MRI image (spin echo; sagittal projection) from the same patient, again demonstrating thickened pericardium (*arrow*). **C:** Short-axis CT image of the heart in another patient, demonstrating calcification of the pericardium. (From Troughton RW, Asher CR, Klein AL. Pericarditis. *Lancet.* 2004;363:717–727. Image provided by Richard D White, Cleveland Clinic Foundation.)

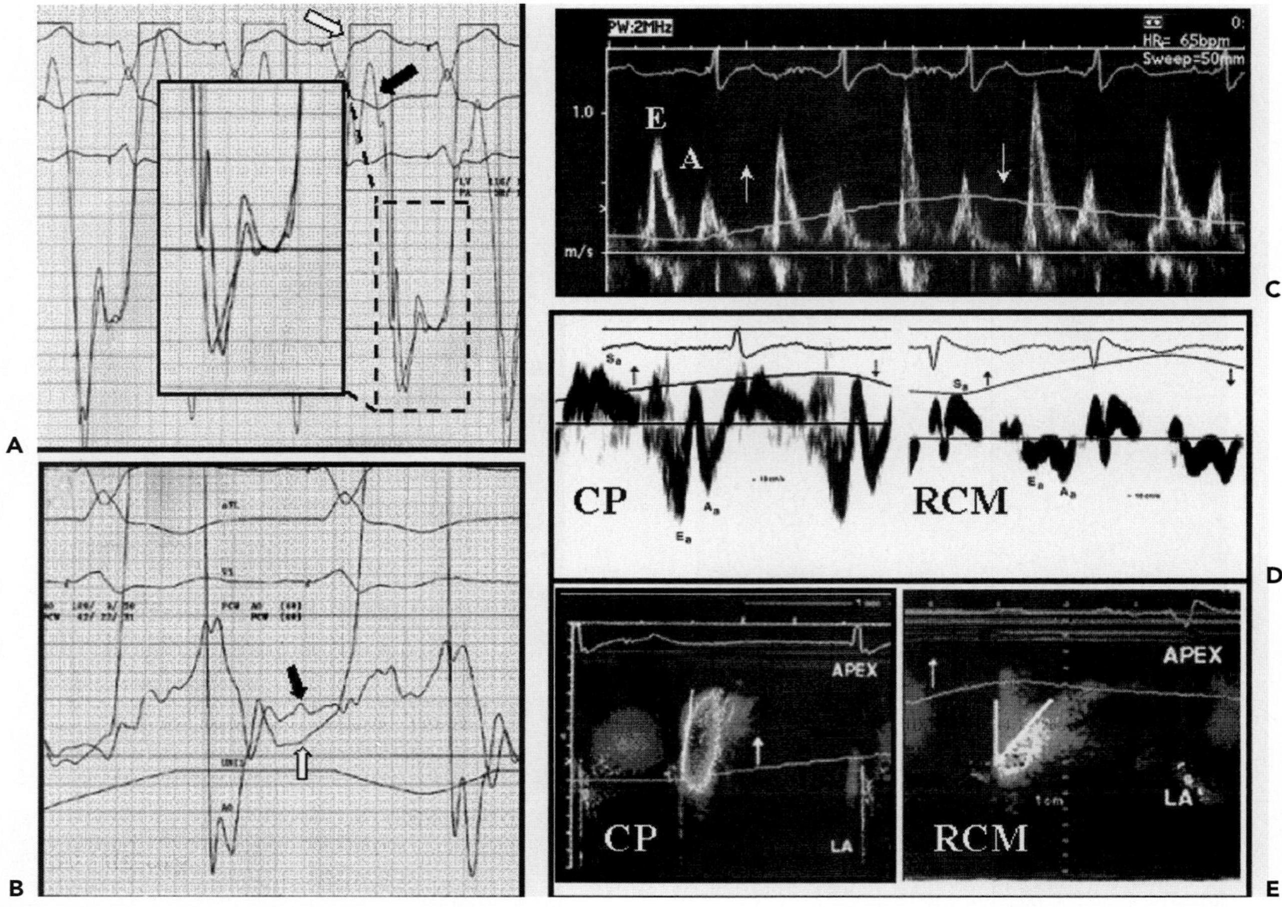


**Figure 53–4** Hemodynamic and echocardiographic findings in constrictive pericarditis. **A:** Simultaneous pressure tracings from the left (*white arrow*) and right (*black arrow*) ventricles, demonstrating equalization of diastolic pressures with the typical "dip-and-plateau" or "square-root" pattern (zoomed box). In the cycle at left, pressure at plateau is 27% of peak right ventricular systolic pressure. **B:** Respiratory variation in simultaneous left ventricular (*white arrow*) and pulmonary capillary wedge (*black arrow*) pressure tracings as a result of dissociated intrathoracic and intrapericardial pressures. **C:** Respiratory variation in early diastolic transmitral flow velocities measured by pulsed-wave Doppler as a consequence of increased interventricular interdependence and dissociation of intrathoracic and intrapericardial pressures. Velocities are 27% lower at the onset of inspiration (*up arrow*) and higher at the onset of expiration (*down arrow*). **D:** Tissue Doppler imaging demonstrating rapid (15-cm/s) peak early diastolic mitral annular velocities (*arrow*) in constrictive pericarditis (CP). By comparison, these velocities are low in a patient with restrictive cardiomyopathy (RCM) as a result of abnormal longitudinal myocardial relaxation. **E:** Color Doppler M-mode echocardiography of diastolic flow from the left atrium (LA) toward the ventricular apex imaged in the four-chamber view. The velocity of propagation (Vp) of early left ventricular flow measured as the slope of the first aliasing contour (*white line*) is steep (110 cm/s; normal range 50–80 cm/s) in constrictive pericarditis (CP) and by comparison is delayed (25 cm/s) in a subject with restrictive cardiomyopathy (RCM), reflecting abnormal myocardial relaxation. (From Troughton RW, Asher CR, Klein AL. Pericarditis. *Lancet.* 2004;363:717–727.)

choice when cardiac tamponade is suspected. Echocardiographic signs of tamponade are as follows (Fig. 53–2):

1. Pericardial effusion is present.
2. Late diastolic right atrial collapse is the most sensitive but least specific finding.
3. Early diastolic right ventricular collapse is less sensitive but more specific.
4. Left atrial collapse is less common but is very specific.
5. Doppler evaluation reveals a decrease in the transmitral inflow by 25% during inspiration. The tricuspid inflow is reduced by >40% during expiration.
6. The inferior vena cava appears plethoric and the diameter is fixed, with no decrease with deep inspiration.

## CONSTRICTIVE PERICARDITIS

Constrictive pericarditis is caused by inflammation and fibrosis of the pericardium that inhibits normal diastolic filling. The most common causes of constrictive pericarditis are postviral or idiopathic, previous cardiac surgery, and chest radiation therapy.

Clinical presentation is nonspecific in the early stages, but patients develop exertional dyspnea and paroxysmal nocturnal dyspnea with disease progression. In advanced stages, patients have edema and abdominal distention with ascites. Physical findings include increased jugular venous pressure that increases with inspiration (Kussmaul sign). On auscultation there are muffled cardiac sounds and a pericardial knock in early diastole (after an opening snap and before an S3 in timing).

### Pathophysiology

The fundamental abnormality in constrictive pericarditis is limited filling and enhanced interventricular dependence of the heart as a result of the rigid encasement of the heart by thickened pericardium, effectively isolating it from the normal respiratory swings in pressure and allowing a finite filling volume for the ventricles. Within the pericardium, the myocardium is intrinsically normal, with no specific abnormality of systolic or diastolic function. In constriction, the ventricle fills abruptly on valve opening. However, in mid-diastole, the chambers reach the maximum volume that the constraining pericardium will allow, and filling abruptly ceases.

### Diagnostic Workup

ECG usually reveals low voltage, and atrial fibrillation is a common finding. Radiography reveals pericardial calcification, and CT scan or MRI reveals increased pericardial thickness (>2 mm in thickness) (Fig. 53–3). Cardiac catheterization in most cases shows the classic findings of ventricular pressure discordance. During peak inspiration there is a decrease in left ventricular (LV) pressure and a concomitant increase in right ventricular (RV) pressure compared to the case in normal pericardium, in which there is a decrease in pressure in both chambers. Ventricular waveforms demonstrate the classic dip and plateau (the square-root sign), with the initial dip reflecting isovolumetric relaxation and the plateau the cessation of flow after early brisk diastolic filling. The end-diastolic pressures in both ventricles are equal.

### Echocardiography

Echocardiography is a key tool today to diagnose constriction (Fig. 53–4). Two-dimensional echo can reveal increased pericardial thickness, atrial tethering, abnormal septal bounce motion, and plethoric inferior vena cava. In both restrictive cardiomyopathy and constrictive cardiomyopathy there is an increased early or E velocity (rapid initial ventricular filling), short deceleration time, and slow velocity during atrial contraction. Differentiating restrictive cardiomyopathy from constrictive pericarditis depends on the respiratory changes in the transmitral flow E velocity. With the first beat of inspiration there is a decrease in the E velocity of the transmitral flow. The opposite is true for right-sided flow profiles. In restrictive cardiomyopathy and other diastolic disorders with a normal pericardium there is no respiratory variation. With constrictive pericarditis, there is increased tissue Doppler annular E wave as well as enhanced color M-mode flow propagation.

### Treatment

The vast majority of patients require pericardiectomy. This is advocated early in the disease process, because perioperative risk increases with worsening clinical condition. Medical therapy with diuretics and a low-sodium diet should probably be reserved for mildly symptomatic disease and those with severe co-morbidities that preclude surgery.

## BIBLIOGRAPHY

**Asher CR, Klein AL.** Diastolic heart failure: restrictive cardiomyopathy, constrictive pericarditis, and cardiac tamponade: clinical and echocardiographic evaluation. *Cardiol Rev.* 2002;10:218–229.

**Bertog SC, Thambidorai SK, Parakh K, et al.** Constrictive pericarditis: etiology and cause-specific survival after pericardiectomy. *J Am Coll Cardiol* 2004;43:1445–1452.

**Klein AL, Asher CR.** Diseases of the pericardium, restrictive cardiomyopathy and diastolic dysfunction. In: Topol EJ, ed. *Textbook of Cardiovascular Medicine.* 2nd ed. Philadelphia: Lippincott Williams & Wilkins; 2002:595–646.

**Lange RA, Hillis LD.** Clinical practice. Acute pericarditis. *N Engl J Med.* 2004;351:2195–2202.

**Troughton RW, Asher CR, Klein AL.** Pericarditis. *Lancet.* 2004;363:717–727.

## QUESTIONS

1. What is the most common cause of constrictive pericarditis in the United States?
   a. Previous cardiac surgery
   b. Irradiation
   c. Tuberculosis
   d. Idiopathic or viral

Answer is d: Idiopathic or viral. In one series (Bertog et al), etiology was idiopathic in 46%, previous cardiac surgery in

37%, irradiation in 9%, and miscellaneous (including tuberculosis) in 8% of the patients.

**2.** A young patient presents with chest pain and ankle swelling. Four weeks earlier, the patient had been diagnosed with viral pericarditis and treated with Ibuprofen. Presently he has no chest pain or shortness of breath. An echocardiogram reveals new findings consistent with mild constriction. What is the next course of management?

a. MRI to better assess pericardium
b. Consultation for pericardiectomy
c. Start steroids
d. NSAIDS and Colchicine

Answer is d: NSAIDS and Colchicine. Acute pericarditis can be followed by mild transient constriction, which usually resolves in 2–3 months. Steroids could be used for resistant cases. Pericardiectomy is not indicated.

**3.** Pulsus paradoxus can be caused by all of the following *except:*

a. Pericardial tamponade
b. Asthma
c. Obesity
d. Constrictive pericardial disease

Answer is d: Constrictive pericardial disease. Pulsus paradoxus is an inspiratory fall in systolic blood pressure >10 mmHg. It occurs most often in pericardial tamponade, asthma, and obesity. It is not usually seen in constriction unless there is an effusive component.

**4.** Central venous pressure examination in tamponade reveals:

a. Prominent X descent (rapid ventricular filling during systole) and absent Y descent (absent diastolic filling).
b. Prominent X and Y descents.
c. Prominent Y but blunted X descent.
d. These waveforms can only be discerned with right heart catheterization.

Answer is a: Prominent X descent (rapid ventricular filling during systole) and absent Y descent (absent diastolic filling).

**5.** Post–MI pericarditis is associated with all the following *except:*

a. Incidence has been reduced by thrombolytic therapy.
b. Most common after inferior MI.
c. ECG manifestations are rare.
d. Associated with atrial arrhythmia.

Answer is b: Post-MI pericarditis occurs more commonly after larger infarcts, usually anterior MI.

# 54 Effects of Systemic Diseases on the Heart and Cardiovascular System

**Bret A. Rogers** **Curtis Rimmerman**

Many inherited and acquired organ system disorders result in clinically significant changes in the heart and cardiovascular system. These changes often demand specific cardiovascular monitoring and therapies in addition to disease-specific treatment. Successfully completing the Cardiovascular Board examination requires an understanding of such clinical situations and appropriate management strategies. In this chapter, the most commonly tested topics are reviewed, categorized by primary organ system.

## INHERITED DISORDERS/GENETIC SYNDROMES

### Marfan Syndrome

Marfan syndrome is an autosomal dominant disorder that primarily affects connective tissues as a result of its associated mutation of the gene that codes for fibrillin-1, an important component of such tissues. Cardiac involvement consists of structural abnormalities of the heart and cardiovascular system. Degradation of the abnormal vascular structural proteins—combined with mechanical stress—results in cystic medial necrosis, which then leads to structural failure of the affected tissues. Mitral valve prolapse, aortic root and aortic annular dilation may be seen, leading to incompetence of the mitral and aortic valves. The aorta itself is at risk for aneurysm formation, intramural hematoma, dissection, and rupture, and this risk increases significantly with pregnancy.

Treatment of these abnormalities consists of $\beta$-adrenergic blockade to minimize aortic wall shear stress and surveillance echocardiography and computed tomography (CT) angiography for timing of valvular and aortic surgical replacement or repair. Aortic surgical intervention may take place at dimensions less than traditionally indicated for non-Marfan causes of aortic dilation, because the risk of catastrophic rupture increases precipitously with increasing aortic size.

### Ehlers–Danlos Syndrome

Ehlers–Danlos syndrome is also an autosomal dominant syndrome that affects the connective tissues and thereby results in similar heart abnormalities. Mitral and tricuspid valve prolapse causing mitral and tricuspid regurgitation, aortic root dilation causing aortic regurgitation, and dissection of the aorta and great vessels comprise the most common cardiovascular complications. Treatment consists of the surveillance measures described above.

### Osteogenesis Imperfecta

The result of a sporadic mutation that causes improper bone formation, osteogenesis imperfecta may cause mitral valve prolapse and aortic root dilation, leading to mitral and aortic valvular regurgitation. Surveillance echocardiography should be used to assess for indications for surgical valve repair or replacement.

### Noonan Syndrome

Noonan syndrome is an autosomal dominant disorder that includes characteristic facies and cognitive impairment in addition to its cardiovascular abnormalities. Heart lesions include pulmonic valve or infundibular stenosis, atrial septal defect, patent ductus arteriosus, tetralogy of Fallot, and hypertrophic cardiomyopathy. Vascular abnormalities include peripheral pulmonary arterial stenosis.

### Williams Syndrome

Williams syndrome, the result of spontaneous mutations, is characterized by cognitive impairment, an elflike facies, hypercalcemia, and dental abnormalities. Cardiovascular manifestations include congenital supravalvular aortic stenosis, atrial septal defect, ventricular septal defect, and peripheral pulmonary arterial stenosis.

### Osler–Weber–Rendu Syndrome

Also known as hereditary hemorrhagic telangiectasia, Osler–Weber–Rendu syndrome is characterized by mucocutaneous telangiectasias (on the tongue, lips, and fingertips) and arteriovenous malformations (AVMs) in the upper and lower gastrointestinal tracts and pulmonary vasculature. These pulmonary AVMs may result in paradoxical emboli in the presence of venous thrombosis.

Treatment consists of screening affected individuals by physical exam, arterial blood gas, and chest radiography, with pulmonary angiography used to direct balloon occlusion of significant lesions.

### LEOPARD Syndrome

Characterized by basal cell nevi, deafness, rib abnormalities, and a broad facies, LEOPARD syndrome affects the heart by causing pulmonic stenosis; surgical repair—guided by echocardiographic evaluation—is the appropriate treatment.

### Kartagener Syndrome

Kartagener syndrome, also called primary ciliary dyskinesia, is an autosomal recessive disorder that primarily affects microtubule function. The phenotype may also result in transposition of the great vessels and dextrocardia as part of situs inversus. Though patients are at risk for chronic pneumonia and bronchiectasis, sinusitis, and infertility, they have a normal life expectancy without need for cardiovascular management specific to the syndrome.

## NEUROLOGIC DISORDERS

### Muscular Dystrophy

The three most common variations of muscular dystrophy—Duchenne, Becker, and Emery–Dreifuss—are each X-linked disorders associated with significant cardiac abnormalities. Conduction disturbances are common, especially atrioventricular nodal block and atrial dysrhythmias; atrial paralysis and atrial fibrillation/flutter are particularly common in the Emery–Dreifuss variant. Each muscular dystrophy syndrome may also result in a cardiomyopathy, leading to heart failure. The cardiomyopathy that occurs in Duchenne muscular dystrophy preferentially affects the posterobasal left ventricle, which may exacerbate heart failure by causing posteromedial papillary muscle–mediated mitral regurgitation.

Treatment of the conduction disturbances and cardiomyopathy is supportive; permanent pacing may become indicated for the former, and patients may require heart transplantation for the latter.

### Friedrich Ataxia

Friedrich ataxia is an autosomal recessive neuromuscular disorder, caused by intramitochondrial iron accumulation, resulting in progressive ataxia, areflexia, upper motor neuron injury, and loss of proprioception. From a cardiovascular perspective, it is associated with a hypertrophic cardiomyopathy. Although fatal ventricular dysrhythmias are rare, the cardiomyopathy itself often causes death, especially in cases that progress to dilated cardiomyopathy.

Recent advances indicate that antioxidant therapies may slow progression, but treatment is generally supportive, using conventional heart failure modalities.

### Myotonic Dystrophy

Myotonic dystrophy, also known as Steinert disease, is an autosomal dominant disorder caused by a mutation in the myotonin gene; the resultant phenotype includes myotonia, weakness, frontal balding, cataracts, and gonadal dysfunction in addition to its cardiovascular manifestations. Electrocardiogram changes include pathologic Q waves in the absence of coronary artery disease or myocardial infarction. It also is associated with conduction disturbances, manifested primarily by atrioventricular block and intraventricular conduction delay. Treatment is supportive.

### Kearns–Sayre Syndrome

Kearns–Sayre syndrome is a mitochondrial encephalopathy characterized by ophthalmologic abnormalities. Atrioventricular block is seen, often requiring pacemaker placement.

### Myasthenia Gravis

Myasthenia gravis is an autoimmune process that reduces the number of acetylcholine receptors present at the neuromuscular junction. Affecting more females than males, it presents as progressive weakness and fatigue that worsens with repetitive muscle use and improves with rest. In addition to the autoimmune effect that it has on the neuromuscular endplate, myasthenia gravis can cause a myocarditis that responds to conventional myasthenia gravis treatment modalities.

### Guillain-Barre Syndrome

Guillain-Barre syndrome (GBS) is an acute, autoimmune-mediated demyelinating disorder of the peripheral nervous system, characterized by ascending motor weakness, paresthesias, and areflexia. The adverse effects that GBS has on the nervous system include autonomic dysfunction involving the cardiovascular system. Hypertension, orthostatic hypotension, resting sinus tachycardia, and potentially fatal dysrhythmias are all potential complications of GBS. Supportive treatment, including plasmapheresis and intravenous immunoglobulin, is the mainstay of care.

## ENDOCRINE AND METABOLIC DISORDERS

### Acromegaly

Acromegaly results from an excess of circulating growth hormone, usually from overproduction in the pituitary gland. The most common cardiovascular manifestation of this excess is hypertension, though premature atherosclerosis and cardiomegaly also occur. The cardiomegaly is out of proportion to the overall organomegaly and results in congestive heart failure and cardiac dysrhythmias, occasionally resulting in sudden cardiac death.

Treatment consists of destruction of the growth hormone source (i.e., the pituitary gland), either via transsphenoidal surgical resection or external-beam radiation. The associated cardiovascular abnormalities generally can be controlled with conventional therapies; hypertensive patients respond favorably to diuretics and sodium restriction.

### Cushing Syndrome

Cushing syndrome is characterized by excess glucocorticoids and androgens, either primarily from adrenal hyperplasia or secondarily from ACTH-producing neoplasms or exogenous administration. Patients with this syndrome are characterized by central obesity with slender extremities and proximal muscle weakness. Associated cardiovascular disorders include hypertension, accelerated atherosclerosis, and dyslipidemia. Cardiac dysrhythmias associated with hypokalemia are seen.

Therapy is directed at the specific cause of the hormonal excess. From a cardiovascular standpoint, efforts should be aimed at controlling hypertension, which is often difficult without first reducing cortisol production and maintaining normal potassium levels.

### Hyperaldosteronism/Conn Syndrome

Usually caused by an aldosterone-secreting adenoma, hyperaldosteronism features hypertension, hypokalemia, and metabolic alkalosis. The hypertension can be severe enough to cause renal insufficiency or stroke. Typical electrocardiogram changes associated with hypokalemia can also occur, manifest as flattened T waves and prominent U waves.

Surgical resection of the adenoma or medical therapy with aldosterone antagonists (e.g., spironolactone, eplerenone) is the treatment of choice, in addition to appropriate potassium replacement.

### Adrenal Insufficiency

Adrenal insufficiency can result from (a) primary adrenal cortex failure (Addison disease), (b) hypopituitarism (secondary adrenal insufficiency), (c) selective/isolated hypoaldosteronism (a hyperreninemic state usually caused by a congenital inability to produce aldosterone with preserved glucocorticoid function), or (d) enzymatic deficiency (congenital adrenal hyperplasia). Cardiovascular effects include hypotension with orthostasis and several possible electrocardiogram changes—small/inverted T waves, sinus bradycardia, prolonged QT interval, low-voltage QRS complexes, and first-degree atrioventricular block. Unlike the adrenal excess states described above, potassium concentration changes in adrenal insufficiency rarely result in electrocardiogram changes.

Treatment consists of replacement with corticosteroids, usually hydrocortisone in daily divided doses.

### Hyperthyroidism

Excess circulating thyroid hormone results in a physiologic state that resembles activation of the sympathetic nervous system. Hyperthyroidism has a peak incidence in the third and fourth decades, and women are four to eight times more likely to be affected.

Cardiac features include palpitations, dyspnea, tachycardia, and systolic hypertension, consistent with the increased chronotropic and inotropic state expected with increased adrenergic tone. Cardiac dysrhythmias and electrocardiogram changes also occur, including atrial fibrillation and other supraventricular tachyarrhythmias, an intraventricular conduction delay, and right bundle branch block. Finally, anginal chest pain and congestive heart failure symptoms can occur, even in a structurally normal heart.

Goals of treatment consist of reversal of the hyperthyroid state and resolution of symptoms. The latter is generally accomplished with $\beta$-adrenergic-blocking agents; the former can be done medically with targeted antithyroid agents such as methimazole and propylthiouracil, radioactively with $^{131}$I ablation of thyroid tissue, or surgically via thyroidectomy.

### Hypothyroidism

A lack of thyroid hormonal effect will also adversely affect the cardiovascular system. Interstitial myocardial fibrosis can result in gross biventricular dilation. Facial and peripheral edema can progress to brawny, nonpitting myxedema, and myxedematous pericardial effusions can be found in as many as one third of patients. Electrocardiogram changes may include sinus bradycardia, low-voltage QRS complexes, a prolonged QT interval, and intraventricular conduction delay or right bundle branch block. Hypertension or hypotension may result. Dyslipidemia (hypercholesterolemia and/or hypertriglyceridemia) is common.

Thyroid hormone replacement should be instituted at a low initial dose, with small increases in dosage at long intervals, especially in elderly patients or those with known coronary artery disease, as abrupt elevation of thyroid hormone levels can precipitate myocardial ischemia and/or heart failure.

### Amiodarone Therapy

Amiodarone has a chemical structure similar to that of both T4 and T3 and contains a large amount of iodine. As such, it decreases peripheral conversion of T4 into T3; its use can precipitate a hypothyroid state. Hyperthyroidism, however, can occur in patients receiving amiodarone as well, especially if concomitant iodine deficiency is present. For these reasons, patients receiving amiodarone on a long-term basis merit follow-up serum thyroid function test measurements.

## CONNECTIVE TISSUE DISORDERS

### Systemic Lupus Erythematosus

Systemic lupus erythematosus (SLE) is a well-described autoimmune disorder characterized by antibodies against cellular antigens, resulting in an inflammatory state that is manifested by effects on multiple organ systems. Most commonly, patients with SLE present with arthritis and dermatitis. The most common cardiovascular complication of SLE is pericarditis, with or without pericardial effusion. The effusion, usually exudative, is characterized by an elevated protein concentration, a low/normal glucose concentration, and low complement. Other cardiac abnormalities seen in SLE patients include early coronary artery disease, caused by both progressive atherosclerosis (with chronic corticosteroid use) and coronary arteritis. Myocardial infarction may occur via embolism of noninfectious (Libman–Sacks) endocarditis vegetations, or via SLE-related antiphospholipid antibody (APLA)–mediated thrombosis. The noninfectious endocarditis tends to cause insufficiency of the aortic and mitral valves more commonly, generally sparing the ventricular surface of each valve. Valvular lesions that can be detected by echocardiography are much more common than clinically significant disease. In those patients with clinically significant disease, the tendency is toward valve repair or replacement with bioprosthetic valves rather than mechanical valves, given the propensity of SLE patients to suffer bleeding complications from associated serositis or cerebritis. In patients with the APLA syndrome, mechanical valves are preferred, since anticoagulation is already indicated. Infants born to female patients with SLE (especially those having anti-Ro or anti-La antibodies) may suffer congenital heart block as a result of fibrosis of the conduction system *in utero*.

SLE-related pericarditis and pericardial effusions should be treated with nonsteroidal anti-inflammatory agents (NSAIDs) initially, with a plan to switch to corticosteroids should more aggressive treatment be necessary. Percutaneous or surgical drainage may be necessary should there be evidence of cardiac tamponade physiology or should medical therapy (corticosteroids and cyclophosphamide) fail to result in resorption of the effusion. Coronary artery disease treatment consists of conventional measures, except in cases of arteritis (which demands an intensive course of corticosteroids) or APLA-mediated thrombosis that requires systemic anticoagulation. In cases of endocarditis, serial echocardiography should be used to monitor for progressive valvular incompetence and indications for surgical valve repair or replacement. Women with SLE who become pregnant should undergo intensive gestational screening; intrauterine dexamethasone has been used successfully to slow progression of congenital heart block.

### Rheumatoid Arthritis

Rheumatoid arthritis is a progressive autoimmune arthritis, resulting in joint destruction, deformation, and immobility. In patients with rheumatoid arthritis (RA), pericardial disease is the most prominent cardiac complication, ranging in complexity from a chronic asymptomatic effusion to constrictive pericarditis. Early coronary artery disease and myocardial infarction can result from the chronic inflammatory state of RA and the long-term use of corticosteroid therapy. Rarely, secondary amyloidosis will occur, causing an infiltrative cardiomyopathy that may be accompanied by conduction abnormalities.

The mainstay of initial treatment is NSAIDs, followed by more intensive immunosuppression if necessary. Pericardiocentesis or surgical drainage of effusions may be required in cases of tamponade or refractory effusion. Coronary artery disease management should follow conventional recommendations.

## Seronegative Spondyloarthropathies

The seronegative spondyloarthropathies—ankylosing spondylitis, Reiter syndrome, and the inflammatory bowel disease arthritides (ulcerative colitis and Crohn disease)—appear to be closely related from a clinical standpoint and are associated with the HLA-B27 antigen. Ankylosing spondylitis results in ankylosis, sacroiliitis, peripheral arthritis, iritis, and aortitis. Reiter syndrome includes asymmetric arthritis, conjunctivitis, and genital ulcers. Aside from the well-described gastrointestinal findings in inflammatory bowel disease, they also feature an asymmetric arthritis and enthesitis. In general, this set of connective tissue disorders also shares a similar cadre of cardiac involvement: a thickened/ dilated aortic root, leading to aortic regurgitation, and atrioventricular conduction abnormalities.

Treatment consists of serial echocardiography for indications for aortic valvular surgical replacement as well as serial electrocardiograms for indications for permanent pacemaker implantation.

## Polymyositis

Polymyositis is an idiopathic inflammatory myopathy characterized by proximal muscle weakness and elevation of muscle enzyme serum levels. Cardiac involvement consists of a myopericarditis that can either be focal or generalized, at times involving the conduction system and resulting in conduction system abnormalities including heart block. Corticosteroids are generally administered if myocarditis is proven on endomyocardial biopsy.

## Scleroderma/CREST Syndrome

Systemic sclerosis, especially when complicated by the CREST syndrome (calcinosis cutis, Raynaud phenomenon, esophageal dysmotility, sclerodactyly, telangiectasias), can cause pericardial effusions and pericarditis. Patchy myocardial fibrosis may occur, as well as conduction system abnormalities at all levels. Pulmonary hypertension can be a prominent feature.

Echocardiography should be used both to assess for pericardial drainage indications and to monitor pulmonary pressures for significant elevations, possibly requiring the institution of vasodilator therapy.

## Takayasu Arteritis

Takayasu arteritis is an idiopathic, large-vessel vasculitis that generally occurs in young people, with a 10-fold female preponderance. Hypertension and aortic regurgitation secondary to aortic annular and aortic root dilation are its most prominent cardiac complications. Involvement of the coronary arteries is exceptionally rare.

Corticosteroids with or without further immunosuppression (cyclophosphamide, methotrexate) constitute primary therapy. Serial echocardiography is used to evaluate for valvular disease requiring surgical replacement. Angiography with invasive pressure measurements in major aortic branches early in disease progression is advisable to verify accuracy of extremity sphygmomanometry, as the most common site of stenosis is at the level of the subclavian artery.

## Sarcoidosis

Sarcoidosis is an idiopathic noncaseating granulomatous disorder that predominantly affects the lungs and mediastinal lymph nodes, causing a restrictive pulmonary physiology similar to that of interstitial lung diseases. Sarcoidosis may involve the pericardium, causing a pericarditis, the myocardium, causing a restrictive cardiomyopathy, or the conduction system, causing varying levels of atrioventricular and intraventricular block. Ventricular arrhythmias, both benign and malignant, can occur in the presence of myocardial sarcoid infiltration. In addition to monitoring for permanent pacing indications, corticosteroids are the mainstay of treatment.

## Relapsing Polychondritis

Relapsing polychondritis is an idiopathic, degenerative, inflammatory disease characterized by destruction of cartilage, which results in damage to organs of special sense (outer/inner ear, eyes, nose) in addition to the musculoskeletal system. Relapsing polychondritis can cause aneurysms of the ascending aorta and subsequent aortic regurgitation (because of its effect on the cartilaginous support structures of the mediastinum) as well as vasculitis of vessels ranging in size from the aorta to postcapillary venules. The vasculitis may result in either thrombosis or thrombotic emboli. Corticosteroids are primary therapy.

## Polyarteritis Nodosa

Polyarteritis nodosa (PAN) is a rare necrotizing vasculitis that affects small to medium-sized arteries. Clinical findings include weight loss, myalgias, neuropathy, testicular pain, elevated diastolic blood pressure, renal insufficiency without glomerulonephritis, and false-positive serum hepatitis B testing. The vessels affected by PAN include the coronary arteries. Coronary arteritis and coronary artery aneurysms are seen, which can lead to an acute myocardial infarction. Atherosclerosis is also accelerated in PAN as a result of the associated hypertension, steroid therapy, and renal failure. Occasionally, patients with PAN develop myopericarditis. Congestive heart failure may occur related to the long-term effects of hypertension, renal failure, and coronary insufficiency. Corticosteroids are primary therapy.

### Behçet Disease

Behçet disease is a chronic inflammatory disease—considered a multisystem vasculitis—characterized by oral aphthous ulcers as well as ulcers of the skin, genitals, and eyes. The vasculitis can result in aneurysms of the arch vessels and the abdominal aorta as well as a proximal aortitis that may cause aortic regurgitation from dilation of the aortic root. Corticosteroids are primary therapy.

### Churg–Strauss Syndrome

Churg–Strauss syndrome is an eosinophilic granulomatous inflammation of the respiratory tract, characterized by a necrotizing vasculitis of small and medium-sized vessels. The eosinophilia results in an association with asthma and other atopic diseases. Eosinophilic myocarditis, causing a restrictive cardiomyopathy, pericarditis with or without an associated effusion, and coronary arteritis characterize the cardiac manifestations of Churg–Strauss syndrome. Congestive heart failure secondary to the cardiomyopathy is the most common cause of death in Churg–Strauss syndrome patients. Corticosteroids are primary therapy.

### Wegener Granulomatosis

Wegener granulomatosis is characterized by systemic granulomatous inflammation of the upper and lower respiratory tract as well as a necrotizing vasculitis of small and medium-sized vessels that may result in necrotizing glomerulonephritis. Its cardiac manifestations include pericarditis (which rarely results in constrictive physiology or tamponade), myocarditis with left ventricular dysfunction (which may cause lethal ventricular dysrhythmias or sinus node dysfunction), and an uncommon valvulitis, most often aortic (which may result in regurgitation with or without leaflet prolapse). Serial electrocardiograms and echocardiography to monitor electrophysiologic and ventricular function are warranted, respectively, to guide supportive therapy. Corticosteroids are primary therapy, and cyclophosphamide may be added for progressive disease.

## HEMATOLOGIC/ONCOLOGIC DISORDERS

### Iron Overload

Iron overload may result from primary hemochromatosis, multiple transfusions, intestinal hyperabsorption, and from diseases characterized by bone marrow failure. The most common cardiac complication of iron overload is a restrictive cardiomyopathy secondary to myocardial iron deposition. Pericarditis, atrioventricular conduction disorders, and angina, despite normal coronary arteries, also occur.

Chelation therapy with deferoxamine can reverse some of these cardiovascular effects. In the setting of bone marrow failure, phlebotomy after successful bone marrow transplantation effectively removes excess iron.

### Anemia

Although there are many different anemias, the effects they have on the heart vary little with etiology. Severe anemias can result in left ventricular dysfunction and ultimately congestive heart failure. Angina may also occur in severe anemias as a consequence of a marked reduction in oxygen transport capacity. Initial treatment consists of transfusion, followed by etiology-specific therapy and possibly intravenous or subcutaneous erythropoietin injections. Transfusion is also the best initial treatment for hemolytic anemias related to prosthetic valves, as increased blood viscosity will reduce valve-related hemolysis.

In sickle-cell disease, myocardial infarction may occur with sickling of cells in coronary arteries, leading to coronary artery thrombosis. Acute mitral regurgitation from papillary muscle involvement can complicate myocardial infarctions in sickle-cell disease. Pulmonary infarction may also occur, either from pulmonary arterial thrombosis or embolization of venous thrombi.

### Polycythemia

In addition to polycythemia vera, other polycythemic states may result in adverse cardiovascular effects. Like polycythemia vera, thrombocytosis, leukocytosis, plasma cell neoplasms, monoclonal gammopathies such as multiple myeloma, and cryoglobulinemia each may cause a hyperviscosity syndrome, leading to vascular thrombosis. Coronary arterial thrombosis may result in myocardial infarction, deep venous thrombosis can lead to pulmonary embolism, and peripheral arterial thrombosis may cause skeletal muscle or organ-specific infarction.

Therapy is focused on reducing the polycythemic load with treatment specific to the involved cell line. Polycythemia vera and thrombocytosis may respond to hydroxyurea. Leukocytoses and plasma cell neoplasms should be treated with appropriate chemotherapeutics, and, in the case of paraproteinemias, plasmapheresis is an important adjunctive therapy.

### Neoplastic Disease

Tumors originating in the heart and those that commonly metastasize to the myocardium are discussed in the Cardiac Tumors chapter. Pericardial disease may take the form of metastatic infiltration causing a constrictive physiology or it may be effusive, resulting in possible cardiac tamponade. Noninfectious, nonmetastatic, thrombotic endocarditis, also known as marantic endocarditis, may occur. Marantic endocarditis generally does not destroy valve architecture or disrupt valvular function but does predispose to peripheral embolism. Myocardial ischemia is a potential complication of thrombotic emboli or extrinsic compression of epicardial coronary arteries. Dysrhythmias are common with metastases to the myocardium. The superior vena cava (SVC) syndrome, caused by extrinsic compression of the SVC by tumor or enlarged lymph nodes resulting in venous stasis in the head, arms, and upper torso, may also complicate malignancies.

Effusive pericardial disease is treated with percutaneous or surgical drainage, whereas infiltrative pericardial disease requires surgical pericardial stripping. The presence of marantic endocarditis requires no specific therapy, though treating ischemic syndromes that may result or occur concomitantly requires anticoagulation that may precipitate further embolic phenomena. The SVC syndrome requires urgent combination therapy with external-beam radiation and chemotherapy, and endovascular stenting has become a common adjunctive treatment.

### External-Beam Radiation Therapy

Patients who receive external-beam radiation (XRT) for chest wall or mediastinal tumors often suffer heart-specific side effects. Pericardial disease may range from an effusion to calcific constrictive pericarditis. Coronary arteries may undergo accelerated atherosclerosis or narrowing, a form of radiation fibrosis. Heart valves may also be damaged, resulting in valvulitis that can cause either stenosis or regurgitation. XRT may also cause a cardiomyopathy from direct myocardial damage, though this can be difficult to distinguish from a cardiomyopathy caused by simultaneously used chemotherapeutic agents.

Pericardial disease is treated with drainage or pericardial stripping. Coronary artery disease should be managed with conventional therapies, and valvulitis requires serial echocardiography to determine timing of surgical repair or replacement. XRT-related cardiomyopathy is managed by usual congestive heart failure therapies.

### Chemotherapy

Anthracycline chemotherapeutics and mitoxantrone (a chemically similar antineoplastic medication) are known to cause a well-described dilated cardiomyopathy that is related to cumulative dose. The cardiomyopathy should be treated with conventional congestive heart failure therapy. These drugs may also cause an acute toxicity, characterized by electrocardiogram changes that include a prolonged QT interval and nonspecific ST-segment and T-wave changes. Other chemotherapeutics are also identified as cardiotoxins. Ischemic coronary syndromes may be precipitated by 5-fluorouracil in patients with pre-existing coronary artery disease. Treatment consists of usual coronary artery disease management. Cyclophosphamide and ifosfamide have been shown to cause a cardiomyopathy similar to that observed with the anthracyclines and should be managed similarly.

## RENAL FAILURE

Although congestive heart failure may lead to renal insufficiency, the reverse may also occur. Uremic cardiomyopathy may result from volume and pressure overload related to insufficient fluid clearance, and circulating uremic toxins have a negative inotropic effect. As with most secondary cardiomyopathies, treatment consists of conventional congestive heart failure management measures.

Accelerated atherosclerosis can result from the hyperlipidemia that constitutes a component of the nephrotic syndrome, which should be treated with aggressive medical therapy. Hypertension can also occur as a result of renal failure, especially in cases caused by arterionephrosclerosis, glomerulopathies, or transplant-associated renal failure. Treatment consists of antihypertensive medications and early hemodialysis as the renal failure progresses.

Calcification of the heart's valvular apparatus, coronary arteries, conduction system, and pericardium may develop as the calcium phosphorus product increases with worsening renal failure. Diet modification and phosphate-binding agents are the treatments of choice.

Further pericardial disease in renal failure ranges from constriction to uremic pericarditis with effusion. Percutaneous or surgical drainage may be required. Effective hemodialysis can reduce the likelihood of developing further effusions.

Because of the rapid changes in electrolytes and pH that accompany dialysis and the high prevalence of underlying heart disease among patients with renal failure, dysrhythmias are common, requiring supportive care and close monitoring of electrolytes both pre- and postdialysis.

## HIV

Among the protean clinical manifestations of HIV, the heart is not spared. Left ventricular dysfunction results as HIV infection progresses to individual cardiac myocytes, causing focal myocarditis. This cardiomyopathy is more common as the CD4+ cell count decreases and tends to occur more frequently in infected children. Treatment consists of usual measures for dilated cardiomyopathy.

As HIV progresses, the release of cytokines to fight opportunistic infections and to signal maximal activation of the immune system compromises endothelial integrity at the capillary level. This results in pleural, peritoneal, and pericardial effusions. The presence of a pericardial effusion markedly increases predicted mortality. Screening echocardiography is a reasonable consideration in the later stages of HIV, and percutaneous or surgical drainage may become necessary in the presence of hemodynamic compromise or to examine fluid for treatable opportunistic etiologies (e.g., tuberculosis, malignancy).

The chronic inflammatory state present in HIV and lipid-raising tendency of protease inhibitors may result in accelerated atherosclerosis of the coronary arteries. Patients on antiretroviral therapy should receive aggressive lipid-lowering therapy, and a high degree of suspicion should exist in even young HIV+ patients presenting with possible anginal syndromes.

A heart-specific opportunistic infection occurring in the setting of HIV is *Salmonella* endocarditis, as the transient bacteremia that may occur after ingestion of affected food will not be effectively cleared. Fungal endocarditis is also included on the list of HIV-associated opportunistic infections. Treatment consists of broad-spectrum antibiotic therapy pending isolation of a specific pathogen.

Finally, HIV-associated malignancies may involve the heart as well, most commonly metastatic Kaposi sarcoma and lymphomas, which may be heralded by pericardial effusions. Treatment is specifically directed at the identified malignancy.

## CONCLUSION

Given the spectrum of noncardiac disease that may significantly affect the heart and cardiovascular system, a working knowledge of these interactions is essential for treatment of patients with cardiovascular disease and for success on the Cardiovascular Medicine Board Examination. Effective care for patients with systemic disease demands cooperation with internists as well as medical and surgical subspecialists.

## BIBLIOGRAPHY


**Barbaro G.** HIV infection, highly active antiretroviral therapy and the cardiovascular system. *Cardiovasc Res.* 2003;60(1): 87–95.

**Harjai KJ, Licata AA.** Effects of amiodarone on thyroid function. *Ann Intern Med.* 1997;126(1):63–173.

**Haskard DO.** Accelerated atherosclerosis in inflammatory rheumatic diseases. *Scand J Rheumatol.* 2004;33(5):281–292.

**Klein I.** Thyroid hormone and the cardiovascular system. *Am J Med.* 1990;88(6):631–637.

**Lautermann D, Braun J.** Ankylosing spondylitis—cardiac manifestations. *Clin Exp Rheumatol.* 2002; 20(6 suppl 28):S11–S15.

**Lowe GD.** Blood viscosity and cardiovascular disease. *Thromb Haemost.* 1992;67(5):494–498.

**McCullough PA.** Cardiovascular disease in chronic kidney disease from a cardiologist's perspective. *Curr Opin Nephrol Hypertens.* 2004;13(6):591–600.

**McKenna WJ.** Inherited disorders associated with cardiac disease. In: Rose BD, ed. *UpToDate.* Wellesley, MA: UpToDate; 2005.

**Metivier F, Marchais SJ, Guerin AP, et al.** Pathophysiology of anaemia: focus on the heart and blood vessels. *Nephrol Dialys Transplant* 2000;15(suppl 3):14–18.

**Sarnak MJ.** Cardiovascular complications in chronic kidney disease. *Am J Kidney Dis.* 2003;41(5):11–17.

**Sondheimer HM, Lorts A.** Cardiac involvement in inflammatory disease: systemic lupus erythematosus, rheumatic fever, and Kawasaki disease. *Adolesc Med Art Rev.* 2001;12(1):69–78.

**Surawicz B, Mangiardi ML.** Electrocardiogram in endocrine and metabolic disorders. *Cardiovasc Clin.* 1977;8(3):243–266.


## QUESTIONS

**1.** Match the syndrome with the phenotype:

| | |
|---|---|
| a. Marfan | 1. Basal cell nevi, deafness, pulmonic stenosis |
| b. Osler–Weber–Rendu | 2. Infundibular stenosis, atrial septal defect, patent ductus arteriosus, tetralogy of Fallot |
| c. Kartagener | 3. Mitral valve prolapse, aortic regurgitation, aortic aneurysm/dissection |
| d. Noonan | 4. Paradoxical emboli |
| e. LEOPARD | 5. Elfin facies, hypercalcemia, supravalvular aortic stenosis, atrial septal defect, ventricular septal defect |
| f. Williams | 6. Dextrocardia, chronic sinusitis, infertility |

Answers: a–3, b–4, c–6, d–2, e–1, f–5

**2.** In a patient with myotonic dystrophy, which of the following is *not* an associated electrocardiographic abnormality?

a. Intraventricular conduction delay
b. Left ventricular hypertrophy by voltage criteria
c. Pathologic Q waves
d. Atrioventricular conduction block

Answer is b: Unlike the muscular dystrophies, myotonic dystrophy is not associated with a hypertrophic cardiomyopathy. It is, however, associated with the electrocardiogram abnormalities above.

**3.** Typically, Guillain-Barré syndrome is *not* associated with which of the following abnormalities?

a. Hypertension
b. Sinus tachycardia
c. Sinus bradycardia
d. Orthostatic hypotension
e. Ventricular tachycardia

Answer is c: The autonomic instability that characterizes the polyneuropathy in Guillain–Barre syndrome may result in hypertension, orthostatic hypotension, and sinus tachycardia;

sinus bradycardia is usually not observed. Ventricular tachycardia may also occur.

4. A 35-year-old woman with rheumatoid arthritis (RA) presents for evaluation of hypertension and resting tachycardia. Her RA is controlled on 5 mg/day of prednisone. She does not experience chest pain or dyspnea. Her vital signs include an irregular apical pulse of 120 beats/min and a blood pressure of 165/70 mm Hg. Serum electrolytes and a complete blood count are within normal limits.

What is the most appropriate initial therapy?

a. Increase the steroid dosage.
b. Discontinue steroid therapy.
c. Transsphenoidal pituitary resection followed by corticosteroid and T4 replacement.
d. $\beta$-Adrenergic blockers and methimazole.

Answer is d: This patient has hyperthyroidism. Her rheumatoid arthritis increases her risk of other autoimmune disorders; the most common cause of hyperthyroidism is Graves disease, an autoimmune disorder characterized by autoantibodies against the thyrotropin receptor. Her associated hypertension and atrial fibrillation are best managed initially with $\beta$-adrenergic-blocking agents, then by antithyroid medications.

5. A 27-year-old white man presents to the outpatient department with dyspnea on exertion. He has no symptoms of chest pain or presyncope, and reports only a migratory joint discomfort on review of systems. Vital signs demonstrate a heart rate of 90 beats/min and a blood pressure of 125/44 mm Hg. His jugular venous pressure is normal, his lungs are clear, and his heart rhythm is regular.

What findings would you expect on further examination and testing?

a. Malar rash, holosystolic murmur radiating to the axilla, positive serum anti-dsDNA antibody
b. Telangiectasias, sclerodactyly, diffuse ST-segment elevations on electrocardiogram
c. Loss of lumbar lordosis, diastolic murmur at the left sternal border, iritis, positive serum HLA-B27 marker
d. Digital ulnar deviation, positive serum rheumatoid factor, electrical alternans on electrocardiogram
e. Atrioventricular conduction block and a restrictive pulmonary function test pattern

Answer is c: This patient has ankylosing spondylitis. The wide pulse pressure results from a regurgitant aortic valve, which would also cause the diastolic murmur. The arthritis associated with ankylosing spondylitis is asymmetric and migratory, and loss of lumbar lordosis occurs with sacroiliitis. The clinical findings listed would not account for scleroderma-associated pericarditis (as in choice b), for rheumatoid arthritis-associated pericardial effusion (as in choice d), or for sarcoid-associated heart block (as in choice e).

6. A 45-year-old woman with a history of Hodgkin disease presents with dyspnea. She underwent chemotherapy and external-beam radiation 10 years ago, and her Hodgkin disease has been in clinical remission ever since.

Which of the following is *not* likely to be the cause of her dyspnea?

a. Complete heart block
b. Coronary artery disease
c. Aortic stenosis
d. Constrictive pericarditis

Answer is a: Complete heart block is not a complication of external-beam radiation. Diffuse coronary artery disease, valvulitis causing aortic stenosis, and constrictive pericarditis may all result from radiation-induced mediastinal damage.

7. Which of the following is *not* a cardiac complication of HIV infection and antiretroviral therapy?

a. Diffuse coronary artery disease
b. Intraventricular conduction delay
c. Pericardial effusion
d. Dilated cardiomyopathy with regional wall motion abnormalities

Answer is b: Although HIV and protease inhibitors may cause diffuse coronary artery disease, pericardial effusion, and focal myocarditis, intraventricular conduction delay is not an associated complication of the infection or therapy.

# 55

# Pregnancy and Heart Disease

*Anjli Maroo* *Russell E. Raymond*

Cardiac diseases, both congenital and acquired, are becoming increasingly prevalent in women in their childbearing years. Improvements in the diagnosis and treatment of individuals with congenital heart disease (CHD) have led to a growing number of adults who survive well past their reproductive years. Whenever possible, these patients should be counseled in advance about the potential risks associated with pregnancy. Advanced maternal age and an overall rise in the prevalence of diabetes mellitus have contributed to a growing number of women with acquired cardiac diseases during pregnancy.

## NORMAL PHYSIOLOGIC CHANGES DURING PREGNANCY

Demands on the cardiovascular system increase steadily during pregnancy, labor and delivery, and in the postpartum period (1). In fact, pregnant women experience major changes in hemodynamics, respiratory parameters, and glucose metabolism throughout pregnancy and into the postpartum period (Table 55–1). Because these changes reach their peak late in the second trimester of pregnancy, hemodynamic deterioration in diseased or structurally abnormal hearts most often becomes clinically manifest at this time.

During normal pregnancy, plasma volume increases 40% to 50%, in part due to estrogen-mediated activation of the renin–aldosterone axis. Because red blood cell mass increases 20% to 30%, hemodilution contributes to an overall fall in hemoglobin concentration (i.e., the relative anemia of pregnancy). Cardiac output rises 30% to 50% above baseline. It peaks by the end of the second trimester and remains at a plateau until delivery. The change in cardiac output is mediated by (a) increased preload due to the rise in blood volume, (b) reduced afterload due to a fall in systemic vascular resistance, and (c) a rise in the maternal heart rate by 10 to 15 beats/min. Stroke volume begins to rise by 5 weeks' gestation and peaks by 31 weeks. In the third trimester, caval compression by the gravid uterus causes stroke volume to fall slightly. However, a compensatory rise in heart rate allows maintenance of cardiac output. The direct effect of pregnancy on cardiac contractility is controversial. Blood pressure typically falls to 10 mm Hg below baseline by the end of the second trimester, as a result of a fall in systemic vascular resistance induced by hormonal changes and by the addition of low-resistance vessels in the uteroplacental bed.

During labor and delivery, wide hemodynamic swings add further stress to the cardiovascular system. Each uterine contraction displaces 300 to 500 mL of blood into the general circulation. As a result, cardiac output can increase up to 75% over baseline during labor. Mean systemic pressure rises from maternal pain and anxiety. During delivery, blood loss (300 to 400 mL for a vaginal delivery and 500 to 800 mL for a cesarean section) can further compromise the hemodynamic state.

During the postpartum period, cardiovascular hemodynamics are altered once again by the relief of vena caval compression. The increase in venous return augments preload and cardiac output, resulting in an increase in renal blood flow and a brisk diuresis. Cardiovascular homeostasis is restored to the prepregnant baseline within 3 to 4 weeks following delivery.

Pregnancy induces marked changes in respiratory parameters (2). The gravid uterus gradually limits diaphragmatic excursion, resulting in reductions in total lung capacity and functional residual capacity. These

**TABLE 55–1**
**NORMAL CHANGES IN HEMODYNAMIC, RESPIRATORY, AND METABOLIC PARAMETERS DURING PREGNANCY**

| Hemodynamic Parameter | Change During Pregnancy | Change During Labor and Delivery | Change Postpartum |
|---|---|---|---|
| Blood volume | ↑↑ | ↑ further | ↓ to baseline |
| Heart rate | ↑ | ↑ further | ↓ to baseline |
| Cardiac output | ↑ | ↑ further | ↑ initially, then ↓ |
| Blood pressure | ↓ | ↑ | ↓ to baseline |
| Stroke volume | ↑ 1st and 2nd trimester<br>↓ 3rd trimester | ↑ | ↓ to baseline |
| Systemic vascular resistance | ↓ | ↑ | ↓ to baseline |
| **Respiratory Parameter** | **Change During Normal Pregnancy by 7–9 mo** | | |
| Thoracic cage | Upward displacement of diaphragm, increase in anteroposterior and transverse diameters | | |
| TLC | ↓ by 4–5% | | |
| FRC | ↓ by 20% | | |
| DLCO | ↔ | | |
| Minute ventilation | ↑ 50% | | |
| Tidal volume | ↑ 50% | | |
| Respiratory rate | ↔ | | |
| **Glucose Metabolism** | **1st Trimester Normal Pregnancy** | **2nd & 3rd Trimester Normal Pregnancy** | |
| Insulin sensitivity | Normal | ↓ | |
| Insulin secretion | ↑ | ↑↑ | |
| Fasting plasma glucose | ↔ | ↓ | |

changes are countered by hormonally induced increases in airway dilatation. In addition, minute ventilation increases 45% via an increase in tidal volume.

Pregnancy is also characterized by a complex series of hormonal and metabolic changes that govern glucose regulation (3). Typically, a state of maternal insulin resistance develops during the second and third trimesters. Insulin resistance is a physiologic response that favors a shift in the glucose supply to the fetus. In normal women, however, insulin resistance is countered by a steady increase in basal insulin secretion and a marked increase in insulin secretion immediately after a glucose load (first phase). In contrast, women with gestational diabetes exhibit impaired pancreatic $\beta$-cell secretory function and demonstrate a blunted first-phase insulin secretion response to glucose loading. The cardiovascular consequences of gestational diabetes can be profound, for both the mother and the fetus.

Normal pregnancy is associated with several signs and symptoms that can mimic cardiac dysfunction (4). Fatigue, dyspnea, and decreased exercise capacity are common. Pregnant women usually have peripheral edema, lateral displacement of the point of maximum impulse, and jugular venous distension. Most pregnant women have audible physiologic systolic murmurs, created by augmented blood flow. A physiologic third heart sound (S3) can often be appreciated. Signs and symptoms that are unusual during normal pregnancy and may signal true cardiac abnormalities include chest pain, orthopnea or paroxysmal octurnal dyspnea, pulmonary edema, a fourth heart sound, and ventricular arrhythmis.

## ASSESSMENT OF RISK IN PATIENTS WITH PRE-EXISTING CARDIAC DISEASE

### Maternal and Fetal Outcomes

Whenever possible, women with known pre-existing cardiac lesions should receive preconception counseling. In particular, they should be given information about contraception, potential maternal and fetal risks during pregnancy, and possible long-term morbidity and mortality after pregnancy. Women with particular cardiac risk factors should be cautioned against pregnancy. For example, women with New York Heart Association (NYHA) Class III and IV symptoms who become pregnant face a mortality rate of >7% and a morbidity rate of >30%. Recently, a risk score, composed of five factors, was found to be predictive of maternal cardiac complications (Table 55–2) (5). Each risk factor was assigned a value of one point. The maternal cardiac event rate associated with 0, 1, and >1 points was 3%, 30%, and 66%, respectively. Newborns whose mothers had NYHA Class II or greater symptoms suffered worse neonatal outcomes.

Although such scores serve as an overall assessment of risk, prepregnancy counseling should be tailored according to specific cardiac lesions. In the following section,

**TABLE 55–2**
**PREDICTORS OF MATERNAL RISK FOR CARDIAC COMPLICATIONS**

| Criterion | Example | Points[a] |
|---|---|---|
| Prior cardiac event[a] | Heart failure, transient ischemic attack, stroke before present pregnancy | 1 |
| Prior arrhythmia | Symptomatic sustained tachyarrhythmia or bradyarrhythmia requiring treatment | 1 |
| NYHA Class III–IV *or* cyanosis | — | 1 |
| Valvular and outflow tract obstruction | Aortic valve area <1.5 cm$^2$, mitral valve area <2 cm$^2$, or left ventricular outflow tract peak gradient >30 mm Hg | 1 |
| Myocardial dysfunction | LVEF <40% or restrictive cardiomyopathy or hypertrophic cardiomyopathy | 1 |

[a]Maternal cardiac event rate for 0, 1, and >1 point is 0%, 30%, and 66%, respectively.
*Source:* Siu SC, Sermer M, Colman JM, et al. Prospective multicenter study of pregnancy outcomes in women with heart disease. *Circulation.* 2001;104:515–521.
LVEF, left ventricular ejection fraction.

congenital and acquired cardiac lesions are classified as low, intermediate, or high risk (Table 55–3) (6).

## Specific Congenital or Acquired Cardiac Lesions

### *Low-Risk Lesions*

#### Atrial Septal Defect

Ostium secundum atrial septal defect (ASD), the most common congenital cardiac lesion encountered during pregnancy, is usually well tolerated (1). An uncorrected ASD does carry a small increased risk of paradoxical embolism. With advancing maternal age (especially >40 years), uncomplicated ASD may be accompanied by a higher incidence of supraventricular arrhythmias (e.g., atrial fibrillation or atrial flutter). Although it is unusual for secundum ASD to cause pulmonary hypertension during the childbearing years, the presence of pulmonary hypertension substantially increases the risk of cardiac complications during pregnancy. A secundum ASD that has been

**TABLE 55–3**
**MATERNAL CARDIAC LESIONS AND RISK OF CARDIAC COMPLICATIONS DURING PREGNANCY**

| Lesion | Low Risk | Intermediate Risk | High Risk |
|---|---|---|---|
| Left-to-right shunt | ASD; VSD; PDA | Large left-to-right shunt | |
| AS | Asymptomatic AS with low mean gradient (<50 mm Hg) and normal LV function (EF >50%) | Mild to moderate AS | Severe AS, with or without symptoms; LVEF <40% |
| MS | Mild/moderate MS (MVA >1.5 cm$^2$, mean gradient <5 mm Hg) without severe pulmonary hypertension | Moderate/severe MS | MS with NYHA Class II–IV symptoms; LVEF <40% |
| AR | AR with normal LV function and NYHA Class I or II | — | AR with NYHA Class III–IV symptoms or LVEF <40% |
| MR | MR with normal LV function and NYHA Class I or II | — | MR with NYHA Class III–IV symptoms or LVEF <40% |
| Cyanotic congenital heart disease | Repaired acyanotic congenital heart disease without residual cardiac dysfunction | — | Complex cyanotic heart disease (TOF, Ebstein anomaly, TA, TGA, tricuspid atresia) |
| Peripartum cardiomyopathy | — | — | Prior peripartum cardiomyopathy with or without persistent LV dysfunction |
| Marfan syndrome | — | Normal aortic root | Aortic root or valve involvement |
| Pulmonary hypertension | — | — | Severe pulmonary hypertension or Eisenmenger syndrome |
| Mechanical prosthetic valve | — | — | Requiring anticoagulation |

AS, aortic stenosis; LV, left ventricle; EF, ejection fraction; AR, aortic regurgitation; NYHA, New York Heart Association; MVP, mitral valve prolapse; MS, mitral stenosis; MVA, mitral valve area; PS, pulmonary stenosis; TOF, tetralogy of Fallot; TA, truncus arteriosus; TGA, transposition of the great arteries.

repaired prior to pregnancy is not associated with any increased risk of cardiac complications. Antibiotic prophylaxis for infective endocarditis is not required (or indicated) prior to delivery.

### Ventricular Septal Defect

Isolated ventricular septal defect (VSD) is also a low-risk lesion that is usually well tolerated during pregnancy. However, VSD accompanied by pulmonary hypertension and/or Eisenmenger syndrome carries a high risk for cardiac complications. VSD can occur in conjunction with other congenital cardiac lesions, including ASD, patent ductus arteriosus, mitral regurgitation, and transposition of the great arteries. The risk associated with a VSD that was repaired prior to the development of pulmonary hypertension is negligible. Antibiotic prophylaxis is recommended at the time of labor and delivery because the turbulent blood flow across a VSD is associated with increased risk for infective endocarditis.

### Patent Ductus Arteriosus

The presence of a patent ductus arteriosus (PDA) during pregnancy is not associated with additional maternal risk, provided that the shunt is small to moderate and that the pulmonary artery pressures are normal. PDAs are usually corrected by either catheter-based closure or surgical ligation. Following repair, women are at no additional risk for complications during pregnancy. Antibiotic prophylaxis is not recommended during labor and delivery in patients who are ≥6 months after repair and who have no evidence of residual shunting on echocardiography.

### Mitral Valve Prolapse

In isolation, mitral valve prolapse (MVP) rarely causes any difficulties during pregnancy. However, MVP accompanied by mitral regurgitation can cause turbulent flow across the mitral valve. Therefore, antibiotic prophylaxis should be administered during labor and delivery.

### Mitral Regurgitation

Chronic regurgitant lesions are generally well tolerated during pregnancy. In chronic mitral regurgitation, the physiologic reduction in SVR partially compensates for the additional volume overload generated by the regurgitant valve. However, the development of new atrial fibrillation or severe hypertension can upset this balance and precipitate hemodynamic deterioration. In contrast, acute mitral regurgitation (e.g., from rupture of chordae tendineae) is not well tolerated and can produce flash pulmonary edema and/or life-threatening cardiac decompensation.

The most common causes of mitral regurgitation are rheumatic heart disease and myxomatous degeneration. Hypertrophic cardiomyopathy and mitral annular dilatation secondary to dilated cardiomyopathy can also result in mitral regurgitation.

Women with pre-existing severe mitral regurgitation may develop symptoms of congestive heart failure during pregnancy, especially during the third trimester. In general, these symptoms can be managed medically with judicious use of diuretics and afterload-reducing agents. Nitrates and dihydropyridine calcium channel blocking agents can serve as relatively safe afterload-reducing agents in pregnant women. Angiotensin-converting enzyme (ACE) inhibitors and angiotensin-receptor blockers (ARBs) are strictly contraindicated during pregnancy. Although hydralazine has been used safely during the third trimester for treatment of pre-eclampsia, its use during the first and second trimesters as an afterload-reducing agent is controversial (6). Women with severe symptomatic mitral regurgitation prior to pregnancy may consider operative repair prior to conception. Although repair is strongly preferred to valve replacement before pregnancy, the success of operative repair is dependent on suitable valve anatomy.

### Aortic Regurgitation

Like chronic mitral regurgitation, chronic aortic regurgitation is also generally well tolerated during pregnancy. In addition to the physiologic fall in systemic vascular resistance, the tachycardia of pregnancy shortens diastole and reduces the aortic regurgitant fraction. Aortic regurgitation may be encountered in women with rheumatic heart disease, a congenitally bicuspid or deformed aortic valve, infective endocarditis, or connective tissue disease (e.g., systemic lupus erythematosus or rheumatoid arthritis). Hormonal effects on the aortic wall during pregnancy render women with bicuspid aortic valves at increased risk for aortic dissection during pregnancy (7). Signs or symptoms of this serious complication should be evaluated expeditiously.

Similar to mitral regurgitation, severe aortic regurgitation generally can be managed medically during pregnancy with use of diuretics and afterload-reducing agents. Operative repair prior to pregnancy is feasible in certain patients, especially when the valve is anatomically bicuspid. However, the long-term durability of repair may not be superior to valve replacement (8). During pregnancy, surgical intervention for both mitral and aortic regurgitation is usually performed only for refractory congestive heart failure, which is a rare occurrence. Antibiotic prophylaxis is recommended for both types of lesions during labor and delivery.

### Pulmonary Stenosis

As an isolated lesion, pulmonic stenosis is well tolerated during pregnancy. Severe, symptomatic pulmonary stenosis may be treated with percutaneous pulmonary valvuloplasty prior to conception. If necessary during pregnancy, percutaneous pulmonary valvuloplasty should be delayed until after the first trimester in order to avoid fetal radiation exposure during the early developmental period.

Pulmonary stenosis frequently coexists with other congenital cardiac lesions that may cause cyanotic heart disease.

### Moderate-Risk Lesions

#### Mitral Stenosis

Mitral stenosis in women of childbearing age is most often rheumatic in origin. Hemodynamic deterioration during the third trimester and/or during labor and delivery is common in women with moderate to severe mitral stenosis. Patients with a mitral valve area $<1.5$ cm$^2$ face a substantial risk of congestive heart failure, cardiac arrhythmia, and/or intrauterine growth retardation during pregnancy (9). Increased blood volume and heart rate during pregnancy lead to an elevation of left atrial pressure, which can result in pulmonary edema formation. Additional displacement of blood volume into the systemic circulation during uterine contractions makes labor particularly hazardous.

Mitral stenosis requires close and regular follow-up during pregnancy. Echocardiography should be performed at the end of the first and second trimesters, and monthly during the third trimester. Medical therapy is indicated in patients who develop symptoms or who have evidence of pulmonary hypertension (estimated pulmonary artery pressure $\geq$50 mm Hg) on echocardiography (6). Beta-blockers and diuretics should be used to control signs and symptoms of pulmonary congestion and to maintain the estimated pulmonary artery pressure $<$50 mm Hg.

Although mild mitral stenosis can often be managed with conservative medical therapy during pregnancy, patients with moderate to severe mitral stenosis should consider correction prior to conception. When pregnancy has already occurred and medical therapy is insufficient to control severe symptomatic mitral stenosis, repair of the valve during pregnancy may be necessary. Percutaneous mitral balloon valvuloplasty (PMBV) is the therapeutic option of choice. Its safety and feasibility during pregnancy have been well established (10). Radiation exposure to the fetus is minimized by abdominal lead shielding, use of transesophageal echocardiographic guidance, and omission of invasive hemodynamic measurements and angiography. When PMBV cannot be performed, open surgical comissurotomy is the preferred surgical correction. Although this procedure is considered safe for the mother, it carries a 2% to 12% risk of fetal mortality. Cardiopulmonary bypass during pregnancy should be performed with normothermic perfusion and high flow volumes, to reduce fetal morbidity and mortality. Women past 20 weeks' gestation should be positioned in the lateral decubitus position during surgery, to avoid uterine compression of the inferior vena cava during surgery. If possible, hyperkalemic arrest should be avoided, because of the potential for hyperkalemic arrest solutions to reach the fetal circulation (11).

The combination of atrial fibrillation and mitral stenosis in the pregnant patient may result in a rapid rise in left atrial pressure and a reduction in forward cardiac output. Clinically, pregnant patients with mitral stenosis and new-onset atrial fibrillation may present with signs and symptoms of decompensated heart failure. Treatment consists of heart rate control with digoxin and beta-blockers plus gentle reduction of blood volume and left atrial pressure with diuretics. Hemodynamic deterioration is an indication for electrocardioversion, which can be performed safely during pregnancy. The development of atrial fibrillation is an indication for the initiation of anticoagulation. The modes of anticoagulation during pregnancy are discussed in greater detail in the section, "Anticoagulation during Pregnancy."

Most patients with mitral stenosis can undergo vaginal delivery. However, hemodynamic monitoring with a Swan–Ganz catheter during labor, delivery, and for several hours into the postpartum period is advisable in patients with symptoms of congestive heart failure or with moderate to severe mitral stenosis. In these patients, epidural anesthesia during labor and delivery is usually better tolerated than general anesthesia. Antibiotic prophylaxis is recommended during labor and delivery.

#### Aortic Stenosis

The most common etiology of aortic stenosis in women of childbearing age is a congenitally bicuspid valve. Other, less common etiologies include rheumatic heart disease, calcific valvular disease, and a unicuspid aortic valve. Mild to moderate aortic stenosis with preserved left ventricular function usually is well tolerated during pregnancy. Severe aortic stenosis (aortic valve area $<1.0$ cm$^2$, mean gradient $>$50 mm Hg), in contrast, significantly increases the risk of pregnancy. Classic symptoms of aortic stenosis such as dyspnea, angina pectoris, or syncope usually become apparent late in the second trimester or early in the third trimester.

Ideally, women with known severe aortic stenosis (mean pressure gradient $>$50 mm Hg) should undergo valve correction prior to conception. Although percutaneous aortic balloon valvuloplasty (PABV) prior to pregnancy can decrease the risk of pregnancy, labor, and delivery, it has limited durability and is unlikely to relieve aortic stenosis long term (12). Therefore, surgical correction is the preferred approach. In contrast to regurgitant valves, stenotic bicuspid aortic valves are usually calcified by age 20 to 30 years and require valve replacement.

Bioprosthetic valves have limited durability; young patients will likely require reoperation in several years. However, implantation of a bioprosthetic valve avoids the need for anticoagulation during pregnancy. Mechanical valves have greater durability but require anticoagulation, which independently increases both the maternal and fetal complication risk during pregnancy. The decision to undergo replacement with a bioprosthetic valve versus a mechanical valve is not simple and should be made in consultation with both a cardiologist and a cardiothoracic surgeon.

Management of mild to moderate aortic stenosis during pregnancy is largely conservative. When severe symptomatic aortic stenosis is diagnosed during pregnancy, PABV should be performed prior to the demands of labor and delivery. Aortic insufficiency that occurs as a postprocedural complication of PABV usually is well tolerated during labor and delivery. Vaginal or assisted vaginal delivery is usually well tolerated, although spinal and epidural anesthesia are discouraged during labor and delivery because of their vasodilatory effects. As with mitral stenosis, invasive hemodynamic monitoring and antibiotic prophylaxis are recommended during labor and delivery.

#### Coarctation of the Aorta

Coarctation of the aorta is a stenosis that can develop just distal to the origin of the left subclavian artery at the ligamentum arteriosum. Coarctation is well tolerated during pregnancy, although hypertension, congestive heart failure, angina, and aortic dissection are possible complications. Coarctation can be associated with intracerebral aneurysms, which can rupture during pregnancy. Hypotension in vascular beds distal to the coarctation can compromise uteroplacental blood flow, resulting in intrauterine growth retardation. Coarctation of the aorta is often associated with a congenitally bicuspid aortic valve, which increases the risk of infective endocarditis. Antibiotic prophylaxis is indicated during labor and delivery.

If at all possible, coarctation of the aorta should be corrected prior to pregnancy with standard surgical repair or balloon angioplasty with endovascular stent placement. Correction of coarctation during pregnancy is indicated in patients with severe uncontrollable hypertension, heart failure, or uterine hypoperfusion. The aortic wall adjacent to an area of coarctation has histologic features of cystic medial necrosis, which renders it vulnerable to dissection. Thus, women who underwent surgical repair of an aortic coarction in childhood remain at risk for complications during pregnancy.

#### Marfan Syndrome

Marfan syndrome is a connective tissue disorder resulting from mutations in the fibrillin gene that are inherited in an autosomal dominant fashion (i.e., 50% of offspring will inherit the disorder, regardless of gender). Thus, women with Marfan syndrome should receive genetic counseling well in advance of pregnancy consideration. The clinical manifestations of Marfan syndrome include skeletal abnormalities, ectopia lentis, and cardiovascular abnormalities, such as aortic root dilatation with or without aortic regurgitation, aortic dissection, and mitral valve prolapse. However, Marfan syndrome is a heterogeneous disorder with highly variable disease penetrance.

It is estimated that pregnancy in patients with Marfan syndrome carries a 1% risk of fatal complications; this risk rises with increasing aortic root dimensions. Women with Marfan syndrome are more vulnerable to aortic dissection and/or rupture during pregnancy because of the additional weakness in the aortic wall imposed by hormonal changes. In addition, women with Marfan syndrome may be more prone to spontaneous abortion and preterm labor (13).

Screening echocardiography should be performed prior to pregnancy. Enlargement of the aortic root $>4.0$ cm increases the risk of aortic dissection and/or rupture from moderate to high. Elective repair of the aortic root prior to conception is advised with a root dimension $\geq 4.5$ cm. The aortic root should be monitored by serial echocardiography throughout pregnancy; progressive dilatation may warrant termination of pregnancy and timely aortic repair or replacement.

Medical management involves the use of beta-blockers throughout pregnancy to reduce the risk of aortic rupture, careful control of blood pressure, and consideration of general anesthesia and cesarean section at the time of delivery to maximize hemodynamic control. Women with Marfan syndrome who do not manifest any cardiac abnormalities have a low rate of complications and can usually tolerate a normal vaginal delivery. Spinal or epidural anesthesia is advised, to minimize the pain and stress of labor. Antibiotic prophylaxis is recommended when significant valvular abnormalities are present.

### *High-Risk Lesions*

#### Eisenmenger Syndrome

The Eisenmenger syndrome occurs in the setting of uncorrected long-standing left-to-right shunts. Over time, pulmonary artery pressures approach and can exceed systemic pressures, resulting in reversal of the shunt flow direction from right to left and cyanosis. Eisenmenger syndrome is a possible common endpoint of multiple congenital lesions, including ASD, VSD, and PDA. Maternal mortality in women with Eisenmenger syndrome ranges from 30% to 50% percent. Mortality is frequently caused by complications of thromboembolic disease. Decompensation occurs most frequently during the first week after delivery. Fetal risk due to maternal hypoxemia is substantial, with a high incidence of fetal loss, premature delivery, intrauterine growth retardation, and perinatal death.

Because of the considerable risk to both the mother and the fetus, pregnancy is not advised for women with Eisenmenger syndrome. If pregnancy should occur, therapeutic abortion is recommended. Women who choose to continue with pregnancy are advised to restrict physical activity. Anticoagulation is recommended during the third trimester and for 4 weeks after delivery, to reduce the risk of thromboembolic complications. Vaginal delivery, facilitated by vacuum or low forceps extraction, is the delivery method of choice. Cesarean delivery is associated with a substantially higher mortality than the vaginal route. Anesthetic management includes maintenance of adequate systemic vascular resistance (SVR) and intravenous volume and prevention of sudden increases in pulmonary vascular resistance (PVR).

#### Complex Cyanotic Congenital Heart Disease

More women born with cyanotic congenital heart disease are surviving to childbearing age. In general, pregnancy is not recommended for women with uncorrected lesions. The most common cyanotic congenital defect is tetralogy of Fallot, which is characterized by a VSD, pulmonic stenosis, right ventricular outflow tract obstruction, and an overriding aorta. Women with tetralogy of Fallot who have undergone successful repair during childhood may tolerate pregnancy well, provided that they have little or no residual right ventricular outflow tract gradient, no pulmonary hypertension, and preserved ventricular function. Ebstein anomaly, characterized by abnormal right ventricular function, apical displacement of the tricuspid valve septal leaflet, and tricuspid regurgitation, is often associated with the Wolf–Parkinson–White syndrome. Pregnancy can precipitate supraventricular arrhythmias that may be rapidly conducted over the accessory pathway. Surgical correction reduces the maternal risk of pregnancy, but does not reduce the risk of congenital anomalies in the fetus. Experience during pregnancy in women with surgically corrected D-transposition of the great arteries, truncus arteriosus, or tricuspid atresia is limited.

#### Cardiomyopathy

Peripartum cardiomyopathy is discussed further in the following section. However, it should be noted that women with a history of prior peripartum cardiomyopathy should be counseled against subsequent pregnancy because of the high maternal mortality. Hypertrophic cardiomyopathy (HCM) is associated with increased maternal morbidity and mortality. Although an increase in blood volume helps to reduce intracavitary or left ventricular outflow tract gradients, tachycardia and a reduction in SVR can exacerbate outflow tract obstruction. Avoidance of volume depletion helps to prevent hemodynamic deterioration in these patients. Vaginal delivery is usually well tolerated. Whenever possible, women should receive genetic counseling prior to conception, because for certain forms of HCM the risk of inheriting the disease may approach 50%.

## CARDIOVASCULAR DISORDERS ACQUIRED DURING OR AFTER PREGNANCY

### Peripartum Cardiomyopathy

Peripartum cardiomyopathy (PPCM) is defined as the development of idiopathic left ventricular systolic dysfunction (demonstrated by echocardiography) in the interval between the last month of pregnancy up to the first 5 months postpartum in women without pre-existing cardiac dysfunction. The incidence of PPCM in the United States is estimated to be 1 in 3,000 to 1 in 4,000 live births; the incidence is thought to be higher in other parts of the world, such as Africa and Haiti. The true cause of PPCM is unknown. However, the following risk factors for PPCM have been proposed: age >30 years, multiparity, multiple fetuses, history of pre-eclampsia, eclampsia, or postpartum hypertension, African descent, history of maternal cocaine abuse, or selenium deficiency (14).

Medical therapy for PPCM is similar to therapy for cardiomyopathies of other etiologies. Digoxin and diuretics may be used safely during pregnancy and while breastfeeding. Beta-blockers may improve left ventricular function and outcomes in patients with cardiomyopathy (15). Beta-blockers are considered safe during pregnancy, although there have been case reports of fetal bradycardia and growth retardation. ACE inhibitors and angiotensin-receptor blockers are strictly contraindicated because of adverse neonatal effects. Hydralazine is an effective afterload-reducing agent, although it is currently is listed as a Category C agent (adequate and well-controlled studies in pregnant patients are lacking, and it should be used only when the expected benefit outweighs the potential risk to the fetus). Anticoagulation with warfarin may be considered after the first 12 weeks of gestation in select patients with severe left ventricular dilatation and dysfunction. When conventional medical therapy is not successful, women with PPCM may ultimately require cardiac transplantation.

The prognosis after development of PPCM is variable. Fifty to sixty percent of women recover completely normal heart size and function, usually within 6 months of delivery. The remainder either experience stable left ventricular dysfunction or continue to experience clinical deterioration. One third of women with PPCM eventually undergo cardiac transplantation. Estimated maternal mortality ranges from 10% to 50%. Women with PPCM who attempt a subsequent pregnancy face a high risk of complications, including deterioration of left ventricular function, symptomatic congestive heart failure, and death. Consequently, they should be counseled *against* subsequent pregnancies, even if the ventricular function normalizes after the initial pregnancy (16).

### Hypertension in Pregnancy

Hypertension during pregnancy can be classified into three main categories: chronic hypertension, gestational hypertension, and pre-eclampsia, with or without pre-existing hypertension. Hypertensive disorders can complicate 12% to 22% of pregnancies and are a major cause of maternal morbidity and mortality.

Chronic hypertension is defined as blood pressure ≥140/90 mm Hg present prior to pregnancy, before the 20th week of gestation, or persisting beyond the 42nd postpartum day. Drug therapy for diastolic blood pressure ≥110 mm Hg has been shown to reduce the risk of stroke and cardiovascular complications. Options for drug therapy are shown in Table 55–4.

Gestational hypertension is defined as hypertension that (a) develops in the latter part of gestation, (b) is not associated with proteinuria or other features of pre-eclampsia, and (c) resolves by 12 weeks postpartum. This condition may portend the future development of chronic hypertension, but is otherwise associated with good maternal and fetal outcomes.

**TABLE 55–4**
**DRUG THERAPY FOR MILD TO MODERATE CHRONIC HYPERTENSION IN PREGNANCY**

| Drug Class | Example | Fetal Risk | Breastfeeding | Risk Class[a] |
|---|---|---|---|---|
| | | **First-Line Agents** | | |
| $\alpha_2$-Adrenergic blockers | Methyldopa | Most commonly used. Drug of choice. Longest safety track record. Avoid in women with prior history of depression. | Safe. | C |
| | | **Second-Line Agents** | | |
| Calcium channel blockers | Nifedipine | Avoid sublingual nifedipine (minimize sudden hypotension). Good safety data. | Compatible. | C |
| | Amlodipine | Has been used effectively, but safety data are lacking. | No data. | C |
| Arteriolar vasodilators | Hydralazine | Possible associations: (a) first-trimester use and hypospadias; (b) third-trimester use and neonatal thrombocytopenia; (c) maternal and neonatal lupuslike syndrome; (d) more maternal hypotension and lower 1-min Apgar scores compared to labetolol or nifedipine (17). | Safe. | C |
| Beta-blockers | Atenolol Metoprolol | Associated with intrauterine growth retardation and newborn bradycardia. | Not recommended because of newborn bradycardia. | C/D |
| $\alpha,\beta$-Blockers | Labetolol | Associated with intrauterine growth retardation and newborn bradycardia. May induce fetal lung maturation. | Safe, but infants should be observed for bradycardia. | C/D |
| Thiazide diuretics | Hydrochlorothiazide | Associated with neonatal hypoglycemia, thrombocytopenia, hemolytic anemia, and with maternal electrolyte disturbances. | Safe, but may suppress lactation. | D |
| | | **Drug Classes to Avoid** | | |
| Angiotensin-converting enzyme (ACE) inhibitors | Captopril Lisinopril | Second- and third-trimester use causes prematurity, intrauterine growth retardation, renal tubular dysplasia and neonatal anuria, severe oligohydramnios, lung and skull hypoplasia, limb contractures, neonatal hypotension. | No data. | D |
| Angiotensin-receptor blockers (ARBs) | Losartan Valsartan | No human data, but potentially associated with fetal renal and skull defects, neonatal hypotension and anuria. | No data. | D |

[a]Risk Class C: Either studies in animals have revealed adverse effects on the fetus and there are no controlled studies in women, or studies in women are not available. Drug should be given only if the potential benefit justifies the potential risk to the fetus. Risk Class D: There is positive evidence of human fetal risk, but the benefits from use in pregnant women may be acceptable despite the risk.

Pre-eclampsia occurs in 3% to 8% of pregnancies in the United States. The classic clinical triad involves gradual onset of hypertension, proteinuria (>300 mg in 24 hours), and edema. Symptoms usually begin in the third trimester and resolve with delivery. The etiology of pre-eclampsia is still unclear. Eclampsia is the development of grand mal seizures in a woman with pre-eclampsia.

Untreated pre-eclampsia is a risk to both the fetus and the mother. When pre-eclampsia is accompanied by risk factors, including seizures, severe hypertension, HELLP syndrome (hemolysis, elevated liver enzymes, low platelets), placental abruption, cerebral hemorrhage, pulmonary edema, renal failure, or liver failure, the fetus must be delivered immediately. Antihypertensive agents are usually initiated after the diastolic blood pressure exceeds 105 mm Hg and the systolic pressure is > 160 to 180 mm Hg. Labetolol, nifedipine, and methyldopa are first-line agents in the treatment of hypertension in pregnant women. Calcium channel blockers, such as amlodipine, are also used. A meta-analysis of trials that compared hydralazine to labetolol or nifedipine found that more maternal and neonatal side effects were associated with hydralazine use (17). Although these results require confirmation in clinical trials, the authors concluded that hydralazine might not be an optimal first-line antihypertensive agent in pregnant women. Hypertension due to pre-eclampsia typically improves within a few days of delivery and should return to baseline by 12 weeks following delivery.

### Coronary Artery Disease

Coronary heart disease during pregnancy is rare, occurring in 0.01% of pregnancies. Most myocardial infarctions occur during the third trimester in women over age 33 years who have had multiple prior pregnancies. Coronary spasm, *in situ* coronary thrombosis, and coronary dissection are possible etiologies of myocardial infarction (in addition to classic obstructive atherosclerosis) (18). Acute myocardial infarction may be the initial clinical manifestation of an underlying hypercoagulable state, such as the antiphospholipid antibody syndrome. The diagnosis and management of acute myocardial infarction in the pregnant patient should follow established guidelines.

Therapy for acute myocardial infarction must be modified in the pregnant patient. Thrombolytic agents increase the risk of maternal hemorrhage substantially (8%). Cardiac catheterization and primary percutaneous intervention must be performed with lead shielding of the patient's abdomen. Medications that are considered generally safe include low-dose aspirin, nitrates, beta-blockers, and short-term heparin. ACE inhibitors and statins are contraindicated during pregnancy.

### Arrhythmias in Pregnancy

The most frequent rhythm disturbances during pregnancy are premature atrial and/or ventricular complexes. They are not associated with adverse maternal or fetal outcomes and do not warrant antiarrhythmic drug therapy. Atrial fibrillation and atrial flutter are not common during pregnancy and can be treated with rate-controlling agents, such as beta-blockers or digitalis, or direct-current cardioversion, which can be performed safely during any stage of pregnancy. Anticoagulation is recommended for chronic atrial fibrillation in the setting of underlying structural heart disease. Atrioventricular nodal re-entrant tachycardia (AVNRT), the most common supraventricular arrhythmia in pregnant women, can be treated with adenosine and/or beta-blockers.

Ventricular tachycardia is rare during pregnancy. However, it may be seen in the setting of underlying peripartum cardiomyopathy, thyrotoxicosis, or hyperemesis gravidarum. Most antiarrhythmic medications used to treat ventricular tachycardia are safe during pregnancy.

Bradyarrhythmias are uncommon during pregnancy. Pacemaker support is recommended only if the escape rhythm has an intraventricular conduction delay, the bradyarrhythmia is symptomatic, or there is hemodynamic deterioration.

Commonly used antiarrhythmic cardiovascular drugs during pregnancy and their potential side effects are shown in Table 55-5.

### Abnormal Glucose Regulation during Pregnancy

In normal pregnancy, hormonally induced insulin resistance is countered by a compensatory increase in insulin secretion. Inadequate compensation caused by dysfunction of $\beta$ cells in the pancreas likely contributes to the development of gestational diabetes. Women who develop gestational diabetes prior to the 24th week of pregnancy face an 80% chance of developing type 2 diabetes mellitus within 5 years. Moreover, women who develop gestational diabetes have a greater risk of hypertension, hyperlipidemia, electrocardiographic abnormalities, and overall mortality. Maternal hyperglycemia is associated with an increase in fetal and neonatal morbidity, including macrosomia, congenital malformations, fetal hypertrophic cardiomyopathy, and neonatal hypoglycemia. Women diagnosed with gestational diabetes require close follow-up for primary prevention of type 2 diabetes, including dietary modification, maintenance of body weight control, and regular exercise. There is some evidence that insulin-sensitizing agents may reduce the rate of conversion from gestational diabetes to type 2 diabetes (3).

## ANTICOAGULATION DURING PREGNANCY

Several conditions require the initiation or the maintenance of anticoagulation during pregnancy, including mechanical prosthetic valves, hypercoagulable states, prior or current deep venous thrombosis, and Eisenmenger syndrome. The three most common agents considered for use during pregnancy are unfractionated heparin (UH), low-molecular-weight heparin (LMWH), and warfarin. The Seventh American College of Chest Physicians (ACCP) Consensus Conference on Antithrombotic Therapy recommended three potential strategies for anticoagulation during pregnancy (Table 55-6): (a) adjusted-dose LMWH administered twice daily throughout pregnancy, (b) adjusted-dose UH administered subcutaneously twice daily throughout pregnancy, or (c) UH or LMWH until the 13th week, warfarin from week 13 to week 35, and UH or LMWH from week 35 until delivery (19). Nevertheless, the choice

**TABLE 55–5**
**ANTIARRHYTHMIC DRUGS IN PREGNANCY**

| Drug | Use | Fetal Risks | Risk Class[a] | Use during Breastfeeding |
|---|---|---|---|---|
| Adenosine | SVT | None reported | C | No data |
| Amiodarone | SVT, VT | IUGR, prematurity, hypothyroidism | C | No data; not recommended |
| Beta-blockers | AF, atrial flutter, SVT, VT | Fetal bradycardia, IUGR | C first trimester; D second and third trimesters | Safe |
| Digoxin | AF, atrial flutter | Low birth weight<br>Prematurity | C | Safe |
| Flecainide | AF | ? Fetal death; limited data | C | Safe |
| Lidocaine | VT | Neonatal CNS depression | C | Safe |
| Procainamide | SVT, VT | None reported; limited data | C | Safe |
| Sotalol | AF, SVT, VT | Fetal bradycardia, IUGR | B first trimester; D second and third trimesters | Safe |

IUGR, intrauterine growth retardation; SVT, supraventricular tachycardia; VT, ventricular tachycardia; AF, atrial fibrillation; CNS, central nervous system.
[a]Risk Class B: Either animal reproduction studies have not demonstrated a fetal risk but there are no controlled studies in pregnant women, or animal reproduction studies have shown an adverse effect that was not confirmed in controlled studies in women in the first trimester (and there is no evidence of risk in later trimesters). Risk Class C: Either studies in animals have revealed adverse effects on the fetus and there are no controlled studies in women, or studies in women are not available. Drug should be given only if the potential benefit justifies the potential risk to the fetus. Risk Class D: There is positive evidence of human fetal risk, but the benefits from use in pregnant women may be acceptable despite the risk.

of anticoagulation regimens depends on the preferences of the patient and physician after consideration of the maternal and fetal risks associated with each drug.

Warfarin crosses the placental barrier freely and can result in warfarin embryopathy (abnormalities of fetal bone and cartilage formation). The risk of warfarin embryopathy has been estimated at 4% to 10%. The risk is reduced if the total daily dose is less than 5 mg (20). Although the highest-risk period is during the first trimester (weeks 6 to 12), warfarin use during the second and third trimesters has been associated with fetal central nervous system abnormalities, such as optic atrophy, microencephaly, mental retardation, spasticity, and hypotonia.

Unfractionated heparin (UH) does not cross the placenta and is considered safer for the fetus. Its use, however, has been associated with maternal osteoporosis, hemorrhage, thrombocytopenia and/or thrombosis (HITT syndrome), and a high incidence of thromboembolic events with older-generation mechanical valves. UH may be administered parenterally or subcutaneously throughout pregnancy. The appropriate subcutaneous dose of UH is based on a 6-hour postinjection activated partial thromboplastin time (aPTT) of 2.0 to 3.0 times the control level or an anti-Xa level of 0.35 to 0.70 U/mL. UH should be initiated in high doses (17,500 to 20,000 U subcutaneously every 12 hours). Parenteral infusions should be stopped 4 hours before cesarean sections. In the event of preterm labor, spontaneous hemorrhage, or significant bleeding during delivery, UH can be reversed with protamine sulfate.

**TABLE 56–6**
**ANTICOAGULATION STRATEGIES DURING PREGNANCY**

| Trimester 1 | Trimester 2 | Trimester 3 | Dosing | Monitoring |
|---|---|---|---|---|
| UH | UH | UH | Subcutaneous: BID with an initial dose of 17,500–20,000 U; intravenous drip | aPTT 2.0–3.0 times control 6 h postinjection; Xa level 0.35–0.70 U/mL |
| LMWH | LMWH | LMWH | Subcutaneous: BID | Xa level 1.0–1.2 U/mL 4 h postinjection |
| Wk 6–12: UH/LMWH | Warfarin | Warfarin up to wk 35, then UH or LMWH | UH and LMWH as above; Warfarin QD | UH and LMWH as above; Warfarin to goal INR 3.0 (range 2.5–3.5) |

UH, unfractionated heparin; LMWH, low-molecular-weight heparin; BID, twice daily; QD, once daily.

Low-molecular-weight heparin produces a more predictable anticoagulant response than UH and is less likely to cause HITT. Its effect on bone mineral density is unclear. LMWH can be administered subcutaneously and is dosed to achieve a 4-hour postinjection anti-Xa level of 1.0 to 1.2 U/mL. Although there are data to support the use of LMWH in pregnant women with deep venous thrombosis, data on the safety and efficacy of LMWH in pregnant patients with mechanical valve prostheses are controversial. In fact, a manufacturer of LMWH recently issued a warning regarding the safety of LMWH in patients with mechanical heart valves (21). Because of the small number of patients on which this warning was based, the true incidence of valve thrombosis in patients receiving LMWH during pregnancy is unclear. Furthermore, it is unclear whether inadequate dosing caused the reported failures of LMWH in pregnant patients with mechanical heart valves. Experience with these agents is still accruing.

Warfarin, UH, and LMWH can be administered safely to nursing mothers. Furthermore, low-dose aspirin (<150 mg/day) has been found to be safe during the second and third trimesters. In certain women with mechanical valves and high risk of thrombosis, the addition of low-dose aspirin to warfarin is advisable.

In summary, anticoagulation in the pregnant patient can be difficult because of the risk profile associated with each drug regimen. In planned pregnancies, a careful discussion about the risks and benefits of warfarin, UH, and LMWH will help the patient and physician to choose an anticoagulation strategy. Unplanned pregnancies are often diagnosed partway through the first trimester. It is advisable to stop warfarin when the pregnancy is discovered and to use UH or LMWH at least until the 12th week.

## REFERENCES


1. Klein LL, Galan HL. Cardiac disease in pregnancy. *Obstet Gynecol Clin North Am.* 2004;31:429–459, viii.
2. Tsen LC. Anesthetic management of the parturient with cardiac and diabetic diseases. *Clin Obstet Gynecol.* 2003;46:700–710.
3. Di Cianni G, Miccoli R, Volpe L, et al. Intermediate metabolism in normal pregnancy and in gestational diabetes. *Diabetes Metab Res Rev.* 2003;19:259–270.
4. Thorne SA. Pregnancy in heart disease. *Heart.* 2004;90:450–456.
5. Siu SC, Sermer M, Colman JM, et al. Prospective multicenter study of pregnancy outcomes in women with heart disease. *Circulation.* 2001;104:515–521.
6. Expert consensus document on management of cardiovascular diseases during pregnancy. *Eur Heart J.* 2003;24:761–781.
7. Immer FF, Bansi AG, Immer-Bansi AS, et al. Aortic dissection in pregnancy: analysis of risk factors and outcome. *Ann Thorac Surg.* 2003;76:309–314.
8. Davierwala PM, David TE, Armstrong S, Ivanov J. Aortic valve repair versus replacement in bicuspid aortic valve disease. *J Heart Valve Dis.* 2003;12:679–686; discussion 686.
9. Hameed A, Karaalp IS, Tummala PP, et al. The effect of valvular heart disease on maternal and fetal outcome of pregnancy. *J Am Coll Cardiol.* 2001;37:893–899.
10. de Souza JA, Martinez EE Jr, Ambrose JA, et al. Percutaneous balloon mitral valvuloplasty in comparison with open mitral valve commissurotomy for mitral stenosis during pregnancy. *J Am Coll Cardiol.* 2001;37:900–903.
11. Pomini F, Mercogliano D, Cavalletti C, et al. Cardiopulmonary bypass in pregnancy. *Ann Thorac Surg.* 1996;61:259–268.
12. Reich O, Tax P, Marek J, et al. Long term results of percutaneous balloon valvoplasty of congenital aortic stenosis: independent predictors of outcome. *Heart.* 2004;90:70–76.
13. Lalchandani S, Wingfield M. Pregnancy in women with Marfan syndrome. *Eur J Obstet Gynecol Reprod Biol.* 2003;110:125–130.
14. Tidswell M. Peripartum cardiomyopathy. *Crit Care Clin.* 2004;20:777–788, xi.
15. Lechat P, Packer M, Chalon S, et al. Clinical effects of beta-adrenergic blockade in chronic heart failure: a meta-analysis of double-blind, placebo-controlled, randomized trials. *Circulation.* 1998;98:1184–1191.
16. Elkayam U, Tummala PP, Rao K, et al. Maternal and fetal outcomes of subsequent pregnancies in women with peripartum cardiomyopathy. *N Engl J Med.* 2001;344:1567–1571.
17. Magee LA, Cham C, Waterman EJ, et al. Hydralazine for treatment of severe hypertension in pregnancy: meta-analysis. *Br Med J.* 2003;327:955–960.
18. Esinler I, Yigit N, Ayhan A, et al. Coronary artery dissection during pregnancy. *Acta Obstet Gynecol Scand.* 2003;82:194–196.
19. Bates SM, Greer IA, Hirsh J, Ginsberg JS. Use of antithrombotic agents during pregnancy: the Seventh ACCP Conference on Antithrombotic and Thrombolytic Therapy. *Chest.* 2004;126:627S–644S.
20. Cotrufo M, DeFeo M, De Santo LS, et al. Risk of warfarin during pregnancy with mechanical valve prostheses. *Obstet Gynecol.* 2002;99:35–40.
21. Lovenox Injection (package insert). Bridgewater, NJ: Aventis Pharmaceuticals; 2004.


## QUESTIONS

(Adapted from the syllabus of The Cleveland Clinic Intensive Review of Medicine, Drs. Raymond and Maroo, year 2005.)

**1.** All of the following lesions are contraindications to pregnancy *except:*

a. Primary and secondary pulmonary hypertension
b. Shunt lesions complicated by Eisenmenger syndrome
c. Mild to moderate mitral stenosis
d. Complex cyanotic congenital heart disease
e. Diminished residual left ventricular function (ejection fraction <50%)

Answer is c: Listed in this question are four clear contraindications to pregnancy, including primary and secondary pulmonary hypertension; shunt lesions complicated by Eisenmenger syndrome, because of the high pulmonary pressures and right-to-left shunting; complex cyanotic congenital heart disease; and residual poor left ventricular function following peripartum cardiomyopathy and other cardiomyopathies. Mild to moderate mitral stenosis is usually well tolerated during pregnancy and can be treated with percutaneous mitral valvuloplasty in the event the patient becomes dyspneic in the second or third trimester.

2. A 28-year-old G3P2 Hispanic woman with known mild mitral stenosis presents to your office after referral by her obstetrician. She is now 18 weeks pregnant and has noted 2 weeks of progressive dyspnea on exertion, which she states is much worse than during her last pregnancy. During physical examination you note 3 cm jugular venous distension at 45 degrees, rales halfway up the posterior lung fields, and a Grade II–III diastolic rumble murmur at the apex. An echocardiogram is consistent with moderate to severe mitral stenosis. All of the following therapeutic modalities are appropriate *except:*

a. Immediate admission to the hospital with plans for urgent open mitral commissurotomy.
b. Initial admission to the hospital including bedrest in the left lateral decubitus position and gentle diuresis.
c. Consider percutaneous mitral valvuloplasty if initial conservative measures such as bedrest and diuresis do not result in complete resolution of her symptoms.
d. The initiation of oral digoxin as prophylaxis against atrial fibrillation.

Answer is a: Pregnancy complicated by symptomatic mitral stenosis is first managed by bedrest and general diuresis as well as the initiation of digoxin for atrial fibrillation prophylaxis. Percutaneous mitral valvuloplasty should be considered if symptoms do not resolve with initial measures. Open mitral commissurotomy is seldom necessary in the modern day of valvuloplasty.

3. A 37-year-old woman presents with dyspnea. She is 2 weeks postpartum status post–uncomplicated delivery of her first child. Physical examination findings include a heart rate of 100 beats/min and prominent jugular venous distention. Inspiratory rales are noted at the lung bases. The apical impulse is diffuse and displaced. Also noted is a third heart sound. On echocardiography, the left ventricle is moderately enlarged and systolic function is reduced, with an estimated ejection fraction of 25%. Mild mitral regurgitation is noted. All the following statements about this patient's condition are true *except:*

a. Predisposing factors include the patient's age and that this was her first pregnancy.
b. Future pregnancies are contraindicated if the left ventricular ejection fraction does not return to 50% in 6 months.
c. Management should be conservative and medical therapy should be instituted immediately.
d. Recurrent problems occur in approximately 50% of subsequent pregnancies.
e. There is a 50% chance of complete resolution of symptoms and left ventricular dysfunction with therapy.

Answer is a: This patient with obvious peripartum cardiomyopathy should be treated conservatively with medical treatment. Risk factors for peripartum cardiomyopathy include a multiparous female, advanced maternal age, twin pregnancy, previous history of peripartum cardiomyopathy, and slight increase with African American ethnicity. Approximately 50% of patients experience complete resolution of left ventricular dysfunction. If left ventricular ejection fraction does not return to >50%, the patient is at higher risk for subsequent congestive heart failure during another pregnancy and should be so advised.

4. A 29-year-old G2P1 with a mechanical mitral valve prosthesis presents with rapidly progressive dyspnea in her 28th week of gestation. She takes coumadin with an international normalizing ratio (INR) of 1.8. Her physical exam reveals a heart rate of 100 beats/min, prominent jugular venous distention, rales up the back, and a displaced apical impulse. The mechanical prosthetic sounds are blunted, in addition to a soft systolic murmur. Echocardiography revealed an 18-mm transvalvular mitral gradient (5 mm prior to pregnancy) and mechanical leaflets that were difficult to visualize. Left ventricular function was normal. All of the following are appropriate treatment options *except:*

a. Cardiac catheterization to measure the mitral valve gradient and coronary angiography
b. Emergency high-risk obstetric evaluation
c. Thrombolytic therapy
d. Emergency cardiovascular surgery
e. Administration of both furosemide and heparin

Answer is a: This emergency situation needs to be evaluated by a cardiac surgeon and high-risk obstetrics specialist. Thrombolysis should be considered emergently unless the patient is at a facility where cardiac surgery is an option. A transesophageal echocardiogram is preferable if it can be performed safely. However, the entire history and physical scenario is consistent with thrombosis of a mechanical prosthesis. Urgent intervention is necessary to save both the mother and fetus. Mild diuresis may be helpful initially. Thrombolysis has been shown to be safe during pregnancy, without adverse effects on the mother or fetus in this emergency situation. If necessary, emergency cardiovascular surgery can be performed, but with an adverse risk primarily to the fetus. Perioperative uterine and fetal heart tone monitoring is necessary.

5. A 32-year-old white woman with suspected Marfan syndrome presents for consultation

during the first trimester of her first pregnancy. All of the following statements are true *except:*

a. There is a nearly 50% risk that her child will inherit this syndrome.
b. Compared to the nonpregnant state, she has an increased risk of aortic rupture and dissection during this gestation.
c. Her risk of aortic dissection increases as the ascending aorta exceeds 4 cm in diameter.
d. Natural childbirth via vaginal delivery with a local anesthetic is appropriate with an aortic root diameter of 5.5 cm.

Answer is d: All of the statements are true except d. Natural childbirth via vaginal delivery is appropriate if the aortic root is <4 cm; otherwise, this patient should be delivered by cesarean section as soon as the fetus is judged to be mature. The risk of aortic rupture or dissection increases substantially >4 cm diameter in the presence of the stress of vaginal delivery.

# Women and Heart Disease

# 56

***Ellen Mayer Sabik***

## EPIDEMIOLOGY/SCOPE OF PROBLEM

Cardiovascular disease (hypertension, cerebrovascular disease, and coronary artery disease) is the number-one killer of women in the United States. Approximately 500,000 U.S. women die annually from cardiovascular disease. Coronary artery disease is responsible for half of those deaths (approximately 250,000 deaths annually in the United States). Although the number of cardiovascular deaths in U.S. men has declined over the years, that for women has remained unchanged or increased. This may in part be due to the lack of awareness among women: Although ultimately 1 in 2.4 women will die from cardiovascular disease, as opposed to 1 in 29 deaths from breast cancer, many women consider breast cancer their greatest health problem. These attitudes are beginning to change as the American Heart Association (AHA) and the National Health Lung and Blood Institute (NHLBI) have undertaken national education campaigns to educate women and their physicians regarding women's risk for cardiovascular disease. One reason that heart disease has usually been thought of as a disease of men is that clinical manifestations typically occur in women 10 years later than in men. Because cardiovascular disease had been traditionally considered a male problem, historically women were markedly underrepresented in the national trials studying risk factors, diagnosis, and treatment for coronary artery disease, heart failure, and arrhythmias. "Optimal care" for treating women with these problems has been extrapolated from data collected on male patients. More recent studies have attempted to improve recruitment of women patients as well as perform separate analyses on specific treatment effects on women patients, specifically to identify possible differences in outcomes based on gender.

## RISK FACTORS FOR CORONARY ARTERY DISEASE

To target populations at risk for coronary artery disease (CAD) and appropriately diagnose and treat these individuals, we need to understand the risk factors for CAD and determine the effect of modifying these factors on risk for disease progression. The standard risk factors for CAD include elevated cholesterol, hypertension, smoking, diabetes, and a positive family history of the disease. The prevalence of risk factors is high in women of all racial and ethnic groups in the United States, with risk factors being more prevalent in socioeconomically and educationally disadvantaged women. Data for U.S. women aged 20 to 74 years in 1991 (National Centers for Health Statistics [NCHS], 1991) showed that more than one third had hypertension, more than one fourth had high cholesterol, more than one fourth were cigarette smokers, more than one fourth were overweight, and more than two thirds had a sedentary lifestyle, considered by many to be a risk factor for coronary disease with the prevalence of obesity and diabetes continuing to rise. Although risk factors for CAD are similar in men and women, the effects of the individual risk factors as well as interventions differ dramatically based on gender.

### Elevated Lipids

Total cholesterol and low-density lipoproteins (LDL) are only weakly associated with CAD in women, and only in women $<65$ years old (there is a stronger association in men). Total cholesterol/high-density lipoprotein (HDL-C) ratio is a more accurate measure of CAD risk in women. The level should be $\leq 4$. In older women, low HDL and elevated triglycerides are strong risk factors for CAD.

Cholesterol levels in women: The average HDL-C level in adult premenopausal women is 20% higher than in age-matched men. Although HDL-C declines following menopause, it still remains higher than in men.

Several secondary prevention studies have been undertaken to assess the effect of treatment of lipid abnormalities in women. The CARE (Cholesterol And Recurrent Events) trial studied pravastatin as treatment in patients with average cholesterol levels and prior myocardial infarction (MI). The outcome was a 46% reduction in death or recurrent MI in treated patients (as compared with a 26% reduction in men). The 4S trial (Scandinavian Simvastatin Survival Study) studied the use of simvastatin in patients with known CAD. The outcome was a 35% reduction in relative risk for coronary events in women (compared with a 34% reduction in men). The LIPID (Long Term Intervention with Pravastatin in Ischemic Disease) trial studied patients with prior MI or unstable angina who were treated with pravastatin. The outcome was a 24% decrease in CAD events.

Primary prevention studies include the AFCAPS/TexCAPS (Air-Force/Texas Coronary Atherosclerosis Prevention Study). Patients were men and postmenopausal women with average total cholesterol and LDL-C levels but below-average HDL. Long-term lipid-lowering treatment decreased the incidence of a first major acute CAD event by 46% in women and by 37% in men. There are no data to support aggressive lipid lowering in premenopausal women without CAD or family history or multiple risk factors.

## Diabetes

Diabetes is the most powerful risk factor for CAD in women: the presence of diabetes eliminates the 10-year gender gap in risk for CAD. Diabetes increases the risk of CAD fivefold, and increases the risk of MI twofold. It also increases the risk for developing congestive heart failure post–MI.

Hyperglycemia decreases estradiol-mediated nitric oxide production, thus causing endothelial dysfunction and platelet aggregation. Diabetes is also associated with abnormalities of platelet function and coagulation factors. Diabetics have elevated levels of fibrinogen, factor VII, and fibrinopeptide A, all markers of a hypercoagulable state. Also, women have increased platelet response and reactivity. Not only are women with diabetes at increased risk of developing CAD and having cardiac events, they are also at higher risk for mortality following these events.

## Hypertension

More than 50 million people in the United States have been diagnosed with hypertension, and >60% of these individuals are women. Hypertension is more likely to cause a cardiovascular event in women and is a risk factor for congestive heart failure in women. Women, however, are more likely than men to be aware of their diagnosis, to receive treatment, and to reach target blood pressure.

### *Etiology*

The origin of hypertension is predominantly essential. Etiologies that are seen exclusively or disproportionately in women include hypertension associated with pregnancy or use of oral contraceptives (especially older agents with higher doses of estrogens and progestins); and renovascular hypertension, which has a female:male ratio of 8:1.

### *Treatment*

There is ongoing ontroversy regarding the ideal treatment of hypertension in women. Thiazides have a benefit in that they enhance bone mineral density and decrease urinary calcium excretion. The Women's Health Initiative (WHI) studied 98,000 women aged 50 to 79 years, 38% with hypertension, 63% treated with medications, only 36% with controlled blood pressure, and found the worst control in the oldest age group. Diuretics achieved best blood pressure control as monotherapy.

Some have proposed that beta-blockers and angiotensin-converting enzyme (ACE) inhibitors may be less effective in women than in men because of low plasma renin activity in women. Perry et al., in a meta-analysis, showed no difference in effectiveness among ACE inhibitors, beta-blockers, and diuretics as monotherapy for hypertension.

## Smoking

Cigarette smoking is the leading preventable cause of death in men and women in the United States. Women who are heavy smokers (>20 cigarettes a day) have two- to fourfold increased risk of coronary disease compared with nonsmokers. Even light smokers (1 to 4 cigarettes a day) have a two- to threefold risk of fatal coronary heart disease or nonfatal MI. Second-hand smoke may increase risk of CAD by 20%.

The prevalence of smoking has declined in the United States since 1965, but more men have been successful at quitting than women. There are multiple factors in women's failure to quit, including fear of weight gain and lack of confidence.

### *Mechanisms by Which Smoking May Increase Risk of CAD*

Chronic smokers are insulin resistant, hyperinsulinemic, and dyslipidemic compared to nonsmokers. (There is a dose–response relationship between number of cigarettes smoked and plasma cholesterol, possibly due to increased lipolysis.)

Second-hand smoke may cause intimal wall damage and accelerate atherosclerotic plaque formation. In young women, the combination of smoking and use of oral contraceptives promotes thrombogenesis.

#### *Smoking Cessation Decreases Risk*

The Nurses' Health Study showed a 30% decrease risk for CAD in 2 years following cessation of smoking. There is continued decline in risk over next 10 to 15 years, and then the risk is at the same level as that of a nonsmoker.

Most studies show a 30% to 50% decrease in risk for CAD in the first 2 years following cessation.

### Obesity and Sedentary Lifestyle

Obesity is an independent risk factor for CAD in women. In the Framingham Heart Study, relative weight in women was positively and independently associated with the development of CAD as well as mortality from CAD and cardiovascular disease. In the Nurses' Health Study, women with a body mass index (BMI) of 25 to 29, had an age-adjusted relative risk for CAD of 1.8, whereas those with BMI ≥29 had a relative risk of 3.3, compared with the leanest women.

Truncal obesity correlates with increased LDL-C and decreased HDL-C and also is associated with hyperinsulinemia and hypertension. Although obesity is associated with diabetes (insulin resistance), hypertension, and hypercholesterolemia, the waist/hip ratio still correlates positively with CAD after controlling for smoking, hypertension, glucose intolerance, lipids, and BMI.

## AHA/ACC GUIDELINES FOR HEART DISEASE PREVENTION IN WOMEN

The American Heart Association/American College of Cardiology (AHA/ACC) guidelines are evidence based and are the first guidelines specifically developed for women based on available data for women, with individual recommendations for a woman based on her individual level of risk.

Women are grouped into high-risk (risk for CHD event of >20% over the next 10 years), intermediate-risk (risk of CHD event 10% to 20% over the next 10 years), and low-risk (risk for CHD event <10% over the next 10 years) categories based on their Framingham Risk Score. The Framingham Point Score Estimate of 10-year risk for women is calculated as a sum of scores based on the patient's age, total cholesterol, smoking, HDL-C, systolic blood pressure (see Tables 1 to 5). Each recommendation is rated based on the strength of evidence supporting the recommendation.

### Clinical Recommendations

#### *Lifestyle Interventions*

1. *Cigarette smoking:* Consistently encourage women not to smoke and to avoid environmental tobacco.
2. *Physical activity:* Consistently encourage women to accumulate a minimum of 30 minutes of activity on most, and preferably all, days of the week.
3. *Cardiac rehabilitation:* Women with recent acute coronary syndrome (ACS) or coronary intervention, or new onset or chronic angina, should participate in a comprehensive risk-reduction regimen, such as cardiac rehabilitation or a physician-guided home or community-based program.
4. *Heart-healthy diet:* Encourage a healthy eating pattern, including intake of a variety of fruits, vegetables, grains, low-fat or nonfat dairy products, fish, legumes, and sources of protein low in saturated fat (e.g., poultry, lean meats, plant sources). Limit saturated fat intake to <10% of calories, limit cholesterol intake to < 300 mg/dL, and limit intake of trans fatty acids.
5. *Weight maintenance/reduction:* Encourage weight maintenance/reduction through an appropriate balance of physical activity, caloric intake, and formal behavioral programs as needed to maintain/achieve a BMI between 18.5 and 24.9 and a waist circumference <35 in.
6. *Psychosocial factors:* Women with cardiovascular disease should be evaluated for depression and referred/treated as indicated.
7. *Omega-3 fatty acids:* As an adjunct to diet, omega-3 fatty acid supplementation may be considered in high-risk women.

#### *Interventions for Major Risk Factors*

1. *Blood pressure:* Target blood pressure is <120/80 mm Hg. Pharmacotherapy is indicated when blood pressure is >140/90 mm Hg, or an even lower blood pressure in the setting of blood pressure–related target organ damage or diabetes. Thiazide diuretics should be part of the regimen unless they are contraindicated.
2. *Lipids and lipoproteins:* Optimal levels of lipids and lipoproteins in women are LDL-C <100 mg/dL, HDL-C >50 mg/dL, triglycerides <150 mg/dL, and non–HDL-C (total cholesterol/HDL-C) <130 mg/dL. In high-risk women or when LDL-C is elevated, saturated fat intake should be <7% of calories, cholesterol <200 mg/day, and trans fatty acid intake should be reduced. Pharmacotherapy, when advised, is based on risk.
   - High risk: Initiate LDL-C–lowering therapy (preferably a statin) simultaneously with lifestyle changes in high-risk women with LDL-C ≥100 mg/dL, and initiate statin therapy in high-risk women with LDL-C <100 mg/dL unless contraindicated. Start niacin or fibrate therapy when HDL-C is low, or when non–HDL-C is elevated.
   - Intermediate risk: Initiate LDL-C–lowering therapy (preferably a statin) if LDL-C ≥130 mg/dL on lifestyle therapy, or niacin or fibrate therapy when HDL-C is low or non–HDL-C is elevated after LDL-C goal is reached.
   - Lower risk: Consider LDL-C–lowering therapy in low-risk women with 0 or 1 risk factor when LDL-C ≥190 mg/dL or if multiple risk factors are present when LDL-C ≥160 mg/dL, or niacin or fibrate therapy when

HDL-C is low or non–HDL-C elevated after LDL-C goal is reached.

3. *Diabetes:* Lifestyle and pharmacotherapy should be used to achieve near-normal HbA1c (<7%) in women with diabetes.

### *Medications*

1. *Aspirin:* The use of aspirin depends on the patient's risk.
   - In high-risk women, ASA (75 to 162 mg) or clopidogrel should be used unless it is contraindicated.
   - In intermediate-risk women, consider ASA (75 to 162 mg) as long as blood pressure is controlled and benefit is likely to outweigh the risk of gastrointestinal side effects.
   - In low-risk women, the routine use of ASA is *not* recommended.

   Note that since the AHA/ACC guidelines were published, the Women's Health Study failed to show any benefit in primary prevention of coronary artery disease with respect to total mortality or cardiovascular mortality in women except in the age group over 65 years. (check exact results)
2. *Beta-blockers:* Beta-blockers should be used indefinitely in *all* women who have had a myocardial infarction or who have chronic ischemic syndromes, unless contraindicated.
3. *ACE inhibitors:* ACE inhibitors should be used in high-risk women unless contraindicated.
4. *ARBs* : ARBs should be used in high-risk women with clinical evidence of heart failure or an ejection fraction <40% who are intolerant to ACE inhibitors.

### *Medications for Prevention of Atrial Fibrillation and Stroke*

1. *Warfarin:* Women with chronic or paroxysmal atrial fibrillation should take warfarin to maintain an internation normalizing ratio (INR) of 2.0 to 3.0 unless they are considered to be at low risk for stroke (<1%/year) or at high risk for bleeding.
2. *Aspirin:* Aspirin (325 mg) should be used in women with chronic or paroxysmal atrial fibrillation with contraindications to warfarin or who are at low risk for stroke (<1%/year).

### *Contraindications to Medications*

Medications that should not be used for prevention of cardiovascular disease in women include the following:

1. Combined estrogen-plus-progestin hormone therapy (or other forms of menopausal hormone therapy) should not be initiated or continued to prevent CVD in postmenopausal women.
2. Antioxidant vitamin supplements should not be used to prevent CVD in women.

## ESTROGEN THERAPY FOR PREVENTION OF CARDIOVASCULAR DISEASE

### Physiologic Effects of Estrogen

#### *Benefits*

- Beneficial effects on lipid profile
- Antioxidant effects
- Reduction of serum fibrinogen
- Inhibition of neointimal hyperplasia, smooth muscle cells, and collagen biosynthesis
- Potentiation of endothelium-derived relaxing factor
- Calcium channel blocking effect
- Increases prostacyclin biosynthesis
- Decreases insulin resistance
- May cause favorable distribution of body fat

#### *Risks*

- Breast cancer: relative risk is 1.35 with >10 years of hormone-replacement therapy (HRT).
- Endometrial cancer: relative risk is 8.22 with >8 years of HRT.
- Risk of DVT/PE is doubled with HRT.
- Risk of gall bladder disease is doubled with HRT.

### Population Data

Observational studies (e.g., the Nurses' Health Study) showed a significant reduction in myocardial infarction or death among postmenopausal estrogen users.

Some randomized controlled trials of HRT for secondary prevention of cardiovascular disease have been undertaken. The HERS (Heart and Estrogen/progestin Replacement Study) was the first randomized controlled trial of HRT for prevention of CHD. It looked at estrogen and progestin versus placebo in postmenopausal women with prior MI, coronary revasularization, or angiographic evidence of CAD. Results showed, over a mean follow-up period of 4.1 years, no difference in the rates of nonfatal MI and coronary death, and a 52% increase in cardiovascular events in the first year of HRT.

The ERA (Estrogen Replacement and Atherosclerosis) trial was the first randomized angiographic-endpoint trial to test the effect of estrogen replacement therapy (ERT) and HRT on the progression of atherosclerosis in postmenopausal women with documented CAD. Neither the HRT (estrogen and progestin) nor the ERT (estrogen only) showed any angiographic benefit on disease progression.

In a randomized controlled trial of HRT for the primary prevention of CHD, the Women's Health Initiative (WHI) studied estrogen plus progestin in >16,000 postmenopausal women ages 50 to 79 years. Primary outcomes were nonfatal MI or death from CHD. Mean follow-up was 5.2 years, but the trial was stopped early because the overall risks exceeded the benefits, with a hazard ratio for CHD of 1.24. The study's conclusions stated: "Estrogen plus progestin does NOT confer cardiac protection and may increase the risk of CHD among generally healthy postmenopausal women, especially during the first year of treatment."

The separate Estrogen Only arm of the WHI was stopped because the hormone increased the risk of CVA and did not reduce the risk of coronary heart disease.

Thus, based on the randomized, placebo controlled trials, hormone replacement therapy (estrogen and progestin or estrogen alone) is not indicated for either primary or secondary prevention of cardiovascular disease in women, and may in fact increase risk.

## CLINICAL PRESENTATIONS OF CAD IN WOMEN

The most common presentation of CAD in women is angina pectoris (typical and atypical), in contrast to men, who present most commonly with MI or sudden cardiac death. Women who present with ACS are more likely to be older and to have more co-morbidities than men, including hypertension, diabetes, hyperlipidemia, and congestive heart failure. Women are less likely to have had a prior MI or revascularization.

The possibility of a referral bias has been explored. In the GustoIIb trial, fewer women than men underwent coronary angiography (53% versus 59%). Women at catheterization had less severe coronary disease than men. Although previously women with abnormal noninvasive test findings suggesting CAD were less likely to be referred for catheterization, this bias has changed so that currently men and women have comparable referral rates for angiography following abnormal nuclear stress tests. Referral rates for revascularization have been comparable between men and women based on coronary anatomy once angiography has been performed.

In MI, both men and women present with chest pain as the most common symptom; however, women are more likely to have atypical symptoms, including shoulder, neck, and abdominal pain. Women may also present with profound fatigue or dyspnea without pain. Atypical symptoms often contribute to delay in women seeking medical attention for acute MI.

During hospitalization for MI, women had more complications and higher 30-day mortality rates than men, but similar rates of reinfarction. In GUSTO IIb, once the data were adjusted for age and baseline characteristics, however, men and women had similar mortality rates. Complications seen more commonly in women include shock, heart failure, recurrent chest pain, cardiac rupture, and stroke.

## TREATMENT RESULTS

### Thrombolytics

GUSTO I showed comparable infarct-related artery patency and significant reduction in early mortality with thrombolytic treatment in women as in men; however, unadjusted 30-day mortality for women was double that for men (13% versus 4.8%.) Multiple factors may be contributing to women's increased mortality: later presentation and diagnosis, more co-morbidities and older age, as well as more bleeding complications (including intracranial hemorrhage), due in part to lack of weight-adjusted dosing. TIMI II and GISSI also showed mortality benefits for both men and women with thrombolytics, however both showed higher 6-week and 1-year mortality rates for women. Data from the National Registry of Myocardial Infarction showed that women have greater mortality with acute MI than men, even when matched for age, both with and without thrombolysis. Women were less likely to receive thrombolytics and were more likely to have major bleeding when they did. Younger women (<70 years of age) had higher mortality rates during hospitalization than age-matched men.

### Primary Angioplasty for Acute Myocardial Infarction

Similar procedural success rates have been found for men and women treated with primary angioplasty. Primary PTCA decreased risk of intracranial hemorrhage seen in women with thrombolytics, and improved survival. Note that women still had higher 30-day and 7-month mortality, although this is likely due to differences in baseline characteristics.

### Noninvasive Evaluation of Women Suspected of Having Coronary Artery Disease

The gender-specific challenges of noninvasive evaluation in women are due to the fact that women are more likely to have single-vessel disease and nonobstructive coronary artery disease than men (who have more multivessel disease or left main disease), and there is a decreased diagnostic accuracy of noninvasive testing in women, with a higher rate of false positives. Therefore it is important to determine the likelihood of disease before testing.

Data support the use of stress testing with stress electrocardiography or cardiac imaging in patients with intermediate risk for CAD, to provide the best chance of determining the presence of disease. In patients at high risk for CAD, cardiac imaging is more useful for determining prognosis and guiding therapy than determining if the disease is present. The use of testing in low-risk patients is more likely to produce a false positive and should be avoided.

Exercise electrocardiograms (ECGs) are less accurate for women than for men. Using ECG alone, sensitivity and specificity are 61% and 70% in women, compared to 72% and 77% in men. Improved accuracy can be achieved by integrating multiple other clinical parameters of the stress test, including Duke treadmill score, heart rate recovery, and maximal exercise capacity, all of which have significant prognostic as well as diagnostic value.

Recommendations based on stress ECG include the following:

1. If the Duke treadmill score is high or high risk stress ECG indicates high risk, there is increased likelihood of obstructive disease, and the patient should be referred for cardiac catheterization.
2. If the Duke Treadmill score is intermediate, further risk stratification using cardiac imaging is recommended.
3. If pretest probability is low and Duke treadmill score is also low, no further evaluation for CAD is usually necessary. Exercise ECG in women has a high negative predictive value in women with low pretest probability.
4. Lower work capacity on exercise tests (average 5 to 7 minutes) challenges the ability of the test to provoke ischemia. Therefore, patients who are expected to perform <5 METs at exercise are better evaluated using pharmacologic stress imaging.
5. Women who exercise at <5 METs are at increased risk of death.

Stress echocardiography can indicate not only the presence or absence of ischemia but may also provide information on overall systolic and diastolic function, valvular structure and function, and the extent of infarct or stress-induced ischemia. Meta-analysis of stress echo studies in women found that mean sensitivity and specificity are 81% and 86%, respectively. Stress echo testing is gender neutral; there is no gender effect on diagnostic accuracy. Echo data provide incremental value over the exercise ECG and clinical variables, and may be the most cost-effective tool to diagnose CAD in women with intermediate pretest likelihood of disease. Use dobutamine echo for patients who are unable to exercise.

Radionuclide imaging, myocardial perfusion and ventricular function imaging, has special features in women. SPECT imaging parameters include perfusion defects, global and regional left ventricular (LV) function, and LV volumes. In women, however, a generally smaller LV cavity decreases the accuracy of the test. Breast attenuation can be improved by using a higher count isotope ($^{99m}$Tc) and less attenuation, allowing gating that improves accuracy.

Vasodilator pharmacologic stress SPECT can be used for patients who are unable to exercise adequately. Because women with suspected CAD are typically older and have diminished exercise capacity, pharmacologic stress is useful. Vasodilator stress perfusion imaging is more accurate than exercise stress, and is the test of choice in men and women with left bundle branch block.

SPECT imaging provides incremental prognostic value to clinical and exercise variables. The annual cardiac event rate for a person with a normal SPECT is <1%. The prognosis worsens as the number of vascular territories with provocable ischemia increases. Rather than a dichotomous result of positive or negative, evaluation of extent and severity of perfusion defects allows gradation of risk.

### Emerging Technologies for the Evaluation of Women with Suspected Coronary Artery Disease

Limited data are now appearing on the use of cardiac computed tomography (CT) and magnetic resonance imaging (MRI) as well as carotid IMT (combined thickness of intima and medial layer of the carotid) in the diagnosis of coronary artery disease in women. These techniques appear promising; however, further studies, which are currently ongoing, are required to determine their role in diagnosis and risk assessment in women.

## WOMEN AND HEART FAILURE

Risk factors for heart failure differ by gender. Hypertension and diabetes mellitus are major risk factors in women (with diabetes in younger women markedly increasing the risk of congestive heart failure), while CAD is a more important risk factor in men. Note, however, that women, especially diabetic women, have a greater risk of developing heart failure post-MI than men. There are also gender-specific causes of heart failure, such as peripartum cardiomyopathy and X-linked cardiomyopathy.

Structural responses to loading differ by gender; women, for example, are more likely to develop concentric left ventricular hypertrophy.

### Heart Failure and Survival

There are discrepancies in the literature as to whether women have a better prognosis with heart failure than men. A problem is that many studies lump different etiologies of heart failure as well as systolic and diastolic heart failure (i.e., patients with impaired systolic function lumped with those with preserved left ventricular ejection fraction, LVEF). In the Framingham Heart Study (controlled for age and etiology of heart failure), and NHANES I, women had better survival than men with congestive heart failure. These were epidemiologic studies and did not assess LV function. The SOLVD (Studies of Left Ventricular Dysfunction) data showed no differences in survival based on gender. These patients had reduced LVEF as enrollment criteria. CIBIS-II showed that women with heart failure had better survival than men, independent of baseline clinical profile and beta-blocker therapy.

Overall, it appears that women have a better prognosis with heart failure than men, even though the mechanisms are not yet clear. Oddly enough, the higher survival rate for women makes it more difficult to detect a mortality benefit in therapeutic trials.

### Treatment of Heart Failure in Women

The large therapeutic trials suffer from the problem of limited numbers of women enrolled as subjects. Attempts to pool data, such as Gali et al.'s examination of the use of ACE inhibitors for patients with decreased LVEF, found no reduction of mortality or combined endpoint of all-cause mortality and heart failure hospitalizations in women. MERIT-HF looked at benefits from the addition of beta-blockers to heart failure regimens, but only 23% of the patients studied were women. A subgroup analysis did not show a mortality benefit for women. It is possible that the study was underpowered to detect benefit.

Thus, the standard treatment for women with heart failure with depressed LVEF (including ACE inhibitors, beta-blockers, spironolactone, and possibly digitalis) is based on overall population benefits shown in studies that predominantly enrolled men. Morbidity and mortality benefits have not been specifically proven for women, and further study is needed. Heart failure in women with preserved systolic function is a different entity seen mostly in older women, often women with hypertension. Only small numbers of clinical trials have addressed treatment of these patients, and thus there is no conclusive data to guide therapy. The 2001 ACC/AHA guidelines for this patient population recommend a physiologic approach to pharmacologic treatment using agents to control blood pressure and heart rate, decrease central blood volume, and treat myocardial ischemia. Further study is required to optimize treatment of this patient population to improve their quality of life.

## BIBLIOGRAPHY


**Gibbons RJ, Balady GJ, Bricker T, et al.** ACC/AHA 2002 guideline update for exercise testing: summary article: a report of the American College of Cardiology/American Heart Association Task Force on Practice Guidelines (Committee to Update the 1977 Exercise Testing Guidelines. *J Am Coll Cardiol.* 2002;40:1531–1540.

**Hochman JS, Tamis JE, Thompson TD, et al.** Sex, clinical presentation, and outcome in patients with acute coronary syndrome. *N Engl J Med.* 1999;341:226–232.

**Mieres JH, Shaw LJ, Arai A, et al.** Role of noninvasive testing in the clinical evaluation of women with suspected coronary artery disease. Consensus statement from the Cardiac Imaging Committee, Council on Clinical Cardiology, and the Cardiovascular Imaging and Intervention Committee, Council on Cardiovascular Radiology and Intervention, American Heart Association. *Circulation.* 2005;111:682–696.

**Mosca l, Apel L, Benjamin EJ, et al.** Evidence-based guidelines for cardiovascular disease prevention in women. AHA Scientific Statement. *Circulation.* 2004;109(5):672–93.

**Wenger NK.** Clinical characteristics of coronary heart disease in women: emphasis on gender differences. *Cardiovasc Res.* 2002;53: 558–567.

**Wenger NK.** Coroanry heart disease: the female heart is vulnerable. *Prog Cardiovasc* Dis. 2003;46(3):199–229.

**Wenger NK.** Women, heart failure, and heart failure therapies. *Circulation.* 2002;105(13):1526–1528.


## QUESTIONS

1. All of the following are true regarding women with a myocardial infarction *except*:
   a. Women are more likely to have complications such as VSD, heart failure, cardiac rupture, and shock than men.
   b. Women are more likely than men to have had a prior myocardial infarction.
   c. Women have unadjusted 30-day and 1-year mortality rates post-MI that are higher than those for men.
   d. Primary PTCA decreased the risk of intracranial hemorrhage that is seen with thrombolytics.

Answer is b: Women who present with an MI are *less* likely to have had a prior MI, and are more likely to have mechanical complications including VSD, congestive heart failure, cardiac rupture, and shock. Women also have higher 30-day and 1-year unadjusted mortality rates compared to men who present with an MI. Primary PTCA has decreased the risk of intracranial hemorrhage that is seen with thrombolytics.

2. Women with hypertension are
   a. Less likely than men to be aware of their diagnosis
   b. More likely than men to reach their target blood pressure
   c. Less likely than men to have a CVA than men with hypertension
   d. Less likely than men to have renovascular hypertension

Answer is b: Women with hypertension are more likely than men to be aware of their diagnosis, to have appropriate treatment, and to reach their target blood pressure. Women with hypertension are more likely to have a stroke than men with hypertension. Women have renovascular hypertension much more commonly than men (ratio 8:1).

3. All of the following are true regarding diabetes as a cardiac risk factor in women *except*:
   a. Eliminates the 10-year gender gap
   b. Increases the risk of CAD fivefold over women without diabetes
   c. Increases the risk for developing congestive heart failure post-MI
   d. Increases the risk of MI 10-fold over women without diabetes

Answer is d: Diabetes increases a woman's risk of CAD fivefold and of MI twofold, not 10-fold, over nondiabetics. The other statements are all true.

4. All of the following are true regarding the use of hormone replacement therapy for prevention of coronary artery disease *except*:
   a. Estrogen therapy increases the risk of breast and endometrial cancer.

b. Hormone replacement therapy is useful for secondary prevention of CAD in women.
c. The HERS trial showed no difference in nonfatal MI or coronary death in postmenopausal women with prior MI or revascularization or angiographic CAD who had hormone replacement therapy.
d. Hormone replacement therapy may increase risk of CAD in healthy postmenopausal women.

Answer is b: Hormone replacement therapy has no role in either primary or secondary prevention of coronary artery disease. It may, in fact, increase the risk of CAD in healthy postmenopausal women. HRT has certain noncardiac risks associated with it, including increased risk of breast cancer, endometrial cancer, and gallbladder disease, as well as increased risk of DVT and pulmonary embolism.

**5.** The use of thrombolytics in women who present with an MI:

a. Is associated with comparable infarct-related artery patency as seen in men
b. Is associated with fewer bleeding complications than are seen in men
c. Did not show mortality benefit as seen in men
d. Is contraindicated in menstruating women or women of reproductive age

Answer is a: The use of thrombolytics in women produces equivalent rates of infarct-related artery as when used in men, as well as mortality benefit. More bleeding complications were seen in women, but this is likely related to the uniform dosing (i.e., not weight adjusted) that was used in the early studies. These bleeding complications included intracranial hemorrhages as well as groin bleeds at the site of catheterization.

# 57

# Preoperative Evaluation of Cardiac Patients for Noncardiac Surgery: Stress Test, Catheterization, or Just Proceed?

***Richard A. Grimm***

The evaluation of cardiac patients undergoing noncardiac surgery plays a vital role in the day-to-day practice of the consulting cardiologist. Unfortunately, poor outcomes can and do occur in high-risk patients. Therefore, predicting risk of potential nonfatal myocardial infarction, heart failure, pulmonary embolism, or death is imperative when managing this group of patients, and several risk prediction indexes having been proposed by various authors (1,2). Despite these concerns, coronary revascularization before surgery to enable the patient to "get through" the operation is rarely necessary and is utilized in only a small subset of patients. In this chapter the American College of Cardiology/American Heart Association (ACC/AHA) Task Force on Practice Guidelines (3) will be used extensively as the primary reference for review of the literature and practice recommendations. These guidelines emphasize the importance of utilizing clinical predictors, evidence-based practice, along with a rational and common sense approach.

Approximately 30 million patients underwent noncardiac surgery in the United States in 2003 (4). Of these, it has been previously estimated that approximately 4% will have diagnosed coronary artery disease, 8% to 12% will have multiple risk factors for coronary artery disease, and approximately 16% will be older than 65 years of age. This group of patients (those diagnosed with coronary artery disease, having multiple risk factors, or >65 years old) accounts for approximately 80% of the estimated 1 million patients who have complications (morbidity and mortality) from noncardiac surgery yearly. These complications account for approximately $12 billion annually in expenditures.

Patients are undergoing these procedures at increasingly older ages (half of individuals >65 years old will undergo major surgery during their lifetime), although investigations have demonstrated that age by itself is at most a minor risk factor for perioperative complications (3). Although the overall risk of suffering a postoperative myocardial infarction is low (<1%), up to 50% of these events can be fatal. Furthermore, a prior history of myocardial infarction (MI) increases the risk of a postoperative MI, with the risk of perioperative reinfarction being highest within the first 6 months of the index infarction. This risk decreases with time. The guidelines published by the ACC/AHA recommend that elective surgery may be performed before the 6-month time period so long as a postinfarction risk stratification has been performed (3). A negative stress test for ischemia or complete revascularization does reduce the risk of reinfarction with elective surgery. Nonetheless, the guidelines suggest that waiting 4 to 6 weeks is prudent before proceeding with elective surgery.

For cardiovascular patients undergoing noncardiac surgery, surveillance for cardiac complications should be performed for at least 48 hours following surgery, as the peak risk of myocardial infarction is within the first 3 days, but may persist for as long as 5 to 6 days. Most postoperative MIs are non–Q-wave MIs, usually detected within the first 24 hours as a result of increased vigilance and surveillance with electrocardiographic and cardiac enzyme testing. Routine acquisition of an electrocardiogram immediately postoperatively was recently shown to be useful in updating risk in both low- and high-risk populations undergoing major noncardiac surgical procedures (5). Patients with evidence of ischemia on the immediate postoperative electrocardiogram (ECG) were found to have a higher risk of subsequent major cardiac complications. Though they are often silent in presentation, postoperative infarctions may also present as new-onset heart failure, hypertension, nausea, altered mental status, or new arrhythmias as their only indication (6).

## PREOPERATIVE CARDIAC RISK ASSESSMENT

Surgical risk assessment encompasses patient-specific, procedure-specific, and institution-specific factors that must be identified in order to estimate individual risk and in turn outline management plans. Risk factors include the type of operation, presence and severity of coronary artery disease, status of left ventricular function, age, presence of severe valvular heart disease, serious cardiac arrhythmias, co-morbid medical conditions, and overall functional status.

### Clinical Markers of Increased Risk

Perioperative cardiovascular risk can be stratified further into major, intermediate, and low risk categories (1,2). Acute or more active conditions carry more weight than stable chronic conditions; for example, decompensated heart failure would be considered a major risk and would likely require further evaluation and therapy, whereas compensated heart failure would be considered an intermediate-risk condition. Major clinic predictors of risk include unstable coronary disease, decompensated heart failure, symptomatic arrhythmias, and/or severe valvular heart disease. Intermediate predictors include mild angina pectoris, prior MI (by history or pathologic Q waves), compensated or prior heart failure, diabetes mellitus (particularly insulin-dependent), and renal insufficiency. Notably, a history of MI is defined as an intermediate risk factor, however, an acute (a documented MI <7 days before the exam) or recent MI (>7 days but <1 month before the exam) is considered a major predictor (3). Minor clinical predictors include advanced age, abnormal ECG, rhythm other than sinus, low functional capacity, history of stroke, and uncontrolled systemic hypertension.

### Procedure-Specific Risks

Procedure-specific risks also need to be considered and can be categorized into high, intermediate, and low risk categories (1,2,7). High-risk procedures include emergency major operations (particularly in the elderly), aortic and other major vascular surgery, peripheral vascular surgery, aortic surgeries, as well as surgical procedures that are expected to be prolonged and associated with large fluid shifts and/or blood loss. Such high-risk procedures are often associated with a perioperative event rate (i.e., heart failure or myocardial infarction) of >5%. Blood loss, large intra- and extravascular fluid shifts, aortic cross clamping (in the case of aortic surgery), duration, and postoperative hypoxemia are factors believed to contribute to this increased risk. The risk of peripheral vascular surgical procedures is thought to be related to the likelihood of associated coronary artery disease in this patient population. Intermediate-risk procedures (cardiac risk generally <5%) include carotid endarterectomy, head and neck surgeries, intraperitoneal and intrathoracic surgery, orthopedic surgeries, and prostate surgery. Examples of low-risk surgeries (cardiac risk generally <1%) include endoscopic surgery, superficial procedures, breast surgery, and cataract surgery.

### Functional Capacity and Stress Testing for Preoperative Assessment of Risk

A patient's functional capacity is a good indicator of his or her ability to safely tolerate noncardiac surgery. Estimating functional capacity can be accomplished using readily available energy requirement correlates of daily activities (Fig. 57–1) (8). In addition, exercise stress testing is a commonly used test for more objectively determining a patient's ability to exercise, as well as to assess the ST-segment response to stress as an assessment for ischemia, particularly in the intermediate-risk category. Unfortunately, studies have shown that a majority of patients in need of risk stratification are either unable to exercise or have an

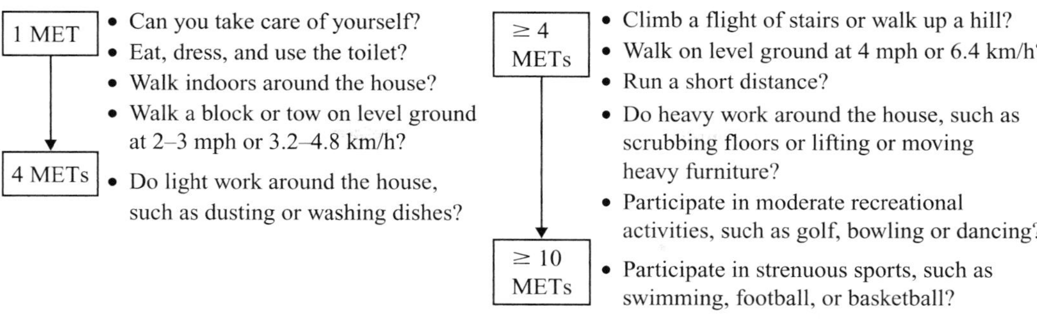


**Figure 57–1** Estimated energy requirements for typical daily activities. [Adapted from Eagle KA, et al. Guideline update for perioperative cardiovascular evaluation for non-cardiac surgery. A report of the American College of Cardiology/American Heart Association Task Force on Practice Guidelines (Committee to Update the 1996 Guidelines on Perioperative Cardiovascular Evaluation for Noncardiac Surgery). *J Am Coll Cardiol.* 2002;39:542–553.]

uninterpretable ECG and therefore are in need of pharmacologic stress testing in order to obtain a "functional assessment." In this patient population, intravenous dipyridamole myocardial perfusion scintigraphy or dobutamine stress echocardiography are commonly employed. The negative predictive value of these tests is high (99% for dipyridamole thallium, and 93% to 100% for dobutamine stress echo), though the positive predictive value of these tests for perioperative events is low (4% to 20% for intravenous dipyridamole thallium and 7% to 23% for dobutamine stress echocardiography) (9). Therefore, incorporating clinical markers of risk is essential for improving the specificity and positive predictive value of these diagnostic studies. As a guideline, noninvasive testing in preoperative patients is indicated if two or more of the following are present: (a) intermediate clinical predictors (Canadian Class I or II angina, prior MI based on history or pathologic Q waves, compensated or prior heart failure, or diabetes), (b) a poor functional capacity (<4 METs), or (c) a high-surgical-risk procedure (aortic repair or peripheral vascular, prolonged surgical procedures with large fluid shifts or blood loss).

The presence of a thallium redistribution abnormality associated with one or more clinical risk factors has been associated with a higher incidence of perioperative cardiac events as compared to a population of patients with a reversible thallium defect but no clinical risk factors. Furthermore, postoperative events increased from 29% to 50% in a population of patients with thallium defects in the group of patients that were found to have three clinical risk factors as opposed to only one or two variables present (1). These data, again, highlight the importance of eliciting clinical markers of risks. Finally, the extent of ischemia (i.e., number of abnormal segments), as well the severity of ischemia, correlates with perioperative cardiac events.

## Which Stress Test Is Best?

For most patients evaluated in the outpatient setting, treadmill exercise ECG testing is best able to provide an assessment of functional capacity, as well as an assessment for myocardial ischemia by ST-segment analysis. This generalization holds true provided the patient is adequately able to exercise and his or her resting electrocardiogram is normal. In patients with abnormal resting electrocardiograms (LVH, LBBB, or digitalis effect), an exercise imaging study is necessary.

In patients who are unable to exercise adequately, pharmacologic stress testing in the form of intravenous dipyridamole thallium (or MIBI) testing or dobutamine echocardiography should be employed. In many locations it is the specific expertise in the local laboratory that determines the test of choice. In most cases, either test, whether it be Dobutamine stress echocardiography or stress perfusion imaging, is appropriate, provided the expertise in a specific institution is satisfactory and commensurate with published investigations. However, certain guidelines should be kept in mind when deciding on the ideal choice of a test. Dipyridamole perfusion imaging should be avoided in patients with significant bronchospasm, critical carotid disease, or in patients with a condition that prevents them from being withdrawn from theophylline preparations. Dobutamine should not be used as a stressor in patients with serious arrhythmias, severe hypertension, or hypotension.

## Indications for Angiography

For patients with suggested or proven coronary artery disease, Class I indicators for proceeding directly to coronary angiography include high-risk results during noninvasive testing, angina pectoris that is unresponsive to medical treatment, unstable angina pectoris in most patients, and nondiagnostic or equivocal noninvasive tests in a high-risk patient undergoing a high-risk procedure. Class II indications include intermediate results during noninvasive testing, nondiagnostic or equivocal noninvasive test in a patient at lower risk undergoing a high-risk procedure, urgent noncardiac surgery in a patient recovering from an acute MI, and perioperative MI.

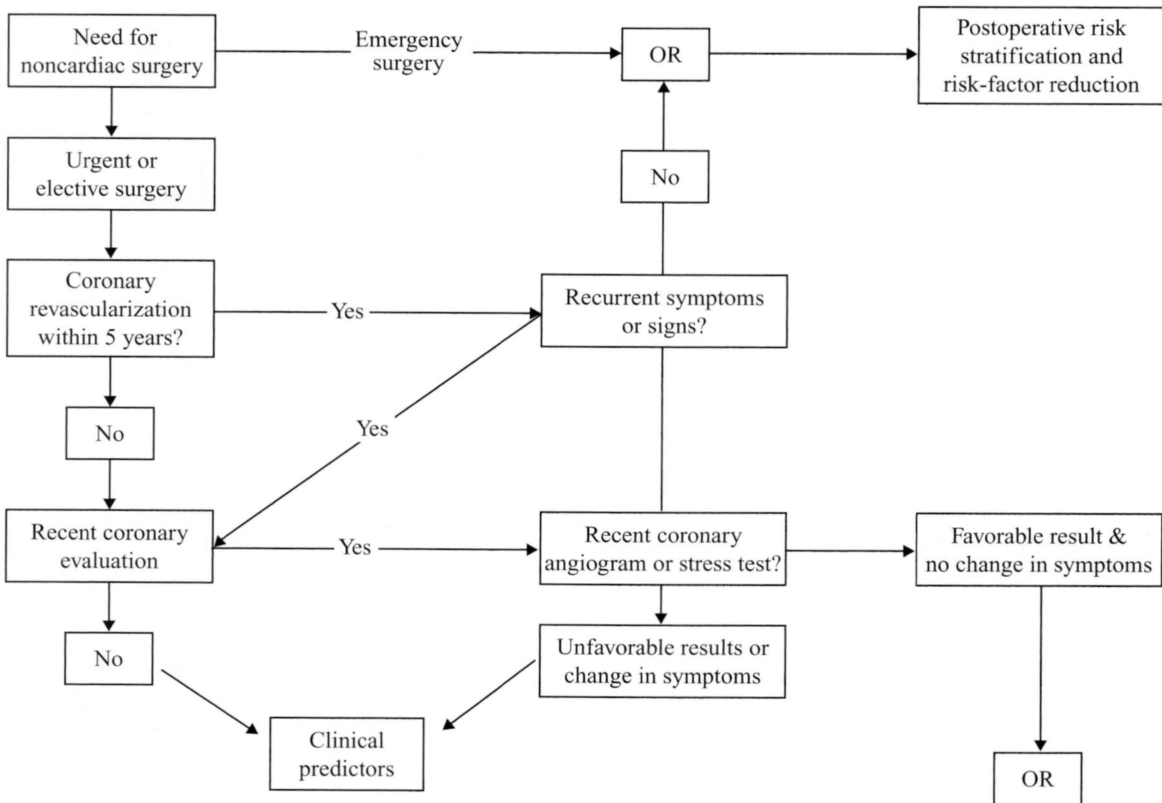


**Figure 57–2** Stepwise approach to the assessment of a cardiac patient undergoing noncardiac surgery. [Adapted from Eagle KA, et al. Guideline update for perioperative cardiovascular evaluation for noncardiac surgery. A report of the American College of Cardiology/American Heart Association Task Force on Practice Guidelines (Committee to Update the 1996 Guidelines on Perioperative Cardiovascular Evaluation for Noncardiac Surgery). *J Am Coll Cardiol.* 2002;39:542–553.]

## GENERAL APPROACH TO SUCCESSFUL PERIOPERATIVE EVALUATION OF CARDIAC PATIENTS UNDERGOING NONCARDIAC SURGERY

The approach to the management of cardiac patients undergoing noncardiac surgery as outlined by the joint ACC/AHA Task Force is based on a Bayesian strategy that relies on clinical markers, prior coronary artery disease evaluation and treatment, functional capacity, and type of surgical procedure being anticipated (3). The following are general guidelines that may be useful in most situations commonly encountered. Since publication of the original guidelines in 1996, several studies have shown that this stepwise approach is both efficacious and cost effective.

The first step is to assess the urgency of noncardiac surgery (Fig. 57–2). When encountering a patient in need of emergency surgery, time often does not allow for a preoperative evaluation. In such cases, proceeding directly to the surgical suite and performing a postoperative risk stratification is most appropriate.

Once the urgency of the situation has been appropriately addressed, one should determine whether the patient has had a coronary revascularization within the past 5 years and whether symptoms and/or signs of ischemia have developed over that period of time. If this history is determined to be negative, further testing is not necessary. If the patient has undergone a coronary evaluation within the previous 2 years (assuming risk was adequately assessed and findings were favorable) and is currently without symptoms, further testing is usually not necessary. The next step in the evaluation is to determine if major clinic predictors of risk (i.e., unstable coronary disease, decompensated heart failure, symptomatic arrhythmias, and/or severe valvular heart disease) are present. Cancellation or delay of surgery until the problem has been satisfactorily identified and treated is usually necessary (Fig. 57–3).

The presence or absence of prior MI (by history or ECG), angina, compensated or prior heart failure, a preoperative creatinine >2 mg/dL, and/or diabetes helps to stratify clinical risk for perioperative coronary events. Functional capacity and level of surgery-specific risk assessment allows for a rational approach to identify patients most likely to benefit from noninvasive testing.

Patients without major predictors but with intermediate predictors of clinical risk (Fig. 57–4), and moderate or excellent functional capacity, generally may undergo intermediate-risk surgery with little likelihood of

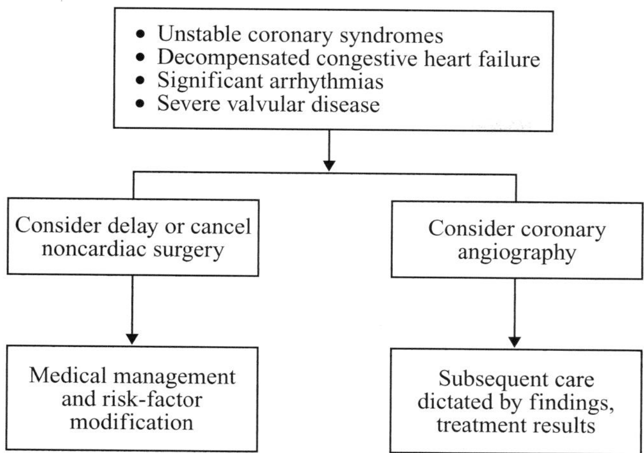


**Figure 57–3** Stepwise approach to a patient with major clinical predictors. [Adapted from Eagle KA, et al. Guideline update for perioperative cardiovascular evaluation for noncardiac surgery. A report of the American College of Cardiology/American Heart Association Task Force on Practice Guidelines (Committee to Update the 1996 Guidelines on Perioperative Cardiovascular Evaluation for Noncardiac Surgery). *J Am Coll Cardiol.* 2002;39:542–553.]

perioperative death or MI. Conversely, further noninvasive testing is often considered for patients with poor or moderate functional capacity undergoing higher-risk surgery or patients with more than two intermediate predictors.

Noncardiac surgery is generally safe for patients without major or intermediate clinical predictors (Fig. 57–5) and a functional capacity of more than 4 METS. Additional testing may be considered for patients without clinical markers but considered to have a poor functional capacity who are facing high-risk operations, particularly those with several minor predictors of risk who are scheduled for vascular surgery. Finally, the results of noninvasive testing should be used to determine further preoperative management.

## MANAGEMENT OF OTHER CARDIOVASCULAR CONDITIONS

### Hypertension

Severe hypertension (systolic blood pressure >180 mm Hg, diastolic blood pressure >110 mm Hg) should be controlled preoperatively when possible. The decision to delay

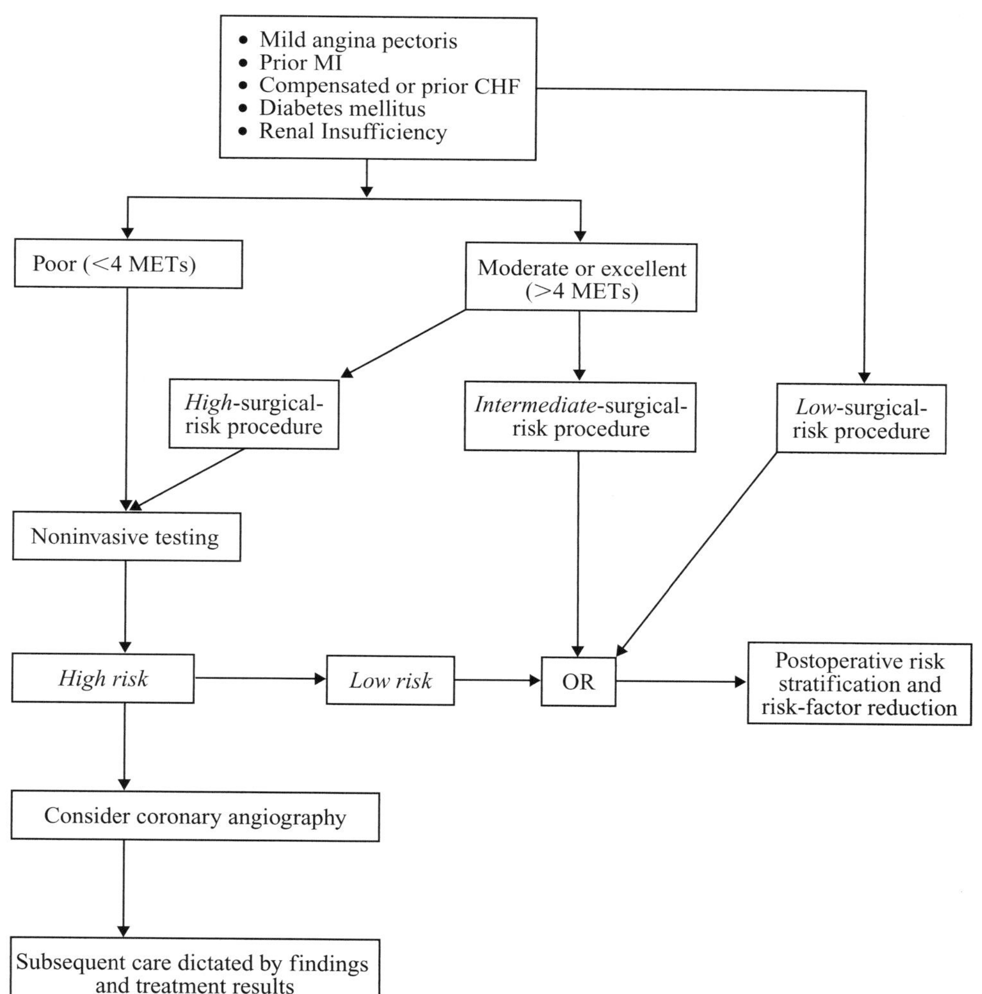


**Figure 57–4** Stepwise approach to a patient with intermediate clinical predictors. [Adapted from Eagle KA, et al. Guideline update for perioperative cardiovascular evaluation for noncardiac surgery. A report of the American College of Cardiology/American Heart Association Task Force on Practice Guidelines (Committee to Update the 1996 Guidelines on Perioperative Cardiovascular Evaluation for Noncardiac Surgery). *J Am Coll Cardiol.* 2002;39:542–553.]

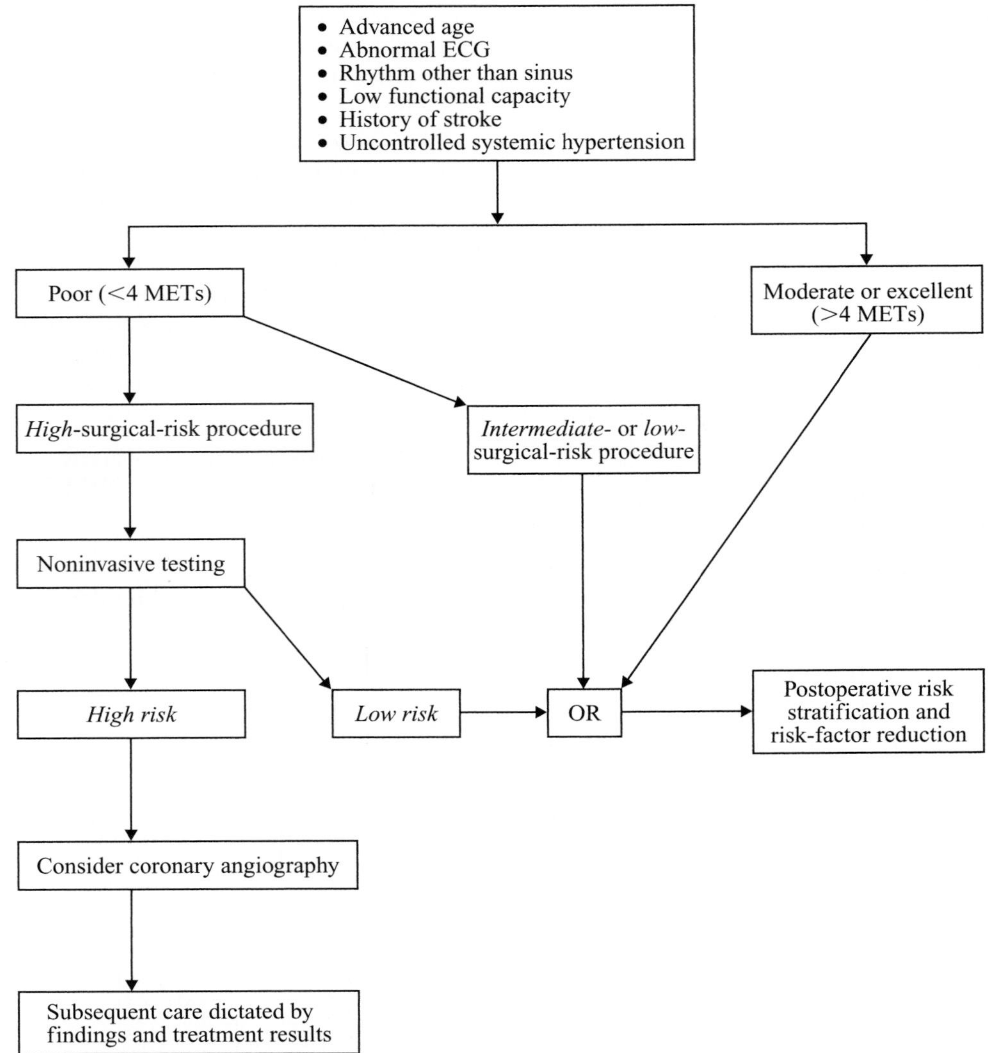


**Figure 57–5** Stepwise approach to a patient with minor or no clinical predictors. [Adapted from Eagle KA, et al. Guideline update for perioperative cardiovascular evaluation for noncardiac surgery. A report of the American College of Cardiology/American Heart Association Task Force on Practice Guidelines (Committee to Update the 1996 Guidelines on Perioperative Cardiovascular Evaluation for Noncardiac Surgery). *J Am Coll Cardiol.* 2002;39:542–553.]

surgery because of severe hypertension needs to take into account the urgency of the noncardiac surgery. Continuation of preoperative antihypertensive treatment through the perioperative period is important.

## Valvular Heart Disease

The indications for evaluation and treatment of valvular heart disease are the same as those in the nonoperative setting. Symptomatic stenotic lesions are associated with an increased risk of perioperative congestive heart failure or shock, and often require balloon valvuloplasty or valve replacement before the cardiac surgery. Symptomatic regurgitant lesions, on the other hand, are usually better tolerated perioperatively and usually can be stabilized preoperatively with medical therapy and monitoring. This strategy assumes normal left ventricular function, and therefore, relatively adequate cardiac reserve. These recommendations are appropriate if a delay in the noncardiac surgery is thought to have potentially dire consequences. In the case of severe valvular regurgitation and left ventricular dysfunction in which cardiac reserve is limited, instability during noncardiac surgery is likely, and therefore, valve replacement prior to noncardiac surgery may be warranted.

## Hypertrophic Obstructive Cardiomyopathy

Patients with hypertrophic obstructive cardiomyopathy generally tolerate surgery well, provided that attention is given to a few critical factors. Anesthetic-associated decrease in peripheral vascular resistance, hypovolemia, and adrenergic stimulation may result in tachycardia and should be avoided if possible. Any of these factors may precipitate hemodynamic deterioration. Ventricular rate control can be key, and therefore a beta-blocker is often helpful in allowing adequate time for ventricular filling, and the negative inotropic effect can help to avoid hemodynamic instability.

### Dilated Cardiomyopathy

Patients with dilated cardiomyopathy also are at increased risk for perioperative heart failure. Management is directed at optimizing preoperative hemodynamics and providing intensive postoperative medical therapy and surveillance.

## PERIOPERATIVE MEDICAL THERAPY

Although few randomized controlled trials have been performed to determine the optimal perioperative medical regimen for patients with cardiac disease who are undergoing noncardiac surgery, all of the data support beta-blocker therapy as a treatment that reduces the frequency of postoperative ischemia, as well as events such as myocardial infarction. Recently, a randomized trial of beta-blocker therapy versus standard treatment in a series of patients with positive dobutamine stress echocardiograms demonstrated a positive benefit to bisoprolol in reducing perioperative death and nonfatal myocardial infarction (10). These data, as well as prior studies, support the use of beta-blocker therapy unless it is contraindicated. Beta-blocker therapy should be initiated days to weeks before the procedure and the dose titrated to a resting heart rate of 50 to 60 beats/min. Nitroglycerine, on the other hand, had not been demonstrated to be effective in this setting.

## PERIOPERATIVE THERAPY OR PREVIOUS CORONARY REVASCULARIZATION

Indications for coronary artery bypass graft (CABG) before noncardiac surgery are identical to those reviewed in the ACC/AHA guidelines for CABG. Unfortunately, there are no controlled trials comparing perioperative cardiac outcome after noncardiac surgery for patients treated with preoperative percutaneous coronary intervention (PCI) versus medical therapy. In the event of a patient undergoing PCI and stent placement, the issue of appropriate timing between the PCI and the noncardiac surgery is problematic. A delay of at least 2 weeks is reasonable, and ideally 4 to 6 weeks to allow for a full 4 weeks of dual antiplatelet therapy and re-endothelialization of the stent.

## POSTOPERATIVE MYOCARDIAL INFARCTION MANAGEMENT

Patients with postoperative myocardial infarction often sustain these events secondary to increased myocardial oxygen demand outstripping myocardial oxygen supply. These are commonly associated with minimal symptoms, nonspecific ST–T-wave changes, and small increases in cardiac enzyme leaks. A significant number of postoperative myocardial infarctions, however, are believed to result from acute coronary thrombosis and occlusion. These are the patients who are thought to be at highest risk for large myocardial infarctions and fatal outcomes. For this reason, some investigators have proposed an aggressive reperfusion strategy for these patients, with coronary angiography, angioplasty, or even coronary bypass surgery. Future studies will undoubtedly be required in order to test this hypothesis satisfactorily.

## AREAS OF CONTROVERSY AND FURTHER RESEARCH

1. The role of prophylactic revascularization in patients with demonstrated myocardial ischemia in reducing perioperative and long-term myocardial infarction and death
2. Establishing improved guidelines for patients with valvular heart disease undergoing noncardiac surgery
3. The efficacy and cost effectiveness of various noninvasive testing methods as a method of determining risk and reducing cardiac complications
4. Establishment of optimal guidelines for selected subgroups of patients undergoing noncardiac surgery, especially the elderly and women
5. Establishment of the efficacy of surveillance and monitoring of patients for myocardial ischemia and infarction perioperatively
6. Establishment of the efficacy of $\alpha_2$-agonists for decreasing the risk of ischemia, MI, and death perioperatively

Despite the above-noted areas of ongoing controversy, the preoperative assessment of cardiac patients being considered for noncardiac surgery has become a largely data-driven process. The recently published ACC/AHA guidelines provide a rational, conservative, and systematic approach for the clinician to utilize, which emphasizes the importance of clinical risk-factor stratification and the premise that intervention is rarely necessary to lower the risk of an operation.

## REFERENCES


1. Eagle KA, et al. Combining clinical and thallium data optimizes pre operative assessment of cardiac risk before major vascular surgery. *Ann Intern Med.* 1989;110:859–866.
2. Goldman L, et al., Multifactorial index of cardiac risk in non-cardiac surgical procedures. *N Engl J Med.* 1977;297: 845–850.
3. Eagle KA, et al. Guideline update for perioperative cardiovascular evaluation for non-cardiac surgery. A report of the American College of Cardiology/American Heart Association Task Force on Practice Guidelines (Committee to Update the 1996 Guidelines on

Perioperative Cardiovascular Evaluation for Noncardiac Surgery). *J Am Coll Cardiol.* 2002;39:542–553.
4. De Frances CJ, Hall MJ, Podgornik MN. 2003 National Hospital Discharge Survey. Advance Data from Vital and Health Statistics. National Center for Health Statistics; 2005:359.
5. Rinfret S, et al. Value of immediate post op eleectrocardiogram to update risk stratification after major non cardiac surgery. *Am J Cardiol.* 2004;94:1017–1022.
6. Mangano DT, et al. Perioperative myocardial ischemia in patients undergoing non-cardiac surgery. II. Incidence and severity during the 1st week after surgery. *J Am Coll Cardiol.* 1991;17:851–857.
7. Hertzer N. Fatal myocardial infarction following peripheral vascular operations: a study of 951 patients followed 6–11 years postoperatively. *Clev Clin Q.* 1982;49:1–11.
8. Fletcher GF, et al. Exercise standards: a statement for health care professionals from the American Heart Association: Writing Group. *Circulation.* 1995;91:580–615.
9. Shaw L, et al., Meta-analysis of intra-venous dipyridamole-thallium-201 imaging (1985–1994) and dobutamine echcardiography (1991–1994) for risk stratification before vascular surgery. *J Am Coll Cardiol.* 1996;27:787–798.
10. Poldermans D, et al., The effect of bisoprolol on perioperative mortality and myocardial infarction in high-risk patients undergoing vascular surgery. *N Eng J Med.* 1999;341:1789–1794.

## QUESTIONS

**1.** You are asked to evaluate a 55-year-old man with a history of prior myocardial infarction in preparation for an abdominal aortic aneurysm repair. A dobutamine stress echocardiogram has been ordered and shows the following.

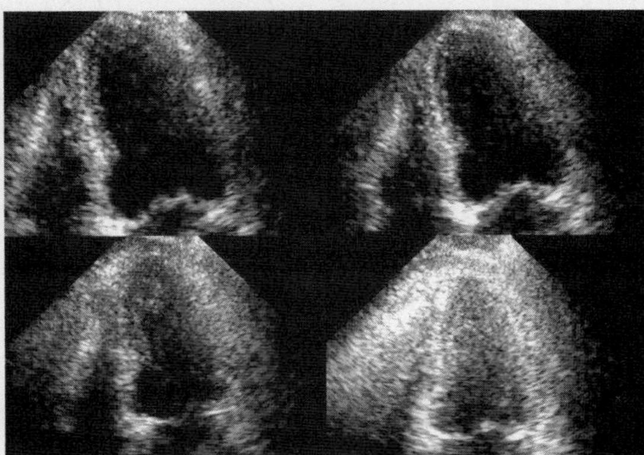

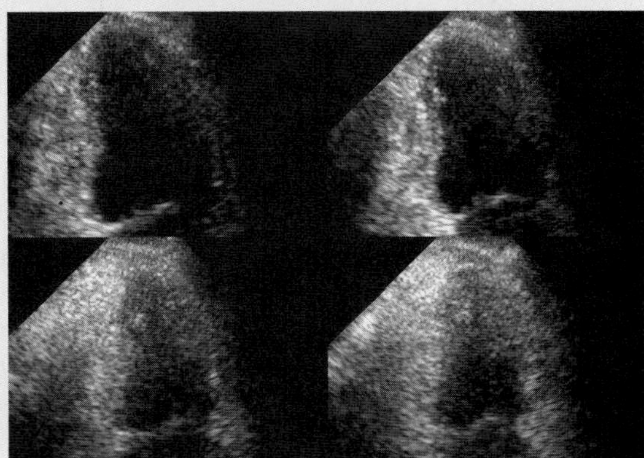

Your recommendation to the referring physician is

a. Clear the patient for surgery with beta-blocker prophylaxis.
b. Stress SPECT thallium nuclear imaging.
c. Coronary angiography.
d. Cancellation of surgery.
e. Stent grafting, in hopes of avoiding major aortic surgery.

Answer is a: The dobutamine echocardiogram demonstrates (still frames at end systole) a fixed regional wall motion abnormality involving the base of the inferior wall and base of the septum consistent with a right coronary artery territory scar. The remaining left ventricular wall segments were contracting normally at rest with a resting ejection fraction of approximately 55%. Peak dobutamine stress images reveal an appropriate improvement in wall motion involving the left anterior descending and circumflex coronary territories with no change in the wall motion involving the inferior and basil septum. These results are consistent with right coronary artery territory scar and no evidence for ischemia. Based on this negative echocardiogram for ischemia, this patient with an intermediate clinical predictor, namely, prior myocardial infarction, may be considered at a relatively low perioperative risk for a cardiac event and therefore could be cleared for his procedure with beta-blocker prophylaxis.

**2.** A 70-year-old man with hypertension and a recently diagnosed solitary pulmonary nodule is scheduled for wedge resection. He is otherwise healthy, active, and regularly plays 18 holes of golf. His ECG reveals left ventricular hypertrophy with secondary repolarization changes consistent with a strain pattern. Your recommendation is

a. Stress echocardiography for risk stratification.
b. Clear the patient for surgery.
c. Coronary angiography.
d. Echocardiogram.
e. Stress SPECT thallium imaging.

Answer is b: This 70-year-old man with hypertension is scheduled for an intermediate-risk surgery. He has a history of hypertension with ECG changes consistent with left ventricular hypertrophy. Other than his age and an abnormal baseline electrocardiogram, this gentleman has no other significant clinical predictors of perioperative risk. Reportedly, he has a very good exercise capacity, which would place him in the moderate to excellent category for functional capacity based on his ability to regularly play 18 holes of golf without difficulty. Based on the absence of significant clinical predictors, as well as a good exercise capacity, this patient can be cleared for his wedge resection with a low perioperative risk of sustaining a cardiac event.

3. An 80-year-old woman with hypertension and a history of "congestive heart failure" recently suffered a hip fracture and is in need of stabilization. She lives with family but is known to be inactive, primarily because of arthritis. Your recommendation is to do the following:

a. Clear the patient for the orthopedic procedure with beta-blocker prophylaxis and careful hemodynamic monitoring.
b. Coronary angiography.
c. Dobutamine stress echocardiography for risk stratification.
d. Echocardiogram, and if left ventricular function is normal, clear the patient for surgery.
e. Exercise stress SPECT thallium.

Answer is c: Because of the one reported critical predictor, namely, the prior history of congestive heart failure, as well as a suspected poor functional capacity, this patient should undergo further risk stratification using a pharmacologic stress imaging study. Stress echocardiography can be considered a good stress imaging modality in a patient with hypertensive heart disease, as the microvascular disease associated with hypertensive heart disease may result in abnormalities in coronary flow reserve that may in turn lead to a false positive result when using nuclear perfusion imaging.

4. A 78-year-old woman with a history of chronic stable angina is scheduled for cataract surgery. Your recommendation is

a. Dipyridamole stress SPECT thallium imaging.
b. Coronary angiography.
c. Clear the patient for cataract surgery.
d. Echocardiogram, and if left ventricular function is normal, clear the patient for surgery.
e. Exercise stress echocardiography.

Answer is c: This 78-year-old woman does have one intermediate clinical predictor of risk, namely, stable angina pectoris. However, she was noted to have good functional capacity and is undergoing a very low-risk surgical procedure, so she can be cleared for the cataract surgery with a low anticipated risk for adverse events.

5. Your patient is a 55-year-old man who is in need of a fem-pop bypass for claudication. What do you recommend for risk stratification?

a. Exercise ECG
b. Angiography
c. Dobutamine stress echocardiography
d. Dipyridamole thallium
e. Clinical evaluation

Answer is e: In any patient undergoing preoperative evaluation, an assessment of clinical predictors of risk is central to initiating an appropriate workup prior to the noncardiac surgery. If this man with vascular disease were found, on clinical evaluation, to have a history of one or more intermediate or major clinical predictors of risk, or were found to be unable to exercise to a moderate level, further risk stratification with pharmacologic stress imaging would be indicated.

# Pharmacology

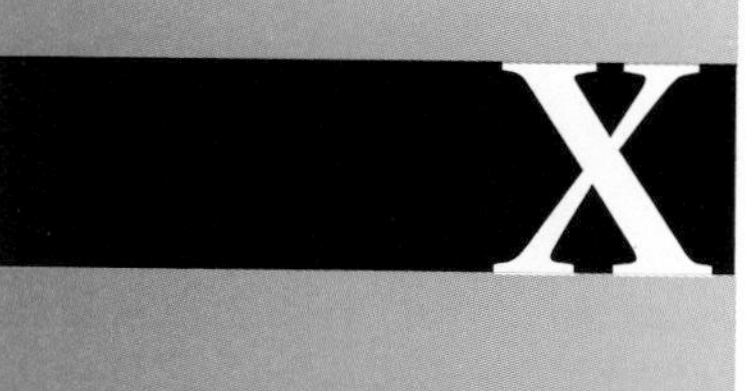

# 58 Pharmacokinetic and Pharmacodynamic Essentials

*Michael A. Militello*   *Jodie M. Fink*

Basic understanding of pharmacokinetic and pharmacodynamic concepts is essential to the design of rational, patient-specific pharmacotherapy. The study of pharmacokinetics was first introduced some 40 years ago and is defined as the time course of drug absorption, distribution, metabolism, and elimination. In basic terms this is described as how the body handles the drug. The concepts of pharmacokinetics can be applied to individual patients in order to maximize efficacy and limit drug toxicities. Drug plasma concentration can help to predict efficacy and toxicity of selected medications. Even though there are limited data for therapeutic drug monitoring for all medications, pharmacokinetic principles can be applied to a wide range of medications.

The primary principle of pharmacodynamics is that a relationship exists between drug concentration at the site of action (receptor) and pharmacologic response. The concentration at the receptor site is most important for elucidating pharmacologic response, with the assumption that serum concentration is directly proportional to receptor concentration. This assumption is not always true. For example, although abciximab has an initial half-life of 10 minutes and second-phase half-life of about 30 minutes, measurement of plasma concentrations of abciximab is not of clinical importance, whereas measurement of platelet activity potentially could be of importance.

The focus of this chapter is to review pharmacokinetic and pharmacodynamic concepts and relate them to specific cardiovascular medications. This chapter does not cover current guidelines for use of medications. Please refer to individual chapters in this review book for guideline reference.

## PHARMACOKINETICS

Pharmacokinetics refers to the concepts of drug absorption, distribution, metabolism, and elimination (known as "ADME"). Such principles can be applied to drug therapy by such examples as determining loading and maintenance doses of medications, adjusting doses for altered elimination (e.g., renal or hepatic insufficiency), and interpreting plasma drug concentrations. The concepts of ADME are reviewed below.

### Absorption

Absorption of medications can occur via multiple routes of administration. Medications administered via the intravenous route are considered to have 100% absorption because the drug is delivered directly into the patient's circulation. Other routes of administration include oral, transdermal, buccal, sublingual, subcutaneous, intradermal, and rectal. Depending on the type of medication, there are advantages and disadvantages of each of these administration techniques related to absorption. For example, the administration of nitroglycerin via the oral route would provide little systemic effect because of the high degree of presystemic clearance through hepatic metabolism. However, when nitroglycerin is administered intravenously, transdermally, or sublingually, the amount delivered is greatly increased, as presystemic clearance is bypassed.

A number of factors affect the amount of drug absorbed. These include:

- Dose administered
- Fraction of the administered dose that is "active drug" ($S$)
- Bioavailability of the drug ($F$)

The equation for amount of drug absorbed is

$$\text{Amount of drug absorbed} = (S)(F)(\text{Dose})$$

The fraction of administered dose that is "active drug" ($S$) is typically described as the salt form of a drug, and varies with different salts. For example, quinidine sulfate has 82% active drug, and quinidine gluconate has 62%. By using the above equation one can convert from one salt form to another salt, assuming you know the bioavailability ($F$). For example, quinidine sulfate is 82% quinidine base with a bioavailability of 0.73, and quinidine gluconate is 62% quinidine base with a bioavailability of 0.7. With this information you can compare the amount of quinidine in each tablet to make your conversion. Below is a comparison of quinidine bases assuming you have 200-mg tablets of both quinidine sulfate (a) and quinidine gluconate (b).

$$\text{Amount of quinidine base absorbed} = 0.82 \times 0.7 \times 200 \rightarrow 114.8 \text{ mg}$$

$$\text{Amount of quinidine base absorbed} = 0.62 \times 0.7 \times 200 \rightarrow 86.8 \text{ mg}$$

Bioavailability ($F$) is defined as the fraction of an administered dose that reaches the systemic circulation of a patient. Values of bioavailability can be found in a number of pharmacology texts and drug reference handbooks. Factors that can alter bioavailability include:

- *Inherent characteristics* of the dosage form administered (e.g., tablet dissolution characteristics).
- *Administration route* (e.g., oral versus transdermal versus intravenous). The bioavailability of most parenterally administered drugs is 100% (i.e., $F = 1$).
- *Issues related to the gastrointestinal (GI) tract.*

The bioavailability of orally administered medications can be affected by gastric pH, GI transit time, gut metabolism, and the presence of food. Certain medications may be unstable in low-pH environments and therefore may be enteric coated in order to prevent breakdown in the stomach. Conversely, certain medications, such as itraconazole, require an acid environment for optimal absorption. Likewise, changes in gastrointestinal motility with promotility agents or patients experiencing diarrhea may have decreased absorption secondary to decreased transit time through the GI tract. Enzymatic metabolism of medications in the GI tract can also alter absorption and can be responsible for drug interactions. A well-described example of this is the fact that administration of grapefruit juice with certain medications may actually enhance bioavailability secondary to preventing GI metabolism of the compound, thereby increasing the amount of drug available for absorption (see Chapter 62). Finally, the amount of bioavailable drug may be reduced as a result of the extent of metabolism before reaching the systemic circulation. Examples of this include metabolism via GI bacteria (e.g., digoxin) or "first-pass metabolism" by the liver.

Drugs are absorbed from the GI tract into the portal circulation, and certain drugs are extensively metabolized in the liver before reaching systemic circulation. These drugs have a high *first-pass effect* or high *first-pass metabolism,* which can significantly decrease the amount of medication reaching the systemic circulation and hence drug bioavailability. Drugs with high first-pass metabolism have much lower intravenous doses compared to oral doses. Examples of medications with high first-pass metabolism are

- Diltiazem
- Hydralazine
- Isoproterenol
- Labetalol
- Lidocaine
- Metoprolol
- Nifedipine
- Nitroglycerin
- Propranolol
- Verapamil

## Distribution

After absorption, medications distribute to various tissues in the body to produce a pharmacologic effect. Not all distribution sites for a given medication produce a therapeutic effect. In fact, some distribution sites may produce no effect or untoward effects. The *volume of distribution* ($Vd$), or apparent volume of distribution, refers to the total amount of drug in the body, assuming the drug is present at the same *plasma drug concentration* ($Cp$) throughout the body. The $Vd$ is expressed in terms of volume (e.g., liters or liters per kilogram) and is a function of the solubility (lipid versus water solubility) and binding (tissue versus plasma protein binding) characteristics of the drug. Actual sites of distribution cannot be determined from the $Vd$ value.

The volume of distribution equation is

$$\text{Volume of distribution} = \frac{\text{amount of drug in body}}{\text{plasma drug concentration}}$$

Factors that tend to increase $Cp$ will decrease apparent $Vd$ and include drugs that have:

- Low lipid solubility
- High plasma protein binding
- Low tissue binding

Factors that tend to decrease *Cp* will increase apparent *Vd* and include drugs that have:

- High lipid solubility
- Low plasma protein binding
- High tissue binding

Volume of distribution can be used to estimate a loading dose needed to achieve a desired plasma concentration rapidly. Medications such as amiodarone, which has a large volume of distribution (66 L/kg), requires a longer duration (weeks) to load adequately, as there is a large number of distribution sites. In contrast, a person receiving procainamide, which has a volume of distribution of 2 L/kg, can be adequately loaded with a single dose in the appropriate amount. Although a loading dose does not decrease the time to achieve steady-state plasma concentration, it does reduce the time to reach a therapeutic plasma concentration or therapeutic range. For many medications there is not a target concentration that is defined, and therefore, loading-dose equations are typically not used. In this circumstance, which is true for most drugs, initial and maximal doses are chosen based on dose ranging, and randomized studies comparing the expected response to the dose. For instance, early trials of metoprolol tartrate used starting doses of 25 to 50 mg twice daily for hypertension, and these doses produced the clinical response desired to obtain the specified endpoints. Therefore, using both pharmacokinetic and pharmacodynamic data can help to establish appropriate dosing of medications when obtaining serum drug levels is not available.

To determine the loading dose, the following equation is used:

$$\text{Loading dose} = \frac{(Vd)(Cp)}{(S)(F)}$$

The target plasma concentration for a given drug is often referred to as the *therapeutic range*, and can be thought of as a range of drug concentrations in which there is a relatively high probability of achieving a desired clinical response and a relatively low probability of developing unacceptable toxicity. *Narrow-therapeutic-range drugs* are ones in which this desired drug concentration range is small (e.g., lidocaine, procainamide, digoxin, quinidine, etc.) and the therapeutic concentration and toxic concentration are similar. This concept will be reviewed later in this chapter under pharmacodynamics.

### Metabolism and Elimination

*Clearance* (*Cl*) is the intrinsic ability of the body (or eliminating organs such as kidneys or liver) to remove drug, and is expressed in volume per unit of time (e.g., liters per hour). Hepatic metabolism of a drug can lead to formation of active or inactive metabolites. Metabolites may contribute to the therapeutic efficacy or toxicities associated with the parent drug (e.g., procainamide and N-acetylprocainamide).

At steady state, the rate of drug administration (*RA*, or dose/time) and rate of drug elimination are equal, and the concentration of drug remains constant. Clearance can be thought of in terms of these factors in the following equation; where *Cpss* refers to steady-state plasma drug concentrations:

$$Cl = \frac{(RA)}{(Cpss)}$$

The relative clearance of drug is an important factor in calculating the rate of administration or maintenance dose to produce a desired average plasma drug concentration:

$$\text{Maintenance dose or } RA = (Cl)(Cpss)$$

Another consideration in determining dosing interval is evaluating the half-life of a medication. *Half-life* ($t_{1/2}$) refers to the amount of time required for the total amount of drug in the body or the plasma drug concentration to decrease by half. Half-life can be calculated with the following equation:

$$t_{1/2} = \frac{0.693 \times Vd}{Cl}$$

Half-life can be used to determine the amount of time it will take to reach steady-state plasma concentrations. Typically, three to five half-lives are required to reach steady state. It takes one half-life to reach 50%, two to reach 75%, three to reach 87.5%, four to reach 93.75%, and five half-lives to reach 97% of steady state. Half-life can also be used to determine how long it will take to eliminate drug from the body after the drug has been discontinued. It takes one half-life to eliminate 50%, two to eliminate 75%, and so on.

Metabolism of medications typically occurs in the liver, producing more hydrophilic compounds to allow for elimination through the kidneys. However, many drugs may undergo exclusive renal elimination without any form of biotransformation or metabolism. Biotransformation may also convert prodrugs (precursors to active drug forms) to drugs with biologic activity (e.g., enalapril, losartan). Other routes of drug elimination include biliary routes.

## PHARMACODYNAMICS

The main principle of pharmacodynamics is the relationship between drug concentration at the site of action (receptor site) and pharmacologic response. Simply stated, pharmacodynamics is the study of plasma concentration and pharmacologic response. This relationship can be described by the equation

$$E = \frac{(E_{\max} \times C)}{(C + EC_{50})}$$

where

$E$ is pharmacologic effect
$E_{\max}$ is the maximum effect the drug can cause (determines efficacy)

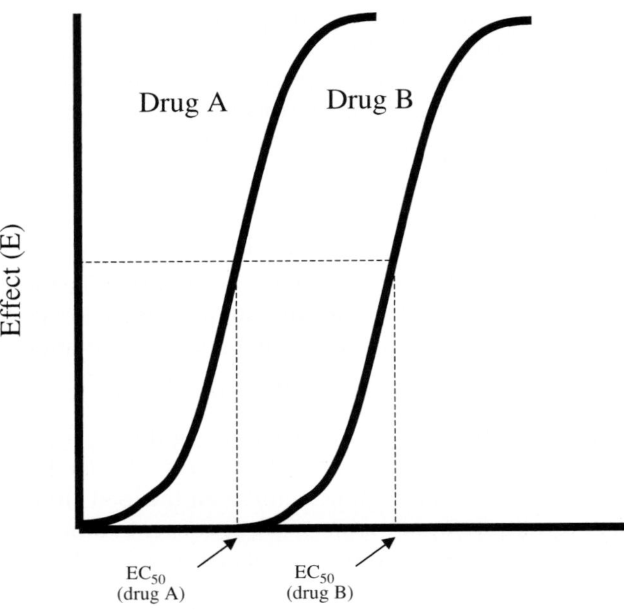


**Figure 58–1** Potency and efficacy curves. Drug A is considered to have the same efficacy as drug B, because the maximal effect is the same. However, drug A is considered to be more potent, because the $EC_{50}$ is less than that of drug B.

$EC_{50}$ is the concentration at which one half of the maximal response will occur (determines drug potency)
$C$ is the concentration of the drug at the receptor site

Drugs with low $EC_{50}$ are considered more potent than the comparison drug (i.e., these drugs elicit the same response at lower concentrations). Drugs with a similar $E_{max}$ are considered to have similar efficacy (Fig. 58–1). Some medications may have the same $EC_{50}$ but very different $E_{max}$ values.

These same efficacy principles can be applied to toxicity and used to evaluate therapeutic ranges or indexes. The dose that produces toxic effects in 50% of evaluated subjects (typically animals) is called the *toxic dose 50* or $TD_{50}$. The ratio of the $TD_{50}$ to the $ED_{50}$ is the typical definition of *therapeutic index*. As this ratio approaches one, the therapeutic index is considered narrow. The risks versus benefits of the therapy as well as the severity of the disease state determine an acceptable therapeutic index. For example, medications to treat chronic diseases or non–life-threatening diseases typically have therapeutic indexes that are large. In contrast, physicians accept a narrower therapeutic index when treating a disease state that has a high mortality (e.g., certain malignancies).

## BIBLIOGRAPHY


**Braunwald E, Zipes DP, Libby P, eds.** *Braunwald's Heart Disease: A Textbook of Cardiovascular Medicine.* 7th ed. Philadelphia: WB Saunders; 2005.

**Evans WE, Schentag JJ, Jusko WJ, eds.** *Applied Pharmacokinetics: Principles of Therapeutic Drug Monitoring.* 3rd ed. Vancouver, WA: Applied Therapeutics; 1992.

**Winter ME.** *Basic Clinical Pharmacokinetics.* 4th ed. Baltimore: Lippincott Williams & Wilkins; 2004.


## QUESTIONS

**1.** Which of the following drugs is the most potent?

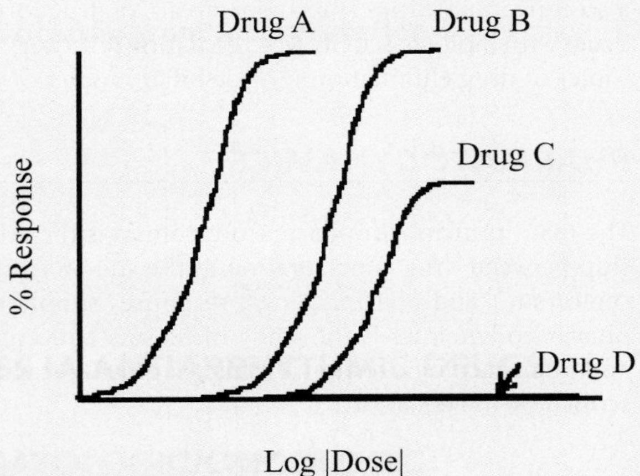


a. Drug A
b. Drug B
c. Drug C
d. Drug D

Answer is a: Drug potency is related the concentration that elicits 50% of the maximal response. Therefore, when comparing drug response to concentration curves, the drug that produces 50% of the maximal response at the lowest concentration is the most potent drug. In the graph above, both drugs A and B will elicit the same maximal response, therefore they have the same efficacy; however, drug A produces its effect at a lower plasma concentration. Drug C would be considered either a partial agonist or a lower-potency and -efficacy drug, whereas drug D would be defined as a receptor antagonist.

**2.** Which of the following is a principle of pharmacodynamics as opposed to pharmacokinetics?

a. Absorption in the gastrointestinal tract
b. Distribution into the central nervous system
c. Metabolism of medications in the liver
d. Tolerance to medication with prolonged exposure

Answer is d: Tolerance to medication with prolonged exposure is a biologic issue reflecting pharmacodynamics, whereas the others reflect concepts that determine how medications are handled by the body (pharmacokinetics).

**3.** What two pharmacokinetic parameters determine the half-life of a medication?

a. Loading dose and clearance
b. Absorption and clearance
c. Volume of distribution and clearance
d. Absorption and volume of distribution

Answer is c: Both the volume of distribution and the clearance determine the half-life of a medication. As can be seen from the equation,

$$t_{1/2} = \frac{0.693 \times Vd}{Cl}$$

either increasing the volume of distribution or decreaseing clearance will increae the half-life of the drug.

**4.** RT is a 42-year-old man with atrial fibrillation after a recent aortic valve replacement. You would like to start IV procainamide in this patient. He weighs 75 kg and has normal renal function. Your target therapeutic level for procainamide is 8 $\mu$g/mL. The volume of distribution of procainamide is about 2 L/kg. What is this patient's calculated loading dose?

a. 1,000 mg
b. 1,200 mg
c. 1,400 mg
d. 1,600 mg

Answer is b: Based on the equation for loading dose, volume of distribution $\times$ weight $\times$ serum drug concentration needed, you can determine the loading dose. Here 2 L/kg $\times$ 75 kg $\times$ 8 mg/L (converted from $\mu$g/mL) gives a loading dose of 1,200 mg. Practically speaking, we would round this to the nearest 250 mg and limit the initial load to 1,500 to 1,750 mg.

**5.** Therapeutic index is defined as the ratio of $TD_{50}$ to $ED_{50}$.

a. True
b. False

Answer is a: This is known as the therapeutic index of a medication.

# 59

# Cardiovascular Medicine—Essential Pharmaceuticals

**Soundos K. Moualla Hanna Ahmed Michael A. Militello**

Cardiovascular disease (CVD) accounts for nearly 50% of all death in Western societies and 25% of all death worldwide. Furthermore, cardiac medications rank second in frequency of use worldwide, after antibiotics. Medical therapy plays an essential role, not only in the management of CVD, but also in prevention.

Pharmacology accounts for about 12% of the questions on the Cardiology Boards. The topic is vast and may be approached in various ways. Pharmacokinetics and dynamics, drug interactions, and antiarrhythmics are addressed in other chapters. In this chapter, we cover most of the available cardiovascular drugs used in clinical practice in the United States. We review names (brand and generic), starting and maximum doses, mechanisms of action, labeled and unlabeled indications, and side effects. When appropriate, we comment on the major clinical trials involving the particular drug. The classes and drugs are classified alphabetically according to mechanistic class and/or therapeutic class, as shown in Table 59–1.

## ADRENERGIC AGONISTS

Before detailing specific medications, we review basic information on adrenergic receptors that is useful for understanding the mechanism and side effects of this class as well as classes discussed subsequently. The adrenoceptors are classified into alpha ($\alpha$) and beta ($\beta$) subtypes. There are two main subtypes of $\alpha$ adrenoceptors, $\alpha_1$ and $\alpha_2$, and three main types of $\beta$ adrenoceptors, $\beta_1$, $\beta_2$, and $\beta_3$. The primary effects of receptor activation are shown in Table 59–2. The adrenergic agonists of cardiac interest in this section are the $\alpha_2$ agonists, which act centrally. In later sections we discuss other adrenergic agonists that stimulate $\alpha$ and $\beta$ receptors, such as epinephrine, norepinephrine, dobutamine, and other inotropes and pressors.

### The $\alpha_2$ Agonists (Clonidine, Guanabenz, Guanfacine)

#### Mechanism of Action

The $\alpha_2$ receptors are presynaptic and are found in the central nervous system (CNS). Stimulation of the $\alpha_2$ receptors decreases sympathetic outflow from the CNS, thus lowering blood pressure and, in some patients, heart rate.

#### Side Effects

Common side effects include sedation, dry mouth, hypotension, dizziness, sexual dysfunction, bradycardia, nausea, headache, and depression. Abrupt withdrawal of therapy causes rebound hypertension. Rebound hypertension can be severe with concurrent administration of beta-blockers secondary to unopposed $\alpha_1$ receptor stimulation.

#### Indication and Precautions

##### Clonidine (Catapres and Catapres-TTS)

Clonidine is labeled for use in hypertension. For patients with severe renal insufficiency (i.e., CrCl <10 mL/min),

**TABLE 59–1**
**MAJOR CLASSES OF CARDIAC MEDICATIONS, LISTED ALPHABETICALLY**

| Drug Class[a] | Subclasses |
|---|---|
| Adrenergic agonists | |
| Adrenergic antagonists | $\alpha_1$ antagonist<br>Selective $\beta$ antagonists (beta-blockers)<br>Nonselective beta-blockers<br>Mixed $\alpha_1$/beta-blockers |
| Angiotensin-converting enzyme inhibitors (ACEIs) | |
| Angiotensin II-receptor blockers (ARBs) | |
| Aldosterone-receptor antagonists | |
| Anticoagulants | Unfractionaed heparin/low-molecular-weight heparin<br>Pentasaccharide<br>Direct thrombin inhibitors<br>Oral anticoagulants |
| Calcium channel blockers | Dihydropyridines<br>Nondihydropyridines |
| Diuretics | Loop diuretics<br>Thiazide diuretics<br>$K^+$-sparing diuretics |
| Inotropic agents and vasopressors | Catecholamines<br>Phosphodiesterase inhibitors |
| Lipid-lowering agents | Bile acid resin<br>HMG CoA reductase<br>Fibrates<br>Other |
| Nitrates | |
| Platelet inhibitors | Cyclo-oxygenase inhibitors<br>Thienopyridines<br>Glycoprotein (IIb/IIIA) inhibitors |
| Thrombolytics | |
| Vasodilators | |
| Miscellaneous drugs | |

[a]Antiarrhythmics are covered in Chapter X.

**TABLE 59–2**
**MAIN EFFECTS OF RECEPTOR ACTIVATION OF ADRENOCEPTORS**

| Receptor Class | Biologic Effect When Stimulated |
|---|---|
| $\alpha_1$ | Vasoconstriction, relaxation of GI smooth muscle, stimulation of salivary secretion |
| $\alpha_2$ | Inhibition of norepinephrine release from autonomic nerves, contraction of smooth muscle, platelet aggregation |
| $\beta_1$ | Increased heart rate and contractility, GI smooth muscle relaxation |
| $\beta_2$ | Bronchodilation, vasodilation, relaxation of visceral smooth muscle |
| $\beta_3$ | Lipolysis |

doses should be reduced by 25% to 50%. Transdermal patches are replaced weekly.

#### Methyldopa (Aldomet) (Oral); Methyldopate HCL (Intravenous)

Methyldopa is labeled for use in hypertension and hypertensive emergency (IV only) and is one of the few drugs that can be used for hypertension in pregnant women. In addition to the general side effects of $\alpha_2$-receptor agonists, methyldopa has specific side effects: peripheral edema, hemolytic anemia, drug fever, systemic lupus erythamatosus (SLE)-like syndrome, nightmares, hepatocellular injury, hepatitis (rare), and anxiety. Positive Coombs tests occur within 6 to 12 months in 10% to 20% of patients.

## ADRENERGIC ANTAGONISTS

This section is divided according to the various subgroups of adrenergic antagonists, based on the adrenergic receptors they block, and include $\alpha_1$-receptor antagonists, $\beta$-receptor antagonists, and nonselective $\alpha/\beta$ antagonists.

### $\alpha_1$-Receptor Antagonists

***Selective $\alpha_1$ Antagonists: Doxazosin (Cardura), Prazosin (Minipress), Terazosin (Hytrin)***

#### Mechanism of Action

Selective $\alpha_1$-receptor antagonists act peripherally and lead to arterial and venous vasodilation.

#### Side Effects

Side effects of $\alpha_1$-receptor antagonists include orthostatic hypotension, dizziness, lightheadedness, drowsiness, headache, dry mouth, and malaise. The first dose should be given at bedtime to limit effects associated with orthostatic hypotension. Tachyphylaxis may develop with long-term administration in patients with heart failure (e.g., prazosin).

#### Indications and Precautions

These drugs are labeled for use in hypertension and benign prostatic hypertrophy (BPH) (terazosin only).

#### Major Clinical Trials

VHeFT I (1). In this trial, hydralazine combined with nitrates and prazosin were compared to placebo for the treatment of heart failure. No effect on the primary endpoint of mortality was observed, and no difference in left ventricular ejection fraction was observed when prazosin was compared to placebo.

ALLHAT (2). This trial was designed to evaluate different antihypertensive medications to reduce cardiovascular events. An interim analysis 2 years before the final publication demonstrated that patients receiving doxazosin had a significantly higher rate of stroke cardiovascular events, and the rate of congestive heart failure was two time higher. The doxazosin arm was stopped early as a result of the findings.

### *Nonselective α Antagonists: Phentolamine (Regitine)*

#### Mechanism of Action

Nonselective $\alpha$-adrenergic antagonist have similar affinities for $\alpha_1$ and $\alpha_2$ receptors, producing vasodilation and an increase in heart rate.

#### Side Effects

Side effects of these drugs include hypotension, tachycardia, arrhythmias, angina, and nausea/vomiting/diarrhea. They may exacerbate peptic ulcer disease (PUD) and produce nasal congestion.

#### Indications and Precautions

Phentolamine is labeled for use in hypertensive crisis in patients with pheochromocytoma and for treatment of skin necrosis in patients with norepinepherine, dopamine, epinephrine, and phenylephrine extravasation.

### *β-Receptor Antagonists*

Beta-blockers were first discovered in 1958 (dichloroisoprenaline). The effects produced depend on the degree of endogenous sympathetic activity and are less dramatic at rest. Beta-blockers are classified as selective and nonselective as well as having $\alpha_1$-blocking properties.

#### Mechanism of Action

Nonselective beta-blockers antagonize both $\beta_1$ and $\beta_2$ receptors, inhibiting the effects of catecholamines on these receptors. Cardiovascular effects include decreases in contractility and heart rate. Noncardiovascular effects mediated through $\beta_2$ blockade include increased peripheral vascular resistance or bronchospasm. Selective beta-blockers antagonize $\beta_1$ receptors to a greater extent than $\beta_2$ receptors, when administered in typical or usual doses. Cardiovascular effects are the same as with nonselective beta-blockers. Both classes generally lead to a decrease in blood pressure, sinus node automaticity, conduction through the atrioventricular (AV) node, and increased AV nodal refractoriness. The antiarrhythmic properties are a class effect. Other pharmacologic properties of selective beta-blockers include intrinsic sympathomimetic activity (ISA). Agents that have ISA are partial $\beta$ agonists during low catecholamine states, preventing resting bradycardia; however, they act as full agonists when endogenous catecholamine levels increase. Beta-blockers without ISA activity have been shown to decrease recurrent myocardial infarction (MI), sudden death, and overall mortality in acute-MI survivors. They also have been shown to reduce mortality and hospitalizations secondary to heart failure. A list of the various beta-blockers that are used is provided in Table 59–3.

#### Side Effects

Side effects of these drugs include fatigue, bradycardia, heart block, bronchospasm, depression, lipid abnormalities, masking the symptoms of hypoglycemia, a rebound effect with abrupt discontinuation, precipitation of heart failure, and impotence.

#### Indications and Precautions

Indications for beta-blockers include hypertension, ischemic heart disease, acute myocardial infarction, stable and unstable angina, heart failure, antiarrhythmia, and stable heart failure (see Table 59–3). Absolute contraindications include hypersensitivity to beta-blockers, asthma, heart block greater than first degree, insulin-dependent

**TABLE 59–3**
**PHARMACOKINETICS OF COMMONLY USED BETA-BLOCKERS**

| Drug | Selectivity | ISA | Lipid Solubility | Dose, Initial–Maximum mg/day | Onset of Action | Half-Life (h) |
|---|---|---|---|---|---|---|
| Acebutolol | $\beta_1$ | + | Low | 400–1,200 mg/d | Oral, 1–3 h | 3–4 |
| Atenolol | $\beta_1$ | 0 | Low | 25–200 mg/d | 1–3 h | 6–9 |
| Bisoprolol | $\beta_1$ | 0 | Low | 5–20 mg/d | 2–4 h | 9–12 |
| Esmolol | $\beta_1$ | 0 | Low | [a] | IV, 2–5 min | 0.15 |
| Metoprolol[b] | $\beta_1$ | 0 | Moderate | 50–450 mg/d | Oral, 1 h<br>IV, 5 min | 3–7 |
| Nadolol | $\beta_1\beta_2$ | 0 | Low | 40–320 mg/d | 1–2 h | 20–24 |
| Pindolol | $\beta_1\beta_2$ | +++ | Moderate | 10–60 mg/d | >3 h | 3–4 |
| Propranolol | $\beta_1\beta_2$ | 0 | High | 30–480 mg/d | Oral, 1–2 h IV, 2–5 min | 3–5 |

[a]Esmolol is an IV-formulated drug. The loading dose is 500 $\mu$g/kg given over 1 minute. Then the maintenance dose is 25–300 $\mu$g/kg per minute.
[b]Metoprolol is available as an immediate-release preparation and as an extended-release preparation. The extended-release product is labeled for both hypertension and heart failure.
ISA, intrinsic sympathomimetic activity.

diabetics with frequent hypoglycemic episodes, and overt heart failure. Relative contraindications include chronic obstructive lung disease, diabetes mellitus, and severe peripheral arterial disease. Beta-blockers have significant interactions with other drugs, including: medications that slow AV nodal conduction such as digoxin, diltiazem, and verapamil, as well as nonsteroidal anti-inflammatory drugs (NSAIDS), other antihypertensive medications, other negative inotropic agents, rifampin, phenobarbital, phenytoin, cholestyramine, and colestipol, to name a few.

### *Combined $\alpha/\beta$-Receptor Antagonists*

#### Mechanism of Action

The combination preparations are specific $\alpha_1$-receptor antagonists, but nonselective $\beta$-receptor antagonists. Labetalol is 7:1 selective $\beta$ to $\alpha$ receptor in the IV preparation and 3:1 in the oral preparation.

#### Side Effects

Refer to side effects of beta-blockers.

#### Indications and Precautions

The labeled indication of labetalol is hypertension.

#### Major Clinical Trials

MERIT-HF (3). Metoprolol CR/XL improved survival and New York Heart Association (NYHA) functional class, and reduced the number of hospitalizations and days in the hospital due to worsening heart failure.

CIBIS-II (4). This trial demonstrated that bisoprolol therapy was well tolerated and reduced mortality and hospitalization rates in patients with stable congestive heart failure.

CAPRICORN (5). This trial showed that long-term therapy with carvedilol, in addition to angiotensin-converting enzyme I (ACE-I) and standard therapy, reduced mortality and recurrent MI in stable patients with left ventricular (LV) systolic dysfunction after acute MI.

COPERNICUS (6). This trial studied the effect of carvedilol on survival in patients with severe chronic heart failure. Carvedilol reduced mortality in patients with severe congestive heart failure (CHF) by 34%, and also reduced the number of days spent in hospital because of CHF and for any cause.

COMET (7). Carvedilol improved survival and LV ejection fraction to a greater degree than immediate-release metoprolol during long-term therapy for heart failure.

BHAT (8,9). The Beta blocker Heart Attack Trial, using propanolol, and the Norwegian Multicenter Study Group, using timolol, both showed a reduction in mortality rate, reinfarction rate, or both with the use of the beta-blocker.

## ANGIOTENSIN-CONVERTING ENZYME INHIBITORS (ACE-I)

The renin–angiotensin system (RAS) is a hormonal system that interacts very closely with the sympathetic nervous system, angiotensin II formation, and aldosterone secretion. It has an essential role in sodium and volume management. Renin, an enzyme, is secreted by the juxtaglomerular apparatus located in the wall of the arteriole of the glomerulus. It is secreted secondary to multiple stimuli, low sodium concentration of the fluid in the distal tubule, stimulation of the $\beta$-adrenoceptors, and circulating prostacyclin and nitric oxide, as shown in Figure 59–1.

The RAS pathway is important in the pathogenesis of heart failure and hypertension, hence all aspects of this pathway are targets for therapy in CHF and hypertension, whether in renin release such as beta-blockers, angiotensin II formation such as ACE inhibitors, or angiotensin II blockade such as angiotensin II receptor blockers (ARBs) and aldosterone antagonists.

### *Mechanism of Action*

Angiotensin-converting enzyme inhibitors (ACEIs) block the conversion of angiotensin I to angiotensin II by inhibiting angiotensin-converting enzyme (ACE), as shown in Figure 59–1. In response to this blockade, there is decreased formation of angiotensin II, leading to vasodilatation. Also, there is a decrease in the breakdown of bradykinins, which may produce additional vasodilatory effects.

### *Side Effects*

Side effects include cough (because of decrease in breakdown of bradykinin), acute renal failure (particularly if there is bilateral renal artery stenosis), angioedema, hyperkalemia, proteinuria, hypotension (which needs to be monitored after the first dose and in water-depleted patients), headache, rash, neutropenia/agranulocytosis, and dizziness.

Angioedema is rare but may occur at any time; when it does occur, however, it is usually early in therapy. Severe hypotension may be seen in volume-depleted patients; hence the volume status of a heart failure patient should be carefully assessed before initiating therapy. Neutropenia and/or agranulocytosis has been reported with many ACEIs and is usually associated with collagen vascular disorders, higher doses, and renal dysfunction.

### *Indications and Precautions*

ACEIs are labeled for use in hypertension, heart failure, LV dysfunction, post–acute myocardial infarction (AMI), and diabetic nephropathy (Table 59–4). ACEIs are contraindicated in pregnancy and in patients with bilateral renal artery stenosis (RAS) or unilateral renal artery stenosis in patients with a solitary kidney.

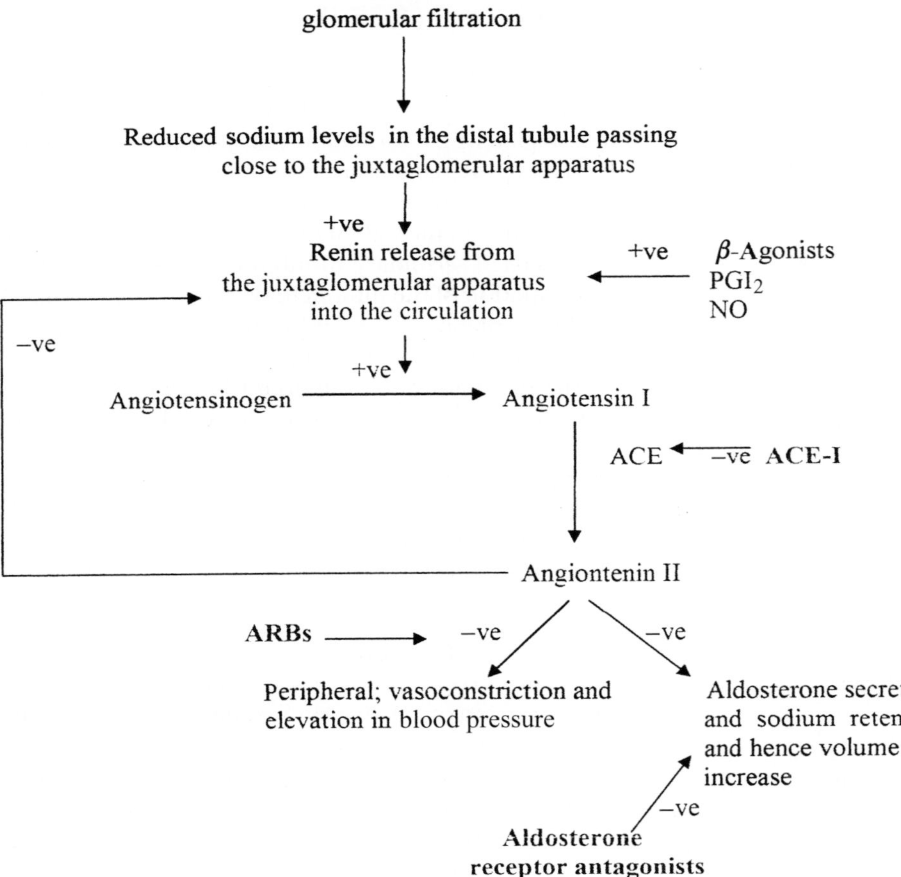


**Figure 59–1** The renin–angiotensin–aldosterone pathway and mechanism of action of angiotensin-converting enzyme (ACE) inhibitors and angiotensin-receptor blockers (ARBs). ACE is a membrane-bound enzyme on the surface of endothelial cells abundant in the lung (+ve, positive or stimulatory effect; −ve, negative or inhibitory effect).

### *Major Clinical Trials*

SAVE (10,11). The SAVE trial showed that the long-term use of captopril in patients with asymptomatic LV dysfunction following acute MI was associated with lower mortality and morbidity.

GISSI-3 (12). This trial showed that lisinopril therapy reduced mortality and improved outcome after MI. The mortality benefit manifested primarily during the early phase (6 weeks), whereas the LV remodeling benefit manifested later.

TRACE (13). The TRACE trial update confirmed that trandolapril reduced death and major cardiovascular complications in diabetic patients after infarction.

HEART (14). The HEART trial showed that in patients with acute anterior myocardial infarction, early use of

**TABLE 59–4**
**PREPARATIONS AND DOSING OF AVAILABLE ANGIOTENSIN-CONVERTING ENZYME INHIBITORS**

| Medication | Side Group | Half-Life (h) | Comments |
|---|---|---|---|
| Benazepril (Lotensin) 5, 10, 20, 40 mg | Carboxyl | 10–11 | |
| Captopril (Capoten) 12.5, 25, 50, 100 mg | Sulfhydryl | 1.7–2 | Best taken on empty stomach; not a prodrug |
| Enalapril (Vasotec) 2.5, 5, 10, 20 mg | Carboxyl | 11 | Also available in IV form (1.25 mg/mL); IV form is not a prodrug |
| Fosinopril (Monopril) 10, 20 mg | Phosphinyl | 12 | |
| Lisinopril (Prinivil, Zestril) 2.5, 5, 10, 20, 40 mg | Carboxyl | 12 | Not a prodrug |
| Moexipril (Univasc) 7.5, 15 mg | Carboxyl | 2–9 | Best taken on empty stomach |
| Perindopril (Aceon) 2, 4, 8 mg | Carboxyl | 10–25 | |
| Quinapril (Accupril) 5, 10, 20, 40 mg | Carboxyl | 2 | |
| Ramipril (Altace) 1.25, 2.5, 5, 10 mg | Carboxyl | 13–17 | |
| Trandolapril (Mavik) 1, 2, 4 mg | Carboxyl | 10–16 | |

ramipril (titrated to 10 mg) attenuated LV remodeling and resulted in swift LV recovery.

AIREX (15). This trial showed beneficial effects of ramipril started early after MI in patients with heart failure, and that the benefit was sustained over several years.

CONSENSUS (16). CONSENSUS studied the effects of enalapril on mortality in severe congestive heart failure. Enalapril reduced mortality and improved symptoms in severe CHF, when added to conventional therapy.

V-HeFT II (17). This trial compared enalapril with hydralazine-isosorbide (H-ISDN) for the treatment of CHF. Mortality with enalapril was significantly lower than in the H-ISDN group.

Stop-Hypertenion-2 (18). This trial showed that ACE-I and calcium channel blockers have similar efficacy in prevention of cardiovascular mortality compared to older-generation antihypertensive drugs (diuretics and beta-blockers) in elderly patients. ACE-I was associated with less MI and CHF than calcium channel blockers, but not compared to conventional therapy with diuretics and beta-blockers.

## ANGIOTENSIN-II RECEPTOR BLOCKERS

### Mechanism of Action

ARBs block angiotensin II (A-II) from binding to angiotensin II type 1 receptors ($AT_1$), thereby inhibiting the vasoconstrictor and aldosterone-secreting effects of angiotensin II (see Fig. 59–1; Table 59–5). ARBs do *not* alter the metabolism of bradykinin or neuropeptides, so they should not cause side effects related to this effect, such as cough. However, there are case reports of angioedema occurring with ARB therapy.

### Side Effects

Side effects include hypotension, acute renal failure (particularly if there is bilateral renal artery stenosis), hyperkalemia, proteinuria, hypotension, dizziness, headache, and angioedema (rare).

**TABLE 59–5**
**FORMULATIONS OF ANGIOTENSIN II-RECEPTOR BLOCKERS (ARBS)**

| Medication | Half-Life (h) |
|---|---|
| Candesartan Cilexetil (Atacand) | 9 |
| Eprosartan (Teveten) | 6 |
| Irbesartan (Avapro) | 11–15 |
| Losartan (Cozaar) | 6–9 |
| Olmesartan (Benecar) | 12–18 |
| Telmisartan (Micardis) | 24 |
| Valsartan (Diovan) | 6 |

### Indications and Precautions

The labeled use for all ARBs is hypertension; however, both candesartan and valsartan are also labeled for heart failure. Losartan is also labeled for hypertension in patients with LV hypertrophy as well as prophylaxis of diabetic nephropathy in patients with a history of hypertension. Additionally, irbesatran also carries an indication for prophylaxis against diabetic nephropathy in patients with a history of hypertension.

### Major Clinical Trials

ELITE-II (19). This trial demonstrated that losartan was not superior to captopril in reducing mortality in patients with CHF who were >60 years of age.

CHARM (20). This trial had multiple arms. The CHARM-alternative looked at candesartan in patients with symptomatic heart failure who were intolerant of ACE inhibitors. Patients were randomized to either candesartan or placebo. There was decreased risk of cardiovascular death or hospitalization from heart failure in the candesartan group compared to the placebo. The CHARM-added trial randomized patients with symptomatic heart failure who were already on ACE inhibitors to either candesartan or placebo. In contrast to the results of Val-HeFT, mortality was significantly reduced by addition of an ARB to an ACE-I compared to the ACE-I alone. The CHARM-preserved arm of the study looked at patients with symptomatic heart failure with preserved ejection fraction. They were randomized to either candesartan or placebo. There was no difference in the primary endpoint (cardiovascular death or hospitalization secondary to CHF).

LIFE (21). This trial showed that losartan was more effective than atenolol in preventing death, cardiovascular accidents (CVA), and MI as a combined endpoint. In terms of single outcomes, the reduction in CVA was significant, whereas the reduction in death or MI was only a trend without statistical significance.

Val-HeFT (22). This trial showed that valsartan reduced the combined endpoint of death and morbidity and improved symptoms and signs of CHF. The benefit was seen only in patients who were not receiving ACE-I. In patients who were on ACE-I and beta-blockers, the addition of valsartan was associated with increased mortality.

RESOLVD (23). This trial showed that both candesartan and enalapril were effective, safe, and tolerated in the treatment of CHF. Combination of candesartan and enalapril reduced LV dilatation greater than either agent alone.

RENAAL (24). This trial showed that losartan preserved renal function in patients with type II diabetes and diabetic nephropathy, as well as decreasing hospitalization for CHF.

## ALDOSTERONE RECEPTOR ANTAGONISTS

### Mechanism of Action

As shown in Figure 59–1, this class of drugs antagonizes aldosterone at the mineralocorticoid receptor, consequently inhibiting aldosterone effects in the late distal convoluted tubule and cortical collecting duct, reducing sodium reuptake (hence the diuretic effect) and reducing potassium excretion (hence the side effect of hyprekalemia).

### Side Effects

Side effects of pironolactone include hyperkalemia, hypotension, fatigue, rash, gynecomastia, amenorrhea, breast tenderness, sexual dysfunction, headache, nausea/vomiting, and diarrhea. With eplerenone, hyperkalemia is the predominant effect, with gynecomastia much less common. Drug–drug interactions are common with eplerenone, especially when concomitant medications increase serum potassium levels and when it is given with potent inhibitors of the CYP 3A4 isoenzyme system.

### Indications and Precautions

Spironolactone islabeled for primary aldosteronism, edema, hypertension, and hypokalemia associated with loop diuretics. Unlabeled use at a dose of 25 mg daily is as an adjunct therapy for patients with Class III–IV CHF. Eplerenone is labeled for use in hypertension and for treatment in patients with LV dysfunction after MI.

It is important to point out that this class of drugs should be avoided in patients with renal dysfunction (creatinine >2.5 mg/dL) or hyperkalemia.

### Major Clinical Trials

RALES (25). RALSES found that the addition of spironolactone to standard-therapy ACE inhibitor, loop diuretic, and digoxin, reduced mortality and hospitalizations due to heart failure, with a 30% decrease in mortality in patients with NYHA Class III or IV heart failure.

EPHESUS (26). This trial was designed to assess the safety and efficacy of eplerenone in patients with CHF after acute MI. The study showed a 15% decrease in mortality in patients with CHF post-MI.

## ANTICOAGULANTS

Anticoagulant drugs are subclassified into unfractionated heparin, low-molecular-weight heparin, direct thrombin inhibitors, and oral anticoagulants. A diagram of the coagulation cascade is shown in Figure 59–2.

### Unfractionated Heparin

#### Mechanism of Action

Unfractionated heparin (UFH) is a thrombin inhibitor that binds to antithrombin, increasing antithrombin's activity to inactivate thrombin in addition to activated factors IX, X, XI, and XII.

#### Side Effects

Common side effects include bleeding, thrombocytopenia (benign type I and more severe type II, which may cause thrombosis), elevation in aspartate aminotransferase (AST)/alanine aminotransferase (ALT), osteoporosis (long-term therapy), and hyperkalemia.

#### Indications and Precautions

Heparin is administered subcutaneously or as an IV preparation. Generally, a weight-based nomogram is utilized that is titrated to a specific activated partial thromboplastin (aPTT) level. It is labeled for use in the treatment and prophylaxis of venous and arterial thrombosis. Heparin-induced thrombocytopenia (HIT) occurs in two forms, type I (non–antibody-mediated reaction) and type II (antibody-mediated reaction—typically IgG). Thromboembolic complications (e.g., deep vein thrombosis, MI, stroke) are associated with type II HIT and can be life threatening. The incidence of thrombocytopenia is 10% to 15%, but the incidence of developing type II HIT is around 1% to 3%.

### Fondaparinux (Arixtra)

#### Mechanism of Action

Fondaparinux inhibits activated factor X through by the neutralization capacity of antithrombin.

#### Side Effects

Common side effects include bleeding, injection site–related bleeding, rash. and pruritis. Asymptomatic increases in AST and ALT may occur.

#### Indications and Precautions

Fondarparinux is used for prophylaxis of deep vein thrombosis in patients undergoing orthopedic surgery. Fondaparinux is contraindicated in patients with a creatinine clearance <30 mL/min and in patients weighing <50 kg. Currently, it should not be used in patients with heparin-associated antibodies or in those in whom heparin-associated antibodies are suspected. As with direct thrombin inhibitors, there is no known antidote for fondaparinux.

### Direct Thrombin Inhibitors: Bivalirudin (Angiomax), Lepirudin (Refludan), Argatroban (Argatroban)

#### Mechanism of Action

These drugs bind directly to thrombin (factor IIa), causing it to be inactivated (see Fig. 59–2). Bivalirudin and

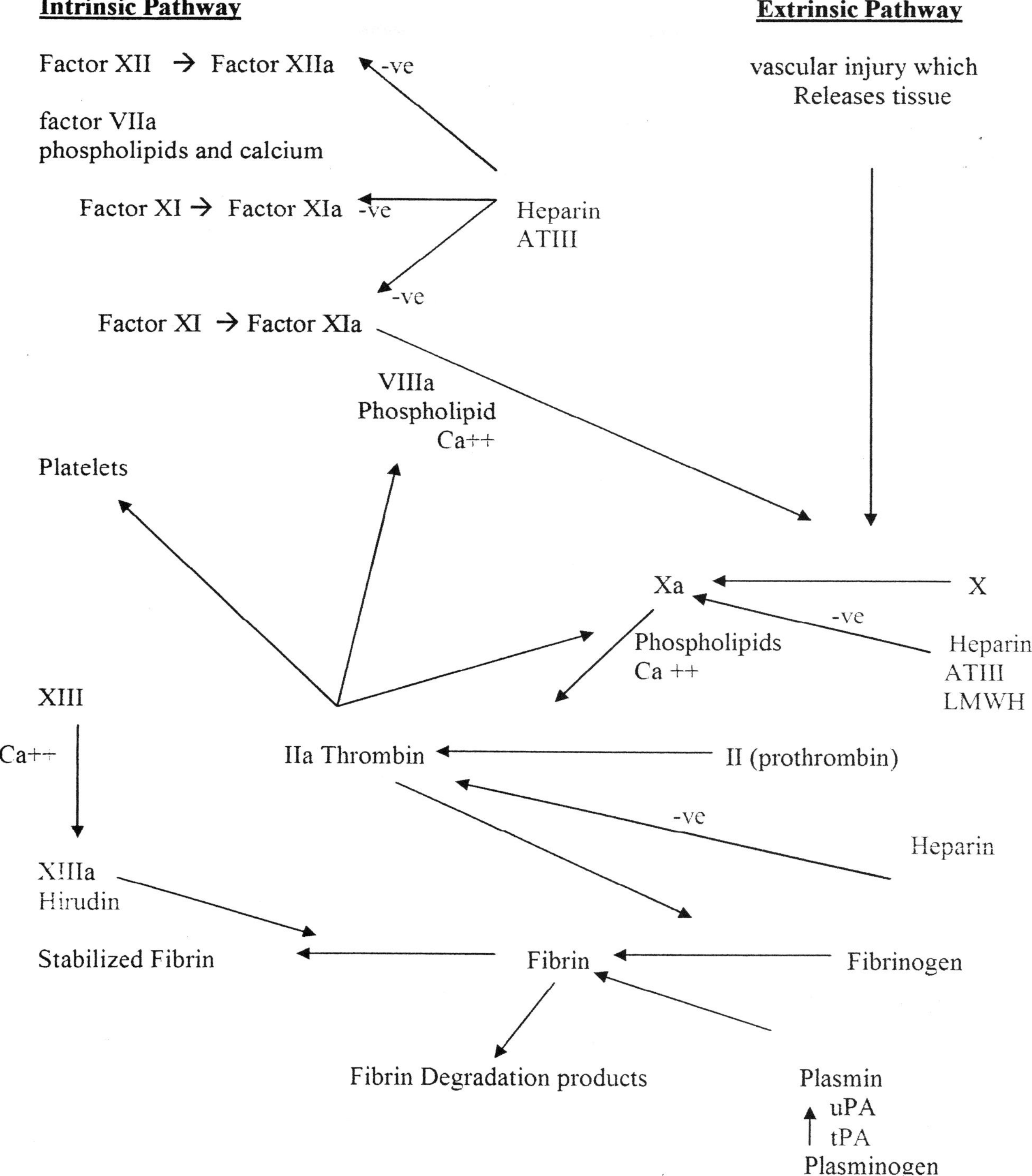


**Figure 59–2** The blood coagulation pathways, intrinsic and extrinsic, and the sites of impact of anticoagulant. When the arrow is not marked, it indicates either a positive effect of a factor on a step in the pathway, or a transformation into another factor. The negative effect is marked on the relevant arrows (+ve, positive or stimulatory effect; −ve, negative or inhibitory effect).

**TABLE 59–6**
**PREPARATIONS, DOSING AND INDICATIONS FOR DIRECT THROMBIN INHIBITORS**

| Drug | Hirudin Derivative | Half-Life | Elimination Route | aPTT | PT | Dosing | Indications |
|---|---|---|---|---|---|---|---|
| Argatroban | No | 21–60 min | Hepatic | ↑ | ↑ | Indication determines dosing (HIT or PCI). For HIT, initial dose is 0.5–2 $\mu$g/kg/min and maximum dose is 10 $\mu$g/kg/min. For PCI, initial dose is 350 $\mu$g/kg/min and maintenance is at 25 $\mu$g/kg/min. Adjustments during PCI are based on ACT | Anticoagulation for prophylaxis of thrombosis in patients with HIT. Anticoagulation for treatment of thromboembolic disease (to prevent further complications) in patients with HIT. |
| Bivalirudin | Yes | 25–210 min[a] | Proteolytic cleavage within plasma (80%) and renal | ↑ | Dose dependent | Initial dose is 1 mg/kg bolus, maintenance dose is 2.5 mg/kg/h for 4 h. If continued for >4 h, infusion rate should be decreased to 0.2 mg/kg/h for 20 h. In the REPLACE 2 trial, the initial bolus was 0.75 mg/kg and the maintenance dose was 1.75 mg/kg/h for the duration of the procedure. | Anticoagulant for patients with unstable angina undergoing PTCA. Unlabeled use is for patients undergoing PCI. |
| Lepirudin | Yes | >80 min[a] | Renal | ↑ | Dose dependent | Loading dose is 0.4 mg/kg over 15–20 s. Maintenance dose is 0.15 mg/kg/h. Dosing should be altered if patient has renal dysfunction. | Indicated for anticoagulation in patients with HIT and associated thromboembolic disease in order to prevent further thromboembolic complications. |

[a] Half-life depends on renal function.
aPTT, activated partial thromboplastin; PT, prothrombin time; HIT, heparin-induced thrombocytopenia; PCI, percutaneous coronary intervention; ACT, activated clotting time; PTCA, percutaneous transluminal coronary angioplasty.

argatroban bind directly and reversibly, whereas lepirudin binds directly and irreversibly.

### *Side Effects*

Common side effects include bleeding. Patients on lepirudin may develop antibodies against lepirudin that decrease the elimination of lepirudin, hence increasing the duration of activity. Recent data demonstrated that patients may develop anaphylactic reactions with administration of lepirudin, and the occurrence is higher in patients who have previously been treated with the drug.

### *Indications and Precautions*

All these preparation are given intravenously; they are listed in Table 59–6. The labeled indication for bivalirudin is for percutaneous transluminal coronary angioplasty in the setting of unstable angina.

### *Major Clinical Trials*

Thrombin Inhibitors Trialist (DTIT) Collaborative Group (27). This meta-analysis reviewed the use of direct thrombin inhibitors in acute coronary syndrome. A total of 5,674 patients were included, of whom 4,603 underwent percutaneous coronary intervention (PCI). Bivalirudin reduced the risk of death and MI by about 30% in the few weeks after procedure compared to heparin.

HERO-2 (28). This trial compared bivalirudin to heparin in patients receiving streptokinase therapy for acute MI. The conclusion of the study was that the use of bivalirudin was associated with reduction of reinfarction rates within 96 hours, but it was not associated with reduction in mortality. It was associated with a slight increase in the risk of bleeding.

HASI (29). This trial showed that bivalirudin is as effective as heparin in preventing ischemic complications in unstable angina or after PCI. It was found to be superior to heparin in reducing immediate post–MI complications. In this study, bivalirudin was associated with increased incidence of bleeding. In an update of the study which that published in (30), bivalirudin was better than heparin in reducing death, MI, revascularization, bleeding (as a combined endpoint) in patients with unstable angina or postinfarction angina who were undergoing PCI. The difference stemmed mainly from a reduction in the rate of revascularization.

OASIS (31). This study compared lepirudin to heparin in acute coronary syndrome. Lepirudin reduced mortality and reinfarction at 3 days after the event compared to heparin, but was associated with an increased cost and risk of major bleeding, which required transfusion.

REPLACE-II (32). In this trial, bivalirudin, given during PCI as an IV bolus followed by an infusion, was compared to heparin and GPIIb/IIIa inhibitors given 12 to 18 hours after the procedure. The study was set to assess for noninferiority for primary endpoint of death, MI, urgent revascularization, or major bleeding. Bivalirudin was found to be associated with a significant reduction in major bleeding compared to heparin and GP IIb/IIIa inhibitor.

### Low-Molecular-Weight Heparin: Dalteparin (Fragmin), Enoxaparin (Lovenox), Tinzaparin (Innohep)

#### *Mechanism of Action*

Each of these three drugs binds to antithrombin, increasing antithrombin's activity.

#### *Side Effects*

Common side effects include bleeding and thrombocytopenia (Type II occurs less often than with unfractionated heparin but is still a concern), rash, hematoma at the injection side, and fever.

#### *Indications and Precautions*

Dalteparin is indicated for prophylaxis of deep vein thrombosis (DVT) in high-risk patients undergoing abdominal surgery, and in unstable angina/non–Q-wave MI for the prevention of ischemic complications in patients on concurrent aspirin therapy. It should be avoided in patients with HIT or suspected HIT. Although there is a lower reported incidence of thrombocytopenia with low-molecular-weight heparin (LMWH) than with unfractionated heparin, it can still occur. Cross-reactivity of patients developing HIT type II on unfractionated heparin to those receiving LMWH is >90%. Because it is cleared renally, it is contraindicated in patients with severe renal insufficiency (creatinine clearance <30 mL/min).

Enoxaparin is labeled for prevention of DVT in patients undergoing hip replacement surgery, during and following hospitalization for knee replacement surgery, or in patients undergoing abdominal surgery who are at risk for thromboembolic complications, as well as in medical patients who are at risk for thromboembolic complications due to severely restricted mobility during acute illness. Other indications include the prevention of ischemic complications of unstable angina and non–Q-wave MI when coadministered with aspirin. Furthermore, it is labeled for use with warfarin for inpatient treatment of acute DVT ± pulmonary embolism (PE) or outpatient treatment of acute DVT without PE when administered in conjunction with warfarin.

Tinzaparin is labeled for treatment of acute symptomatic DVT with or without pulmonary embolism when administered in conjunction with warfarin sodium. The safety and effectiveness of Innohep were established in hospitalized patients. The same precautions apply as for other LMWH products.

## CALCIUM CHANNEL BLOCKERS

This class of drugs is chemically and pharmacologically diverse. Before we classify the drugs, we will review some information on the various calcium channels. The main ports of entry for calcium into the cell are via voltage-gated calcium channels, which open when the membrane depolarizes. Another is a sodium–calcium channel, which moves one calcium out in exchange for three sodium ions entering into the cell. The electrical balance within a cell is accomplished by the sodium/potassium ATP channel. Calcium is normally stored the sacroplasmic reticulum which also helps control the level of intracellular calcium. There are three types of calcium channels, L, N, and T. They differ in distribution in various tissues, duration of opening, and voltage range. Only L and T are of interest in cardiology.

### L-Type Channels

L-type channels are found in heart muscle and in parts of the conducting system, smooth muscle, brain, adrenals, and kidneys. Although all calcium channel blockers bind to the calcium channel receptor, they have different binding sites. Blocking the L channels or receptors inhibits inward calcium currents into the cell, thus reducing the concentration of calcium needed for muscle contraction, which leads to smooth muscle dilation, decreasing contractility of heart muscle, slowing of the sinoatrial (SA) node firing rate, and increasing AV nodal conductance time.

### T-Type Channels

T-type channels are found in blood vessels, adrenals, brain, kidneys, the heart conduction system, and in heart muscle under pathologic conditions such as cardiomyopathy. There is only one identified binding spot for medications, and blocking this receptor leads to dilation of peripheral and coronary blood vessels, thus decreasing systemic vascular resistance (SVR) and increasing myocardial blood flow. Also, blockade of T-type channels produces a lowering of heart rate.

### Mechanism of Action

The various classes of calcium channel blockers and the drugs in each class, as well as their mechanism of action, are shown in Table 59–7.

#### *Side Effects*

The side effects as well as contraindications for calcium channel blockers are shown in Table 59–8.

#### *Indications and Precautions*

The various preparations and respective doses along with the labeled uses are shown in Table 59–9.

#### *Major Clinical Trials*

In a recently published trial (33), the calcium channel blocker amlodipine was compared to atenolol as an antihypertensive regimen in patients with risk factors for coronary artery disease other than hypertension. The study was stopped early because the all-cause mortality rate was significantly lower with the amlodipine strategy than with the atenolol strategy. The amlodipine-based regimen was associated with reduced rates of strokes, cardiovascular death, and new-onset diabetes, and also total cardiovascular events and procedures.

## DIURETICS

By definition, diuretics (except osmotic diuretics) are drugs that lead to a net loss of sodium ($Na^+$) and water from the body. These drugs (except spironolactone) work primarily in the kidneys, acting from within the tubular lumen. Hence, for these drugs to reach their target, they are secreted into the proximal tubule. The sites of action for these drugs are shown in Figure 59–3.

### Loop Diuretics

Loop diuretics are the most powerful diuretics, causing about 15% to 20% of sodium in the tubule to be excreted, hence the name "high-ceiling diuretics."

#### *Mechanism of Action*

Loop diuretics act in the thick segment of the ascending loop of Henle and inhibit the transport of sodium out of the lumen of the nephron by blocking the chloride ($Cl^-$) component of the sodium/potassium/2 chloride ($Na^+/K^+/2Cl^-$) pump in the luminal membrane of the tubule. The net outcome is sodium and water loss. It is important to remember that loop diuretics gain access to the lumen of the nephron by organic acid pumping, without relying on glomerular filtration.

#### *Side Effects*

Common side effects of loop diuretics include hypokalemia, hypomagnesemia, hypochloremic metabolic alkalosis (with overdiuresis), ototoxicity (when given in high

**TABLE 59–7**
**CALCIUM CHANNEL BLOCKERS**

| Subclass | Drugs Available in Subclass | Mechanism of Action |
|---|---|---|
| Dihydropyridines | Amlodipine (Norvasc)<br>Felodipine (Plendil)<br>Isradipine (Dynacirc)<br>Nicardipine (Cardene)<br>Nifedipine (Procardia, Adalat)<br>Nimodipine (Nimotop)<br>Nisoldipine (Sular) | Blocks $Ca^{2+}$ channel in smooth muscle, which leads to vasodilatation of peripheral and coronary arteries. Effect on sinus and AV nodes is negated by reflex increase in sympathetic tone. |
| Nondihydropyridines | Diltiazem (Cardizem, Dilacor, Tiazac)<br>Verapamil (Calan, Isoptin, Verelan) | Blocks $Ca^{2+}$ channel in smooth muscle, which leads to vasodilatation of peripheral and coronary arteries as well as decrease in heart rate and prolonging conduction across the AV node. |

AV, atrioventricular.

**TABLE 59–8**
**SIDE EFFECTS, CONTRAINDICATIONS, AND MAJOR DRUG INTERACTIONS OF CALCIUM CHANNEL BLOCKERS**

| Subclass | Side Effects | Contraindications | Drug Interactions |
|---|---|---|---|
| Dihydropyridines | Headache, peripheral edema, flushing, reflex tachycardia (short-acting agents have higher incidence), rash, dizziness, hypotension, gingival hyperplasia (nifedipine) | Hypersensitivity to the medications; short-acting agents should not be used for hypertensive urgencies; acute myocardial infarction; acute stroke | Grapefruit juice with certain dihydropyridines.<br>Fentanyl has been reported to cause severe hypotension when given with certain calcium channel blockers. This reaction may occur with all calcium channel blockers, but data are not available.<br>$H_2$-receptor antagonists may increase the bioavailability of many of the dihydropyridine calcium channel blockers. |
| Diltiazem and verapamil | Negative inotropic effects, nausea, bradycardia, dizziness, peripheral edema, hypotension, heart block, constipation | Acute myocardial infarction; heart block >first degree; heart failure; pulmonary edema | $H_2$-receptor antagonist may increase bioavailability of diltiazem.<br>Beta-blockers may increase negative inotropic and chronotropic effects.<br>Inhibit metabolism of carbamazepine, cyclosporin, digoxin, quinidine, theophylline. |

doses and in conjunction with other ototoxic drugs), hyperuricemia, allergic reaction, azotemia, hypocalcemia, and photosensitivity. They are contraindicated for use in patients with severe sulfonamide allergic reaction and anuria.

**TABLE 59–9**
**PREPARATIONS, DOSING, AND LABELED USES FOR CALCIUM CHANNEL BLOCKERS**

| Drug | Indications |
|---|---|
| Amlodipine | Hypertension, stable and vasospastic angina |
| Felodipine | Hypertension |
| Isradipine | Hypertension |
| Nicardipine | Hypertension and stable angina |
| Nifedipine | Hypertension and vasospastic angina; unlabeled uses include prevention of migraine headaches, primary pulmonary hypertension |
| Nisoldipine | Hypertension |
| Diltiazem[a] | Hypertension, angina, and supraventricular tachyarrhythmias |
| Verapamil[a] | Hypertension, angina, and supraventricular tachyarrhythmias; unlabeled uses are for migraine and cluster headaches, exercise-induced asthma, and hypertrophic obstructive cardiomyopathy |

[a]Diltiazem and verapamil are available as IV formulations that can used in the acute management of atrial fibrillation and supraventricular tachyarrhythmias.

### *Indications and Precautions*

This subgroup of diuretics is labeled for use in edema to enhance diuresis. Furosemide and torsemide are also labeled for use in hypertension. Common uses are in heart failure, acute renal failure, hyperkalemia, anion overdose, and acute pulmonary edema.

## Thiazide Diuretics

### *Mechanism of Action*

Thiazide diuretics decrease active reabsorption of sodium and accompanying chloride by binding to the chloride site of the $Na^+/Cl^-$ cotransport system in the distal convoluted tubule. Furthermore, they increase calcium reabsorption in the same region of the nephron. Drugs of this class are effective at low doses, for which reason they are called "low-ceiling diuretics."

### *Side Effects*

Side effects of thiazide diuretics include hypokalemia, hypouricemia, glucose intolerance, hyperlipidemia, hyponatremia, allergic reaction, weakness, fatigue, and photosensitivity.

### *Indications and Precautions*

The various drugs in this subgroup are shown in Table 59–10. Thiazides are not effective in patients with clearance <30 mL/min. Patients may be allergic to the drug if they are allergic to sulfonamide derivatives. Thiazides should

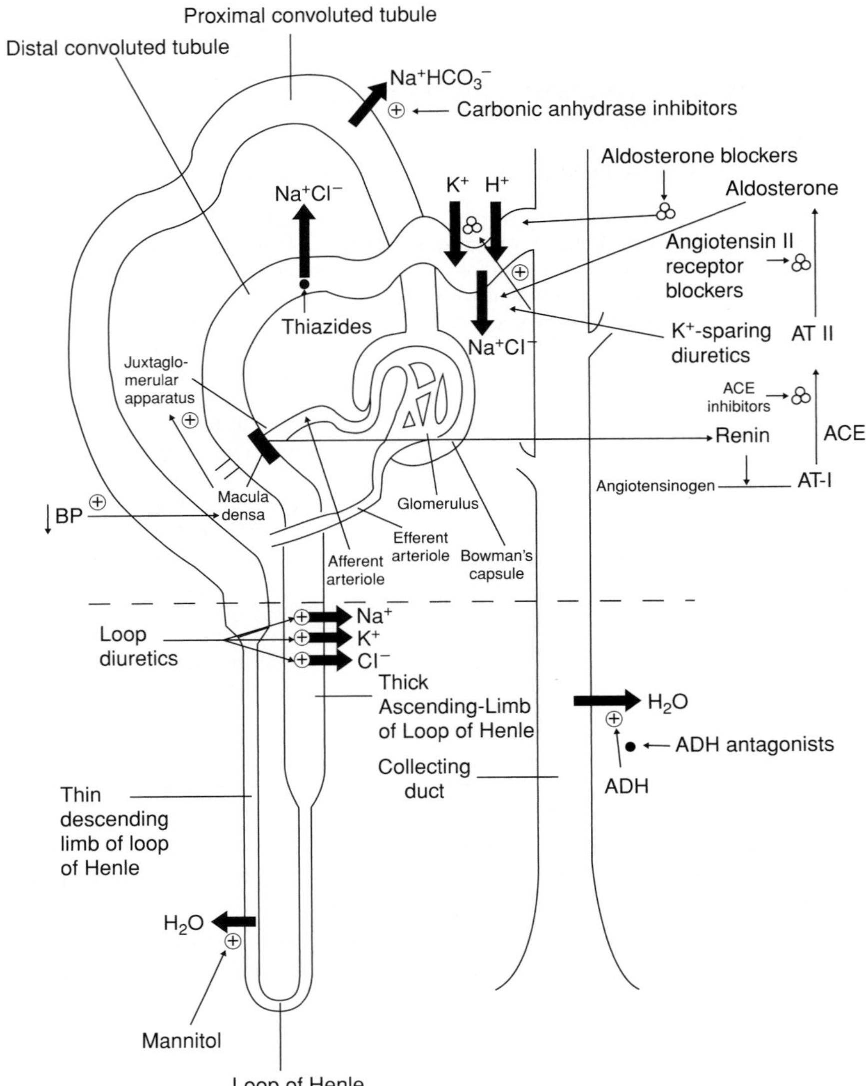


**Figure 59–3** The human nephron and the sites of action of diuretics.

be avoided in patients with elevated serum calcium levels. They have known drug interactions with lithium, NSAIDS, probenicid, digoxin, and calcium supplements.

### *Major Clinical Trials*

ALLHAT (2,34). In ALLHAT, 42,419 people with stage 1 or 2 hypertension were randomized to a diuretic (chlorthalidone), an ACE inhibitor (lisinopril), a calcium channel blocker (amlodipine), or an $\alpha$ blocker (doxazosin). After 3 years, the doxazosin arm was discontinued because of an increase in heart failure. At the end of the study at 6 years, there was no difference in primary endpoints (fatal coronary heart disease and nonfatal MI) or all-cause mortality among ACE inhibitors, diuretics, and calcium channel blockers. In secondary endpoints (stroke, heart failure),

**TABLE 59–10**
**PREPARATIONS, DOSING, AND INDICATIONS FOR THIAZIDE AND THIAZIDE-LIKE DIURETICS[a]**

| Drug | Indications |
|---|---|
| Chlorothiazide (Diuril)<br>Chlorthalidone (Hygroton)<br>Hydrochlorothiazide (Hydrodiuril)<br>Indapamide (Lozol) | Labeled: hypertension and edema; synergistic diuresis when added to loop diuretics |
| Metolazone (Zaroxolyn) | Unlabeled: diabetes insipidus, prophylaxis of renal stones in hypercalcemia |

[a]Agents are available only as oral preparations.

however, the diuretic proved to be better than the ACE inhibitor at preventing strokes and heart failure, and was also noted to be superior to the calcium channel blocker in preventing heart failure. The diuretic was also noted to have better overall outcomes in African American patients.

### $K^+$-Sparing Diuretics

The $K^+$-sparing diuretics spironolactone and elperenone were discussed earlier, under aldosterone antagonists. Triamterene and amiloride are not covered in this chapter.

## INOTROPIC AGENTS AND VASOPRESSORS

The maintenance of tissue perfusion in the body depends on the availability of adequate arterial pressure, which in turn depends on adequate cardiac output and vascular tone. We will approach this group of drugs from two perspectives, that of the inotropic agents and vasopressor agents. The goal of inotropic agents is to improve contractility of the ventricle to enhance cardiac pump function. Vasopressors, as the name suggests, are aimed at supporting the failing circulation by causing vasoconstriction. Many catecholamines have both of these properties.

### Inotropic Agents

Physiologically, the mechanism of inotropic response is mediated via increases in intracellular cyclic AMP (cAMP). Hence, increasing the level of cAMP directly with catecholamines, or decreasing its degradation with phosphodiesterase inhibitors, will increase the contractility of the myocardium. However, because cAMP inhibits calcium-mediated contraction of arterial smooth muscle, vasodilatation of arterial vasculature may occur.

#### *Dopamine (Intropin)*

##### Mechanism of Action

Dopamine has mixed $\alpha$-, $\beta$-, and dopaminergic ($DA_1$)-agonist effects. Through the $\alpha$ effect ($\alpha_1$) it leads to vasoconstriction. Through the $\beta$ effect ($\beta_1 > \beta_2$) it increases cAMP and cardiac contractility. Through the $DA_1$ and $DA_2$ effects it leads to increased renal perfusion and some peripheral dilatation (at low doses).

##### Side Effects

Common side effects of dopamine include tachycardia, arrhythmias, hypertension, headache, and nausea.

##### Indications and Precautions

Dopamine is labeled for use in hypotension, cardiogenic shock, septic shock, and trauma. It should be given by central line because skin necrosis may occur with extravasation. It has a graded dose–response curve, with lower doses causing renal vascular vasodilation, moderate doses having predominantly $\beta_1$-adrenergic effects, and higher doses causing vasoconstriction and elevations in blood pressure.

#### *Dobutamine (Dobutrex)*

##### Mechanism of Action

Dobutamine is a relatively selective $\beta_1$ agonist, but it has much less effect on $\beta_2$ and $\alpha_1$ receptors.

##### Side Effects

Common side effects of dobutamine include tachycardia, hypo- or hypertension, ventricular arrhythmia, nausea, headache, and myocardial ischemia.

##### Indications and Precautions

Dobutamine is labeled for use as a short-term inotropic support in patients with acute cardiac decompensation. Tachyphylaxis may occur with prolonged use. Chronic use has been associated with increased mortality.

#### *Epinephrine (Adrenaline)*

##### Mechanism of Action

Epinephrine is a mixed $\alpha$- and $\beta$-receptor agonist ($\beta_1 = \beta_2 > \alpha$). Hence it leads to increased myocardial contractility and vasoconstriction.

##### Side Effects

Common side effects of epinephrine include tachycardia, flushing, hypertension, restlessness, exacerbation of narrow-angle glaucoma, and ventricular arrhythmia.

##### Indications and Precautions

Epinephrine is indicated for use in ventricular standstill (cardioplegia or cardiac arrest) and shock (particularly anaphylaxis).

#### *Isoproternol (Isuprel)*

##### Mechanism of Action

Isoproternol is a nonselective $\beta$-receptor agonist ($\beta_1 > \beta_2$). It has the most potent inotropic effect of any inotrope.

##### Side Effects

Common side effects of isoproternol include tachycardia and ventricular arrhythmia (the reason it is used in the electrophysiologic laboratory to stimulate tachycardia), hypotension, myocardial ischemia, mild tremor, nervousness, and flushing.

##### Preparation, Dosing, Indications, and Precautions

Isoproternol is labeled for use in shock, heart block, Adams–Stokes attacks, and bronchospasm. Unlabeled uses include for bradycardia and for torsade de pointes until temporary pacing can be established.

### *Milrinone (Primacor)*

Mechanism of Action

Milrinone is a phosphodiesterase inhibitor that results in increased levels of intracellular cAMP by blocking its degradation, thus increasing contractility as well as vasodilatation because of its effect on arterial smooth muscle.

Side Effects

Common side effects Milrinone include hypotension, ventricular arrhythmia, supraventricular tachycardia, angina, chest pain, headache, and thrombocytopenia.

Indications and Precautions

Milrinone is labeled for short-term use in the management of CHF. Similar to dobutamine, it was found to increase mortality with long-term therapy, secondary to increase ventricular arrhythmias.

## Vasopressors

### *Norepinephrine (Levophed)*

Mechanism of Action

Norepinephrine is a mixed $\beta$ and $\alpha$ agonist ($\beta_1 = \alpha > \beta_2$). Its primary effect is vasoconstriction.

Side Effects

Common side effects of norepinephrine include hypertension, headache, trembling, and ventricular arrhythmias.

Indications and Precautions

The labeled used for norepinephrine is hypotension. It should be administered via a central line because of the risk of skin necrosis with extravasation. It should also be used with caution in patients with hepatic dysfunction or ischemic bowel, because it leads to splanchnic and hepatic vasculature constriction.

### *Phenylephrine (Neo-Synephrine)*

Mechanism of Action

Phenylephrine is a pure $\alpha$-receptor agonist that has a vasoconstrictor effect.

Side Effects

Common side effects include: bradycardia, hypertension, and myocardial ischemia.

Indications and Precautions

Phenylephrine is labeled for use in hypotension, particularly when associated with septic shock (vasodilatation), and anesthetic hypotension. Furthermore, it may be used to counter hypotension due to vasodilatation in severe obsructive hypertophic cardiomyopathy (see Chapter X on risk factors for CAD).

## NITRATES

Nitrates are a group of drugs that are a source of nitric oxide, which produces vasodilatation in the coronary circulation as well as arterioles and veins. Nitric oxide mediates vasodilatation via cAMP. These effects contribute to their antianginal properties as well as their role in heart failure. Nitrates that are in use are summarized in Table 59–11.

**TABLE 59–11**
**NITRATES: MECHANISM OF ACTION, SIDE EFFECTS, DOSING, AND INDICATIONS**

| Drug | Mechanism of Action | Side Effects and Precautions | Dosing and Indications |
|---|---|---|---|
| Isosorbide dinitrate (Isordil, Sorbitrate) | Biotransformation of nitrates releases nitric oxide, causing vasodilatation through cAMP. Venous dilation predominates. | Headache, hypotension (large doses), flushing, dizziness, rash, nausea, methemoglobinemia, reflex tachycardia | Labeled: prevention of anginal attacks<br>Unlabeled: heart failure, in combination with hydralazine) |
| Isosorbide mononitrate (Imdur, Ismo, Monoket) | Same | Same | Labeled: prevention of anginal attacks |
| Nitroglycerin paste (Nitrol) | Same | Same; inconvenient for long-term therapy secondary to ointment formulation | Labeled: prevention of anginal attacks |
| Nitroglycerin patch (various) | Same | Same | Labeled: prevention of anginal attacks |
| Nitroglycerin SL (Nitrostat, Nitrolingual spray) | Same | Same | Labeled: acute treatment or prophylaxis of anginal attacks |
| Nitroglycerin IV (Tridil) | Same | Same; methemoglobinemia may occur with high doses<br>— May increase intracranial pressure<br>— IV formulation is poorly soluble | Labeled: perioperative hypertension, congestive heart failure with acute myocardial infarction, angina<br>Unlabeled: hypertensive crisis, pulmonary hypertension |

Some of the major trials studying the role of nitrates in the treatment of heart failure are the following.

V-HeFT I (1). The addition of hydralazine and isosorbide dinitrate to standard therapy (digoxin and diuretics) improved mortality and LV function compared to placebo or prazosin in patients with heart failure.

A-HeFT (35). The addition of a fixed dose of isosorbide dinitrate (ISDN) and hydralazine to standard therapy for heart failure, including neurohormonal blockers, is efficacious and increases survival among black patients with advanced heart failure.

## PLATELET INHIBITORS

Thrombus formation is a complex process that involves platelets, the vasculature including collagen and tissue factors (primary hemostasis), as well as the coagulation pathways (secondary hemostasis), as shown in Figure 59–2. The initiation of thrombus formation in the arterial system mainly involves platelet aggregation with a small amount of fibrin (white clot), whereas in the venous system it is composed mainly of fibrin and red cells (red clot). The primary functions of the platelets are to form a plug by adhesion and aggregation, as well as providing a phospholipid surface to facilitate procoagulant reaction.

For the platelets to participate in coagulation, they have to be activated. This usually happens with exposure of the platelets to collagen in the vasculature (injury). Platelets adhere to the collagen via glycoprotein Ib-IX, leading to change in shape and granular release of ADP and thromboxane. Thrombin (from the coagulation pathway), angiotensin II, norepinephrine, and contents of granules released from platelets (including ADP and serotonin) stimulate the endothelium to release calcium and hence allow platelet activation. Factors that inhibit platelet activation are prostacyclin and nitric oxide. When platelets are activated, arachidonic acid in the endothelium is transformed to thromboxane A2, by cyclo-oxygenase enzyme (COX). Thromboxane leads to more platelet activation. This step is the target for aspirin use as an antiplatelet therapy. Serotonin, thrombin, and ADP bind to receptors on the endothelium, and via secondary messengers lead to release of calcium from the endoplastic reticulum. The binding of ADP to receptors on the endothelium is the site of action for clopidogrel and ticlopidine as antiplatelet therapy. As mentioned earlier, when platelets are activated, thromboxane (TXA2) is released. TXA2 leads to the expression of glycoprotein GP-IIb/IIIa receptors, which allows linkage of adjacent platelets (aggregation) by fibrinogen and van Willebrand factor (vWF) to the GP-IIb/IIIa. The GP-IIb/IIIa receptors are the site of action of IV antiplatelet therapy (abciximab, tirofiban, and eptifibatide).

### Oral Antiplatelet Therapy

#### *Cyclo-oxygenase Inhibitor/Aspirin*

##### Mechanism of Action

Aspirin irreversibly acetylates platelet cyclo-oxygenase, decreasing the formation of thromboxane $A_2$ from arachidonic acid.

##### Side Effects

Side effects include bleeding, gastric ulceration, nausea/dyspepsia/heartburn, hemolytic anemia, and tinnitus (large doses or overdose).

##### Indications and Precautions

Aspirin is labeled for analgesic, antipyretic, and anti-inflammatory use and for myocardial infarction, transient ischemic attacks, and cardiovascular accidents.

#### *Clopidogrel (Plavix)*

##### Mechanism of Action

Clopidogrel acts by inhibiting adenosine diphosphate receptors, which decreases the expression of the GP-IIb/IIIa receptors on the platelet cell surface and thereby prevents platelet aggregation.

##### Side Effects

Common side effects of clopidogrel include diarrhea, headache, dizziness, abdominal pain/nausea/dyspepsia, purpura, rash, and sometimes thrombocytopenia.

##### Indications and Precautions

The drug is labeled for use in acute coronary syndrome and to reduce the risk of MI, stroke, and/or peripheral arterial disease in patients with a completed MI, stroke, and/or peripheral arterial disease. Unlabeled use is as adjunctive therapy after coronary artery stent placement. Most side effects when compared to aspirin in clinical trials were less in the clopidogrel-treated group. Maximal effects are seen 3 to 7 days after initiation of therapy. Eleven cases of thrombotic thrombocytopenic purpura (TTP) have been reported. Recent data demonstrate that clopidogrel should be continued for 12 months after coronary artery stenting with a drug-eluting stent, though the American College of Cardiology recommendation is for 3 months for Cypher stents and 6 months for Taxus stents (61).

#### *Ticlopidine (Ticlid)*

##### Mechanism of Action

See clopidogrel.

##### Side Effects

Common side effects of ticlopidine include bleeding, diarrhea, nausea, vomiting, anorexia, rash, neutropenia, and purpura. Severe neutropenia occurs in 0.8% of patients and has been associated with death. A complete blood count with differential should be measured at baseline and every

2 weeks for the first 3 months of therapy. Case reports of TTP have been reported with ticlopidine.

#### Indications and Precautions

The labeled use for ticlopidine is to reduce the risk of thrombotic stroke in patients with completed thrombotic stroke or stroke precursors. Unlabeled use is as adjunctive therapy for coronary artery stent placement and as an alternative to aspirin in patients who are unable to take aspirin or clopidogrel. Patients should be monitored for fevers or other signs of infection. Maximal effects are seen 3 to 7 days after initiation of therapy.

### *Cilostazol (Pletal)*

#### Mechanism of Action

The mechanism for intermittent claudication in not fully known. However, as an antiplatelet therapy, cilostazol acts as a phosphodiesterase III inhibitor, suppressing breakdown of cAMP and thus leading to vasodilation and platelet inhibition.

#### Side Effects

Common side effects of cilostazol include headache, palpitations, diarrhea, peripheral edema, and dizziness.

#### Indications and Precautions

Cilostazol is labeled for use to reduce symptoms of intermittent claudication. Unlabeled use is an adjunct to aspirin in patients receiving coronary stenting. It should be taken on an empty stomach and should not be used in patients with CHF because phosphodiesterase inhibitors have been associated with increased mortality rates in CHF patients.

### *Major Clinical Trials of Antiplatelet Medications*

ISIS-2 (36). Aspirin and streptokinase independently reduced mortality in patients with acute myocardial infarction. The combination of the two drugs was better than either alone (synergistic effect) in terms of mortality, without increasing the risk of hemorrhagic stroke.

Antithrombotic Trialists' Collaboration (37). This was a collaborative meta-analysis of randomized trials of antiplatelet therapy for prevention of death, myocardial infarction, and stroke in high-risk patients. It found that aspirin is protective in patients who are at increased risk of acute myocardial infarction or ischemic stroke, or who have unstable or stable angina, previous myocardial infarction, stroke or cerebral ischemia, peripheral arterial disease, or atrial fibrillation. Low-dose aspirin (75 to 150 mg daily) is an effective antiplatelet regimen for long-term use, but in acute settings an initial loading dose of at least 150 mg aspirin may be required.

CURE (38). The study's goal was to assess the efficacy and safety of clopidogrel in addition to aspirin in patients with acute coronary syndrome (ACS) without ST elevation. The study found that the long-term use of clopidogrel with aspirin reduced the risk of events in patients with ACS. The use of clopidogrel was associated with an increased risk of bleeding.

CURE-PCI (39). This trial looked at the effects of pretreatment with clopidogrel and aspirin followed by long-term therapy in patients undergoing PCI. The results showed that long-term use of clopidogrel after PCI was associated with a lower rate of cardiovascular death, myocardial infarction, or any revascularization.

CREDO (40). This trial showed that, after PCI, long-term (1-year) clopidogrel therapy significantly reduced the risk of adverse ischemic events.

CLASSICS (41). This study showed that the combination of aspirin and clopidogrel was superior to the combination of aspirin and ticlopidine in terms of safety and tolerability. There was no difference in terms of impact on cardiac events.

ISAR-REACT (42). This trial evaluated the efficacy of abciximab in 2,159 patients undergoing elective PCI. From the clopidogrel point of view, all patients were pretreated with 600 mg of clopidogrel at least 2 hours before PCI. There was no significant difference among groups that received clopidogrel at various intervals.

CLARITY-TIMI 28 (43). This trial randomized 3,491 patients (<75 years of age), presenting within 12 hours of symptoms of STEMI, to either clopidogrel (300 mg loading dose and 75 mg daily thereafter) or placebo. Clopidogrel was given after receiving aspirin and thrombolysis. The clopidogrel group had higher rates of vessel patency at angiography as well as lower rates of reinfarction at 30 days. A subgroup analysis of this study (44) looked at patients who had PCI and stenting within a few days after the clopidogrel loading and fibrinolysis. Early clopidogrel loading after fibrinolysis in patients who subsequently proceeded to PCI was associated with lower risk of cardiovascular death, MI, or stroke at 30 days.

## Intravenous Antiplatelet Therapy/ Glycoprotein IIb/IIIa Inhibitors

Refer to Table 59–12 for details.

### *Major Clinical Trials*

PRISM (45). This study compared the effects of tirofiban with aspirin versus heparin with aspirin on clinical outcomes in patients with unstable angina. There was no difference between the two groups in terms of the combined endpoints at 30 days. Mortality alone was significantly reduced in the tirofiban group.

RESTORE (46). The study focused on the effects of tirofiban on adverse cardiac events in patients with

**TABLE 59–12**
**GLYCPROTEIN IIb/IIIa INHIBITORS: PREPARATIONS, MECHANISM OF ACTION, AND SIDE EFFECTS**

| Drug | Mechanism of Action | Side Effects |
|---|---|---|
| Abciximab (Reopro) | Murine-derived monoclonal antibody Fab fragment to the human GP-IIb/IIIa receptor on the platelet surface, inhibiting platelet aggregation | Bleeding, thrombocytopenia, hypersensitivity reactions |
| Eptifibatide (Integrilin) | Heptapeptide antagonist that reversibly inhibits G-IIb/IIIa receptor on the platelet surface, inhibiting platelet aggregation | Bleeding, thrombocytopenia |
| Tirofiban (Aggrastat) | Nonpeptide antagonist that reversibly inhibits GP-IIb/IIIa receptor on the platelet surface, inhibiting platelet aggregation | Bleeding, thrombocytopenia |

unstable angina who were undergoing PCI. The study showed that tirofiban reduced the primary outcome, which was a composite of death, MI, PCI failure, and CABG. However, the reduction in emergency revascularization seen early in the study was no longer significant at 30 days.

TARGET (47). TARGET compared tirofiban and abciximab for prevention of ischemic events with PCI. Abciximab was more effective than tirofiban in preventing nonfatal MI as well as in the composite endpoint of death, MI, or urgent target vessel revascularization.

TACTICS-TIMI-18 (48). This trial compared early invasive to conservative therapy in patients with ACS treated with tirofiban. The study showed that the strategy of early catheterization and revascularization was associated with fewer major cardiac events than the conservative approach.

PURSUIT (49). This study aimed to determine the effects of eptifibatide in patients with ACS between those undergoing PCI versus those being managed conservatively. The study found that eptifibatide reduced the composite endpoint of death or MI at 30 days with either strategy of management.

ESPIRIT (50). This study was aimed at assessing the efficacy and safety of high-dose eptifibatide in elective coronary stent implantation. The study showed that eptifibatide reduced ischemic complications after elective stent placement, as well as the combined endpoint of death and MI.

IMPACT-II (51). This study aimed at assessing eptifibatide impact on the prevention of ischemic complications following PCI. The study showed that the use of eptifibatide was associated with reduced early abrupt closure and reduced the rates of 30 days ischemic events without increasing the risk of bleeding. However, there was no effect on reduction of 30-day mortality or MI, or 6-month cumulative ischemic event rate.

EPIC (52). This study showed that abciximab bolus and infusion at the time of PTCA improved outcomes for as long as 3 years. It also showed that there was reduction in non-Q wave myocardial infarction (NQWMI) and distal embolization in patients undergoing PCI on saphenous vein grafts.

EPILOG (53). This trial was aimed at studying whether the clinical benefit of abciximab on reducing ischemic complications in patients undergoing high-risk PCI, can be extended to all patients undergoing PCI. Furthermore, the study looked at whether adjusting the heparin dose reduced the hemorrhagic complications associated with abciximab. The study showed that abciximab with low-dose heparin reduced ischemic complications in patients undergoing PCI without increasing the risk of bleeding.

EPISTENT (54). The purpose of this trial was to compare the outcomes of stenting with or without the use of abciximab, and the outcomes of PTCA with abciximab. The study showed that abciximab significantly improved the outcome of PCI. Furthermore, PTCA and abciximab was better and safer than stenting without abciximab.

CAPTURE (55). Abciximab infusion started 18 to 24 hours before PCI and continued for 1 hour after PCI reduced the rates of periprocedural MI and the need for revascularization in patients with unstable angina having PTCA, without affecting the rates of MI.

RAPPORT (56). This trial showed that abciximab in the setting of primary PCI for acute ST-elevation MI did not alter the primary endpoint at 6 months—a composite endpoint of revascularization (elective or urgent), death reduction, or reinfarction. There was an increased risk of bleeding.

ADMIRAL (57). This trial compared the effects of early administration of abciximab before primary stenting to stenting alone without IIb/IIIa-inhibitor therapy. The results showed that early abciximab (before primary PCI for ST-elevation MI) improved vessel patency before and after stenting and at 6 months follow-up after the procedure. It was associated with improved clinical outcomes and LV function preservation compared to primary PCI alone.

## THROMBOLYTICS/FIBRINOLYTICS

When the coagulation pathways are activated, there is a naturally occurring counterprocess of "clot dissolving" that begins spontaneously (Fig. 59–2). This process involves plasminogen activators, tissue-type plasminogen activator (t-PA), and urokinase-type plasminogen activator (u-PA). t-PA is the major player in fibrinolysis, whereas u-PA is involved in cell migration and tissue remodeling. These activators break down plasminogen to plasmin, which in turn breaks down fibrin (thrombus) to fibrin degradation products. Fibrinolytics are drugs that mimic biologic activators and hence increase the level of plasmin, which in turn enhances thrombus breakdown. The goal of this therapy is to establish reperfusion to the myocardium, brain, or lung in acute MI (ST-elevation MI), CVA or pulmonary embolism, respectively.

### Alteplase/t-PA (Activase)

#### *Mechanism of Action*

t-PA binds to clot-bound plasminogen to catalyze conversion to plasmin. The specificity for clot-bound plasminogen decreases systemic fibrinolysis.

#### *Side Effects*

Common side effects of t-PA include bleeding, intracranial hemorrhage (0.7%), hypotension, nausea/vomiting, and epistaxis.

#### *Indications and Precautions*

The labeled use of t-PA is for acute myocardial infarction, pulmonary embolism, and acute ischemic stroke. Acute MI patients should receive aspirin and heparin during t-PA infusion. In pulmonary embolism, heparin should be started at the end of the alteplase infusion. It is considered superior to streptokinase, but the risk of intracranial hemorrhage is greater than with streptokinase. Age >65 years and weight <70 kg are independent risk factors for intracranial hemorrhage.

### Reteplase, r-PA (Retavase)

#### *Mechanism of Action*

r-PA is a single-stranded mutant of wild-type t-PA with action similar to that of t-PA, with less high-affinity fibrin binding but increased potency.

#### *Side Effects*

Common side effects include bleeding and intracranial hemorrhage.

#### *Indications and Precautions*

The labeled use is for acute myocardial infarction. Combination of half-dose reteplase and full-dose abciximab was evaluated in the GUSTO-V trial and found not to be inferior to full-dose reteplase, but there was no mortality benefit, and risk of bleeding was increased.

### Streptokinase (Streptase)

#### *Mechanism of Action*

Streptokinase binds to clots and circulating plasminogen; this complex then catalyzes the conversion of plasminogen to plasmin. It is not specific for clot-bound plasminogen and therefore produces a systemic fibrinolytic state.

#### *Side Effects*

Common side effects of streptokinase include bleeding, bronchospasm, periorbital swelling, angioedema, anaphylaxis, hypotension, rash, intracranial hemorrhage (0.2%), fever, and urticaria.

#### *Indications and Precautions*

Labeled uses of streptokinase are acute myocardial infarction, pulmonary embolism, deep vein thrombosis, arterial thrombosis or embolism, and occlusion of AV cannulae. Patients should not receive streptokinase if they have received anisoylated plasminogen streptokinase activator complex (APSAC) or streptokinase within the last 12 months. Heparin is not given with streptokinase; if it is needed, the heparin is initiated 4 hours after streptokinase infusion.

### Tenecteplase (TNK-ase)

#### *Mechanism of Action*

Tenecteplase binds to clot-bound plasminogen to catalyze conversion to plasmin.

#### *Side Effects*

Common side effects of tenecteplase include bleeding and intracranial hemorrhage. Hypotension may occur.

#### *Indications and Precautions*

Tenecteplase is labeled for use in acute MI. It has the same rate of intracranial hemorrhage as t-PA, but it should not be used with enoxaparin in patients >75 years old. The advantage is that it can be given as a single weight-adjusted bolus injection over 5 to 10 seconds.

### Major Clinic Trials

GUSTO-I (58). This trial found that the mortality in patients with acute ST-elevation MI was lower in patients who received t-PA and IV heparin than in those who received streptokinase with either IV heparin or subcutaneous heparin. Furthermore, early PCI when appropriate led to improved survival of patients with MI with cardiogenic shock at 30 days.

GUSTO-III (59). Reteplase did not show superiority over alteplase in terms of mortality benefit. The two therapies had comparable rates of hemorrhagic strokes.

GUSTO-V (60). In this trial, half-dose reteplase was given with a 12-hour infusion of abciximab. This combination was not superior to the standard dose of reteplase in terms of mortality. The combination therapy was associated with an increased risk of bleeding complications.

## VASODILATORS, MISCELLANEOUS

In this section we discuss a more diverse group that does not fall into any specific pharmacologic class.

### Hydralazine (Apresoline)

#### *Mechanism of Action*

Hydralazine works by direct relaxation of the arteriolar smooth muscle, causing a fall in blood pressure, reflex tachycardia, and an increase in cardiac output. The exact mechanism of action at a cellular level has not been determined completely.

#### *Side Effects*

Common side effects of hydralazine include: palpitation, tachycardia, flushing, myocardial ischemia, nausea, vomiting, anorexia, hypotension, and drug-induced lupus-like syndrome with prolonged use.

#### *Indications and Precautions*

Hydralazine is used for hypertension and hypertensive urgencies and in congestive heart failure.

### Fenoldopam (Corolpam)

#### *Mechanism of Action*

Fenoldopam is a dopamine ($DA_1$) receptor agonist that causes smooth muscle relaxation, leading to vasodilatation and increased renal blood flow.

#### *Side Effects*

Common side effects of fenoldopam include hypotension, headache, flushing, tachycardia, and, rarely, hypokalemia.

#### *Indications and Precautions*

Fenoldopam is labeled for use as short-term therapy for hypertensive emergencies and urgencies. It is very expensive while having similar efficacy to nitroprusside in terms of hypotensive effect.

### Minoxidil (Loniten)

#### *Mechanism of Action*

Minoxidil acts as a vasodilator, primarily affecting arterial smooth muscle. It antagonizes the effect of ATP on the ATP-sensitive channel, which leads to hyperpolarization and muscle relaxation.

#### *Side Effects*

Common side effects of minoxidil include significant reflex tachycardia, sodium and water retention, weight gain, hirsutism in women, breast tenderness, gynecomastia, and headache.

#### *Indications and Precautions*

The labeled use for minoxidil is hypertension, and usually it is the last resort in treating hypertension that is not responsive to other medications. It should be used with beta-blockers to reduce the reflex tachycardia, and diuretics to reduce sodium and water retention.

### Nitroprusside (Nipride)

#### *Mechanism of Action*

Direct vasodilatation occurs secondary to the liberation of the nitroso group from the nitrosocyanide structure. Nitroprusside has a balanced effect on both veins and arteries.

#### *Side Effects*

Common side effects of nitroprusside include hypotension, headache, nausea, confusion, and metabolic acidosis. Less common side effects are thiocyanate and cyanide toxicity.

#### *Preparation, Dosing, Indications, and Precautions*

The labeled use for nitroprusside is hypertensive urgencies and the management of acute CHF. Patients with hepatic failure are at increased risk for developing cyanide toxicity, and this should be suspected in patients with metabolic acidosis, venous hyperoxemia, increased serum lactate levels, air hunger, confusion, seizures, and ataxia. Patients with suspected cyanide toxicity should receive inhaled amyl nitrite while being given 300 mg of sodium nitrite IV, followed by 12.5 mg of sodium thiosulfate IV. If symptoms reappear, then administer half the amounts of sodium nitrite and sodium thiosulfate again. These modalities shift cyanide conversion to thiocynate. Cyanide levels are not helpful acutely, because it may take up to 5 days to achieve results. Thiocyanate is a neruotoxin that causes confusion, psychosis, lethargy, tinnitus, convulsions, and hyperreflexia. Hemodialysis removes thiocynate from the blood. Levels are not typically monitored unless infusion of >3 days or when high doses are used in patients with renal failure.

### Bosentan (Tracleer)

#### *Mechanism of Action*

Bosentan is an endothelin-receptor antagonist (ET-A and ET-B), which leads to vasodilatation (endothelin is a potent vasoconstrictor).

### Side Effects

Common side effects of bosentan include severe hepatotoxicity (11% of patients), teratogenicity, headache, flushing, hypotension, fatigue, pruritus, edema, and anemia.

### Indications and Precautions

Bosentan is labeled for management of pulmonary hypertension in patients with Class III or IV symptoms. It is necessary to monitor the liver function tests (LFTs); if there is three- to fivefold increase in these, dosage reduction or discontinuation is required. It is available only by direct shipment from the manufacturer and costs about $3,500 per month.

## Nesiritide (Natrecor)

### Mechanism of Action

Nesiritide is a recombinant human b type of BNP or rhBNP. It binds to guanylate cyclase receptors in vascular smooth muscle and endothelial cells, increasing the intracellular level of cGMP and thereby causing venous and arterial vasodilatation, resulting in dose-dependent reduction in pulmonary capillary wedge pressure (PCWP) and systemic blood pressure. It also causes mild natriuresis.

### Side Effects

Common side effects of nesiritide include hypotension, headache, dizziness, and renal dysfunction.

### Indications and Precautions

Nesiritide is labeled for use in acutely decompensated heart failure patients who have dyspnea at rest or with minimal activity. It should be avoided in patients with cardiogenic shock, aortic stenosis, and severe hypotension (systolic blood pressure <90 mm Hg).

## Epoprostenol (Flolan)

### Mechanism of Action

Epoprostenol is prostaglandin $I_2$. It is a vasodilator of the systemic as well as pulmonary arteries. It also inhibits platelet aggregation.

### Side Effects

Common side effects of epoprostenol include jaw pain, hypotension, headache, rash, diarrhea, joint pain, and noncardiogenic pulmonary edema.

### Indications and Precautions

The primary use for epoprostenol is for pulmonary hypertension, and pulmonary hypertension secondary to scleroderma. The half-life of the drug is very short, 3 to 5 minutes, hence abrupt cessation is not well tolerated by patients.

## Digoxin

Digoxin, a digitalis glycoside, is used as adjunctive treatment for heart failure and to slow ventricular rate in patients with atrial fibrillation. Digoxin inhibits the sodium–potassium pump on the cell membrane, blocking sodium transport out of the cell, thus increasing intracellular sodium concentrations, and eventually resulting in increased intracellular levels of calcium. This results in an increase in cardiac contractility. Digoxin enhances parasympathetic tone, leading to an increase in AV nodal refractory period, as observed by increases in the P–R interval.

Dosing of digoxin can be challenging, as one needs to consider patient weight, renal function, and concomitant medications. The inherent half-life of digoxin is 36 hours in patients with normal creatinine clearance. In patients with impaired renal function, the half-life of digoxin increases, and it will prolong to about 5 days if the patient has end-stage renal disease. Concomitant medications may alter digoxin levels, and therefore when initiating new medications or discontinuing medications, one needs to assess the dose. Common drug interactions include those with amiodarone, quinidine, diltiazem and verapamil, erythromycin, and clarithromycin, to name a few.

The most common side effects related to digoxin include atrial and ventricular arrhythmias, blurred vision, anorexia, nausea and vomiting, and visual color distortion.

Digoxin no longer first-line therapy in the treatment of heart failure unless the patient has underlying atrial fibrillation and rapid ventricular response. Patients with continued symptoms of heart failure or with frequent admissions to the hospital may be considered candidates for digoxin after they have been maximized on therapies that improve survival.

## Intravenous Nitroglycerin

Nitroglycerin liberates nitric oxide (NO), which activates guanylyl cyclase, increasing intracellular cGMP levels. The resulting effect produces smooth muscle relaxation leading to vasodilation. Standard doses of nitroglycerin primarily produce venodilation, leading to a decrease in ventricular wall tension by lowering left ventricular end diastolic volume. Nitroglycerin, by decreasing myocardial oxygen demand, is typically used to treat chest pain associated with acute coronary syndromes and to relieve dyspnea associated with congestive heart failure.

Nitroglycerin is rapidly metabolized in the liver to less active and inactive metabolites. Because of extensive first-pass metabolism, nitroglycerin cannot be given orally for a therapeutic effect. Sublingual, transdermal, and IV administration of nitroglycerin bypass portal circulation, avoiding first-pass metabolism. Chronic use of nitroglycerin or isodorbide di- and mononitrates without interruptions in therapy frequently leads to tolerance. Multiple mechanisms of tolerance have been described and include cellular sulfhydryl group depletion, volume expansion, free-radical generation, and neurohormonal activation. The exact mechanism is unknown, but daily nitrate interruptions (8 to 12 hours) will restore the efficacy of nitrates.

The most common side effects include headache, hypotension, tachycardia or bradycardia, dizziness, and rash.

## REFERENCES


1. Cohn JN, Archibald DG, Ziesche S, et al. Effect of vasodilator therapy on mortality in chronic congestive heart failure. Results of a Veterans Administration Cooperative Study. *N Engl J Med.* 1986;314:1547–1552.
2. Major cardiovascular events in hypertensive patients randomized to doxazosin vs chlorthalidone: the antihypertensive and lipid-lowering treatment to prevent heart attack trial (ALLHAT). ALLHAT Collaborative Research Group. *JAMA.* 2000;283:1967–1675.
3. Hjalmarson A, Goldstein S, Fargerberg B, et al. Effects of controlled-release metoprolol on total mortality, hospitalizations, and well-being in patients with heart failure: the Metoprolol CR/XL Randomized Intervention Trial in congestive Heart Failure (MERIT-HF). MERIT-HF Study Group. *JAMA.* 2000;283:1295–1302.
4. The Cardiac Insufficiency Bisoprolol Study II (CIBIS-II): a randomised trial. *Lancet.* 1999;353:9.
5. Dargie HJ. Effect of carvedilol on outcome after myocardial infarction in patients with left-ventricular dysfunction: the CAPRICORN randomised trial. *Lancet.* 2001;357:1385–1390.
6. Packer M, Coats AJ, Fowler MB, et al. Effect of carvedilol on survival in severe chronic heart failure. *N Engl J Med.* 2001;344(22):1651–1658.
7. Poole-Wilson PA, Swedberg K, Cleland JG, et al. Comparison of carvedilol and metoprolol on clinical outcomes in patients with chronic heart failure in the Carvedilol Or Metoprolol European Trial (COMET): randomised controlled trial. *Lancet.* 2003;362: 7–13.
8. A randomized trial of propranolol in patients with acute myocardial infarction. I. Mortality results. *JAMA.* 1982;247:1707–1714.
9. A randomized trial of propranolol in patients with acute myocardial infarction. II. Morbidity results. *JAMA.* 1983;250:2814–2819.
10. Moye LA, Pfeffer MA, Braunwald E. Rationale, design and baseline characteristics of the survival and ventricular enlargement trial. SAVE Investigators. *Am J Cardiol.* 1991;68:70D–79D.
11. Pfeffer MA, Braunwald E, Moye LA, et al. Effect of captopril on mortality and morbidity in patients with left ventricular dysfunction after myocardial infarction. Results of the survival and ventricular enlargement trial. The SAVE Investigators. *N Engl J Med.* 1992;327:669–677.
12. GISSI-3: effects of lisinopril and transdermal glyceryl trinitrate singly and together on 6-week mortality and ventricular function after acute myocardial infarction. Gruppo Italiano per lo Studio della Sopravvivenza nell'infarto Miocardico. *Lancet.* 1994; 343:1115–1122.
13. Gustafsson I, Torp-Pederson C, Kober L, et al. Effect of the angiotensin-converting enzyme inhibitor trandolapril on mortality and morbidity in diabetic patients with left ventricular dysfunction after acute myocardial infarction. Trace Study Group. *J Am Coll Cardiol.* 1999;34:83–89.
14. Pfeffer MA, Greaves SC, Arnold JM, et al. Early versus delayed angiotensin-converting enzyme inhibition therapy in acute myocardial infarction. The Healing and Early Afterload Reducing Therapy trial. *Circulation.* 1997;95:2643–2651.
15. Hall AS, Murray GD, Ball SG. Follow-up study of patients randomly allocated ramipril or placebo for heart failure after acute myocardial infarction: AIRE Extension (AIREX) Study. Acute Infarction Ramipril Efficacy. *Lancet.* 1997;349:1493–1497.
16. Effects of enalapril on mortality in severe congestive heart failure. Results of the Cooperative North Scandinavian Enalapril Survival Study (CONSENSUS). The CONSENSUS Trial Study Group. *N Engl J Med.* 1987;316:1429–1435.
17. Cohn JN, Johnson G, Ziesche S, et al. A comparison of enalapril with hydralazine-isosorbide dinitrate in the treatment of chronic congestive heart failure. *N Engl J Med.* 1991;325:303–310.
18. Hansson L, Lindholm LH, Ekbom T, et al. Randomised trial of old and new antihypertensive drugs in elderly patients: cardiovascular mortality and morbidity the Swedish Trial in Old Patients with Hypertension-2 study. *Lancet.* 1999;354:1751–1756.
19. Pitt B, Poole-Wilson PA, Segal R, et al. Effect of losartan compared with captopril on mortality in patients with symptomatic heart failure: randomised trial—the Losartan Heart Failure Survival Study ELITE II. *Lancet.* 2000;355:1582–1587.
20. Pfeffer MA, Swedberg K, Granger CB, et al. Effects of candesartan on mortality and morbidity in patients with chronic heart failure: the CHARM-Overall programme. *Lancet.* 2003;362:759–769.
21. Dahlof B, Devereux RB, Kjelsen SE, et al. Cardiovascular morbidity and mortality in the Losartan Intervention For Endpoint reduction in hypertension study (LIFE): a randomised trial against atenolol. *Lancet.* 2002;359:995–1003.
22. Cohn JN, Tognini G. A randomized trial of the angiotensin-receptor blocker valsartan in chronic heart failure. *N Engl J Med.* 2001;345:1667–1675.
23. McKelvie RS, Yusuf S, Pericak D, et al. Comparison of candesartan, enalapril, and their combination in congestive heart failure: randomized evaluation of strategies for left ventricular dysfunction (RESOLVD) pilot study. The RESOLVD Pilot Study Investigators. *Circulation.* 1999;100:1056–1064.
24. Brenner BM, Cooper ME, de Zeeuw D, et al. Effects of losartan on renal and cardiovascular outcomes in patients with type 2 diabetes and nephropathy. *N Engl J Med.* 2001;345:862–869.
25. Pitt B, Zannad F, Remme WJ, et al. The effect of spironolactone on morbidity and mortality in patients with severe heart failure. Randomized Aldactone Evaluation Study Investigators. *N Engl J Med.* 1999;341:709–717.
26. Pitt B, Zannad F, Remme WJ, et al. Eplerenone, a selective aldosterone blocker, in patients with left ventricular dysfunction after myocardial infarction. *N Engl J Med.* 2003;348:1309–1317.
27. Direct Throbin Inhibitor Trialists' Collaborative Group. Direct thrombin inhibitors in acute coronary syndromes: principal results of a meta-analysis based on individual patients' data. *Lancet.* 2002;359:294–299.
28. White H. Thrombin-specific anticoagulation with bivalirudin versus heparin in patients receiving fibrinolytic therapy for acute myocardial infarction: the HERO-2 randomised trial. *Lancet.* 2001;358:1855–1863.
29. Bittl JA, Strony J, Brinker JA, et al. Treatment with bivalirudin (Hirulog) as compared with heparin during coronary angioplasty for unstable or postinfarction angina. Hirulog Angioplasty Study Investigators. *N Engl J Med.* 1995;333:764–769.
30. Bittl JA, Chaitman BR, Feit F, et al. Bivalirudin versus heparin during coronary angioplasty for unstable or postinfarction angina: final report reanalysis of the Bivalirudin Angioplasty Study. *Am Heart J.* 2001;142:952–959.
31. Comparison of the effects of two doses of recombinant hirudin compared with heparin in patients with acute myocardial ischemia without ST elevation: a pilot study. Organization to Assess Strategies for Ischemic Syndromes (OASIS) Investigators. *Circulation.* 1997 Aug 5;96(3):769–777.
32. Lincoff AM, Bittl JA, Harrington RA, et al. Bivalirudin and provisional glycoprotein IIb/IIIa blockade compared with heparin and planned glycoprotein IIb/IIIa blockade during percutaneous coronary intervention: REPLACE-2 randomized trial. *JAMA.* 2003;289:853–863.
33. Dahlof B, Sever PS, Poulter NR, et al. Prevention of cardiovascular events with an antihypertensive regimen of amlodipine adding perindopril as required versus atenolol adding bendroflumethiazide as required, in the Anglo-Scandinavian Cardiac Outcomes Trial-Blood Pressure Lowering Arm (ASCOT-BPLA): a multicentre randomised controlled trial. *Lancet.* 2005;366:895–906.
34. ALLHAT Officers and Coordinators for the ALLHAT Collaborative Research Group. Major outcomes in high-risk hypertensive patients randomized to angiotensin-converting enzyme inhibitor or calcium channel blocker vs diuretic: the Antihypertensive and Lipid-Lowering Treatment to Prevent Heart Attack Trial (ALLHAT). *JAMA.* 2002;288:2981–2997.
35. Taylor AL, Ziesche S, Yancy C, et al. Combination of isosorbide dinitrate and hydralazine in blacks with heart failure. *N Engl J Med.* 2004;351:2049–2057.
36. ISIS-2 (Second International Study of Infarct Survival) Collaborative Group. Randomised trial of intravenous streptokinase, oral aspirin, both, or neither among 17,187 cases of suspected acute myocardial infarction: ISIS-2. *Lancet.* 1988;2:349–360.
37. Antithrombotic Trialists' Collaboration. Collaborative meta-analysis of randomised trials of antiplatelet therapy for prevention of death, myocardial infarction, and stroke in high risk patients. *Br Med J.* 2002;324:71–86.

38. Yusuf S, Zhao F, Mehta SR, et al. Effects of clopidogrel in addition to aspirin in patients with acute coronary syndromes without ST-segment elevation. *N Engl J Med.* 2001;345:494–502.
39. Yusuf S, Mehta SR, Peters RJ, et al. Effects of pretreatment with clopidogrel and aspirin followed by long-term therapy in patients undergoing percutaneous coronary intervention: the PCI-CURE study. *Lancet.* 2001;358(9281):527–533.
40. Steinhubl SR, Berger PB, Mann JT 3rd, et al. Early and sustained dual oral antiplatelet therapy following percutaneous coronary intervention: a randomized controlled trial. *JAMA.* 2002;288(19):2411–2420.
41. Bertrand ME, Ruprecht HJ, Urban P, et al. Double-blind study of the safety of clopidogrel with and without a loading dose in combination with aspirin compared with ticlopidine in combination with aspirin after coronary stenting: the clopidogrel aspirin stent international cooperative study (CLASSICS). *Circulation.* 2000;102:624–629.
42. Kandzari DE, Berger PB, Kastrati A, et al. Influence of treatment duration with a 600-mg dose of clopidogrel before percutaneous coronary revascularization. *J Am Coll Cardiol.* 2004;44(11):2133–2136.
43. Sabatine MS, Cannon CP, Gibson CM, et al. Addition of clopidogrel to aspirin and fibrinolytic therapy for myocardial infarction with ST-segment elevation. *N Engl J Med.* 2005;352:1179.
44. Sabatine MS, Cannon CP, Gibson CM, et al. Effect of clopidogrel pretreatment before percutaneous coronary intervention in patients with ST-elevation myocardial infarction treated with fibrinolytics: the PCI-CLARITY study. *JAMA.* 2005;294:1224–1232.
45. The Platelet Receptor Inhibition in ischemic Syndrome Management (PRISM) study investigators. A comparison of aspirin plus tirofiban with aspirin plus heparin for unstable angina. *N Engl J Med.* 1998;338:1498–1505.
46. Effects of platelet glycoprotein IIb/IIIa blockade with tirofiban on adverse cardiac events in patients with unstable angina or acute myocardial infarction undergoing coronary angioplasty. The RESTORE Investigators. Randomized Efficacy Study of Tirofiban for Outcomes and REstenosis. *Circulation.* 1997;96:1445–1453.
47. Topol EJ, Moliterno DJ, Hermann HC, et al. Comparison of two platelet glycoprotein IIb/IIIa inhibitors, tirofiban and abciximab, for the prevention of ischemic events with percutaneous coronary revascularization. *N Engl J Med.* 2001;344:1888–1894.
48. Cannon CP, Weintraub WS, Demopoulos LA, et al. Comparison of early invasive and conservative strategies in patients with unstable coronary syndromes treated with the glycoprotein IIb/IIIa inhibitor tirofiban. *N Engl J Med.* 2001;344:1879–1887.
49. Kleiman NS, Lincoff AM, Flaker GC, et al. Early percutaneous coronary intervention, platelet inhibition with eptifibatide, and clinical outcomes in patients with acute coronary syndromes. PURSUIT Investigators. *Circulation.* 2000;101:751–757.
50. ESPRIT Investigators. Novel dosing regimen of eptifibatide in planned coronary stent implantation (ESPRIT): a randomised, placebo-controlled trial. *Lancet.* 2000;356:2037–2044.
51. Randomised placebo-controlled trial of effect of eptifibatide on complications of percutaneous coronary intervention: IMPACT-II. Integrilin to Minimise Platelet Aggregation and Coronary Thrombosis-II. *Lancet.* 1997;349:1422–1428.
52. Topol EJ, Califf RM, Weisman HF, et al. Randomised trial of coronary intervention with antibody against platelet IIb/IIIa integrin for reduction of clinical restenosis: results at six months. The EPIC Investigators. *Lancet.* 1994;343:881–886.
53. Platelet glycoprotein IIb/IIIa receptor blockade and low-dose heparin during percutaneous coronary revascularization. The EPILOG Investigators. *N Engl J Med.* 1997;336:1689–1696.
54. Randomised placebo-controlled and balloon-angioplasty-controlled trial to assess safety of coronary stenting with use of platelet glycoprotein-IIb/IIIa blockade. The EPISTENT Investigators. Evaluation of Platelet IIb/IIIa Inhibitor for Stenting. *Lancet.* 1998;352:87–92.
55. Randomised placebo-controlled trial of abciximab before and during coronary intervention in refractory unstable angina: the CAPTURE Study. *Lancet.* 1997;349:1429–1435.
56. Brenner SJ, Barr LA, Burchenal JE, et al. Randomized, placebo-controlled trial of platelet glycoprotein IIb/IIIa blockade with primary angioplasty for acute myocardial infarction. ReoPro and Primary PTCA Organization and Randomized Trial (RAPPORT) Investigators. *Circulation.* 1998;98:734–741.
57. Montalescot G, Barragan P, Wittenberg O, et al. Platelet glycoprotein IIb/IIIa inhibition with coronary stenting for acute myocardial infarction. *N Engl J Med.* 2001;344:1895–1903.
58. An international randomized trial comparing four thrombolytic strategies for acute myocardial infarction. The GUSTO investigators. *N Engl J Med.* 1993;329:673–682.
59. A comparison of reteplase with alteplase for acute myocardial infarction. The Global Use of Strategies to Open Occluded Coronary Arteries (GUSTO III) Investigators. *N Engl J Med.* 1997;337:1118–1123.
60. Topol EJ, GUSTO Investigators. Reperfusion therapy for acute myocardial infarction with fibrinolytic therapy or combination reduced fibrinolytic therapy and platelet glycoprotein IIb/IIIa inhibition: the GUSTO V randomised trial. *Lancet.* 2001;357:1905–1914.
61. Smith SC Jr, Feldman TE, Hirshfeld JW, et al. ACC/AHA/SCAI 2005 guideline update for percutaneous coronary intervention: a report of the American College of Cardiology/American Heart Association Task Force on Practice Guidelines (ACC/AHA/SCAI Writing Committee to update 2001 Guidelines for Percutaneous Coronary Intervention). *Circulation.* 2006;113(7):e166–286.

## SUGGESTED READING

**Antman et al.** Management of patients with STEMI: executive summary. ACC/AHA guidelines for the management of patients with ST-elevation myocardial infarction. *J Am Coll Cardiol.* 2004;44:671–719.

**Braunwald E, et al.** ACC/AHA 2002 guideline update for the management of patients with unstable angina and non-ST-segment elevation myocardial infarction—summary article. *J Am Coll Cardiol.* 2002;40:1366–1374.

**Braunwald E, et al., eds.** *Braunwald's Heart Disease: A Textbook of Cardiovascular Medicine.* 7th ed. Philadelphia: WB Saunders; 2005.

**Gibbons RJ, et al.** ACC/AHA 2002 guidline update for the management of patients with chronic stable angina—summary article. *J Am Coll Cardiol.* 2003;41:159–168.

**Griffin BP, Topol EJ, eds.** *Manual of Cardiovascular Medicine.* 2nd ed. Philadelphia: Lippincott Williams & Wilkins; 2004.

**Hunt SA, et al.** ACC/AHA 2005 guideline update for the diagnosis and management of chronic heart failure in the adult—summary article. *J Am Coll Cardiol.* 2005;46:1116–1143.

**Kloner RA, Birnabaum Y.** *Cardiovascular Trials Review.* 7th ed. Darien CT:Louis F. Le Jacq; 2002.

**Kloner RA, Birnabaum Y.** *Cardiovascular Trials Review.* 8th ed. Darien, CT: Louis F. Le Jacq; 2005.

**Opie LH, Gersh BJ.** *Drugs for the Heart.* Philadelphia: Elsevier; 2005.

**Topol EJ, ed.**, Califf RM, Isner JM, et al., assoc. eds. *Textbook of Cardiovascular Medicine.* 2nd ed. Philadelphia: Lippincott Williams & Wilkins, 2002.

## QUESTIONS

**1.** A 54-year-old African American woman with a history of ischemic cardiomyopathy and congestive heart failure is on stable doses of lisinopril, carvedilol, furosemide, and digoxin. She was admitted to the hospital with shortness of breath, orthopnea, and lower-extremity edema. Her jugular venous pressure was 15 cm $H_2O$, with bilateral basilar crackles on lung examination. She was 5.6 L in negative fluid balance over 48 hours of hospitalization, and her symptoms were much resolved. On the third day of hospitalization, the patient described orthostatic dizziness, with vitals showing hypotension as well as orthostasis. Which of the following is the best next step?

a. Add an ISDN/hydralazine combination to her drug regimen because she is African American and this drug combination has been shown to increase survival among black patients with heart failure on standard therapy.
b. Stop lisinopril.
c. Stop digoxin.
d. Reduce or decrease furosemide dose.
e. Discharge home with no change in medication.

Answer is d: Though the addition of ISDN/hydralazine has been shown to improve survival in black patients with congestive heart failure who are on standard therapy (beta-blockers, ACE-I, digoxin, and diuretics), it is not the appropriate time to do so when the patient has decreased filling pressures. Even though the patient is orthostatic, it is not advisable to stop ACE-I, considering that it has been shown to reduce morbidity and mortality in CHF whereas furosemide has not been shown to have that effect. Digoxin does not have much effect on blood pressure. It is not advisable to discharge the patient home on her current medications (including diuretics), considering how symptomatics he is from reduced filling pressure.

**2.** A 64-year-old man presented to the emergency room with crushing chest pain that he had been experiencing for the last 20 minutes. Electrocardiogram (ECG) showed 3-mm ST elevation in leads V1–V3 with reciprocal ST depression in the inferior leads. The patient received aspirin and was started on a heparin drip in the emergency room and forwarded to primary angioplasty. The patient was found to have an acute occlusion of the middle of the left anterior descending artery (LAD). The patient underwent PCI with a Cypher stent (sirolimus-coated stent) to the middle LAD. How long should you recommend the patient take clopidogrel?

a. The patient should take 75 mg of clopidogrel for at least 6 months.
b. The patient should take 75 of clopidogrel for at least 3 months.
c. The patient should take 75 mg of clopidogrel for at least 12 months.

Answer is b: Though the current guidelines recommend taking 75 mg of clopidogrel for 3 months after stenting with a sirolimus-eluting stent and for 6 months after a paclitaxel-eluting stent, many physicians are recommending therapy for 1 year after drug-eluting stent placement. The recommendations may change pending new guidelines.

**3.** A 62-year-old man has a history of hepatitis C infection and chronic hepatitis with a liver function test 10 times the normal level. He has had an aortic valve replacement with a St Jude mechanical prosthetic valve. In addition, he has a history of heparin-induced thrombocytopenia (HITT) complicated with pulmonary embolus. In anticipation of an elective abdominal surgery, warfarin was discontinued. The patient's INR is now <2. Which if the following choices for anticoagulation would you recommend?

a. Argatroban, 2 $\mu$g/kg per minute
b. Lepirudin, 0.4 mg/kg bolus, then 0.15 mg/kg per hour
c. Heparin bolus and drip per weight normogram
d. Enoxaparin, 1 mg/kg SC every 12 hours

Answer is b: Argatroban is not recommended because the patient had chronic liver disease and argatroban is cleared hepatically. Choice b, lepirudin, is cleared renally, and the patient is not known to have renal dysfunction. Heparin is contraindicated because the patient has a history of HITT and is at increased risk for thrombotic complications, particularly with prosthetic valve. Enoxaparin is not advised because there is a significant degree of cross-reactivity with unfractionated heparin with regard to HITT.

**4.** A 65-year-old woman has a history of dilated cardiomyopathy, an ejection fraction of 20%, and is NYHA Class III in terms of symptoms. Currently, she is on a home regimen of ramipril, long-acting metoprolol, spironolactone, and furosemide. She presented to the emergency room with shortness of breath and four-pillow orthopnea, and PND. On examination, she was tachycardic at 110 beats/min, blood pressure was 100/50 mm Hg, and there was evidence of fluid overload. The patient was admitted to the intensive care unit for pulmonary artery catheter-guided therapy. The cardiac index was 1.7 L/min/m$^2$, PCWP was 25 mm Hg, and pulmonary artery pressure was 70/40 mm Hg. Which of the following inotropic agents would be most appropriate for this patient?

a. Isoproterenol
b. Dobutamine
c. Milrinone
d. Dopamine

Answer is c: Milrinone is an inodilator (it has positive inotropic effect and vasodilator effect). It will allow improved cardiac output as well as decreasing pulmonary artery pressure without affecting the heart rate much (the patient is already tachycardiac). Dopamine, dobutamine, and isoproterenol cause tachycardia, which in this patient will increase the heart rate to even more than 110 beats/min and worsen the patient's hemodynamics. In addition, milrinone will lower pulmonary artery pressure and LVEDP in a more predictable fashion than the other agents.

5. Which of the following diuretic agents can be used in a patient with a sulfa allergy?

   a. Furosemide
   b. Toresmide
   c. Ethacrynic acid
   d. Bumetanide

Answer is c: Ethacrynic acid is the only agent listed that does not have a sulfa moiety.

# 60 Cardiovascular Drug Interactions

***Michael A. Militello*** ***Christine L. Ahrens***

Drug interactions occur when the combination of two or more medications alters the pharmacokinetic parameters or changes the pharmacologic response of either drug. These changes can produce undesirable responses including exaggerated or reduced pharmacologic effect or an added toxic response. It is clear that with the aging population and the increasing number of prescribed medications, the likelihood of having a significant drug interaction increases. In general, drug interactions account for a reported 7% to 17% of all adverse drug events and are probably higher considering underreported events.

Drug interactions are categorized as either pharmacokinetic or pharmacodynamic. Pharmacokinetic interactions occur when combining two or more medications results in an alteration of the drug's disposition in the body. Examples include the use of amiodarone with warfarin resulting in an increased international normalizing ratio (INR), or itraconazole decreasing the metabolism of certain HMG-CoA reductase inhibitors. Pharmacodynamic interactions occur when the addition of a medication leads to changes in the pharmacologic response of either medication. Examples include the addition of digoxin for heart rate control to beta-blockers or nondihydropyridine calcium channel blockers, which may lead to an unacceptable lowering of heart rate.

This chapter outlines typical types of drug–drug interactions observed in clinical practice and includes information on selected food–drug interactions that are commonly encountered.

## PHARMACOKINETIC DRUG INTERACTIONS

As reviewed in Chapter 58, the basic characteristics of pharmacokinetics include absorption, distribution, metabolism, and elimination. Alterations in one or more of these characteristics may lead to a significant drug interaction. Many of the documented interactions occur as a result of changes in metabolism or elimination of medications.

Absorption-related interactions result in decreases or increases in the amount of drug absorbed as well as delays in absorption. The presence of food or certain types of food may change medication absorption characteristics, leading to either a decrease in the extent or an increase in absorption time. Certain medications must be taken on an empty stomach for adequate bioavailability. For example, captopril, a non–prodrug angiotensin-converting enzyme inhibitor, is a prototypical drug that must be taken on an empty stomach because food may decrease the bioavailability by 25% to 50%. Additional medications that should be taken on an empty stomach are listed in Table 60–1. In addition, other medications such as bile acid binders and fiber laxatives may alter absorption of medications. Bile acid binders such as cholestyramine interfere with the absorption of a number of medications, and as a general rule medications should be taken 2 hours before or 2 hours after the bile acid resin to minimize a decrease in absorption. Another mechanism that may alter absorption is chelation, whereby di- or trivalent cations such as calcium and aluminum bind and decrease bioavailability. Tetracycline and quinolone antibiotics are prototypical for chelating interactions. Also, medications that may increase gastric motility, such as metoclopramide and erythromycin, may alter the bioavailability of medications because gastrointestinal transit times are hastened.

Certain medications require either an acidic or basic gastrointestinal pH for absorption. Alterations in pH may change the bioavailability of these medications. For example, itraconazole requires an acidic pH for optimal absorption, and medications such as $H_2$-blockers and proton

**TABLE 60–1**
**CARDIOVASCULAR MEDICATIONS THAT SHOULD BE TAKEN ON AN EMPTY STOMACH**

| | |
|---|---|
| Captopril | Moexipril |
| Felodipine | Perindopril |

pump inhibitors may decrease bioavailability and possibly result in treatment failure. Finally, antibiotics can alter the flora of the gastrointestinal tract and may change the bioavailability or efficacy of certain medications. Digoxin is metabolized in the gastrointestinal tract by the bacteria *Eubacterium lentum* in approximately 10% of patients. Both tetracycline and erythromycin can decrease the levels of this bacterium, therefore increasing the bioavailability of digoxin. Antibiotic-induced vitamin K depletion may interfere with warfarin. Gut flora that produce vitamin K may be killed, leading to an increased sensitivity to the effects of warfarin.

Alterations in protein binding may also play a role in drug–drug interactions. Drugs that are highly protein or tissue bound are more affected by other drugs that displace the original drug from the protein-binding site. Levels of the unbound fraction of drug will increase either transiently or permanently when the two medications are given concomitantly. These interactions are more difficult to identify, and medications with high protein binding such as warfarin and digoxin should be taken into consideration when adding or discontinuing medications.

Drug metabolism occurs via phase I or phase II reactions. Phase I reactions include oxidation, reduction, or hydrolysis and convert parent compounds into more water-soluble compounds such as losartan. These metabolites may be inactive, have more activity than the parent compounds (pro-drugs), or have less activity than the parent compound. Phase II reactions typically result in development of inactive compounds via glucuronidation, sulfation, or addition of other endogenous substances such as lorazepam.

Most phase I reactions occur via the cytochrome P450 (CYP) enzymes found in the liver, gastrointestinal tract, brain, kidneys, and other organs throughout the body. The vast majority of the enzymes are hepatic; however, there are large concentrations in the gastrointestinal tract as well. The CYP enzymes are a group of heme-containing compounds located on the membrane of the endoplasmic reticulum. The nomenclature for CYP includes a lead number referring to the family, followed by a letter referring to the subfamily, and finally an additional number that refers to the individual enzyme. Examples include CYP3A4 or 2D6. Most drug metabolism occurs via enzymes in the families 1, 2, and 3. CYP3 enzymes account for nearly 70% of the total CYP in the liver.

An individual drug can be a substrate, inhibitor, or inducer for a specific enzyme. A drug may act as an inhibitor of one or more groups of enzymes and may be a substrate for one or more groups of enzymes. For example, amiodarone is a substrate for CYP3A4 and is an inhibitor of CYP2C9 and 2D6 enzymes. Genetic variation also exists in the expression of certain CYP enzymes. Polymorphism is seen with both CYP2D6 and 2C19, and expression of the enzyme can be variable. Between 3% and 10% of Caucasians and 2% of Asians and African Americans have either low or no activity of CYP2D6. Patients with low or no activity of a particular isoenzyme are known as "poor metabolizers." Some individuals are also poor metabolizers of medications that are eliminated through the CYP2C19. Many commonly used cardiovascular medications are eliminated through the CYP system. Table 60–2 lists the drugs and the enzyme(s) responsible for their elimination as well as other enzyme(s) they may inhibit.

Besides being inhibitors or substrates, medications can also be inducers of the CYP enzyme system. Inducers increase metabolism of medications that are eliminated by these enzymes (Table 60–3). Enzyme inducers increase the activity of certain CYP isoforms and may require dosing increases of affected medications. Ethanol and smoking can influence metabolism of medications. The amount of ethanol intake and the number of cigarettes smoked daily directly influences the degree of enzyme induction. However, caution must be exercised with patients who are binge ethanol users. Although chronic ethanol intake will induce hepatic enzyme metabolism, acute or binge use of ethanol will inhibit metabolism of medications.

## PHARMACODYNAMIC DRUG INTERACTIONS

Interactions classified as pharmacodynamic do not alter the medication's disposition in the body but instead alter the expected pharmacologic response. The addition of a second agent may act synergistically to increase the response of the first drug, as in the addition of digoxin to a beta-blocker to control ventricular rate in patients with atrial fibrillation. Adverse reactions may be additive, as in the case of adding a medication that prolongs the QT interval to a regimen already consisting of a Class III antiarrhythmic agent such as sotalol. Table 60–4 contains a truncated list of medications that prolong the QT interval.

Sildenafil, tadalafil, and vardenafil enhance the effects of nitric oxide to produce their pharmacologic response. Nitrates that produce similar effects are considered contraindicated, as the additive effects of the combination may lead to life-threatening hypotension.

## FOOD–DRUG INTERACTIONS

Food may increase or decrease the extent of medication absorption. These types of interactions may depend on the

## TABLE 60–2

## COMMONLY OBSERVED DRUG–DRUG INTERACTIONS WITH CARDIOVASCULAR MEDICATIONS[a]

| Cardiovascular Drug | Interacting Drug | Mechanism | Considerations |
|---|---|---|---|
| Amiodarone | Warfarin | Amiodarone inhibits CYP2C9 and increases warfarin levels | Monitor closely; consider decreasing warfarin dose early |
| | Digoxin | P-glycoprotein inhibition | Monitor closely; consider decreasing dose by 50% when initiating amiodarone |
| | Simvastatin, lovastatin | Amiodarone inhibits CYP3A4, leading to elevations in levels | Use lower doses of statins to decrease risk of rhabdomylosis; atorvastatin not as significant, as less is metabolized through 3A4 |
| | Diltiazem, verapamil | Amiodarone inhibits CYP3A4, increasing levels of verapamil and diltiazem; amiodarone also slows heart rate | Both pharmacokinetic and pharmacodynamic interactions occur with amiodarone and diltiazem and verapamil |
| | Cyclosporine | Amiodarone inhibits CYP3A4, increasing levels of cyclosporine | Monitor cyclosporine levels closely |
| | Metoprolol | Amiodarone inhibits CYP2D6, increasing levels of metoprolol; amiodarone also slows heart rate | Both pharmacokinetic and pharmacodynamic interactions occur with amiodarone and metoprolol |
| Digoxin | Amiodarone | P-glycoprotein inhibition | Digoxin levels may be increased with the addition of these agents; Consider dosing adjustment when adding or discontinuing medications to digoxin |
| | Clarithromycin | P-glycoprotein inhibition | |
| | Cyclosporine | P-glycoprotein inhibition | |
| | Diltiazem | P-glycoprotein inhibition | |
| | Erythromycin | P-glycoprotein inhibition | |
| | Itraconazole, ketoconazlole | P-glycoprotein inhibition | |
| | Propafenone | P-glycoprotein inhibition | |
| | Quinidine | P-glycoprotein inhibition | |
| | Verapamil | P-glycoprotein inhibition | |
| | Beta-blockers | Additive effects | Pharmacodynamic interaction with additive effects on slowing heart rate; also occurs with other rate-controlling medications such as diltiazem and verapamil |
| Dofetilide | Cimetidine | Inhibition of renal tubular secretion and CYP 3A4 metabolism | Contraindicated to give concurrently |
| | Hydrochlorothiazide | Inhibition of renal tubular secretion | Contraindicated to give concurrently |
| | Itraconazole | QT-prolonging effects possible; inhibition of CYP3A4 | Contraindicated to give concurrently; dofetilide has minimal metabolism through 3A4; itraconazole may prolong QT interval |
| | Ketoconazole | Inhibition of renal cation transport system; additive effect on QT prolongation | Contraindicated to give concurrently |
| | Trimethoprim (alone or in combination with sulfamethoxazole) | Inhibition of renal tubular secretion | Contraindicated to give concurrently |
| | Triamterene | Inhibition of renal cation transport system | Contraindicated to give concurrently |
| | Verapamil | Unknown; however, may increase absorption of dofetilide | Contraindicated to give concurrently |
| | Prochlorperazine | Inhibition of renal tubular secretion | Contraindicated to give concurrently |
| | QT-interval–prolonging drugs | Additive effects on QT interval | Contraindicated to give concurrently; many drugs, such as Class Ia and III antiarrhythmics, certain antipsychotics, certain quinolones, phenothiazine, many others |
| | Megesterol | Inhibition of renal tubular secretion | Contraindicated to give concurrently |

(continued)

**TABLE 60–2**
**COMMONLY OBSERVED DRUG–DRUG INTERACTIONS WITH CARDIOVASCULAR MEDICATIONS[a] (CONTINUED)**

| Cardiovascular Drug | Interacting Drug | Mechanism | Considerations |
|---|---|---|---|
| Statins<br>Simvastatin<br>Lovastatin<br>Atorvastatin | Amiodarone | CYP3A4 major metabolic pathway of statins listed on left | See amiodarone |
| | Bosentan | CYP3A4 enzymes are induced by bosentan | May require higher dose for pharmacologic response |
| | Cyclosporine | Cyclosporine inhibits CYP3A4 | Product literature recommends not to exceed 10 mg of simvastatin daily |
| | Diltiazem, verapamil | Both verapamil and diltiazem are inhibitors of CYP3A4 | Reduce dose of listed statins |
| | Itraconazole, ketoconazole | Inhibits all CYP enzymes | Avoid statins during therapy with these antifungals |
| | Gemfibrozil | Increased risk of myopathy and rhabdomyolysis | Product literature recommends not to exceed 10 mg of simvastatin daily |
| | Erythromycin, clarithromycin | Certain macrolide antibiotics inhibit the CYP3A4 | Avoid statin use during therapy with these antibiotics |
| | Nefazodone | Nefazodone decreases CYP elimination of certain statins | Avoid statin use |
| | HIV-protease inhibitors | Certain protease inhibitors decrease metabolism of statins | Avoid statin use |
| Warfarin | Amiodarone | See Amiodarone | See Amiodarone |
| | Bile acid binders | Concomitant use decreases the absorption of warfarin | Take warfarin 2 h before or 2 h after a bile acid binder |
| | Antiplatelet medications | Increased risk of bleeding | Monitor for signs and symptoms of bleeding |
| | Metronidazole | Inhibition of warfarin metabolism | Change antibiotic if possible; if not, consider reducing dose of warfarin and monitor INR more frequently |
| | Gemfibrozil | Inhibition of warfarin metabolism and protein-binding displacement | Monitor INR more frequently while on therapy; consider alternative therapy; interaction may be seen with fenofibrate as well |
| | Trimethoprim and sulfamethoxazole | Inhibition of warfarin metabolism and protein-binding displacement | Avoid use if possible; if not, consider reducing warfarin dose and monitor INR more frequently while on therapy |
| | Rifampin | Increased metabolism of warfarin | Monitor INR more frequently, as patients will need higher doses. |
| | Phenobarbital | Increased metabolism of warfarin | Monitor INR more frequently, as patients will need higher doses. |
| | Phenytoin | Increased metabolism of warfarin | Monitor INR more frequently, as patients will need higher doses. |
| | Azole anifungals | Decreased metabolism of warfarin | Monitor INR more frequently, as patients will need lower doses. |
| | Macrolide antibiotics | Decreased metabolism of warfarin | Monitor INR more frequently, as patients will need lower doses. |
| | Cyclosporine | Unknown mechanism, probably reduced warfarin metabolism | Monitor INR more frequently, as patients will need lower doses. |

[a]This table provides a limited list of medications and interactions, and is by no means complete. A review of the complete medication list for drug interactions should be performed frequently, especially when adding or discontinuing medications, to avoid unnecessary adverse drug events.

**TABLE 60–3**
**TRUNCATED LIST OF MEDICATIONS THAT INDUCE CYP**

| Drug | CYP Enzyme(s) Induced |
|---|---|
| Phenytoin | 1A2, 3A4, 2D6, 2C9 |
| Phenobarbital | 1A2, 3A4, 2D6, 2C9 |
| Carbamazepine | 3A4, 2D6, 2C |
| Rifampin | 1A2, 3A4, 2D6, 2C9 |
| Ritonavir | 1A2, 2D6 |
| Smoking | 1A2 |

characteristics of the medication and the meal. Considerations of food vitamin and electrolyte content can be as important as significant drug–drug interactions. Increased risk or toxicities may occur, as in the case of high-potassium foods or salt substitutes with angiotensin-converting enzymes inhibitors, or treatment failures as in the case of warfarin and excessive vitamin K intake. Finally, there have been occurrences of gastrointestinal interactions with CYP3A4 and P-glycoprotein. P-glycoprotein is a drug efflux pump found in high concentrations in the villi in the gastrointestinal tract, which is responsible for transporting lipophilic compounds from the enterocyte back to the intestinal lumen (reverse transport). Hence these two enzymes work together to change the amount of medication that reaches the systemic circulation.

Grapefruit juice is the classic example of a drug–food interaction, with inhibition of gastrointestinal CYP3A4 and P-glycoprotein leading to an increase in medication bioavailability. Grapefruit juice may increase the levels of certain dihydropyridine calcium channel blockers, statins, cyclosporine, and other medications. This interaction may be observed with as little as 200 mL daily, with an effect possibly lasting hours after ingestion. Medications that interact with grapefruit juice have increased toxicities, as in the case of felodipine, for which there can be two times the amount of drug absorbed, increasing the hypotensive risk. Other calcium channel blockers, such as amlodipine, are less affected by grapefruit juice. A similar case can be made for co-administration of certain statins with grapefruit juice. Simvastatin, lovastatin, and to a lesser extent atorvastatin will have increased levels with the co-administration of grapefruit juice and have an increased potential for the development of adverse events.

**TABLE 60–4**
**TRUNCATED LIST OF MEDICATIONS THAT PROLONG THE QT INTERVAL**

| | |
|---|---|
| Amiodarone | Ketoconazole |
| Disopyramide | Procainamide |
| Dofetilide | Phenothiazine antipsychotics |
| Droperidol | Quinidine |
| Erythromycin | Quinolone antibiotics |
| Haloperidol | Sotalol |
| Ibutilide | Tricyclic antidepressants |
| Itraconazole | Ziprasidone |

## BIBLIOGRAPHY

**Åsberg A.** Interactions between cyclosporin and lipid-lowering drugs: implications for organ transplant recipients. *Drugs*. 2003;63(4): 367–378.

**Ferrari P, Bianchi G.** The genomics of cardiovascular disorders: therapeutic implications. *Drugs*. 2000;59(5):1025–1042.

**Haddad PM, Anderson IM.** Antipsychotic-related QTC prolongation, torsade de pointes and sudden death. *Drugs*. 2002;62(11):1649–1671.

**Hunter AL, Cruz RP, Cheyne BM, et al.** Cytochrome p450 enzymes and cardiovascular disease. *Can J Physiol Pharmacol*. 2004;82:1053–1060.

**Kane GC, Lipsky JJ.** Drug-grapefruit juice interactions. *Mayo Clin Proc*. 2000;75:933–942.

**Kuhlmann J, Mück W.** Clinical-pharmacological strategies to assess drug interaction potential during drug development. *Drug Safety*. 2001;24(10):715–725.

**Michalets EL.** Update: clinically significant cytochrome P-450 drug interactions. *Pharmacotherapy*. 1998;18(1):84–112.

**Ozdemir V, Shear NH, Kalow W.** What will be the role of pharmacogenetics in evaluating drug safety and minimising adverse effects? *Drug Safety*. 2001;24(2):75–85.

**Schelleman H, Stricker BH, de Boer A, et al.** Drug-gene interactions between genetic polymorphisms and antihypertensive therapy. *Drugs*. 2004;64(16):1801–1816.

**Schmidt LE, Dalhoff K.** Food-drug interactions. *Drugs*. 2002;61(10): 1481–1502.

**Stone SM, Rai N, Nei J.** Problems and pitfalls in cardiac drug therapy. *Rev Cardiovasc Med*. 2001;2(3):126–142.

**Trujillo TC, Nolan PE.** Antiarrhythmic agents: durg interactions of clinical significance. *Drug Safety*. 2000;23(6):509–532.

**Zhang Y, Benet LZ.** The gut as a barrier to drug absorption: combined role of cytochrome P450 3A and P-glycoprotein. *Clin Pharmacokinet*. 2001;40(3):159–168.

## QUESTIONS

1. Amiodarone increases the levels of all of the following *except*:
   a. Digoxin
   b. Simvastatin
   c. Pravastatin
   d. Metoprolol

Answer is c: Hepatic CYP metabolism is a minor elimination pathway for pravastatin clearance. Amiodarone can increase the levels of digoxin, simvastatin, and metoprolol. Also, amiodarone can cause bradycardia and may have additive effects with other medications that slow heart rate.

2. Which of the following induces the CYP450 3A4 enzyme?
   a. Rifampin
   b. Amiodarone

c. Grapefruit juice
d. Warfarin

Answer is a: Rifampin is a known inducer of multiple CYP enzymes. Amiodarone and grapefruit juice are inhibitors of this system, whereas warfarin dose not inhibit or induce the CYP3A4 enzyme. Other common inducers include phenobarbital, phenytoin, and carbamazepine.

**3.** Which of the following additions will significantly elevate the INR in patients on a stable dose of warfarin?

a. Digoxin
b. Metronidazole
c. Cholestyramine
d. Aspirin

Answer is b: Metronidazole decreases the metabolism of warfarin, leading to increases in the INR. Cholestyramine may decrease the absorption of warfarin when taken with it, and as a general rule, medications should be taken 2 hours before or after a dose of a bile acid binder. Aspirin does not change the pharmacokinetics of warfarin; however, because of the antiplatelet effects, it may increase the risk of bleeding when the two are taken concomitantly.

**4.** Simvastatin and lovastatin levels can be increased by all of the following medications *except*:

a. Verapamil
b. Diltiazem
c. Sotalol
d. Cyclosporine

Answer is c: Sotalol is cleared renally and does not affect the levels of either simvastatin or lovastatin. Verapamil, diltiazem, and cyclsporine can inhibit the CYP3A4 enzyme, increasing the levels of these two statins. However, most statins will reach increased levels when used with cyclosporine, and close monitoring is recommended.

**5.** Quinidine, a potent inhibitor of the CYP2D6 enzyme, can inhibit the analgesic response to which of the following:

a. Morphine sulfate
b. Hydromorphone
c. Fentanyl
d. Codeine

Answer is d: Quinidine is a potent inhibitor of CYP2D6, and codeine as a prodrug needs to be converted through this enzyme to morphine for full analgesic effect.

**6.** Which of the following groups of drug interactions are considered pharmacodynamic?

a. Warfarin and amiodarone
b. Warfarin and metronidazole
c. Warfarin and clopidogrel
d. Warfarin and rifampin

Answer is c: Pharmacodynamic interactions are those that do not change the disposition of medications in the body but may alter the pharmacologic response. In this case, the addition of clopidogrel to warfarin increases the risk of bleeding, as one is an anticoagulant and the other is a potent antiplatelet medication. The other combinations may have pharmaocokinetic interactions, in which one drug will affect the levels of the other.

**7.** Which of the following medications interact with sildenafil?

a. Isosorbide dinitrate
b. Amiodarone
c. Erythromycin
d. All of the above

Answer is d: The answer is not as straightforward as it seems. The interaction between sildenafil and nitrates is well known and is avoided. However, sildenafil is metabolized through the CYP3A4 enzyme system, and agents such as amiodarone and erythromycin can increase the levels of sildenafil. Caution should be used when prescribing these drugs together, and lower initial sildenafil doses should be used.

# Index

Page numbers followed by *t* indicate table; those followed by *f* indicate figure.